YOU CAN
CONQUER
CANCER

YOU CAN CONQUER CANCER

The ground-breaking
self-help manual, including
nutrition, meditation
and lifestyle
management techniques

~

IAN GAWLER

Thorsons

HarperThorsons
An imprint of HarperCollins*Publishers*
1 London Bridge Street
London SE1 9GF

www.harpercollins.co.uk

First edition published in Australia 1984
Revised edition published 2001
Second revised edition published 2004
Third revised edition published 2013
First published in the United States by Tarcher/Penguin 2015
Copyright © 1984, 2001, 2004, 2013 by Ian Gawler
Published in Great Britain by HarperThorsons 2015

1 3 5 7 9 10 8 6 4 2

Copyright © 1984, 2001, 2004, 2013 by Ian Gawler

Ian Gawler asserts the moral right to be identified as the author of this work

A catalogue record of this book is available from the British Library

ISBN 978-0-00-811760-3

Book design by Tanya Maiboroda

Printed and bound in Great Britain by Clays Ltd, St Ives plc

MIX
Paper from
responsible sources
FSC www.fsc.org **FSC® C007454**

FSC is a non-profit international organisation established to promote
the responsible management of the world's forests. Products carrying
the FSC label are independently certified to assure consumers that they
come from forests that are managed to meet the social, economic
and ecological needs of present and future generations.

Find out more about HarperCollins and the environment at
www.harpercollins.co.uk/green

The advice in this book is designed to complement medical advice. Always consult your doctor. The author of this book does not dispense medical advice or prescribe the use of any techniques as a form of treatment for physical or medical problems without the advice of a physician, either directly or indirectly. The intent of the author is only to offer information of a general nature to help you in your quest for emotional and spiritual well-being. In the event you use any information in this book for yourself, the author and the publisher assume no responsibility for your action.

*This edition is dedicated
to the health, healing and well-being
of all who read it.
May you all live long and happy lives!*

Contents

The Big Picture

What Is Possible and How

IT IS A GREAT FEELING TO HAVE RECOVERED FROM CANCER—TO HAVE BEEN through it all and to be living a full, happy life again. I have done it. I have seen others do it and know many more will repeat the process in the future. This book, then, is offered with a sense of excitement and joy—the joy in having done it and the excitement of being able to help others to do it.

We all share a common goal. We all want to enjoy good health along with long, happy and meaningful lives. And we can. However, when a diagnosis of cancer comes into a family, all this is severely threatened. There is the real threat of life cut short, along with fear, distress and potential suffering.

Good news. We can turn all of this around. I have done it myself and I have seen many, many others do it as well. You can conquer cancer. That is a fact. It is possible. There is a process by which you can combine your own resources with those of the medical and allied health professions so that you can transform the experience of cancer and recover. This book examines the patient's role in disease and healing. It is intended as a self-help manual that provides the signposts along the path to well-being and long-term health.

Currently, of all the people diagnosed with cancer, Western medicine helps around 65 percent to be alive five years later. For someone whose prognosis predicts they are likely to be in that 65 percent, this approach will mobilize your own inner resources, along with those who support you, and give you every chance of becoming a long-term survivor.

For those with a poor prognosis from the medical point of view, take heart. You too can do it. I did. At my lowest point in 1976 my surgeon thought I would only live for a few weeks. So it is wonderful not only to still be alive, but to have raised a family, had the good fortune to be able to help many thousands of others and, importantly, to have seen many, many others recover using these methods.

For more than thirty years now, people have continued to ask me the same question. It is a good question and it is as relevant to the start of this book as it is to every person who asks it.

"When it comes to cancer, what is the most important thing that will help me, or the person I love, to recover?"

I never tire of this question. Is it the food? Is it all in the mind? Is it some new medical breakthrough or some ancient herb? Is it the meditation? What is it? What is *the* thing that helps the most?

Well, in my experience it is a combination of things. You need the best of all that is available.

You can conquer cancer. But you do need to work at it. This is not a casual business. You need to learn what to do and you need to do it. And when you do, you are bound to feel better in ways that right now you may not even imagine. There is the real prospect of becoming cancer free and enjoying a whole new phase of your life.

WHERE THERE IS A RHYME, THERE IS A REASON

My right leg was amputated with osteogenic sarcoma (bone cancer) in January 1975. While there were no signs of the cancer anywhere else in my body at that time, I was told that only 5 percent of patients could expect to be alive five years after such surgery. If my cancer reappeared, it would be expected to be rapidly fatal. In those days, most people died within three to six months of developing secondary growths of this form of bone cancer.

In fact, my cancer did reappear in November 1975. By March 1976, my specialist thought that I would live for only two more weeks. My subsequent recovery ran the full gamut of available treatments and, in June 1978, I was declared free of active cancer.

Over the next few years, my former wife, Gail (who later changed her name to Gayle and then Grace), and I had four children. I began a new veterinary practice, took up a thirty-seven-acre farm, developed vegetable gardens and orchards, and built a new house.

In 1981, Grace and I initiated the Melbourne Cancer Support Group. This lifestyle-based support group was one of the very first of its kind anywhere in the world. It began with an initial urge to pass on the benefits of my own rather extraordinary experience of recovering against the odds. Having been through it all myself, I understood the problems cancer patients face. Furthermore, being a rather pragmatic veterinarian, I had enough medical knowledge to understand my own position at the outset, evaluate my progress, and assess critically the wide range of treatments considered. Fortunately, I was blessed with an open mind, so I was ready to consider anything that worked toward my aim. That aim was to create the right environment in which my body would heal itself. To think that the body can play a major part in healing itself was a novel approach way back in the mid-seventies, but is one that we now know to be full of possibilities.

When my cancer had recurred and the situation looked hopeless from the medical viewpoint, I remained confident that there *was* another way. Already I had been introduced to the idea that cancer involved a state of immune deficiency, a weakness in the body's healing defense system. To explain: it is known that throughout the lifetime of every healthy person, cancerous cells develop in their body. This is a medically accepted fact. It also is accepted that the body normally recognizes these abnormal cells as a potential threat to its health and acts quickly to isolate and destroy them. It does so before any physical symptoms become apparent. However, in people who go on to develop cancer this does not happen and the growths continue unopposed. The body offers no resistance and symptoms of cancer are the result.

So I began with the attitude that it was possible to restimulate the body's natural defenses—in particular, the immune system. This being so, it followed that the body itself could destroy and remove all traces of the cancer. As an extension, if the immune system remained intact and functioning properly, there should be no worry about the cancer reappearing. An exciting prospect!

That attitude was my starting point, my basic premise. All I did was directed toward that end. So, while I explored many avenues of treatment, every one was a part of the process of finding the right balance for me. Now more than thirty years later, and having worked with many thousands of people intent on dealing with their own cancer challenges, what this book is able to present are the key principles that will be helpful, as well as exploring some of the more peripheral options.

This attitude of being empowered and learning how to overcome the many challenges cancer can present is so very different to the fear that normally surrounds the word.

FEAR AND THE FOUR MISCONCEPTIONS OF CANCER

Probably no other word strikes as much emotional fear in the community today as does *cancer*. While over the years the intensity of this fear may have lessened to some degree as more people have come to realize there is something constructive they can do in response to cancer, for most the fear is still very real.

When *You Can Conquer Cancer* was first published in 1984, it was regarded as somewhat provocative and revolutionary. First, there was the title, *You Can Conquer Cancer*. Conquer? Maybe "get help with," maybe "manage," maybe "live with" would have fitted the expectations of the day better. But "conquer" and "you can" in the same sentence? You can conquer cancer? Is that for real?

Actually the title was quite deliberately chosen to confront what many people believed back then and what some people still do believe: you get cancer and you die. This of course is the primary fear cancer engenders. But there is more to it. The fear of cancer is based on four basic misconceptions:

1. The cause of cancer is unknown.
2. Cancer is generally associated with pain and an untimely death.
3. There is nothing patients can do to help themselves except hand over responsibility for their well-being, and indeed their lives, to a doctor.
4. Treatments are unpleasant and probably will not work anyway.

It is the work of this book, of the Gawler Foundation and of other like-minded practitioners and groups to dispel these fears, to replace them with a positive attitude, and then to show how people can make a decisive contribution toward restoring their own health. Supporting the mind and body when undergoing treatment prescribed by a medical practitioner is a step we can all take.

GOOD NEWS • Cancer Is a Process That Can Be Reversed

This book presents the good news on cancer. It is not a book about dying gracefully with cancer. It is about a process of living—living to the fullest.

The starting point is seeing cancer as a process. We must realize that most of the causes of cancer are now known and that cancer is not a chance happening of random fate. Once the causes are identified it becomes possible to plan appropriate action. To do this satisfactorily we need to expand our horizons. We need to consider the roles of those three aspects of our human condition that we know as *physical, psychological* and *spiritual.*

While personally I recognize the overriding importance of spiritual factors, I do not confuse these with religious issues. Religious preference is something different and personal to the individual, and therefore I talk little of this. Some prefer to leave religion alone, others take their religion seriously indeed, and it is my experience that whatever their choice, people explore that avenue for themselves. The techniques talked about in this book have no religious loadings, nor do they interfere or impose on patients' preferences in any way. However, the majority of people do find the techniques an aid in their search for their own spiritual reality.

Most people, and people diagnosed with cancer in particular, are concerned with the basic questions: Who am I? Where did I come from? Where am I going? These fundamental spiritual questions are often prominent in the mind of someone diagnosed with cancer and are certainly worth exploring later in the book.

In these pages we shall consider also the role environmental and psychological factors play in the causation and treatment of cancer; for herein lies the key to success. We can identify the majority of the causes of cancer. I contend that there are techniques which provide effective antidotes to those causes. The techniques center on appropriate diet, exercise, positive thinking, stress management and meditation—all in conjunction with suitable specific therapies. By utilizing all these means, the body's natural healing urge can be helped to reassert itself.

A body with properly functioning defenses cannot have cancer.

WHAT IS POSSIBLE?

I have experienced the pleasure of working with other people who have been able to repeat the process I went through and become free of a supposedly terminal illness. But just as exciting and pleasing is the fact that these techniques have consistently produced a deeper love for life coupled with a profound acceptance of the outcome of that life.

So, while I have seen and continue to see many recoveries, I accept that not everyone is going to become free of their physical problems. Sadly, some may die of their illness. But it has been part of my joy to know that the great majority of those who used these same techniques and did not recover were able to die with great dignity, and a poise that often surprised and always impressed themselves and their families. In this way, too, cancer was truly conquered. So, although the aim is always first and foremost to help people back to full health, this approach is of great value to those who face dying.

While in general the earlier in the course of the illness a person begins using this approach, the easier they will find it and the better their result, for those making a later start there is still the real prospect of overcoming cancer. There are always genuine grounds for hope, plus the bonus of overcoming fear and the problems associated with the disease. For many others there is the exciting prospect of using this approach to prevent cancer. I have found that, indeed, you can conquer cancer.

A COMMITMENT TO WHAT WORKS

This is a book about what works. The essence of this book has been distilled in the cauldron of major disease. People faced with cancer take life seriously— very seriously. They want answers. They want to know what works. They need to know what works.

What you are reading in *You Can Conquer Cancer* represents the accumulated wisdom of thousands of people over several decades who were all focused on these question: What are the best things to do? How best to respond to the many challenges cancer presents? How to recover physically? How to transform what for many at first diagnosis was shock and fear? How to transform the potential suffering of this illness into good health and long-lasting well-being?

The reality is that between the thousands of people I have worked closely with, we have tried many things. In fact, between us, we have tried most, if not all, the things you could think of, and probably quite a few you could not! My job has been to collect, distil and communicate the lessons learned from all this experience—this experience of what works. It is presented here in the hope that you too will benefit from the experience of so many others, and from the knowledge that comes out of it.

Of course, both myself and the many people I have worked with as group participants and colleagues value science and its evidence base. I love research, read lots of it, take it into account, and highly value it. But then science needs to be tested in the real world. So in this book, the focus is on what works in practice, what I can share with you based on so much practical experience. As such, I have deliberately chosen not to attempt to document what I present with more than rudimentary research evidence. This book is not intended for research scholars it is intended for practical use.

I first wrote this book back in 1984, and have thoroughly rewritten it in 2012. On both occasions I had in mind what I would say if I was speaking personally to the most valued person in my life. What follows is the best I can offer. It is informed by research; much of the book is validated by research. But unashamedly I suggest its real strength is that it is the product of shared human experience.

The accumulated experience of all the people I have been blessed to work with, gathered together here in this one book, can save you a lot of time. It may even save your life!

This book, then, focuses upon the principles of self-healing. What you can do to restore natural health, what you can do to help someone you love and care for. As a bonus, for those still well, the book can guide you directly with how you can prevent illness and experience lasting good health.

You Can Conquer Cancer presents an integrated approach, a guide to health and well-being.

GRATITUDE

There is nothing like sitting and talking with a room full of people whose lives are on the line to clarify what is important and what works. This book is a tribute to all the thousands of people affected by cancer who over three decades have helped to test, trial and debate the possibilities. The strength of the book resides in the fact that what it presents has been tested in the crucible of human experience, intense human experience, the intensity of aiming to overcome cancer and all the challenges it presents. So my gratitude, and respectfully I would suggest, your gratitude as the reader, needs to go to those people whose experiences the book reflects. This book stands as testament to their commitment and achievements.

There is a need to acknowledge and thank my two main meditation teachers, Dr. Ainslie Meares and Sogyal Rinpoche. It is useful to be aware that it was only a few decades ago that medical innovators like Dr. Meares began to identify the health-promoting possibilities of the ageless forms of meditation and adapt them to modern, everyday problems. Dr. Meares' first major contribution in this area was popularized in his international best seller *Relief Without Drugs,* first published in 1967.[1] I was fortunate indeed that at the time when my cancer recurred in 1975, Dr. Meares was putting forward his hypothesis that intensive meditation may help people with advanced cancer to recover. I was then equally fortunate to meet the great Tibetan lama Sogyal Rinpoche in 1985 and I continue to learn from him. Rinpoche, as he is known, is the author of the international classic *The Tibetan Book of Living and Dying*[2] and has been at the forefront of bringing the ancient wisdom of the Tibetans into a vibrant, modern context. What I can offer regarding meditation stems largely from these two great teachers, Dr. Meares and Sogyal Rinpoche, along with the many people who have taught me as I attempted to teach them.

You may be able to imagine that working in this field has its challenges. I have so much gratitude to my wife, Ruth Gawler, for all that she does to support me both professionally and personally. Ruth is an extraordinary doctor, a wonderful meditation and yoga teacher, and she has had a profoundly positive impact on so many people she has counseled. She has taught me what real love is and it is a delight to be married to her.

I have also been fortunate to work with many extraordinarily talented and compassionate colleagues. I think of the many people who volunteered to sit on the Gawler Foundation's board and the many staff I have worked with. Of course things go up and down a little when you work with lots of people, but one thing that has been a constant is the clarity of purpose all the staff have taken to their work which manifests as their unfailing capacity to work together for the interests of those attending programs and to create a caring, nurturing, transformative environment. This capacity is truly wonderful.

As to the book itself, I am deeply grateful to the Brady Foundation for supporting me in a very direct way and providing the opportunity to concentrate on the writing. Particular thanks is due to Ross Taylor, himself a long-term remarkable cancer survivor, who has encouraged and inspired me personally, as well as a multitude of other people dealing with cancer.

Then to thank my publisher, Michelle Anderson, who has been a tireless advocate for the book and become a very supportive friend in the process. Robina Courtin brought her formidable skills as an editor to bear on the book and contributed significantly to the end result. Pam Cossins did great work transferring my handwriting into type, while David Johns did his best with his photography to make me look good for the front cover. Great photography at least! Ruth also made a significant contribution reading and assisting with many drafts, and thanks to Maia Bedson, Michelle Anderson, Professor Gabriel Kune and Rohan Erm for reading some or all of the book and offering useful feedback and suggestions. As with the first edition, John Simkin contributed the index.

Finally, a thank-you to the critics. Criticism provides the opportunity to reexamine what you take to be correct, to reconsider how you can express things more clearly or in a more accessible way, and to check how what you say resonates with others. While destructive skepticism has little merit, constructive criticism is always welcome.

THE BENEFIT OF THE YEARS

Given the years since the first edition back in 1984, I now have even more confidence in these principles because I have observed them at work for so long. They can transform your life! For many people, they have been lifesaving. For others they have sustained and prolonged life, then helped them with a dignified, honorable death. For all who do use them, these principles bring more inner peace, more joy, more happiness.

One of the personal delights in writing this new edition has been to reaffirm that the essence of what worked over thirty years ago is very similar to what it is today. While this new edition represents a very thorough rewrite when compared to the original, there is a fundamental truth here. Your lifestyle affects your health. Your lifestyle can produce disease and your life-style can produce healing. So while this new edition is updated, the language more current, the stories often more recent, the basic principles have stood the test of time and remain constant. The reason for this? What is presented here is how you can use your own resources to get the best from your body's potential to heal. These things are constants: good nutrition, exercise, sun-light, healthy emotions, the power of the mind, meditation—your lifestyle. Do not be confused by the simplicity of the theory. What we will be talking of here are things you can control for yourself and apply in your own healing journey. They can be highly therapeutic. The book will explain how!

A FINAL WORD

There is no magic bullet in this book. No wonder drug or herb that can be taken three times daily and which, leaving all else unchanged, will offer you a cure.

You *can* conquer cancer using a process—a healing process that takes effort, perseverance and does require changes to be made. It is a process through which our natural state of health can be regained. For those pre-pared to walk this road, I know that cancer can be prevented or overcome. My wish is that more and more people will do it.

For the benefit of others, I offer this book.

Ian Gawler
The Yarra Valley, 2013

CHAPTER 1

The First Step

How to Begin

WHAT YOU DO WILL MAKE A DIFFERENCE. THERE IS A COMPELLING LOGIC TO this. If you, or someone you love, have been diagnosed with cancer, it makes good sense to get all the outside help you can. But then, as with everything else in life, how you respond, how you react, what you actually do—all this will affect the outcome significantly.

For those willing to take up the challenge that cancer has put to them, there is a road back to health.

What to do? There is so much information available these days. Advice from friends, opinions from medical and other health professionals, lots of great books and so much information on the Internet. This book will distill the benefits of years of experience and gathered knowledge, present it in logical, sequential form, help you to evaluate the many choices available, and then support and guide you along the way.

We will begin in the first two chapters by working through the options, from first diagnosis to long-term survival. Then come the details you will need to convert a good idea into a practical reality. You can conquer cancer. What follows spells out the process of how to do it.

HOPE IS REAL

The starting point is having hope. And hope has a compelling logic to it. No matter how dark it may seem as you start on this road, you need to be assured recovery is possible. It may not always be easy, it may well take a good deal of planning and commitment, but it definitely is possible.

At my worst I was expected to live for only a few weeks. That was early in 1976! After I recovered, Dr. Ainslie Meares said a very important thing: "It only has to be done once to show that it is possible." But these days there are many documented cases of people who have recovered against the odds. I have helped to publish two books recounting the lives, the methods and the recoveries of some of these people. The first, *Inspiring People*,[3] gathered the stories of forty-four people who had attended groups I ran in the early years and went on to become long-term survivors. Out of print now, that book was replaced by *Surviving Cancer*,[4] which recounts the remarkable journeys of twenty-eight people. Written by Paul Kraus, himself one of the longest-known survivors of mesothelioma, his is a wonderful book to read and then dip into from time to time whenever inspiration is needed.

FEATURES OF LONG-TERM SURVIVORS

There are two important features I observe in the many long-term survivors I have worked with and come to know well. First, they really applied themselves—they did many things. Second, the main things that they did they had in common, while many varied some of the minor details.

Let me explain. Some years back, I surveyed thirty-five long-term survivors. These were all people who had been given short-term prognoses by good medical people. But they went on to turn their difficulties around and were alive many years later. In the survey, they were asked to consider all the things that may have helped them to recover and to rank their importance on a sliding scale. They were asked to reflect on the importance any medical treatment had played, any natural therapies, overcoming fear of dying, forgiveness, nutrition, meditation—all the options you could think of.

The first thing that stood out in this survey was that most people valued most things highly. What this indicated was they did do a lot. Turning around a major illness is not a casual affair. It does take work. These people were committed. They did a lot, and they rated highly the value of many things that they did do.

These people were then asked to think back over their recovery and to identify what they considered to be the three most helpful things they did. Interestingly, quite a number took the trouble to write on the survey that they did not like the question! They had done so much, and found so many things to be helpful, that choosing just three was quite challenging.

Anyway, they did choose three, and the results were fascinating and important. Three things stood out way and above the others. They were the diet, the meditation and the development of their spiritual life.

Now, many of these people were alive ten years after they had initially been predicted to die. So next I asked them what they would recommend to people newly diagnosed. Here four things stood out. The diet and meditation again, but then the advice was to attend a well-run, lifestyle-based self-help group (presumably to learn these techniques and be supported in applying them) and to aim to find meaning and purpose in life.

So what is it with the spiritual life and the meaning and purpose? What our survivors are pointing out is the importance of the mind and its key role in all we do. What inspires you? What motivates you? Why do you want to get well? How important is getting well to you? How much are you prepared to do? How much effort do you want to make? What can you learn through this illness? What meaning and purpose does it clarify for your life? What will you do with your good health? What will you do with your life once you are well again?

These are all questions for our mind. They come under the heading of spirituality, meaning and purpose. It is well said that if you have a "reason" to do something, you will find a "how." If the desire to live is strong and you follow a logical approach, there is every reason to expect a good outcome.

Have enough courage to believe in the possibilities. Then take the next step.

THE FIRST BIG QUESTION • Do I Really Want to Get Well Again?

You may say I am crazy to ask a question like this. However, the fact is some people diagnosed with cancer do accept their condition as terminal and cannot imagine themselves getting well again. For many of these people, this reflects their lack of any real hope. In some cultures there is still a pervading belief that you get cancer and you die. Some families, some individuals still hold this view, either as a result of some morbid fear or maybe as the product of experiences they have had with people they knew who did not do so well.

The antidote? Hope. People in this situation need inspiration—they need to realize the possibilities. This is where groups can be helpful, especially if they contain long-term survivors who can be met, seen, and touched! Even hearing stories of recovery or reading of them in *Inspiring People* or *Surviving Cancer* can help reawaken lost hope and help people to move forward.

However, there is a deeper issue. Some of the people whom I have known had given up on life itself. Some of these people had enough clarity to tell me that life was just too hard. We will examine this possibility in more detail in the chapter on the causes of cancer, but some people, when you come to know them really well, confide that they have lost their zest for life. Perhaps through past trauma, maybe through a variety of accumulated reasons, the future just seems too difficult. It is almost as if they have had enough of life and if cancer is the way to go, then they are not going to fight it.

The antidote? Like our survivors said, find the meaning and purpose in life. What ignites your passion? What inspires you? What have you got to live for? Is there something from years gone by that you put aside that now can be rekindled? Could you change your circumstances to make life seem worth living again? It is so extraordinary to be a living human being. Even the tough times are extraordinary. When we reflect on it, there really is so much to live for.

But what to do right now? If you are clear you want to recover, then no problem, go for it. Move on to the next step, the next question. If you have doubt, if you are unsure about survival, first examine the question of hope and seek inspiration. If there are deeper doubts or fears, or a lack of motivation, look into your heart, seek inspiration, and seek solutions. This may well be the time to talk to a trusted friend or an experienced counselor who can assist you to reach a point of clarity.

So while there is nobility in a good death and while the prospect of a good death is important for all of us as certainly we will all face it one day, the majority of *You Can Conquer Cancer* focuses on the process of getting well and being well.

THE SECOND BIG QUESTION • Who Is Responsible for My Decisions?

This question is best characterized by imagining a visit to your doctor. Do you go to them and say, "Here is my diseased body. You fix it. You tell me what is wrong. You decide what treatment I will have. I will accept whatever you say. The responsibility is yours."

Or, do you go to them and say, "Here is my diseased body. What can we do to get it better again?" With this latter approach, the relationship becomes a more equal one. Instead of handing responsibility for your well-being— and your life—to someone else, you are embarking upon a shared quest for health, a collaborative venture.

Now, in all probability, as time goes on, you are likely to work with a range of health professionals. Their technical skills and their communication skills are bound to vary. Some will be excellent; however, whether through lack of time, lack of aptitude, interest or training, some may well be poor communicators. For the same reasons, some may have a narrow range of expertise. Being practical, it may well serve you best to use some doctors and other health professionals almost mechanically. You take advantage of their technical skills, you take their treatment while accepting that to attempt a deep and meaningful discussion may be rather futile.

What is paramount is to identify the key person in your healing team. I suggest the ideal person for this could well be a general practitioner (GP) or family physician. This implies the need to find and work with a broadly trained, open-minded doctor you can respect and trust. Someone you can talk with freely. Someone who is interested in and takes account of your own, unique situation. Your hopes and your beliefs. Someone who is prepared to set out your options, explain the possibilities and the risks and then give time for questions. Someone who is not afraid to offer a considered opinion, to tell you what they would recommend if you were their own partner, parent or child. And then encourages you to make your own choices and supports you in them.

Currently, many hospitals are working in a more integrated way. They are setting up teams of doctors and allied health professionals who can come together to discuss individual cases and make specific recommendations. This is all to the good, but the questions still remain, who do you talk to? Who coordinates your management? Who is the focal point?

While encouraging you to take ultimate responsibility for your own decisions, the key question remains, who will be your chief adviser?

You may be fortunate and find a cancer specialist who can fill this role. However, experience tells us this is not so common. While I regard the role of doctors as pivotal, it is a sad fact that many patients and their families bemoan the communication skills of their specialists. This criticism has been around for many years and while it does take good training and committed practice to be able to give bad news well, one would hope the quality of communication improves soon.

In some hospitals, nurse-practitioners fill this coordinating confidante role. However, maybe a GP who is trained in and enthusiastic about the integrative approach remains the best choice.

Statistics tell us the average GP sees around three new people diagnosed with cancer each year. Only three. So it is a big thing for them when it happens. However, GPs are very well placed to understand both the medical treatments and your other options. They can provide time for discussion, and they may be specifically trained and experienced in counseling.

You may well have a long-standing relationship with a GP who can fill this role. Unfortunately, what often happens for many people is that they go to the GP with the initial complaint and have their help during diagnosis. Then often they will be referred to specialists, spend plenty of time with them and not revisit the GP. So you may need to remember to go back to your GP for this coordinating role, or you may need to seek a doctor who is more suitable for your current needs, and make ongoing appointments.

Do make it a priority to identify the coordinator of your healing team. Then tell them everything. Tell them about any other treatments you are having. Any and all the supplements or herbs you are considering or taking. Seek their advice to ensure you avoid doubling up or using things that conflict with each other. And seek their support and encouragement. A good GP in this situation can be invaluable, providing clarity, confidence and stability. They can be like a life coach, a healing coach. It is well worth keeping in regular touch with them.

So assemble a good team, seek their advice and support, and make your own decisions.

THE THIRD BIG QUESTION • What Is Most Likely to Heal Me?

Essentially there are three main sources of healing: conventional medicine, natural medicine, which has three components, and your own resources, best expressed here as lifestyle medicine.

Conventional or Orthodox Medicine

Conventional medicine generally describes medical interventions that are taught at medical schools, generally provided at hospitals and meet the requirement of peer-accepted mainstream medicine and standards of care.

Natural Medicine—Made Up Of:

COMPLEMENTARY MEDICINE

Complementary medicine refers to a medicine or therapy that is used in addition to, or complements, conventional medicine. Complementary medicine is increasingly taught in medical schools and practiced in hospitals and is steadily gaining widespread support. More research is needed to better evaluate it.

TRADITIONAL MEDICINE

Traditional medicine includes well-documented or otherwise established medicine or therapies that are based upon the accumulated experience of many traditional health care practitioners over an extended period of time.

Traditional therapies include traditional Chinese medicine, traditional Ayurvedic medicine, Western herbal medicine and homeopathic medicine. These traditional medical systems represent a different paradigm of health care when compared to conventional Western medicine.

ALTERNATIVE MEDICINE

Alternative medicine is the term widely used by many medical authorities to describe modalities that they regard as being on the periphery, being unproven and unwelcome. We will investigate what all these different modalities have to offer in the later chapter on healing.

What is helpful to understand now is that all four—conventional, complementary, traditional and alternative medicine—generally involve seeking help from the outside and having things done to or for you. This makes good sense. You go to a surgeon, massage therapist or acupuncturist for the help they can provide. You take the drugs, herbs or supplements recommended for you and receive their benefits. You have things done to or for you. But then there is another completely different possibility—what you can do for yourself.

Lifestyle Medicine

Lifestyle medicine focuses on what you can do for yourself in the context of your daily life. This is what we focus upon in this book. Lifestyle medicine can be highly therapeutic. It can improve your quality of life and increase your chances of long-term survival dramatically.

Lifestyle medicine involves attending to physical, psychological, social and spiritual factors. The actual techniques include nutrition, exercise, sunlight, stress management, social support, emotional health, the power of the mind, relaxation, imagery, mindfulness and meditation.

It is strongly recommended that anyone diagnosed with cancer attend to their lifestyle right from the start. If you have conventional treatment, lifestyle medicine is likely to minimize any side effects and maximize the benefits. If no curative conventional medical treatment is available, then lifestyle medicine still offers real hope.

INTEGRATIVE MEDICINE • Finding a Suitable Doctor

It is worth emphasizing one more term: integrative medicine.

Integrative medicine refers to a style of medical practice that is holistic and integrates the best and safest of conventional medical care with lifestyle advice and evidence-based complementary medicines and/or therapies. It aims to use the most appropriate of all available modalities and to help each individual patient make informed choices. Integrative medicine is an umbrella term that aptly embraces all styles of medical practice, including lifestyle medicine.

Integrative medicine is becoming a major specialty and many doctors now describe their approach to health, healing and well-being as being integrative. Simply put, perhaps this is what good medicine has always been—taking full regard of the patient as a whole and working collaboratively with a comprehensive range of allied health professionals.

When seeking a medical practitioner to head your healing team, a good starting point would be a doctor who is an advocate of integrative medicine, and preferably a member of an integrative medical association.

Most people start their cancer journey by consulting a doctor. So now, let us take a logical approach and consider how to manage diagnosis, prognosis and treatment options.

START AT THE BEGINNING • Seek an Accurate Diagnosis

Diagnosis is something modern medicine is very good at. Establishing whether you have cancer or not, what type it is, where it is, how extensive it is—all these facts modern medicine generally gets right. Sure, as in anything, mistakes sometimes are made, and particularly in unusual cases second opinions may be worthwhile, but generally the diagnosis can be taken as a fact and as such warrants being accepted.

The Reaction to a Diagnosis of Cancer

Some people accept a cancer diagnosis quite calmly, but I have seen people of all ages and from all walks of life go into deep shock on hearing the fateful words: "You have cancer." A strong emotional reaction is common, completely understandable and needs to be taken in context. Quite often the reaction is one of disbelief and numbness. Sometimes an outpouring of grief. Often confusion, uncertainty and fear. While any or all of these are understandable and common, none of them are good states of mind to be in when making important decisions.

A strong word of advice: Following a diagnosis, give time to adjust emotionally and take your time before making any major decisions. Contrary to common belief, there are very few decisions in cancer medicine where waiting to make them, waiting to act for a week or two, will affect the overall outcome. Many people think that the need to receive treatment for cancer is like when you are hemorrhaging—it needs to be done now, as soon as possible. While it is sometimes true that there can be medical emergencies involved that do demand urgent attention, in the main, a short delay of a week or two will not affect the long-term outcome. Taking your time could have you in a far better state of mind to make crucial decisions and to work well with the treatments you do accept.

This then is a time to be close to family and good friends, particularly those who have the capacity to stay present and offer their stability amid turbulent emotions. Here it is important not to be confused. Many people think the need is to be "positive," which is true, but some think to be "positive" is to be unemotional, which is not true. I have met people who were so afraid of their emotions that they thought it was almost as if they were to cry even once, it would take a week or two off their lives. Of course if one were to cry all day, every day, that may well be a problem, but it would be perfectly natural and normal to have a few, tough emotional days as you take in a cancer diagnosis and what it means for your life and the lives of those around you.

What to Do with the Emotions

Healthy emotions are natural emotions. Unhealthy emotions are when wild emotions control you, or, as is often the case with people affected by cancer, when emotions are suppressed.

Everyone feels emotions. It is how we express them that is the issue. The observable fact is that people vary quite naturally in their range of emotional expression. Some are naturally very expressive, some quite reserved. This is influenced by a variety of factors. Some cultures are very emotionally expressive—Italians often come to mind in this regard. Some keep their emotions under pretty tight control—my culture of origin, the English, seem pretty good at this.

The point is, with emotions, as with all else, individuals do vary. Your aim is to be authentic. To allow yourself to be natural and to be comfortable with your own emotional expression.

Emotions are so important we have two specific chapters on them later, but for now, recognize that allowing your natural emotions to flow is natural, normal and healthy. While the emotions that result from a cancer diagnosis may be painful, do what you can to let them out, either on your own or in the company of those you trust. Once they have been released, it will feel like a real weight has lifted and you will be in a much better place to move on with treatment, using your own resources and taking the steps to recovery.

If you are in doubt about your emotions, if none come or if they seem to be going on forever, do be brave. This is a time to seek help, talk with a professional counselor or an experienced, trusted friend and check your situation out.

Experience says it is very difficult to think clearly, to make good decisions, to really commit to what you need to be doing, if your emotions are all over the place. Once the immediate emotional response to a diagnosis is felt, expressed, and showed, usually the intensity goes out of it. Maybe emotions will arise again in the future. Again that would be natural and normal. But be authentic. Be comfortable with your own degree of emotional expression and realize emotions·are another natural part of a healthy life.

So do take time. Sit with those you are close to. Be with them. Maybe in silence. Maybe with tears. Maybe with talking and discussion. Take it in. Let it out. Allow yourself to settle. And then begin to plan. To move forward again.

CHAPTER 2

Keeping Hope Alive

Prognosis and Looking into the Crystal Ball

WHILE DIAGNOSIS IS BASED ON FACT, PROGNOSIS IS BASED ON SPECULA-tion. With a prognosis comes an attempt to predict the future, to give an informed estimate of what the diagnosis, along with any treatment, is likely to lead to.

The problem with a prognosis is that it can have power in its own right.

In the ancient culture of the indigenous Australian Aborigines there is a phenomenon called the "pointing of the bone." This culture is the oldest continuous culture on the planet and its roots stretch back in time for at least forty thousand years. Many of the Aboriginal tribes lived in small nomadic groups that thrived amid extremely harsh environments. To survive and flourish they had quite strict laws that everyone recognized and generally adhered to. One of the ultimate penalties for transgressing these laws was the pointing of the bone. Here is how it works.

If a person broke a major law, they would be very aware of it themselves. They would know something serious was wrong and they would be aware of the likely consequences. Once the transgression was recognized by the tribe, the senior people would confer, and if all agreed, the punishment of pointing the bone would be carried out by the senior law holder. This person, often referred to as a man of high degree, would dress up in ceremonial garb and the instrument of the punishment literally would be a bone—a human thigh bone.

But there was no beating or physical assault with the bone. It was "pointed." Amidst the ritual of the process, the bone was pointed at the transgressor along with the words—the curse, if you like—the threat, the promise, that the person would die.

Interesting things would begin to happen immediately. First, the law-breaker, the person who had been pointed, would go into a rapid decline. Then, all of the tribe would withdraw and avoid contact with them. The person would become depressed, lose all interest in life, then they themselves would withdraw and become listless, apathetic.

At this point there are frequent records of Western medicine attempting to intervene. No conventional treatment has been shown to prevent the ongoing decline toward death.

As death approaches, another significant observation. The tribe members, sensing the closeness of the end, gather around again. This time they go into pre-mourning rituals and, in the process, seal the fate of the wretched victim of this extraordinary punishment.

So the pointing of the bone is invariably fatal in this Aboriginal context.

Now let us make some unnerving comparisons. A person knows they are not well, that something serious is wrong. They go for help. Senior people confer. Then comes the consultation where the key figure dresses up in ritual garb, with white coat and stethoscope, and makes a pronouncement.

When bad news is given badly, there are all the hallmarks of the pointing of the bone.

"You have only three months to live and there is nothing we can do about it."

In days gone by the message was often given this bluntly. These days, many doctors attempt to be more subtle and compassionate, but even so, many people get the take-home message: you have cancer, you will die.

All too often what happens next is that they go home in shock, they withdraw and then so do their friends. Often friends, even family, are unsure of what to do, how to respond, how to help. Many of these people, well-meaning, kind and considerate in their nature, have told me how they were deeply concerned about doing or saying the wrong thing and so they thought it safer to do nothing, to stay away.

However, if a person with cancer does decline and seems close to death, it is common for people to gather around to say their good-byes. This is natural and we will discuss how to do this in a healthy, constructive way in the chapter on death and dying, but here again, done badly it can fit exactly into the pointing of the bone process.

The message is simple. If bad news is given badly, if a prognosis is given bluntly and taken to heart, the person affected may well have two life-threatening conditions to deal with. The first is the actual illness. The second is the "pointing of the bone." And we know both have the potential to be fatal.

Traditional Aborigines have survived the pointing of the bone. There are accounts where Aboriginal elders or today's doctors have used their own rituals to persuade the person who has been pointed that the punishment has been countered or reversed. No medicine will do this. It all needs to come through the mind of the individual who has been pointed.

Therefore, we need to take heed of all this. For a start, let us use our logic again. In reality, offering a prognosis is a bit like setting the odds on a horse race. While in cancer medicine this process will involve high levels of technical skill and clinical expertise, setting a prognosis remains a process of making an informed guess. One takes into account all the factors one can and then makes the best estimate possible.

Now, we know that in horse racing the reality is that favorites win quite often. Yet we all know long shots get up from time to time. The only way to find out the result of a horse race is to wait until the race is run. Just the same in life. Just the same with cancer.

A prognosis is a bit like setting the odds. It can be helpful in giving all involved a sense of the degree of difficulty the diagnosis implies. Obviously, the odds of recovering from a cold are very high. No one who develops a cold takes it too seriously and fears dramatically for their future. The prognosis with a cold is usually pretty good and we can afford to treat it rather casually. If someone is diagnosed with a widespread aggressive cancer, obviously that is a vastly different matter and makes for a situation that requires the focused attention of everyone concerned.

YOU ARE A STATISTICALLY UNIQUE INDIVIDUAL

But let us go a little deeper. Here is some more good news. Human beings are statistically unique events. What does this mean and why is it so important?

Easy to explain. Consider a game of chance like Two-up. Two-up is where you take two coins, each with heads and tails on either side, throw them into the air, and bet on whether they land with two heads up or two tails. If they land with one head and one tail, you throw them again. Imagine now that two heads have come up five times in a row. Most people instinctively feel the next throw is now more likely to produce two tails. Surely, the odds predict this, we think. Not so. Each time you throw two coins, you have a statistically unique event. There is no connection, no link between one throw and the next! Statistically unique. Sure, if you throw two coins one thousand times you are highly likely to have around five hundred heads and five hundred tails. On average, over large numbers, statistics are relevant and work well. But individual events like tossing coins are unique.

So too with people. People diagnosed with cancer are statistically unique. On average, statistics are useful to predict what might happen, to set the odds. That has some validity and some use, but you will never know the outcome for a unique individual until time moves on and the race is run.

Before my own secondaries were diagnosed, I had been into the medical libraries and had not been able to find a record of anyone surviving my type of metastasized cancer (osteogenic sarcoma) for more than six months. If I had accepted this fact, accepted my prognosis, I could very easily have withdrawn, become passive, and died on time. What a blessing in retrospect that I was "crazy" enough to believe it was possible to recover—"crazy" in that to aspire to recovering I went against all the prevailing evidence of the day. However, there is real logic to what I did and how any other person with cancer needs to approach their prognosis.

When one looks at the range of outcomes for nearly all situations in life, they commonly vary quite a deal. In cancer it is just the same. The evidence is clear that faced with similar diagnoses, some people will live a long time and some not so long at all. This is often referred to as normal distribution and expressed graphically via the bell curve. The bell curve records how, if, say, a thousand people were diagnosed with a similar cancer, as time goes on, some die soon, most die in average time, and some do live on for a much longer time.

The Bell Curve or Normal Distribution
Where the numbers shown represent the percentage of the whole

The time factors will differ for different cancers and the exact shape of the curve may vary too. But the idea is clear. When a large number of people with a given cancer are tracked, most die around the same time. This is the statistic most prognoses are based upon. Maybe if the doctor is optimistic, it is pushed a little to the right; pessimistic, a little to the left. But the message is clear. This represents statistics.

If you or someone you love have been diagnosed with the same cancer as many other people, their history is interesting and points to what is possible, but not to what is certain. You are a statistically unique event. You could fall anywhere on the curve. That is a statistical fact. That is reality.

The big question then is, what affects where you end up on the graph? Is it simply a matter of statistics and random chance, or will what you do influence the outcome?

Back to horse racing again. If you were interested to back a horse in a race and you knew it was not being fed well, how would you feel? What if it was not well trained? How about if it was one of those horses that did not enjoy racing? Surely, these factors affect the outcome.

So too with cancer. If you embrace a good treatment, what direction will that head you in? If you eat well, will that take you right or left on the graph? Eat badly? If you remain filled with fear and dread, or if you develop a positive, committed approach, what is likely?

Given that everyone is a statistically unique event, everyone therefore deserves to be treated uniquely, to be regarded uniquely. Whether you have been diagnosed with cancer or are helping someone through cancer, your situation is unique. No one else has exactly the same situation as you. No one else has exactly the same body. Your emotions will be different, the state of your mind is bound to vary, and your spiritual realities differ. You are unique.

So two women diagnosed with breast cancer may be described as having the same disease, breast cancer. Just as two men with prostate cancer may both be said to have prostate cancer. Same label, very different situations, very different possibilities. Maybe it is more useful to say one woman by the name of Jane who is diagnosed with breast cancer has Jane's disease, another Mary's disease—they could well be that different.

Again, while statistics are useful to generalize, you need a large group for statistics to be useful. The key point is this:

Individuals do not behave statistically. Individuals behave individually.

We are all individuals. If you want an average outcome, do what the average does. If you want a unique outcome, an extraordinary outcome, be logical, regard yourself as you are, unique, and do something extraordinary!

CHAPTER 3

What Treatments Will I Use?

Attending to Individual Needs

MOVING ON FROM DIAGNOSIS AND PROGNOSIS, WHAT ABOUT THE TREATment options? How do you develop a comprehensive treatment plan that is most likely to work and take account of your individuality, your personally unique situation? How to move beyond generalizations and standard treatments, to taking account of individual needs? How do you personalize the appropriate response for your particular situation?

Again, we rely on logic for the framework and then aim to draw on experience, wisdom and insight for the details.

Nearly everyone in the Western world will be diagnosed and consider initial treatment within the conventional Western medical framework. This makes good sense and is as it should be.

Given that the diagnosis and prognosis will be provided by the best medical people available, it is they who will recommend an initial treatment plan. This too makes good sense. Certainly if there were a simple, medical solution to cancer, one piece of surgery, one pill we could take that ensured a cure, we would all do it. You would be a fool not to. But it is not so simple.

DEFINITIONS • Curative Treatment, Palliative Care or Living with Cancer?

While the medical treatment of cancer tends to focus on one of two outcomes, to be curative or to be palliative, there is a third option. Let us be clear with the definitions.

Curative Treatment

Curative treatment involves more than what many people imagine it to be, which is to be free of cancer after five years. Actually, curative treatment aims to render the person clinically free of detectable cancer and restore the person to their normal life expectancy.

Palliative Care

On the other hand, palliative care is an umbrella term for assisting those approaching death—a fundamental need and right. It is generally used in the context that death is imminent and inevitable and aims to make dying as easy and comfortable as possible.

PALLIATIVE TREATMENT—LIVING WITH CANCER

Palliative treatment is a specific but integral part of palliative care. Palliative treatment can be more interventionist. It is noncurative by definition but aims to extend life, ameliorate symptoms, and increase quality of life in situations where a cure is not medically feasible.

The lines between palliative care and palliative treatment can often be blurred, but these days, palliative treatment is often called living with cancer.

While overall survival rates in the conventional management of cancer may not have improved all that much, in recent years many people are living longer with cancer. This can involve significantly slowing the progression of the disease, minimizing any side effects and maximizing all the quality of life issues. Palliative chemotherapy often plays a significant part in conventional medicine's management of palliative treatment.

WHAT TO DO WHEN A MEDICAL CURE IS LIKELY

Now the logic. If a person is offered medical treatment for cancer where there is a high probability of a cure, then, in my view, what to do is fairly straightforward. Embrace that treatment as your main focus while you go through whatever it entails. The common treatment options are surgery—which often comes first—then maybe chemotherapy and/or radiotherapy.

However, right at the start or even better still, before you start your treatment there is more to do. As soon as possible, review your lifestyle and do whatever you can to complement and support the treatment with your own efforts. The details of what this entails follow in the subsequent chapters. Lifestyle medicine will have your body and your mind in the optimal state to get the best out of any treatments and to minimize the potential for any side effects.

When it comes to the complementary, traditional and alternative options, there may well be useful things to consider that will support your body's healing capacity, minimize or manage side effects and have other useful benefits. These options will be discussed in later chapters as well.

THE CHOICES WHEN A MEDICAL CURE IS NOT SO LIKELY

However, what if a cure is not so likely from the medical point of view? What if at first diagnosis, or further down the track, it becomes clear that a medically based cure is improbable? What if palliative care or living with cancer is all that remains medically? There are three options.

1. Acknowledge Death as the Likely Outcome

This is probably not the option you are opting for if reading this book. However, we do need to recognize and accept that some people do accept their prognosis and do acknowledge death as the likely outcome. They then may choose to focus on what can be done to garner the best from whatever time remains, to live with cancer as long as possible and to prepare for a good death.

Yes, prepare for a good death. Death is like everything else in life. We can stumble into it, hoping for the best, or we can prepare for it and, in all likelihood, have a good death. To be open about this, when I started working in the early eighties with others affected by cancer, I knew little of death and I was preoccupied with the desire to help people to recover. I admit to being apprehensive about what would happen if and when people died of their cancer. While many did recover, others did go on to die of their disease. Over the years I have worked closely with many of these people and it has been incredibly heartening to observe how consistently the people I have known who prepared for death were able to die well. What they learned and what they did stood them in good stead, and the quality of their deaths was exceptionally high. We will speak more of this in a later chapter.

For now, it needs to be said that some people faced with the situation where there is no medical cure on offer do accept death. Some are content to focus on living with cancer and are keen to utilize palliative care when the time comes. Again, that is a perfectly reasonable and logical choice. However, if for whatever reason you are not ready, if you do not accept death, and if you are still intent on getting well, you need to be logical. If medicine cannot cure you, what will? Can anything?

2. Seek a Cure from the Nonconventional Medical Options

Remember the different styles of medicine: conventional, traditional (TM), complementary and alternative (CAM). If conventional medicine says a cure is beyond them, do any of the others have a solution? I have the personal knowledge of many individuals telling me that individual TM or CAM therapies were very significant in their recoveries. But I do not have the experience of consistency in this. It seems that from time to time, for some individuals, individual TM and CAM modalities fit really well with that particular person and are highly effective. But I am not aware of a TM or CAM therapy that reliably will be of major benefit to a wide range of people. I do not know of a magic bullet in the realms of traditional, complementary or alternative medicine.

3. Seek a Cure Within—Recovering Against the Odds

Even when conventional medicine says there is nothing more we can do toward a cure, I do believe there still is real hope on offer. Where the "magic bullet" actually does reside is within you. In the face of difficult odds, a cure may be much more likely through mobilizing your own inner healing than through chasing after some elusive external TM or CAM treatment.

Remember, it only has to be done once to show that it is possible. You only need one person to use their own inner resources to recover without the aid of external, curative medical treatments and you know that it is possible. Just one case demonstrates that there is the potential for the body to react, to reject the cancer within it, and to heal. And if it can be done once, it can be done again. And the truth is it has been done many more times than once. What I have been studying and teaching for over thirty years is what makes this most likely to happen.

Clearly, if you aim to recover against the odds, it is not likely to be easy. There is no point misleading anyone here. If it was easy, everyone would be doing it and no one would be dying. My experience is, as we have discussed already, those who do become remarkable survivors make a good deal of effort. They dare to hope, they seek out good information, they rally support, and they put good intentions into action. Then they persevere. They deal with the ups and downs. They learn from what others might judge to be mistakes, are prepared to experiment, try new things, and in doing so, develop an inner confidence. They learn through their process, often see it as a journey and commonly come to enjoy the challenge and reflect warmly on their achievements. And in all probability, they have a little good luck as well!

Recovering against the odds is not a casual business. It takes focus, energy and commitment. What then is the main thing to focus upon? Clearly if conventional medicine has said it cannot cure you, it is not that. In my view TM or CAM therapies cannot do it reliably either. The focus in this situation needs to be on inner healing, and to support this inner healing with the best of what conventional medicine, TM and CAM have to offer. Maybe more surgery or chemotherapy is useful to minimize the amount of cancer your body needs to attend to. Maybe you use medical, TM or CAM treatments to boost your immunity and your healing capacity, or to minimize symptoms. But in the situation where no medical cure is on offer, you may be wise to focus on your potential, the lifestyle medicine as we call it, and support that with all else.

HOW TO COMBINE THE BEST OF WHAT IS AVAILABLE • A Summary

When Curative Treatment Is a Real Prospect

Focus on the medical treatment, and support that with all the other options available to you. Lifestyle medicine will always be useful; use TM and CAM judiciously.

When No Curative Conventional Medical Cure Is on Offer

The choices are

i) Palliative care—accept the diagnosis and the prognosis, and plan for a good death. Lifestyle medicine is likely to be of great benefit for extending life as well as preparing for a good death. Use conventional medical treatments and CAM judiciously.

ii) Living with cancer—accept the diagnosis and the prognosis, then accept that your real goal is to live as long as possible, as well as possible. Quality of life becomes the focus—along with whatever is likely to extend your life. So again, the lifestyle factors set out in this book warrant being the focus of your plans, supported by good medicine and whatever TM and CAM therapies may be helpful.

iii) Accept the diagnosis and reject the prognosis. Dare to recover. Focus on developing healing within by employing lifestyle medicine—and support that with all else. Use conventional medicine, TM and CAM judiciously.

WHAT SPECIFIC TREATMENTS WILL YOU ACCEPT? HOW TO DECIDE WHAT TO DO

Before we examine in detail how to activate the healer within, let us pause to investigate what external forms of treatment, if any, to which you will be wise to commit. Let us begin with the medical options.

The logical way to assess any proposed form of medical treatment would be to ask your doctor the following questions:

(a) What does the future hold for you if no treatment is given, and in such circumstances what range of life expectancy would you have? The best way to ask this question is statistically. Ask if there were one hundred patients just like you and they had no treatment, what would be a reasonable estimate for the following:

  i) How many people would be alive after one year and what would their health be like?

  ii) How many people would be alive after five years and what would their health be like?

(b) What range of life expectancy would you have if given the proposed form of treatment? Again, ask for the answer to this question in statistical terms. If there were one hundred people like you who had the same condition and they received the proposed treatment, what would be a reasonable estimate for the following:

  i) After one year, how many people would be alive and what would their health be like?

ii) After five years, how many people would be alive and what would their health be like?

Note: These statistical ranges should be available in virtually all medical situations, barring those that involve very rare cancers or experimental treatments including chemotherapy trials. If they are not provided upon request, I would seek another opinion. If you are considering an experimental treatment or a trial, you can only assess it on its possible merits.

In other words, through these first questions you are aiming to find out the anticipated benefits of the treatment, expressed in statistical terms.

(c) What are the side effects of the treatment? It will be most useful to obtain the answer to this question in statistical terms as well so that you obtain a real sense of any potential risks. So again, ask:

i) If there were one hundred people like you who had this treatment, what side effects are possible and how many people are likely to be affected by those side effects? Do 5 percent or 95 percent have nausea? Do 5 percent or 95 percent lose their hair?

ii) And how long are those side effects likely to persist? For a few minutes, weeks, years? Will they be permanent?

iii) How might they be managed if they do occur? For example, there are many good treatments available these days for the side effects of chemotherapy, and hair that falls out because of chemotherapy commonly grows back fairly quickly.

(d) What impact will my own response to the treatment have on the outcome? In truth, the answer to this question may be harder to define than the previous three. The medical system is very good at evaluating its results. This is made easier by the fact that a single intervention, such as a drug therapy, is relatively easy to study and accurately evaluate. By contrast, the human being is incredibly complex—the role of emotions, mind and spirit are extremely interwoven. They are not so amenable to the standard double-blind, crossover trials used to research and evaluate so many drugs.

What does seem clear, however, is that how you respond has the potential to affect the outcome of anything you do. If in cancer treatment you are treated with chemotherapy, full of fear and loathing, preoccupied with potential side effects and the possibilities of damaging your immune system, you are highly likely to undermine the potential benefits of that treatment. If, on the other hand, you think it through and decide to accept the treatment, regard it as in your best interest and do all you can to work with it, you are likely to get the very best from that treatment.

THE KEY TO GREAT OUTCOMES • Embrace Everything You Do

This is why you are strongly advised to make conscious decisions about all you do. Nearly always, there are pluses and minuses to consider when making medical decisions. Take your time and think things through. If you need help with this, a very useful decision-making technique that draws on both the intellect and intuition is presented soon in the first chapter on mind training (chapter 7).

Once you do come to a decision, the strong recommendation is to embrace all that you do. Embrace! Not just put up with, not just tolerate, nor even just accept it. Embrace it! Understand that this is what you have chosen to do. It is in your best interest—like when you would take antibiotics for pneumonia. Know that whether it be having chemotherapy, changing your diet or practicing meditation, the more you welcome it into your life, the better you feel about doing it, the more you support your choice, the more you embrace it—the better it will work.

When you embrace what you do, you release all the positive potentials of your mind, emotions and spirit. My belief is that when you embrace a treatment and really work with it in positive expectation, then you can reasonably hope to get the best possible results with the least side effects.

However, given all this, you may still have a very difficult decision to make.

The reality is that most current treatments for cancer are hard on the patients—sometimes very hard. It is a fact that most of the conventional therapies are toxic to the body. Radiation and chemotherapy frequently impair the body's own immune system along with other components of its defense mechanism. This reduces the body's ability to heal itself. Often this impairment is severe and side effects can be marked. Radiation burns, vomiting and loss of hair are obvious problems that can follow. Tiredness, lethargy, "foggy" thinking, depression and loss of memory are all observed as regular consequences of cancer treatments.

The impact of many medical treatments upon the rest of the body can be less obvious, but nevertheless more drastic in nature. Minor infections that previously would have been of no consequence can assume major proportions. Most important, the body's own ability to fight the cancer is frequently lessened.

However, while the side effects of conventional treatment require careful consideration, chemotherapy or radiotherapy may still be the best medical treatments that are available at present. It may well be that it is in your best interest to use them. If this is the case and if you are having a toxic form of therapy, it is all the more important to concentrate on those self-help techniques that aim to boost the immune system and help the body to help itself. These techniques are discussed in later chapters.

Be Brave—Communicate!

Here again, good communication with your doctor is essential. The ideal is to be able to discuss all your concerns freely and easily with your main doctor. If this is not the case, talk with that doctor about the communication problem. We all know how some personalities clash and there are some people we just do not seem able to get along with. If you cannot find a way to correct the situation and communicate well, then request a referral to someone more suited to your temperament. No one should be offended by this. It will make life easier and more constructive for everyone. (For more detailed recommendations, see Appendix A.)

The final choice regarding what conventional treatment to accept may still be difficult. Again recognize the value of making this decision with clarity and confidence and the imperative of committing to what you do decide to do. A reminder then of the value of taking your time. Better to avoid a rushed, hasty decision that may later cause you doubt or regret. Best to take your time, seek expert opinion, discuss the options with those you value, contemplate, give due regard to your intuition and then commit.

Maybe in the final analysis it is the level of confidence and trust you place in the doctor(s) involved that decide it for you.

If surgery is what seems necessary, it seems wise to leave the details of the surgery to your surgeon. If chemotherapy is something else that you decide to commit to, again it would seem wise to leave the choice of agents to your chemotherapist.

You may desire, however, to know more or less of the details of your treatment and you can reasonably expect to have your questions answered in an open, cooperative manner.

Whatever the final choices you make, the next step is to do all that you possibly can to make sure the treatment works to full effect. We will discuss the means to achieve this throughout the book.

How to Enhance Surgery, Chemotherapy or Radiotherapy

The majority of people diagnosed with cancer will have one or more of the conventional treatments recommended to them, and decide to commit to the treatment. With the intention of minimizing any side effects and maximizing the benefits, it is important to be well prepared and to do the best possible to work with any treatments. While the details of what to do unfold in the coming chapters, a quick summary of the recommendations regarding how to prepare for medical treatments forms Appendix B.

Activating Your Inner Healer

Based upon many years of clinical experience and supported by the most recent research, the way to activate healing through your own efforts is easy to define. Your body's capacity to heal is directly affected by what you eat, what you drink, and whether or not you smoke. Sunlight, vitamin D and exercise all play important roles, as does your emotional life and state of mind. How you manage stress, your capacity to relax, to be mindful and to meditate—along with the way your spiritual view impacts on your life and those around you; all these factors impact on the inner healer.

While I have to say it strikes me as a somewhat bland term, all these elements are best described as being under the banner of lifestyle medicine— they are to do with the things you can control and do in the course of your daily life. And the key? It is your mind. Again, it is your mind that decides what you eat and drink. It is the mind that helps you to adopt a healthy, healing lifestyle or remain stuck in old unhelpful habits. Truly, it is the mind that changes everything and so we will begin the road to recovery with the mind.

To embark on the healing journey, to embrace outer help with conventional medicine, TM and CAM, to begin to activate the inner healer—all this is best achieved by being in a stable state of mind, clear and confident. What meditation promises and reliably delivers is a stable, clear mind. As stability becomes more constant, clarity more natural, and confidence more assured, it becomes easier to go from the broad recommendations regarding what to eat, how much to exercise and so on, and to be able to personalize those recommendations. Therefore, in seeking a stable, calm and clear mind, we begin with meditation.

To Those Interested in Prevention

If you are well, just how well are you? Are you just symptom free or are you as fit as your true potential allows?

When this book was first written in 1984, the statistic quoted was that "one in three people alive in the United States today will get cancer during their lifetime. One in five in Australia will die from it." Now the figure is closer to one in two people alive today will develop cancer and currently one in four Australians dies of cancer. This is not scare-mongering. This is fact. Cancer is a lifestyle disease. Are you prepared to learn the lesson of this disease and take up on a lifestyle aimed for optimal health? A lifestyle that is highly likely to prevent the majority of cancers?

These techniques we talk of can save the lives of people affected by cancer. We have seen them work for many other disease conditions as well. Also they can make a basically well person a picture of health. Back in 1981, in his landmark work, *The Causes of Cancer*,[5] Professor R. Doll gave the medical evidence that 85 percent of all cancers could be prevented by changes in lifestyle! The challenge is there. It takes effort; it requires commitment and an ability to be open to change. Again, it can be done. Our natural state *is* health. Please take up that challenge. It would be wonderful to see people learning from the difficulties of others and not having the need for change forced upon them by physical disease. While it is wonderful to help people to recover from cancer, how much better—and wiser—not to get sick in the first place.

Four Features of Long-Term Survivors with Advanced Malignancy

Throughout this book you will pick up many features of long-term survivors and gain insights into what they did to recover. However, reflecting on a long and illustrious career as a cancer surgeon, Professor Gabriel Kune highlighted special characteristics of a particular group—people with advanced malignancy who became unexpectedly long-term survivors, and I quote:

1. They seek a wide exposure to conventional medical opinion and treatment.

   They take "control" of their health. They will decide for themselves what advised treatment to have and what treatment not to have. They are often critical of their medical management.

2. They seek a wide exposure to nonconventional opinion and treatment. Again, they will decide for themselves what they will choose to have and they are often critical of nonconventional management.

3. They operate at an intuitive level.

   They are usually not "thinkers" or intellectuals. They tend not to operate at a rational level as their main guide for making decisions and appear to make decisions "intuitively."

4. They are at peace with themselves.

   One often gets a sense of tranquility, peace and spirituality while in their presence. They are not at all fearful.[6]

Now, in my own experience I would agree with all this generally, and while I certainly recognize the importance of the intuition in decision making, many of the long-term survivors I have known have also been very smart and drawn on their intellects well. Where people can get into trouble is when they think too much, get lost in the range of options, lost in doubt and worry, and as such do not access their intuition, do not make clear and confident decisions, do not commit to what they are doing.

Maybe we can summarize Professor Kune's four points by saying that long-term survivors have a calm and clear mind. This enables them to think clearly, to make good decisions and to be at peace with the world and themselves. Given all the challenges cancer can present, how do we avoid fear and even panic? How do we develop a calm and clear mind? Meditation provides a well-proven solution, plus it has real healing benefits in its own right. In the next chapter we will begin to unlock meditation's secrets.

CHAPTER 4

Meditation

The Principles Behind the Silent Healer

MEDITATION IS THE SINGLE MOST POWERFUL SELF-HELP TOOL THAT ASSISTS recovery from disease and leads to a life of maximum health. It provides all the basic ingredients. It has direct physical effects ranging from relief of physical tension to reactivation of the immune system. Meditation reliably leads to a calm and clear mind, the ability to think clearly, to make good decisions, and to see them through to completion. On top of this, meditation aids the development of emotional and mental poise, generates a positive attitude, and most important, leads automatically and effortlessly to a heightened level of well-being.

Currently, more than six thousand scientific studies published in the medical and scientific literature around the world attest to meditation's capacity to positively affect physical and psychological health and well-being. Little wonder then that it has enjoyed such a rise in popularity as a self-help technique! When coupled with dietary considerations and active efforts to utilize the benefits of positive thinking, it forms the pillars upon which to build our capacity for healing and total health.

In the past, meditation has been used by most major religions as one part of a complex process intended for developing a heightened level of consciousness. Today the word "meditation" is used to describe many different processes. The specific form of meditation that interests us here, with its emphasis on being used as a therapy, relies on learning how to relax profoundly in body and mind. We call it mindfulness-based stillness meditation (MBSM). This form of meditation is disarmingly simple to learn and apply in our daily life, and has played a major part in transforming the health and lives of many people I have known.

My initial introduction to this form of meditation, and its therapeutic application, came through the great Australian psychiatrist Dr. Ainslie Meares. Interested in pain management, Dr. Meares first became interested in meditation as a means to relieve pain. However, he soon realized meditation had much more to offer and he began to experiment with meditation as a means for helping people to cope with anxiety and stress-related symptoms such as phobias, high blood pressure, allergies, nervous tension and pain intolerance. Then he wrote the world's first book on the therapeutic benefits of meditation, *Relief Without Drugs*, in 1967.

One of Dr. Meares' major contributions has been that he recognized the importance of stillness. A still mind, in a still body. He suggested that in this stillness, the body has the opportunity to return to its natural state of balance. He also observed that when meditation was practiced regularly, this refound state of balance persists throughout the day, helping the person to return automatically to that condition of balance we call health! Just as a cut finger heals itself automatically without us dwelling upon it, so meditation can reactivate natural healing mechanisms that operate automatically and have profound effects. It is to his great credit that Dr. Meares was able to perceive this and then devise a simple and quick technique that leads to that point of stillness and balance without, say, twenty years of rigorous concentrated study and practice of Zen discipline.

To understand why meditation is so helpful for so many health conditions, and for cancer specifically, we need to understand the role stress plays in our lives, in our health, and in our capacity to heal. This will then provide us with vital clues as we plan our self-help program.

MEDITATION, STRESS, ANXIETY AND RELIEF

To understand how stress does affect us, let us look at the simple case of what happens when we get a sudden fright. Suppose that a bolt of lightning were to hit the ground near where you were standing. Your body would react very quickly, almost instantaneously. With a gasped "Oh!" you instinctively would take a sharp breath in and your muscles would contract with a jerk. Your body chemistry would change almost immediately as an array of hormones was released. Adrenaline would flow and cortisol levels rise. Your heart would race, your blood pressure would increase, and your blood would be diverted to the muscles of action. You would have been readied for immediate action, thanks to the automatic changes produced by what is called the fight-or-flight response. In our example, if you were quick, you may have dove under cover. But then, also quite quickly, you would have realized that the big bang really was just lightning, it had missed you, and everything was all right. "Ah!" would have come the response. The tension would be released and you would relax.

The events in this sequence are very important. The challenge gave rise to a bodily reaction that immediately prepared you for physical action. In the normal course of events, a period of physical activity would follow, which in turn would be completed and be followed by release. The sequence can be summarized:

1. Challenge
2. Bodily reaction with changes in body chemistry
3. Appropriate physical action with a clear beginning and end
4. Release and relax
5. Body chemistry returns to its usual, daily balance

This is a perfectly healthy sequence that was developed in earlier times when life was simpler and very physical in nature. The fight-or-flight response was then, and remains to this day, a vital aid for self-preservation. So if, for example, in older times, a saber-toothed tiger came charging over the hill toward you, intent upon making you dinner, the threat was very obvious! That threat produced rapid changes in your body chemistry and you were immediately prepared for action. This would lead to your doing the appropriate thing. If you felt you had a chance, you stood your ground and fought it out; if not, you ran. Either way, the challenge was resolved by a period of intense physical action that was followed through to a definite conclusion. You would then be free to relax, either licking your wounds or basking in success.

This sequence flowed with the rhythm of a simple life and it left no adverse aftereffects. Any fears that did remain were healthy ones based purely on instinct and self-preservation. Such fears did little to lessen the quality of life or lead to any physical symptoms. Animals in their natural state still demonstrate the appropriateness of this fight-or-flight response in a physically oriented world.

However, for us humans living in modern times, things are no longer so simple. The challenges we face now are rarely of a purely physical nature and frequently are complex indeed. Most, if not all, of our challenges nowadays are emotional or mental in their origins. However, an even greater problem is that frequently they are difficult to resolve.

So when the boss is overbearing and demanding, or the neighbor disturbs our sleep early on Sunday morning with his lawn mower, we react in the same old way. We take that short little gasp and tense our muscles. Our body chemistry changes rapidly, preparing us for action. But can we punch the boss's nose or wrap the neighbor's lawn mower around his ears? Not if we want the paycheck that we need to meet our commitments; not if we want to remain socially acceptable in our community! Often then, taking the action we might feel inclined to take instinctively is inappropriate and so our response is stifled. Worse still, we can have the situation where we do act reasonably, we do take what seems to be the appropriate action, and yet, even so, the challenges in our lives remain unresolved. We do all we can to reduce the mortgage, but it still remains, nagging away and causing us fear and worry.

When we do have an unresolved challenge, people tend to react in one of two general ways. The first is to accept the situation, let it go, and get on with life. No problem. The other is to stew on it, hang on to it, worry over it. Big problem! Common problem!

If we are one of the many people who do stew on things, then the problem is that every time we face that same situation or even think about it, the physical changes in our body chemistry are reinforced. Feeling that there is no obvious resolution or conclusion to our problems, having no way of finding an adequate release, there is no return to our basic, healthy body chemistry. We are locked into a situation where the fight-or-flight changes in our body chemistry persist.

A crucial point here is that the changes in body chemistry we are discussing and that are associated with the fight-or-flight response are fine in the short term. They are an appropriate preparation for a short period of intense activity. Where they are not appropriate is when they persist for long periods.

This brings us to another important point. Some people who are intent on de-stressing and getting well worry if they get an occasional fright or a even a brief moment or stress. Let us be really clear about this. In the short term, the fight-or-flight response is no problem and, in fact, can be quite helpful. It is when the biochemical changes that accompany the response become chronic and stay with us long term that we develop real problems.

If the changes in our body chemistry persist, we experience what is known as destructive stress. This type of stress is a challenge that leads to a prolonged untoward effect on a person. Stress occurs when there is an inability to take appropriate action in response to a challenge and so release it. Therefore, stress is an unresolved challenge.

It is easy to appreciate that stress is a very personal thing. It is really determined by how we respond to a challenge, rather than by the nature of the challenge itself. What may be an easily resolved challenge for one person may produce profound stress for another.

STRESS AND CANCER

The next key is that persistent stress affects the body chemistry in such a way that the body's immune system is depleted. It is the changes in hormonal levels particularly that reduce the body's immune function, along with its ability to maintain and repair itself. And so, with time and other factors such as poor diet, stress leaves the way open for many diseases to precipitate. The American Academy of Physicians states that stress-related symptoms lead to two-thirds of all visits to American family doctors. Stress is a major contributor, either directly or indirectly, to absenteeism, coronary heart disease, lung conditions, accident injuries, cirrhosis of the liver, suicide and a host of lesser ailments. I am convinced that stress is a major causative factor in cancer.

Virtually all the many thousands of cancer patients I have asked believe stress was a major factor in the development of their disease. Most recognize that first there was a chronic level of stress in their lives. But, more important, they generally identify readily with a psychological profile common to cancer patients. In about 95 percent of patients asked, this profile involves one particularly severely stressful experience precipitating a drastic drop in their well-being. The stressful event invariably occurred well before the cancer was diagnosed but its untoward effects continued. This highly significant factor will be discussed in detail in the chapter dealing with the causes of cancer (chapter 15).

RECOGNIZING STRESS

For the moment, though, how do you know when stress is a problem? If it is not patently obvious, as it often is, muscular tension is a good guide. If you suffer from stress, one of the body changes it will produce is physical tension. Your body can be your guide. If you are free of muscle tension, feeling relaxed and well, then you almost certainly have no problems! If your brow is knotted, your jaw clamped shut, if you have a persistent knot in your stomach, your shoulders are rigid or your hands clenched tightly, if you feel physical tension—beware! It is a warning signal. However, with appropriate action we can transform this, avoid future problems and generate healing.

RELIEVING STRESS WITH MEDITATION • The Theory

Understanding the stress cycle makes it easy to understand how to deal with stress. It is not necessary to avoid stress totally, just deal with it appropriately. What we need is a means to release it. All successful people who cope well with potentially stressful situations have their personal means of finding release, of relaxing, of letting go.

But based on more than thirty years of experience assisting people with cancer, the easiest, the safest and the most reliable method—the best method for relieving muscular tension and stress—is the specific meditation technique we call mindfulness-based stillness meditation (MBSM). Because this type of meditation concentrates on a profound relaxation of the body and mind, it provides the opportunity for release—it allows us to let go! It allows us to regain a healthy balance in our body chemistry.

To learn how to achieve this, we begin by meditating formally and learning how to relax body and mind. The release found in these initial periods of meditation soon flows on to become an integral part of our life. As we return to a more relaxed state, we return to that healthy balance of body chemistry that is essential for promoting healing and maintaining good health.

Moreover, once we understand the stress cycle, we can understand why meditation for healing needs to be so simple and so uncomplicated. We can understand why it needs to begin with the relaxation of body and mind, and advance to include the release that comes with inner stillness.

For it is by entering this state of simple stillness that we enter a state of profound rest. When we are still, everything comes to rest—profoundly! And in that state of deep rest, we return to a natural state of balance. It is this state of balance we call good health. Good health is a state where we are in balance—a state where balance involves body, emotions, mind and spirit.

For many people, then, meditation has been enough in their quest for sustainable good health. Practiced regularly, meditation frees them from the bondage of stress, allows them to relax, to regain balance, and so enjoy life to the fullest. Do use this basic self-help technique and make it a part of your life. The benefits will repay the initial effort.

THE TRADITIONAL ROLE OF MEDITATION

As we seek to adapt this ancient technique into a modern context, and apply it specifically in a therapeutic setting, it may well be helpful to understand meditation in its historical context, to consider and be informed by some of its traditional techniques.

Meditation has been practiced for thousands of years in all major cultures and traditions, primarily as a major tool on the spiritual path. It has been well said that meditation provides a reliable means through which we can come to know our own minds more fully. Meditation is an ideal technique to call upon when we are interested to examine the question of who we really are, and delightfully, history tells us that reliably it does lead to satisfying answers. Appendix C offers an insight into the traditional role of meditation and some of its key techniques. The book I cowrote with my colleague Paul Bedson, *Meditation—An In-depth Guide,*[7] is a good reference point.

Personally, I feel very grateful for having close contact with and learning from a wide range of extraordinary meditation teachers over many years. Initially there was Dr. Meares, and more recently Sogyal Rinpoche, an authentically trained Tibetan master of meditation who has provided me with the rare opportunity to access ancient and authentic wisdom teachings that marry so well with modern needs. Then, too, I have learned so much from the many thousands of people who I have taught to meditate over the years. What I can offer here is a testament to all these great teachers.

WHAT DOES MEDITATION OFFER TO THOSE WITH CANCER?

I had been fortunate to develop my cancer at a time when Dr. Ainslie Meares first contemplated the use of meditation for people affected by cancer. I had an emerging interest in the traditional forms of meditation and felt that these principles should be able to restore the inner harmony I felt I had lost. I believed if I could regain that inner harmony, it would be reflected on the outer physical level. Dr. Meares' idea was that the meditation would relieve anxiety and stress. This would lead to a reduction in the levels of cortisone in my body and so allow my immune system to operate normally. Then my body would remove the tumors itself. It would return to normal. Putting it all together sounded good to me!

As I have practiced meditation more and come to see others benefit from it too, there do appear to be two broad areas of benefit. Meditation increases quality of life and quantity of life. In my experience, people who meditate regularly do feel better, and they do live longer.

Considering quality of life first, we see benefits on all levels of human experience. There are physical, emotional, mental and spiritual gains.

Physical Benefits

Chronic physical tension is a symptom of stress that we know inhibits the body's natural function. Meditation relieves physical tension. Many people are struck by how good their body feels once this tension is removed. They realize just how much tension they had before learning to meditate in this way. While previously they had come to accept the tension as normal, now they realize just how unpleasant it really was.

Athletes have found meditation can increase their performance and certainly most people find their general efficiency in day-to-day tasks goes up extraordinarily once they begin to meditate. Consistently, heart rates go down, and even severely elevated blood pressure can return to normal. A typical example was Dr. Colin, who joined our group not with cancer but as an interested observer, and found much to his surprise that meditation and diet brought his severely elevated blood pressure back to normal within two months.

Emotional Benefits

Emotionally, our own level of ease is greatly improved through meditation. People find that they feel better about themselves. They feel more able to accept their limitations and to use their strengths positively. In so doing, they are more able to relate to other people in an open, honest and meaningful way.

Any cancer patient knows that being just that—a cancer patient—has its problems. Before cancer was diagnosed, you may have been a doctor, a teacher, a housewife, whatever. So often after diagnosis, to your friends you are now a cancer patient first and foremost, and everything else comes a poor second. This can cause much awkwardness and can become quite a cause for anxiety in itself. However, it is remarkable how meditation reliably leads to an acceptance of the situation and an openness that is infectious, putting everyone at ease.

Also, many people find meditation reduces any feelings of guilt and negative emotion they may have. As a consequence, they develop a greater capacity for loving. While this often results in an improved quality of sexual love, it also improves that more erudite, selfless love and compassion for all. People find they are able to feel good about themselves to a higher degree and, in doing so, give of themselves more safely and freely, and to be of more help to those around them.

Mental Benefits

Mental anxiety, if present, hinders all aspects of our being. Its causes are endless, often unidentifiable. Frequently, psychiatrists have spent long hours raking over the traumas of the past in a quest for the elusive cause of present anxieties. From the womb, to birth, the formative years, adolescence and beyond, all manner of incidents can be identified as potential causes for anxiety and stress. Even if the cause is identified, treatment often remains difficult.

Here is a vivid example. The Lancaster bombers of World War II had their rear ends protected by tail gunners. These men climbed into the tail section of the plane via a ladder. They lay down in the cramped fuselage and then had a Perspex bubble slammed tight around them. Their only communication with the rest of the crew was by headphone. They then set off on an incredibly rough ride with little to dwell upon except their solitary machine guns and the fact that on average they could expect to survive about two missions. An extreme and obvious cause for anxiety. It was not surprising then to find that after the war those who did survive frequently felt great tension when they were confined in small spaces. Many of these men found great difficulty in relaxing enough to urinate when in the narrow confines of a toilet! Frequently they knew the cause of their problem as did all who tried to relieve their anxiety. What happened? The problem remained and invariably they needed to leave the toilet door open!

There are two principles operating here. First, just knowing the cause of a problem is not necessarily enough to relieve it; an appropriate technique is also important. Second, if those men could not have related their inability to go to the toilet to their wartime experiences, they would have felt a great deal more anxiety and suffered greater distress.

Actually, it was with these very tail gunners that Dr. Meares began his foray into the realm of stress and anxiety. He found the standard psychiatric techniques of the postwar period were of little help to these men, but that hypnotherapy brought rapid relief. Dr. Meares went on to become a world authority in hypnotherapy and it was through this interest he came across meditation and pioneered its therapeutic use.

What he realized was that in seeking health, we need to understand as much about our situation as possible, as well as having appropriate techniques to deal with it. We benefit greatly from our own realization of what a constant effort it is to live with the pressure created by persistent anxiety. It is like trying to keep the lid on a pressure cooker all the time. It tires us physically, emotionally and mentally. However, once that anxiety is relieved, we feel benefits all through and our physical symptoms soon respond.

Perhaps Dr. Meares' greatest contribution has been to show that meditation reliably treats stress and anxiety regardless of cause, and, more important, it works even if what caused it is unidentified. Meditation is so effective because it short-circuits the stress cycle. It provides a reliable means of moving quickly and easily from those changes in body chemistry that are an integral part of the physical effects of stress. Releasing stress in this natural way heralds a return to normal function and health.

This rationale explains further why we benefit from starting the meditation technique with relaxing the physical body and why the "release," or the relaxation of body and mind, promotes a return to normal health. Once we trigger that state of release, the body chemistry returns to normal and the normal state means health. What we really need to do quite simply is to let go!

Spiritual Benefits

Spiritually, many people find meditation leads to a peace of mind they had not imagined possible. A member of our group, Cathy, recently told me that her body had never been worse but she had never felt so good! Her face was shining, full of enthusiasm and she said she was experiencing a quality of life she had never known before.

This peace of mind comes at a level so fundamental that it becomes in reality a true, direct experience. Many people who have firm religious beliefs to begin with are surprised by the depth of this experience. While some are apprehensive that meditation may conflict with their beliefs, the usual experience is that it leads to a heightened appreciation of their particular religious tradition and a greater level of personal joy.

This experience is often even more noticeable in people with no fixed religious views. I am sure that we all would like confirmation that there is more to life than just this mortal coil. In the past, most people seem to have relied on the word of others that this was or was not so. By contrast, in modern times there has been a common disenchantment with formal religion and an urge to seek direct experience. Frequently, however, as the immediate material world is explored more fully, it is found to be exciting, but lacking. There has to be something more. Meditation often leads to a direct experience of that something more. You only have to see the smiles on the faces of many of the people I have known who have learned to meditate to realize that this is a fact.

Does Meditation Lead to Survival?

How long am I going to live? That question can lurk in the recesses of our minds to catch our breath whenever we are unaware. If we are a cancer patient, that question can be a constant nagging fear unless we reach acceptance, unless we regain our peace of mind. This does happen.

There is plenty of evidence from recent research that lifestyle factors do extend how long we live, as well as how well we live. Regarding meditation specifically, there are many studies confirming the quality-of-life benefits. Remarkably, while meditation has been shown to be therapeutic for many illnesses and enhance or lead to recovery from them, to date there have been no good outcome trials with meditation and cancer. What we can say is that many long-term survivors greatly valued their meditation and believe it to be a major factor in their recovery. My own case attests to this and so do the stories of many of the people in the book *Surviving Cancer*.[8]

There is no doubt in my mind that these techniques work. I am consistently surprised by the large number of people who tell me their lives are the better for having had cancer and responding to it in the way they have. Speaking personally, I now feel my whole quality of life to be vastly better than before I had my leg amputated. I meditate because I want to. Meditation is a regular part of my day. As Judy, another person with cancer, said recently, "Cancer changed my life for the better. It has taught me so much and I have gained so much through it. I cannot imagine myself having done it all without the prompting cancer gave me."

A SUMMARY

Meditation is so important because it leads to

1. A clear mind

This enables us to think clearly and to make good decisions.

2. A calm mind

This frees us from stress and reestablishes balance in body, emotions, mind and spirit. Inner peace and contentment follow, along with a quiet confidence in all we do.

3. Healing

This flows naturally from the balance we experience in deep, natural peace.

4. The truth of who we really are

As we relax deeper and deeper, our awareness opens in such a way that we experience our inner essence, the truth of who we really are. Now the confidence and the smile come from deep within, and they last throughout the ups and downs of life.

CHAPTER 5

Meditation

The Practice

HOW DO WE DO IT? HOW DO WE MEDITATE IN THIS WAY?

It is such a simple thing this meditation, and yet we are used to great complexity in our modern lives. How do we relearn simplicity? How do we learn to be still? How do we "let go"?

It helps to understand something of the process. The type of meditation that will help us most to heal is very specific. In meditation that is intended to be therapeutic and lead to recovery, the intention is for the body to be deeply relaxed and for the thinking brain to relax, to become calm and to become still. But what is this meditation really like?

We can explain a great deal of the nature of meditation, how it works and what it does. But the true essence of meditation needs to be experienced to be fully comprehended. Dr. Meares asked a venerated Yogi in Nepal what it was like to meditate. The Yogi replied by asking him how he would describe the taste of a banana. You can use words to make comparisons and descriptions, but in the end the only way someone else can really know that taste is to peel a banana and try it! It is a matter of direct experience.

I hope these words give you the impetus and the confidence to try meditation. I trust they will leave you free to enter into this experience with an open, willing mind, knowing you are embarking on a very personal, exciting venture.

I have felt meditation transforming my life for the better and I have seen it happen often in others. It is probably the most pleasant thing I can do on my own and the most beneficial. Meditation has a place in everybody's life.

As we set out the techniques, we are aiming to deeply relax our body and our mind. We are seeking to let go and regain our balance at a very deep, fundamental level.

The technique we shall use is set out in four easy steps: preparation, relaxation, mindfulness and stillness. Each of these steps is easy to learn; each has healing benefits in its own right and each flows quite naturally into the next.

STEP 1 • PREPARATION

Start with the Right Attitude

The attitude with which we begin and then continue to practice our meditation is very important. In modern society we are used to striving for achievement. If we want something, we normally expect to have to work or struggle for it. Not so in meditation. Once we actually start the procedure, we need to abandon any sense of striving, for if we sit down with the intention to "meditate or bust," we can be sure of an unhappy result! The only striving may be in making the time to do it, exerting the will to say, "This is my time for meditation and nothing else takes precedence." That can be effort enough, but once we commence, the accent is on effortlessness. It needs to be a focused but relaxed process.

Use an Affirmation

Next, to reinforce the attitude that this is a health-promoting procedure, many people find it helpful to begin with an affirmation. Nothing rigid or forced, just a gentle statement of intention. Usually, when I lead a meditation I begin with:

Let your eyes close gently.
Turn your thoughts inward.
Remember that this is a time for healing.

However, for you at home, simply repeating the last line works very well.

Some people feel comfortable following this with prayer and, of course, prayer can be highly beneficial. Something brief like "Not as I would, O Lord, but as Thou will" seems particularly appropriate, while many repeat longer prayers. Of course, prayer can have real benefits in its own right. More advice and a summary of interesting research in this field forms Appendix D.

Where to Meditate?

It makes obvious sense to be in as conducive an environment as possible. You will find it easiest when you feel secure, free from the prospect of interruptions and distractions and when you are in a quiet, comfortable space. A group of people all doing the same thing is very supportive, but meditation can easily be embarked upon in private.

Choose a room where you feel comfortable, preferably a room that is away from any bustle. If necessary, ask other people to leave you undisturbed. Be prepared to ignore the front doorbell or telephone should they ring. Initially it is good to use the same place regularly and to practice at the same time each day, if possible.

Posture

Now, what position should we use? The position you choose needs to satisfy only two criteria—it needs to be a position that is symmetrical, and a position that has an element of discomfort in it.

Discomfort—why should we be uncomfortable to begin something that is intended to be relaxing, pleasant and beneficial? Using this technique, the mild, initial discomfort soon fades from our awareness. It is essential to begin with it, however, as it makes us concentrate more. This works to make the relaxation more profound. The more uncomfortable we are when we begin, the deeper our level of relaxation has to be for us to regain a feeling of comfort and ease. Please just try this, as experience will soon show that this mild discomfort is a really useful ingredient in the process.

For most people what works well is to simply sit in a fairly upright chair, feet flat on the floor, just a little apart, hands resting comfortably on your thighs or cupped in your lap. Not much discomfort in that, but enough to be useful. Ideally, it is helpful to have your back fairly straight, although if the need is strong, you can lie down. As a beginner, closing the eyes is an effective way to start, but as you advance, they may just naturally open a little. As you meditate more, you may even like to experiment with sitting cross-legged on a cushion on the floor. However, the main thing is to take up a position you can relax into and stay in for the period you wish to meditate.

STEP 2 • RELAXATION

Now we are ready to use our body as the tool to guide us into the experience of meditation. We do this by training our body to relax, feeling what that relaxation is like, and letting it flow into our mind.

In the beginning we use a simple, formal procedure to capture the feeling of relaxation. Once we have done that and can reproduce the feeling, we can speed up the technique and simplify it, but every time we begin a session of meditation, we do take the time to consciously relax.

Remember that what we concentrate upon in this technique is a feeling—in this case, the feeling of relaxation.

Start by Becoming Familiar with Relaxing Individual Muscles

Be assured, this is a very simple technique. How it works is that we concentrate on one area of the body at a time. First we feel whatever sensations we can notice in that area. We simply notice how that particular area is feeling at this particular time. Then we contract the muscles in that area and make them tense. As we do this we notice the different feeling created by the tension. We feel the tension and then we relax the muscles. By repeating this technique through all the areas of the body we quickly learn how to relax the body very deeply indeed.

To do this as a complete exercise, first we need to go through the different areas of the body, learn how to feel them, create tension within them and then relax them.

We begin with the feet. Having taken up our chosen position, we let our eyes close gently and put all our attention on our feet. To do this exercise really effectively, we shift our center of awareness. Normally, our center of awareness is in our head, around about the space between our eyes. We feel as if that is the central point of everything for us. Now, by closing our eyes and concentrating on our feet, we feel as if they have become our center—almost as if we are "in" our feet. We then find that the feet do have a particular "feel." If you find that hard to realize at first, the second step makes it more obvious. You now contract all the muscles in the feet to impose tension on that area. In effect, you are making the feet rigid so they are tense and immovable. The feeling of tension is quite different to the feeling of relaxation. Feel that difference. Next you let the muscles relax, and you pay attention to the feeling of the muscles relaxing, the feeling of letting go.

So there is the simple process. Feel the area, contract the muscles, and let them go.

Learning to Relax the Muscle Groups in Our Body

Another necessary step in learning this technique is to familiarize yourself with how to contract the different muscle groups. Remember that this is the introductory part of the technique and that if you follow it, you will soon experience meditation proper.

When it comes to relaxing physically, the forehead and the hands are particularly important, as over 60 percent of the body's nerve endings are in these two areas. The more nerve endings we relax, the more the message goes back to the brain to relax. Therefore, the more we feel the relaxation, the more we become truly relaxed.

As the body first relaxes, often it begins to feel very heavy. It is so loose and relaxed—it feels as if it could just melt into the floor. Then, as it goes deeper into the process, it begins to enter a phase that we describe as "letting go." A new lightness comes over it. Sometimes there can be a tingling, a sensation of warmth; invariably there will be a sense of comfort, pleasure and ease. If we let our mind go along with this feeling, we soon lose all awareness of our body and surroundings. Noises seem far away and inconsequential and we are left with an expansive, floating feeling. This feeling of "letting go" can be likened to a sensation that is similar at first to floating peacefully in warm water. Then it is as if we were dissolving out into that water. We feel as if we are taking up more space than just the normal confines of our body.

The Progressive Muscle Relaxation Exercise

Having become familiar with contracting the various muscle groups and relaxing them, we are ready for our first meditative exercise—the progressive muscle relaxation (PMR). We need to go with this a little, to trust in its simplicity and allow ourselves to move into it. The body is the guide. As we feel the body relaxing, we notice our thinking processes winding down, and as the body enters the state of "letting go," we allow the mind to flow with it.

To lead ourselves through this technique based on physical relaxation, we speak quietly to ourselves. In our mind, we talk ourselves through the

Contracting and Relaxing the Muscles

Sit symmetrically, let your eyes close gently, and contract the muscles of the feet. If you find it hard to work out how to make the muscles move, pull the toes back toward the heels while at the same time resisting any movement. This locks all the muscles tightly and gives a good impression of what tension is like in that area.

Then relax the muscles.

The calves: Imagine someone was going to pull your ankle in any direction and you wanted to resist. This locks all the calf muscles as desired. You may notice some of the muscles in the thighs become involved and that they also contract. Keep this to a minimum but do not be concerned by it, while it is helpful to concentrate as much as possible on what is happening in the calves.

Next, the thighs: These are the largest muscle group in the body and it is easy to feel the tension in them. If you need help to make these muscles contract, try to lift the feet off the ground while at the same time holding the thighs down with the hands. The tension is then obvious.

The buttocks: These are contracted by squeezing the big muscles of the backside and so lifting a little off the chair. However, we want to be aware of the whole pelvic area, so feel the relaxation flowing right through that region of the body, including all around the pelvis.

The tummy: We begin with this area by contracting the tummy muscles as well as those of the lower back. If we imagine that we are lying on our back and someone is about to drop a heavy ball on our tummy, the right muscles will be working! With the tummy, the need to feel the relaxation all through the area we are focusing upon is even more evident. So when we relax, we feel the muscles relax and also feel that inside the tummy is relaxing as well as all through the lower sections of the spine. There is no need to try to imagine a relaxed liver, a relaxed spleen, etc.—just feel that same deep relaxation all through the tummy, in a general, nonspecific way.

(continued)

(continued)

The chest: The same principle applies as with the tummy. We contract all the chest muscles and make the chest tight like a rigid barrel. Then we relax the muscles and feel the relaxation all through the chest and around and through the upper spine.

The arms: We do the arms as one unit. Make them completely rigid as if resisting movement in any direction. Stiffening them produces the feeling of tension very readily; then feel the relaxation.

The shoulders: This includes the neck and the throat as well. Here we contract the muscles by lifting the shoulders and pulling the head down. Feel the relaxation then in the shoulders, neck and throat.

The jaw: Grit the teeth and feel the tension in the big muscles we use for chewing. Relaxing, feel it in the mouth, lips and cheeks as well as the big muscles at the side of the jaw.

The eyes: Closing the eyes in a squint makes the tension obvious. Relax and feel it in the eyes and across the nose.

The forehead: Some people find it easier to frown than others! Contract the muscles, feel the tension and let it go. Maybe you raise and lower the eyebrows. Feel the forehead smoothing out.

exercise using the simple, abstract phrases reproduced opposite. In the group situation, I lead people by saying these words aloud. At home you can begin by learning them, then repeating them quietly to yourself, or you could use a CD or download with the words recorded.

The words need to be repeated slowly and rhythmically. Many people find it helpful to repeat one phrase every second breath. That is, you breathe in and say a phrase as you breathe out; then breathe in again, breathe out, breathe in and say another phrase as you breathe out the second time.

You will notice in the exercise that follows, each phrase is separated by a number of dots. These are to remind you to breathe, to proceed slowly and steadily. You will find that as the relaxation progresses, your breathing is likely to slow down automatically. There is no need to emphasis the breathing at all. It will adopt its own slow and steady rhythm in a natural way.

Now we are ready to give our attention to this key exercise. So when you are ready, take up your position and begin.

The Progressive Muscle Relaxation Exercise

Let your eyes close gently . . . Turn your thoughts inward . . . And remember that this is a time for healing . . .

Turn your attention to the feet . . . really concentrate on the feet . . . perhaps move them a little . . . really feel what they are like at the moment . . . now contract the muscles of the feet . . . feel the tension . . . feel the difference . . . and let them go . . . feel the muscles relaxing . . . feel it deeply . . . completely . . . just simply letting go . . .

The calves . . . feel them . . . contract the muscles . . . and let them go . . . feel it deeply . . . it is a good feeling . . . a natural feeling . . . feel it deeply . . . feel the letting go . . .

The thighs . . . contract the muscles . . . and let them go . . . feel it all through . . . the legs feel heavy . . . as if they could merge down into the floor . . . more and more . . . deeper and deeper . . . letting go . . .

The buttocks . . . contract the muscles . . . and let them go . . . and feel it all through the hips and the pelvis . . . sometimes it helps to imagine there has been a belt or a band around the hips that has just been released a little . . . just simply letting go . . . letting go . . .

The tummy . . . contract the muscles . . . and let them go . . . feel it all though the tummy . . . it is a good feeling . . . a natural feeling . . . feel it deeply . . . feel the letting go . . .

Now the chest . . . contract the muscles . . . and let them go . . . feel it all through . . . more and more . . . deeper and deeper . . . letting go . . .

The arms . . . contract the muscles . . . and let them go . . . and feel it in the hands particularly . . . maybe you notice a warmth or a tingling flowing down into the hands . . . calm and relaxed . . . maybe a feeling of lightness . . . as if they could be just floating there . . . just going with it . . . letting go . . .

The shoulders . . . contract the muscles . . . and let them go . . . deeply . . . completely . . . and feel it up through the neck and throat . . . more and more . . . deeper and deeper . . . letting go . . .

(continued)

(continued)

Now the jaw . . . contract the muscles . . . and let them go . . . feel the jaw drop a little . . . feel it deeply . . . the tongue, soft and loose . . . feel it all through the mouth . . . it is a good feeling . . . a natural feeling . . . feel the letting go . . .

And feel it up over the nose and across the cheeks . . . now the eyes . . . contract the muscles . . . and let them go . . . deeply . . . completely . . . feeling it all through the eyes . . . almost like the eyes could be floating in their sockets . . . more and more . . . letting go . . .

And feel it around the ears . . . the back of the head . . . up over the top of the head . . . calm and relaxed . . . just going with it . . . calm and relaxed . . .

Now the forehead . . . contract the muscles . . . and let them go . . . feel it in the forehead particularly . . . feel the forehead smoothing out . . . feel it all through . . . more and more . . . deeper and deeper . . . letting go . . . letting go . . .

After a period of silence, we usually finish by saying, "That's good . . . Let your eyes gently open now."

And so what happened? Most people, on first doing the PMR are struck by the deep sense of physical relaxation it produces. They find this a new and exciting sensation they want to repeat more often. Just recently, David, a cancer patient who is fifty-eight, said he had worked hard all his life and enjoyed doing so, but on trying this exercise for the first time, realized he had never before known the joy and pleasure of being so simply, so deeply relaxed.

As a beginner, what is recommended is to start with this PMR exercise and use it as your main meditation practice for some weeks at least. Actually, for many people I helped in the early days this was all they used. However, in current times, people often find it useful to take the time to learn how to simplify and deepen the relaxation aspect of the PMR, and then proceed, giving added emphasis to the mindfulness and the stillness. The explanation for all of this follows and the main meditation practice to move on to once you have mastered the PMR is at the end of the next chapter.

STEP 3 • MINDFULNESS

As we do come to feel more relaxed, we actually become more aware. This is another key point. We relax our body, feel the relaxation in our body and feel that relaxation flowing into our mind. But this is not a sleepy thing. We keep our awareness awake and, in fact, it becomes more vivid. It is like we are awake, aware and at the same time deeply relaxed.

How we do this is expressed in the word *mindfulness*. Now *mindfulness* may be a new word for some but it is very simple, both in concept and in practice. Mindfulness describes how we concentrate in a particular way. It helps us with the next step, what to do once our body is deeply relaxed and our mind calm.

Mindfulness has been defined by Jon Kabat-Zinn[9] as paying attention, deliberately and nonjudgmentally, to our present moment experience. Another way to say this is that mindfulness is concentrating on what is going on right now, in this particular moment, in a way that is focused and non-judgmental. It is to do with observing, with being aware of what is happening right now, without judging what is happening as being good or bad, right or wrong. It is to do with simply being really interested, really curious, really attentive to what is going on right now, in this very moment.

This then is the ability to be mindful. It is as simple as being able to give your full attention to whatever you are doing. And doing this in a way that is not distracted by old thoughts, doubts or fears from the past, or anxious wondering about how things will turn out in the future.

Mindfulness cuts through stress and anxiety by focusing on what we are doing now. And think of it: If we give our full attention to what we are doing now, how can we do any more? With mindfulness, we learn to give our best, to give our full attention, to whatever we do. This is why developing mindfulness is so valuable for more than meditation and healing. Mindfulness frees the mind to engage fully in sport, business, relationships, creativity, feeling good and being well! You name it—everything goes better when you do it mindfully.

Sometimes it is helpful to have the contrast and to realize what mindlessness is. Mindlessness is the opposite of mindfulness. Mindlessness is when you are not paying attention, when you are spaced-out as if no one is home.

It is like when you do something, know you actually did it, but have no memory of it at all. Like you get home after being out, travel home, arrive at your front door and have no real memory of the trip. Or you plan to listen to something like the weather on the radio, it comes and goes and there is no memory of it. It is like you missed it altogether. That is mindlessness and we all do it pretty regularly.

Mindfulness is where we begin to change that and we learn to be present more often, more fully. Where we learn to give our full attention; where we learn to give our best to whatever we do.

Now what most people do notice when they start to become aware of mindfulness is how often they are mindless! This is why this practice, this mind training is so useful. Not only does it help us to learn to be more mindful, more often, but it teaches us how to go easy on ourselves.

There is this natural tendency to judge ourselves harshly, so now we want to change all that. What is known from experience is that many people have a history of feeling badly about what they do and do not do. Most of us when we begin these mind-training practices do tend to notice our mindlessness, and as a result we feel awkward, unhappy, sometimes embarrassed or even ashamed. Why am I like this? Why do I do this? We tend to judge ourselves as meditators, judge our capacity to be mindful.

Now of course, we do not want our meditation to become another source of stress. So what to do? Well, it is simple. Everyone has fairly frequent moments of mindlessness, unless they have trained their minds. All of us as human beings have the tendency to be lazy, to be forgetful, to be mindless, to be judgmental. This is normal. So while it may be a bit disappointing as a beginner to even notice all this, go easy on yourself.

Be inspired! Isn't it wonderful that there is a part of us that can actually become aware of all this and do something about it! Any progress is a step in the right direction and becoming more mindful helps to let go of the judgments of others and of ourselves. The thing is to persevere. Do not be put off by what is the common starting point for so many people. We can all learn these new skills. We can learn to master our minds and feel the benefits. Here then is how we add the next step and begin to practice and develop mindfulness.

Relax and Become More Aware

As we begin to experience the relaxation, quite naturally our thoughts settle a bit and we just simply start to notice what is going on around us a little more clearly. This is the beauty of this technique. It simply unfolds from one step to another. So as we relax, we become more aware, more mindful.

Perhaps it is the sounds we notice first. We notice any sounds that may be around about us. And what we aim to do is to simply notice these sounds as they come and go. We let go of any judgment, let go of commentary. So we aim to avoid thinking about the sounds. It is fine to be aware of what is making the sound; for example, an ambulance may pass by in the street. But we avoid wondering where it is going or will we be in an ambulance one day. We simply register there is an ambulance passing by and let it go. Simple as that.

Then maybe we become a little more aware of the sensations in our bodies, and again we choose to notice these things more nonjudgmentally. We aim to let go of any sense of good or bad, right or wrong, and focus our awareness on just simply noticing what it is that we are aware of. We take up the stance of being an impartial observer; a nonjudgmental observer. We are aware, we are interested, we are curious. What is happening right now? What is our body feeling like at this particular moment? We are coming into the present moment with awareness. This is mindfulness.

And so then we might take some time to focus our mindfulness more deliberately. To begin with, it can be very helpful to focus our awareness more particularly on our breath. We feel the breath coming in. Feel the breath going out, and we feel the natural release, the relaxation, the letting go that flows quite effortlessly, quite naturally with the out breath. Almost with a sigh of relief we can let go, we can relax a little deeper.

Now it can be helpful to bring the focus of our mindfulness more particularly to our body. Again with that open curiosity, we notice the sensations in our body. We scan our attention through the body, starting from the feet and moving up to the head. If any area does feel a little tight or tense, sore or painful, we simply notice that, aiming to be free of any judgment, free of reaction, free of commentary. Maybe there is the feeling of letting go a little. That natural feeling of relaxing, releasing, letting go. Quite effortlessly. Effortlessly. We feel the natural ease of it all.

We are content to relax, to be aware, to be mindful.

STEP 4 • STILLNESS

Having prepared well, relaxed deeply and become more mindful, now we begin to notice something really interesting—we begin to become aware of a deeper stillness. In time it becomes more apparent that this stillness is like an all-pervasive background. It is like when all the activity stops, the stillness is naturally revealed.

This is just like being in a room full of people, all talking, all busy. While initially it may be the noise and movement that is most obvious, we know there is a potential silence in the room all the time; it is just with all the activity it is not so easy to notice it. If we were to ask everyone to tell the others to be quiet so we could hear the silence, they might all rush around anxiously and the noise become louder! Some people attempt this with their meditation. They spend their time trying to tell their minds to shut up and just get caught up in one form of mental activity after another.

This is why the mindfulness is so useful. We let go of trying to do any-thing other than to be aware. This is the key to it. Do it effortlessly, in a kindly, nonjudgmental manner. Just be curious to notice whatever happens and quite naturally the activity will settle and the stillness will become more obvious.

It is like having a glass full of muddy water. If you continue to stir the water, you just get more and more muddy water! But when you put the glass down and leave it undisturbed, the nature of water is that it clears. The mud settles to the bottom and you are left with the clear water. The mind is just the same. Leave it undisturbed and it settles.

So what is this like in practice? As we relax, our body and our mind set-tles. As our mind settles, thoughts invariably continue to come and go. So now, we choose to observe the thoughts. No need to try to push any thoughts away or to dwell on any thoughts in particular. We just simply notice them, again free of reaction or judgment. We are curious. What thoughts are com-ing into my mind right now? What am I actually thinking about right now? We turn our mindfulness to being aware of our thoughts.

We can understand what this mindfulness of thoughts is like is if we consider what happens when we watch a movie. We go into the movie theater, sit down and wait for the film to start. We are conscious of being in our seat, in the theater with other people around about us. We are watching the screen and then the lights dim and the movie starts. Almost invariably, we soon forget we are in our seat and it is like we are in the movie, lost in the projection of light and sound that is the movie. Then from time to time it is like we snap out of the movie and remember we are in our seat, observing the movie. Mindlessness is when we are caught up in the movie. Mindfulness is where we have our awareness, we are the impartial observer, and we are aware we are watching a movie. When we can adopt this attitude with our thoughts, we give them no strength. If we allow them to just roll on, to come and to go like scenes in a movie we are watching, they do just that—and soon they slow down and settle.

What becomes obvious as we relax and become more mindful is that as we go with all this, we become a little calmer and importantly, our thoughts do quite naturally begin to slow down. Again, we do not need to do anything more than what we have been doing for this to happen. This is a process based on relaxation—focused relaxation, it is true, but relaxation, mindfulness and natural ease. We just focus on doing the exercises, go with the flow as they say, and by doing so we progress quite easily and reliably.

And as we do this, a remarkable thing unfolds. As we notice our thoughts more clearly, we notice how each individual thought has a starting point, a middle and an end point. Obviously each and every thought we have has to start somewhere, and to finish somewhere. And as we relax more, as we become more mindful, this fact just becomes more obvious. We notice when we first become aware of a particular thought, we notice it passing through our awareness, and we notice when it finishes.

Then another really useful observation. As our thoughts begin to slow a little and we notice them more clearly, we notice that after one thought finishes, and before another thought starts, there is often a small gap.

Now in the gap between our two thoughts, there is obviously a moment of silence, a moment of stillness. So now we turn our attention, our awareness, to noticing the gap between the thoughts. And again, when we do this mindfully, free of judgment, just with an open curiosity, not only do we notice the stillness but often enough it lasts a little longer; there is a bigger gap before the next thought comes. But again we make no effort to force this or to manipulate it. We just notice it. We are patient. We are the impartial observer. Just simply curious to notice what happens.

More stillness? Another thought? What is it? We take the attitude of a patient, curious, impartial observer and do just that, we observe. We aim to treat the stillness and the thoughts in just the same way. Nonjudgmentally. With curious awareness. So we notice the stillness. We notice if and when another thought comes. We remain aware and undistracted.

And what we do notice is that the thoughts do come, and they do go. Thoughts are just like white clouds drifting across a blue sky. They come when they are ready. They go when they are ready.

The blue sky is there all the time. Vast. Pure. Pristine. Always there. The clouds just come and go. And even on the cloudiest of days, we know the sky is still there, we just cannot quite see it because of the clouds.

Meditation is like getting into an airplane on a cloudy day. When we take off, all we can see are the clouds everywhere. We fly up through those clouds, break through, and there it is again, like a big canopy stretching above us, the vast, blue sky. It was always there, it was just that we could not see it from the ground. We needed the plane. We needed to learn how to fly.

So it is with our thoughts. Sometimes our mind is full of them. Sometimes it may even seem as if we have a raging storm going on inside. But we can always use meditation to reconnect with that other aspect of our mind, that deeper stillness.

Sure our thoughts can be really useful, but sometimes they can be too much, too problematic. Sometimes we can suffer from excessive thinking! What a relief to know that there is a way out. That there is always the possibility we can turn our attention from the active thoughts, to the stillness. It is like on a cloudy day, we choose to focus on what we can see of the blue sky rather than what we can see of the clouds.

And in our meditation, as we move our attention from the thoughts to the stillness, we come to realize that the stillness is just like the sky is to the clouds. The stillness is ever present. It is there all the time. Vast. Pure. Untouched. The thoughts come and go but the stillness, like the sky, is always there.

Now be reminded once again that while thinking can obviously be very useful, there is great benefit in letting go of the thinking for a while—of going beyond the thinking into that deep natural peace of this stillness where balance is restored and sustained for body, emotions and clarity of mind. We may even reconnect with the essence of who we really are in that stillness.

And there is another powerful truth here. You must have noticed that even after the darkest clouds, the worst storm, sooner or later it does actually clear and the blue sky reemerges. And despite the worst storm, the sky is never stained.

Sure, there is a part of us that can feel pain, we can be ill, we can have troubling thoughts. Our personal storms can take many forms. But this is one of the really wonderful discoveries that comes with meditation: No matter how difficult things have been or may be now, no matter how stormy, there is always a part of us that is unstainable, untouchable and inviolable. There is this inner essence, this core of our being that is good, pure, whole and unstainable.

Knowing this brings a deep inner satisfaction and contentment. To experience the truth of who we really are, to directly experience that in our essence we are whole, pure and good—this is the real heart of meditation. This is what brings a confidence to all we do. This is what helps to bring out the best in all we do. This is what brings a gentle smile to the face of so many meditators. This is the truth of who we really are and the truth of how we can be.

SUMMARY • HOW TO MEDITATE

To put it really simply: Having prepared well, we relax. Relaxing more deeply, we become more mindful. As our mindfulness develops, the stillness naturally reveals itself. We rest in open, undistracted awareness. Easy as that.

This is the essence of mindfulness-based stillness meditation, and this, the main meditation technique that is recommended, is set out at the end of the next chapter.

Time to Practice

Finally then, what level of commitment is required? Quality of life or quantity of life? Your aims and priorities must be very clear. Any time allocation has to be balanced by your needs, your beliefs and your other commitments.

Quality of life is vastly improved by doing ten to twenty minutes once or twice daily. To make an impact on quantity of life, to aim for recovery, three longer sessions per day from forty minutes up to one hour each are recommended.

I feel it very important to set yourself a goal in this regard. Work out your priorities and set a goal for the coming week. It is far better to set a conservative goal to begin with and succeed in meeting it than to fall short of an overambitious target.

So having set your goal, practice for a week. Then assess your results, reassess your goals and priorities, and reset your target. Remember that it is probable that you will have what seem to be good sessions and ordinary ones to begin with. The more meditation you do, the more repeatable and the more satisfying it becomes.

When I first began, my situation was critical and I did about five hours a day for three months. I then did three hourly sessions for the next year, then around an hour each day ever since. Also, for many years I have continued to regularly attend (or give) more intensive meditation retreats. This is obviously a big time commitment. I did it when I was ill because it felt good and it gave me results. I continue to do around an hour each day for the same reasons.

If quality of life is your aim, and time appears short, ten to twenty minutes twice a day will help you a lot. I remember the story from many years ago of a man who had been estimated to have three weeks to live. He went to Dr. Meares full of enthusiasm for his ideas around meditation and was keen to begin. However, on being told he would need to spend three hours a day at it, he replied, "Oh, I haven't time for that" and left!

I am sure meditation improves both quality of life and quantity of life. Only you can do it.

CHAPTER 6

Meditation in Daily Life

Calm, Clear and Relaxed

THE BODY'S NATURAL ABILITY TO HEAL ITSELF IS REALLY QUITE PHENOM-enal. While we often take it for granted, this ability is nothing short of miraculous.

For example, take the healing of a broken leg. First there is a trauma, a solid bone is broken in two and the shattered ends displaced. There will be torn muscles, probably internal bleeding—a lot of damage. Surgery is often required to stabilize the situation, and perhaps a steel pin is inserted to fix the broken bones together and keep them stable. Yet, once the right conditions are created, that bone will automatically reunite itself, the muscles will regenerate, and normal function return. In six months' time an X-ray will show the bone to be healed, and actually often where the break was, the bone will now be even stronger. What an amazing process!

RELAXATION, BALANCE AND HEALING

Let us see this process in perspective. First, the right conditions were created and then the body healed itself. The medical intervention was necessary to provide those right conditions. However, the doctors did not actually heal anything. What they did achieve is that by realigning the bones, they created the first requirement for the healing of a fracture to proceed. The patient then had to look after the leg and make sure the healing process could continue. The patient did not have to think of the intricate process of the bones reuniting. The body's natural healing power was what returned the leg to normal. The body, given the right conditions, healed itself—automatically.

The body's normal state is health. It has a tremendously varied and complex set of mechanisms to maintain it in good health. Whenever the body is out of balance, these mechanisms swing into action to re-create health. If those mechanisms are thwarted or unsuccessful, then we have disease.

So, what is the problem in cancer? Why does the body appear unable to cope? It is just the same as with the broken leg!

If we are able to provide the right conditions, the body has the potential to heal itself.

In the acute situation of a broken bone, the medical intervention is a very obvious first step. Surgery provides the right conditions by realigning and stabilizing the bones. The patient maintains those conditions by keeping the leg still and having a diet and an environment that permit the normal healing functions to proceed.

However, cancer is a chronic, multifactorial, degenerative disease. It takes a long time to develop and has a multiplicity of contributing factors, as we shall discuss later. While surgery and other medical treatments clearly have their place in treating cancer, correcting the causes of the disease is more involved; while providing the correct environment to allow the body's potential for healing to proceed is also more involved. All of this requires consideration of far more than the body mechanics involved in surgically repairing a broken leg. It involves consideration of the whole person—body, emotions, mind and spirit.

What we are concerned with here is investigating the potential for each of us to be directly involved in re-creating our own health. What we seek is the ideal environment for healing in general and cancer in particular. What we know is that this all comes back to that simple principle of balance. Balance equates with good health, and good health does not include cancer. Balance equates with healing.

Again, a healthy body cannot have cancer. There was a man in America who had kidney failure and was given a kidney transplant. Unbeknown to anyone, the kidney he was given in the transplant was already cancerous. Naturally, he was placed on immune-suppressant drugs to prevent his body from rejecting his new kidney and this meant his body's normal defenses could not operate properly. In a very short time, not only was the new kidney engulfed by the cancer, but it had spread throughout his lungs. With his life threatened, the immune-suppressant drugs were ceased, the new kidney was removed, and he was returned to a dialysis machine. What happened? The immune-suppressant drugs wore off, his normal bodily defenses rapidly reasserted themselves, and all the cancer in his chest disappeared—automatically, with no outside intervention. His body's normal ability to heal itself did just that. His body, with its immune system working again, had the ability to recognize the cancer should not have been there and so eliminated it.

We want to create the conditions in our body so that it can do the same thing. We want to reactivate our own immune system and provide the right conditions where healing can take place. We can do it.

There is a very close link between the function of our body and the function of our psyche. That is, if we are relaxed and easy in mind and emotions, our body will be relaxed. If, on the other hand, we have anxiety or are affected by stress, our body will suffer from subtle but far-reaching changes in body chemistry and it will also show up as physical tension. I believe that this reflex is a key factor which we can use in the process of getting well.

Equate stress, anxiety and tension with immune-suppression and illness.
Equate relaxation and balance with health and healing.

If our body and psyche are relaxed, we will be in a state of balance, and that balance means health. If we are deeply relaxed, our body's natural tendency will re-create health for us—true, deep, meaningful health, including a healthy body.

The first step, the starting point that we can readily appreciate and learn, is to lead the body into deep relaxation. Relieving emotional and mental stress is hard to begin with, as causes of anxiety are difficult to isolate and often difficult to treat using conventional means. However, if we relax the body, that reflex produces relaxation of emotions and mind.

Mental anxiety, stress and physical tension are intricately connected and interdependent. They are all disease-producing factors. However, truly break that connection at any one point and relaxation spreads all through. Healing begins.

Pause to consider a cat. A lithe, graceful cat. Watch it on the move. It moves with an ease and smoothness that is a joy to watch. In slow motion it is a sight to behold. Yet, if it has to react in a hurry, it can—in an instant. It will pounce in a flash, or turn and run with amazing speed. So too, it will often stop, consider a situation at length and then go on with its business. Concentration and relaxation are mutually supportive. All so easy, so relaxed.

This, to me, shows what relaxation is all about. It is being physically relaxed and so being free to make an appropriate response.

If we are relaxed we react appropriately. We do not rush into things and overreact; neither are we sluggish and unable to take appropriate action. What we do is simply appropriate.

There is no need to avoid the problems of everyday life. Life should have challenges and a zest of endeavor. Such challenges become causes for stress only when we do not handle them appropriately.

If we do not react to challenges well, tension and anxiety cloud our normal processes. They interfere with judgment and reactions, so that responses become inappropriate. If our mind is confused or anxious, we have great difficulty thinking clearly and are highly likely to make poor decisions. However, the more relaxed our being, the more calm and clear is our mind, the more likely we are to make good choices and to do the appropriate thing.

COMMON FORMS OF RELAXATION

Where then, do we find this relaxation? Some of the common ways we relax in a healthy way are through sleep, exercise, hobbies and holidays. All have their place.

Sleep

Sleep is an excellent way of dealing with acute stress. Even sleep imposed by drugs will often provide the time and space necessary for adjusting to and dealing with a major, temporary stress. We certainly need a regular amount of natural sleep to avoid fatigue and added stress.

As an aside, here is an important tip. We can significantly improve the quality of our sleep by doing our relaxation exercises when we go to bed. When you get into bed at night, spend five minutes, perhaps ten, doing your relaxation. This is important. If you have muscular tension when you get into bed, your body is like a spring and you will spend half the night unwinding. Researchers have observed people sleeping and documented the muscles of tense people struggling to unwind. In a series of jerks and twists, the body tries to get itself relaxed. For some people this can take most of the night and so they wake up without having much profitable relaxed sleep. So do spend a few minutes before you go to sleep and practice the progressive muscle relaxation exercise. As you get that good relaxed feeling all through, you will find that you can put yourself to sleep. You could well find that you need less sleep than you used to, as well as waking feeling the better for it.

In chronic stress situations, however, while sleep may provide some relief, it changes very little. We wake up with the same problems and responses that accompanied us to sleep. We need to look further.

Exercise

Exercise is well worth considering. In the right amounts, it helps to relax physical tension by tiring the muscles and so creating a natural form of relaxation. Also, it certainly invigorates and makes the body feel better, as well as being well proven to relieve depression, promote well-being and aid the healing process generally. Exercise warrants being a feature of our healing program and more detail on the best forms of exercise for recovery comes in the next chapter.

Hobbies and Holidays

These can be very pleasant diversions. They also provide an opportunity to relax, to release and to let go a little. They can certainly aid our general level of well-being. They are well worth considering, but frequently they produce little change in our overall situation.

Meditation and Deep Relaxation

The practice of meditation has the potential to produce the most profound and effective levels of deep relaxation. Another reason the specific meditation technique we recommend for healing works so well is that it starts with deep physical relaxation. Then, relaxing the mind enhances the effect.

However, let us be clear about this. While meditating once or even three times a day is clearly beneficial, if we get up from our meditation and spend the rest of the day just as tense and uptight as ever, the benefits will be relatively small. What we need is to take the relaxation, along with the calm and clear mind, from the meditation into our daily life.

This is most important. The relaxation we feel during our formal meditation periods needs to become a way of life for us. We need to aim to be as relaxed as possible because except when we are faced with an immediate threat, relaxation is our hallmark of the balance we seek.

This is not to say we will be sluggish or lethargic. On the contrary, we will react quickly and be sharp and alert but, like the cat, be relaxed at the same time. There are a number of ways to achieve this.

INTEGRATING RELAXATION INTO DAILY LIFE

The Automatic Flow-On Effect

As you begin meditating, you will notice the calm you feel during your formal sessions of practice remains with you for a short while after. Meditating regularly in this way throughout the day enhances this effect, so that one session's benefits soon begin to flow on to the next. This is why it is useful to spread a number of meditation sessions throughout the day. While initially you will seem to have good and bad sessions, soon you will notice a cumulative effect that means you get more benefit from each experience of meditation.

This effect can be increased still further by improving the quality of the meditation and by becoming more aware of relaxation throughout the day.

Speeding Up the Process of Relaxation

Initially, as we learn to relax and meditate, the progressive muscle relaxation (PMR) is a very helpful technique. Using the physical act of contracting muscles and letting them go leads to a very reliable experience of relaxation and helps us to appreciate what it feels like to be deeply relaxed. But we can then progress and learn to relax more quickly and, in fact, more deeply. Here is how we do it.

The next step is to experience the same level of relaxation we did through using the full PMR, only this time we do so without physically contracting the muscles. We simplify and speed up the process. So now, we focus our attention on the muscles in each area of the body, and using the same sequence as we did with the PMR, this time we feel those muscles relaxing without having contracted them first. Once we have mastered this step and can feel that same deeply relaxed body we felt with the first technique, we go even further.

Now we learn to relax the legs as one unit, rather than the feet, then the calves and the thighs. We learn to relax the torso as another "block," and then the head and neck. Ultimately, it is like we can sit to meditate, bring our attention to our bodies, and, almost like throwing a switch, feel the whole body relax as one unit. Now we have arrived at that ultimate point where we do not even need to spend time relaxing individual areas. We can just sit down and feel a wave of relaxation move throughout the body, producing that total, deep calm.

However, there is no hurry to speed up the procedure. We need to feel confident at each phase before advancing. The accent is on ease. No effort, no striving, just a natural progression to a faster, easier way. Again, the point to emphasize is that we arrive at the end point where the body will be deeply relaxed and so will the mind. If we do need to employ the PMR exercise to achieve this, we do so. If we can relax just as effectively but more quickly, we do so.

Using Discomfort to Deepen Relaxation

Once we begin to develop the capacity to relax at will, we are ready to use a more uncomfortable starting position. What, more discomfort? Yes, just a little at a time. Why? Well, a measured element of discomfort makes the physical relaxation a little harder to achieve and this makes us focus more on what we are doing. Undoubtedly, this in turn heightens the effect of the meditation. It is like when you go to the gym, work out, and develop your physical muscles. Here, we develop our "relaxation" muscles. You really do need to try this, the results will be obvious.

The suggestion is that if you began learning to relax and meditate in an armchair, once the technique is working well, try it in an armless chair. The change is very little, but I am sure you will notice a different effect. Once you are comfortable with that and it has become easy and effortless, go on to trying it on a stool. Harder still, but still fairly easy and, again, a greater benefit. Then you could go on to experiment with sitting cross-legged on the floor, or going outdoors. In the open air the sounds and smells increase the potential distractions while adding to the naturalness of it.

In my own situation, I generally meditate sitting cross-legged on the floor or on a chair in the morning and at lunchtime. My back can often be tired after a day on one leg, so frequently I lie on a hard surface in the evening, as this allows it to relax better. I notice that lying down produces more benefit in terms of relaxing my body, but there is no doubt sitting cross-legged produces a better overall effect, particularly when it comes to the mind.

Using Imagery to Focus Relaxation—The Radiant Light Imagery Exercise

We will be examining the benefits and techniques of imagery in chapters 8 and 9; however, when it comes to deepening our relaxation and meditation, there is a particular form of imagery that is easy to learn and can be of great benefit. This is what we call the "radiant light" imagery exercise. This is an "extra" technique worth experimenting with. If you warm to it and find it helpful, continue on with it; if not, simply move on to the next step. What you may discover is that this exercise has the added advantage of leading on to a heightened body awareness. Using this technique you will be in better touch with your body and more responsive to its messages. Similarly you will be able to control it better.

To practice this technique takes around thirty minutes. It can be done in any position, but I find this particular exercise does work best if you lie down on a hard surface. The floor is ideal. Choose a carpeted area, or place a blanket underneath yourself to begin with. Lie flat on your back, hands loosely by your sides. Legs should be out straight, just comfortably apart and the feet allowed to flop loosely outward. Some find a pillow under the knees quite helpful.

When you have taken the time to practice this a little, and you can do it well, you will have a means to relax yourself deeply and revitalize yourself amazingly. Practicing this technique regularly, once a day for a few weeks, will produce a new dimension in body awareness and relaxation.

The clarity of visualization, how clearly you "see" the different body parts, is not so important. Obviously, someone with detailed anatomical knowledge will be able to build up a more detailed image than others. The important thing is to feel that close contact and awareness of each part of your body. So, in a large complex area such as the abdomen, you feel as if your mind is moving through the whole area. You feel the deep sense of relaxation and then the glow.

When it comes to areas affected by cancer or other disease, just do the same thing. No effort or striving, just feel your mind moving through the area, relaxing it and letting the light build up to the same level as in the rest of your body. This produces a feeling of uniformity throughout the body—a vital, healthy uniformity and it promotes the healing response.

Sometimes, relaxing areas affected by disease causes some initial dis-

The Radiant Light Exercise

Begin by putting all your attention onto just one big toe. Form an image in your mind of your toe and travel through it, examining each part in your mind. It is as if in your mind, you travel around the skin, under the nails, through the joints, tendons, ligaments and muscles. As you do so, you aim to relax each part in minute detail. So this is a process to take slowly. You really do dwell on each part of the toe, feel into it and feel it relaxing deeply and completely.

You may well notice feelings of warmth flowing into the areas you relax in this deep way; maybe even a light tingling almost like mild pins and needles. This is a sign blood is flowing more freely through the area and relaxation is deepening.

Next, you build up an image of radiant white light suffusing each area of the toe. It is as if that toe was a light globe with a dimmer switch. You turn on that switch and gradually increase the light until the toe is full of vibrant white light. You will find it feels marvelous. When you do it well, you will be thinking of nothing else, just experiencing the vibrancy of it all.

So, having begun with one toe, then move to the next and so on, until the whole foot is "lit up." You may find that at the first session attending to just one toe takes all your time. That would be fine. Next session you will find that you can recapture the feeling in that toe more easily and more quickly and so you can start with the next toe. At each session work on more areas until you can capture the feeling throughout the body. It is the feeling of relaxation, lightness and vitality that is the main thing. You aim to complete the exercise feeling deeply relaxed, filled with the radiant, healing, vibrant light.

comfort. This is because we often have long-standing tension in the region around them as a defense mechanism. These exercises relax that tension and often produce sensations of temporary discomfort, occasionally tingling, even brief muscle spasms or jerks. Be assured this soon gives way to a feeling of warmth and ease. Also, this radiant light technique is very helpful for pain relief, and we will discuss this in detail soon (chapter 10).

The aim of the radiant light exercise is to lead us to a point of profound relaxation, with an accompanying sense of wholeness and vitality. So this exercise really serves to add another means of reaching the stillness of passive meditation. It is that end point which is the really important thing.

Relaxation Trigger Points

As you become more aware of your body, you will almost certainly find that some areas feel more tense than others. Common areas of tension are the muscles of the forehead, jaw, shoulders, tummy, hands and lower back. You will find that when you are placed in a stressful situation, one or more of these areas may tense up first. Just watch what happens next time you are "pushed." These areas are called trigger areas and they are very useful! Remember the reflex?

> Anxiety + Stress = Muscular tension
> Muscular relaxation = No anxiety, no adverse effect from stress

Having identified localized areas where tension shows up, we can concentrate on relaxing those areas, and when we succeed in doing so, we are well on the way to being relaxed. This is a very good defense mechanism to use if you feel stress is still affecting you. If you feel a situation is causing stress to build up, concentrate upon relaxing your trigger areas. You will find that if you keep your body relaxed, the whole situation will be defused.

Relaxation in Daily Life

Once you have experienced the "feel" of relaxation in your formal exercises, you will be able to recapture it at will during the day. Soon it will become your natural state. Free from tension, you will be able to react appropriately and will not be affected by stress.

Ideally, we aim to be relaxed all day and impervious to potentially stressful situations. Practicing these techniques goes a long way toward this end and we can do still more to achieve it. At every opportunity through the day, at every idle moment, take the time to check your level of relaxation. Do an internal inventory. Start with the trigger areas and make sure they are relaxed.

When you begin doing this, you may find that every time you think of your trigger areas, they need help to be more fully relaxed. That is fine. It is good to simply notice such a fact; and then to realize you can do something about it! That is why we practice. That is why we persist with these exercises. Relax. Smile. Know that the worse the tension to begin with, the more benefit you will get in the long run by relaxing!

Seek to experience the feeling of relaxation at every opportunity. After a while you will stay relaxed and you will feel a wonderful difference.

Relaxing Moments

Use your time wisely. When in the car, do not just waste those precious seconds at the red lights. Relax as much as you can and feel how good it is. Maybe take a deeper breath in; breathe out, and let go. The muscles softening and loosening. The feeling of relaxation all through.

And then remember the cat. Relaxed but alert. As we watch a cat in slow motion, the foreleg flows gracefully forward. All the muscles at the front of the leg are contracting to draw the leg forward. The muscles at the back of the leg are relaxed. There is nothing to hinder the flow of the leg or stilt the action. Look at a tense person walking—they jerk along in a most ungainly way. The relaxed cat flows. When the leg moves backward, the muscles at the back of the leg contract, and those at the front relax.

So even while driving along, be aware that your trigger areas are relaxed. Ideally, your whole body is inherently relaxed. And at the same time, you are quite alert, focused and mindful, ideally poised in body and mind for the driving.

The key to this is the principle that you use only the muscles you need for any given task of the day. To avoid stress, to maintain a relaxed state, muscles are either working at a specific function or at rest. They do not need to hold any residual tension.

I have seen many people take on a new elegance and charm merely by learning to relax properly. Perhaps this was most marked in Edna, an elderly patient. As she learned to relax, the worry and tension left her face. Coupled with the benefits of the diet, a new vitality and vigor came over her, producing a genuine, radiant glow that was obvious to all.

Very soon, using these techniques, your body will be relaxed, your mind also, and the benefits of the meditation will have entered your daily life. You will be reacting appropriately and you will be heading toward profound healing and long-term good health.

PUTTING IT ALL TOGETHER • The Main Meditation Practice:
Mindfulness-Based Stillness Meditation

This completes all the background and preliminaries we need to be aware of
and to have practiced so that we are ready for the main meditation practice
of mindfulness-based stillness meditation (MBSM).

Remember the simple summary: having prepared well, we relax. Relaxing more deeply, we become more mindful. As our mindfulness develops,
the stillness naturally reveals itself. We rest in open, undistracted awareness.

Here is the "script" we can learn to lead us through mindfulness-based
stillness meditation:

The Mindfulness-Based Stillness Meditation—Main Practice

Take a few moments to adjust your body . . . and then, when you are
ready . . . relax into your posture . . .

Now, let us begin by letting go of what we have been doing
recently . . . and bringing our attention more particularly to this
present moment . . .

To do this, it may help to bring the focus of our attention to the
breath for a few moments . . . to simply be aware that as we are
breathing in, we are breathing in . . . and as we are breathing out,
we are breathing out . . .

And as you do bring your attention more particularly to the
breath . . . you will probably notice that as you do breathe out, there
is a natural feeling of relaxing a little with the outbreath . . . of letting go a little . . .

Breathing out . . . and letting go . . . relaxing . . . releasing . . .
letting go . . .

Feeling it deeply . . . completely . . . and feeling it all through the
body . . . and the mind . . . it is a good feeling . . . a natural feeling . . .
just going with it . . . calm and relaxed . . . calm and relaxed . . . going
with it . . . quite effortlessly . . . effortlessly . . . letting go . . .

And just allowing your breath to take up whatever rhythm feels comfortable for you at the moment . . . breathing out . . . relaxing . . . releasing . . . letting go . . . breathing out, and the breath becoming longer . . . finer . . . subtler . . . then a pause . . . and simply allowing the breath to come back in of its own accord . . . quite effortlessly . . . effortlessly . . . going with it . . . relaxing . . . releasing . . . and feeling the ease of it all . . . the ease of it all . . .

And now, it might help to take your attention to that point between the eyes, a little into the forehead . . . and notice there what is like a still, quiet center . . . a point of stillness . . . and relax your eyes . . . and soften your gaze . . . and hold your attention lightly, on that point of stillness . . .

And if you do notice any sounds coming to your awareness . . . just let them come when they are ready . . . and go when they are ready . . . a bit like white clouds, drifting across a blue sky . . . they just come when they are ready . . . go when they are ready . . .

Holding your attention lightly on the stillness . . . and simply letting go . . . letting go . . .

And if any sensations in your body do come to your awareness . . . just the same . . . just simply notice them . . . free of any judgment . . . free of any reaction, or commentary . . . and feel the letting go . . . your body relaxing . . . and releasing . . . holding your attention lightly on the stillness . . . and simply noticing whatever may come to your attention . . . simply being aware . . . a gentle focus on the stillness . . . and letting things come when they are ready . . . go when they are ready . . . letting go . . . letting go . . .

And if you do notice any thoughts coming to your attention . . . just the same . . . just let them come when they are ready . . . go when they are ready . . . gently holding your attention on the stillness . . . and feeling the ease of it all . . . the ease of it all . . . just simply letting go . . . letting go . . .

And then it is almost as if you can merge into that stillness . . . relaxing . . . releasing . . . simply resting in the stillness . . . aware . . . free of any judgment . . . free of any commentary . . . and feeling the ease of it all . . . the ease of it all . . . just simply letting go . . . and

(continued)

> *(continued)*
>
> resting in the stillness . . . quite effortlessly . . . effortlessly . . . letting go . . . letting go . . .
>
> LONG GAP—for your meditation
>
> And if at any stage you do notice your mind wandering or becoming distracted . . . as soon as you become aware of that . . . gently bring your attention back to that point of stillness . . . relaxing . . . releasing . . . just going with it . . . melting . . . merging . . . simply resting in the stillness . . . quite effortlessly . . . effortlessly . . . letting go . . . letting go . . .
>
> LONG GAP—for your meditation
>
> That's good . . . good . . . good . . . When you are ready now . . . just let your eyes gently open once again.

MEDITATION CONCLUSION

The aim of our meditation is to relax deeply and to rest in the balance of deep natural peace. In any given session of meditation, we do the simplest things that will help us to this end. So if we need to, it may be wise to start by taking the time to go through the complete progressive muscle relaxation exercise. But if we have practiced enough and it works for us, it may be enough to simply take a deeper breath or two and feel the body relax quickly and deeply.

Once we feel the body to be relaxed, we become more mindful. We notice whatever does come to our awareness, free of any judgment or commentary. We just allow things to come when they are ready, go when they are ready, and we remain in undistracted awareness.

As time goes on a deeper stillness becomes apparent. Sounds may come and go, thoughts may come and go. They do not disturb us. We rest in deep, natural peace. And as we do so, there is the knowing that we are in a state of deep, natural balance. And the healing flows.

Happy meditating. Happy healing.

CHAPTER 7

Mind Training 1

Positive Thinking: The Conscious Mind at Work

IT WAS HENRY FORD WHO SAID, "WHETHER YOU THINK YOU CAN OR YOU think you cannot, you are right!"

What is the most important thing when it comes to any treatment you may be considering, whether it be a medical or a nonmedical treatment? Clearly, it is your mind, as your mind will decide whether you agree to that treatment or not. Your mind will decide whether you continue with the treatment or cease it. Further, your mind has the very real potential to significantly influence the outcome by reinforcing or sabotaging the treatment.

What is the most important thing when it comes to the food you eat? Clearly it is the mind, as it is your mind that will decide what you eat and how much you eat, as well as what you drink, and whether you exercise along with that.

Clearly, the mind is responsible for the choices we make, the knowledge and experiences we remember, the habits and the beliefs that shape our lives. However, everyone who has studied the mind, from the ancient mystics to the modern neuroscientists, says we use barely a fraction of our mind's potential. In these next three chapters we will learn how to train the mind and how to activate its potential for restoring health and for maintaining well-being.

To provide some structure and so that we can understand the various aspects of the mind and their potential for healing, here is an outline of what we will cover:

THE FOUR WAYS IN WHICH THE MIND INFLUENCES HEALING

1. Consciously—Via Positive Thinking

We will learn that positive thinking is about making good decisions and following them through. Positive thinking recognizes that it is the mind that shapes our world through the choices it makes. Our health and our healing, in fact all that we do, will be dramatically affected by whether we make constructive or destructive decisions, and whether we follow through on those decisions or not.

2. Unconsciously—Via Our Habits and Belief Systems

i) The beliefs we hold have the potential to significantly influence the outcome of everything we do. We will examine the powerfully positive placebo response and the incredibly destructive impact of the "pointing of the bone." Together, these two phenomena graphically reveal the mind's capacity to influence healing directly. Then we will learn what we need to do to gain the full benefit from the power of belief.

ii) The habits we live with will directly affect our potential to heal. Are you lazy in some ways? Do you have trouble exercising regularly? Are you habitually bound to eating certain things? Do you have difficulty sticking to what you know you need to do? Habits can be changed. We will learn how to identify what, if anything, does need changing, and then how to make necessary changes in a way that is empowering, sustainable and actually fun! This is a crucial element of recovery.

3. The Mind-Body Connection

Here we will examine how the mind can be mobilized to directly activate healing. We will learn more about how to apply the techniques of imagery and affirmation.

4. Meditation

Meditation establishes an ideal state of balance. From this balance healing flows free of effort, almost automatically. We have covered meditation thoroughly in the previous chapters.

Let us begin.

THE CONSCIOUS MIND, POSITIVE THINKING AND HEALING

Imagine a loving mother who is giving her all to being the best mother that she can be. Do you imagine she ever feels that she is managing 100 percent? But do you imagine she ever gives up trying? Of course she does not. That is what positive thinking is all about—always aiming to do the best we possibly can, acknowledging our strengths and weaknesses, being comfortable with what we do achieve and knowing we will become better and better at whatever we turn our attention to.

Positive thinking is all about using our mind intelligently. Specifically, positive thinking involves understanding how our mind works, and then getting the best out of its vast potential.

The crucial point in this field of mind training is to realize there is a big difference between positive thinking and wishful thinking.

Wishful thinking is where you hope for the best and do nothing about it.

Positive thinking is where you hope for the best and do a lot about it.

This is a fundamental distinction and opens up our understanding to the truth of what "positive thinking" really is. Positive thinking is way more than just that optimistic hope—"If he can do it, so can I." That hope is real enough. It is true; it has to be done only once to show that it is possible. But what did she do to achieve what she did? And what are you prepared to commit to, to achieve the results you are after?

Positive thinking begins when we use our mind to choose a specific goal. But then we must act on that goal. We need to use our mind to commit to that goal and embrace all we need to do to give ourselves the best chance of realizing that goal. This is a very active process. Wishful thinking is a passive process that involves little active effort and clearly is not likely to make a big difference to anything we do. By contrast, positive thinking regularly results in the extraordinary.

Your Mind at Work

How then does positive thinking work? Let us begin with the role of the conscious mind. In practical terms, the mind is well described as a goal-orientated, decision making tool.* Here is how it works.

---

* For a more expansive definition of the mind, see Appendix E.

Imagine you ask me to come and share a meal with you and I agree. You say you live in Australia or Canada or France. Big places. A lot of homes to look for you in. So maybe you are a little more specific and you give me the district you live in—the Yarra Valley, the Rockies, the Bordeaux region. I am getting closer, but it is still going to be a while before I find you. So you give me a full address: street name and number, town, city, country. Now I will find you. I can use a map, a GPS, ask the locals. If I persevere, there is only one address that matches your home and I will find you.

The mind is goal oriented. The more specific the goal, the more potently it functions and the more reliably it works. If I have only your local region, it will be easy for me to be confused, to become disheartened, to give up. But with a specific goal, the prospect of success becomes very realistic.

However, clearly the specific goal is just the beginning. Once I decide to pursue that goal, to come to your address, I need to decide how best to make the journey and I need to actually complete the journey. So if I decide to come by car and the battery in the car is flat, I can either give up at that point or persevere. Having managed to start the car, I am then faced with many choices. As I begin to drive forward, I need to decide which direction to take, and I base that decision on what is most likely to lead me to your address. So I choose left, right or straight ahead, over and over, at one intersection after another, until I find you.

That is how it works. It is simple. The thinking mind is a goal-oriented, decision-making tool.

We are all positive thinkers. We all use our minds in this way many times over, day after day. However, some people become overwhelmed. "You want me to come to dinner? I don't know about traveling on the roads just for a meal. What if I get lost? What about all the dangerous drivers on the road? Maybe it will be dark on the way home and I get scared in the dark." Some people manage to talk themselves out of even simple things.

Of course, the truth is some people do set out in their cars each day fully expecting to reach their journey's end and do not make it. Fatal car accidents are real. People do get lost, have flat tires, run out of gas and have minor accidents. Does this mean we stay at home and do nothing? Well, some do, but not so many when it comes to simple journeys. We accept the risks and persevere.

Consider this. Healing from a major illness like cancer can well be described as a journey. Often it is a lengthy journey, with many choices to deal with, many decisions to make, and often enough there are unexpected turns for better and worse. In my experience, some people do sense the scope of this particular journey and decide "to stay home." Some may be paralyzed by fear. Others are deeply concerned by the fear of failure. What if I make all this effort and it does not work? Will I feel like a failure? Will I have let myself down or let down those around me?

Face the Fear and Do It Anyway!

The fear of failure is related to the notion of false hope. In many of the early media interviews that focused upon my work, presenters would ask if I was concerned about giving people false hope. Some doctors have also expressed a related concern—what happens to people who try hard to recover and still end up dying?

The answer to this is simple. Any major endeavor carries some risk. Recovering from a difficult diagnosis is not easy. If it was easy, everyone would be doing it and it would be commonplace. We know it is possible, but we do need to be realistic; it requires a good deal of effort. And the truth is I have seen people who have tried hard and still died of their disease. Long-term recovery is not easy, but it is possible.

When I had widespread secondary bone cancer in 1976 and was expected to live for a few months, I could have just accepted the disease as my fate and sat by hoping for the best, waiting to see what happened. My guess is that if I had done so, I could have died quite easily. But I dared to believe recovery was possible and, being realistic, knew that if I was to recover, I would need to do something dramatic. I knew I needed to do the best I possibly could with everything I took on.

When I became sicker before I began to recover, I simply became even more determined, more thorough. I knew I did not want to die with regret. I did not want to be near my last breath wondering if things would have been better if I had an extra carrot juice, or meditated a bit longer. Now, obviously there is a limit to how much carrot juice one should or could drink, and a balance in how much meditation to do. What all of us need to do is to decide for themselves how much carrot juice we drink, how much meditation we do, and then do it. That is the essence of positive thinking.

Commitment and Outcome

What can be said after many years helping people to face difficult situations is that these people fall into three broad categories. A number find that all this positive thinking and the lifestyle-based approach is simply not for them and they drop out. By contrast, most people recognize the truth in what is on offer, and the possibilities. However, even among these people, there are two types. We call them the 100 percenters and the 70 percenters.

The 100 percenters set clear goals and do them, 100 percent! Maybe they miss a little here or there, but essentially they do what they turn their mind to. By contrast, the 70 percenters consistently fall short of their goals. Maybe they set unrealistic goals, maybe for a multitude of reasons they just cannot persevere. But the gap between what they plan to do, what they set as their own personal goals, and what they actually do creates an inner tension. This tension commonly leads to unhelpful emotions like anger, blame, shame or guilt.

Now this latter situation is where help is urgently needed. I often suggest to people that if there is a big gap between what they believe is best for them to be doing and what they are actually doing, they need to treat that situation as if it is a medical emergency. It requires urgent attention. Either the expectations need to be brought into line or the questions of commitment and discipline addressed. To remain with a significant gap or disparity between your beliefs and your actions, between what you believe you need to be doing and what you actually are doing, for any length of time is an invitation to misery and poor outcomes. One way or the other, it needs to be resolved. More on how to do this is coming soon.

Once beliefs and actions are in sync, people invariably do well. Giving 100 percent to what they do has resulted in many people making a full recovery. But perhaps not too surprisingly, even those who give 100 percent and still go on to die of their disease, they do well too. They invariably have a good death. Maybe there is a natural disappointment and a sense of regret about dying itself. But there is no regret about having not done all that was reasonable. There is no guilt or shame. No anger or resentment. They do not die wondering. We will discuss this more in the chapter on death and dying (chapter 18), and no, it is not being "negative" to discuss dying. We will all die one day, so let us plan for a good death. That certainly is possible and perhaps a good death is a testament to a good life, a life lived well.

However, we are focused here on getting well, then living well and dying a long time later! So for those who are keen, we need to observe that positive thinking can be an innate trait or a learned skill. This is more good news. I have seen really pessimistic, "negative" people learn the three simple principles of positive thinking and transform their health. However, before we learn these three principles and clarify how to apply them, there are some really useful preliminaries.

Positive Thinking 101—Choose to Be Positive

We begin our move toward becoming more positive by giving attention to our basic state of mind. The first question is, just how positive are you? Are you content with your current attitudes, or do you need to work at being more positive?

If you already have a positive state of mind, count your blessings. You have the starting point in place to develop the power of your mind more fully.

If you doubt your own level of positivity, or know it to be lacking, the first step is actually one of clear-cut choice. You are either positive or you are not. This may seem somewhat simplistic, but it is a fact: you can choose to be positive, hold that intention, and then follow through with the steps that develop it. This act of choice is a crucial one.

We literally can choose to be positive. It is that simple. This is one of those basic choices in life that can be made consciously. We can decide, we can have the intention to be positive, commit to what is effectively a state of mind we choose, and then carry it through. To do this, the intention needs to be one that is firm and one that we strengthen at every opportunity.

One of the best ways to reinforce this intention to be positive is with the aid of contemplation. Contemplation is a reliable way to think something through in a way that brings clarity of mind, understanding and confidence. To do this, we begin by taking up our usual meditation position and consciously relax the body as normal. Then, instead of aiming for a still mind, we actively think about what positivity means to us. We consider it from every viewpoint. We think of how we would define what it is to be positive, we compare it with negativity, think of positive people we know, think of positive aspects of our own character. Think of why we want to be more positive, why we need to be positive.

A hint here to assist your contemplation. Positive thinking may be as simple as being clear about what you are aiming for and being confident you can achieve it.

As we reflect and contemplate more, we will generate a very comprehensive understanding regarding positivity and what it means. This may take one or more sessions and so we repeat the contemplation until we have thought it through and gained real insight into what being positive means to us, why it is helpful and why we choose to adopt the positive approach.

What If I Do Not Feel So Positive? Use an Affirmation

Be reassured. Many people start this program knowing they are not very positive. Others have been rocked by their diagnosis, had their confidence undermined by all that can be a part of cancer. More than thirty years of experience tells us many people have turned all this around. That is why we learn how to train our mind. That is the joy of using positive-thinking techniques.

So to consolidate and to reinforce our intention to be positive, we use an affirmation. An affirmation is a short statement that accurately reflects our goal, our intention. We will discuss them more in the next chapter, but it will be very useful to begin to build your positivity straight away. The affirmation in this case is: "I am a positive person now." What we do is to repeat this short statement, this affirmation, over and over until it has been imprinted onto our mind and carries conviction.

Affirmations are wonderful things. They work! By using such simple, positive statements and repeating them regularly, we can condition our thoughts so that they lead on to the actions we intend.

So, when you first get up in the morning, repeat to yourself, "I am a positive person now," for a couple of minutes. Make time to do it again at least twice more during the day. Especially when driving in the car, say it out loud—even sing it if you like! Adding a sense of fun can be helpful, so put it to different tunes; be theatrical and keep doing it.

What will start to happen quite quickly is that when a new decision needs to be made, you will now have a little voice in the back of your mind saying, "I am a positive person now." And bingo! To satisfy that inner voice you will make a positive decision! As you become more positive, you see the system work and it becomes that much easier to be positive the next time. As the intended actions are put into practice, the cycle of positivity is completed and all of this will steadily help to build healing and a better life.

You will soon find that you have a new feeling, a feeling of being responsible for your own situation. You will be doing everything because you feel positive about it. You will want to do it; it is your choice. You will feel in control of your situation and you will find that your inner resources will be strengthening and developing rapidly.

You will come to recognize that if you were not positive before, you almost certainly suffered from "victim consciousness." This is the "Why me?" syndrome, the attitude that leaves people feeling a powerless pawn of random fate that has slated them for doom! It is the most negative and destructive attitude in which you could have become stuck. If you recognize it from your new vantage point of positivity, be gentle with yourself. You are a positive person now. Quietly remind yourself that is not the way you are now. Seek out how you can change those negative aspects and not repeat them again.

You can reasonably expect to have ups and downs, so you need to be prepared to persevere. When you do act positively, congratulate yourself. Quietly, of course! But happily. Reaffirm your new attitude and seek the next opportunity to practice it.

Armed with our positive attitude we are now ready to sort out all the challenges cancer presents and set ourselves clear goals. The next step provides us with a major key with which we can unlock the power of the mind.

THE THREE PRINCIPLES OF POSITIVE THINKING

Before the details, a short summary of the three principles:

Principle 1. Set a clear goal. Remember, the mind is a goal-oriented, decision-making tool, so the starting point is a clear goal. When it comes to healing, there are many choices. We will explore reliable methods for good decision making and for setting clear goals.

Principle 2. Do whatever it takes. Once we have a clear goal, we need to accomplish it. Sometimes the commitment required will flow easily, other times we will need to work at it. We will investigate how best to take a good idea and put it into action, how to do whatever it takes.

Principle 3. Choose to enjoy doing it. Those things we enjoy doing we tend to persevere with; we keep doing them. Things we do not enjoy doing we tend to avoid, forget, become disenchanted with, find excuses to let go of. The value in enjoying what we are doing is obvious enough and we will discover how simply and effectively we can achieve this final key to positive thinking.

But we begin with the first principle, goal setting.

THE FIRST PRINCIPLE OF POSITIVE THINKING: SET A CLEAR GOAL

Step 1. Who Decides?

When it comes to setting your goals, when it comes to deciding what to do, who tells you what to do? Is it some external authority figure like a doctor, a counselor, a natural therapist, a parent, a child or a partner? The lady over the back fence? Or is it you?

Who decides?

Authority figures can be really useful; genuine experts are invaluable. It is always sensible to consider seeking help from people who are knowledgeable, passionate and confident in what they recommend and what they do. But who takes the ultimate responsibility for what is done to you, or what you do for yourself?

Here we need to talk of fear again. Fear has this uncanny knack of disempowering people. Often when fear is strong, we feel so anxious, so uncertain of what to do, we want someone else to fix it, to tell us what to do. This is perfectly understandable and maybe in times of crisis it is wise to defer decisions to the people we trust the most.

However, if you value your own integrity and prefer to take more responsibility for your own choices, this tells you that making big decisions when fear is strong is fraught with danger. Fear commonly causes us to overreact and become frenetic, or to underreact and become too passive, too inactive. Again that reminder, it is wise to give yourself time for major decisions. Particularly allow time for any shock to settle so that you will be more relaxed and be in a better place with fear. Then with a calmer, clearer mind you will be able to gather all the information you need, make your choices and set your goals.

Step 2. Use Both Sides of Your Brain to Make Good Choices in the Decision-Making Process

The human mind has intelligence and wisdom. We think logically and also we can think more abstractly, more intuitively, more wisely. Clearly, both logic and wisdom are useful; in fact, logic without wisdom can be dangerous.

However, in the world we live in, where science has such a high value, it makes sense to begin by assessing things logically. Then we need to add the wisdom. Wisdom in its most ordinary form may be as simple as "common sense," but we will investigate developing wisdom more fully soon.

START WITH GOOD INFORMATION AND LOGIC

Ideally, it is wise to obtain the best opinions, the best advice from the most experienced experts in whatever field you are considering. It is wise to ask them for an opinion. What would they do in your position? What would they recommend or where would they send you if you were their child, their parent or their partner? Then, informed by this expert opinion, do whatever additional research you consider warranted or within your capabilities.

But consider this, and a warning, if you do not want your head messed with a little, perhaps it will be wise to skip the next paragraph!

There was a major study carried out some years ago in the United Kingdom with the aim of developing best practice recommendations for women with breast cancer. Two hypothetical case histories were formulated: one for a typical woman with primary breast cancer, the other for a typical woman with a recurrence. These were circulated to all the major cancer hospitals and treatment centers around the UK seeking consensus as to the best treatment to recommend. The results were somewhat disconcerting. While the recommended treatments had some similarities from all the centers, there were enough variations for the study to report that a number of different recommendations were received. For the women with primary breast cancer, the number of treatments regarded to be different was put at thirty-five! For the typical case of secondary breast cancer, the woman with a recurrence, the number was forty-five! So if the woman with primary breast cancer had been a real woman rather than an hypothetical case and if she had gone to one major cancer hospital, then decided she wanted a second opinion, she could have gone to thirty-five other centers before finding a match. What do you do with that if you only use your logic?

In real life, a woman with a breast lump is likely to start with her family doctor. If breast cancer is suspected or confirmed, she is likely to be referred to a specialist. She may have known the local doctor for years or not, she will almost certainly have no prior experience with the specialist.

The logic of what the specialist has to say regarding her condition and treatment options will be really useful information. It is likely to form the basis of the decision-making process. But logic also says there may be other ways to consider treating her condition. Is it worth seeking thirty-five other opinions? Of course not. These days, many major cancer centers aim to resolve this potential problem by using a team approach. There is a trend toward gathering together surgeons, oncologists, radiologists and other health professionals to discuss the individual needs of individual people.

But what of the person him- or herself? I strongly suggest there is more to decision making than pure logic. If we talk of a broken leg with major damage, the logic is compelling to have surgery and a cast. In that situation one does not need to dwell on the choices too much. But in cancer medicine, the choices are not always so clear. The reality is that many cancer treatments are tough on the patient. Often the risk of side effects is considerable and the potential gains debatable. Unfortunately, in this and many other situations, logic does not always provide an obvious answer.

However, with almost all decisions, it will make obvious sense to gather the best information you can, based on the best evidence available. An example of how to achieve this was given in chapter 3, where we discussed how to decide what treatment to commit to.

ADD CONTEMPLATION—DEVELOP CLARITY, CONFIDENCE AND WISDOM

Contemplation is a methodical way to think something through and to gain a deeper understanding of it. Also, contemplation provides a way of directly tapping into our intuition. All this helps to dispel doubts and reliably builds clarity and confidence. As a consequence, commitment develops more strongly and it becomes easier to follow through with our decisions.

Contemplation is easy to do and comes highly recommended for all our major decisions, and for setting all our positive-thinking goals.

So we can investigate and learn how this technique works. We will use the example of reviewing our eating habits and deciding on what sort of diet to follow. Here are the steps.

Goal Setting Using Contemplation

1. Decide what the issue is (e.g., in our example, to set dietary goals) and determine to reach a conclusion.

2. Express the issue as a question (e.g., What will be best for me to eat?).

3. Do the research. Use your intellect and your logic. Read the books, get on the net, speak to the experts, discuss it with friends, listen to CDs. Ideally, make notes. This person said that, this book the other, etc. With food it is usually easiest to write lists of the different recommendations.

4. Set a time for the decision to be made. There are two ways to do this. If you were to buy a new washing machine, probably you would wait until you gathered all the relevant information. Presuming you have determined your price range, you could find out the makes and models available and collect all their details within a reasonable period of time. However, with food you could collect information indefinitely. So you probably need to say to yourself something like, "I will collect all the information I can in the next two weeks [this two weeks is just an arbitrary figure I have used—there is no need to take me literally on this one—choose your own time frame] and then I will make the best decision I can."

5. On the day when the decision is to be made, give yourself some time—half an hour to an hour is ideal—and some space—either where you meditate regularly or in any quiet area. Make sure you can be free from the telephone and other possible distractions. Take with you any notes you have made and any other material you have gathered. Also, take a pen and some paper in case you want to write on it.

(continued)

(continued)

6. When you sit down, begin by reviewing your research material and in this way refresh all the knowledge you have of your subject. If you do not have written material go straight to the next step.

7. Consciously relax your body and calm your mind. This will be a familiar process if you have some experience of meditation. The aim is to relax your body and to calm your mind so you are in a better state of mind to progress into contemplation.

8. Once relaxed in this manner, focus your attention on consciously reviewing the facts as you remember them.

9. So, in our example, you might recall the style of food you have been eating, the broad issues relating to why you are considering changing your diet, what different people have recommended to you, what you have read in different books and so on.

10. If at any stage you become distracted or your mind wanders off onto other thoughts, as soon as you recognize this, be gentle with yourself and simply come back to concentrating on issues relating to food and diet.

11. This first part of the process then is clearly a rational, "left brain" exercise. You actively think about the topic and all issues relating to it. You are actively focusing on the topic and thinking it through.

12. What happens next, as you continue to concentrate on the topic, is that at some point your mind will automatically shift into more abstract, intuitive, "right brain" contemplation. It will be as if all the facts you have been reflecting upon and analyzing, all the pieces of the jigsaw puzzle as it were, come together and now you can clearly see the bigger picture. This will give you a new sense of comprehension and understanding and usually leaves you with a clear sense of what to do. This can all come with a moment of clear insight, almost like an "Aha! I've got it," moment of revelation.

13. The more you practice this technique, the more reliable it becomes. It is a wonderful and dependable way to solve problems, develop creativity and instigate lateral thinking. (As another aside, this is an excellent way to prepare for and complete creative writing.)

14. Once the sense of clarity dawns, usually it is best to write the ensuing insight down. Perhaps you can remember having the experience of a moment of insight like this before. Perhaps you were in the shower, or was it when you were half asleep, and suddenly like a bolt out of the blue, it seemed as if you had the perfect solution to a problem you had been wrestling with. Yet by the time you got dressed and ate breakfast, it had flown from your memory! Insight during contemplation sometimes comes like that too, so it is best to write it down. I always do this exercise with pen and paper close by and as soon as the answer begins to form write it down.

This contemplation technique can be used to solve any problem. It leads to a clarity that is backed by a deep sense of your own inner wisdom. As a result, the directions that come with it, the goals that emerge from this exercise, will feel very "right" for you.

So when it comes to contemplating food, we may think through specific issues like whether we will eat tomatoes or not, and whether we will cook them or not. Or we may arrive at a more comprehensive overview and, for example clearly understand why eating organic food makes sense and come away deeply committed to doing just that.

People often ask me, "How can I trust the result of an exercise like this?" Well, if you come out of this exercise with no clarity and are still clouded by doubt, all that has happened is you have spent time simply thinking about the issue. No harm done, but no profound insight, either! The insight we are talking of has as one of its features the confidence of certainty. It comes with a deep inner knowing and no doubt. You really know what to do with the tomatoes! No one else will need to confirm such an insight for you; it will be easy to feel confident about, easy to commit to, and it is highly likely to work well.

But what if you do all this and you still have doubts?

Step 3. When in Doubt, Do Something!

It would be nice to think we will arrive at a point of certainty before making all the decisions in front of us. Maybe we will. But doubt remains a real possibility—and does that mean you are unable to set a goal effectively?

One of the benefits of contemplation is that it does clarify the choices. When you reflect on this, with most things you either do them or you do not, or you put them off. Now, while there is the old Irish saying, "If you put something off long enough it will take care of itself," maybe we need to be a bit more proactive when it comes to cancer.

Faced with lingering doubts, what many people find works well is to accept the doubts and make a decision anyway. With a decision made in this way, it is still useful to decide to commit to whatever it is you are planning, make the commitment, and to embrace it. But then it is always healthy to review your progress from time to time and adjust accordingly.

Here it is helpful to appreciate another facet of how the mind works. As we have established, the mind is a goal-oriented, decision-making tool. In this regard, however, it is more like a heat-seeking missile than an arrow. Pardon the warlike images but they serve as useful metaphors here. When an archer takes aim and lets fly an arrow, the arrow is at the whim of the archer's aim and the elements. If a wind begins to blow the arrow off course, it has no self-righting mechanism. A heat-seeking missile is quite the opposite. A heat-seeking missile locks on to its target, and then receives feedback. If the target moves, the heat-seeking missile adjusts its course.

Step 4. Make Friends with "Mistakes"

Our mind functions like a heat-seeking missile. The mind is designed to manage the complexity and changing nature of our lives. It is designed to receive feedback, to compare our progress to what we are aiming for, to adjust, to change course regularly and to persist until the goal is reached.

Some people feel badly about mistakes. Some mistakes are regrettable, and we will consider later how to transform common feelings of guilt, shame, embarrassment and blame that often accompany mistakes (see healthy emotions, chapters 16 and 17).

However, here is another possibility. Mistakes are feedback. Mistakes can be really useful feedback. It is reported that Thomas Edison made ten thousand experiments before discovering how to produce a lightbulb that worked. When asked what it felt like to make 9,999 mistakes, Edison replied that he had not made 9,999 mistakes. He had completed 9,999 attempts to achieve his goal and with each experiment he learned something. In the end, courtesy of all he learned from what appeared to be his "mistakes," he revolutionized the world with his 10,000th attempt.

Be brave. Make a start. Stick to your goal. And be flexible with how you achieve that goal. Respond to feedback. Be prepared to hold to the big goal and be prepared to be flexible when it comes to how to get there.

Step 5. Rambo or the Martial Arts?

Pardon me again but we need to discuss the state of mind that goes with our positive thinking. While what we do is of great importance, the state of mind we do it in can be even more significant.

Most people are familiar with the Rambo image. Isolated, tough, uncompromising, resolute. Very driven, a fair bit on edge, high energy. Not much inner peace or calm. Contrast this with a martial artist. There is the same resolve, the same willingness to do whatever it takes, but there is a deep calm, a palpable inner peace. Meditation leads directly to this inner peace. Meditation can provide the background, the milieu, the atmosphere for our positive thinking, so that we will find it easier to make good decisions, easier to follow them through, easier to enjoy doing what we need to do to achieve them.

Step 6. Your Primary Goal—How Healthy Can You Imagine Yourself?

When it comes to cancer, what are you aiming for? What can you imagine as the best possible outcome? Whatever that is, that becomes your primary goal.

Can you imagine yourself fully recovered? Free of cancer, with a normal life expectancy again, fit and well? Is that easy to imagine, or a struggle? Is it easier for you to imagine yourself living well with cancer? Is it just a good quality of life you are after and you do not want to focus on the disease itself? Can you imagine your illness becoming stable? Or is there a deep sense of fear, or maybe an acceptance that dying of the disease is a likely outcome?

Challenging questions. Doubts are OK. Most people have doubts. Positive thinking is not about denying doubts. Or denying fears. Positive thinking is about recognizing the doubts and the fears, and using our minds intelligently to move through them, past them, and to accomplish our goals anyway.

The limit in positive thinking is what you personally believe is possible. Not what someone else believes. What *you* believe. Some people do accept they will probably die of their cancer; we spoke of this earlier. But maybe at the moment the limit of your belief is that you can genuinely only imagine the cancer becoming stable. If you consider that prospect for a moment, we know cancer tends to multiply, to increase in size exponentially. That is why once it is large enough to be detected, it commonly grows quite rapidly. (Please note, this is a broad generalization. Some cancers do grow very slowly indeed.) Therefore, when a cancer becomes stable, it is a sign of real progress. Maybe once stable, you can imagine the cancer receding a little.

Positive thinking works well with progressive goals. While some people go for an all-out, big goal like total recovery right from the start, others find it more manageable, more realistic and effective to advance in stages.

Step 7. Write Down Your Goals

With any significant goals you have, write them down in a journal, in a special notebook or simply on paper you can easily refer to. The writing will lead to even greater clarity, and you have a good chance of remembering what is written!

Step 8. Finally, Decide How Important Each Goal Is

Once you have clarified your goals, the next question is simple. How important is each goal to you? Is it a casual thing? If it works out, would it be nice but no big deal? Or is it a matter of life and death? Something you choose to give your all to?

When my secondary cancers appeared, I became totally uncompromising. For the next few years, until it was clear that I was well again, everything I considered, everything I did, needed to get past the first big filter.

Will this help me to recover?

If it did not pass that test in the affirmative, I was not interested. Of course, having fun passed that test. Some people seem to be of the impression getting well is tough work, which it can be, and unpleasant, which it has no need to be at all. In fact, I had a wonderful time during my recovery. There was this fabulous excuse to do all the things that were good for me, all the things that caused me joy and happiness. I had cancer. I could change whatever I liked, do whatever was needed. I had a great reason, a great excuse, and when I did it all in this uncompromising fashion, I was fortunate indeed: I fully recovered.

Positive thinking is a measure of what you are committed to and how committed to it you are. The first principle, having a clear goal, leads naturally to the second principle.

THE SECOND PRINCIPLE OF POSITIVE THINKING: DO WHATEVER IT TAKES

The three principles of positive thinking tend to flow on, one to the other, fairly naturally. When we have a clear goal, it often seems easy to commit to doing whatever it takes to achieve that goal. If so, it is as easy as that. If not, if it seems hard to do whatever it takes, then planning and concerted effort makes sense—all in the right state of mind!

Step 1. Embrace All That You Do

When it comes to positive thinking, the key recommendation is to embrace all that you do. To think through your options, decide upon your goals and embrace them. So to not just passively accept a treatment, or put up with dietary changes. Not just go along with things because someone else wants you to do it. Take ownership. Take control. Embrace everything you do. Welcome it. Commit. Believe in what you are doing. Then your mind will be activated and the placebo response will be working courtesy of your conscious mind, your conscious commitment.

Jill was a lady who came to our groups in a heightened state of anxiety. She was having chemotherapy for secondary cancer and was deeply concerned for her own future and the fate of her two young children. Amid the emotionally safe environment the group created, for the first time she shared her fears and cried openly. Quiet understanding supported Jill as she released her deeply held pain. She reported feeling as if a weight had lifted from her shoulders.

Up to this point Jill had been experiencing major anticipatory nausea even before she went into the hospital for her regular chemotherapy treatments. It transpired she was quite undecided in her own mind regarding this treatment. There was the hope of some benefit and another deep fear for the potential side effects. Once the emotion had cleared, Jill subsequently talked through her choices regarding the chemotherapy.

Now, with her mind somewhat clearer, she could think more logically and she decided she was doing the right thing for her. She embraced her treatment and went to the hospital looking forward to doing something she considered to be in her own best interests. She embraced the lifestyle program, ate well, meditated regularly, exercised and so on. When Jill arrived at the group, she had not been responding to her treatment. Two months later her tests had improved dramatically. Her main doctor remarked on this and encouraged her, saying whatever she was doing, she should stick to it!

Step 2. Check Your Clarity

This is a major point. In my experience, the most common factor behind a lack of commitment is a lack of clarity. The answer? Revisit the first principle! Set a clear goal.

Step 3. Use Ideals Wisely

A great deal of what is presented in this book is made up of ideal ways to use our lifestyle, our own inner potential along with our actions to generate healing. Remember, however, ideals are just that, ideals. As such they may be unattainable in their entirety. However, ideals do give us a goal, they do give us a sense of direction, and they do give us a strong sense of what to aim for. Obviously, we will be the better for any step we make toward an ideal.

So as we lay out these lists of things to do, these ideas, be comfortable with where you are, start where you can, do what you can. It is obvious. If you are really tense and anxious to begin with and you relax 10 percent of what is ideally possible, you are 10 percent better off. That is quite a good start! It will serve you well to be pleased that you are 10 percent more relaxed, rather than to worry about being 90 percent short of being fully relaxed. Positive thinking is acknowledging the 10 percent gain, focusing on that as progress, and being committed to making even more progress as time goes on.

Step 4. Seek Inspiration

Emphasis has been given to the pivotal role of hope. Many people find it useful to collect a "bank" of inspirational material to read, view or listen to when they need inspiration. Perhaps at the place where you meditate, you keep photos of inspiring people or landscapes, whatever inspires you the most. Even simply bringing inspiring people to mind can powerfully lift your spirits and these people may be family, friends, community leaders, spiritual or religious figures.

Step 5. Develop Constructive Discipline

The discipline we are talking of here is best described as a "personal kindness." This type of discipline is not a discipline imposed by someone else, it is a self-discipline. This self-discipline is based upon having the clarity of mind to understand what is in our own best interests, what is needed for our own welfare and well-being. This self-discipline is about having the resolve to actually do whatever is good for us. It is the capacity to do what is appropriate. That is what it is to be kind to ourselves. Simple as that. It may not always be easy, but it is always kind.

So when we wander off track we need to notice, to be vigilant and to gently and firmly bring ourselves back to what we know is good for us.

There is a very useful and practical recommendation here. Do something each day purely as an exercise in discipline. Perhaps go without a piece of food you would have had for pleasure's sake; do exercise as an act of discipline; even do as I do—finish your daily shower by turning the hot tap off and the cold full-on. This for me takes great discipline! Although it is extremely invigorating and I have been doing it for years, it still takes effort for me to do it. Practicing discipline by choice makes it a little easier to use self-discipline when it is more important—such as persevering through the ups and downs of the healing process.

Another way to develop personal discipline is to develop the capacity "to go without." Perhaps simply to go without that piece of cake. Perhaps to fast through one meal or one day. Build your discipline muscles!

Step 6. Develop Your Communication Skills

As a group, people affected by cancer tend to keep their thoughts and especially their emotions to themselves. Reversing this can help to change the dynamics of the illness.

- Start with a diary. Research has actually shown this is good for your immune system. When you write, aim to be brief on fact, long on personal detail. It is helpful to record what happens day by day, but the real benefit from writing a diary comes when you elaborate and recount how you felt, how you were affected by what happened. This helps "get it out," to express your feelings in a safe, private environment. And writing it down makes everything clearer and that little bit easier. I made diary entries virtually every day of my recovery and found doing so to be very helpful.

- Letter or e-mail writing can flow on from keeping a diary. What many people find useful these days is to set up a personal blog or Facebook page where news can be shared. This can help to reduce time spent by the patient or the family retelling the same details of what has happened recently. Also, it means that phone calls or face-to-face meetings can be used for more personal exchanges.

- Decide who your "listening post" will be. Seek a safe environment. Maybe a group, maybe an experienced counselor, maybe a trusted friend can become your listening post. This is someone or some group who is stable enough to listen to you. They do not need "an answer" for your problems. They do not need to fix anything. Their job is to listen in an open, nonjudgmental way and by doing so, allow you to express thoughts, feelings and emotions that otherwise may remain bottled up inside. To be able to provide this service of being a compassionate, nonjudgmental listener is a great gift if you are supporting someone with cancer.

Be increasingly open with family and friends. Brian had a brain tumor with a poor prognosis. He wanted to protect his eleven-year-old daughter and thirteen-year-old son and so only told them he had migraines. He reported that the son became increasingly hostile toward him and the daughter withdrew. Brian's wife, Kath, was deeply concerned and felt great pressure attempting to secretively manage phone calls to doctors, the friends who called in, the discussions she wanted to have with Brian and the children. The whole family was suffering. Brian became increasingly anxious and, as time went on, it was increasingly clear he had been withholding from the children. On discussing the dilemma, he finally decided to tell the children. They took it well, his son later confiding to Kath that he had known for quite a while. Kath reported both children soon appeared much more at ease and welcomed being able to discuss what Dad was doing.

Step 7. Laugh and Be Selective

Laughter is good for just about everything. There is a good deal of research to prove it, even if your common sense does not know it already! The trick is, how do we manage to laugh when things are grim?

First, avoid the grumps in your life. Avoid the people who feel compelled to tell you about Uncle Ted who had the same cancer as you, tried everything, and died anyway. Tell those people to take a holiday. Do not call us, we will call you.

Then hang out with the people that make you feel good. Use a simple test. If a guest leaves you feeling worse when they leave than when they got there, strike them off the invite list. You want to be with the people who can be serious when needed, but lift your spirits and ideally make you laugh.

Lighten up. It is bad enough being sick, there is no benefit in feeling miserable as well. So develop a store of funny DVDs and books. Read humor. Watch the comedy channel. Maybe even join in with a laughter club from time to time. People are different. Find out what gets you laughing.

Step 8. Recognize Your Sexuality May Change, and Adjust

Cancer has the potential to impact upon every facet of life and our sexuality is no exception. Treatments may directly affect sexual function and some people find the worry and concern they feel affects their interest in sex or their capacity to engage with it.

The important thing to be aware of is that sexuality and sexual function is another area that needs to be discussed and sorted out. While meditation is very effective in alleviating worry and helping people to be more open and loving, many find that they do need to adjust their sexual life. Of course with couples this may well necessitate both people adjusting, so communication is vital. Many couples do work this out in their own way, but it may be helpful to seek couples counseling if needed. Like everything else, satisfying solutions are found when we communicate and plan accordingly.

Step 9. Monitor the TV

Looking back, one of the best things I did at the start of my illness was to give the TV away. In those days I would watch anything. I was used to working an eighty-hour week as a veterinarian, training for the decathlon a couple of hours each day and then collapsing in front of the TV. I used it as an anesthetic. It was a second-rate way of relaxing and attempting to clear my mind. However, by giving it away, I freed up hours of my time. Without the TV I read two to three books each week, I meditated, I even talked to some people!

If you can manage the TV and regulate what you watch and how often, then of course there are some good things on it. But if the TV becomes a distraction, or at worst a barrier to communication between you and those you are close to, reconsider your options.

Step 10. Exercise Regularly and Within Your Limits

Exercise is profoundly therapeutic as demonstrated by research with several major cancers. Also, exercise is a powerful antidote against depression and leads to a generally more positive state of mind. Aim to exercise for about half an hour each day and then if you miss one session occasionally you will still receive the benefits.

Exercise that is helpful therapeutically is best if it is on the moderate to gentle side. There are two criteria that help you to monitor how hard to go at your exercise, taking into account your own level of fitness and health.

First, when you finish your exercise, you need to feel better than when you began. This means you come back feeling refreshed and invigorated. If you were training for a marathon, it would make sense to extend yourself and to need time to recover, but if healing is your motivation, you have overdone it if you need to lie down for half an hour after exercising.

Second, while exercising you need to be able to keep up a conversation. If you are walking up a hill and puffing so much you cannot string a sentence together, you are overdoing it. Slow down, take a rest, get your breath back.

Step 11. Get Creative

Creativity is another proven method for improving your state of mind and prospects of healing. Maybe you already paint, knit, play music, or build things. Keep doing it and know it is doing you good. Maybe you had a hobby in the past you felt passionate about. Anything that becomes a vehicle for creative passion is highly beneficial and is to be engaged with enthusiastically.

Step 12. Immerse Yourself in Nature

Nature is healing. Fresh air, tall trees, open spaces, the seaside—nature inspires us, comforts us, shares her natural healing gifts freely with us. For those living in cities, find the best parks nearby. Make the effort to travel into the countryside or to have a day by the water. Relax into nature. Sit with your eyes open. Contemplate. Meditate. Feel the deep natural peace and the healing qualities so ever present in nature.

Step 13. Develop Patience

Many people I have met approached an initial diagnosis of cancer with gusto. As if preparing for a sprint, they used a lot of energy to do all they could to overcome the challenges and gain the benefits. For some, recovery actually turned out to be relatively easy and quick, but for many others, more like a marathon.

So be patient, use the chapters on healthy emotions and overcome any tendencies to lapse into destructive, negative states of mind, while building the ability to be resilient, to endure, to persevere and to prevail.

Step 14. Practice Gratitude

Before bed each night, reflect on your day and find three things to be grateful for. They may be simple things like the sun was shining or the rain was falling. They may be acts of kindness you experienced or lessons you learned through the circumstances of the day. This simple practice of gratitude is a proven antidote to depression, but more significantly, it can really warm your heart and result in a positive attitude to all you do.

Step 15. Meditate

Out of the balance of meditation, a positive state of mind naturally arises. Maybe this is to do with the clarity that comes with meditation, the inner confidence, the natural optimism. Maybe the fact is that our natural state is to be positive and the balance of meditation simply reasserts that state.

Step 16. Consider Using Affirmations and Imagery

These will be explained in the next chapter.

Step 17. Celebrate What Is Good

Aim to find joy in what is healthy, positive and wholesome! This is a crucial point. If you do all the so-called right things in a grumpy, resentful and miserable state of mind, you will undermine the benefits and you run the risk of becoming quite miserable!

Find joy in doing what is good for you. How? This recommendation links directly with our third principle of positive thinking—choose to enjoy doing it. Remember, when you are aware you can decide your state of mind. Become informed regarding your choices. Decide what is in your own best interests and choose to be diligent; choose to enjoy doing it! Celebrate life.

DO WHATEVER IT TAKES • Where to Start

Quite a list! Obviously it is not possible or recommended to aim to be doing them all tomorrow. Besides, some you are bound to be doing already and others will just leap out and you will recognize their immediate value. Start with them. This whole art of positive thinking is something we can continue to develop and continue to gain more benefit from.

THE THIRD PRINCIPLE OF POSITIVE THINKING: CHOOSE TO ENJOY DOING IT

We have delved into the first two principles of positive thinking in some detail, learning how to set a clear goal and do whatever it takes. The third principle concerns the attitude with which we do the things we do, given that what we enjoy we tend to persist with, and what we do not enjoy, we tend to let go of.

Now another key principle, one that has transformed the lives of many people. The operative word in the third principle is "choose." We "choose" to enjoy doing whatever it is that we do. This is one of the great lessons the mind can teach us. We can choose how we respond to our circumstances.

Many people are literally slaves to what is happening in their lives. "Of course I am angry, look at what he did to me." "Of course I am sad, she left me, didn't she?" "Of course I am laughing, listen to this!" "Of course I am miserable, don't you know how sick I am?" There is no freedom in being a slave to your circumstances. You can rise above your situation and decide how you will respond to it.

Viktor Frankl was a world-renowned psychiatrist who was confined in the Nazis' concentration camps in the Second World War. He survived and wrote *Man's Search for Meaning*,[10] which highlighted two powerful observations. What Frankl realized first was the power of the will to live. In this toughest of environments, it was easy to die. Frankl observed that those who had a reason to live seemed to do so more often than those who lost it. Whenever anyone gave up hope, they seemed to die quickly.

So consider this, what inspires you to live? Why do you want to recover? What will you do when you regain your good health? The more heartfelt that motivation, the more Frankl would say you are likely to survive.

The second observation is more directly relevant to our discussion. Frankl was in a concentration camp where every effort was made to deprive the captives of their freedom. This was carried through ruthlessly and thoroughly. Most human freedoms can in fact be stripped away. Yet Frankl observed that there was one freedom that no one could take away if the individual had the state of mind to recognize it and to preserve it. That ultimate human freedom is the freedom to decide how we respond to our circumstances. So in the camps, that may have been the freedom to decide how to go into a gas oven. Would one go in kicking and screaming, or walking with their head held high? Either would be understandable. No one could decide which it would be other than the person involved and no one could take away the freedom to choose how to do it, if that person was clear-minded.

Marjory had experienced a blessed life. In her early seventies, still married to her teenage sweetheart, her three children all doing well, she developed an aggressive, painful cancer. Marjory had a strong Christian faith. A regular member of her local church, she was active across her community. She had led a charmed life free of any real suffering. So why this tough illness? What sense did it make? It really challenged Marjory's Christian view and caused her deep introspection. "Why me?" seemed a profound mystery to her.

Marjory's response was extraordinary. She decided that her faith in God, which she had believed to be strong, had never been tested. Having had such an easy life, for Marjory it had been easy to have faith. Now it was not so easy. Marjory decided the test was to find out if she could suffer well, if her faith could withstand a real test.

What anyone else might think of this response is to miss the point. Marjory's illness progressed steadily, attended by bouts of serious discomfort and pain. But a strange thing happened. She grew in strength. Her faith shone through and she only had one problem. As her illness advanced and her physical condition deteriorated, more and more of her friends wanted to spend time with her. Her family told me they felt Marjory was demonstrating how to suffer well and how to die well.

Maybe you do not think this is such a positive story, but I suggest that again, this would be to miss the point. As Marjory approached her death, her body became increasingly frail, yet her spirit shone through. It was there for all to see. In my experience of this, Marjory found her own way to conquer cancer. She died with a deep satisfaction, a deep peace. Marjory died knowing she had chosen how to respond to her situation and she had seen it through without wavering. She died with her faith stronger, her confidence assured.

And her family? They felt the loss deeply. But they told me how meaningful the experience was for them also. They had the mixed emotions of grief and elation, and the knowing they had been a part of something extraordinary.

So choose to enjoy doing it! Sure, if things are tough you may need to work at it and revisit all the items we listed for reinforcing your good intentions. But it can be done. It is an act of choice. You can choose to be positive. You can choose to enjoy doing whatever you turn your mind toward and remarkable things can be accomplished.

FINALLY, A SUMMARY

Positive Thinking Requires:
- A sound understanding of how the mind functions, particularly the three principles of positive thinking.
- A commitment to be positive.
- Good information on which to base our decisions.
- A calm clear mind that is free to make the best choices possible. To have a calm and clear mind we need:
  - freedom from stress and confusion;
  - freedom from conflicting emotions;
  - freedom from unhelpful habits and prejudices;

- the ability to draw on the rational, logical mind, as well as our intuition and inner wisdom.
- The most reliable technique that delivers a calm and clear mind is meditation.
- Diligence—the capacity to commit to our goals, to embrace them, to persevere and to accomplish them.
- Good support.

Put all this together and extraordinary things are possible; in fact, what seems extraordinary can become commonplace!

However, some of us will be familiar with the New Year's resolution syndrome. This is when we have a good intention that makes really good logical sense, and yet we struggle to do it, or even worse, just forget all about it. So in our next chapter on mind training we need to investigate and understand the power that beliefs and habits can have in our life, and put them to good use, as well.

CHAPTER 8

Mind Training 2

Habits and Beliefs, Affirmations and Imagery: The Unconscious Mind at Work

THE UNCONSCIOUS MIND IS THE STOREHOUSE FOR OUR BELIEFS AND OUR habits. Our beliefs and our habits powerfully shape our lives. We know that what we often describe as "negative" beliefs and habits can be powerfully destructive, while when we use them effectively, strong beliefs and healthy habits can set us free and catalyze profound healing.

For example, if our belief is that cancer always proves fatal and there is nothing we can do about it, we are in deep trouble once diagnosed. If we believe we can overcome cancer, then that outcome becomes a real possibility. If we conclude we need to change our way of eating to give ourselves the best chance of recovery, and yet we are stuck in our old habits and cannot change, again we are in real trouble. If changing unhelpful habits or adopting new ones comes naturally, or we learn how to do it, then the whole process of change can be enjoyable and a source of pride, as well as being highly beneficial to ourselves and to those around us.

Our beliefs and our habits can bind us, or set us free.

The potential that the unconscious mind holds is another crucial factor in recovery and so in this chapter we aim to understand its role and how we can use it to best effect. The focus will be on developing beliefs and habits that actively support the process of recovery, along with the use of affirmations and imagery. To begin with, we will investigate how beliefs have the remarkable power to both destroy life and to restore it. Please note that my own book *The Mind That Changes Everything*[11] is recommended as a companion piece for these chapters on the healing power of the mind.

THE DESTRUCTIVE POWER OF BELIEF • The Pointing of the Bone Effect

One of the most extreme examples of the destructive power of the mind comes from the ancient peoples of Australia. As we discussed in chapter 2, the pointing of the bone is a potent ritual that involves no direct physical force, yet it routinely results in death. The only known cases of a traditional Australian Aborigine successfully surviving being pointed is when an antidote in the form of another ritual has been applied and, in doing so, convinced the victim that the second ritual had more power than the first.

When we examine it closely, the key element in the first ritual, the bone pointing is that it creates hopelessness, a powerful belief that there is no other hope, no other expectation, than to die. What the antidote provides is a satisfactory rationale, congruent with the belief system of the victim that validates the real possibility of recovery. The antidote replaces hopelessness with hope.

Knowing about all this provides two more keys to recovery—the power of hope, and the power of the placebo.

THE HEALING POWER OF BELIEF • The Placebo Response, Hope and Recovery

If the pointing of the bone demonstrates the negative impact of beliefs, placebos clearly reveal their positive effects.

When new drugs are tested, people believe they may be useful. It is well-known in the medical world that this belief on its own can produce very positive results, so a sugar-coated pill with no active ingredients is used to measure how much benefit that belief will produce. Then, the results gained with the new drug are compared to those of the placebo to measure the new drug's real value. The sugar-coated pill is called a placebo. In many conditions, "treatment" with a placebo manages to produce a 30 percent improvement. With pain, placebos given with enthusiastic conviction, "this will really help reduce the pain," have regularly produced pain relief comparable to heavy-duty narcotics. Just what the mind is capable of when beliefs are activated effectively is literally extraordinary.

Take the incredible story of an American "hillbilly" with a difficult throat cancer that had little prospect of a medical cure. This story is as extreme as the pointing of the bone, only in this case the outcome was extremely positive. Diagnosed by his local doctor, the patient was told that he was being referred to a large city hospital to have a new form of ray treatment that would cure him. Arriving in awe at the hospital, he was given a basic checkup. When a thermometer was put in the naive man's mouth, his clinician was astute enough to realize that the patient thought this was the new wonder treatment. After several sessions of this "treatment," the cancer disappeared completely! While we might smile at the mental picture of a simple "hillbilly" being cured by a thermometer, let us not lose sight of the importance of the principle he demonstrated so well.

The message is that the placebo works. Maybe in cancer medicine we could call the role the mind has through the power of belief "placebo medicine." For while it is clear that we can explain a good deal of how the mind has such positive effects in very practical ways, such as how it leads to good choices and commitment, it is also clear the mind on its own can dramatically affect our chances of recovery. What we are seeking through studying and using the power of belief is to avoid any downside comparable to the pointing of the bone effect, while we access the positive benefits demonstrated by the placebo response. However, rather than being "tricked" by a placebo, we seek to use our intelligence to harness that same potential.

How do we do it? The answer is simple. The more we believe in whatever we do, the more we will get the best out of any treatment we have, the more we are likely to reduce any potential side effects, and the more we will gain from all the self-help techniques we utilize.

Jim's story provides a glimpse of what is possible. Jim was diagnosed with widespread cancer of the prostate and given months to live. He plunged into feelings of despair and hopelessness. A self-made man, Jim stopped work and spent his days at home behind drawn curtains. He did this so no one would glimpse how he spent those days—crying! When it came time in the evening for his wife and children to return home, he did his best to pull himself together, attempted a brave face and struggled on. Jim said what he was really doing was simply waiting to die; he felt hopeless and he felt miserable.

One day, not long after this book was first released in 1984, Jim's gaze fell on the title at his local newspaper shop. *You Can Conquer Cancer.* Maybe there was something he could do for himself after all. He bought the book and then he asked his wife to take a look. This was all happening in Melbourne, and Jim's wife, Angela, knew of the groups I was running not far from where they lived. He came, but remained confused for the first few weeks. Jim could not comprehend at first how attending to his diet, becoming positive, using the power of his mind and meditating could achieve what the doctors could not. But hope was kindled.

Soon the curtains were open, the tears gone. Jim began talking to his wife and three boys. They enthusiastically embraced the dietary changes and supported him fully as he began to meditate regularly. The first sign of real progress was when the pain subsided. Jim said later that when the meditation brought him pain relief, it helped him to believe in what he was doing. It gave him the confidence to persevere and then to intensify what he had begun somewhat tentatively. Jim went on to have a complete, long-term remission.

The important conclusion we must take from all this is that if we do feel hopeless, if we do have doubts or fears, at the very least they have the capacity to undermine whatever we do, or worse as in Jim's case, render us passive, depressed and miserable. In extreme situations, they could have the same impact as the pointing of the bone.

WHAT IF MY BELIEFS ARE FRAGILE? • Building Hope

Doubts and fears are normal to begin with. Reread Jim's story above. Nearly everyone who ever came to one of the cancer groups came with some degree of fear, doubt, confusion, and uncertainty. That is normal. That is where most people begin. It is because we know this to be true that we need to address all these issues. This is not something of itself to be fearful, but it is something to act upon. The good news is that we can do something about it; the bad news is that those who do not know about all this, or do not act on it, severely limit their possibilities and often have a miserable time.

Here is what will help.

Step 1. Hope

To restate it, the starting point is hope. Hope is real. It only has to be done once to show that it is possible, but in fact we do know recovery happens quite regularly. Maybe this is a good time to revisit our discussions in earlier chapters around hope, statistics and individuals (see chapter 2), and not only dare to believe in what is possible, actually reconfirm the logic in the possibility of recovery.

However, what we hope for and believe to be possible is a combination of the knowledge we hold and the emotional overlay that affects that knowledge. We are all bound to know some people whose emotional life overrides their logic and whose hopes are more about emotion than reason. This is not always a problem, but if for example, fear overrides your sensibility, then that may well be a big problem.

Step 2. Clarity

To build hope, clarity is vital. Clarity begins with clearing our emotions and we will discuss how to manage this in the chapters on healthy emotions (see chapters 16 and 17). What we also need to appreciate is that clarity comes with knowledge and so we do need the best information possible. This is challenging amid the information-saturated age in which we live. We need to revisit the earlier sections on decision making that addressed how to sort out our choices, how to decide who and what to trust, who and what to believe (see chapter 3). The crucial point is to make the time to set clear goals and to commit to them.

Step 3. Action

Once we have hope, we need to do something with it. Do be reminded, however, that hoping for the best and doing nothing about it is what we call wishful thinking and we know that particular state of mind is a far cry from the potency of positive thinking. To convert hope into reality we need to act.

So next we need to apply the positive-thinking skills of the previous chapter. The eight steps that support the first principle of positive thinking— to set a clear goal—are where we begin. Following these guidelines helps us to make good choices and to develop confidence in those choices. Then we use the second principle, to do whatever it takes to follow through.

So do be reassured. The doubts and fears are normal to begin with; hope can be rekindled, the confidence and certainty we call belief is something that can be developed—reliably!

BELIEFS AFFECT ALL THAT WE DO

The next key point is that the benefit of whatever we do is a product of the actual thing itself, and the overarching and additional impact of our beliefs. Will you add the pointing of the bone effect or the placebo effect?

If we sit in front of a fantastic, really healthy organic salad, and the only thought going through our head is "Oh no, not another salad. I must be crazy to be eating this stuff!" then it is easy to imagine the physical benefit of the good food is significantly undermined by our state of mind. If on the other hand, we sit in front of the same salad and we think, "Wow! This is terrific! This is really going to do me good. I can feel myself healing," then not only do we gain the benefit from the good food, we gain the benefit that our mind has to offer.

So the message is to think through all that you do. Decide what is the best you can do. Accept that. Believe it to be true—it is the best you can do. Commit to it. Do all you can to reinforce it. Hang out with those that support what you are doing. Read books that reinforce what you are doing. Use all the positive-thinking techniques. This is how we utilize the power of belief and how we can be assured of getting the best out of whatever we do.

Next, we need to address the role habits play on the road to recovery.

THE HEALING POWER OF HABITS • Getting the Job Done

Habits are really useful. Imagine if we were not in the habit of cooking. Then, at each meal we would need to start from scratch. We would need to think about everything we planned to do and there would be a huge amount of information and technique to sort out. It would take forever. By contrast, most of us do cook pretty much on automatic—we do a lot of it by habit and it is quick, easy and satisfying. So a habit provides us with a fairly automatic way of doing something that often is learned by repeating that thing over and over.

The main point is that on the healing journey, habits can really free us up and support us to do the things we enjoy and that are good for us, or they can severely restrict us. We need to break free of any limitations and to ensure our habits do work for us. Good habits make for good health.

BREAKING FREE OF OLD HABITS AND REALIZING YOUR GOALS

I imagine most of us at some time in the past have suffered from what we can call the New Year's resolution syndrome. You know the one: this year I am going to give up smoking; or this year I will exercise every day; or this year I will transform my anger. These good intentions always make so much sense. They are logical choices, obviously in our best interests. Everyone around us it seems would welcome and support the changes. It should be so easy! Yet how often is it that only a week into January, rather than enjoying having made the changes, there is that nagging, recurrent guilt born of not only not having made the change, but often enough, not even being able to remember exactly what the resolution was.

One of the major challenges in using your own efforts to heal is that you are the one who has to do most of the work. You need to make the time to meditate. You are the one who needs to eat a healing diet, to exercise and so on. It is clear that on the healing journey what we need to do is develop and maintain healthy habits. Often this will require us to change our habits, and often to do this effectively, we will need to overcome the New Year's resolution syndrome.

It must be easy for each of us to reflect on times when goals seemed easy to achieve, when we decided to do something and just simply did it. But almost certainly we will have had other times when we seemed content (in a funny sort of way) to give up on a good idea all too easily and all too soon. We need to be aware of how the mind has the potential to restrict us, to bind us to old patterns, and notice too those magical times when the mind sets us free.

The question is, does all this happen at random or can we have some control? What we need now is to investigate the workings of our mind a little more deeply, to understand how our habits develop and how when we need to, we can change them in a way that is easy, sustainable and even enjoyable!

HABITS AND BELIEFS HAVE A LOT IN COMMON

Just as habits are a fairly automatic, somewhat unconscious way of doing things, beliefs could be said to be fairly automatic, somewhat unconscious ways of thinking about things. We can consciously remember, identify and discuss our habits and our beliefs, but both are held in the domain of the unconscious mind.

So that we can use both habits and beliefs to better advantage we need to establish how they develop and then learn the techniques of affirmations and imagery. What is to come is really empowering as it holds the potential to set us free from binding, limiting beliefs and habits, while enabling us to do what we need to do!

HOW HABITS AND BELIEFS DEVELOP • The Five Steps

Step 1. Habits and Beliefs Are a Product of Our Experiences

Our habits and beliefs begin to develop early in life. We have a range of life experiences that we take in, learn from, and use to form our habits and our beliefs. We become aware of these experiences, these life lessons via our five senses. So we see things, we hear them, we touch, smell and taste them.

What is important for us to realize is that what we do perceive with our five senses we generally take as being real. However, we often see something, hear something, feel something which we take to be real, only to find out later that we were wrong. If our perception is inaccurate and it concerns a major life issue, we could develop an inaccurate belief that affects our life in a major way. Further, our perception is not only affected by the physical senses.

Step 2. Our Perception Is Colored by Our Emotions and Our State of Mind

The perception of our experiences, the meaning and the relevance we place on them, is affected by our emotional and mental state. For example, it is claimed that when angry, our capacity to perceive and take in the truth of events happening around us is diminished by up to 90 percent. Furthermore, we will all know of people with befuddled minds. Minds that lack clarity for one reason or another. Maybe drugs, old age, limited knowledge or intelligence—all these things can dramatically affect perception and the capacity to develop really useful belief systems.

So sometimes we only see something once, or have something happen to us once, and because it is so emotionally charged it makes a deep impression. Other times things happen of little moment in our lives and we forget them almost as soon as they happen. Some things happen over and over so that we cannot help but remember them. Some things stick, others do not.

Step 3. Our Experiences Are Stored in Our Memory

The things that do stick, those experiences are stored in the unconscious realm of the brain as memories. The emotions that accompany memories have a big bearing on how important they are to us. Generally speaking, the more dramatic, the stronger the emotions, the more prominent the memories.

Step 4. Memories Are Stored as Images

When we analyze them, we find that memories are actually made up of images—primarily pictures, sounds (words) and feelings. Taste and smell can be involved to a lesser degree.

Step 5. Memories Accumulate to Produce Habits and Beliefs

As we accumulate memories, they steadily build up to produce our habits and our beliefs. The beliefs we have developed will be the reflection of the full range of our life experiences and these beliefs will lead to both positive and negative expectations. If you notice yourself saying, "This is too good to be true," or "That always happens to me," or "It is not like me to have done . . ." then you are voicing an expectation, a direct expression of your belief system.

Our beliefs and our habits can limit us or set us free.

THE IMPACT OF UNHELPFUL HABITS AND BELIEFS

Julia was a very likable lady. Her outgoing personality had led her into a successful designing career but her personal life was dogged by emotional distress, and she had cancer. Amid the safety of a residential cancer program, Julia spoke with frustration of the many relationships she had been in with what appeared to her to be highly suitable men. Yet time after time these relationships had turned sour.

Julia quickly came to realize she had a huge problem with not allowing intimacy into her life and that she had put barriers up against deepening relationships. She realized her relationship breakdowns had not "just happened." In fact more often than not she had actively destroyed them by the way she had acted.

Then Julia made the mind connection. As a young girl she had grown up in the country amid a large family. Here, there seemed to have been much of the best of country life—close contact with nature, an easy lifestyle, lots of friends and time with her parents and extended family. Then at the age of seven, Julia had been diagnosed with measles. In the family's large farmhouse, the only place Julia could be isolated was in the rather large pantry. Julia went from living in the midst of a very large, open, loving family to being confined by her parents in an internal room with no windows, poor ventilation and quite a few rats! Julia wondered what she had done wrong. Her seven-year-old brain concluded she must have been very bad, that no one really loved her, that she was not even worthy of love!

Looking back as an adult, Julia could reason that her family really did love her, but she also realized that this one powerful childhood experience had been anchored deep inside her unconscious mind and that it had shaped her behavior dramatically. Julia came to realize her deeply held belief of being unworthy of love had sabotaged all her relationships.

Then Julia made another crucial observation. All her life she had been driven to succeed. Now she realized that her burning ambition was motivated by repeated attempts to prove her self-worth to herself, and to others. While she had become quite successful, Julia was beginning to realize the cost she had paid for that success. It was time to find another way. Julia knew that what she needed was to change the inner beliefs she held about herself.

HOW HABITS AND BELIEFS CAN BIND US • Or Set Us Free

As human beings we have a fundamental commitment to act in accordance with our beliefs. The reality is that when we are doing what we believe in, we feel comfortable and satisfied—we have peace of mind. When our actions do not match our beliefs, we feel uncomfortable, we have a deep sense something is wrong, and we become highly motivated to do something about it.

What this means, what makes our beliefs so important, is that what we believe in becomes a yardstick for our actions. This is because we are constantly striving to fulfill our beliefs, to live true to our beliefs.

So if we happen to believe eating fast food or junk food is OK, and if we are in the habit of eating it and we like eating it, we are really stuck with it. Perhaps you think this is an extreme example, but I suggest we may all have things we believe in and are in the habit of doing, things we feel comfortable with, that are not all that healthy and that could well make it more difficult for us to get well and stay well. When we do not manage to change our unhealthy old habits and beliefs and to adopt and sustain healthy ones, recovery is given a major boost!

HOW TO CHANGE HABITS AND BELIEFS

Remember, habits and beliefs are stored in our unconscious mind and are the accumulated balance of our life experiences. Happily, we can learn how to replace unhelpful habits and beliefs with helpful ones.

What makes it possible to achieve this—in fact, what makes it easy—is that the unconscious mind cannot distinguish between a real-life experience (and the set of images that go with it) and artificial, positive experiences we can choose to generate (through the use of affirmation and imagery).

To establish, change or reinforce habits and beliefs in such a way that they will be effectively anchored in our unconscious mind and responded to, we need to learn how to use the techniques of affirmation and imagery.

HOW DO THESE TECHNIQUES WORK IN REAL LIFE?

Betty was a senior lady whose life had been lived helping others. She had supported her husband in his work, raised a fine family and contributed to her community. But now she had cancer with secondary spread, and in medical terms, a hopeless prognosis. There was no medical treatment offered or given to her. But Betty loved life and felt she had more to do. She came to our groups with her rather reluctant, but duty-bound husband. Phillip took all the sessions in, while he remained somewhat distant and aloof.

Betty's condition appeared to deteriorate at first, her pain became worse, and despondency set in. Sitting in her armchair one evening, tears began to well up in her eyes. Phillip, sensing Betty's mood, asked her what was wrong. She spoke gently of how perhaps it was all too much, perhaps she should face reality, accept her fate and give up on getting well.

As it turned out, up until now, Betty had always been a rather negative person. She explained later that a string of events early in life had not worked out as she hoped. She had taken those experiences in and developed a pessimistic view. At a deep level, Betty had come to believe that things always went wrong for her.

Fortunately for Betty, her husband had been paying attention during the group sessions. He had taken in the discussion on beliefs, affirmations and imagery, and he knew Betty was working on becoming more positive with the affirmation "I am a positive person now!" So Phillip, seeing his wife sitting there with gloom hanging over her head and pervading her very being, said to her, "That's strange. What are you now?"

"What do you mean?" responded Betty rather gloomily.

"Oh, I thought you were a positive person now."

Betty told me later this was a magical moment in her amazing recovery. With her husband's words, it was as if some inner switch was thrown.

"Yes," she said. "You are right. I am a positive person now!"

From that moment on, Betty's focus was on the positive side of life. Instead of the old half-empty glass she had been dealing with, now she truly saw the glass half full. She looked for the positive aspect in every situation, found it and, in the process, discovered a wonderful inner peace. Her physical recovery was quite remarkable and over twenty years later her calm and joyful manner was a delight to all who knew her.

The strong suggestion is to spend time reflecting on these principles that have the power to transform old unhelpful beliefs and establish new, healthy, healing belief systems and habits. The more you understand all this, the more you contemplate and take to heart how it all works, the easier it will be to use the techniques and the better they will work.

Once you have this solid framework of understanding, move on to put it all into practice. It is the use of affirmations and imagery that provides us with the technology of the mind to change our mind. One of the delightful things about affirmations and imagery is that they are rather simple to use. And they work! By following a fairly easy number of steps, we can develop a practice that has the potential to bring major benefits into our lives. First affirmations, then imagery.

How to Develop Affirmations

Affirmations are short, precise statements that summarize a specific goal. By repeating the affirmation over and over, it replaces any old, contradictory habits or beliefs and imprints the new one onto our unconscious mind.

Then, when we are faced with a new situation that requires us to respond, we check our unconscious and the affirmation guides us with what to do. Betty's story from above is a great example of an affirmation at work.

For affirmations to be effective they must satisfy three essential points, and then there is some fine-tuning to do.

STEP 1. THE THREE ESSENTIAL POINTS

Affirmations need to be expressed in the first person, present tense, and they need to be goal-oriented.

First person, present tense means we start our affirmations with words like "I am . . . ," "I do . . . ," "I have . . . ," etc.

Present time is the only time the unconscious responds to. What this means is that when we check with our memory to retrieve a habit or a belief, we are looking for what to do. If what comes out is "I am hoping to be a little more positive some time off in the future and I hope I will be, but probably I won't because I tried that before and it did not work so well, but I guess I better give it a go anyway," our mind is going to recognize our confusion for what it is and not act upon it. We will remain befuddled. If, on the other hand, our unconscious tells us, "I am a positive person now," then everything we do will need to satisfy that criteria for us to feel happy to commit to it. We will inevitably become more and more positive. Therefore affirmations need to indicate the goal is already achieved or reached. The aim is to give the mind a target to lock on to—the target is the end goal, hence, "I am a positive person now."

STEP 2. THE FINE-TUNING
Be Positive

Indicate what is needed, not what is not. The mind is goal-oriented, it locks on to targets. It needs a positive direction to aim for, not something to avoid. So, rather than saying, "I am not a negative person now," for an affirmation we use "I am a positive person now."

Avoid Comparisons

There is no need to say, "I am as good as . . . ," or "I am better than . . ." Your capacity, your potential, may be to be better, or it may be to be worse.

Aim to develop affirmations that encourage the development of your own full potential.

Unless Essential, Do Not Specify a Time for Completion

As with comparisons, specifying time may slow you down or frustrate you. Part of the joy in using affirmations is that they release the power of our creativity and inner wisdom. The fact is that this aspect of our being has a wonderful talent for getting us into the right place at the right time, and if we go with it, we will be content and at ease.

Do Be Specific, Accurate and Accountable

The mind needs a specific target. The more precise the goal, the greater its clarity, and the more confident you can be of success.

Be Realistic—*Expect a Discussion!*

You will be limited by what you believe is possible. However, it is normal to expect some reaction to using affirmations.

"I am a positive person now," you say. "No, you're not," comes that little doubting echo. That is normal. The echo is the old belief having its say. If it were not there, you would have very little need to use the affirmation in the first place.

Remember, this process directs or redirects the mind's attention and mobilizes all its power and creativity. This is a process for making change, for replacing one belief with another, as well as simply establishing a new belief or goal. So do not be surprised by the echo. As long as the affirmation has more energy, more expectation, more hope, more determination, more *oomph* than the echo, and it is repeated, it will gradually replace it and soon become the guiding force for your mind.

Consider Setting Ongoing Goals

You will need to stay within the bounds of what you can believe is reasonably possible. Some people, for example, can imagine themselves fully recovered and can set that as their goal. Others may be more confident of their condition becoming stable and recognize this is a big step in itself. Set goals you can commit to and then as you observe yourself nearing completion of one goal, look for what comes next. Extend your planning and make new resolutions.

Use Action Words and Add a Sense of Excitement

The feeling, the emotion that goes with an affirmation has a lot to do with how quickly it will imprint and be accepted by the unconscious. Affirmations, therefore, work better when said with zest and excitement. One way to do this is to add "Wow!" on the end of them: "I am a positive person now—Wow!" Saying "Wow!" encapsulates that positive, expectant feeling. If "Wow!" does not suit you, use another word or phrase from your own vocabulary to enliven your affirmation.

Similarly, look for ways of expressing confidence, ease, naturalness and joy in all you aim for.

Be Precise with the Use of Your Words

Words used in affirmations are definitely words of power. Pay great attention to how they might be interpreted. You can cover your bets by adding words like "in a harmonious way." Be as clear and precise as possible, consider all angles and choose your words wisely. Meditating and contemplating on your choice of affirmations before you use them is an excellent way to check their meaning and their validity—for you.

Keep a Balance

Affirmations can have a profound effect upon your direction in life. Consider again the range of goals you are setting. Take heed of your physical, emotional, mental and spiritual needs and those of your family, friends and community. Affirmations are exciting tools to use. Aim to maintain that sense of balance.

Some Sample Affirmations for Personal Development

These are some favorite, well-tested affirmations that can act as a guide for your own needs:

FOR HEALTH

"Every day in every way I am getting better and better."

This is one of the oldest and most famous affirmations. It was first used over a century ago by a Frenchman, Emile Coué, and recorded in his book *Self-Mastery Through Conscious Autosuggestion.*[12]

It remains an extremely powerful and effective tool for mobilizing our inner drive toward better health.

"Actively engaged with healing, I experience life fully and give myself every chance of recovery."

FOR RELATIONSHIPS

"I greet this person with love."

FOR SELF-ESTEEM

"I am worthy of being here."
"I am worthy of being happy."
"I am worthy of being loved."

OVERCOMING FEAR, FACING DYING

"Prepared for death, I transform fear."
"Prepared for death, I live well, and when my time comes, die well."

Before discussing the finer practical details of how to combine the practical use of affirmations, imagery and feelings, let us examine how to develop imagery.

HOW TO DEVELOP IMAGERY

While affirmations focus on the use of words, imagery involves using inner pictures to imprint a new goal on our subconscious mind and so stimulate our motivation and creativity to achieve that goal.

Choose the Type of Imagery That Suits Your Needs

There are three classifications for the types of images we can use—literal, symbolic and abstract.

Literal Images

With this type of imagery, we aim to see an image of the behavior, event or goal literally. This means you visualize your goal the way you are intending it to happen and you repeat it over and over in your mind's eye, a bit like rerunning a video or DVD. This literal imagery is very practical and can be applied in any situation where there is a clear understanding of the goal. This literal style is widely used in sport and has well-established benefits for changing habits and beliefs.

So if you have a very tangible goal like becoming less anxious and more positive, the use of literal imagery can be a great asset. Imagine yourself in situations where you used to be negative, only now you see yourself calm and relaxed, making positive choices, acting in a way that you consider to be positive, and feeling a sense of pride and achievement. Combining this with an affirmation such as "I am a positive person now" and persisting with the repetition of both virtually assures a change in the behavior.

While literal images are highly effective in sport and for making personal changes, when the goal is clear but the mechanism for achieving it is uncertain, highly complex or to do with healing, symbolic or abstract imagery is often far more appropriate.

Symbolic and Abstract Imagery

Symbols can be used as a vehicle to convey our conscious intention into the subconscious in a way that the intention can be recognized and acted upon. Take healing, for example. The complexity and timing of the healing process is beyond most, if not all, conscious minds. However, one does not need sophisticated instruments to learn how to influence the body's healing functions directly. Imagery in either the symbolic or abstract form is probably the most powerful tool for this purpose and we will investigate and learn these specific techniques in the next chapter.

HOW TO PRACTICE AFFIRMATIONS AND IMAGERY

Affirmations are best repeated with positive expectation, with power, confidence and good feeling. If you have a fair degree of confidence when you first begin to use a particular affirmation, you will only need to repeat it for a minute or two a few times a day and that mind-set will soon become established. When you have a more challenging belief to establish, or if your mind is cluttered, you will need to practice more often and for longer periods.

The imagery that accompanies affirmations is used similarly and the time you will need to practice it will depend on the ease and clarity that accompanies the image. While an individual session of symbolic imagery usually takes about ten minutes, abstract imagery can be used for longer times. For instance, a session of the white light healing imagery (which will be described in the next chapter) can easily occupy thirty to sixty minutes. Also, abstract imagery can be an excellent prelude to letting go into the simple silence of deeper meditation.

Affirmations and imagery can be used together. This is the most direct and effective way. However, sometimes you may feel it more appropriate to use an affirmation or imagery on its own.

For example, an affirmation on its own may work well to begin the process of changing an undesired long-standing state of mind such as low self-esteem. You may find it more effective to begin by repeating, "I am worthy of love now" as an affirmation. Then, once some confidence in the accuracy and reality of that statement is established you may enhance the affirmation by adding related and supportive images. In the case of building self-esteem, you could remember situations where previously you had felt awkward, underconfident, and vulnerable, and now you re-create those same situations in your mind and imagine yourself to be calm, at ease, confident and feeling good about yourself. Similarly, many healing situations appear to respond well to the direct use of imagery.

With the repetition of affirmations and imagery, our aim is to imprint a consciously chosen goal onto our unconscious mind so that it becomes anchored as a habit and/or a belief. This belief will then act as a target that our mind will do all possible to direct us toward.

The process of imprinting occurs most easily and most effectively when there is a close connection between the conscious mind and the unconscious. A good example of this is when we are in that reverie state just before going to sleep. It is when our mind is relaxed, not dwelling on anything in particular, and at peace. That state of reverie before you get out of bed in the morning, or as you go to bed at night, can serve as an excellent time to practice affirmations and imagery.

Also, singing or joking with affirmations loosens the power of the conscious mind and its conditioned responses, and so facilitates the imprinting process. Making up jingles for your affirmations and singing them out loud can be useful and fun!

Looking directly into your eyes via a mirror and saying your affirmations out loud with power and conviction is extremely effective if you can do it.

Best of all is to combine imagery with your meditation. The meditation provides a poise and balance and has a stabilizing effect on the whole process.

HOW TO COMBINE RELAXATION, IMAGERY AND MEDITATION

(a) Sit in a slightly uncomfortable, symmetrical position.

(b) Relax physically, inducing the relaxation response wherever possible.

(c) Then begin the imprinting—using affirmations and imagery in combination or separately.

(d) Let go of the imagery and rest in the natural peace and stillness of meditation before finishing the session.

SUPPORT YOUR GOOD INTENTIONS, RESPOND TO FEEDBACK

Reinforce your good intentions, your affirmations and imagery with these powerful supports:

- Develop a support network. Discuss your goals with family and friends. Get them on your side. Consider enlisting the new technologies and activating your social media contacts.
- Seek out allies who can support you wholeheartedly. Avoid those who challenge you too directly or too strongly.
- Read books, listen to CDs and DVDs and attend workshops that support your goals.
- Attend a support group or meditation group that is relevant to your needs.
- Tell others of your goal—be accountable.
- Be prepared for setbacks. Changing habits can take time. Be prepared to persevere.
- Be gentle on yourself. Determine to be patient and reward yourself as you notice progress.

- Do seek feedback. Be prepared to reassess your situation, make adjustments and move on.
- Smile regularly! All of this needs to be fun to be sustained. Enjoy being alive. Change is a feature of life. If you were not changing you would be dead. Enjoy the changes by celebrating your successes.

DEALING WITH SETBACKS

While you may move steadily and uneventfully toward your goals, it may also be that life goes up and down a little along the way. Setbacks can cause you to reassess your whole situation, strengthen your resolve and lead to useful modifications and changes.

The best insurance against disappointment is to give whatever you do your best, to do everything to 100 percent of your ability. Then if you have a setback, there will be no regrets, no guilt, no wondering "What if . . . ," or "If only I had . . ." At least you will have the comfort of knowing you have been giving it your all. Then there will be a level of acceptance and acknowledgment that leaves you free from looking backward. You will be free to look forward for fresh solutions.

With this approach, answers to questions and solutions for setbacks seem to come very reliably. When I was ill, often the answers to setbacks came via books. Often when faced with another setback (there were many in my own road to recovery), it would seem as if I was drawn almost intuitively, almost magnetically, to a particular book. I would open it and there would be the answer on the page in front of me! Often too, old friends would appear unannounced and have the answers. The more I trusted in the process, whenever a question or problem presented itself, the more I expected an answer, the more rapidly it appeared. Synchronicity at work! Or is it manifestation?

ESTABLISH YOUR GOAL • Move Toward the Moment

While your new goal and the changes that go with it are bound to require your conscious effort to begin with, it is to be hoped that after a while it becomes effortless, a natural part of your life. As a part of this natural flow, be prepared to move on from using active creative imagery techniques into the quieter stillness of meditation.

Be prepared for new qualities in your imagery and meditation.

As time goes on, your practice of imagery will develop and your quality of meditation will improve. You may discover that this leads to feeling more in tune with your life and the world around you. You will move steadily into a better experience of current time. You may well find there is then less need to practice imagery and that the process of goal setting and achievement begins to flow naturally, easily and powerfully with your passage through life.

A FINAL STORY, AND A GIFT

A high-powered corporate accountant involved in management takeovers and restructuring, Robert admitted to being a tough number cruncher. He hardly knew his children, fought regularly with his wife and, despite material success, was deeply unhappy. His cancer diagnosis was devastating. He had the sense of impending doom and feared the happiness he hoped he would always get to later in life was going to elude him. He rapidly plunged into the depths of despair and strong suicidal thoughts filled his mind.

Amidst this depression Robert came to our groups and realized there was hope. He leaped at the possibilities and with his usual flair, vigor and commitment proceeded to turn his life around. He changed his attitude, he changed his lifestyle, and he changed his job. His health changed and he became another person to experience a medically unexplained and quite remarkable recovery.

Many years later, Robert thanks the cancer for what it has done for him. Like so many others, he says it was as if before his diagnosis he was living his life on automatic. He was putting up with so many compromises in his life and hoping that some time off in the future he might find happiness and might have time to be happy. The cancer changed all that. With the diagnosis, his future became uncertain.

Realizing he may not have long to live, Robert felt he had to address what was happening now. The old compromises became unacceptable; he realized the value of relationships. He set about healing the relationship with his wife and began getting to know his children better. He sought work where he could live his real ethics and sense of values. So much changed for the better as a result of the cancer, that Robert thanks it for helping him to reassess his priorities and values and for putting them in order.

It is an unhappy observation that for many of us it takes a major trauma before we deeply question our habits and our beliefs. So often it seems we take life for granted, put up with the compromises and hope to find happiness later. Perhaps this is one of the great gifts on offer from the many people I have worked with who have been diagnosed with cancer. Why wait? Why put it off? Life is so precious. And so uncertain. Why not take time now to reconsider what you really value and what your true priorities are?

There is a wonderful exercise (below) that is a real gift, as it provides the mechanism for working with these ideas.

The beauty of this exercise, which has been popularized more recently as "the bucket list," is that it can provide clarity and direction for everyone. For those who are well, it can provide the benefit of a life-threatening illness, without having to get sick!

The "What If?" Exercise

Give yourself time and space and sit down with pen and paper. Fantasize. Imagine that for the next three months, everything in your life will stay the same. You will have all the same possibilities, all the same limitations. At the end of this time, your life (your life alone) will end. There is no bargaining, no extensions. This is a fantasy exercise and the first question is:

If you had three months to live, what would be the ten most important things that you would do?

Take time to contemplate this question. Then write your answers down. Review them, perhaps you can rank them in order of priority.

The second part to the exercise is to consider how much of your time currently is being given to these priorities? If you are like many people, you may well find that the top priorities are getting very little time. Commonly, they are being put off. So, the second question is:

"What would it take to fulfill the priorities you have set?"

Contemplate that question.

CHAPTER 9

Mind Training 3

The Mind-Body Connection: Using the Power of the Mind for Healing

SANDY WAS IN HER LATE THIRTIES AND HAD TWO YOUNG CHILDREN AND A husband who was very successful in business. Her diagnosis of breast cancer devastated the family, particularly as the cancer had already spread into her bones. After breast surgery, her ovaries were removed in the hope this might slow down the progress of the disease.

When Sandy came to our cancer support group many years ago, she changed her diet, learned to meditate and began to use imagery. Sandy had difficulty seeing pictures to use in imagery. She was one of those people who found "visualization" difficult. However, with a little experimentation and discussion, we soon found Sandy was strongly kinesthetic—she *felt* her images. She also had a strong Christian faith. So Sandy imagined the presence of God in the sky above her. She then prayed in a way that led to her feeling connected to her God. Then, immersed in this feeling, she felt a stream of healing energy flowing down through her head and into her body.

Sandy had seen her bone scan. She had two secondary cancers in her bones—one located in the left hip, the other in one of her ribs. When she saw the scan, her attention had focused on the lesion in her hip; she had not really taken in the one in her ribs.

About eight weeks after diagnosis, Sandy and her family were required to make a major move to follow her husband's work. Sandy was keen to find out how her cancer was progressing, as this information may have affected their choices. Her doctors felt at best her condition may be the same, they strongly implied it was likely to be worse. They were quite unprepared for what they found! The lesion in the ribs had remained unchanged—no worse, no better. Yet the lesion in the hip was not only better, the cancer was gone and the bone had regenerated completely. It was fully healed!

Sandy was delighted to share her good news with the group. But then came her realization that she had formed a clear mental picture of the hip lesion, based upon what she had seen of her scan. With the imagery, she was able to feel this flow of energy, coming from its divine source, and as it came into her body, she felt a flow of warmth come with it. She said that for her, she knew the healing was flowing whenever she felt the warmth. Sandy realized, however, that while she had done this clearly and powerfully for the hip, she had neglected the ribs almost completely.

Obviously, the next step was for Sandy to direct the healing energy to her ribs. She went home to put this into practice but rang me a few days later very concerned. In attempting to focus on her rib, she found strong feelings rising up that in doing this she was neglecting the hip and that the cancer would recur.

Reflecting on this for a moment, I asked Sandy how big her God was. She said her God was infinite. So I asked her to consider that she was drawing healing energy from this infinite source and then feeling there was not enough to go around! She laughed at the limitation she was imposing, and recognized the logical flaw in her feeling of inadequacy. Interestingly enough, however, it still took her about two weeks of practice before she felt fully comfortable with the notion of healing the second lesion while she adequately covered the rest of her body.

Given what was essentially good news, with one lesion completely healed, Sandy and her family decided to go ahead with their move. This involved the usual pressures of packing and unpacking, major change, readjustment, saying good-bye to friends, renewing old relationships and making new beginnings. Shortly afterward and, conscious of the potential effects of stress, Sandy had more tests to reassess her situation. No change—the hip all clear, the ribs still affected. Three months later, a well-settled Sandy had her next tests. All clear—healed hip, healed ribs—a remarkable recovery.

Sandy's story is a dramatic example of many cases where the use of specific forms of imagery brought specific results. Coincidence? Well, maybe, but there does seem to be a lot more to it.

Sarah had a similar background and problem to Sandy—except that Sarah had eleven bony secondaries that were diagnosed three years after her treatment for primary breast cancer. Sarah had seen her bone scans, fixed that image in her mind, was very visual in her imagery and imagined each lesion healing. She received excellent support from her family and her local doctor who was actively involved with mind-body techniques and integrative medicine. Three months later, all the cancer was gone—except for one lesion in her hip. Sarah and her GP were puzzled by this until they checked with the original scan. Sarah had missed seeing that particular lesion in her hip! She had retained a clear picture of all the other spots but had missed this one. Sarah adjusted her imagery. Three months later, at her next scan, the hip was clear too.

Steven's diagnosis of lung cancer led to major chest surgery with removal of the lower section of one lung in an unsuccessful attempt to rid him of the cancer. At the point where the windpipe (bronchus) was severed to remove the lung, staples were used to seal it shut. Not long after the surgery, these staples popped open creating a bronchopleural fistula—a large cavity filled with air in the chest. A CAT scan demonstrated that a large triangular area was affected.

Steven sought several opinions, hoping the lung might heal itself or that further surgery would fix it. His doctors were convinced the breakdown had resulted from the activity of cancer that had been left after the surgery. They told Steven that the area remaining was like a buttery mass in his chest, that it could not heal itself and further surgery was dangerous and unwarranted. They offered to wait and see, and that if it did unexpectedly improve, then perhaps they could staple it again later. Steven pressed the doctors, asking if they were sure it could not heal on its own. "Absolutely. There is no way!" they stated emphatically.

Now Steven had some previous experience of meditation with Dr. Ainslie Meares. This had helped him through a period of stress some twenty years earlier. Although he had let the practice slip, there was an experience, a foundation to build upon—and a sense of the possible. After coming to our residential program, Steven returned to intensive meditation and also began a new practice—imagery. Every day, he began his meditation sessions with ten to fifteen minutes of imagery. As a bonus, Steven found that the imagery flowed easily and naturally into the stillness of meditation. The imagery enhanced his meditation.

For his imagery, Steven brought the CAT scan to mind. In a very visual way, he saw the lesion fairly literally. Then on a microscopic level, Steven imagined filling in the hole, using symbolic bricks of a wobbly, rectangular shape that for him represented new lung cells. In his mind he envisaged these bricks slowly building up, one on top of the other, re-forming healthy lung tissue and closing the gap. Three months later, a rather incredulous doctor showed Steven a healthy CAT scan, with the report that the bronchopleural fistula has spontaneously healed! Spontaneously! Steven is in no doubt that the meditation and the specific imagery work was what did it.

So how can we explain these cases, these anecdotes? Are they just coincidences? Is it just mind over matter—or is there more to it? I believe that there is a simple theoretical basis behind these remarkable true stories. While it will be wonderful when these observations and hypotheses are followed up by serious research, this theory is based upon good science and when converted into practice through the use of imagery there is the potential to help many people overcome a wide range of illnesses.

THE RATIONALE OF HEALING IMAGERY

To put healing imagery in its full context, we need to go back to basics. The body has an extraordinary ability to heal itself. It is exquisitely well designed to cope with both trauma and disease. The body's basic urge is to maintain itself in the dynamic state of balance we call health.

To understand this a little more we need to appreciate how these healing mechanisms are controlled. In the late sixties and seventies, when I went through my veterinary training, not much was known about all this. We did know, for example, that the immune system played a major role in the body's defenses. As well as the immunity made active by our white blood cells, we knew there was cellular immunity too—that the cells of the body themselves had some capacity to resist infection and even cancer.

However, these healing mechanisms were thought to operate largely independently, and in a way that was removed from any central nervous system or mind control.

Current knowledge has come a long way! It is now well-known that the brain regulates healing in two major ways—the first by the wide variety of chemicals it produces, the other via direct nerve pathways.

What we now know is that different states of mind, different feelings and different emotions produce different and quite specific chemicals in the brain. These chemicals—called neurotransmitters, neuropeptides or, more simply, messenger molecules—are then released into the bloodstream. Traveling in the blood they then flow to cells of the immune system. There they attach onto specific receptor sites on the outer membranes of those cells. By doing so, they then trigger changes within the cells that dramatically affect their function.

This, then, is another key point. It is not only a matter of how many immune cells you have, it is a matter of how actively and effectively these cells are functioning. For a long time it has been known that white blood cells are the front line for the immune system. Also, for a long time it has been known that having too many of these cells is a problem, just as it is to have too few. More recent research, however, has revealed you could have the right number, but they could still range in function from inactive and so ineffective to highly active and highly effective. Clearly an active, vibrant immune system made up of the appropriate number of cells is a strong pre-requisite for both good health and active healing.

One of the key principles in mind-body medicine is that what we commonly characterize as negative thoughts readily depress immune function, while so-called positive thoughts enhance it. What this means is that if you are depressed, suffer unresolved grief or bottle up your emotions, you are highly likely to release specific chemicals from your brain that will directly suppress immune function.

Happily, on the other hand, when you are inspired, feel a surge of hope or love, or when you have a good laugh, other different but similarly specific messenger molecules are released from the brain, travel via the bloodstream, attach to immune cells, and activate them markedly.

Furthermore, quite remarkably, it is now known that cells of the immune system, the white blood cells, produce their own messenger molecules that they too release into the bloodstream. These molecules return to the brain, giving feedback and completing the loop of communication between the mind and the healing functions of the body. This is another key principle that helps us to understand how mind-body medicine works.

THE HEALING CENTER IN THE BRAIN

What all these recent discoveries point to is that there is a healing center in the brain that has a great capacity to control and regulate healing throughout the body.

This notion of a healing center is very similar to the fact we have a running center in the brain. By this I mean when you decide to go for a run, the idea starts as a conscious thought in your mind. However, when it comes to the actual process of the running, that is a very complex process. Fortunately, when you go for a run you do not need to consciously think how to move this leg and that, how to combine the movement of your legs in rhythm with your arms, and how to regulate your heart rate and your breathing. That complexity is controlled by the automatic part of the brain.

The process of going for a run begins with the conscious thought "I will go for a run." Then that conscious thought goes down into the unconscious, automatic part of the brain where "the running center" picks up the message, recognizes it, and says, "Sure, I know how to do that. How fast do you want to go?" Again, using conscious intention, we may give the message to speed up or slow down, while the actual process of running remains under automatic direction.

Now, everyone it seems has needed to go to the trouble of learning how to connect the conscious desire to run, with the automatic center that actually does it for us. I love watching young children learning to walk and run. You see them struggle up onto their feet, usually hanging on to a chair or table leg. And you see the thought form: "I'm going to walk across the room." And off they go, full of hope, full of expectations. A few tottery steps and crash! Down they go. Now I have yet to see a toddler just lie there, give up, and say, "Well, I guess I am going to be one of those kids who never learns to walk!" No, it seems so natural. They get up, try again, and again, and finally master it.

So it seems most of us have taken the time to learn how to connect the conscious mind with the brain's running center. What I suggest is that the same potential is there to control the healing center. It is just that most of us have not yet learned how to consciously connect with it.

What we need, then, is a reliable mechanism that will connect the conscious intention "I want to heal" with that automatic, unconscious part of the brain that regulates healing. We need a link between the conscious mind and the unconscious. Sound familiar?! Obviously, what provides such a link is the creative use of imagery.

In healing, as elsewhere, imagery provides a link between the conscious intention and the automatic function.

We can use imagery as a vehicle to carry a specific message concerning a need to heal in a specific way from the conscious mind, through the healing center and on directly to the body's wonderful array of healing mechanisms.

IMAGERY OR MEDITATION?

Before we move into the techniques that make all this possible, here is another important reminder of the value of meditation and balance. Do remember that in the simple silence of mindfulness-based stillness meditation (MBSM) we return to a profound sense of balance and in that state, healing is free to flow naturally.

So the question often arises when it comes to healing, is meditation enough or should I do imagery only? Or a bit of both?

I encourage everyone who is engaged actively in healing to practice simple, stillness meditation. It provides that deep sense of balance, a stable foundation from which to work and within which to heal.

About three-quarters of the people affected by cancer that I help take up the practice of imagery. What I have found through this experience is that imagery is particularly helpful for people when recently diagnosed, particularly if they have their own fears and anxieties for the future, or have been given bad news poorly and had their hope taken away. Also, imagery is usually easy for people who have active minds. As an added bonus, it combines particularly well with any form of treatment, providing a direct means to support that treatment with the active and creative power of the mind. Imagery is a reliable, intelligent way to harness the potential that the placebo response establishes.

The principles to have strongly in mind with the use of healing imagery are that as for other imagery exercises, the images need to be accurate, complete and feel good to use. This latter point is of particular importance. Often when you begin imagery you know it could be better, you have the sense that as a beginner you are learning, but it feels good. You feel confident with where you are with it, against the background of knowing with time and more practice the actual technique will improve. This sense of feeling content and basically confident with your imagery is a vital ingredient in its successful application.

WHAT TYPE OF IMAGERY TO USE FOR HEALING

Remember, too, that when it comes to technique, we can use three types of imagery—literal, symbolic or abstract. Obviously, as has been explained earlier, healing is an area where the actual physical reality is that it involves a complex interaction of many processes that really are far better suited to being regulated by the automatic, unconscious healing center of the brain rather than by direct conscious act of will. So literal images have very limited use, although, as the examples we have already used demonstrate, semiliteral images (such as CAT scans, X-rays, photographs of immune cells, etc.) can provide a useful starting point for healing imagery.

The fact is that while healing imagery is a technique that has helped many and offers great promise, it needs to be well thought through and thoroughly planned. Let us move on then to consider how we can put all this into practice.

First, here is a summary of the necessary steps for the use of symbolic imagery.

HOW TO USE SYMBOLIC IMAGERY FOR HEALING • The Principles

Step 1. Develop symbolic images that represent:
  (a) the illness
  (b) any treatment
  (c) the immune system and other aspects of the body's healing mechanisms
Step 2. Combine these images into a sequence of action in a way that removes the image of the illness and replaces it with a symbol of fully restored health.
Step 3. Check that these symbols are accurate and complete and that you can feel good using them.
Step 4. Support your practice with meditation, other imagery exercises where necessary, and the general principles of positive thinking.
Step 5. Assess your progress, and modify or adapt your imagery as required. You may well find that over the longer term the urge to practice imagery declines and you feel more fully satisfied with the ongoing practice of meditation.

SYMBOLIC IMAGERY FOR HEALING • The Practice

Step 1. Develop the Images

When using your own symbolic images for healing they need to represent the illness for you in a way that is acceptable intellectually and, even more important, intuitively. Symbolic imagery is very personal, so the best images are the ones that you can identify with directly. The best measure for assessing that you have good, useful images is that they feel good.

There are four main ways to derive images for healing:

BY BEING INSPIRED BY OTHER PEOPLE'S IMAGES

Sometimes as you read of other people's imagery or listen to others discuss it, you are inspired and your own image springs to mind, based upon what you have read or heard. Having said that, in my experience it rarely works if you try to take on someone else's images just because they worked for them.

An excellent example of what we are discussing here involved an elderly lady who came to me having read the Simontons' excellent book *Getting Well Again*[13] (a highly recommended read if you are using healing imagery). Margaret was a small woman. Petite, well dressed, conservative and polite to a fault, she had a warm, gentle and kindly quality that was very endearing. Margaret had taken in the Simontons' recommendation to use aggressive images. She latched onto their suggestion to imagine the cancer as being like lumps of meat in the body and the immune system as being a pack of savage, hungry dogs that were let loose to race around the body and greedily gobble up the meat (alias the cancer). As Margaret described these dogs in detail, I recoiled at the terrifying picture she presented. Asking her what she felt about these dogs, Margaret replied, "Well, actually, they scare me to death!" When I asked her how she felt about being scared to death by an image that represented her own immune system, she realized she needed to change the picture.

Talking on, it became apparent Margaret's passion in life was her garden. So, together we worked out she could imagine her body to be a beautiful garden, the cancer would be a particular form of weed and her immune system was a very wise and diligent old gardener. Margaret's chemotherapy would be a weed killer that had a very selective action. It would kill the weeds (cancer) very effectively, but the rest of the garden (her body) would be unaffected by it. Then the gardener would add compost to the garden, representing the good food that made up Margaret's new diet. With all this, the garden would thrive.

We now had an accurate image Margaret could feel good about and that was consistent with her nature and life. However, to me there was a sense what she was proposing to do may still be incomplete. Being a gardener myself, my experience is that once a new weed comes into the garden, you may well get rid of it, but often it comes back. Questioning Margaret on this, I found her experience matched mine. So to offset the subtle implication in the image, and the real possibility of natural recurrence, we added to the imagery sequence. After spraying the weeds, Margaret's gardener was then sent on regular patrol, to seek out any new signs of weed growth and to eliminate them before they developed into any serious problem. He also was to constantly tend and support the garden, making it healthier and stronger—so healthy that illness had no part in it.

THE USE OF SEMILITERAL IMAGES

All the examples at the start of this chapter featured the use of semiliteral images based upon scans or X-rays. For Sandy, Sarah and Steven, what they had literally seen as a representation of their cancers (the scans and X-rays) formed the starting point for very effective imagery. However, each one of them was encouraged to regard their CAT scan or X-ray as a representation or symbol of their cancer, which of course it really is. Therefore, they were using what we call semiliteral images.

It is hard to predict who will be best suited to which type of imagery, but it is easy to imagine that more literal, left-brained people may be drawn to this type of semiliteral imagery; whereas the more creative types prefer the symbols like the ones Margaret used. While there have been plenty of exceptions to these rules, people with a medical background often find the semiliteral approach appealing and easy to work with.

Tom was a specialist surgeon who had a rather rare and particularly nasty cancer intertwined around his spine. He was well aware of his poor medical prognosis and the fact his treatment was regarded to be purely palliative. However, Tom had a very detailed anatomical knowledge of the area affected by the cancer. He studied his X-rays and scans to form a clear picture of the extent of the cancer and the damage it had done to his spine.

He then formed a very clear picture in his mind of what the area would look like when healed again. Tom proceeded to imagine the cancer shriveling and the healthy tissue regenerating. He had a remarkable response to his "palliative" treatment: the cancer disappeared and normal function of his spine returned. Tom is alive and well many years later.

We have found it often helps people with their imagery and healing when they develop a strong image of what healthy, healed tissue looks like. For example, it may sound a little weird at first, but many people with liver disease have been helped by going to the butcher and actually asking to see a healthy liver. This image can then be held in mind as the end goal.

OUT OF THE STILLNESS OF MEDITATION

Very often once people have learned the background to imagery, it works well to contemplate the principles, reflect on them deeply, and then wait for the images to arise spontaneously. This is a reliable process that has worked for many people.

Henri had prostate cancer with multiple bony secondaries. He found great comfort in using imagery as a lead-in to meditation. He would imagine he was on a large flat rock, beside a river near his childhood home, then relax and let go into the feeling, the ease and the comfort of that place. As he learned about healing imagery and was considering applying it in his own situation, a spontaneous image came to mind.

While he was meditating one day, Henri imagined sitting on his rock as he often did to relax his mind and transition into meditation. However, this time a spontaneous sequence of healing imagery arose in his mind as if he were actually doing it. He felt himself taking one of the affected bones out of his arm and in his mind he had no trouble imagining washing it in the river! Next, he took a large bottlebrush from beside the rock, pushed it up through the marrow of the bone, washed out all the cancer and then rinsed the bone in the river. He saw the cancer as a dark red stain that the river washed away, and he enjoyed seeing the color trailing away downstream. Once the first bone was sparkling white and clear of cancer, he put it back and moved on to take out and clean the next. Henri went on to have a remarkable long-term recovery.

HAVE THE BODY PRODUCE THE IMAGE

Charles was an accountant who had led a highly stressed, if fairly successful, business life. When bowel cancer was diagnosed with inoperable liver secondaries, Charles attended our residential programs more out of desperation than conviction. During meditation sessions, we sometimes apply light touch in the way of Dr. Ainslie Meares. This helps people to relax more directly and often helps focus their attention on particular areas. Sometimes it helps people to form an image of their illness.

Charles had been having little success with his meditation or imagery. His busy mind seemed to be ever active, that is, until he felt the gentle hands on his shoulders while he was meditating. At first he knew they belonged to one of our therapeutic team. He felt deeply reassured by the touch, deeply calmed. His thoughts settled, he could feel his state of mind changing. Then these initial hands felt as if they lifted from him, only to be replaced by two more hands. Two hands that had an even stronger quality. Charles, a long-time agnostic, swears they were the hands of Christ! They filled him with a sense of unconditional love. They brought heat and energy to his liver. He began to sweat, he began to smile. He was deeply moved. He felt that healing had begun.

The feeling of the hands stayed with Charles as part of a powerful image. The whole experience transformed his attitude; he began on a healing path, he began the spiritual journey. Many years later, Charles had survived liver secondaries longer than anyone his experienced specialists knew of.

For others, putting their own attention into the area of their cancer, or touching the area lightly themselves, is effective in drawing forth an image from the cancer itself.

Images derived in this way are invariably very relevant, very powerful and, when used in this way, very effective.

Step 2. Practice the Sequence of Healing

This is where all the principles of imagery come into action. Most people are able to see their imagery sequence as you might watch a DVD or a cartoon sequence. Some talk their way through the healing sequence too, either just describing to themselves what is happening or repeating affirmations as the pictures run. Whenever possible, it is ideal to add a physical sensation to the imagery. For some, this means having a sensation of a flow of energy; for others, feelings of warmth attend the healing.

Ideally, it is best to imagine the healing sequence taking place in the location of the illness itself. This means rather than imagining the healing pictures are running (literally) through your head, or on an imaginary screen in front of you, aim to focus your attention where the lesions are and super-impose the images on that place within the body. Many people find it help-ful to put their hands on or over the affected areas, so the sense of the imagery taking place at that point is strengthened.

To reiterate, the aim of the healing sequence is to start with an image of the illness, for the treatment and immune system to combine to remove the illness, and for the healthy tissue to regenerate. Steven's sequence was an excellent example of an image that powerfully symbolized the healthy tissue regenerating and completing the healing.

Step 3. Check That the Images Are Accurate, Complete and Feel Good

A risk with these practices is that they may be inaccurate or incomplete, reflecting poor technique or deeper issues of doubt or self-sabotage. Very commonly the people I work with find their first attempt at healing imagery produces useful images that remain at the core of their practice. However, it is very common that these initial images have limitations and that they can be improved upon.

One of the best ways to check healing imagery is to draw your imagery sequence. All you need are a few sheets of paper and either colored pencils or crayons. The aim is to draw a series of pictures, like a storyboard or cartoon sequence. These pictures need to start with the symbol of the disease and then demonstrate the way any treatment interacts with that disease, as well as the way your body's defenses and healing capacities are both imagined and inter-act. You then finish with an image that represents you in total good health.

Ideally, you do this drawing exercise with a therapist who is experienced in the field, although a smart friend may well suffice. You explain your intention with the imagery, what the symbols mean and how they interact. Against the need for accuracy and completeness, most outsiders will pick any deficiencies.

Nancy had stomach cancer with liver secondaries. The stomach had been cleared with surgery, but the liver remained a major problem. Nancy asked me to check her imagery, as she was committed to getting well and keen to pursue every possible avenue. She had seen a scan of her liver and had a clear picture of the extent of the three lesions in it. In her imagery, Nancy repre-sented her immune system and other healing qualities with the symbol of Pac-Man. Her Pac-Man characters had two legs and big teeth! She knew she needed the right number of them and for her this meant she needed a team of twelve. With this very personal imagery, Nancy imagined her twelve Pac-Man characters lived behind her liver. Three times a day she did her practice, bringing up the images in her mind and seeing them eat up the three cancer lesions before she put them back to rest behind her liver.

This imagery was accurate enough but clearly incomplete. Nancy was directing her healing to be active three times a day for about five minutes each time—the time she was actually doing the imagery. For the rest of the day, she was instructing her immune system to rest! Clearly, Nancy needed to have her healing operating twenty-four hours a day. This is how it normally operates, anyway. However, faced with this suggestion, Nancy was deeply concerned that her Pac-Man characters, the symbols for her immune system, would become tired and ineffective if they worked all day! After discussing this apparent dilemma, what Nancy decided she could imagine were two more teams of twelve. She set up a rotating roster, with each team working a shift while the other two rested! For Nancy, this satisfactorily represented her immune system working fully and effectively. Nancy lived for many years, longer than her doctors had ever thought possible.

Step 4. Support Your Healing Imagery Practice

Imagery becomes a vehicle for positive expectations. It puts those hopes and beliefs into practice. Therefore your imagery practice will be supported by anything that builds your confidence, develops your belief in the possibility of healing, and anything that generates faith. So far in this book we have discussed many helpful things that have the potential to help in this regard—the benefits of simple meditation and specific positive-thinking exercises with the use of affirmations and other forms of imagery. Do recognize the value of an integrated approach and be reminded of the impact the company you keep can have on your state of mind.

The attitudes, hopes and beliefs of those around you can influence your own situation strongly. We have witnessed this repeatedly with young children battling cancer. Jane had an eighteen-month-old child, Nathan, who was not responding to his cancer treatment. His doctors told Jane and her husband, Roger, that they were sorry, but nothing seemed to be working and they did not expect Nathan to live long. Jane changed Nathan's diet to simple wholesome food, while she and Roger learned to meditate and practice imagery. At least twice a day when Nathan was asleep, one or both of his parents would cradle him in their arms, enter their own state of meditation, and imagine their meditative state was also encompassing Nathan. They imagined him wrapped in a warm blanket of loving, healing light that was all around, and all through him. As his treatment continued, they did specific healing imagery for him, imagining the imagery projected onto his tiny body. Remarkably, his condition began to improve. To his doctor's amazement, Nathan went on to make a full recovery and is now a healthy young adult.

A Caution and Some Advice for Partners and Health Professionals

Partners can share meditation and imagery with the one they love, with the patient. This needs to be done as free of ego as possible—as free of desire and longing as possible. It is a big ask to let go of the selfish motives, and to move into a space of unconditional lovingkindness, but here is an important and necessary caution. If you attempt to do this type of exercise for someone you love or care for, and find you are doing it with a sense of desperation or urgency, you may be better to leave it. You need to have a perspective that understands that in doing this exercise you are not taking on exclusive responsibility for the outcome. In other words, this exercise can help but it is only one factor. Whether your partner gets well or not will depend on many issues. What is being said here is to do your best, but do not set yourself up for mental anguish or guilt. Do the best you can, that is all you can do.

Be aware, too, that the beliefs or images held by other key people around you could also have an effect. Larry Dossey's excellent book *Healing Words*,[14] discusses the power of prayer and the impact of thought on healing. It is quite conceivable that if your doctor has a strong belief as to the outcome of your disease, then those thoughts will have some impact. It is highly recommended for people with cancer who are aiming for recovery to seek out key medical people who can imagine them as long-term survivors. I regularly suggest patients discuss this sensitive issue with their doctors and persist until they find practitioners who can support them in this very important way without compromising their medical integrity.

Step 5. Assess Your Progress, Adapt as Necessary

When you set yourself specific goals, it is important to assess your progress. With healing, assessments can range from easy to difficult, depending on what types of tests may be needed for useful feedback. How often to seek this feedback therefore will depend upon how quickly it seems the condition can change and how invasive any tests may be. I am a strong advocate of backing up your feelings and intuition with a reality check in the physical world. While mind, heart and spirit have a major and profound impact on our lives, it is still a physical body we live in, so I value physical assessments and reassessment.

Quite often imagery does change with time and with healing progress. Tessa had secondary spread of breast cancer in the lymph nodes under her arm. She had a Pac-Man image (no legs, big teeth!) that represented her healing. Three times a day she reinforced the sequence of healing characters by imagining the characters gobbling up her cancer. Then one day, as she prepared to begin the imagery, the characters went on strike! They literally refused to do anything and stayed motionless.

Tessa was deeply concerned, so I recommended she go for a checkup immediately. All her cancer had disappeared. She was in remission and it appeared her Pac-Man characters were not prepared to waste their time! They were quite happy, however, when Tessa responded to our discussion and sent them off on patrol, roaming Tessa's body to target any loose cancer cells and to make sure no relapse could become established.

Another major issue with healing, and the repeated practice of imagery, is the question of whether or not the image needs to change with each session. For example, Judy had breast cancer that had been treated by surgery and radiotherapy. Now she had secondaries in her liver and was using imagery to assist her healing. She had an excellent healing sequence that finished with an image of her liver being clear of cancer, returned to full health. What bothered her deeply was when she went to do her imagery at the next session (she was doing it twice each day), there was the cancer again. Sure, she could imagine getting rid of it, but by going back to the beginning each time she did her imagery practice, was she re-creating it? Should it get smaller each time she imagined it, or should it disappear altogether after just one effective imagery exercise? Judy was confused.

This is a common problem for many people beginning healing imagery. The practical answer is that you are using the imagery to convey the conscious intention "I want to heal" directly to the healing center, that automatic part of the brain that controls the healing process. To achieve this goal, you are rehearsing the complete sequence of healing. What the healing imagery sequence represents therefore is the complete process of healing, from what is known of the disease at the start, to the end point of complete health.

This is similar to the way we rehearse in our mind a physical journey from one place to another. We start at the beginning, imagine all the steps along the way and finish at the destination. In the case of healing, we are using the healing sequence to instruct the automatic healing center in the brain what to do. We want it to take us from disease to health. We entrust the details of how to complete this healing journey to the healing center. What we are aiming to do is to give it a very clear message of what we want—healing—so each time we do rehearse the whole sequence.

As feedback is not as easy to obtain on the healing journey as it is when compared to a literal journey, usually we need to wait for reassessment via medical tests that we only take from time to time. Then, based on this new evidence we may modify or adapt the imagery. Sometimes, as Tessa's story indicates, the images will change spontaneously and predict or point to a change in the physical reality of the illness.

A FINAL NOTE ON SYMBOLIC IMAGERY IN HEALING

Many people have found imagery to be a vital part of their healing journey. It seems fair to me to say that for many people it has played a pivotal role in catalyzing remarkable healing. I have seen it happen often.

I always recommend people who use active imagery in this way, to reinforce it, to balance it with the practice of simple meditation. What I then notice is that very commonly, over time—perhaps six to twelve months—people come to feel they have done enough imagery, that the meditation seems complete in itself and it is the meditation which forms the basis of their ongoing daily practice. Often as time progresses, people find imagery is something they value, enjoy to use, but that they only do it from time to time when the need feels ripe. Often too, the imagery they do persevere with tends to be of the more abstract type. So let us conclude this section by considering abstract imagery.

Abstract Imagery for Healing

With abstract imagery we move from personally significant symbols to more abstract and archetypal symbols. Archetypal images are those that are interpreted with the same meaning by the majority of people. When asked for their major images of healing, nearly all cultures respond with water and light. Therefore, the abstract healing images that are recommended involve the use of water and light. The two techniques I have found to be most effective are the white light healing imagery exercise using the breath, and the white light healing imagery exercise using energy flow. These exercises will be detailed soon.

It needs to be emphasized that these are excellent exercises for people who are healthy, as well as being powerful tools for healing. For well people, becoming familiar with white light healing imagery provides ready access to a major energy boost. When tired, you can do the exercise, draw on an infinite source of energy and rapidly revitalize your system. For example, I have used this technique often on long car trips and find it works very well for me.

For healing, the white light healing imagery exercises are the most common ones people use after coming to our programs. They are simple in their technique, combine the best of imagery principles, are relatively free of complication, work well for many, and always offer the added bonus of the very real prospect of a direct and profound spiritual experience.

When used for healing there are a few details to be aware of. An image for the illness is still required. Using a CAT scan image or X-ray for this often does link naturally with the image of water and/or light. Many people prefer to imagine the body in outline with the illness as a colored lump.

This technique is highly applicable for use with cancer, multiple sclerosis and many other diseases. Once an image is formed for the disease, the light is drawn into the body with the breath, or flows in via the top of the head, and then proceeds to wash away the symbol of the illness.

WHITE LIGHT HEALING IMAGERY USING THE BREATH—THE THEORY

Using the breathing-based technique, you imagine the breath as a white vapor, seeing and feeling it (perhaps with a sensation of warmth or tingling) flowing toward the illness. Usually in this context when you imagine and feel into the illness, the area associated with the illness will feel harder and denser to you than the rest of the body. A common sensation is that it has some pain associated with it. It may also feel warmer than the rest of the body (occasionally some people feel it cooler). Usually the illness will have a color associated with it.

White Light Healing Imagery Using the Breath—The Exercise

Once you are comfortably seated, let your eyes close gently . . . turn your thoughts inward . . . and remember that this is a time for healing . . .

Feel your body relaxing . . . feel the muscles becoming soft and loose . . . feel your weight begin to settle down into your chair, your muscles relaxing . . . feel any tension releasing . . . feel yourself relaxing deeply . . . completely . . . more and more . . . deeper and deeper . . . letting go . . . feel it all through the body . . . feel it deeply . . . feel the letting go . . . completely . . . it is a good feeling . . . a natural feeling . . . feel the letting go . . . letting go . . .

And as you feel yourself relaxing more deeply, imagine as if it is in the sky above you, whatever embodies or symbolizes the highest source of power that you know.

So this may be the image of Christ, or Mother Mary; a particular saint; the Buddha; or a figure from another tradition. Or you may have a more abstract view and imagine a ball of light like the sun which represents an infinite source of energy and healing power, as well as love, compassion, all that is life affirming and that has your own best interests at heart.

Imagine you are in the direct presence of this embodiment of all you value most . . . feel that presence and relax into it . . .

Maybe you choose to say something, like a prayer or a request . . . speaking quietly under your breath as if you are speaking to this presence . . .

Maybe there is a response or something said for you . . . so you can listen for that.

And as you feel yourself connecting more directly with this presence, become aware of your breathing . . . simply giving your breathing your full attention . . . and allowing your breath to take up whatever rhythm feels comfortable for you at the moment . . . the breath moving in and out . . . quite effortlessly . . . effortlessly . . .

And as you continue to hold your attention on your breath, imagine that you are breathing in a pure white vapor that stems from the very heart, or the center of the image in the sky above you . . . so, with each breath in, see this pure white light moving down through your nostrils . . . down into your chest and filling it with a pure white light . . . and as you breathe out, imagine that you are releasing gray light, a gray vapor, that carries with it anything that is old, worn, or unwanted . . . anything you need to be free of . . .

As you breathe in again, imagine that you are breathing in the pure white light . . . bringing with it all that is pure, and fresh and vital . . . breathing out and releasing the old and the worn and anything unwanted in your system . . . breathing it out and releasing it . . . anything at all that you want to be free of . . .

And allow yourself to settle into a rhythm . . . breathing in the pure white light . . . seeing it streaming down into your chest . . . and breathing out all the gray . . . in with the white and pure . . . out with the gray, the old and the worn . . .

And as you continue, feel the white light coming down steadily into your chest, and the strength of the light in your chest growing stronger . . . and brighter . . . and purer . . . displacing any old and worn and gray areas . . . filling your whole chest with a pure white light . . . a symbol of wholeness . . . purity . . . vitality . . . and healing . . . you may be feeling the light as a warmth . . . perhaps it even tingles a little as it flows throughout your body . . .

With each new breath, draw in more white light . . . until your chest feels like it is aglow . . . filled with this pure white light . . . so that it feels like it is radiating pure white light . . . and, as you breathe in again, you feel the white light beginning to flow over . . . traveling down into your tummy . . . as you breathe out now, you can direct the white light, down into your tummy . . . and as you see the white light flowing down, feel it relaxing . . . feel it releasing . . . feel it healing . . . purifying . . . and feel the warm white light traveling down . . . relaxing . . . releasing . . . feel the warmth, the relaxation, the softness . . . releasing any old and worn energy . . . releasing any areas that are uncomfortable, painful . . . feel them being filled with the white light, with its comfort and ease . . . releasing . . . relaxing . . . letting go . . .

(continued)

(continued)

And as you breathe in now, draw in more pure white light from its source . . . see it traveling down into your chest . . . and, as you breathe out, radiate that white light down . . . down through your abdomen . . . down into your pelvis . . . releasing any tension . . . softening . . . bringing warmth . . . and relaxation . . . feeling it deeply . . . completely . . .

And now, breathe in more white light and see it traveling down into your legs . . . down your thighs . . . softening . . . releasing . . . filling with a new strength . . . purity . . . bringing healing . . . and wholeness . . . breathing in more white light . . . seeing it passing down now, into your calves . . . down into your feet . . . releasing any tension . . . releasing any old and worn areas . . . and bringing a new vitality . . . bringing healing . . . strength . . . so that now your legs too are filled with this pure, bright white light . . .

And as you breathe in again, direct the white light now down through your arms and feel the relaxation, the release . . . the softening, as your muscles loosen still more . . . right down . . . feel the light flowing right down into your fingers . . . feel them soft and loose . . . see them filled with the pure white light . . . symbol of purity . . . a feeling of natural vitality . . .

As you breathe in again, draw more of the pure white light from its source . . . see it filling your lungs . . . and now see it traveling up your neck . . . into your head . . . and, as it moves upward, feel the muscles relaxing . . . feel them becoming soft and loose . . . feeling the ease of it all . . . any worn areas . . . letting go . . . any diseased areas being freed, and replaced with a pure white light . . . symbolic of new strength . . . of purity . . . of healing . . . of whole vitality . . .

So, now feel your whole body filled with this pure white light . . . and, with each new breath in, draw more white light from its source . . . and see it filling your whole body with still more white light . . . so that your whole body is glowing intensely with the pure white light . . .

And, as you breathe in more, see the white light expanding out . . . beyond your body . . . to encapsulate you, like an egg . . . like a cocoon of bright, pure, white light . . . filling you with strength and vitality . . . feel it as a whole . . . feel its unity . . . feel yourself to be at one with it . . . allow yourself to merge in the purity of the white light . . . feel its energy moving through you . . . feel yourself to be at one with it . . . feel yourself at peace . . . be still . . . feel it all through . . . deeply . . . completely . . . all through . . . feel yourself at one . . . and be still . . .

As you feel its sense of wholeness through you, you may now like to direct that white light to someone you care for . . . to share that feeling with them . . . and so imagine this person as if they were in front of you . . . and imagine, that as you breathe in . . . the white light passes through you . . . and as you breathe out, it radiates like a searchlight to this person you care for . . . and see it fill them with its whiteness . . . see their body glowing white . . . and see them surrounded in a cocoon of pure white light . . . a symbol of purity . . . of wholeness . . . of healing . . . of renewed vitality . . .

And, as you breathe in . . . draw in more white light and radiate it to this person . . . feel it flowing through you . . . and see them filled with a new wholeness . . . a new sense of balance . . . purpose . . . seeing them whole and healthy . . . pure and vital . . . and share your experience with them . . . feel them filled with this same pure white light . . . and add your blessing . . .

Now bring your attention back to your own body once again . . . Allow yourself to merge again with the feeling of purity and wholeness of the light . . . breathe in . . . breathe in more white light . . . see it streaming down from the embodiment of your own truth . . . pouring into you like a funnel . . . a funnel coming down through your nose and filling your body . . . and this time, imagine that as you breathe out, the light radiates out from your own body . . . spreading out around you . . . and flowing through the place you are in . . . see this white light filling the space around you . . . everyone nearby . . . filling them with purity, wholeness, health and vitality . . . feel your love flowing with it . . . feeling that warm, happy feeling going with it . . .

As you breathe in more, draw in more of this energy . . . as you breathe out, radiate it beyond the space you are in . . . to the people

(continued)

(continued)

around you . . . to the buildings around you . . . feel it moving off, across the country . . . breathing in more white light . . . drawing it down, like a funnel . . . drawing it down from the image above you . . . then through your body, and out across the land . . . spreading out, so that you can imagine the whole country bathed in this pure white light . . .

Breathing in more white light . . . breathing it out, and feeling it traveling right around the globe . . . wrapping the whole planet in a pure white light . . . and now share your feeling of peace and unity with the whole planet . . . radiate that feeling out, and feel it traveling right around, so that the whole planet is held like a ball of pure white light . . .

As you breathe in more, feel that white light streaming down . . . feel yourself again merging with it . . . feel it entering every part of your being . . . feel yourself at one with its purity . . . at one with its peace . . . one with its healing . . . feel yourself at one with its vitality . . . and realize that this white light symbolizes love in action . . . allow yourself to merge into that feeling of love, that pure love, streaming down and filling your whole being . . . feel it all through . . . feel its peace . . . and be still . . . feel yourself merging with the stillness, to allow it to be all through you . . . deeply . . . completely . . . be still . . .

As the white vapor of the breath reaches the illness, most commonly it swirls around the outside of the mass, dissolving it or perhaps causing it to burn or smolder, releasing a gray vapor. This gray vapor, representing the residue of the illness, is then breathed out and released from the body.

White light (vapor) accompanies the in breath, representing healing and all the life-affirming qualities coming in; gray light (vapor) flows with the out breath, representing the disease breaking down and being released, along with anything else, old, worn or unwanted you need to release.

Many people find it helpful to breathe in the white vapor and to direct it into the center of the illness, imagining the illness breaking down from the inside out, rather than from the outside in (as above). As another option, it may help to focus a beam of light almost like a laser, and to imagine this concentrated shaft of light accentuating and accelerating the healing process.

WHITE LIGHT HEALING IMAGERY USING ENERGY FLOW—THE THEORY

Using the energy flow technique for white light healing imagery is similar in some respects to the exercise we have just done that focuses on the breath, except that now the light is imagined to have liquid properties as well. The liquid white light then flows down into the body and filters through it, quite slowly—a bit like water filtering down through dry sand. Again, this warm liquid white light gently but effectively washes away anything old, worn or unwanted! Often the disease can be imagined as a particular color that can be seen to be washed away by the liquid light—a bit like a stain being rinsed from dirty clothes under a water tap. Also, the liquid white light can be directed readily to any areas that may need it more. This technique also can be done in a similar way to a laser, where a beam of liquid white light either washes or burns the disease away from the outside in, or from the inside out.

With these forms of abstract imagery, sometimes the disease, especially when it is cancer, will be seen to clear completely in a particular session. Other times, and for other people, it may seem that only partial progress is made. This can be fine as long as you (yourself) feel confident with the amount of progress in any given session, and you avoid any temptation or tendency to worry. Ideally, to repeat, the aim is to do these exercises with a good feeling and plenty of confidence.

Please be aware that these healing imagery techniques and principles apply well to pain control, which will be discussed in detail in the next chapter.

A Final Note on Abstract or Archetypal Images

If you reflect on this for a moment, probably the most abstract imagery of all would be to use the simple silence of meditation. To accomplish this, you begin by reminding yourself that when you enter the stillness of meditation, your immune system will return to its natural balance and in that state it will be fully activated and empowered to heal you. Then, having affirmed

White Light Healing Imagery
Using Energy Flow—The Practice

Take up your position, relax physically (see the earlier directions when using the breath).

Imagine now, as if it were in the sky above you, the highest source of power that you know. The embodiment of your own truth. It may be an image that symbolizes God, or it may be the figure of Christ, Mother Mary or a particular saint. Or you may prefer a more abstract image such as the sun that could represent the source of universal energy. Whichever of these symbolic images you find most helpful, imagine that as well as a source of energy and healing power, this is a source of love and compassion, of lovingkindness, of a presence that has your own best interest at heart.

As this image forms in your mind, allow yourself to imagine what it would feel like to come into the presence of this infinite source of energy. What would it be like to feel yourself in the presence of God? Or Christ? Or the source of universal energy?

Sometimes as you feel yourself coming closer to that presence, you may wish to say something—a prayer, an explanation, a request . . . sometimes, something may be said to you, or for you . . . so you could listen for that.

Once you feel this presence as if it is in the sky above you . . . imagine that a beam of white light begins to flow from its very center, down toward you . . . an outpouring of energy and loving-kindness . . . if you are focused upon a figure . . . imagine this light flowing from its very heart . . . if you are using the sun, imagine the shaft of light flowing from its very center . . .

Now as this beam of warm, liquid, white light reaches your head . . . it not only flows down around your body . . . but also it flows through your body . . . warm . . . liquid . . . white light . . . slowly flowing down through your body . . . almost like water filtering down through dry sand . . .

Warm, liquid, white light . . . flowing from that infinite source . . . and flowing down through every part of your body . . . like having a wash on the inside . . . it washes away anything old or worn or unwanted . . . it brings with it a new energy . . . a vitality . . . a sense of healing and wholeness . . . you can feel it filling your body and your being . . .

You may see this quite visually or you may have it as a feeling experience . . . like feeling a flow of energy or a sensation of warmth moving down through your body . . .

When the light does flow down to the ends of your arms . . . it will flow out the end of the fingers . . . when it does reach the end of your legs . . . it will flow out through the feet, washing away with it anything old, worn or unwanted . . .

When this light comes to difficult, tense, painful or blocked areas . . . it washes through them . . . clearing them . . . relaxing them . . . letting them go . . . You may see the affected area as having a particular shape . . . maybe a particular color . . . when the light reaches such an area . . . you may see that color being washed away like a stain being washed away from clothes held under running water . . . you may see the area dissolving from the outside in . . . maybe you find it helpful to imagine the light being concentrated almost like a laser . . . this then burns away the affected blockage . . . either from the outside in or the inside out . . .

See and feel this warm liquid light filling every part of your body . . . feel the same all over . . . your body filled with the vigor . . . the vitality . . . the radiance of the warm liquid white light . . .

As this feeling becomes all-encompassing . . . it is as if you merge with it . . . almost as if you dissolve into the light . . . you feel it through your body . . . and your mind . . . it is as if you become at one with it . . . given that it stems from an infinite source, this can feel like merging or reuniting with the infinite . . . go with it . . . feel it all through . . . all through . . .

You conclude by merely resting in the presence of that light and the universal energy it represents and carries.

And when you feel it is time to conclude, move your feet a little, your hands and then, when you are ready, just let your eyes open gently.

this strong intention, once you do enter the deeper stillness of meditation you will be activating subtle but powerful imagery forces. When you do this you will in fact be using the most abstract imagery of all. It is my belief that when the two elements of abstract imagery and the stillness of silent meditation are combined in this way, remarkable and profound healing becomes a strong possibility.

CHAPTER 10

Pain Control

It Is Only Pain!

IMAGINE HAVING MORE CONTROL OVER YOUR OWN EXPERIENCE OF PAIN. What a relief that would be! How empowering. Transforming our experience of pain is another very real possibility that comes with training our minds and it leads to a whole new level of personal freedom and comfort.

We will all have experienced the distressing aspects of significant pain. While many people rely on external help for their pain management, and pain management as a medical specialty has improved dramatically over recent decades, what we are talking of here is our personal management of pain. How we can learn to experience pain in a way that does not even hurt! This radical approach to pain management has transformed the lives of many who have developed it. It has freed them from the fear of pain, from the hurtful experience of pain and it has left them with a life skill that is incredibly satisfying.

The crucial point is that to convert these good ideas around pain management into reality, we need to work at it a little. We need to train ourselves, starting with understanding the theory, and then we need to practice the techniques.

FIRST, THE THEORY

The basic premise centers around the fact that pain has two aspects. Pain involves a physical sensation that is overlaid with a psychological reaction. When we learn how to experience the physical sensation free of the psychological reaction, we take the hurt out of pain. Pure pain, free of any psychological reaction, does not hurt! Interested?

REDUCE THE FEAR, REDUCE THE PAIN

We have talked of fear being a basic hurdle to overcome in the process of getting well again. Cancer is associated with two main fears: the fear that it will cause pain and the fear that it will lead to an untimely death. These fears are the primary reason why society dreads hearing or relating to the word "cancer." In fact, we have created a culture that commonly regards pain and death with undue horror, and commonly treats them as unmanageable, negative events. As a result, they are often approached with a sense of panic as individuals feel powerless to help themselves through situations where either is involved. This often leads people to rely on external aids that often do little for their quality of life.

The influence of fear extends beyond the patients themselves, as often relatives and friends become preoccupied with whether their loved ones are "in pain" or not. This concern is natural and reasonable, but in my experience, is usually accentuated and often clouded by the relatives' own personal fears. This leads to an unnatural preoccupation and is frequently a cause for tension and anxiety that in turn prevents dealing with problems on a more satisfactory level. Pain needs to be managed, but total quality of life remains of paramount importance. There is no answer in being a society of pill-poppers rushing for the analgesics at the slightest twinge.

What is needed is a fresh approach that develops the individual's ability to manage most, if not all, of the pain that may come our way. Of course, we do not need to be a cancer patient to derive benefit from such an approach. I see this as a fundamental prerequisite in self-defense and well-being. When pain can be handled without fear or difficulty, it is a great thing.

There is such a concept. It makes the self-management of pain a very real possibility, but it involves techniques that are totally new to most people. However, first a warning.

PAIN IS A SIGNAL THAT SOMETHING IS WRONG

It is important to know what is behind any pain we experience, to heed any warnings and to take such appropriate action as is necessary. People can learn to be unaffected by pain so that headaches do not bother them, so that back pain does not inconvenience their movement. That is fine if the pain is chronic and the person can be sure that it does not indicate a need for other or more treatment.

Anne had three collapsed vertebrae in her spine. She used the methods we are about to learn to such effect that all the initially excruciating pain was gone and her mobility returned to normal. She then had to be extremely careful not to overdo her exercise, as her back was very unstable. Similarly, it is important to know before you turn a headache off that it is just a simple headache and does not have a more serious cause.

Always investigate and clarify the cause of any pain before setting about its management.

THE MEDICAL MANAGEMENT OF PAIN

It was not so long ago that unmanageable pain was a real concern for people with cancer. There is no doubt that if you do feel pain and it persists, then that pain can easily consume your interest and demand your attention. Everything else rapidly becomes secondary to it. If pain is a reality for you, its treatment requires top priority.

Therefore, it is important to know that these days the medical management of pain is a highly developed area of expertise. Cancer pain can be relieved reliably by external means if you cannot do it yourself. There is no need to feel bad or guilty in seeking such aid. If you are experiencing pain that is above a reasonable threshold for you, it is very appropriate to seek suitable relief. Once the situation is under control, you will be able to redevelop your own resources. It is comforting to know that most large hospitals now boast pain-control clinics where the full range of possibilities are explored. One such large clinic in England reported that in one year they admitted four hundred patients with a specific pain problem; only ten could not be relieved satisfactorily.

The range of medical options used to relieve pain usually begins with analgesic drugs. They certainly have their place, but can have their side effects. Some have the potential to become addictive, while some affect our normal thinking processes and lessen our quality of life. The additional help of counselors, hypnotherapists, acupuncturists and physiotherapists with mechanical aids such as transcutaneous electrical stimulators may well be warranted. Even surgeons can contribute by cutting nerves to problem areas.

Palliative care teams are often experts in pain management and can be called upon for their expertise in this field.

There are less drastic but more experimental methods that have possibilities. Some medical practitioners report consistent pain reduction following large intravenous doses of sodium ascorbate, better known as vitamin C. Iscador, a German mistletoe extract, has been used by injection, again with considerable results. The controversial Laetrile (an extract from apricot kernels) also has been associated with many cases of pain reduction.

At home, I found two great aids, the ever-faithful hot-water bottle applied over the affected area and the generalized effect of coffee enemas. (More will be said of coffee enemas in discussing the dietary principles. See Appendix F for details of their preparation.) Also, many people have found that transferring to a really healthy way of eating significantly decreased their experience of pain. Removing any toxic load in the body leads to further reductions.

PERSONAL PAIN MANAGEMENT USING THE MIND

Before we investigate the radical notion that true pain does not hurt, we need to be aware that there are two main ways in which the mind can change our perception of pain. They are dissociation and a version of mindfulness. We will begin by considering the very real usefulness of dissociation.

DISSOCIATION

Dissociation (dis-association) is where we move our attention away from the pain and onto something more pleasant, more manageable. We may do this in an almost unconscious way by simply becoming distracted, or we may dissociate quite deliberately using a technique based on imagery or hypnosis. Distraction is a reliable way of minimizing, avoiding or even forgetting the pain.

Vera attended a meditation group seeking relief from her painful scoliosis, a chronic recurrent back condition marked by persistent pain. Vera reported how important being busy was to her:

> When I go to work and have to interact with people, it takes my mind off my back. The more involved I am, the quicker the time passes. The busier it is, the better. The worst part of the day is when I go to

bed. I spend ages trying to find a comfortable position. That is when the pain is strongest.

This experience is a common one. Being busy, especially when we are engrossed in the busyness, or being distracted, like when we go to a good film, are both ways of dissociating. What we are giving our attention to comes into the foreground of our mind, and it is as if the pain slips into the background.

It is last thing at night, with all the activities of the day completed and with nothing else for our mind to dwell on, that pain often comes to the fore. There are no more distractions and our mind is free to fantasize. *How long will the pain go on for? Will it be better or worse tomorrow? What if it gets worse?* And so on. With no distractions, no dissociation, the psychological reactions of the mind and emotions are free to run riot. The pain seems more obvious, stronger and more distressing.

Understanding how this works, how the impact of dissociation and distraction affects our perception of pain, gives us more confidence to manage it. Clearly, it can be useful to use dissociation. When we engage in a pleasant and engaging activity we can experience genuine pain relief. Also, we can use the principle of dissociation in some very good mind-body medicine techniques that provide effective pain relief.

It is not the intention of this book to discuss techniques like hypnosis and self-hypnosis. It is enough to acknowledge that these are also useful applications and to say that, commonly, when hypnosis is used for pain, the principle that makes it work is often dissociation. The mind is distracted from the pain. It is paying attention elsewhere.

DISSOCIATION USING IMAGERY FOR PAIN RELIEF

We can apply this same principle of dissociation for ourselves through the use of imagery. One of the most reliable ways we have found to do this is to utilize a technique where we create a mental image of a place where we feel particularly peaceful and comfortable. This place becomes an inner sanctuary, a place to which we can retreat, give all our attention to and rest in the feeling of its space and comfort. In this exercise we move the focus of our attention quite deliberately from the pain to this inner sanctuary.

The whole intention of this exercise is to imagine yourself to be as fully as possible in your inner sanctuary. Aim to use all of your senses—see the place through your own eyes as if you were actually there, hear the sounds, notice whatever there is to smell, and feel the physical sensations. Perhaps there may even be something to taste (for example, when a person imagines themselves to be in the ocean). The intention is to transport yourself from your normal conscious reality to this place of inner peace and comfort.

Here, then, is the exercise (opposite). You might like to read it and learn it well enough so that you can lead yourself through it, or you might find it useful to have someone else read it to you in a slow, steady and relaxed tone of voice. The exercise is recorded on my CD *Effective Pain Management*.

Many people find this exercise gives them a reliable way to dissociate from pain and to find a comfortable inner haven. Children are particularly good at it, and as a technique it is very useful when there is a short-term need for pain relief.

Marty was a nine-year-old boy who needed repeated injections for cancer tests and treatment. The most challenging were lumbar punctures, where Marty would have to lie still while a needle was passed between the bones of his lower spine and into his spinal canal to collect fluid. Just one of these procedures would have been harrowing enough, but as more and more were required he began to react with great distress.

Two techniques transformed Marty's experience. First, Marty was taught how to "go all floppy." This is childspeak for relaxing the body. In a few moments, Marty was taught to make his body all stiff, and then to relax it, to make it go all floppy. Children are terrific at learning the essence of the progressive muscle relaxation exercise in this very quick, simple and effective way.

Second, Marty was taught to go to his own personal inner sanctuary. No real-life place for him, Marty created a Disney-like fantasy castle full of interesting and fun characters and animals. There was plenty to entertain and distract him.

Marty's medical staff cooperated by giving him time to do his preparations before each new procedure was performed. When Marty was advised that the procedure was about to begin, first he made his body go all floppy, then it was as if he left his body there on the table while the procedure was

The Inner Sanctuary

Settle into your posture and take a few moments to relax your body in your own way.

Allow an image to form in your mind of a place where you feel particularly peaceful and comfortable . . . it may be a place you have been to before, or it may be a fantasy place . . . just allow an image to form in your mind in a way that you can explore it in more detail . . .

What can you see in this place? . . . what is close by? . . . what is further off in the distance? . . . what can you see? . . . what shapes? . . . what sizes? . . . what colors? . . . what shades of color? . . . what time of day is it? . . . if you can see the sky, are there clouds, or is it clear? . . . what movement do you notice in this place . . . or is it quite still? . . . what can you see in this place?

Now notice what sounds you can hear in this place . . . are there any sounds coming from nearby? . . . are there any sounds coming from farther away? . . . what sounds can you hear in this place?

Give your attention now to noticing what you may be able to smell in this place . . . what fragrance? . . . what odor? . . . perhaps just the quality of the air itself . . . what can you smell in this place?

What sensations can you feel in this place? . . . you will probably be aware of the temperature . . . is it warm? . . . or cool? . . . or neutral? . . . can you feel a breeze on your skin? . . . or the warmth of the sun on your face? . . . notice too your position and what you are in contact with . . . is it hard or soft? . . . damp or dry? . . . what physical sensations are you aware of in this place?

Is there anything you might like to change to make this place even more peaceful and comfortable? . . . if so, you could do that now . . .

Now dwell on the feelings that come with being in this place . . . allow these feelings to build within you and rest with those feelings . . . just simply letting go . . . relaxing . . . releasing . . . letting go.

carried out. Instead of being present for the harsh realities of what was going on, Marty was happily off in his own magical space. When the procedure was completed, he quite readily and easily took leave of his inner sanctuary and brought his attention more particularly back to his body. These relatively simple steps transformed Marty's experience.

Therese was an older woman who had chronic rheumatic pain that had distressed her and restricted her movement for many years. When Therese attempted to meditate, she found the hurdle of her pain was too much to manage. She simply could not relax or find any peace. Even in the group setting she made little progress. However, with this inner sanctuary imagery exercise, Therese found instant relief. After her first experience of it, she explained:

> It was wonderful. I went to a tropical beach that I visited not long after I was married. We were so happy there. I could feel the warmth and I relaxed on the sand. I just seem to drift off in that place. It is the most relief I can remember experiencing for so long.

What Therese did next was even more useful for her. She was able to remember the feeling of her inner sanctuary and to keep that feeling with her.

While this inner sanctuary exercise can be a great way to dissociate from pain, by its nature it involves dissociating from life itself. To do it, we need to move our attention from our present moment, worldly reality to an inner fantasy, an inner reality. Many people like Marty find this really useful for short-term pain relief. Some, like Therese, use it to work out a method that brings long-term relief. Therese again:

> What I did was to find such comfort in that inner sanctuary, such peace and relief, that it really left its mark. I did not want to forget it. So in some way after I come out of the experience, the feeling stays with me. It is like I remember that feeling and it becomes a new part of what I experience during the day. Perhaps it is the comfort of knowing I can go back to that lovely beach any time I want to. It is like it is always there. And I feel it. I really feel it and it gives me a lot of comfort. My pain is much easier to manage than it used to be.

Dissociation, then, has its place and can be quite useful. But it does involve dis-associating—losing our association with what is actually happening in our current moment experience.

So what of the other possibility? How about, rather than avoiding the pain, we give it our full attention? What happens then?

This brings us back to the proposition of learning how to feel the pain as a purely physical sensation, free of any psychological reaction.

MINDFULNESS-BASED PAIN MANAGEMENT

This is a comprehensive system of pain management that does take a little while to learn, understand and practice. However, the time we spend doing this will be repaid when we have acquired a profoundly effective way of managing both acute and chronic pain. While as the name suggests, this technique does draw on mindfulness, there is more to it. We begin by understanding more about the nature of pain.

THE TWO ASPECTS OF PAIN • The Physical and the Psychological

The more radical premise we will now investigate is that true pain does not hurt! You will come to see that this apparently extravagant claim is true. To begin with, however, it may be well removed from your normal experience of pain. We all know from past experience that when we feel a pain that goes beyond a certain level, it jolly well hurts. Whether the pain is coming from a physical cause, such as a cut finger, or a psychological cause, such as a broken romance, if we feel pain we normally experience it as a hurt.

So, having said that, the normal experience is that pain hurts, and myself having gone through some very tough times with what reputedly is one of the most painful types of cancer, how can I say that true pain does not hurt? *True* pain does not hurt. Not many people have experienced true pain. Once we do understand the nature of pain and its basic components we can come to experience it ourselves and learn that pain does not have to hurt.

ANIMALS PROVIDE A CLUE

I recall a little puppy that came into my veterinary surgery some years ago. It was four months old and owned by a policeman. He rushed into the surgery with it, saying that the puppy had been hit by a car and he thought he ought to shoot it, but first he wondered if we could do anything.

When I first saw the animal, I could not imagine what the problem was because all I could see was a little puppy looking around the surgery with a smile on its face and wagging its tail. It reacted just like any exuberant puppy would, trying to give me a lick and wagging its tail. When I looked at its front legs, however, I found all the skin had been stripped right off them and both wrists were broken. The two open joints were just hanging loose. I am sure that, for a human, the shock alone would have put them in a very precarious position, but here was this puppy looking around the surgery as if nothing had happened.

When I went to examine him, I needed to move his legs. His initial response was to try and pull out of the way. When he could not get away from me he tried to nip me. Not very seriously, but he was definitely trying to tell me that he would rather I did not do what I was trying to do. So, the nurse held his head. Once he would not get out of the way and could not bite us, he immediately accepted his position and allowed us to examine him. His tail stopped wagging and he looked a bit unhappy about it all, but soon we had finished looking at his legs and put them back down on the table. His tail started wagging again and he went back to looking around the room as if nothing had happened.

Later, we gave him an anesthetic to clean him up as best we could and to keep his legs still while the plaster casts we used set hard. About two months later, the casts came off and that puppy was walking around again. Over the next month, all the hair grew back on his legs. He was a normal dog again!

To me, that experience really shows us what is involved with pain and how to deal with it. It was a remarkable demonstration of how pain in its proper context does not hurt. Pain is a stimulus. For the puppy, his pain was a warning signal. It told him that if he moved or was moved, his legs hurt more. He avoided movement. He did all he could to remain still. He made the appropriate response to the stimulus. If he had been in the wild, and could have kept still long enough, his legs may well have healed just as they did in our plaster casts.

The pain was a warning stimulus—not pleasant, presumably, but still for the puppy, only a stimulus. When he was in a position of minimal discomfort, he was quite ready to accept that stimulus and make the most of his situation.

THE PSYCHOLOGICAL COMPONENT OF PAIN AND HUMAN SUFFERING

Contrast the puppy's reaction with what might happen if we were to break a leg. We would have the initial physical pain of the event that caused the break. But in the same instant our mind would start to race. "Hell, I think I have broken my leg! Will I ever walk again? Is my insurance up to date? Who's going to do my work for me? How will I pay the bills while I'm in the hospital?" And on and on it goes. This is the *psychological* aspect of pain— the worry and the anxiety, the mind's response, the fear that goes with the physical reality.

The key principle that has the potential to free us from the distress of pain is that true physical pain does not hurt. It is merely an unpleasant stimulus. Psychological pain can be excruciatingly hurtful. Understanding the difference between the physical and psychological aspects of pain is fundamental to dealing with pain in the most appropriate manner.

Consider a day of 107 degrees Fahrenheit. Hot, uncomfortable—but painful? Very few people would consider it to be so. We know that the pure physical effect of such a temperature is not likely to be harmful and, anyway, it will probably be cooler tomorrow. We tolerate it and go on with our business as best we can.

Yet imagine what would happen if people started dying when the temperature reached 109 degrees. The psychological component of pain would swing into action. Faced with a reason to fear the temperature, people would no doubt become preoccupied with the weather and limit their activities dramatically. I am sure that as a consequence 107 degrees would suddenly become a very painful temperature indeed.

This psychological component of pain is very strong in humans. Surely it accounts for that wonderful phenomenon we discussed earlier, the placebo effect. Many trials have shown the effectiveness of placebos in controlling even the most severe pain just as there is ample scientific evidence of their dramatic benefits for many medical conditions.

We need to appreciate what the placebo is demonstrating. If a sugar pill can relieve pain for us, surely we can learn to do it for ourselves and derive the satisfaction that we otherwise laughingly bestow on the placebo. A placebo is an external agent that we can accept as a treatment for the nonphysical aspect of our condition. We can learn to harness the placebo effect and put it to work for ourselves. We can experience pain in its true, pure, nonhurtful and manageable form.

This to me is a basic technique in self-defense that everyone should know. Through it, we can become free of the fear of pain and improve our level of well-being enormously.

I used to have a very low pain threshold. In my athletic days, when I was fit I could run a reasonable four hundred meters, but my performance was poor at any farther distance. It hurt too much! To run a fast 1,500 meters or mile, or especially something like a marathon, you require a very high pain threshold indeed. I could not handle it. In the past, even just having stitches taken out was for me an acutely painful experience. I also remember that after my leg was amputated, I avoided analgesics wherever possible. I was afraid I might become conditioned to them. The bone cancer I had is normally very painful and, not knowing any better then, I was quite afraid of what the pain might be like if the cancer recurred. What would I do if the analgesics did not work? How could I handle chronic, severe pain?

I learned through experience and by training in pain. Seriously, we train in so many things to increase our ability in that area. In athletics I used to train hard to improve my performance. No one would consider it strange to go through the rigors of what on one level could be fairly described as quite painful training. So why not train ourselves to better our performance in dealing with pain?

By doing so myself, I have freed a whole area of my life. I no longer have fear of pain. Whereas before I used to be scared stiff of visits to the dentist, now I see it as an opportunity to confirm my freedom from the stranglehold that pain held me in. I have been able to suture my own cuts without anesthetic and again marvel at how pain, true pain, really does not hurt.

CHILDREN AND HOW WE LEARN THAT PAIN HURTS!

If a child falls over and cuts himself, comfort and treatment may well be required. However, there is no need to overreact. Children are conditioned by the emotions of those around them so quickly. Just watch the influence of a group of adults reacting to a small child's fall. "Oh, my goodness!" they cry, as the hands fly up in horror. "You poor thing, where does it hurt?"

I have seen society's effects on my own children. The eldest, Rosemary, initially had a remarkable pain tolerance. The normal bumps and scrapes she went through were only an annoyance to her. She was far more interested in getting back to learning, experiencing and doing other things like having fun than to worry about pain. Up she would get and carry on, as I struggled to contain my own anxieties.

Reinforced by her obvious lack of hurt, I was soon able to react in an appropriate way and the everyday minor accidents became nonevents. After turning two, however, it took only a couple of episodes with doting elders gushing over some minor falls for her to begin reacting in the stereotyped way. Soon these same falls became a cause for tears and apparently genuine hurt. Interestingly, however, the worse the accidents, the less the reaction. Now it was as if the minor incidents were an outlet for pent-up emotions. It then took several years for her to relearn how to accept pain and deal with it appropriately.

When she was four, Rosemary had a plantar wart deep in her foot. It was quite irritating for her. Finally, being used to watching me work in the veterinary surgery, she declared she was going to cut it out. Did she think that would hurt? "No, Daddy. I'll just make myself all floppy." Rosemary had learned how to relax herself and she is an expert at it. She made herself go "all floppy"—deeply relaxing herself so her muscles were loose like a rag doll—and then she proceeded to take to the wart with some surgical scissors and excised it completely. The hardest thing was for me to control my own reactions. Surely, it was a reasonable thing for Rosemary to cut out this annoyance and clearly it can be that easy. Perhaps we should not be surprised to see the theory at work!

THE UNDERLYING PSYCHOLOGICAL FACTORS IN OUR PERCEPTION OF PAIN • Transforming Fear and Self-Gain

For most of us, by the time we reach an early age our psychological reactions to pain are deeply ingrained. These psychological reactions commonly are the product of our fears or our attempts at self-gain.

The fears are easier to understand. There can be personal fears such as "Why am I hurting?" "Is it going to get worse?" "Will I recover?" "Am I going to die?" There can be financial fears: "Can I pay my medical bills?" "Will I be able to work again?" "Will I get my job back?" There can be social fears: "Will I be rejected?" "What will my family do?" "What will my friends think?" "Am I to be an outcast?" It does not take long to run up a list of horrors that are all too real in any disease and in cancer especially.

There are many ways available to us to transform fear. These techniques form part of chapters 16 and 17 on emotional health. But for now, perhaps one of the greatest needs in dealing with fears specifically related to pain is to learn how to accept our situation as it is, yet to still be able to act decisively, as and when we need to. This is what mindfulness teaches us: how to avoid worrying about what tomorrow may or may not bring, and how to have the clarity of mind and commitment to do what we need to do now. Also, regular meditation and actually putting the principles of positive thinking into practice consistently leads to a deep level of peace of mind, acceptance and commitment. Many people, therefore, have found that learning to be more mindful, learning to meditate and to be more positive has led to a significant lessening in their pain almost without thinking about the pain itself.

However, another aspect of the psychological reaction to pain is the fact that often we have an ulterior motive in feeling pain. We are getting, or at least trying to get, something through the pain. This idea of pain having secondary gains is often a hard one to look at in our own life. However, it is also most certainly adding some component to any pain we might feel.

Here is one challenging possibility. Many people feel guilty about being sick and so some accept that they "should be suffering." For these people, having cancer and being "in pain" is all part of their expectation and the punishment they accept. Our personal reaction to pain is very much a product of our attitudes, emotional state and level of well-being. There is no need to punish ourselves by accepting pain. Again, use the positive-thinking principles, giving close attention to concentrating on pleasant activities. Laughter beats aspirin any day!

However, secondary gains frequently involve the other people in our life. By being "in pain," relatives and friends rally to us and often fill an emotional need we feel. Again, there is no need to feel guilty about realizing this—unless you are doing it consciously! There has to be a better way. We will discuss how to do this more in the chapters on healthy emotions, when we explore ways to fulfill our needs without the involvement of sickness and pain.

The psychological aspect of pain is therefore rather complex. To deal with it appropriately we need to understand our nature honestly and to look openly at what our goals are in life and how we want to achieve them. Again, this makes cancer an exercise in self-discovery and self-development.

I remember a young man, John, who had a deep fear of the pain of injections. Being on chemotherapy, his fear caused great difficulties. Each time he was to be injected, he would reflexively pull his arm away with a rapid jerk. Often it took many attempts to get the needle into his vein, causing anguish all around. After learning to relax and to cope with pain appropriately, John told me that not only did he stop the jerking, he did not even feel the needle going in. This transformation in his way of experiencing his pain and his treatment gave John a whole new level of confidence in his own abilities. This in turn helped him to transform his disease and his life. How is this possible?

We need to learn how to experience pain in an entirely different way. First we will clarify how it is possible to experience pain free of hurt, then we will examine the amazing possibilities when we learn more specific techniques using imagery, mindfulness and awareness.

TRAINING TO EXPERIENCE PAIN FREE OF HURT

Step 1. Separate the Psychological Reaction from the Physical Sensation

We begin by accepting that physical pain is real, but that it is just a sensation. While the intensity of that sensation can vary, we know that of itself, it is still just a sensation. What we also know is that the psychological reaction to pain can be deeply distressing. Recognizing this, we aim to drop the reaction and to experience the pain in its pure form—free of hurt. To be able to do this we need to learn the theory and then we need to practice the techniques. What we are aiming for is to experience the reality of hurt-free pain.

We can do this in a set exercise by detaching ourselves from the psychological aspect of pain and then applying a controlled painful stimulus. To avoid any psychological loadings we need to feel secure, to be in control of the situation and divorced from the influence of our mind and emotions. We meet all these criteria admirably by doing the initial exercises while meditating. Here is how.

THE BULLDOG PAPER CLIP EXERCISE

Preparation

We begin by choosing a suitable stimulus. We do not want to cause ourselves any bodily injury and so a paper clip of the "bulldog" type works well as these can be purchased from any office-supply shop. They come in different sizes, so when selecting one, you may like to try them out. Actually, while the big ones look most impressive, the small ones tend to create a sharper sensation. Some would say they hurt more! Select the size you feel you can work with.

Remembering that everyone has a different pain threshold to begin with, find a convenient place on your arm or hand where the clip can be put to produce a tolerable stimulus. The upper part of the forearm has quite thick skin and is fairly tough. If the clip does not cause much reaction there, try the inner, softer part of the arm. If need be, try the webbing between the fingers, or use just one corner of the clip. The aim is to produce a strong but acceptable stimulus. Putting it on ourselves leaves us in control. We know that we can stop the stimulus whenever we want to.

Relax, Apply the Stimulus and Observe

Now we take up our normal position for meditation and proceed to relax our body thoroughly. We let the mind come to rest also. Once settled, we open our eyes a little if necessary, and apply the clip. What reaction does it produce?

If you feel any hurt you will probably notice an automatic reflex. Your muscles will tense up. Probably those in the hand and arm will contract first. If you react a lot, the whole body may stiffen. Now, if you can impose relaxation on the body again, a strange thing happens. The hurt gradually diminishes, leaving a pure stimulus. In the calm, you can experience true pain. The more you try this experiment and become confident with it, the easier it is to experience true, non-hurtful pain.

The significance of this reflex is so important to us, we must appreciate it fully. Not only do anxiety and stress lead to tension, but by doing so, they also lead to hurtful pain. Similarly, relaxation relieves tension, defuses anxiety and stress, and takes the hurt out of pain. Relaxation is again the key. When we learn how to keep our body relaxed, free of tension, we will find pain is well on the way to being controlled. This is why these exercises are easier and most effective if they are done while we are practicing meditation each day in the standard simple way.

Experiment in More Challenging Situations

Following these early, easy experiments, we need then to go on to bigger and better things. Increase the level of stimulus first by using more powerful clips. Alternatively, lie on your back with a rock under your shoulders or look for other ways of experimenting with pain.

Next, and importantly, advance to more real-life situations by relinquishing control of the exercises. Have someone else apply the clips when you are meditating and so add the element of the unknown. This will teach you more control over the psychological aspect. Similarly, going outside and sitting near a rotating water sprinkler provides another type of unforeseeable stimulus. Perhaps the ultimate test is meditating where flies or mosquitoes are active! Create the opportunities to experience the reality of true pain.

Step 2. Experiment in Real Life

Having gained confidence through the formal exercises, now it is time to experiment with the use of our new skills in real life.

For example, if you have injections, relax yourself during the procedure and enjoy not having them as hurtful experiences. Consider having dental work done without anesthetic!

I remember well my first trip to the dentist after having resolved to not have an anesthetic. I felt the techniques should work, but I had yet to test them—to know for sure. Needing a sore tooth attended to, I organized a light workload for the morning of the big day. I made sure that I practiced my meditation more than usual for days beforehand and practiced several times before setting off. Arriving unusually early at the dentist's office, I sat and meditated some more in his waiting room. My name called, I scampered into the chair to relax myself and get into meditation as quickly as possible. Mumbling that I wanted no anesthetic, the dentist did little to reassure me by replying in a startled voice, "Are you sure?" Unwaveringly, I said I was sure, and the drilling began.

The result amazed me. Not only did I feel no pain, I virtually felt nothing at all. In response to my questions, the dentist said that yes, it should have been a painful procedure. The decay was near the tooth's nerve. Definitely I should have felt it. I was elated. For the first time, a trip to the dentist had been a positive experience for me. I walked out without half my mouth feeling numb and lopsided. I had no pain or discomfort whatsoever and the tooth was repaired.

I then had a great deal of restorative dental work done, including the fitting of crowns. As I gained confidence, I found the "great meditation buildup" was no longer necessary. One morning I managed to cut one of my fingers with an electrical saw. I was lucky I did not cut it off! I sewed up the gaping wound myself without an anesthetic. And that same afternoon, I had six fillings replaced in an hour-and-a-half session at the dentist's office, again without anesthetics or any particular preparation. I could feel it all, but there was no pain in it, just a stimulus that for preference I would still rather not have had. And remember, it was not long before this that I was known as having a poor tolerance of pain.

Step 3. Take the Benefits into Meditation

Another happy side effect of these exercises with pain is that they deepen our meditation. Using pain in this way focuses our attention very well and makes sure we are attending to our stated aim. If we do happen to let our mind run free, the pain soon asserts itself and reminds us to get it right. This is a bonus from the exercises that makes them doubly worth practicing.

These pain management exercises are ideally done when we feel well. Then we can take our time and there is no urgency to succeed straightaway. Over time, we will learn to perceive pain differently and we will experience a whole new way of living and being.

Be reminded that if pain is distressing in current time, it makes sense to gain relief where best we can. There is a great deal that can be done through the medical system, and through our own efforts. Many people do learn how to train in pain management in the way we have just explored, but there is another equally amazing possibility that is highly recommended when pain is strong and present.

DISSOLVING PAIN WITH IMAGERY AND AWARENESS

Warwick was a commercial fisherman. Used to hardship and having a fairly stoic nature, he was embarrassed to be crying in pain. Warwick was attending a residential program and I found him between sessions distraught due to the relentless pain created by a cancerous lymph node in his groin that was causing his right leg to swell. Warwick also suffered from chronic back pain, a legacy of his life at sea.

The exercise we are about to share often continues to amaze me, despite years of witnessing its transformative effect. I have to admit that when I saw Warwick in such distress, at first I was a little tentative, but I suggested we do an imagery exercise together. He was ready to try anything but I know he had no idea that within five minutes all—yes, all—his pain would be gone, and several months later he told me that while it sometimes recurred, it was minor and manageable. His back pain had been present for around fifteen years and resisted all previous attempts to manage it—now it too was insignificant.

What did we do that produced such remarkable results?

If you are experiencing significant pain, the following exercise can be remarkably transformative.

Option 1. The Exercise for Dissolving Pain

Many people have found the exercise opposite to be truly remarkable, leading to rapid and profound pain relief.

There are several additional techniques that build upon this exercise and are worth mentioning, as some people find they bring additional benefits.

Option 2. Repeated Scanning

It may be necessary or useful to repeat the exercise above and to continue to scan the body, locating and examining the pain using the guidelines as given.

To aid this process, and particularly for someone in distress, you could

The Exercise for Dissolving Pain

1. Sit or lie in a symmetrical position and close your eyes.
2. Relax as completely as you can without giving this step too much attention. Do not try to force yourself to relax; do it as easily and as deeply as you can. If you have already established a practice of meditation, aim to recall the feeling of deep relaxation.
3. Move your attention through the body, seeking out an area that feels different—an area that is painful, tight, under pressure, etc.
4. Be aware of where the sensation is in your body, for example the tummy. Be as specific as possible (e.g., close to the skin, deep in the abdomen). In the upper or lower region, etc. Where is it?
5. Be aware of its shape. Is it shaped like a ball, a sphere, a rod? What is its shape?
6. Be aware if its size. How long is it? Is it three-quarters of an inch or 1½ inches, and how wide is it? Is it three-quarters of an inch wide? One? And how deep is it? What is its size?
7. Be aware of its density . . . is it hard like a rock? . . . or soft like a sponge? . . . and is it harder on the outside, harder on the inside or the same all the way through? . . . What density does it have?
8. What is its surface texture? Is it soft and fuzzy or hard and smooth? What does it feel like?
9. What temperature is it? Is it warm? Or cool? Or neutral?
10. What color is it? If it did have a color, what might that color be?
11. Now hold this area in your attention . . . and as you breathe in next time, imagine you are traveling with the breath . . . right to that area you are focusing your attention on . . . and then imagine the breath gently washes around the outside of it . . . and as you breathe out, the breath just gently ebbs away again . . . a bit like an ocean wave coming into the shore, washing around something in the sand and then just going out to sea again with the out breath.
12. And do that for three more breaths . . . so each time you breathe in, the breath comes in and washes around the outside of the

area . . . with the out breath, the breath just gently ebbs away again.

13. Now the next time you breathe in, imagine that your breath flows right into the very center of this area . . . and as you breathe out, the breath just gently ebbs away again. Do that for three more breaths . . . so breathe in and the breath goes right into the center of this area . . . and then, with the out breath, it just gently ebbs away again.

14. Good . . . Now as you breathe in again, imagine flowing with the breath as it goes to this area once again and washes around the outside of it . . . and then, as you breathe out, the breath gently ebbs away . . . Do this again for three more breaths, breathing in and the breath goes around the outside of the area . . . breathing out and it just gently ebbs away.

15. Good. And now just gently scan your attention through the body again. Notice if there is a particular sensation that your mind is drawn to. If there is, you can repeat the whole process again like this:

16. Notice where that sensation is localized . . . Which part of the body? . . . Is it close to the surface or deeper into the tissue?

    And then be aware of what shape it has . . . round like a ball, or oval like an egg? . . . a rod? . . . What particular shape does it have?

    And then notice more particularly what size it is . . . How long is it? . . . How wide? . . . How deep? . . . How many centimeters or inches? . . . What size is it?

    And then be aware of its density . . . is it hard like a rock? . . . or soft like a sponge? . . . and is it harder on the outside, harder on the inside or the same all the way through? . . . What density does it have?

    And then the surface . . . Notice whether the surface is rough or smooth . . . What is its surface like?

    And what temperature is it? . . . Is it warm? . . . or cool? . . . or neutral? . . . What temperature is it?

    And color . . . If it had a color, what color would it be?

    And now, as you hold your attention on this area, the next time you breathe in, follow the breath in and around the area . . .

(continued)

(continued)

the breath washing around the outside . . . and then with the out breath, gently ebbing away . . . and do that for three more breaths.

Good . . . Next time you breathe in, follow the breath right into the very center of the area . . . then breathe out, the breath just gently ebbing away once again . . . and do that for three more breaths.

17. Good . . . and now you can simply rest with the feeling you have right now . . . or you can continue with this exercise and repeat step 16 once again . . . but you might like to just let go of the exercise and simply rest with the feeling . . . just simply letting go . . . going with it . . . just simply letting go . . . quite effortlessly . . . effortlessly . . . more and more . . . deeper and deeper . . . just simply letting go . . . letting go . . . letting go . . .

---

ask a relative or friend to read you the exercise. They would need to read slowly in an even tone, and you would be wise to reply out loud to the questions as they are read to you: Where is the pain located? Specifically? What size is it? And so on. This process is further enhanced if the support person breathes in time with the person in pain and talks in a quiet, slow and confident manner. They may need to relax themselves first and establish their own inner calm before beginning.

Another very helpful option is to be led by my voice on the CD I have recorded of this exercise (see the details at the back of the book). When using the CD, you could answer the questions quietly to yourself, or even better, get over any awkwardness you might feel and reply out loud.

Once pain is fully experienced in this manner, it will often simply fade away.

Option 3. Imagery Along with Internal Relaxation

Another option, a different way of releasing pain, is that once you have developed your own image for the pain as described above, put your center of attention inside that image and consciously relax it. Doing this may cause an initial increase in discomfort as you concentrate fully on the pain. There is no avoidance here. This is a process that will enable you to pass through the pain and become free of it.

Having already established a practice of meditation, a familiarity with consciously relaxing your body will make this technique easier; however, it can work very well for beginners. Usually, as you relax the pain from the inside, it feels like a bubble bursting in slow motion as the outer shell of the pain breaks down and a wave of warmth and relaxation spreads from the inside out. This wave usually feels as though it extends out into the rest of the body and feels very pleasant.

Option 4. Triggering Endorphins

Sometimes while this process of concentrating upon a pain and releasing it is being practiced there can be a natural release of endorphins, the brain's opiate-like pain relievers.

This is the same effect experienced by many long-distance runners. Commonly, after eight or nine miles, runners experience their "second wind" or "break the pain barrier," a stage that involves the body releasing its own pain-relieving chemicals which produce a powerful sense of euphoria. This is one of the body's natural mechanisms for dealing with protracted pain and it can bring profound relief. In fact, it often produces a deep sense of well-being.

Some people have learned how to trigger this response consciously and so top up their pain management.

Option 5. Talking to the Pain

Some people find that they can talk to their pain. This may sound unusual at first, but sometimes an image of the pain arises spontaneously during meditation or the imagery exercise above and communication can be established with the person, animal or object that appears.

What is happening here is that the creative unconscious is using an image to enable us to talk to our own inner wisdom. This often leads to an insight into the nature of the pain and to its resolution.

So you could ask:

"Is it all right to talk to the pain?"

If the answer is yes, you could then ask any or all of the following:

"What is causing you (the pain)?"

"What is your purpose?"
"What is needed to make you go away?"

Option 6. The Secret of the Stillness

Remember too that as our experience of meditation develops, we become more aware of what we call the stillness. As we become more familiar with the stillness, we learn to give our attention to that stillness and to simply allow the pain to be there—while we remain undistracted.

This technique has a number of elements. It begins with the preparation that gives us a positive mind-set with which to approach pain. It draws huge support from the physical relaxation that we practice. Then, in a way, the stillness can be compared to the ultimate quiet place or inner sanctuary. This stillness is an ever-present source of peace and calm. In fact, the more we experience the stillness, the more we realize there is this inner part of us that is completely free of pain. In the stillness comes the direct experience of that part of us that is more permanent, more enduring and, just like the metaphor of the blue sky, unstainable, inviolable. We realize that there is this part of us that cannot be hurt. This can come as a source of great comfort and relief.

Option 7. The Role of Partners and Caregivers

Support people can also be of great help in the control of your pain. Touch works wonders. The comfort produced by a loving hand reaches us on a psychological level and such contact can ease many situations.

Talking through the progressive muscle relaxation we use as a lead-in to meditation can have a profound effect. This is a particularly helpful technique if someone is restless or distressed. It works best if the patient's given name is used while talking through the exercise. So, it could be said: "Feel your toes, Ian. Contract the muscles, Ian—and let them go." The name need not be used with every phrase, but including it regularly does aid the process. The exercise needs to be talked through in a slow, steady, unemotional tone and the one who is in pain does need to follow the directions. The exercise then finishes with an instruction for the person being guided to rest quietly and to allow any thoughts that do come into their awareness to simply be there, just allowing them to come and go, while remaining undistracted.

In a similar manner, it can be very helpful to have a support person read through the inner sanctuary exercise, or the exercise for dissolving pain.

RECOMMENDATIONS

This mind-based approach to pain control has no element of avoidance in it. It is a means by which the pain can be experienced as it is, free of fear or false imaginings. Commonly, when this is done, particularly in conjunction with the practice of mindfulness and meditation, the pain can be experienced as a sensation which, while it may be unpleasant, is certainly free from distress.

This technique has great merit as once established it requires little energy to maintain it. The pain can be acknowledged and accepted, and life can carry on free from its effects.

Start where you are at. Maybe analgesics are necessary to make life bearable. Maybe you can use more natural self-help methods to take the edge off the pain. Of course you will benefit from working with all the tools discussed in chapters 7 to 9 on positive thinking to improve your self-image and level of well-being. Do not overlook the role of laughing and indulging yourself in purely pleasurable activity. Likewise, aim to reach acceptance of your situation, especially if it does, or is likely to include, pain. If you can accept and flow with the pain rather than resisting and struggling against it, it will cause significantly less inconvenience.

Then, maybe by simply practicing your meditation, any pain eases and becomes more manageable. Maybe you will benefit from the extra learning that can come courtesy of a bulldog paper clip. Maybe there is something else in the range of possibilities we have covered that speaks to you more directly. The imagery and awareness exercise can be extraordinary. And then there is the deep comfort to be found in the stillness.

It is important to be prepared to experiment a little and to find what does work best for you personally. Just knowing that genuine pain relief is a possibility is a starting point. For many who have worked at this, a genuine change in their experience of pain has transformed their life for the better.

Finally, maybe it is obvious, but surely the best time to learn pain management skills is when you are pain free. Why wait until the need is strong? This is a life skill from which everyone can benefit. Use the techniques, practice, and remember, the more reliably you experience the stillness and its deep calm, the more confidence you will have in the face of pain. Why not experiment and find out the truth of the matter for yourself. You might just transform your experience of pain in the process.

Perhaps the greatest comfort I have gained through my cancer is learning that true pain does not hurt. Pain is a physical response; suffering is a conscious reaction that we can choose to do without. Knowing this to be real, experiencing it in daily life has been profoundly liberating.

CHAPTER 11

Nutrition 1

The Principles: A Logical Approach

THERE HAS TO BE AN APPROPRIATE DIET THAT WILL HELP PEOPLE AFFECTED by cancer to get well again. This is something to get positively excited about!

If you were diagnosed with heart disease, at the very first consultation it would be incumbent upon your doctor to talk to you about what you eat. The doctor would also be required to discuss other lifestyle matters: what you drink, whether you smoke or not, your levels of exercise, how you manage stress and, these days, how you relax and probably whether you meditate or not.

If you were diagnosed with type 2 diabetes (T2D), even more so. The link between what you eat, your lifestyle, the diagnosis and your capacity to recover are patently obvious. Heart disease and T2D are chronic, degenerative, lifestyle-related diseases. They respond well—as in you can recover from them—when you attend to what you eat along with your lifestyle more generally. Cancer is just the same.

Virtually all the remarkable, long-term cancer survivors I know value what they ate as a major factor in their recoveries. Same as me. Virtually all the thousands of people I have assisted for well over thirty years found giving considerable attention to nutrition and food produced significant benefits.

However, we live in a technological age. Current-day robots are capable of delicate and intricate surgery, even when the human surgeons directing their movements are on line and at a distance from the actual patient. Computers have phenomenal memories and wonderful capabilities to help us function. Medicine is becoming more and more complex and often when we are seeking healing we think it has to come through some complex technology.

Yet every human being lives in a physical body. While that body in its way of functioning is incredibly complex and could well be described as a technical marvel, it is very much dependent upon the food it eats and the fluids it drinks. Now while it is true that our digestion and all that happens in our body is affected by our emotions and our mind, clearly what impacts on the function and structure of our body most directly is the physical reality of the fuel we provide it with.

WHAT FUEL GOES INTO YOUR TANK?

One recent, very hot summer's day, I pulled into a station for gasoline. Beside me, a hot, sweaty, overweight and grumpy man approached a nearby pump for his fuel. He had three choices—low, medium and high octane—and he seemed clear on which to choose.

Seeing his foul mood, the mischievous part of me thought to suggest he take out his grumpiness on his van and put the wrong fuel in it. The more logical part of me rapidly decided this was not such a good idea. Not to be outdone, the mischievous part rose up with: "*Tell him to do a really good job of it and fill up with diesel instead of gasoline.*" No came the response, you will get hit for sure if you say that!

So I held my tongue and watched. Very attentively this man put the right gasoline into the simple combustion-engined van he was driving. Then he went into the shop, bought all sorts of junk and proceeded to put absolute rubbish into the highly sophisticated, super complex, combustion-engined body in which he was living. My guess is that as well as being so particular regarding the fuel he put into his van, this fellow was like the rest of us and regularly attended to his vehicle's service timelines.

Why the disconnect with the body? Surely, it is common sense that food builds our body and is the mainstay of running and repairing it. If you want a junk body, eat junk food. Want a healthy body? Eat healthy food. Want a body that just manages to function? Well, feed it whatever. Want a body that is capable of remarkable healing? Surely it makes sense to fill it up with the best fuel possible. Again, get excited!

THE HOPE THAT GOOD FOOD OFFERS

For me, food is another major piece of good news following a cancer diagnosis. Understanding the clear role nutrition plays in the causes of cancer helps to make more sense of the disease. Understanding the role changing your diet plays in recovery provides real hope—it gives inner confidence and feeds optimism. Understanding that improving the diet of your family, and who knows, maybe even having a positive influence on friends and others you care for, brings reality to the wish that others will not get cancer or any of the other chronic, degenerative diseases. Eat well and you can be really well!

The aim of the diet chapters is to provide hope, clarity and confidence. We will focus on what works nutritionally to support recovery and long-lasting good health, as well as how to make eating healthy food easy and tasty, practical and enjoyable.

How we will achieve this is by first examining the role our mind and our culture plays in our food choices. Then we will use our logic to investigate how food and nutrition can help us to heal. Experience tells me that when we understand the principles involved in good nutrition, the details follow fairly naturally. The intention is to understand what we do and why, and to enjoy eating for recovery.

Let us begin by examining the principles that connect food, cancer and survival.

WHAT DO THE DOCTORS KNOW?

You will have no trouble in finding cancer specialists who will tell you what you eat is very important. You will have no trouble finding other specialists who tell you it will make no difference whatsoever. Why such a big disparity?

My wife, Ruth, who is a GP with a master's in general practice psychiatry, studied at the highly respected University of Sydney's medical school, where there was not one specific lecture on nutrition in six years of medical training. Not one! This is the norm for medical education. No wonder so many doctors have no knowledge of or interest in nutrition and its relevance to healing.

Having trained as a veterinarian, I find this continuing error of omission in my colleagues' education staggering. One of my daughters, who is currently studying veterinary science, is required to complete four full semesters of study on nutrition. In veterinary science, they study seven main animal species. What is so special about the human species, the human body, that leaves medical educationalists believing that what it eats is of no importance?

I find this oversight in medical education deeply concerning. Also, what this knowledge clearly indicates is that unless your doctor has completed post-graduate education in nutrition, they will be grossly underqualified to comment on this vital area.

This problem is compounded by the food industry's infiltration of the psyche of the community and the health professions. Dietitians generally seem to believe nutritional requirements are solved by formulated and standard eating patterns of the day. In my view many of them represent the food industry far more directly than the real needs of the community.

What we do know for sure is that the current, average Western diet contributes significantly to six of the ten major causes of premature death in modern society: heart disease, diabetes, obesity, hypertension, diverticulitis and, of course, cancer.

World authorities, professors Sir Richard Doll and Sir Richard Peto, in their book *The Causes of Cancer*, first published way back in 1981, stated that the best current estimate was that diet is a major contributing factor in 35 percent of all cancers. August bodies such as the American Academy of Sciences put the figure at 40 percent for men and 60 percent for women. However, medical confirmation of the diet-cancer link had only come in the few years before Doll and Peto's work was first released. Prior to this, the connection had been vehemently denied in most quarters, as was the thought that diet could help a person to get well.

What is apparent, however, is that there is an emerging number of doctors actively counseling people affected by cancer on dietary principles. They get results that are plain for all to see, and the interest grows. Yet diet in the sense in which we are talking is still frequently, if incredibly, considered by some medical authorities to be an "alternative" area of treatment. Some would dismiss it altogether. So you will need to make up your own mind and set a clear path.

Having said that, I strongly recommend that any major dietary changes are best supervised by a qualified and experienced health professional with the necessary skill and knowledge of nutrition. This is particularly important if the disease is directly impacting on the digestive tract or there has been significant surgery in that area. Ideally, this supervision would be provided by a doctor who is qualified and experienced. Some naturopaths are very knowledgeable. In my own experience, people in a stable condition find getting their diet organized to be a safe, relatively easy, and certainly reward-ing experience. It is necessary, however, to be open to change and prepared to learn. For those in a less stable condition, a word of caution and a repeti-tion: seek suitable, qualified guidance and recognize that you may need to make an intense personal effort to begin with.

EVALUATE THE EVIDENCE

Naturally we want to make the best choices possible with our food and all else that we do. For this we need the best evidence, a clear mind to evaluate that evidence and the motivation to follow through on our choices. If it is helpful, revisit the major section on goal setting and contemplation in chapter 7.

As we investigate the role of nutrition in cancer medicine, it will be use-ful to digress a little and take the time to understand what evidence-based medicine (EBM) is, why it is so valued by the medical profession, and how in my view, it is commonly distorted.

EBM is a logical and very useful principle. Simply put, it says that all medical decisions need to be based on the best evidence available. No one would argue with that proposition. However, it is helpful to understand that EBM is commonly distorted in current usage. To understand the problem we need to turn to the definition. The definition of EBM that has most wide acceptance was published in the *British Medical Journal*[15] in 1996:

> EBM is the conscientious and judicious use of current best evidence in making decisions about the care of individual patients. The prac-tice of evidence based medicine means integrating individual clinical expertise with the best available external clinical evidence from sys-tematic research. By individual clinical expertise is meant the profi-ciency and judgment that individual clinicians acquire through clinical experience and clinical practice.

However, the problem is that frequently in medical circles where the emphasis is on "being scientific," the research from published journals is overemphasized and the clinical experience (what happens in the real world) is diminished.

Of course, the science is important. Of course, research is important and it would be wonderful to have more research funding used to investigate the foods that help to heal cancer. However, while clearly there is a great deal of knowledge and research concerning nutrition in general, when we do examine the current research evidence relating to food being used as a therapy for cancer, the first thing to notice is how little of it there is. There are multiple reasons for this as with most things, but significant facts are that nutritional research is very complex and expensive. Doctors who have no undergraduate training in nutrition and therefore no belief in its relevance are hardly likely to drive research in this area, and food is unpatentable, so only government, philanthropic donors or food industry people are likely to fund these inquiries. Unfortunately, the fruit and vegetable growers do not seem to place a high value on investigating the merits of their produce in cancer research.

However, in the absence of compelling, published research, EBM says we need to examine the best level of evidence that is available, and with cancer, nutrition and healing, that evidence comes from clinical experience.

Here is where this book comes in. My background is in veterinary science. I received a thorough, if basic, training in nutrition. I recovered from a very difficult cancer, very much against the odds, using food and nutrition as one of my major platforms for healing. I have over thirty years' experience working closely with people affected by cancer who took what they ate very seriously. It is fair to say that myself along with the foundation I helped to establish have a great deal of clinical evidence regarding what to eat when you have cancer, and that this volume of evidence probably compares favorably with anyone or any organization on the planet.

To be clear about all this, I do value the research highly. I continue to study nutrition and read widely. However, in my experience, what happens in practical reality is the real test of any diet that is proposed. What follows is the best and most practical information I can offer currently based on the accumulated experience of thousands of people and informed by the best of modern evidence.

GOOD NUTRITION STARTS WITH THE MIND

What is the single most important factor when it comes to what you eat? Clearly it is the mind. The mind decides what you will eat and how much of it. The mind will decide what you drink and regulate your levels of exercise. Your mind and its attendant emotions have the potential to completely disrupt or enhance your digestion. Obviously when under stress, our eating habits can suffer. Many people eat to fill an emotional hole. Many eat out of habit, false beliefs, neurosis or food addiction. Most of us are heavily influenced by advertising and by what those we hold in authority, like our doctors, have to say on the subject.

The aim we have here is to break free of destructive mind states regarding food and to eat for enjoyment and genuine good health. This is why we start with meditation. The calm and clear mind that meditation delivers will leave you confident to make good dietary choices, in the right state of mind to digest your food well, and confident to develop and sustain healthy eating habits. Happy meditating equals happy eating! However, along with meditation, it makes good sense to use our logical minds to examine the influences our society and our own unconscious exerts on us, and how we can use these energies to our advantage.

DECIDE WHO TELLS YOU WHAT TO EAT

There is a key question when it comes to what to eat, how much to meditate, what treatments to have and so on. Who tells us what to do? When it comes to diet, will it be a doctor, a dietitian, a naturopath, the lady over the back fence, a book—or will it be you?

Who to believe? My guess is that most people would prefer to work it out for themselves. Yet for many, when it comes to actually doing this, the choices appear complex and often confusing. If we are to take full responsibility for our own decisions and to work it out scientifically ourselves, there is an incredible amount of work to do—references to find, differences to sort out, so much learning. Clearly the amount of information available on food is vast and quite complex. The interactions of different foods that we might eat are complex. People's reactions to food are complex. So how do we simplify it?

My sense of it is that if we were to wait and not eat another meal until all the facts were clear, all the research completed and the debates settled, we would be old and gray indeed. And probably pretty hungry! There is an immediate imperative to make the best choices we can now, to do the best we can. This is what this book aims to help you with—a logical, step-by-step approach to eating for recovery.

GOING NUTS OVER FOOD DOES NOT ONLY MEAN EATING LOTS OF ALMONDS

We need to recognize the complex states of mind and the emotional turmoil that can exist for some people around food.

All of us are creatures of habit and we have discussed the role of conditioning and habitual thinking in chapter 8. But many of us could well be described as neurotic around food, while some are clearly afflicted by dietary-related addictions.

At the risk of laboring the point, it is obvious that our psychology can dramatically affect our food choices as well as our ability to actually do what we choose to do.

We need our mind to support our healing, not to sabotage it. Therefore we need to be honest with ourselves, talk of these issues, maybe even seek help through professional counseling if necessary, and make sure we use our food well.

UNDERSTAND THE INTERNAL FORCES GOVERNING OUR EATING HABITS AND ESTABLISH HEALTHY ONES

We receive training in the rights and wrongs and the dos and don'ts of food from many quarters. Family, friends, school, books, magazines, the media—all are sources of information. The problem is how to differentiate between false or inaccurate information and that which is correct. And how to take account of any biased information that may come your way. For example, the Dairy Board in Australia has created an excellent impression in many people's minds that the only way to get enough calcium is to consume regular and substantial quantities of dairy products. Yet, when you check the analysis of our nondairy, vegetable-based diet via the tables in Appendix M, you will find that it is more than adequate, containing over twice the recommended daily intake of calcium.

The reality is that to develop a healthy diet most people will benefit from clarifying what factual information they have learned already and from learning more.

Next, it only takes a little reflection to realize that our dietary choices are influenced by far more than pure information. There is the culture we grow up in, the social structure and the habits we develop. In a psychological sense, some people appear quite addicted to certain foods while others are dramatically affected by their emotions. Some people eat to excess to fill an "emotional hole," while others provide reward or punishment via food. Commonly, many of us feel the need to rebel and so we eat, smoke or drink something really daft to demonstrate our independence.

Advertising and peer pressure influence and condition the choices made by many people. Anorexia and bulimia are powerful extremes, but most children these days are growing up with their dietary choices heavily influenced by the food industry generally and the fast-food industry more particularly.

If you are embarking upon dietary change, it is really important to bring some awareness to these subtler, yet very powerful issues. These issues help to explain some of the difficulties you may experience. To change your diet is to change a major habit.

To ensure a future life, a healthy life, it may well be necessary to recognize any negative conditioning you have picked up and to develop a healthier way of thinking, a healthier way of eating. This is why we gave consideration to positive thinking in chapter 7—so that you could understand more of how the mind works, how conditioning has the potential to bind us into negative, unhealthy habits and yet how it is possible to transform all this, to make a new start and to rebuild your own good health and the health of those you love and care for.

WHO ARE YOU EATING FOR?

To clarify the psychology around food still further, we need to consider what external influences may be involved. Are you trying to please your partner? Your family? Your doctor? The advertising gurus? Or are you eating to meet your own particular health needs? Obviously the people around you are important and need to be taken into consideration; however, you do need to be clear on your own motivation.

If you do need to change your diet, it is bound to have an impact on your family and friends at least. How they react to your needs, how they support you and how you in turn deal with their reactions, could significantly affect what you do, how long you do it, and how well you do it.

This is why it is so important to communicate with those who you value. Once you have reached a decision as to what to do in the dietary arena, it is highly recommended that you write your dietary choices out as clearly as possible. You will find the charts in chapter 14 helpful for this. Then, using your written plan as a basis, discuss it with the important people in your life, emphasizing what you intend to do and why.

Regarding the family, it is clear that prevention is better than cure. It is well established that a healthy diet can prevent many illnesses, including cancer. So, as a minimum, the Wellness Diet is recommended for all the family. As an extra bonus, when others in the family are eating the same thing, it provides a sense of tangible support and makes meal preparation easier. Doing these things together assists in the healing process and helps to develop lifestyle patterns that will ensure long-term good health for everyone.

HOW MUCH CLARITY AND COMMITMENT DO YOU HAVE?

This really is a summation of what we have discussed so far. Food can help with healing, it can prevent disease, and it can make you feel good. There are many issues you will need to focus on—practical ones like cost and availability, factual considerations, emotional states, mental conditioning and habits. For many, their spiritual view, religious traditions, sense of ethics and responsibility to the environment play a prominent role in deciding their food choices.

So with all this, be clear on why you are eating and what you are eating. It makes good sense to take the time to resolve as many of these questions as you can. Many more questions are likely to arise as you proceed. Welcome this. Work with the questions, stay with them and seek your own answers.

DIFFERENT STAGES • Different Eating Patterns

It may be helpful to realize that for most people, and especially those dealing with cancer, the diet is best regarded as having different stages. When you first pay attention to your diet, it is highly likely that you will decide to make some, if not many, changes. So, there will be a transition—a transitional time where you are saying good-bye and letting go of past habits and adjusting to and welcoming new habits.

Often if illness is a major issue, people benefit from a stage of paying attention to their diet intensively. Then as the outlook improves there comes a stage of modification, experimentation and adaptation. Then it may be time to settle into the maintenance phase—that stage where you are eating in a normal, healthy, ongoing pattern.

My own experience is that food helped me tremendously during my recovery. While I am sure that it has been a major factor in my ongoing survival and good health, I now eat in the way I do because it helps me to feel the best that I can. I enjoy my food. I enjoy the fact that it is good for me and I enjoy the fact that I feel really good after I have eaten. I enjoy the fact that I am well.

ENJOY • The Message of the Big Mac and the Salad!

Is it better to eat a Big Mac and enjoy it, or a garden-fresh salad and loathe it? Is what you eat more important or the state of mind in which you eat it? Is it better to do what is good for you regardless of whether you enjoy it or not, or is it better to do what you enjoy whether it is good for you or not?

Have you read Yogananda's mind-blowing *Autobiography of a Yogi*?[16] It recounts his years as a young spiritual seeker searching through mystical India for his teacher, his guru. In ancient times, before the days of calling cards and websites, spiritual leaders needed to demonstrate their prowess to validate their capacities and to attract followers. There were different ways to do this, but commonly they developed siddhis, or signs of spiritual accomplishment. Yogananda describes many amazing feats he witnessed including "the poison eating saint." This fellow's demonstration was to eat poison and broken glass and remain unaffected—that is, as the story goes, until he repeated his siddhi on a day when he was in an agitated state of mind and unceremoniously died.

My experience of these matters is that there is a spectrum as in most things. Some people do have strong minds and strong constitutions and can manage on a wider range and quality of foods. However, it is a high level of accomplishment to be able to eat any old rubbish and be unaffected by it— especially long term.

For most of us mere mortals our health and our capacity to heal is dramatically affected by what we eat. Healthy eating leads to long-term good health and eating particularly well has the potential to assist us to recover from major illness.

The trick with food therefore is twofold. How can you be sure of what is good for you? And how do you enjoy eating it so you keep on eating it?

Easy. You need good information and the right state of mind.

Everything starts with the mind. It is our mind that decides what food to buy, how to store and prepare it, how much to eat and what state of mind we are in when we eat it.

How then to use the mind to good effect? We need to use our mind, our wits, to gather good information, then we need to train our mind to serve us—to follow through on our good choices and lead the way in deciding what we eat and how much we enjoy eating it.

Here is the kicker. Here is the real secret that so many people I met in the past were not aware of, but who on learning of it changed their lives dramatically for the better. Here is the secret to enjoying what the theory says is good for us:

Anything you do often enough you get used to. Nothing is difficult once you get used to it. Anything you choose to, you can put your mind to and enjoy doing it. It is not such a great accomplishment to decide upon the state of mind you will do something in. With just a modicum of willpower, most people can do it.

So use your intelligence. Choose the salad and choose to enjoy it!

This whole arena of nutrition is full of excitement, controversy and the definite prospect of being helpful. It is essential to be clear in your own mind as to the relevance it has for you. You need to feel good about your choices. It is very necessary to think about the whole area and to come to definite conclusions.

In the final analysis, food needs to be enjoyed. You need to be able to sit down before it, give thanks for what you have to eat, know that it is appropriate for your situation, and eat it with a smile on your lips and a song in your heart!

Let us move on now to consider how to put these principles into practice. What to put on the plate tonight?

CHAPTER 12

Nutrition 2

Foods That Heal: Clarifying Your Choices

IF YOU HAVE BEEN READING MORE WIDELY, YOU WILL KNOW THERE ARE different opinions offered regarding what is best to eat. Most books include a list that features what to avoid and what to eat, then they claim their list works well for those who use the list. So you check—you read another book or visit another authority and receive their list along with the assurance that this list works well too. Only problem is, the lists are different! So you go to the third book, the third authority, to find out which is correct, only to be enthusiastically provided with yet another list. What to do? How to make sense of it?

Many of the lists I read are actually correct—for some people. Where the confusion arises is that we often overlook the fact that people are different. One list can work really well for one group of people, another different list works well for another different group of people. The vital question is: Which group do you fit into? What will work best for you?

There is an answer. To clarify any confusion, we begin by identifying general food principles that apply to most people. Then we develop a process whereby it becomes possible to establish a way of eating that is best suited to your own individual situation and needs. We take two key steps. First, we establish what we call healthy boundaries. Then we establish personal food awareness.

ESTABLISH HEALTHY BOUNDARIES • The Wellness Diet

The first step in establishing a way of eating that will have therapeutic benefits against cancer, and will suit us specifically, is to establish healthy boundaries. The simple principle behind healthy food boundaries is that these boundaries aim to define what we are wise to avoid and what we are best to concentrate upon eating.

These healthy boundaries then form the basis of the Wellness Diet. The Wellness Diet is nutritionally sound, relatively easy to implement and will bring a great deal of benefit very quickly. This way of eating provides a good, general starting point for anyone with cancer and it provides sound guidelines for every member of the family. It is reasonable to say that if the community generally followed the Wellness Diet, overall health would improve dramatically and chronic, degenerative diseases reduce significantly. The details of the Wellness Diet form the next chapter.

DEVELOP PERSONAL FOOD AWARENESS • The Healing Diet

The second step is to develop our own personal food awareness so we can go from the general recommendations of the healthy boundaries, to the specific needs we have as an individual on the Healing Diet. This we will learn to do with the assistance of mindfulness and meditation, along with developing our knowledge of food, and increasing our personal sensitivity and responsiveness to what we eat.

The starting point is to develop your awareness. The deep stillness of pure and simple, uncomplicated, mindfulness-based stillness meditation (MBSM) leads naturally to clarity of mind and heightened awareness. This is another of the automatic and positive flow-on benefits that come with regular meditation. The more you meditate, the more you become aware. The more aware you are, the more you notice what is affecting you and how you are reacting. So as you meditate more, and become more aware, you become more likely to notice whether you react well or badly to any given food you eat. Also, as you meditate more you are likely to feel well within yourself. This means you are more likely to make good decisions. So not only are you more likely to notice what foods agree with you, you are more likely to respond to that observation and to actually enjoy eating what is good for you.

YOUR BODY AS YOUR GUIDE

However, there is more to this. Your body can become a major ally when it comes to making good food choices. It is quite possible that you can help your body to become more sensitive to what you are eating—in a way that it will help you to be able to discriminate between those foods that are good for you and those foods that are not.

We often think of this principle with animals. When they are sick, instinctively they seem to know what to eat, what serves them best. The suggestion is that as human beings, we too can regain this instinctive or insightful capacity. It is possible to help your body to develop to the point where it can assess how the food you are providing it with is affecting you. Even more important, your body can let you know what is helping it and what is not. In this way, it becomes possible to develop a really personalized diet.

Clearly, if you do want your body to be able to assess your food, you will be using it like an instrument. For an instrument to be useful, to be accurate and readable, it needs to be clean. So, if your body is full of junk, then it is hard to imagine how it would be sensitive enough to discriminate. This then is another reason to recommend a period of dietary cleansing or detoxification. Once the body has been purified it will be far more sensitive to what you put in it, and far more likely to give you helpful feedback.

How to cleanse or detox the body will be explored soon in chapter 14. It is enough for now to say that the approach that we recommend is quite similar to an allergy elimination diet, which is an approach used in mainstream food sensitivity and allergy testing.

THE HEALING DIET • A Summary

The Healing Diet is based on the principles of the Wellness Diet, but it involves applying those principles more diligently and then guides us as we develop our own specific program. Here is how we do it:

1. Start with the mind. Meditation leads to clarity and inner peace. This enhances what we learn intellectually, helps us to make good choices, and develops our awareness of what works personally and what is best avoided. Meditation also helps us to be unaffected by any potential stress that changing our diet may involve. We aim for clarity, confidence and enjoyment.

2. Establish healthy boundaries, using the Wellness Diet to ensure we have the basic elements of our food correct.

3. Go from the general to the specific by using:
  1. More meditation and contemplation—and the heightened awareness they bring.
  2. A mono diet or partial fasting for short periods of time to heighten our food sensitivity.
  3. A process of experimentation based upon elimination and reintroduction of sensitive foods.
4. Regularly use foods known for their anticancer properties.
5. Establish a cancer-unfriendly environment in our body by manipulating our own metabolism (through the use of appropriate foods) to make life difficult for the cancer.
6. Use fresh juices to increase the vital nutrients required for healing.
7. Consider using supplements. In my view, there is a hierarchy when it comes to using nutrition to heal cancer. Food is the number one priority, juices come second and supplements third.
8. Continue on the Healing Diet until cancer free, and then modify it toward the Wellness Diet.

The details of the Healing Diet form chapter 14.

As I am frequently asked to detail what I did regarding food and juices during my own recovery, I have summarized my own experiences with the Healing Diet and with the Gerson Therapy specifically in Appendix G.[17] But do remember, just like you, I am an individual. What I did may well be interesting and informative, but it is for each one of us to discover what will work best for us personally.

HOW THOROUGH DO WE NEED TO BE?

When we were developing as a fetus inside our mother's abdomen, both of us had very specific nutritional requirements. As a child and adolescent, we needed about 25 percent more food on a weight-for-weight basis to take account of our growth rate. Some parents would say for teenage boys it is way higher. Certainly if we are engaged in physically demanding sport or work, we need significantly more than someone who sits behind a desk all day.

When we are basically well, it is what we eat mostly that is important. The fact is that as human beings, our bodies are reasonably adaptable. If you eat well at home through the week and then go out on the weekend and play up a little, there is little likelihood of harm. If you play up every night, then the risks begin to build fairly rapidly.

So again, when we are well, what we eat mostly is important. However, when we are dealing with major illness, what we eat all the time is important.

This statement is made based on my years of clinical experience, and is reinforced by Dean Ornish's randomized, lifestyle-based prostate cancer trial.[18] Ornish first won international acclaim in the nineties for publishing research that demonstrated it is possible to reverse coronary artery disease using a basically vegan diet, exercise, meditation, yoga, emotional healing and group therapy—a program very similar to the one we developed at the Gawler Foundation. Ornish then went on to investigate the same program with men diagnosed with early prostate cancer who were in what essentially in those days was called the "watchful waiting phase."

The results were compelling. Not surprisingly, the cancer advanced for most of the men in the control group, their PSAs (a blood marker of prostate cancer activity) went up, the aggressiveness of their cancers went up and several required major medical treatments. Those men who made modest lifestyle changes stabilized their condition, a significant benefit in its own right. However, those who made major lifestyle changes and diligently maintained them were able to reduce their PSAs, reduce the aggressiveness of their cancers and, after one year, none had required medical intervention. After three years, the benefits were still highly significant, although a small number of the diligent men (significantly less than in the control group) had required more medical treatment.

In nearly all areas of life, how we apply ourselves will make a difference. Do nothing and the natural course of events is likely to follow. Do nothing in response to cancer and it is highly likely to progress. Intervene, use your own resources, and remarkable outcomes become possible.

So when faced with active cancer, the recommendation is to take what you eat seriously.

But if you think, "I will eat well long enough to get well, and then go back to junk food," you are missing the point. The first thing when faced with cancer is to recover. Then we aim for a long, happy and healthy life. What we eat provides the raw ingredients for healing and a healthy old age.

CLARIFY YOUR CHOICES • Make a Decision

Having read what has been presented so far, maybe it is time to begin to make some broad but important decisions. Regarding nutrition and our way of eating, there would seem to be four options worth considering:

1. Make no change.
2. Adopt the Wellness Diet.
3. Follow the Healing Diet.
4. Commit yourself to a specific intense diet such as Gerson's and seek professional help with it—preferably in a suitable clinic.

Dietary Choices—Make No Change

If you are happy with your diet as it is and feel it cannot be improved, that is fine. Skip the next two chapters and go on with the other things available to help you back to health.

However, I am convinced that dietary considerations are one of the basic tools for getting well. Most of the dietary factors associated with a risk of increasing the incidence of cancer are prominent in our Western diet. These factors are a high content in the diet of fat, protein, salt, sugar, refined foods and foods with a low-fiber content, as well as too many calories, and drinking excessive alcohol. It is likely, then, that most people need to consider making changes.

Dietary Choices—The Wellness Diet

This is a relatively easy step. It is how we establish healthy boundaries. It requires eliminating from the diet those things associated with a health risk and concentrating on what is known to be good for us.

The Wellness Diet can be described in simple terms as a plant-based, whole-food diet.

For many people, then, this type of diet does involve a significant change in eating habits, but it still fits readily into most daily routines.

The Wellness Diet is ideal for those with cancer who want to improve their way of eating without giving food a great deal of attention. It is a sound "bottom line." It is an excellent consideration for those in remission, being an ideal way to eat for those who are basically well, as well as for those who are interested in preventing disease and in maximizing their health. I feel confident in putting it forward as a basic, sensible and sound diet.

The Healing Diet

This is the more intense approach recommended for people with active cancer. The Healing Diet includes learning to develop a personalized and specific dietary program and requires a good deal of commitment. It is for those who intend to take what they eat seriously and are intent on using nutrition for recovery.

Specific Intensive Dietary Programs

I do not recommend these unless they are supervised by qualified personnel. My attitude is that a knowledgeable doctor needs to be involved in any such program.

MAKE A PLAN

Eating for recovery requires you to set clear goals. Here is how you can establish a good plan that will make it easy for you to eat for recovery.

1. Set a time limit for collecting information on the dietary possibilities.
2. Take what is written here, and add more information from all sources available to you.
3. Assess this body of information. Remember the value of contemplation to enhance the information and use the contemplation technique detailed in chapter 7.
4. Make a decision and plan a course of action.
5. Enlist the support of your family, friends and colleagues.
6. Commit yourself to a period of time to experiment with your diet.
7. For the given period of time, adhere as thoroughly as possible to your plan. Give it a chance to produce an effect.
8. At the end of that period, reassess and plan again.
9. Repeat steps 7 and 8 regularly.

There is a great deal that can be done, and remember: Diet is not the total answer to cancer, but without a good diet, there is no answer.

WHAT I SUGGEST

At the very least, the Wellness Diet is easy and reliable. Committing to this approach will avoid most problems and be significantly helpful. When the need is to recover from cancer and you want to do the best for yourself and those around you, the Healing Diet makes more sense to me. However, the choice needs to be yours. Consider the options. Meditate. Contemplate. Discuss the possibilities with those you value.

When you are ready, move on to the next chapters where we define the Wellness Diet and clarify the Healing Diet.

CHAPTER 13

Nutrition 3

Healthy Boundaries: The Wellness Diet

THE WELLNESS DIET IS BASED UPON A SIMPLE PREMISE. IT AIMS TO AVOID foods that are known to be unhelpful; it concentrates on using the foods that are known to be healthy and enjoyable. By doing this well, we have a diet that is highly anti-inflammatory and highly regenerative. It is a diet that will prevent the majority of chronic degenerative diseases, will be enjoyable to prepare and eat, will provide a sound basis for recovering from illness, and is easy to understand and commit to.

While we could say the Wellness Diet provides logical guidelines for anyone interested in eating well, another way of explaining it is via the concept of healthy boundaries. When you avoid the things that are unhelpful and eat the healthy foods, you are in safe territory.

For many who are basically well, this diet is ideal. For those embarking on recovering from cancer it provides a quick and reliable starting point. By following these guidelines you immediately take out of your diet the things that could aggravate your illness, and you immediately incorporate many things that will help you to regenerate and to heal. Once you have settled into this first step of the Wellness Diet, then you can go on to individualize your eating pattern and to gain the additional benefits available through the Healing Diet.

As we move into clarifying the detail of the Wellness Diet, we will begin with more principles. Remember the key point; by understanding the principles, we gain confidence in what we are doing and the details tend to follow on fairly easily.

Wellness Rule 1: Understand the principles to simplify the details.

So as we discuss the principles of fats, proteins, soy and so on, we will do so in a practical way. The rationale behind what to eat and what to avoid will be explained. As we examine each food or aspect of food, we will consider three questions:

- Quantity—how much, if any, of a given food to eat,
- Quality—what type of the food is ideal if there are choices available, and
- Preparation—including storage and cooking techniques.

FATS AND OILS

Making intelligent choices regarding the quantity, quality and preparation of the fats you consume is one of the most powerful ways to improve your nutrition, your health and your capacity to heal.

Nutritional Information

What is the difference between a fat and an oil? Essentially oils are liquid fats. Fats and oils have a similar chemical structure and from the body's perspective, they both have similar functions. We call those fats that tend to be solid at room temperature fats—such as lard or animal fat—while those fats that are liquid at room temperature, like olive oil, we tend to call oils. To simplify things, we will mostly use the word "fats" during this section.

Fats fulfill a wide range of functions in the body, being a source of energy and a major means to store energy. Fats also act as a buffer—they protect us from trauma, insulate us from temperature changes and importantly are a repository for dangerous material. When the body has an excessive load of toxic material or even unsafe bacteria coming into it, rather than allowing that material to impact on our vital organs, the body in its cleverness shunts the offending matter into our fat stores. There it remains until it can be metabolized and eliminated from our system. This is important to realize, as it means that eating fat from polluted, unhealthy or toxic sources means we accumulate their rubbish.

But also, if we are unhealthy and overweight, and then we lose weight rapidly, we can have a significant toxic overload to deal with as our fat breaks down and releases the offending material into our system.

On a happier note, fats also play a positive role in healthy skin and hair, and are essential aids for the transport and metabolism of the fat-soluble vitamins A, D, E and K. Fats also play a vital role in the integrity of our cell membranes or walls, which we will investigate further soon.

Quantity

Currently the average American acquires over 40 percent of their caloric intake via fats. In Australia it is in the low 30s and yet the ideal is around 15–18 percent. So for the average person, halving your fat intake would be about right. It is worth noting that to reverse coronary artery disease or atherosclerosis, the fat intake needs to go down to about 11–12 percent, which is quite difficult to do. This would require avoiding things like avocados which, while they are about 50 percent fat, do actually fit in nicely with the Wellness Diet.

How do we reduce our fat levels? Simply avoid hidden fats and use modest amounts yourself. Those who do have a high fat intake acquire a great deal of their fats hidden in fried foods, dressings, fast foods, pastries and the like, so we avoid all those unhealthy foods.

The quantity of fat that is ideal is one of the many principles that takes care of itself by adopting the Wellness Diet. What is meant by this is that when you follow the Wellness program and eat in the way recommended, the fat levels will automatically be close enough to ideal. This means you need not be concerned to measure, weigh or add up what actual fats you use. This is something you can trust.

Quality

Understanding the different types of fats available and choosing the best ones is crucial to our health and to our capacity for healing. There are several classifications to be aware of and respond to.

Saturated vs. Unsaturated Fats

Fats fall into these first two major categories: saturated and unsaturated. Saturated and unsaturated fats have one major difference—saturated fats have many more double bonds connecting the molecules that make up their structure. This fact makes them harder, more brittle and more angular in their shape. This in turn accounts for saturated fats being solid at room temperature—like lard (animal fat) and coconut oil (one of the few saturated vegetable fats). This chemical structure also explains why unsaturated fats are liquid at room temperature and why we use the names animal fats and vegetable oils.

To understand the principle behind using unsaturated fats and avoiding the saturated ones, we need to understand how these fats are incorporated into our own bodies. Our body is made up of many, many cells, each with a similar basic structure. Each has a cell membrane, or external wall within which are contained those more fluid, internal elements of the cell that are responsible for the cell's functions. Each cell membrane has what is called a double lipid layer much as a wall could have bricks or timber. Lipids are fats; we are talking of a double layer of fats being an integral part of the membrane of each cell in your body. Now the crucial point.

If you are eating mostly saturated fats, the lipids in your body will be mostly saturated; eat mostly unsaturated fats and the lipids will be unsaturated. Cell membranes composed of saturated fats will be hard, brittle and have what effectively are spiky edges. A direct consequence of this is that saturated fat cell membranes will be dense and not very permeable. This means it is harder for nutrients to get into the cell and harder for waste products to get out. The whole metabolism of the cell is compromised.

By contrast, when our cell membranes are made up of mostly unsaturated fats; those cells will be more pliable, more permeable, more efficient.

This issue is of great importance for your red blood cells. Red blood cells transport oxygen and other nutrients around your body. They can be visualized like balloons filled with water. If their outside membrane is made up mostly of saturated fats, they will be quite rigid and inflexible, as well as sticky because of the angular nature of saturated fats. This has two very unhelpful consequences. First, the blood cells cannot change shape so easily and they will find it harder to squeeze through the tiny capillaries that are intended to bring them into close contact with the other cells of your body. Even more problematic, they tend to stick together a bit like Velcro does, because of their angular shape. This increases the risk of blood clots and thrombosis—a real problem at any time, but an added risk during chemotherapy.

Most people will know of someone who has high blood pressure, or who had heart disease and was put on blood thinners. Sticky blood is a major health risk. Sticky blood refers to how thick your blood is and how easily it flows. Compare a tomato sauce bottle with tomato sauce in it, to one with water in it. Upend the two bottles; the water flows, the sauce sticks.

If your blood is sticky, it does not flow well. It is much harder for your heart to pump it around your body. It is much harder for the blood to get into and through the tiny pipes that are your small blood vessels. Hence sticky blood raises blood pressure and aggravates heart disease, as well as increasing the risk of developing a blood clot or an embolism (significant potential side effects of chemotherapy).

The best way to have thin blood that flows well is to avoid saturated fats; only use unsaturated fats and follow all the other principles in the Wellness Diet.

Wellness Rule 2: Avoid saturated fats; instead, use unsaturated fats or oils.

What are the saturated fats? All animal fats are saturated—whether from beef, chicken, sheep or pig. There are two vegetable-based ones—palm oil and coconut oil.

Palm oil is a disaster for the environment and human health. It is widely used in prepared foods, so read the labels. Most cookies and many candies and pastries contain vegetable oil. If the actual oil is not specified, it will almost certainly be palm oil. Palm oil is very cheap and, being a saturated fat, makes cookies crisp and crunchy. Some commercial cookies use olive oil, which is healthier, and they will always be labeled as such due to olive oil being more expensive.

Vast tracts of ecologically sensitive land, mostly in tropical areas, are cleared daily for more palm oil. Curiously, it is the environmentalists who are leading the push to reduce the world's consumption of palm oil and they are making useful inroads. One cannot help wonder where the dietitians have been when the health risks to people have been known for a long time.

Coconut oil has some advocates, as it is a shorter chain saturated fat and has a high resistance to cooking temperatures. I still recommend against its use, as there are better oils to choose. To understand which ones are recommended we move on to consider:

Omega Fatty Acids

There are three main classifications of omega fatty acids—the 3s, 6s and 9s—and your body needs some of each. However, the consequences for your immune system vary dramatically depending upon which one predominates in your diet.

The omega-3 fatty acids are the good guys—they act as a very positive tonic for your immune system and many other healing functions. The omega-6s are the baddies—they actually weaken your immune system and have other unhelpful consequences—while the omega-9s are neutral for immune function but do have other redeeming features.

Wellness Rule 3: Use omega-3 fatty acids regularly, omega-9s modestly and avoid the omega-6s.

Which is what? The two main omega-3s are fish oil and flaxseed oil. Flaxseed oil is highly recommended. When you hear of the benefits of eating fish, those benefits mostly relate to the fish oils. Of course, to obtain oil from a fish, you need an oily fish! Sardines and tuna qualify, but almost all varieties of canned tuna have the oil removed as the oil is worth more in a capsule than a can. Be extra careful, as several producers put unhealthy oils back in the can. More details of this soon. Also, see Appendix H for details on sustainable fish species that meet health standards.

The main sources of the omega-6's fatty acids are sunflower and safflower oils and they are best avoided. Also, it is best to avoid canola oil.

The omega-9s predominate in olive oil, avocado and most nuts.

To understand exactly what to do, there is one more vital issue with fats.

Preparation

Healthy fats have many benefits but they all share a common problem. Fats all have a high tendency to oxidize and become rancid. Rancid fats are seriously dangerous both in the short and long term. Short term they are highly toxic, long term they are carcinogenic—that is, they cause cancer.

Fats oxidize and become rancid when exposed to air, heat or light.

Wellness Rule 4: Protect your oils from air, heat and light.

This means buy oils in cans or dark bottles, which are protected from the light.

Use cold-pressed or virgin oils because they have not been heated during the extraction process.

Buy flaxseed oil from a refrigerator, not off the shelf, and store it at home in the refrigerator. Once opened, use all oils within two months ideally, three months at most.

Learn to cook without oils. Cooking can easily overheat oils and lead to oxidation. The best solution is to cook oil free and only add oils to your meals at the table. Oil is good to add to food, just do not cook with it. While this does take some adjustment, once established, it is a really healthy and enjoyable habit. As a positive side effect, it makes the washing up easier!

If you really must use some oil in cooking, olive oil has a high resistance to heat (flaxseed is very low). And if using a wok, adding water (before heating the oil) helps protect the oil.

Avoid roasted nuts or cooking with nuts or seeds, as this overheats the oils. Many nuts have around 50 percent oil content, so this is a real issue—more on nuts soon.

FAT RECOMMENDATIONS

On the Wellness or Healing Diet, the amount of fat to consume will be taken care of by following the general guidelines:

- Avoid all animal fats thoroughly (including dairy).
- Learn to cook oil free.
- Include two tablespoons of flaxseed oil daily in your food—best added to meals after cooking, although some do take it off a spoon (not me!).
- Use olive oil for variety. While it is neutral for your immune system, it has other useful properties in its own right.
- Read labels; avoid palm oil and coconut oil.

PROTEINS

Protein is another essential ingredient in the human diet.

Nutritional Information

Proteins are involved in virtually every process in our body, as well as being a major contributor to our structural integrity. Proteins are vital for our immune system and for healthy muscle activity. They make up significant parts of the enzymes that regulate our metabolism, as well as the messenger molecules such as the neuropeptides that transfer information internally around our bodies.

Proteins are made up of amino acids, some of which are called essential amino acids because we need to obtain them directly in our food, while others are nonessential amino acids and can be manufactured in our own body.

Quantity

Virtually everyone who specializes in nutrition, along with the broader mainstream authorities, agrees that the ideal quantity of protein to consume is less than what many in the general public understand.

Speaking personally, being an athlete before I was diagnosed with cancer in 1975, I was encouraged to eat a very high-meat diet. These days, most athletes train on a high-carbohydrate diet with only modest protein levels, as it is known this brings better results. Interestingly, Carl Lewis, perhaps the greatest athlete known, claimed that being a vegan led to his greatest performances. Murray Rose, one of Australia's greatest ever swimmers, was competing as a full vegan and winning Olympic gold medals back in the 1950s.

In the seventies, it was not unusual for people to be averaging 120gms of protein per day. Now the recommended level is around 55–60gm/day for the average-size person; so again, like with the fats, this may be around half of what many have been used to. We will clarify what 55–60gms looks like in the preparation section.

Wellness Rule 5: Eat modest amounts of protein—around 55–60gms/day for the average-size person.

Quality

Why is it that so many authorities who are really serious about nutrition, and especially nutrition for healing, recommend a vegetable-based diet with little or no meat?

To understand, we need to divert a little and consider dogs, cows and digestive systems.

Digestion

There are three types of animal digestive systems: carnivore, herbivore and omnivore. A classic carnivore like a dog is designed to eat a high-meat diet. A classic herbivore like a cow runs on grass, and us human beings—well, we are omnivores trying to get the best of both worlds. Knowing about our own digestive system, and how it compares to the others, helps us to understand what we are wisest to eat, and what makes best sense when we are eating for recovery.

The Carnivore

A dog has a very specific anatomical setup to enable it to manage the food it eats. Here is the key point regarding meat. Digestion of virtually any food produces waste products. We eat a food like meat or a particular vegetable, we take what we can use from that food and we eliminate the leftovers, the waste products. With meat, the waste products are somewhat problematic; they are rich in nitrites and other potentially toxic by-products of their digestion. Vegetables do not produce these problematic waste products.

If the metabolic waste products from meat stay in the bowel for long, they can be directly toxic to the lining of the bowel, or they can be absorbed through the bowel and become toxic to the rest of the body.

Now, the dog is essentially a scavenging meat eater with a matching anatomy. It has sharp canine teeth for biting and ripping its potential meal into big pieces. Then it swallows quickly before anyone else can steal its share. Therefore, it has modest chewing teeth at the back of its mouth and actually does little chewing unless on a bone or equivalent. Next it has just one, relatively compact stomach that secretes almost pure hydrochloric acid to liquefy the lumps of food it has gulped down.

Then the key point: because of the potentially toxic nature of the metabolic waste products that come from the digestion of meat, the dog needs to get rid of them quickly. Therefore, every dog has a very short bowel, and as a result, what we call a rapid transit time. The transit time measures how long it takes food to go through the system, from front to back, or top to bottom. Hence, short bowel, rapid transit time.

The Herbivore

By contrast, a classic herbivore like the cow has a very different digestive challenge. It is eating vegetable matter and with grass, needs to be able to digest cellulose. The cow therefore has a very different anatomy. First, there is a need to start the digestive process by grinding the food very finely. As a result, the cow has no serious biting teeth, but very serious grinders! While the dog's back teeth are permanent and static, in the same way that adult human teeth are, the cow's back teeth constantly grow. Cows do so much chewing that they need to continually replace what has been ground down.

Next, the cow has four stomachs! Four. The first is like a huge tank that mixes the finely ground grass with water and saliva and literally ferments it. In the process, cows produce large amounts of methane. So these days, aware conservationists are joining the push to reduce meat consumption as the volumes of methane produced have a major impact on the atmosphere. Also, to grow an equivalent amount of beef protein compared to vegetable protein requires around eighteen to twenty times more land area. Given the huge problems with the clearing of forests and utilization of land, this is another major environmental rationale for less meat and more vegetable protein consumption.

Back to the cow. After the four stomachs the cow has a very long digestive tract and a much slower transit time than a dog.

The Omnivore

As humans, we are trying to manage eating just about anything, so our anatomical set up is a compromise. We have teeth that can bite and chew. We have one stomach with high acid content and an intermediate length of bowel. While the dog's transit time is around six to eight hours, the cow's two to four days, the ideal human transit time is eighteen to twenty-four hours.

For people, there is another relevant issue. Fiber in our diet does two important things that are relevant to this discussion. First, fiber adds bulk and regulates transit times; low fiber, longer transit time. Second, fiber acts as a sponge or a buffer. If we do eat something, or have some potentially toxic metabolic waste products form in our bowel, high levels of fiber act as a sponge to absorb the toxic material and usher it quickly out of our system.

Now, you probably know that the average Western diet has been high in meat and low in fiber. This means more toxic waste products, less buffering or absorption from fiber and slower transit times—a great recipe for provoking all bowel diseases and some others in the body generally.

Clearly, humans can manage eating meat, but anatomically, we are better designed for vegetable proteins.

Wellness Rule 6: On the Wellness Diet, reduce or preferably avoid meat consumption. On the Healing Diet, it is preferable to avoid meat altogether.

Let us now look at the various protein sources.

Vegetable Proteins

Many vegetables contain useful amounts of protein. The next issue to clarify relates to the quality of those proteins. Proteins are made up of amino acids and our bodies need quite a number of them. Some the body can make itself and these are called the nonessential amino acids. Others the body can only obtain directly from the foods we eat and they are called the essential amino acids. In general, most individual vegetables are described as being incomplete sources of protein because they do not contain every one of the essential amino acids. By contrast, meat is often touted as a complete protein because it does contain all the essentials. The two notable vegetarian exceptions are the soybean (whose popularity is partially based on the fact that it is a complete protein) and quinoa.

The protein quantity and quality in tofu (the cheese-like soy protein) is very comparable to that of chicken—both are nearly 30 percent protein and both contain all the amino acids we need. Common grains such as rice and wheat are incomplete proteins; however, they do have around half the amount of protein in them when compared to chicken, which is still a very useful amount. Legumes or pulses are the protein-rich vegetables like peas, beans and lentils.

Quinoa warrants a special mention as it is an old grain whose nutritional properties have recently come to the forefront and increased its popularity.

An alternative to use in place of rice or couscous, quinoa has a high-protein content (around 18 percent), importantly is a complete protein, is gluten free, easy to digest and just mildly laxative. It can be cooked like rice and is well suited to sprouting; it is highly recommended for regular use.

It is important to understand that the diets of many large cultural groups around the world are largely vegetable based and they know the secret to obtaining complete protein from vegetables. If they only ate one source of vegetable protein over an extended period of time, they would soon have a problem. However, mix any two grains together, or eat a grain with a pulse, and you almost always end up with a complete protein. This mixing is commonly done in the same meal, but is still adequate if done over a day or so. So most vegetarian-based cultures have their staples that manage this. The classic example is in India and other countries where rice and lentils (or dahl) are eaten together regularly.

> Wellness Rule 7: When relying on vegetables for protein, eat cooked soybeans (ideally as tofu) and quinoa regularly, or combine two grains and/or legumes in one meal or one day.

Fish

The metabolic waste products from the digestion of fish fall between the toxicity from meat and the ease of vegetable proteins. Oily fish has the advantage of being a source of omega-3 fatty acids.

Increasingly, fish presents serious environmental and production issues. Intensive fish-farming practices (where antibiotics are being used more commonly) are only somewhat better than those for the intensive rearing of chickens, pigs and cattle (where what goes on can be quite problematic). So, wild fish are highly preferable; but then there are the questions of pollution (particularly for the fish that live close to the shore or built-up areas), environmental degradation (as from bottom dredging), overfishing and wastage (as from longline fishing).

Knowing where your fish came from is now a necessary step in selecting which fish to buy. Then there is the fact that the smaller species of fish are less likely to accumulate pollutants when compared to larger predator fish. Seafood like oysters, prawns and scallops are notorious for picking up pollutants, so where these foods come from is also well worth knowing before you eat them—if you eat them. Farmed prawns are better for the environment, as netting the wild ones can be very harsh on the seafloor.

> Wellness Rule 8: If you eat fish, avoid farmed fish in the main and eat the smaller, sustainable wild fish varieties that come from nonpolluted areas (see Appendix H for more details) and eat seafood only occasionally. On the Healing Diet, fish is preferably avoided.

Eggs

How eggs are produced commercially is a real concern. If you do eat eggs, only use genuine free-range eggs. Many people are also unsure when it comes to the cholesterol in eggs. Cholesterol is very useful in the body and we need some in our diet. The Wellness Diet generally is low in cholesterol and so a few eggs each week are fine inclusions. Be mindful of how you cook them; the frying of eggs is to be avoided altogether.

> Wellness Rule 9: Two to four genuine free-range eggs per week are OK on the Wellness Diet. Most people find eggs are better avoided on the Healing Diet (more on this later).

Dairy Products

It is obvious that before the development of agriculture, milk was not part of the human diet after weaning. Given how long it takes the body to adapt to major changes like this, some critics pose the logical question regarding how well our digestion is suited to consuming a food source that traditionally we never ate. Looking around, you would have to notice many cultures eat dairy, and many people seem to manage just fine. Dairy-based cultures like the Swiss and the French seem to do quite well in the longevity stakes; certainly they are comparable to many other less dairy-focused cultures.

However, there are serious concerns with dairy products that warrant consideration. Over the years, based on the research and clinical experience of working with people adding or subtracting dairy from their diets, I have become increasingly convinced the best approach is to minimize or avoid dairy on the Wellness Diet and leave it out altogether from the Healing Diet. Why? The first and most obvious issue is that natural dairy products contain a large amount of saturated fat. This can be minimized in low-fat milk, but many cheeses actually concentrate the fats and butter (nearly 50 percent saturated fat).

Wellness Rule 10: If you do use dairy products, use the low-fat varieties.

Next, we need to understand that the protein in human milk is a short-chain protein. This means it is a small molecule. By contrast, cow's milk is comprised of a long-chain, large and angular molecular protein. When a young child is introduced to cow's milk early in life, the contrast with human milk is stark. The child's developing immune system will not be sure if this large molecule is a food that needs to be digested or an invader that must be attacked. As it is, it seems many mount a low-level immune reaction to milk—a reaction that results in chronic, low-level, generalized inflammation. While this reaction may not amount to much in ordinary daily life, given extra stress, through environment, unsuitable food, disease, emotional or mental stress, and the inflammation may flare. Children who suffer from recurrent ear infections or tonsillitis often find their conditions clear up when taken off all dairy products.

For adults, consuming dairy products may seem manageable with no obvious consequences. However, faced with stress or disease, or simply wanting to be at our best, it may well be better to leave dairy out of the diet.

What about goat's or sheep's milk? They have smaller chain proteins so that issue is lessened. Many children with full-blown allergies to cow's milk can manage goat's milk. However, these sources of milk are high in fat and naturally homogenized. That means that the fat is suspended in the liquid of the milk, does not naturally settle out and is not so easy to separate. Therefore, goat's and sheep's milk tend to be high in saturated fat with all the related issues. They too are best avoided or minimized.

Nuts

Nuts are a good source of protein but care needs to be taken with their oils, as they go rancid easily and quickly. Nuts like walnuts, pecans and Brazil nuts are all best bought in their shells and eaten within a few months of being picked to reduce the risk of rancidity. Some can be purchased vacuum-packed, which is a great advantage. When nuts taste bitter, that is the sign they are dangerously rancid. Almonds are best bought with their brown skins intact, as this protects their oils from the air and from the light. Also, it is best not to cook with nuts or to eat the roasted varieties.

Chestnuts and especially almonds are relatively low in protein and quite low in oil and are suitable for eating regularly. Because chestnuts are so low in oil they are one nut which is OK to cook and, besides, they really are terrible raw. Almonds make great snacks between meals and, interestingly, have been proven by research to help the overweight lose weight. There is no indication they cause people with a healthy weight to lose more, so they are highly recommended—ten to twenty per day.

> Wellness Rule 11: Eat up to ten to twenty almonds per day, chestnuts when they are in season, and eat the other nuts occasionally, when fresh and not roasted.

Preparation

The Wellness Diet derives a good deal of its protein from the grains we will discuss next in the carbohydrates section. What is needed is to add a modest amount of protein from the high-protein sources covered in the previous section on quality.

What to prepare, therefore, and what it looks like in practice depends on which of those protein sources you choose to use.

VEGETABLE PROTEINS

If these constitute a major source of protein for you, eat them regularly. With tofu, two slices the size of fish sticks are recommended three or four times weekly, and if you have a couple of rice and lentil dishes throughout the week, the protein levels are likely to be quite adequate.

COOKING LEGUMES OR PULSES

There are many different peas and beans. Some can be eaten raw, but most need to be cooked. French beans, runner beans, peas, snow peas, soya, kidney, lima and mung beans, chickpeas and lentils require cooking.

The dried seeds of plants we know as beans are easy to store and a good source of carbohydrate and protein—especially when combined with equal amounts of rice, wheat, etc. Most beans require special cooking because uncooked they contain alkaloids and glycosides that are detrimental to digestion, so never eat them raw. Ideally, beans are best soaked in water eight to sixteen hours and then simmered in boiling water until cooked—usually for two hours. Another cooking method is to pour boiling water over the beans, allow to soak two hours, then cook as above.

With legumes it is wise to throw out the soaking water if you use it, and replace it before boiling, as well as discarding the water used to boil them. This also means that you do not cook legumes (including lentils) in soup; cook them separately and then add them.

Sprouting many legumes before cooking can work well and also makes digestion easier, but this usually takes several days. If sprouted, legumes need only to be blanched before eating.

FISH, IF YOU EAT IT

Once or twice a week is OK. Cooking methods apart from burning are not significant, although steaming works very well.

EGGS

Two to four per week, if you eat them. Do not fry; any other cooking method is OK.

DAIRY

Avoid or just eat on special occasions if you really like cheese, for example. Remember, it is highly recommended not to cook or heat any food in a microwave (especially any dairy products).

NUTS

Eat ten to twenty almonds per day; chestnuts when in season, and eat the other nuts raw, occasionally and when in season.

MEAT, IF YOU EAT IT

Back in the seventies, again, meat was the feature on a dinner plate, the vegetables appearing more like condiments on the side. These days, if you do eat meat, the reverse is the aim—lots of vegetables with a small piece of meat. Cooking methods do not matter much except char grilling or burning;

burned bits contain hydrocarbons, which are highly toxic, so avoid these methods. When using a barbecue, this means it is necessary to use a hot plate and be careful to avoid burning the food.

If you do eat meat, the lean white meats are preferable. Rabbit may be best, veal could be considered, but chicken requires real caution. Commercially raised chicken has overwhelming problems related to what they are fed, how they are housed and the routine use of low-level antibiotics as growth promoters. If you do eat chicken, it is mandatory in my view to only eat genuine, free-range, organically fed birds.

When it comes to red meat, lean is best, while things like fatty sausages and salami are the very worst. Avoid meat that has been through a feedlot; seek organic meat.

Protein Recommendations

- Eat a modest amount—2 ounces/day for the average person.
- Follow the hierarchy of protein sources. The more thorough you choose to be, the more you commit to the Healing Diet, the higher up this hierarchy you stay (e.g., the vegetable proteins are the ideal).
    - Vegetable proteins, known collectively as legumes or pulses: soybeans, tofu or bean curd, quinoa, lentils, chickpeas, any of the beans or peas.
    - Fish (preferably small deep-sea ones).
    - Eggs: two to four per week if agreeable; duck eggs may be suitable if hen eggs are not.
    - Dairy products: especially low-fat yogurt, cow's milk if suitable, soft cheeses. Goat's milk may be suitable if cow's milk is not.
    - Meat, in descending order of preference again: lean white meat such as rabbit or veal, free-range chicken, lean red meat, fatty meats.
- Minimize or avoid meat and dairy products, especially on the Healing Diet.
- Two to four genuine free-range eggs can be eaten weekly; eggs may be better avoided on the Healing Diet.
- Eat almonds regularly; the other nuts need to be fresh and uncooked.
- All grains have reasonable protein levels and warrant regular inclusion.
- Avoid burning all foods, and high-protein sources particularly.

CARBOHYDRATES

This is where we discuss grains and sugars. Grains are the main source of carbohydrates and receive fairly universal acceptance as a major part of any dietary approach. Grains certainly figure prominently in the Wellness Diet and the Healing Diet. However, as they are closely allied to the sugars, which receive a good deal of bad press, a little more explanation is warranted.

Nutritional Information

Carbohydrates are divided into four groups based upon their chemical structure. These groups are called monosaccharides, disaccharides, oligosaccharides and polysaccharides. Of more practical relevance, these are further divided into two groups that we hear of quite a deal, the simple carbohydrates or sugars (monosaccharides and disaccharides) and the complex carbohydrates or starches (oligosaccharides and polysaccharides).

Keeping it simple and avoiding going into a great deal of biochemistry, the complex carbohydrates are made up of aggregates of the simple carbohydrates. The simple carbohydrates include various sugars such as glucose (cane or white sugar), fructose (fruit sugar) and lactose (milk sugar). They provide a ready source of energy and are used to build the nucleic acids that make up our DNA.

Importantly, both sucrose from sugar and fructose from fruits are polysaccharides. What this means is that they need to be converted in the body to the monosaccharide glucose before being used as a source of energy. The speed of this conversion in the body is the crucial point—as the more rapidly it occurs, the more we experience a spike in our blood sugar levels and the more insulin is activated. Insulin, as well as regulating our blood sugar levels, is now recognized as playing a role in the modulation of the immune system and other aspects of healing. Insulin becoming overactivated by glucose spikes is increasingly recognized as a serious problem. Also, the insulin connection may well explain the long clinical experience of too much white sugar being a bad thing and why it is avoided strongly in many healing diets, including ours.

The rate at which all carbohydrates are metabolized into glucose will vary depending upon the source of the carbohydrate. Generally, simple sugars break down much faster than complex starches but fruit sugars are slowly metabolized, while processed or refined starches are fast.

The glycemic index (GI) and insulin index provide ways of assessing these metabolic rates in more detail, but in my clinical experience, there is no need to concern ourselves with these. I have observed some people becoming unnecessarily obsessive, even neurotic about these indices, and we aim to avoid stress and enjoy our food.

The crucial point is that sucrose from white sugar is metabolized very quickly and causes glucose spikes. In practice, fructose from fruit sugars and the more complex carbohydrates like starches do not metabolize so quickly and therefore are much safer to use.

In both animals and plants, energy is stored by combining simple carbohydrates into complex ones. In plants, these complex carbohydrates are commonly known as starches and we find them very commonly in the grains like wheat, rice, rye and so on. At the table they are predominant in bread, pasta, potatoes, corn (or maize) and cereals.

In animals and humans, the complex carbohydrates are stored as glycogen. This stored glycogen then requires a series of metabolic conversions to get back to the usable energy form of glucose. Interestingly, the body can obtain all its energy from fats and protein and do without carbohydrates altogether, but in most cultures, carbohydrates actually are a major source of energy.

Quantity

Major health bodies recommend about 45 percent to 65 percent of dietary energy comes from carbohydrates with the great majority of this coming from complex carbohydrates. The less simple carbohydrates or sugar we consume, the better.

One way of describing the Wellness Diet is to say it is high in fruit, vegetables and grains. It is best not to fixate too much on exact quantities, but to include a significant amount of grains in most meals. Two to three pieces of fruit per day are encouraged in both the Wellness Diet and the Healing Diet. The concerns some people raise about eating fruit sugars in my view are well satisfied by knowing that the conversion of fructose (fruit sugar) to glucose is a far slower process than that of sucrose (white sugar) to glucose. Fruit has many benefits and is recommended highly.

Wellness Rule 12: Use grains and fruit regularly.

Quality

As well as fruit, we need plenty of unprocessed complex carbohydrates. This includes good quality whole-grain bread made from wheat, rye or spelt, whole-grain pasta, or whole-grain rice. Processed carbohydrates such as those made from white flour and white rice, as well as being nutritionally poor, are digested very rapidly and cause significant, unhelpful blood sugar spikes.

Preparation

The digestion of most complex carbohydrates, as with grains, is improved by cooking. For example, while eating raw cereals such as muesli is fine if your digestion and energy level generally are robust, for those who are more fragile or delicate, porridge is easier.

Good-quality breads are widely available these days, but do check the ingredients. Avoid white flour and artificial or chemical additives. Also avoid the addition of seeds like sunflower or flaxseed in breads or other cooking, as they will have been oxidized by the heat of the cooking process. Spelt is a good bread flour and sourdough an ideal method of preparation. Flat or unleavened breads are also recommended.

Potatoes are best eaten with their skins, as are all vegetables and fruits where practical.

Rice is best cooked by the absorption method. Add about 50 percent more water than rice and boil in a saucepan with a lid on. When cooked, all the water will be absorbed.

Wellness Rule 13: Avoid processed foods generally and processed carbohydrates particularly. Eat plenty of whole grains and fresh fruit, eating the skins wherever possible. Prepare meals from raw ingredients as much as possible.

CARBOHYDRATE RECOMMENDATIONS

- Complex carbohydrates in grains along with in fruits are recommended as daily staples.
- Avoid processed or refined foods; eat whole grains, leave skins on wherever possible.
- Remember that grains do provide protein, as well as carbohydrates and their associated energy.

FIBER

Fiber was discussed under the section on digestion. Fiber is important in maintaining regular bowel motions, as well as acting as a sponge to absorb toxic material, including the waste products from digestion, and usher them through to elimination.

Quantity

A high-fiber diet is strongly recommended unless there are specific contra-indications from an active disease process or as a consequence of major bowel surgery.

In America 20 to 35gms of dietary fiber is recommended per day. While the average American consumes around 12 to 18gms, or half the recommended level, this amount is readily achieved using the Wellness Diet and the Healing Diet.

Quality

There are two main types of fiber, so-called soluble fiber and insoluble fiber.

Soluble fiber is able to be fermented in the large bowel, producing useful metabolic substances and some gas. Soluble fiber has a good range of benefits. It is known to reduce the risk of heart disease, helps to stabilize variations in blood sugars, may reduce the risk of developing diabetes, and may reduce glucose and insulin levels for those with clinical diabetes. Soluble fiber is commonly found in oats, (bran, rolled oats and oat flour), barley (the bran and barley flour) and psyllium husks.

Insoluble fiber is as it sounds, inert. It does not break down but can absorb water and is useful in aiding bulk to our stools and stimulating movement through the bowel. Insoluble fiber is known to alleviate constipation and has been closely linked to protecting against colon cancer. A good source is organic wheat or corn bran, while other sources are nuts, seeds (including flaxseed), potato skins and some vegetables.

Both types of fiber contribute to an increased feeling of being full and therefore may help to reduce appetite and stabilize healthy weight levels.

One major study of people aged from fifty to seventy showed that a high-fiber intake reduced the risk of dying over a nine-year period by nearly one quarter. Those on the high levels had significantly lower risk of heart disease, infections and respiratory diseases and lower cancer rates (especially among the men).

Preparation

Wherever possible eat whole foods. The husks of seeds removed during refining or processing are rich in fiber, as is the skin of most fruits and vegetables. It is particularly important to leave potato skins on both for the fiber and as the skins help to reduce the sugar spike peeled potatoes trigger.

It may well be useful to add a teaspoon of wheat bran and barley or oat bran to the daily diet and the easiest way to do this is to add them to morning oatmeal.

There is a caution with too much fiber. If you are not used to it, if you suddenly increase the amount of soluble fiber in your diet, there can be a rapid increase in gas production, with bloating and discomfort to you and maybe those around you! Also, if not enough water is taken with a high-fiber diet, it is possible to create constipation, which links nicely to the next section on fluids. So if you have been used to a low-fiber diet, all you need to do is to adapt slowly over a week or two.

FIBER RECOMMENDATIONS
- Eat a diet high in fiber by using whole grains and eating the skins of all suitable fruits and vegetables.
- Consider supplementing with a teaspoon of both wheat bran and barley or oat bran—most easily taken when cooked with oatmeal but possible to add to breads or other foods.

FLUIDS

Quantity

Generally it is recommended that the average person drink eight glasses of fluid in total each day. Many do not and as such are only partially hydrated.

> Wellness Rule 14: Drink at least eight glasses of fluid in total each day, ideally at times apart from meals.

Water

Fresh, pure water is an essential part of a healthy diet. Ideally, it is chlorine free, as chlorination is linked to a heightened risk of bladder cancer. As unchlorinated water has even greater risks (through infection) in most public water systems, this recommendation is not practical unless you have your own water supply or a water filter. The latter is highly recommended if you are on a chlorinated, public water system and most commercially available water filters do an adequate job. They have the added benefit of removing fluoride that remains contentiously linked to increased cancer rates and immunological impairment. I am not totally convinced by the antifluoride argument, but as adults we do not seem to need it and the chlorine risk seems well established; therefore, the filters make sense.

If you collect your own rainwater at home as we do, you need to be able to regulate its collection. We have a valve that we open after about an hour of heavy rain, which is how long it is said to reasonably clean the atmosphere and the roof, thereby ensuring good quality water is collected.

Juices

These are a feature of the Healing Diet and as such will be discussed in the next chapter.

Teas and Coffee

Black and green tea, along with coffee, contain caffeine. Caffeine is also found in cocoa, which is a major component in chocolate (and chocolate drinks), as well as Coca-Cola and of course the high-caffeine drinks like Red Bull. In the plants it comes from, caffeine serves as a pesticide, protecting the plants from being eaten by insects.

In humans, caffeine is mildly addictive. It is a potent stimulant of the central nervous system and it is the world's most widely consumed, legal psychoactive substance. It can help keep us awake and increase physical performance.

Some people are very sensitive to caffeine's effects, others adjust to them and notice very little. One of the best pointers to the downside of regular caffeine usage is the size and range of withdrawal effects. Within one to two days of stopping the use of caffeine, many people experience some or all of the following: headaches, irritability, lack of concentration, difficulty sleeping despite feeling sleepy, and aches and pains in the stomach, upper body and joints generally.

Most people I know who do cease drinking or eating caffeine report feeling much better for it. I certainly recommend avoiding or minimizing caffeine intake, especially on the Healing Diet.

Instead, use decaffeinated coffee along with herbal coffee substitutes and herbal teas.

Refer to Appendix I for the relative caffeine levels in teas, coffee and chocolate.

Alcohol

Alcohol consumption generally has been associated with a higher risk of several of the cancers of the digestive tract. The cancer link is a serious issue requiring consideration with beer. Chemically brewed beers have been directly linked to an increased incidence of colon cancer. Therefore, drink only naturally brewed beers if you drink any. There are very low alcohol, naturally brewed beer options that taste good. In Australia, Coopers Birell brand is excellent.

Of real concern is the fact that the metabolism of alcohol requires a good deal of liver activity. Alcoholics develop cirrhosis of the liver due to the excess strain involved. To recover from cancer, we need our livers to be functioning at their best, so we avoid alcohol on the Healing Diet.

See Appendix J for the approximate levels of alcohol in commonly used drinks.

ALCOHOL RECOMMENDATIONS
- On the Wellness Diet, social drinking a few days per week is acceptable.
- Ensure regular alcohol-free days.
- Consider using very low alcohol, naturally brewed beer.
- On the Healing Diet, alcohol is not recommended, primarily because of its effect on the liver.

OVERALL FLUID RECOMMENDATIONS
- Drink eight glasses of fluid, combined from all sources (water, tea, juices, soups) per day.

- Make healthy choices—with water, tea and coffee substitutes and alcohol.
- Add juices to the Healing Diet and consider their use on the Wellness Diet.

CONDIMENTS

Now we can consider those things we add to our food for taste and variety.

Salt

It is essential to know that the average diet more than meets the recommended daily allowance for salt. Unless one is working or exercising very hard in very hot conditions, there is no dietary need for additional salt.

Salt is a compound that consists of sodium chloride. The recommendation for sodium consumption for the average person is 1,500 to 2,300 milligrams per day.

Too much salt is linked with high blood pressure, stroke, heart disease and heart failure. Too little is associated with muscle cramps, dizziness and more general electrolyte imbalances that in extreme deficiencies can lead to neurological problems and even death.

More relevant to the cancer situation, and our health generally, is to understand that one of salt's primary roles in the body is to regulate the balance of water. A simple way to understand how this works is by knowing that salt, or more specifically sodium, is hydroscopic. That means salt draws water to it.

If we consume excess sodium via salt it does not accumulate in our blood. The levels of sodium and other ions in the blood are crucial for the healthy functioning of the body and as such, they are tightly regulated within fairly narrow boundaries. Our body will do its best to excrete the excess, but some will build up in our cells. Once in the cells, the extra sodium draws water into those cells, making them effectively "soggy." This is like having a water-logged garden; everything suffers. So excess sodium negatively affects the healthy metabolism of a wide range of our cells, contributing to a general malaise and significantly impairing regeneration and healing.

Finally, some people tout salt from exotic locations claiming special benefits for their product. All salt is made up of sodium chloride, regardless of its origin. Salt is salt. Avoid adding it to your food.

Wellness Rule 15: Adopt a low-salt diet; avoid salty foods and do not add salt to food.

Peppers and Chilies

These foods warrant special mention as they are in such popular use. Green pepper is the natural form of pepper but it is rarely used. Black pepper has been cooked and dried, while white pepper has been "refined," having the shell taken from the same type of seed that is the raw product for all peppers. White pepper tends to have a milder taste.

The use of pepper dates back to antiquity and it has been suggested to have a wide range of mildly medicinal purposes. It does have mild antioxidant properties and maybe some mild anticancer action. Caution is required by anyone with an irritated or inflamed bowel and probably any cancer affecting the bowel, because pepper is an irritant in its own right. It makes sense not to use pepper when on chemotherapy, as that treatment frequently affects the lining of the bowel, making it even more sensitive.

Chilies come from the capsicum family, and have a similar history of use to pepper. Chili also has some positive but minor health claims made for its use. However, it is far more irritating than pepper and as such has a strong potential to aggravate the lining of the bowel and impair digestion. Chili is not recommended for use at all.

Herbs and Seasonings

Garlic has been shown to be a natural antibiotic and antifungal agent, to decrease blood pressure, to have anticancer properties and is a chelating agent.

Ginger, like garlic, also makes an excellent seasoning while having special properties. Ginger stimulates stomach acid production, so aiding digestion. Ginger is particularly useful for people changing from a heavy meat-based diet to a more vegetarian way of eating.

Turmeric has many good anticancer properties, such as targeting cancer stem cells. It is best taken with black pepper to increase absorption.

Other acceptable seasonings are allspice, anise, bay leaves, celery seeds, coriander, dill, fennel, mace, marjoram, rosemary, sage, saffron, tarragon, thyme and summer savory.

Most herbs that are made into teas have medicinal properties and need to be used wisely. Any of the mints make a good refreshing drink and can be used cold in summer. They have a tannin content, so do not overdo them. However, peppermint is particularly useful to aid digestion, soothe the bowel and decrease flatulence. Chamomile, a mild sedative, aids sleep, soothes upset stomach and bowel, and decreases flatulence. Chamomile can be useful before bed.

Coltsfoot is excellent for chest complaints, particularly if mucus needs to be cleared—it is a good expectorant. Prepare by adding two tablespoons of leaves to one pint of boiling water, stand for about ten minutes, strain, then add one teaspoonful of honey and the juice of a quarter of a lemon. Drop the squeezed lemon into the drink also.

Roasted dandelion root coffee (some people call it dandelion tea) is an excellent liver tonic. One to three cups each day are well worth considering. Boil or percolate as for normal coffee, then strain. Add honey or a suitable "milk" if preferred.

Sea Vegetables

Sea vegetables are an important source of iodine, a common deficiency in many soils and hence the food grown on them. It is wise to use sea vegetables regularly, including kelp powder for stews, and nori for salads and rolls.

Sprouts

Sprouts are recommended as an integral part of the diet. We use them regularly in our programs and they are easy to prepare—see Appendix K.

Broccoli seed sprouts are available in many supermarkets these days and have very strong anticancer properties.

CONDIMENT RECOMMENDATIONS

- Add no salt to food unless you're hot and sweaty!
- Use pepper but not chili on the Wellness Diet. Avoid both on the Healing Diet, especially if having chemotherapy or you have a sensitive bowel.
- Most culinary herbs and spices are suitable.
- Use ginger, garlic and turmeric (with black pepper) regularly.
- Use sea vegetables (seaweeds) regularly.
- Consider the regular consumption of sprouts.

SPECIFIC CONSIDERATIONS

Fresh vs. Stored

One of the quickest, most effective ways to improve your diet rapidly is to eat meals that are prepared from fresh, raw ingredients. This means avoiding processed foods. Doing so will save you and your family many potential problems, but then raises the questions of cooking, convenience and storage.

For convenience, the solution is to develop a core group of simple, quick whole-food, plant-based recipes that can be varied easily and endlessly by altering the raw ingredients. So, whether salads or cooked meals, you have your basic recipes that you eat most of the time, and the more elaborate recipes you trot out on special occasions. One problem I find with many recipe books is that they focus on the "party food," what you would prepare for honored guests, and not the day-to-day stuff. On my blog are a group of very simple recipes to get started with that take twenty to thirty minutes maximum to prepare, and all good and very tasty. *The New Gawler Foundation Cookbook* contains many well-tested, easy-to-prepare, tasty recipes.[19]

Regarding storage, of course the refrigerator is very useful and OK. Ideally, and especially when facing active illness, it is best to start every meal with fresh, whole and vital ingredients. When you are really well, that is the ideal to aim for, but most people have occasions where a particularly quick meal is convenient or longer storage is necessary. Sun drying works well for things like apricots, sultanas and currants. Freezing is also an option and good details are available on the BBC's Good Food website, as well as stilltasty.com. Cans of precooked, organic chickpeas, other legumes and tomatoes can be useful to have on hand for when time is at a premium.

Avoid artificially preserved foods thoroughly. This may come under the heading of too much information, but undertakers say that just a few decades ago, dead bodies left in the heat would begin to deteriorate within a matter of hours. Now, due to the high content of preservatives in our food, commonly they last for three or four days, sometimes even more! That cannot be good.

Cooked vs. Raw

On the Wellness Diet, a balance of cooked and raw food is recommended. This balance is influenced by climate, availability and personal metabolism. In a tropical environment, a largely raw diet can work well all year round. In a cold winter, many people struggle on raw food and require a much higher level of cooking. In broad terms, for healthy people, a significant proportion of the diet is raw, the rest cooked. This statement is deliberately vague, as the diet does vary greatly depending on individual circumstances.

When it comes to those dealing with cancer, many Western practitioners who have focused intensively on treating this disease nutritionally recommend an all-raw diet. By contrast, most practitioners of traditional Chinese medicine (TCM), which has a history going back thousands of years, recommend a mostly cooked diet. In my experience, people are different. Some do well on cooked food, some on raw; many are best suited to a mixture. How to solve this and what to do on the Healing Diet will be addressed in the next chapter.

Cooking

For utensils, use stainless steel, cast iron, glass, tin, enamel or earthenware. Do not use aluminum or plastics, and avoid nonstick materials like Teflon.

To cook your food, use steaming, dry baking, a wok, or sautéing in water only. Boil rice and other grains, bake bread and slow stew on low heat. Do not cook with oils, especially avoid deep-frying and do not use microwave cooking.

Prepare your food with love and joy. Enjoy!

Organic Produce

We live in polluted times. Choosing organic produce wherever possible is good for us and good for the environment. Go organic and consider establishing a vegetable garden—or delight in the one you have!

If commercial food is used, most surface pollutants can be washed off in a 1 percent solution of white vinegar.

If juicing, chemicals and pollutants have been shown to concentrate more in the fiber of fruits and vegetables, so juicing actually helps remove some of them. Therefore, if you need to make a choice, eat the organic produce and juice the commercial produce.

Chemical Additives

There are a myriad of artificial colorings and flavorings used these days. It is said that around a hundred years ago, there were only about two hundred food chemicals in use around the world. Now the figure is put at more than eighty thousand! The average person is estimated to have more than a thousand food chemicals in their body at any one time. It begs belief that this is not a major problem. It makes sense to avoid chemicals whenever possible and to consider the detoxing principles we will cover in the next chapter.

> Wellness Rule 16: Read the labels of all commercially prepared food and use a chart that explains the number codes for the additives. Wherever possible, prepare food from natural, organic ingredients and minimize exposure to, or intake of, chemicals and additives.

Plastics

Plastics have been a mixed blessing. With so many uses, their pollution issues are beginning to become overwhelming. Of real concern is that some of the chemicals in plastics, particularly some of the plasticizers used to soften and mold plastics, mirror female sex hormones. These can accumulate in the fats or oils we eat and then build up in our own fatty tissue. There is suspicion this may aggravate breast cancer.

> Wellness Rule 17: Keep plastic out of your kitchen, do not buy or store food wrapped in plastic, especially the plastic cling wraps. Go back to simpler times. Use wooden spoons; ceramic, wooden or stainless steel bowls. Keep plastics away from your food!

Supplements

These will be addressed in the next chapter.

Food Allergies and Intolerances

Food allergies are acute, often severe reactions to food, whereas food intolerances lead to more common, low-level chronic reactions. So someone who has an allergy to seafood may eat an oyster and have an acute reaction that requires hospitalization. Almost always, people know when they have a genuine food allergy, and happily not many people do have them.

Far more common, however, are food intolerances. These can be associated with physical symptoms such as irritable bowel syndrome (IBS) or simply reduced efficiency in digestion. Some individual foods can be identified as causes of intolerance, quite a number of artificial chemical food additives and colorings are well-known problems, while some chemicals that occur naturally in foods are closely linked.

Cow's milk is an example of a food that has a strong capacity to produce both allergy (usually not severe), as well as intolerance (more common), while MSG is a chemical that can produce mild to severe reactions. Significantly, as well as being a common additive in Chinese cooking, MSG occurs naturally in small amounts in many foods.

Of the chemicals that occur naturally in foods and are known to cause intolerances, salicylates pose the biggest issue. Salicylates occur to some degree in nearly all foods, although there is not much in the high-protein foods. Salicylates are linked with flavor; generally the more flavor, the more salicylates, and they are intimately linked with the plants' self-defense systems. Common major sources of salicylates are strawberries, tomatoes (where concentrating the tomatoes into juice, paste and sauce leads to large increases in the salicylate content), fruits (citrus particularly), berries and wine.

Symptoms of food intolerances can include itchy skin, abdominal pain, bloating, diarrhea or constipation, swelling in the face particularly, but also the hands and feet, headaches, hyperactivity, poor concentration, depression and fatigue. Inflammatory processes including chronic ear infections, cystitis and tonsillitis have been linked by many people. Quite a list!

What to do? If you have a chronic history with the symptoms listed above, be aware that food intolerance may be the issue. In mild cases, it may be enough to simply avoid the major known causes of intolerance and eat their substitutes—(see the chart below). Accurate testing can be carried out by medical specialists in this field and involves using elimination diets and food challenges. However, over the years, many participants in this program have solved food intolerance issues by developing their own food

Foods associated with significant food intolerances	Alternatives
Wheat	Use other grains.
Cow's milk	Goat's milk may be suitable.
Hens' eggs	Duck eggs may be suitable.
Chocolate	Use carob.
Shellfish Pollen Strawberries, tomatoes, citrus	Avoid if necessary.

sensitivity and awareness. Further discussion of how to do this will be found in the next chapter.

On Eating Itself

Avoid processed and refined foods such as white flour, white rice and margarine. The diet needs to be low in salt, sugars, fats and proteins. Concentrate on fresh vital foods, primarily vegetables, fruits and grains. Wherever possible, use foods that are in season and grown within approximately 800 kms (about 500 miles) of where you live.

Aim to prepare and eat your food with a sense of joy and the expectation that it will help you back to total health. Take a short time before you eat to be still, relax and be thankful.

Do not overeat. Do chew your food well—to the consistency of mashed ripe bananas. Digestion begins in the mouth and is aided by a happy, positive disposition. Smile!

Recipes

Once you are clear on what you will and will not eat, studying recipe books becomes easier. Some recipes can be easily modified—leaving out, adding or substituting where necessary.

The best recipe book to begin with is the *New Gawler Foundation Cookbook*.

Binges and Breakouts

If you are basically fit and mostly eat this way, you have some leeway. When you are well, what you eat mainly is most important, what you eat occasionally is not such an issue. When your health is fragile, what you eat all the time is important.

THE WELLNESS DIET • The Final Word

In the next chapter we will be considering the Healing Diet. Charts containing recommendations for a large range of foods from asparagus to zucchini will be presented for you to consider and use as the basis for your personalized plan.

Remember, the Wellness Diet aims to establish healthy boundaries. The intention in this chapter has been to provide enough information to give you clarity and confidence to begin to establish a sound, accessible and healthy pattern of eating.

The Healing Diet aims to examine the prospects of using nutrition therapeutically and to help you to individualize your choices. So read on, consider the information in the next food chapter and then put your plan together.

CHAPTER 14

Nutrition 4

Eating for Recovery: The Healing Diet

THE INTENTION OF THE HEALING DIET IS TO NOURISH OUR BODY WITH THE best possible combination of foods. Eating for recovery aims to use nutrition therapeutically and as such offers considerable cause for hope, a very real means of activating our own personal resources, and the prospect of making a significant contribution to recovery from cancer.

On the Wellness Diet what you eat mostly is important. On the Healing Diet what you eat all the time is important. The crucial point of the mind, however, emphasizes that we choose to enjoy what we do, and so we need to monitor stress, be clear on our motivation, overcome any destructive emotions or habits and cultivate a sense of optimism, joy and delight in being able to use our nutrition, what we eat, to powerfully affect our chances of becoming well and staying well. Therefore, on the Healing Diet:

Wellness Rule 18: Be particular about what you eat. Eat for recovery and enjoy it!

There are two ways to take up the Healing Diet, the gradual approach and the rapid approach.

THE GRADUAL METHOD FOR ADOPTING THE HEALING DIET

This is a systematic approach that will suit the needs and disposition of many people. The aim is to progress steadily, taking the big, obvious steps first and then attending to the finer details. These general guidelines are based on existing research and the clinical experience I have developed over thirty years working with many people who have taken their nutrition very seriously.

This gradual method involves six steps:

Step 1. Adopt the general guidelines of the Healing Diet.
Step 2. Add regular juices.
Step 3. Regularly consume foods with known anticancer properties.
Step 4. Create a cancer-unfriendly environment in your body by eating foods that positively manipulate your metabolism.
Step 5. Consider the uses of supplements and other natural products.
Step 6. Once the above five steps are in place, progress to develop your awareness, to experiment and establish a personalized pattern of eating for recovery.

THE RAPID APPROACH TO THE HEALING DIET

This is an option for those who are keen, who maybe have more severe disease, and those who like to dive headlong into things that are good for them. This rapid method is similar to the gradual method, but begins more intensively.

Step 1. Heighten your awareness, meditate, start the process with a detox, then adopt the Healing Diet and be vigilant regarding what food agrees with you and what does not.
Steps 2–6. The same as steps 1–5 above.

First we will elaborate the gradual method, then the rapid method.

THE HEALING DIET, OPTION: THE GRADUAL METHOD

Step 1. Adopt the General Recommendations of the Healing Diet

We need the very best nutrition to fuel recovery. So where there are foods that have reservations raised about them, and which on the Wellness Diet we might eat occasionally, on the Healing Diet we leave them out altogether.

Examples of this are meat, dairy products and eggs. Also, we are more thorough in avoiding salt, sugar, refined foods and so on.

Full details are provided in the following lists. The lists build on, and in many instances, summarize what was explained in the previous chapter.

Do be reminded again that these lists are offered as an introductory guide only. Each person needs to pursue their own research, using these lists as a starting point.

What to Avoid and What to Do

	Avoid	What to Do
1	**Unhealthy Fats**	**Use Fats Wisely**
	(a) Saturated fats, omega-6 fatty acids and rancidity	1–2 tablespoons of cold-pressed vegetable oil (use linseed [flax], oil or olive oil) per day is maximum to add to diet. Avoid sources of saturated fat (e.g., animal fat, palm and coconut oils). Store and prepare oils carefully.
	(b) Oils overheated in cooking	Avoid cooking with oils. Preferably sauté with water instead of frying and only use those oils that are most stable if you do choose to cook with them (e.g., olive oil).
	(c) Oils used for repeated frying	Avoid deep-frying, especially with the same oil.
	(d) Unshelled nuts and seeds	Ideally, buy nuts in shells. Do not use shelled sunflowers seeds, which have had long storage times (see Nuts in the previous chapter). Do not cook seeds or nuts.
	(e) Wheat germ oil begins to go rancid one week after processing.	Do not use it.
	(f) Flour begins to go rancid three days after milling.	Use your own home flour mill or obtain flour freshly ground at health food store, co-op, etc.
	(g) Vegetable oils stored in clear containers	Buy them in amber glass or tin containers. Flaxseed oil needs to be refrigerated.
2	**Unhealthy Proteins**	**Eat Modest Amounts of Protein**
	Meat and dairy products are better avoided on the Healing Diet (minimized on the Wellness Diet).	There are many low-protein sources in the diet that add to the overall total, the most notable of which are the grains. Add to this a maximum of 3 pounds, 3 ounces, in total per week of high-protein foods.
		On the Healing Diet, vegetable proteins are the best to use. On the Wellness Diet, there is a hierarchy, vegetable = best, down to fatty meats = worst. Revisit all the details in the last chapter and choose wisely.
3	**Unhealthy Sugars**	**Keep Sugar Intake Low**
	White sugar and refined carbohydrates provide empty calories and should be avoided.	About 1 teaspoonful of natural honey or pure maple syrup is daily maximum. Use whole-grain products.

	Avoid	What to Do
4	**Added Salt**	**Adopt a Low-Salt Diet**
	No extra is needed in cooking or at the table. (Possible exception being people who work very hard in hot weather and sweat profusely.)	Leave it out and watch your taste buds redevelop. Or, substitute by using vitamin C (only the sodium ascorbate version of vitamin C) in equivalent amounts.
5	**Alcohol**	**Little or No Alcohol**
	Best avoided on the Healing Diet as it stresses the liver, but a small amount on the Wellness Diet is OK.	On the Wellness Diet, stick to social drinking and have regular alcohol-free days.
6	**Caffeine**	**Go Caffeine Free**
	Is in coffee, tea, chocolate. A controversial area but, in balance, we prefer to avoid caffeine.	Use herb teas, fruit juices, etc. It is also wise to avoid other artificial soda drinks.
7	**Tobacco or Marijuana**	**QUIT! (If Necessary)**
	These are self-destructive habits—find a better one! Thirty percent of all cancers are directly attributable to smoking.	Stop! Find a more appropriate way of gaining pleasure and dealing with stress. Marijuana is hard on the immune system and is associated with mental illness.
8	**Aflatoxins**	**Be Careful with Peanuts and Mold**
	Aflatoxins are a fungus that can contaminate peanuts especially, and other carbohydrates—mostly in tropical areas and are linked with liver cancer.	Restrict the use of peanuts unless aflatoxin levels are known. Peanuts are also high in oil and are probably best avoided or kept for special occasions only. Avoid any part of food with signs of fungus or mold on it anywhere. (Such growth may not be aflatoxins, but it can be dangerous.)
9	**Ionizing Radiation**	**Avoid Sunburn and Minimize X-Rays, Especially CAT Scans**
	(a) Excessive exposure to sunlight (ultraviolet rays are the problem and cause skin cancer).	Refer to the section on vitamin D. Cover your skin, wear a hat. Use sunscreen lotions sparingly. Fair-haired, pale-skinned people in the tropics require extra caution to avoid excess sun contact.
	(b) Excessive X-rays. Any X-ray is associated with a risk—the more X-rays, the more risk.	While modern X-rays have low exposure, their benefits need to be weighed against the risk. Pregnant women and young children need to be extremely careful. CAT scans have very high radiation levels and need to be used very wisely.
10	**Pollution**	**Go Green**
	Particularly the end products from the combustion of fossil fuels are suspect.	Be aware of caring for your environment.

Problems and Solutions—What to Do

	Problems and Solutions	What to Do
1	**Start Your Meals with Raw Ingredients**	
	Processed and convenience foods commonly have food preservatives, additives and colorings and they lack vitality.	Learn to prepare quick, simple and tasty whole-food meals from raw ingredients; the benefits will be immediate.
2	**Use Healthy Cooking Techniques**	
	Smoked food, charcoal broiling and barbecuing can all cause pyrolysis and lead to production of dangerous polycyclic hydrocarbons.	Use steaming, dry baking, Chinese-style wok cooking, or cook over a low heat with minimal water that should not be discarded. Do not eat food that has been burned black.
3	**Combine Foods Wisely**	
	Imagine your stomach trying to sort out lobster bisque, beef Stroganoff with a side salad, watermelon, all washed down with coffee, then cheese!	To avoid internal warfare consider the food combining chart—Appendix L.
4	**Maintain High-Fiber Levels**	
	Fiber hastens elimination and its bulk protects the bowel from many problems.	Always use whole-meal grains. Avoid peeling vegetables; merely wash and scrub with brush.
5	**Use Chemical-Free Foods**	
	Some artificial colorings are still used in Australia despite being removed from U.S. markets because of possible associated risks. Flavorings such as monosodium glutamate (MSG) are suspect, as are some preservatives, particularly the nitrites. There are too many doubts about chemical additives. It is practical to avoid many of them.	Read labels. Aim to eat fresh, whole unprocessed food. If not always possible, it is preferable to avoid chemical additives but make sure the food has been properly stored or preserved. There is good evidence that adequate use of preservatives and refrigeration actually decreases the incidence of stomach cancer.
		Use suitable herbs and seasonings, but avoid regular use of hot spices, chili, commercial mustards and sauces.
6	**Use Chemical-Free Products**	
	We live in such a polluted environment that it is wise to avoid whatever chemicals we can. Many chemicals are low-level toxins or carcinogens. Together they become a formidable cocktail.	Do all you can to minimize the chemicals in your environment. Use natural health care products and chemical-free products in the kitchen, home and garden.
7	**Go Organic**	
	A huge range of chemicals is used in commercial food production and it is not possible that the effects of all of them are fully understood.	Seek out organically grown food and encourage its supply. The less chemical unknowns in your diet, the better. Wherever possible, establish your own veggie garden.
8	**Drink Pure, Clean Water**	
	Fluoride is helpful for children's teeth but questionable for cancer patients. Chlorine is definitely best to avoid.	Preferably use spring water or rainwater. Consider a purifier for your main's water.

	Problems and Solutions	What to Do
9	**Keep Aluminum and Plastic Away from Foods**	
	There is no clear-cut evidence, but many questions and doubts persist concerning aluminum cookware and deodorants—some may contain up to 20 percent aluminum. Plastic is a real problem.	Use stainless steel, glass, enamel, cast iron, earthenware or tin cookware. Keep plastic away from your food, including avoiding buying food wrapped in plastic. Use aluminum-free deodorants. Read labels.
10	**Aim for a Lean Weight**	
	The overweight develop more cancers than lean people. Being lean may aid recovery. As so many people are overweight, losing some weight can be healthy.	Be on the lean side. Better to undereat than overeat. Most people on this type of diet tend to a lean optimal weight. Exercise regularly.
11	**Sex Is Fun, Avoid Excesses!**	
	Too much or too little is a problem! Late age at first child's birth or little or no breast-feeding is associated with an increase in breast cancer for women, while there is an increased risk of cervical cancer if a male partner is promiscuous.	Moderation in all things. Mothers are recommended to exclusively breast-feed their babies for the first six months of life, if possible.
12	**Enjoy Life, Minimize Stress**	
	An inability to cope with stress appropriately is a common factor in the lives of many people who develop cancer.	Avoid stress where possible, but also learn how to cope with it. Meditation, contemplation and positive thinking work wonders.

The Use and Preparation of 39 Vegetables and 28 Fruits

Here are detailed charts that set out the recommendations regarding what vegetables and fruits to use and how to prepare them. The recommendations for the Healing Diet and the Wellness Diet are included. Under the Healing heading, vegetables that need to be cooked for easy digestion are identified, and, of course, if you were on an all-raw diet they would not be eaten unless raw.

List of Vegetable Uses

*J = juice   R = raw   S = steam   B = bake   Sa = sauté in water, wok

Vegetable	Healing	Wellness	Preparation*	Comments
Artichoke—Globe	Yes	Yes	S	Good for diabetics. Low-allergenic food.
Artichoke—Jerusalem	Yes	Yes	S B	Highly recommended—be careful with bloating—try a little first if they are new to you.

Vegetable	Healing	Wellness	Preparation*	Comments
Bell peppers	Yes	Yes	J R S B Sa	Red has more vitamin C than green. Juice good for sore throat.
Beetroot	Yes	Yes	J R S B	Good blood builder. Combines well with other juices. Anticancer folk remedy.
Beetroot tops	Yes	Yes	J R S	Do have a little oxalic acid, but a good source of potassium.
Broccoli	Cooked	Yes	R S Sa	All brassicas are associated with cancer-protecting factors.
Brussels sprouts	Cooked	Yes	S Sa	Brassica.
Cabbage	Yes	Yes	R S Sa	Brassica. Small amount of cabbage juice is good for ulcers and upset stomachs. Is acid forming. Can be gas producing, especially for older people—not so bad steamed.
Carrot	Yes	Yes	J R S B Sa	Excellent juice. Highly recommended. Source of vitamin A. Combines well with other juices.
Cauliflower	Cooked	Yes	R S Sa	Brassica. Caution with gas, if raw. Good source of calcium.
Celery	Yes	Yes	J R S Sa	Good source of potassium and excellent tonic for urinary system. Avoid the tops.
Chayote	Cooked	Yes	S B Sa	
Chicory	Yes	Yes	R S	Steam in other greens.
Chili	No	No		Too stimulating.
Cucumber	Yes	Yes	J R	Juice aids treatment of kidney and gallstones. Avoid "apple" varieties—too acidic. Lebanese or Burpless are best, more alkaline.
Eggplant	Caution	Yes	S B Sa	Can aggravate arthritic conditions and may be unhelpful on Healing Diet.
Garlic	Yes	Yes	R S Sa	Good condiment, flavoring, dressing. One clove of garlic in carrot juice works well. Worm treatment. Blood cleanser. Can be pickled. Sauté leads to less aromatic acids. Chelating agent for heavy metals. Recommended for chemotherapy patients. Regulates blood pressure. Has anticancer properties.
Ginger	Yes	Yes	J R	Use regularly and preferably fresh. Excellent addition to vegetables, particularly for vegetarians. Good to stimulate stomach acid and spleen function. Can add to carrot juice. Use for flavoring.
Horseradish	Yes	Yes	R	Aids lung conditions, emphysema. Condiment.
Kohlrabi	Occasional	Yes	B	
Leek	Cooked	Yes	S B Sa	

Vegetable	Healing	Wellness	Preparation*	Comments
Mushroom	Occasional	Yes	R Sa	
Okra	Cooked	Yes	S Sa	
Onion	Cooked	Yes	R S B Sa	High in aromatic acids. Good for helping with weight reduction. Better cooked than raw.
Parsnip	Cooked	Yes	S B	High calcium source.
Potatoes: Common	Yes	Yes	S B	Skins good for potassium. Baking especially recommended.
Potatoes: Sweet	Yes	Yes	S B	
Pumpkin	Yes	Yes	R S B	Easily digested.
Pumpkin seeds	Yes	Yes	R S B	Excellent for zinc.
Radish	Occasional	Yes	R	Stimulant—use moderately.
Rutabaga	Cooked	Yes	S B	
Spinach	Yes	Yes	J R S	High oxalic acid content—use 2–3 times per week at maximum.
Squash	Cooked	Yes	R S B	
Sweet corn	Yes	Yes	R S B	Can be baked in husk (475°F).
Swiss chard	Yes	Yes	J R S	High oxalic acid content—use 2–3 times per week at maximum.
Tomato	Yes	Yes	J R S B Sa	Solanum. Excellent source of vitamin C. 1 gram per large naturally ripened tomato. Less acidic varieties are the cherry types and Roma.
Turnip	Cooked	Yes	S B	
Watercress	Yes	Yes	J R	Good for arthritis.
Zucchini	Yes	Yes	R S B Sa	

List of Fruit Uses

Fruit	Healing	Wellness	Preparation*	Comments
Apple	Yes	Yes	J R B Sa	Cook in juice or water.
Apricot	Yes	Yes	J R Sa	Good sun-dried (soak before eating). Kernels can be source of B_{17}, eaten with fruit. Start with 5, add 1 each day up to 15, or, if headache occurs, decrease.
Avocado	Occasional	Yes	R B	High fat content. Tastes terrific!
Banana	Yes	Yes	R B	Excellent source of potassium. Gentle on upset stomach. Common allergen. Eat when ripe.
Berries:				
Strawberries	No	Occasional	J R Jam	Make into jam with honey. Blood builders. Acidity can be a problem and very high in salicylates (major cause of food intolerance).

Fruit	Healing	Wellness	Preparation*	Comments
Blueberries, Raspberries	Yes	Yes	J R	Raspberries have powerful anticancer activity.
Cherry	Yes	Yes	J R Sa	Good source of iron.
Citrus fruits	Yes	Yes	J R	Grapefruit, limes, mandarins, lemons. Good to start day with. Oranges require care with their acidity.
Fig	Occasional	Occasional	R S	High sugar. Excellent laxative.
Grapes	Yes	Yes	J R	Very good blood cleanser. Excellent tonic. See "The Mono Diet" later in this Chapter. Red grapes build blood, white cleanse intestines.
Mango	Yes	Yes	J R	Very palatable!
Melons	Yes	Yes	J R	Cantaloupe, watermelon, honeydew. Good kidney tonics. Eat on own—not with other fruits, foods (see food combinations Appendix L).
Nectarine	Yes	Yes	J R S	
Papaya or Pawpaw	Yes	Yes	J R	Excellent source of papain, a potent digestive enzyme.
Passionfruit	Yes	Yes	R S	
Peach	Yes	Yes	J R S	
Pear	Yes	Yes	J R S	Juice is a gentle laxative.
Persimmon	Yes	Yes	R	Must be ripe.
Pineapple	No	Occasional	J R	Contains bromelain, an enzyme reputed by some to take the outer layer off tumors. But require care with acidity.
Plum	Yes	Yes	J R S	
Pomegranate	Yes	Yes	J R	Powerful anticancer properties.
Prune	Yes	Yes	J R S	Laxative. Improves blood iron.
Rhubarb	No	Very occasional	S	High oxalic acid content.

Step 2. Add Regular Juices

Eating a lot of fresh, vital food gets the healing process in motion. It is accentuated by the use of freshly prepared juices.

JUICING 101

Juices are an ideal source of easily digestible nutrients in a well-balanced package. Freshly made, they are also full of oxidative enzymes. Authorities like Gerson believed they could help reoxygenate cancerous tissue and revitalize the rest of the body. Gerson advocated drinking juices on an hourly basis, twelve each day—hence the time commitment for those on his diet. I would recommend the need for moderation, depending upon the individual situation.

In my experience, most people on the Healing Diet find that seven per day is manageable and effective.

Wellness Rule 19: Drink seven juices daily.

The general recommendation is seven 200ml (7 oz.) juices to be taken daily.

Start the morning with citrus, preferably one-third lemon juice in two-thirds water. Other citrus may be OK, but be careful with oranges, particularly because they are quite acidic and people with brain tumors have reported them to be problematic over the years.

Next, have apple, grape, carrot, beetroot (one-third each of beetroot, carrot and celery) and two green juices. Two good options to consider for use when available or for variety and good effect are pomegranate juice (that is very good against prostate cancer and is protective against radiotherapy side effects) and the Australian blend of anticancer juices called Dr Red's ginger punch (order via the Internet).

Apple and grape, along with pomegranate juice, can be bought if pure, organically grown juices are available, while the others are best made fresh. The green juices can be made from a combination of celery (not the leaves), green pepper, lettuce, a little cabbage, beetroot tops, Swiss chard or spinach and a little parsley.

The recommendation is that ideally you do make all the green juices freshly. However, for convenience you can use commercially prepared barley juice that comes as a powder, prepared by the rapid dehydration of the juice of young barley shoots. This powder is excellent to take traveling—all you need to do is add water.

Most juices have an acceptable taste, and some are positively pleasant. Orange, apple, grape and carrot are all old favorites. The taste of green juices requires more explanation before they can be relished. Gerson claimed that the oxidative enzymes in these juices were able to enter into the bloodstream and exert a direct effect. Certainly the chlorophyll molecule, the main constituent of green plants, is very similar in structure to hemoglobin, the main constituent of red blood cells. Chlorophyll has a central magnesium molecule, hemoglobin iron; otherwise they are identical.

Wheatgrass

Wheatgrass is a special green juice that may be a great aid to restoring the degenerated metabolism of people affected by cancer. Freshly sprouted wheat is cut off when the shoots are four to five inches high and juiced. This juice is hard to extract without a specialized juicer, but a good alternative is to chew the shoots, swallow the juice, and spit out the fiber—delicately, of course.

Liver Juice

Gerson also placed great value on raw liver juice. This may sound a trifle revolting, and the taste is certainly nothing to rave over, but again, it makes sense especially if your blood count is down or you have other blood disorders. The liver is recognized as the best nutritional source of the components that build the blood. Based on its nutrient content, dietitians would certainly rate it as one of the best individual foods. So, why not cook it and eat the whole lot? Why the need to have it as a fresh raw juice? Cooking can affect the vitamins, enzymes, cofactors and other suspected, but as yet unidentified, beneficial substances in liver. Also, the fiber in it is very tough and the digestion of a person with cancer is often incapable of dealing with it well. It could undergo delayed passage through the bowel, putrefy and then add to the toxicity of the body. So, the juice avoids the fiber while saving all the goodness.

Liver juice, like wheatgrass, is hard to make, and chewing the liver in pieces, swallowing the juice and leaving the fiber is a possibility. Chewing raw liver is even less joy than drinking liver juice, so a minimum of cooking—thirty to sixty seconds grilling each side—is a fair compromise. Still, spit out that fiber! Combining the lightly cooked liver with well-grilled tomato improves the taste, while sucking a lemon afterward clears the palate if you feel the need.

Juice Machines

The normal commercial juicer uses a centrifugal action that shreds the food, then spins it at high speed. This is a fine way to separate the pulp from the juice, and the juice is packed with nutrients, vitamins and minerals. However, it is claimed that the centrifugal action of these machines creates static electricity that destroys some of the oxidative enzymes in the juice. Gerson asserted this and claimed he saw better results when using a machine that had no static in it. He recommended a machine that separately grinds and then presses the juices out by hydraulic action. Fine in theory, but expensive in practice. The Norwalk machine he preferred now costs around $2,400! The Champion juicer seems like a reasonable alternative, costing around $550 and is like a mechanized meat-mincer in its action. These machines do also extract more juice from the same amount of ingredients than the standard machines and are easy to operate and to clean. So, if you are serious about juices, the Champion is well worth considering.

Step 3. Focus on Foods with Known Anticancer Properties

Over one thousand chemicals possessing anticancer properties have been identified in the foods we eat. Of course, some of these chemicals are quite mild in their action, but fortunately some are quite potent. It makes obvious good sense to identify and regularly consume the potent anticancer foods.

First, however, let us be clear, a diet that is rich in fresh, organic and judiciously cooked vegetables and fruits will contain a myriad of anticancer agents. While these agents are being researched more (often with the motivation of identifying the active ingredient and marketing that), it is quite probable many are synergistic. That means they could support each other's benefits and create a sum total of benefit far above their individual merits. The opposite effect of this is well researched in the causes of cancer. For example, as we will discuss further in the next chapter, smoking tobacco and drinking alcohol together create a far greater risk of developing cancer than the sum of the risks associated with one factor on its own.

> Wellness Rule 20: Consider your Healing Diet as a whole to have general anti-cancer properties. On top of this, take advantage of the potent anticancer foods and consume them regularly.

Traditionally, folk medicine in Europe highly recommended asparagus and beetroot for their anticancer properties. Asparagus is known to be a good antioxidant and high in vitamin C, folate and potassium. Beetroot is also rich in antioxidants, vitamin C, magnesium, potassium, boron and betaine. Older beetroot produces betanin, especially in its roots, and this is unpleasant to taste (bitter) and causes red stools and urine, which can be distressing if you do not know what caused it! Despite all this, there are no scientific studies supporting the known anticancer properties of asparagus or beetroot, but I ate a good deal of both while recovering, and continue to do so.

Anticancer Food Recommendations

1. Eat at least one generous portion of brassicas daily.
2. Consume half a medium Chinese or ordinary green cabbage every few days.
3. Eat one or more of raspberries, pomegranates, tomatoes and beans daily. Make sure one of these four is in the daily diet and rotate them around.
4. Use turmeric and/or garlic and ginger daily. Rotate their use.

Step 4. Create a Cancer-Unfriendly Environment—How to Stimulate Healing via Metabolic Change

All living organisms have preferred conditions that support their life. This is very obvious in the garden where camellias, for example, thrive in acid soils but struggle and even die in an alkaline environment.

Vegetables do poorly in acid soils and thrive in more alkaline conditions, so it makes sense if we have acidic soil and intend to grow healthy vegetables that we add lime to make the ground more alkaline. The key point is that if we put vegetables in soil that is too acidic, they will die; put camellias in alkaline soil and we can kill them.

> Wellness Rule 21: Make the food choices that inhibit cancer and promote healing.

One of the elegant ways we can influence cancer is to use this principle and learn how to manipulate our metabolism in a range of ways that work against the disease. Here is how we do it.

Anticancer Diet Recommendations

This is an area of great possibility. From what follows, make an action list that clarifies the anticancer approach you will adopt and delight in eating for recovery. Bon appétit!

Ten Top Anticancer Foods—And How to Use Them

Food	Main Active Ingredients	Action	Usage
1. Raspberries	Ellagic acid	Inhibits cancer cells from dividing. Powerful antioxidant.	½ cup daily. Frozen is OK.
2. Pomegranates	Ellagic acid—about 50 times more concentrated than raspberries	Same as raspberries.	A small amount of fruit or juice daily. Very good against prostate cancer.
3. Turmeric	Curcumin	Antioxidant, anti-inflammatory. Induces apoptosis. Some positive phytoestrogenic activity. Slows cancer cell division. Attacks breast cancer stem cells.	Use in similar ways and amounts as you would ginger.
4. Garlic	Allicin—antibiotic Phytoncide—antifungal Sulfur compounds Allixin—antioxidant and anticancer	Known to be highly preventative. May regulate blood sugar. Acts as a blood thinner.	Raw garlic is more potent. Use either liberally. Note: Garlic is regarded as a stimulant, so some spiritual traditions recommend not using it.
5. Tomatoes	Probably lycopene The benefits of tomatoes are known, the active ingredients are unclear.	Antioxidant. Anticancer properties suggested, particularly for prostate cancer.	Cooking does help to release the lycopene. Use raw or cooked liberally.
6. The bean family, especially soybeans	Isoflavones—the best-known and most potent of which is genestein	Phytoestrogenic activity—beneficially regulate sex hormones and metabolism generally. Mildly regulates cancer cell division and angiogenesis.	Miso has higher concentration than tofu. Use regularly. Supplements of genesteine are not recommended.

Food	Main Active Ingredients	Action	Usage
7. The brassicas—broccoli, cabbage, cauliflower, Brussels sprouts	Glutamine Anti-inflammatory Indole-3-carbinol 3,3 Diindolylmethane	Boosts DNA repair. Blocks cancer cells from dividing. Creates oxidative stress in cancer cells.	Use regularly—best when cooked.
8. Chinese cabbage and probably green cabbage	Brassinin High in vitamin C High in glutamine	General brassica effects. Angiostatin. Anti-inflammatory.	Use ½ medium cabbage every 4 days—raw, lightly cooked and/or juiced.
9. Broccoli sprouts	Sulphoraphane—this is in all brassicas but very concentrated in broccoli sprouts.	Inhibits cancer growth. Enhances tumor suppressant proteins and other anti-cancer metabolites.	Use fresh (do not cook) and liberally
10. Green tea	Epigallocatechin gallate	Induces apoptosis.	Does have caffeine but useful occasionally. Does not combine well with ellagic acid (raspberries), so is the least recommended of these ten.

Stimulate High Cellular Oxygen levels

The metabolism of cancer is anaerobic; it runs on low oxygen. High oxygen levels are cancer unfriendly. What we need is plenty of oxygen being breathed in, and then good quality, nonsticky, free-flowing blood to get the oxygen around the body. Therefore, breathing is very useful! Physical exercise, yoga and qigong all stimulate oxygen uptake and circulation.

1. Exercise three to four times per week. It has many benefits and is covered in chapter 7.
2. Strongly consider learning yoga or chi gong and practicing one of them daily. I received a great deal of benefit from daily yoga practice throughout my recovery.

Create a High-Potassium, Low-Sodium Balance in the Diet

Cancer does best metabolically with a low-potassium, high-sodium balance. This is an easy way to turn the tables on the disease. The Healing Diet generally is rich in potassium and we already know to leave sodium (or salt) out. If you are new to this diet, bananas are one of the richest sources of potassium and warrant being eaten regularly. Also, the area just below the skins of potatoes concentrates potassium, so this is another reason not to peel potatoes.

Develop an Alkaline Balance in the Body

The body has what we call an acid base balance, base referring to its alkalinity. Again, cancer is like camellias in the garden (only not so beautiful!) and prefers an acidic environment. Quite easily we can make life more difficult for cancer by alkalizing the body via an alkaline diet. The Healing Diet as a whole is highly alkaline and very suitable for this purpose.

There is much debate regarding the relative acidity or alkalinity of particular foods. It is accurate to say meat, dairy and most processed and refined foods have an acidic effect, while most fruits, vegetables and grains are alkalizing.

What is being discussed here is the effect the food has at a cellular level, which paradoxically for some foods is different to how they are before being eaten. For example, we would regard lemon juice as acidic, but in the body it has the effect of being mildly alkaline. In my view, it is best not to labor which individual foods are acidic, which alkaline; simply be confident that overall the Healing Diet is alkaline to a very useful degree.

Eat Modest Amounts of Protein
The rationale for this was covered in the last chapter.

Avoid Simple Sugars, Use Complex Sugars and Complex Carbohydrates
This also was explained in the last chapter.

Avoid Free Radicals, Eat a Diet Rich in Antioxidants
Why do we hear so much about the value of antioxidants? One of the main reasons is that they neutralize excessive free radicals. Free radicals are unstable molecules that chemically are highly reactive. Some are necessary for good health but too many can lead to cell damage and death, and cancer is linked to DNA mutation from free radical damage. Free radicals can form naturally in the body, are created by ionizing radiation and from poor nutrition.

Our intake of free radicals is reduced by avoiding fatty foods and, especially, fried foods. Microwaves create free radicals, especially when used to heat dairy and fatty foods. Both the Healing Diet and the Wellness Diet are rich in antioxidants as are some supplements. The latter will be discussed soon.

Minimize the Toxic Load on the Body
Pollutants can aggravate genetic mutation, hinder our metabolism and make life easier for cancer. Reverse this with the use of organic foods, aiming to use natural cleaners and personal hygiene products and eliminate plastics from your food cycle. Garlic is touted as being good for helping the body to detox and eliminate pollutants—another good reason to use it.

Eat Food That Is as Fresh and as Vital as Possible
Vitality is a good test for the foods you buy. If you buy fruit and vegetables that already look dead, how can they serve you well? This is a powerful bonus of the home vegetable garden—freshness and vitality.

Commit to This Highly Anti-Inflammatory, Regenerative Way of Eating
The overall effect of the Healing Diet is to be highly anti-inflammatory, highly regenerative. We know from research that cancer is aggravated by

inflammation. Researchers in this field claim that chronic inflammation is associated with the development of about one-quarter of all cancers.

Of even greater significance to any one actually diagnosed with cancer is that chemicals produced in the inflammatory process stimulate cancer growth. The clear message? Avoid inflammation. Have your teeth and gums checked regularly by your dentist, and treated if necessary, especially if on chemotherapy, which often precipitates gum disease. If you have inflammation of the skin (dermatitis), the tonsils, or any part of the body, take it seriously and have it attended to promptly and thoroughly. Then know that both this diet and the meditation are highly anti-inflammatory and actually support healing in many ways.

Step 5. Consider the Use of Supplements and Other Natural Products
SUPPLEMENTS
The question of supplements is a vexed one indeed. When considering your options, you will find that at one end of the spectrum are those who say that none are needed as "the average diet contains all you need." At the other end of the spectrum are those who recommend taking vast amounts of every known vitamin, mineral and just about everything else that can be made into a tablet and swallowed.

What is reasonable? There is good evidence that the "average" diet is frequently deficient in vital nutrients. A survey that examined the vitamin and mineral content of the diets of new patients in a Melbourne medical practice revealed startling results. The patients whose diets were examined presented for a wide range of everyday problems. They could reasonably be said to represent the average in an affluent society wherein one would expect people to lack little. Yet their diets were grossly deficient. And, significantly, the deficiencies showed up in factors directly involved in the normal functioning of the immune system, zinc being a good example.

The case for supplementation is further increased by the growing body of evidence that extra doses of some minerals, and particularly some vitamins, can be dramatically helpful for some cancer patients.

Maintain High Levels of Vitamin D

This is like a free hit. If your vitamin D levels are low, as they are for many people, particularly those living further away from the equator, your immune system and capacity to heal will be markedly compromised.

Vitamin D deficiencies are strongly implicated as a causative factor in cancer. Currently in Europe, it is estimated that one-third of all the breast cancers in women are directly linked with low vitamin D levels. The link is established with quite a number of other cancers and as research progresses in this rapidly expanding field it seems highly likely that high vitamin D levels aid in recovery and prolong survival times.

Vitamin D is manufactured in the body after sunlight, and more specifically the ultraviolet B (UVB) in sunlight, activates chemical precursors under your skin. There is a limit to how much vitamin D can be activated per day and it takes only a short while in the sun to acquire all the vitamin D you can for that day. What this means is that to develop and sustain vitamin D levels you need to get as much skin as decently possible into the sun regularly, but only for a short period of time. The more UVB when you are in the sun, the less time you need. So a hot summer's day and maybe five to seven minutes is enough; a cool winter's day, maybe twenty to thirty minutes. Clouds reduce the UVB significantly; glass and sunscreens block it out. Clothing produces a range of reduction from a little to a lot.

Vitamin D levels are easily checked by routine blood tests. Recent solid research evidence has led to the realization of just how important the role of vitamin D is for healthy immune function, as well as our health and well-being generally (it leads to happier moods and reduces depression). This has led in turn to the recommended blood levels being increased. Currently, it seems the best advice to aim for is between 100–150 nmol/l.

Many people in our groups, which are well south of the equator and experience cold, cloudy winters, record levels in the 20s, 30s and 40s. This really helps cancer! What can we do?

Vitamin D from the sun is best—if there is sunlight and warmth available. Exercising outdoors in light clothing or short periods of sunbathing (both sides) works well. The aim is to avoid the skin going red and beginning to burn. People with dark skin need longer periods of exposure to get the same amount of vitamin D compared to those with light skins. All colors of skin can burn and this needs to be avoided.

Vitamin D supplements are practical and all indications are that they work well. If you have low levels you will need significant supplementation to return to healthy levels; then you can use a maintenance dose. Check with your doctor, but with a level of 30–40nmol/l you may need 150–250,000, even up to 500,000 IU units of vitamin D to reach the recommended blood levels. While large doses can be taken in one day, it is probably preferable to only take 50,000 IU per day for five to seven days, and then after two to four weeks have another blood test.

A useful maintenance guide is 5,000 IU per day, but the ideal level is best decided in consultation with your doctor and adjusted once you experiment for a while and observe your blood levels. We have found people can create and metabolize vitamin D quite differently—some very efficiently and so needing lower supplementation or sun exposure, others not very efficiently at all and so needing good support.

Wellness Rule 22:   Ensure adequate blood levels of vitamin D.

The Special Case of Vitamin C

Examining the available information on vitamin C demonstrates the controversies surrounding some supplements. While some studies say it makes little or no difference, others point to its wide range of beneficial activities. Again, Doctors Pauling and Cameron refer to an increase in the body's natural resistance in their work *Cancer and Vitamin C*.[20] They cite an improved level of well-being, as measured by improved appetite, increased mental alertness, decreased requirement for pain-controlling drugs and other clinical criteria.

Most animals make their own vitamin C. Not so we humans. We rely on our diet for all we get. It has been claimed by some authorities that an ideal, fresh food diet would provide 8 to 10 grams of vitamin C daily. Some claim this is a reasonable maintenance level, and ideally, such an amount would be obtained in the diet itself. But, in fact, most people would require supplementation to achieve this level. By contrast, the official minimum recommended daily allowance is currently 45 milligrams per day. Our Wellness Diet as analyzed (see Appendix M) contains around 560mgm per day. Gerson's diet contains 930 mgm.

Another consideration is the level required to bring the body to "saturation point." It has been suggested that, at saturation, vitamin C exerts its maximum effects. It has also been suggested that at levels below this its effect may be minimal. To explain: a person in normal health may be at saturation with a total intake of, say, 10 grams. The stress of an impending cold, however, may increase the need for vitamin C so much that 50 grams may be required to reach saturation. If the person is only getting 10 grams, the cold may develop as normal. Giving 50 grams may prevent it developing at all. Likewise, exposure to "flu" may create a need for 200 grams. Giving 10 or 50 grams would be ineffective, whereas 200 grams may be effective.

Experience tells us that the amount of vitamin C required to reach saturation varies widely with individuals and individual situations. Doctors working with this approach often use what is called the bowel tolerance test. They find that once the body is saturated, a little extra vitamin C produces a mild diarrhea, which stops once the supplementation is reduced a little. This makes the point of bowel tolerance a useful signpost to the individual's maximum requirements. So they recommend that their patients find their own level of bowel tolerance, drop the dose just a little, and keep to that, adjusting according to stress levels. Many cancer patients find this requires their adding 18 to 20 grams of vitamin C to their diet daily. Some take 30 grams or more by mouth each day. Such high levels of vitamin C are said to leach magnesium, zinc and vitamin B from the body, and so supplements of these are then required.

Often even higher doses of vitamin C are given intravenously with some good effects. A common, almost uniform, result is the lessening of pain. Some tumors also do regress. In my veterinary days, I treated confirmed cases of lymphosarcoma in cats with intravenous doses of 1 gram per kilogram of body weight on five successive days. Four out of four treated cases went into total remission. The few dogs I treated in the same manner did not respond so well.

The special case of vitamin C amply demonstrates the complex and really rather confusing issues involved with supplements.

My Own Experience

I hope it is obvious that I am only discussing the options, and avoiding making specific recommendations. Supplements pose many complex questions. Their role is not one I find easy to resolve.

My own experience with them runs the full gamut. I did take all the supplements Gerson recommended when I was using his regime. His was an integrated approach. I then dropped various factors off as I began to feel the need for them had passed—relaxing toward the Wellness Diet. At another time during my illness I did try megavitamin therapy, taking huge numbers of vitamin tablets. Apart from learning the art of swallowing thirty pills in one go, I felt it did little for me. However, for quite some time during my recovery and the ensuing years, I did continue to take a general purpose multivitamin and some extra vitamin C.

Some Cautious Suggestions

My overriding attitude is that natural sources of nutrition are the best. It seems clear to me that in an ideal world, when we are eating well, when we are happy, stress free and joyous, there would be no need for extra supplements. However, not many people with our modern, busy lifestyles seem to be in such an ideal situation. Therefore, if the diet is not ideal, if there is the hint of stress around, when we are traveling, or experiencing difficult times, it seems reasonable that basic supplements could help our bodies to cope better.

Staying with the natural is the best principle. If extra nutrients are required on top of what we eat, the next recommendation is to use juices. Juices concentrate nutrients in a form that is natural, well balanced and easily absorbed by the body. However, in many situations, particularly when facing major stress or major disease, even more help from supplement tablets may be beneficial.

A Summary of the Supplement Options

When considering the options regarding extra nutrition, consider the following choices:

- Take no extra supplements—not many people I have worked with have done this.
- Use fresh juices as a source of concentrated nutrition that is provided in a natural balanced form. This approach is highly recommended to anyone with active illness. The juices also seem to be of great help when recovering from surgery, or when undergoing chemotherapy or radiation.

- Self-medicate: Take a good quality general multivitamin and mineral supplements along with extra vitamin D and maybe vitamin C. This is what many people find helpful and it gives them the security of knowing that their requirements for vitamins and minerals are well covered. This is particularly important when preparing for, or recovering from surgery, or when undergoing chemotherapy or radiotherapy. It is at these times that the body is under an increased load and requires extra nutritional help.

- Vitamin C can be taken in the form of 500 milligrams or 1gm tablets with bioflavonoid (which help its function) after each meal. If, along the lines we discussed earlier, you choose larger doses of vitamin C, use sodium ascorbate powder dissolved in water or juices, and again, take it after meals.

- There is a real caution regarding vitamins A and E, which have been shown via large meta-analysis studies to shorten life span in people who are basically well and have taken them over long periods of time. I know of no studies being published regarding the long-term use of vitamins A and E by people affected by cancer, and maybe they are OK short term, but the caution needs to be stated.

- Seek expert advice. Take larger, therapeutic doses of individual vitamins, minerals and/or other dietary supplements. This appeals to many, and if you choose to do this, I strongly recommend that you seek the personalized help of a suitably qualified practitioner. Many doctors are now well trained in nutritional medicine and some naturopaths can be helpful. As always, you are well advised to seek out the qualifications and experience of anyone you are considering consulting. Particularly in this field, it is wise to obtain personal recommendations and feedback from people whose opinions you value and who can help to guide your choices.

COFFEE ENEMAS

The stark reality is I found these really helpful and know many, many others who experienced equally positive benefits. Often I wish this was not so! The notion of using coffee as an enema always seems a little weird and I like my credibility. Of all the things I have ever been criticized for, this is the easiest to understand as a source of mirth.

However, I am committed to sharing what works, so here we go.

I thought coffee enemas to be the funniest thing I had ever heard of when it was suggested that they could help me. I am sure Spike Milligan's crazy genius could not have produced a more comical idea. But, like everyone else I know who has tried them, I felt an immediate benefit from them, and amid some hilarity, persisted with them. What do they do, and how do they work?

Coffee Enemas Stimulate Liver Function

Gerson named the liver as the major organ of detoxification and placed great importance upon restoring and maintaining its efficient activity. He believed liver juices aided liver function and he also recommended the use of liver extract injections.

His main method for stimulating liver function, however, was through the use of coffee or caffeine enemas as they are sometimes known. Caffeine introduced into the rectum by enema is absorbed by the rectal veins and then passes into the portal vein, and on directly to the liver. There it stimulates liver function, including bile flow. Bile is a major means of eliminating toxic material from the body. Coffee is a readily available source of caffeine, and it also makes a convenient enema, therefore, it is coffee enemas that are recommended.

Coffee Enemas Provide Significant Pain Relief

Coffee enemas are remarkably effective in combating and relieving pain. When pain was a problem for me, I found them more useful than the narcotic analgesics I was having. Dr. Meares told me that he believed they have an effect because to hold an enema for ten to fifteen minutes while the caffeine is being absorbed requires quite a degree of relaxation—relaxation in an area you might otherwise not relax so well. I believe this is an added benefit, but they certainly have an immediate physical effect as well.

For many years, I have encouraged researchers I know to investigate why and how coffee enemas work. Perhaps not surprisingly, there has been little enthusiasm for such a project! However, Dr. Candace Pert, a famous researcher in the field of mind-body medicine and author of the wonderful book *Molecules of Emotion*,[21] told me of a distinct possibility.

Dr. Pert published much of the pioneering research on neurotransmitters or messenger molecules—those chemicals that the body produces in one part which, when released, influence how the body functions elsewhere. She has been particularly interested in how our state of mind affects the production of these chemicals and how they in turn affect our immune system and health generally. Dr. Pert was the first to discover that white blood cells, the front line defenses for our immune system, have opiate receptors on their surfaces. The brain is capable of producing natural opiates, such as endorphins and releasing them into the bloodstream. When this happens, we feel pain relief and well-being, as if we had had an injection of morphine. As well, these opiates attach to the white blood cells and enhance their activity, improving the effectiveness of our immune system.

Now the link to coffee enemas. Not only are these natural opiates produced in the brain, they are also produced in cells that line the bowel. It had always puzzled me why coffee enemas produced such good pain relief and such a heightened sense of well-being. Dr. Pert suggested that it may well be that this happens through a direct interaction between some component of the coffee enemas, probably the caffeine, and the endorphin-producing cells lining the bowel.

Again, if the explanation of how they work is inadequate, the pragmatic fact is that many do find them helpful (see Appendix F for details of preparation and administration).

Of all Gerson's treatments, this is the one I kept on with for longest. In the early days I used to try stopping them and I would become obviously jaundiced in one or two days. A coffee enema would clear the yellowness from my skin in about fifteen minutes.

Alternatives to Coffee Enemas

Dr. Alex Forbes, who pioneered the Bristol Cancer Help Center in England, told me that they obtained just as good results using herbs that stimulate liver function. As these herbs can be taken "down" rather than "up," they have a greater esthetic appeal! I have no personal experience of using such herbs, but Dorothy Hall, Australia's leading herbalist, feels that individual patients require individual treatments. She recommends seeking personal advice from a qualified herbalist if you are considering this type of assistance.

Roasted dandelion root coffee has been recommended for centuries as a safe but useful liver tonic, and we have found it to be a gentle and reliable aid for improving liver function—a useful but probably less potent alternative to the enemas. However, I do recommend its regular use at up to three cups per day.

The principle to reaffirm is that generally the liver will profit from active support and it becomes a matter of determining the most appropriate way of providing this assistance.

COMPLEMENTARY AND ALTERNATIVE THERAPIES (CAM)

The intention of this book is to focus on lifestyle medicine—what we as individuals can do for ourselves. There are many options in the CAM arena and some may well be useful. It can be very helpful to locate a doctor engaged in integrative medicine and who sees people with cancer regularly, or a sound naturopath. We are all unique and CAM treatments are similar to conventional medical treatments—they need to be prescribed individually in full knowledge of the individual's situation and preferences. Both conventional and CAM options will be discussed more in chapter 19 on healing.

Step 6. Move from the General to the Specific

Now we need to advance from the general recommendations to the specific needs we have as individuals. We need to personalize our way of eating. Once steps 1–5 are in place, we can proceed and begin to develop a pattern of eating that is tailored to our particular needs and conditions.

Here is how to do it.

STEP 1. DEVELOP YOUR FOOD KNOWLEDGE

It makes good sense to read, study and learn more about nutrition. It is a vast subject and, when dealing with cancer, one needs to prioritize. So if you feel what is in this book meets your needs, study that. Reread each section, put the principles into practice, and come back to the book's theories again and again. Rereading this main text over and over will make good sense.

> Wellness Rule 23: Study nutrition but avoid fixating. The need is to decide on an approach, a dietary plan, and to stick to it for a while; observe the results and readjust if necessary.

STEP 2. HEIGHTEN YOUR FOOD AWARENESS

Our mind is a great ally when we harness its knowledge and its awareness. We have talked of this regularly—meditate and we become more aware.

Practice mindfulness specifically and we do notice more clearly what works for us and what is unhelpful.

> Wellness Rule 24: Meditate, be mindful, and respond to what you may have once called intuition or a "gut feeling."

STEP 3. LET YOUR BODY BE YOUR GUIDE
Helping your body to become more sensitive to the foods you eat heightens the prospect of reliably being able to determine what foods suit your needs best. This can be achieved using one of three methods.

Simply Meditate
Over months or even years, meditation will clear your mind and you are highly likely to make more appropriate food choices. In theory this will work, although I know a significant number of people who have meditated for years and still eat poorly.

Meditation can involve the body or it can be more of a "head trip." People who meditate in their bodies, who consciously relax their bodies and feel integrated with their bodies, are much more likely to notice what goes on in that body and to treat it well. This is another reason why we emphasize the relaxation phase in MBSM meditation.

Follow the Wellness Diet
Put bluntly, the Wellness Diet eliminates the junk from your diet and adds the good stuff! With this, a gentle detox and transformation takes place over weeks to months and heightens and enhances the body awareness we have been advocating.

Thoroughly eliminating salt, sugar and chili from the diet greatly accelerates this process as those three overwhelm the taste buds and severely impair our capacity to discriminate.

This approach is very reasonable for people who are well and are seeking a really sound, personalized diet. It is also very practical and manageable for those dealing with cancer and other diseases who choose to take their nutrition seriously, but elect to move steadily into a better way of eating.

Actively Detoxify the Body

If our car is overdue for a service, we are highly likely to become nervous, maybe even anxious. We know we are not treating it well and fear mechanical trouble. Detoxing the body is a bit like changing the oil in our car. The notion of detoxifying the body recognizes we live in a polluted world and especially if our diet has been below par, the body may well be carrying an inordinate toxic load.

THE DETOX PRINCIPLES

Detoxification has been a major principle in many cultures over many years and is highly valued among modern-day naturopaths. Modern medicine is more equivocal but surely it makes sense. If our body carries a toxic load, its general metabolism and capacity to regulate healing will be impaired. Also, to develop our individual food sensitivity, we are asking our body to measure the value of the foods it consumes. If we are attempting to use a ruler covered in mud to measure a distance, the result will be highly suspect. We need a clean instrument. We need a clean body.

As explained in the last section, detoxifying will occur slowly and steadily over months on the Wellness Diet. However, what we have found most effective for those who want a more rapid process that will produce results in days or weeks is the mono diet.

The Mono Diet

A mono diet is where just one simple, low-allergenic food is eaten consistently for a fixed period of time. It is preferable to fasting on water (a traditional method for purification and detoxifying), as the mono diet does provide some basic nutrition. Clearly, a mono diet is not a complete dietary package, but that is the point. The gentle metabolic stress induced by eating just one food over a period of time triggers the body to shed its toxic load.

However, the partial nutritional content of one food means that the body is not too stressed as it may be during a more rigorous water fast. At the same time, any food that we may react adversely to is cleared from the body. It is as if the body is returned to a clean, uncomplicated state.

What we do after completing a mono diet is to gradually reintroduce a broader range of foods. By having the patience and the willpower to do this gradually, it becomes relatively easy to establish which foods agree with you and which do not.

We can tell when a food is suitable—we feel fine! When we eat something we may be better to avoid, our body will let us know. We may notice an obvious digestive upset—feeling like we ate something that was "off"—biliousness, nausea, even diarrhea. However, commonly the signs are a little more subtle. Feelings of tiredness are common, sometimes headaches or joint pain, sometimes flu-like symptoms, or with dairy products particularly, inflammatory reactions like tonsillitis, sinusitis, bronchitis—even cystitis.

When we are prepared to respond to these signals and modify our diet appropriately and when we do take time to sort out any internal influences that may be affecting our choices, then we will find that we will be free to make the fine tuning to our diet and develop what is a truly individualized nutritional program.

It is worth noting that several people have recommended that a mono diet may be helpful for people with cancer if carried on for an extended period. In her book, *The Grape Cure*,[22] Johanna Brandt recounts how she used a mono diet of grapes, backed up by periods on raw foods, as the basis for recovering from her own cancer. Macrobiotics, the Japanese style of cooking based on their philosophy of balance, recommends that a mono diet of whole brown rice helps people with cancer to rebalance their system.

Consistently I have found that people who do follow a mono diet for a relatively short period receive a good deal of benefit. They invariably experience what they describe as "feeling lighter," their taste buds clear, and their food begins to taste better. Eating the one thing for a few days certainly works to focus the attention on dietary considerations. It doubles as a good exercise in willpower. This is a major benefit as once you have done ten days eating just one food you can achieve just about anything you put your mind to! Many also find that it does develop the sensitivity we are seeking.

Mono Diets Are Not Advised While Having Chemotherapy

If having chemotherapy, it is best to wait about two months after the treatment is finished and energy levels are reasonable before starting a mono diet. Doing so at this time may well help to rid the body of any residue from the treatment. I did a ten-day mono diet on grapes about a year after completing chemo, and despite being on a good diet and meditating regularly during that intervening period, on days six and seven, I passed the same color and smell in my urine as I did when I was having the chemotherapy. I then did ten days on rice in the winter and ten days on grapes in the summer for several years.

There is new research emerging that suggests actual fasting for a day or two around the time when chemotherapy is administered has a significantly beneficial effect. It seems while the cells in the human body can manage fasting for a while quite well, cancer cells do not manage at all well.

When Considering the Mono Diet, There Are Two Variations:

The Summer Mono Diet

In summer, when it is warm and fruit is in season, the ideal is ten days eating organic grapes only. Ten days has been recommended as a good aim but this can be a struggle for some. A minimum of three days is required to experience tangible benefits. I suggest it is best to set your goal in advance—from three to ten days—and then stick to it.

While doing this, eat as many grapes as you want. Use whatever variety you prefer, but do not mix varieties at one sitting. Drink as little as you feel comfortable with, and when you do, take only pure water or grape juice (which may be diluted fifty-fifty with water).

If grapes are not available, then do just three days using one pound of only one fruit at each of three meals, or one half-pound at each of six meals. Again, drink only pure water or fruit juices and do not mix different juices and fruits together. Eating only three pounds of fruit in a day has more of a fasting element than eating unlimited amounts of grapes, but the former is only recommended for three days.

The Winter Mono Diet

In winter, the ideal is ten days on organic brown rice. The rice needs to be cooked by the absorption method. One volume of rice plus two volumes of water is slowly boiled until the water is absorbed. The rice will then be tender. It should be chewed thoroughly—to the consistency of mashed ripe bananas. This may take up to thirty, even up to fifty chews per mouthful, so do not be in a hurry! Do eat as much as you want, without adding anything else to the rice.

Again, keeping fluids to a minimum is recommended, and only water should be taken.

Generally, the rice is relatively easy, but if you do struggle, some vegetable broth could be added. Exercise needs to be kept well within your limits and many people find it best to stay close to home, concentrating on the task in hand. If the cold of winter is a problem, warm baths are the best way to warm up thoroughly.

Coffee enemas are recommended during a mono diet to assist the cleansing process. Again, appropriate supervision is highly desirable. The more thorough you are, the better, but never overlook the need to keep within your physiological and psychological limits.

Challenge Yourself by Reintroducing Foods Slowly

Following a mono diet, the way to reintroduce foods is important. You can just go back to eating as before and hope your sensitivity can manage the variety. While this is an option, it is not so effective. To be thorough, to really give yourself the best way of fine-tuning your diet, it makes sense to reintroduce foods individually.

This process is quite similar to the elimination diets used in mainstream food sensitivity and allergy testing. There, where people are suspected of adverse food reactions, they are put on very bland low-allergy diets from three to fourteen days. This is how long it can take for reactive foods to clear the body. Then foods are reintroduced one by one—the "challenge."

If you have the motivation, the energy, the time and the support to do this it is highly rewarding.

So, in warm weather, after the transition on grapes or fruit, begin by starting with other fruits. At first stick to the one new fruit at each meal. It only takes a few days to try each of the fruits, and then go on to add the salad vegetables. Then add grains and other things until a total spectrum emerges.

In cold weather, after a rice transition, add in steamed or baked vegetables first, other grains, then raw vegetables followed by fruits. Follow the scale of cooked grains, cooked vegetables, raw vegetables, cooked fruit, and raw fruit. Steadily test all the elements of the Healing Diet. Soon a daily program will emerge.

An important tip here is that chewing our food really well enhances our sensitivity to its suitability. When we do take the time to chew food to a really fine, watery consistency, it does seem to make it easier to have the inner knowing of whether it is good for us or not. Try this, you may be surprised how helpful it can be.

Then what one does is to continue to be aware of the foods you eat and any changes in your situation. Maybe for a while you feel the need to eat lots of carrots and go off eggplant altogether. Then broccoli seems really attractive, or beetroot. As you pay more attention to your body and respect its needs, this way of eating becomes more and more natural, effortless and effective.

Speaking Personally

As I came off the Gerson Therapy I experienced a range of sensitivities. I only had to look at eggplant to know it did not suit me. Then I noticed an even stronger reaction to raw onions and avoided them completely. However, once cooked, the aromatic acids in onions are altered and I could eat the cooked form happily. With hens' eggs I experienced a powerful physical reaction—I became liverish and sometimes even showed signs of jaundice, and also my state of mind was affected and I became quite grumpy and felt miserable. Cow's milk was tricky as I quite liked it, but I had to notice every time I ate any dairy products I experienced an inflammatory reaction that usually centered on my throat, so I was better off not eating it. Of course there are good theoretical reasons to avoid cow's milk anyway.

So perhaps my own experience helps to demonstrate how our personal awareness and sensitivity to what we eat can develop.

Recommendation

Seriously consider taking the time and effort to follow the mono diet for ten days and then gradually reintroduce individual foods and test your sensitivity. The reward is you will know what is good for you and what is not, and you will have a very personalized diet that will be well suited for recovery.

THE HEALING DIET, OPTION 2: THE RAPID METHOD

This is simple. You begin with step 6, the detox and then follow through with steps 2–5 as above.

For most people, establishing the Healing Diet first using steps 1–5 in the gradual method is very manageable. Maybe after several weeks, once you have become familiar with the basic Healing Diet, then it makes sense to fine-tune and personalize the diet by using the mono diet and food testing.

Certainly it is wise now to make a plan and consciously seek the foods and the support you need to put your plan into action.

Sample Menus

These are very broad guidelines intended as examples only.

Wellness Diet

The juices are optional, depending on your situation and preferences.

Summer	Spring/Autumn	Winter
On Arising		
Glass of lemon juice (1/3 lemon juice, 2/3 water)	Glass of lemon juice	Orange juice
Breakfast		
Unlimited amount of one fruit, (e.g., watermelon, cantaloupe)	One or more well combined fruits plus 2 tablespoons yogurt and 10–20 almonds, maybe dried fruit like currants or sultanas 1–2 pieces toast with natural jam	Hot porridge—any combination of rolled oats, rye, buckwheat, millet, rice, barley, triticale, (possibly wheat) or homemade muesli **PLUS** 2 tablespoons yogurt, 10–20 almonds, 1 tablespoon currants or sultanas, 1 stewed apple or equivalent 1–2 pieces toast with natural, sugarless jam Cup herb tea
Mid Morning		
Piece of fruit	Piece of fruit	Piece of fruit
+/- almonds	+/- almonds	+/- almonds
+/- juice	+/- juice	+/- juice
Midday		
2 salad sandwiches with 4–6 vegetables and sprouts	2 salad sandwiches with 4–6 vegetables and sprouts	Soup—miso or vegetable broth Salad of 4–6 vegetables with bean spread
And kelp powder	And kelp powder	+ /-bread
Mid Afternoon		
Juice	Dandelion coffee +/- whole-meal cookie or cake	Dandelion coffee +/- whole-meal cookie or cake

Summer	Spring/Autumn	Winter
Evening		
Juice	Juice	Juice
Salad of 4–6 vegetables and sprouts, and sea vegetables (e.g., nori and tofu or beans or a hot meal)	Side salad of 3–4 vegetables and sprouts, followed by dry-baked veggies and rice or pasta dish	Hot meal (e.g., 50–50 steamed vegetables, plus tofu and rice, or whole-meal pasta and veg/tofu sauce, or veg pie and rice)
		Use your flair! Be creative!
Before Bed		
Juice	Juice	Herb tea
May substitute herb teas or equivalent for juices.		

Warm-Weather Healing Diet

AM	
7:00	Arise
	1 tablespoon lemon juice in lukewarm water
7:10	Breathing exercises (e.g., yoga or chi gong)—preferably barefooted on grass (glasses removed if normally worn)
7:30	Breakfast: fruit
	Any one fruit—I frequently used watermelon or fruit salad with appropriate combinations.
8:15	Meditate. Ideally, one hour.
9:15	Juice. Then, exercise in open (e.g., walking for 30 minutes). Smile!
10:30	Juice or piece of fruit or almonds plus herb tea
	Then meditate, ideally one hour before lunch.
PM	
12:00	Juice
	Then prepare lunch.
12:30	Lunch. Salad featuring 4–6 salad vegetables, or as a sandwich, or with a rice/pasta salad, almonds, sprouts.
1:15	Exercise, gardening, reading, free time
3:00	Juice
	Then free time
4:15	Breathing exercises (e.g., yoga or chi gong)—check you are still smiling (optional if done in the morning)!
4:30	Meditate. Ideally, one hour.
5:30	Juice
	Then prepare dinner.
6:00	Dinner. 4–6 salad vegetables, plus rice, pasta or baked potatoes, sprouts.
Before bed	Juice or herb tea
	Physically relax in bed and go to sleep with a prayer and/or a positive thought.
	Jump out of bed the next morning feeling that little bit better!

Cold-Weather Healing Diet

The same basic program is used but extra cooked food is included with an emphasis on rice. Half the evening meal can be rice, the rest steamed or baked vegetables. Breakfast for the first week can be porridge, for the second week fruit, third week porridge, and fourth week fruit again.

Recipes

To repeat, the best available recipe book to begin with is the *New Gawler Foundation Cookbook* and the recipes in it will fit nicely into the programs set out above.

A FINAL WORD ON DIET

I have always enjoyed ice cream and gelato. You could almost say that when I was young, I was addicted. I am just about cured of ice cream as it has so many additives, but I still do delight in gelato. I am happy to indulge in something that pleases me.

There was a time when I felt I was so ill that I needed to concentrate 100 percent on everything that I ate. I did not have ice cream or gelato for over two years. Now I seek out natural ice cream, or preferably gelato. I recognized that it is probably full of sugar, and perhaps other things that are short of ideal.

I know, however, that the way I eat at home is close to what I regard as ideal. We have a large organic vegetable garden and orchard. The bulk of what I do eat is homegrown or bought having been organically or biodynamically grown.

I know that what you are wise to eat when you are well really is different compared to when you have active illness. When you are well, it is what you eat "mostly" that is important. Eat well most of the time and the occasional gelato is fine! When you are dealing with major illness though, what you eat all the time is important. So now that I have been so well for so long, I feel well blessed, and as I savor my gelato, I give thanks for its wonderful taste and swallow it with a smile.

Wellness Rule 25: In your own mind, be clear about what you will eat when, and enjoy doing it! Use the three principles of positive thinking with your nutrition.

Set Clear Goals

On the Wellness Diet, be clear about your boundaries. Be clear about what you will eat when; when you are at home, when you are out, when there is a special occasion. Remember, when you are well, it is what you eat mostly that is important.

On the Healing Diet, be clear about what you will eat when. Remember, when you are eating for recovery, what you eat all the time is important.

Do Whatever It Takes

Ensure you have a collection of tasty recipes that convert your choices into delightful meals.

Choose to Enjoy Doing It

Bon appétit!

CHAPTER 15

The Causes of Cancer

It Is All in the Mind—Or Is It?

WHILE NUTRITION AND FOOD ARE OFTEN PROMINENT IN THEIR THOUGHTS, ask most people diagnosed with cancer the question that first went through their mind after they accepted their diagnosis and you are highly likely to receive a common answer:

"Why me? Why did it happen to me? Why have I got this thing?"

The question is always there. Sometimes it is voiced out loud with anger. Often it remains inside, unexpressed but smoldering with an attendant sense of injustice.

This response is understandable, for there is a popular misconception that the causes of cancer are not known. Therefore those who are diagnosed frequently feel as if they are the victims of a random, vindictive fate. Invariably they find themselves looking around and making comparisons.

"Why not him? Why not old George down the road? He smokes like a chimney, drinks like a fish. Never got a kind word for anyone, never helps anyone; but there he is, eighty years old and still going. Well, I mean I know that I'm no saint, but I sure have been trying to do my best all these years. Why *me*?"

Those who are brave enough to express this vital question out loud to their doctors or friends often hear in response: "I am sorry, we don't really know the causes of cancer." Or, worse still, they are told: "It's just one of those things. Bad luck, I suppose."

IS IT BAD LUCK OR DOES IT HAVE A CAUSE?

Bad luck! Can something as serious as cancer be just "bad luck"? The whole of the universe as we know it is governed by laws. A fundamental one is that for every action there is an equal and opposite reaction. Everything in the physical world is ruled by this law of cause and effect. The investigative skills of modern technology probe from the smallest atoms to the largest stars and find no exceptions. Can man, the central figure in our universe, be excluded from a similar governing law? Can cancer really be the product of mere chance?

If the causes of cancer are not identified, then cancer patients are hapless victims of external influences beyond their control. People who feel this to be the case inevitably regard themselves as victims. Such victim-consciousness is probably the most negative emotion in which we can indulge. It allows us to feel as if we had no part in the development of the disease itself, as if the disease just happened and we had nothing to do with it.

Worse, it leaves us feeling helpless, powerless to resist an external force that we can neither understand nor deal with.

To call yourself a "cancer victim," or to be described as one, conjures up all the worst negative images associated with cancer. Those words, "cancer victim," must be avoided totally. "Cancer" itself is not a dirty word and we need to feel free to use it. "Cancer patient" is fine. Being a patient—someone undergoing treatment—is fine. In another sense, being patient and showing patience, the calm endurance of a situation with attendant perseverance, is a fine attribute. Being a "victim" is totally inappropriate. Perhaps you would rather be described as a "person with cancer" or a "person living with cancer." I was quite content to be a "cancer patient" although these days being someone who "had cancer" is even better!

However, the exciting fact is that there is no reason for using the word "victim." Most of the causes of cancer can now be identified.

For years it seems as if everyone has been looking for the one cause: the one agent, the one food, one chemical, one virus. One anything! Just let there be one thing to blame for the whole problem. It is now obvious that it is not so simple. Cancer has many contributing factors.

This is the exciting fact. If we are prepared to broaden our horizons and take account of the full spectrum of possibilities we can understand the nature of cancer. There are many factors, not just one, which are involved in producing those final physical symptoms we describe as cancer.

To understand the causes of cancer we must explore our physical, emotional, mental and spiritual realms. Not one factor, but many, combine to produce cancer.

CANCER IS A CHRONIC, MULTIFACTORIAL, DEGENERATIVE DISEASE

Like the camel's back, the body must be laboring under the weight of many burdens before one final straw can break it and allow cancer to develop. This is probably the best news that people diagnosed with cancer can have. For once the causes of the problem can be identified, it makes it so much easier to take the appropriate action to rectify the situation. If we remove the causes, lift the load off that broken back, then we have gone a long way toward creating a healing environment. It may be challenging but it can be done. Virtually all the known causes can be remedied.

Cancer is a dynamic process. It is responsive to the influences acting upon it. It is not a one-way, downhill street. It has causes, and those causes produce effects. Remove the disease-producing causes and replace them with health-promoting influences, and recovery is under way.

It is as if there were a set of scales with influences that create health and influences that create disease hanging in the balance. When one side prevails—health results; when the other is down—disease. Once the disease scale is down with cancer, it requires an intense effort to tip the balance again. Attending to the sheer physical realities can often require top priority. But by understanding the disease process we can set about a rational self-help program based upon removing the cancer-producing causes and replacing them with health-promoting factors.

THE KNOWN CAUSES OF CANCER

The starting point is recognizing that there is such a process involved, and understanding what set it in motion. Professor Gabriel Kune, one of the world's leading authorities on the causes of cancer claims that nine out of ten cancers are due to noninherited causes—or, in other words, only 10 percent of cancers are related to inherited factors. This may be in conflict with what many people assume or fear, but it is thoroughly confirmed by modern research. What also comes from the research is the clear fact that the majority of the known causes of cancer relate to lifestyle issues. Kune's book, *The Home Health Guide to a Cancer-Free Family,*[23] is an excellent and readable resource for anyone wanting more detail on the known causes and how they relate to particular cancer types.

Professors Sir Richard Doll and Sir Richard Peto were two of the earliest and most highly respected investigators of the physical causes of cancer. Their research, published in *The Causes of Cancer*,[24] established that it is reasonable to attribute the causes of cancer (excluding cancers of the skin) as follows:

- 35 percent to dietary factors
- 30 percent to smoking nicotine
- 10 percent to infections
- 4 percent to occupational hazards
- 3 percent to alcohol
- 3 percent to geophysical factors
- 2 percent to pollution
- 1 percent to medicines and medical procedures

Less than 1 percent of all cancers are attributable to each of food additives and industrial products.

Doll and Peto's research is now over thirty years old and their figures have been confirmed by many more studies. The one major new causative factor that has been identified and needs to be highlighted is the lack of sunlight and vitamin D. In Europe these days, it has been estimated that around 30 percent of all new breast cancer cases in women are directly linked to lack of sunlight and its related vitamin D. This deficiency has also been associated with an increased risk of colorectal, prostate and pancreatic cancers.

STATISTICS AND INDIVIDUALS

What these statistics mean is that if there were one hundred cancer patients in a random group, we could expect thirty-five of them to be the products of an inappropriate diet. However, exactly which thirty-five may be difficult to determine. Being more specific, we do know that a high-fat diet is associated with an increased risk of breast cancer. But for an individual woman who does happen to have breast cancer, it is not so easy to say her breast cancer was caused just by a high-fat diet, even if she happened to have been on one.

The high-fat diet is just one identifiable, and of course very easily rectifiable, factor. However, that particular woman may also have been eating a lot of other "junk" food, drinking alcohol, been emotionally uptight, financially insecure and so on. The high-fat diet may have been the final "straw" that precipitated her breast cancer. For another woman with the same background burden of risk factors, but without a high-fat diet, being a smoker may have been the final straw, or "trigger factor," that meant she developed lung cancer instead of breast cancer.

RISK FACTORS ARE OFTEN SYNERGISTIC

Another significant issue we need to be aware of is that many physical factors known to cause cancer interact with each other and in combination produce greatly increased risk factors. This is amply demonstrated by the research on smoking tobacco. Someone who smokes 30 grams of tobacco or more per day has about eight times the risk of esophageal cancer compared to someone who does not smoke. Drinking 40–80 grams of alcohol per day results in seven times the risk of esophageal cancer compared with someone who does not. Now if a person does both, what is their risk? Eight plus seven, or fifteen times greater? Unequivocally no! The evidence is clear-cut. The two risks do not simply add together—they are synergistic—the effect is more like multiplication. The combined risk of smoking and drinking together, at that level, is put at thirty-six times that of doing neither.

Similarly, asbestos workers who smoke are diagnosed with ten times more asbestosis when compared with those who do not. Cigarette smokers in the cities have twice the lung cancer of their country counterparts. What extra synergistic factors are involved here? Pollution? Stress?

The basic contention is that cancer is a chronic, multifactorial, degenerative disease. The causes of cancer are often subtle, usually multiple, frequently synergistic and generally build up over a long period! So a person may have a "background" of low-level cancer risk factors that are present in the way they live their life over many years. Then there may be the one more obvious, more identifiable trigger factor, like the high-fat diet or the smoking, which is like the final straw that actually precipitates the specific type of cancer.

But there is still more to all of this.

THE SYMPTOMS AND THE DISEASE

The end point of cancer, and the physical symptoms that go with it, is not so subtle. Once it becomes apparent, cancer is generally very obvious and often acute. Some cancers, once they do appear, are very fast moving and potentially life threatening. Faced with this crisis, the temptation is to regard cancer as a purely physical problem, to focus on treating the symptoms and to overlook or neglect the underlying disease and its collection of causes. While this is understandable, it makes no sense to continue to smoke or to continue to eat badly if those things have contributed to the cancer's onset. At the very least, by adopting a healthy lifestyle we remove a large part of the burden of the cause—but also, by doing so we are creating the basis for recovery.

NOT ALL SMOKERS GET CANCER • What Else Is Going On?

We all know the "old George" type who smokes and drinks and does not get cancer. It seems fairly obvious that just one trigger factor, such as being a smoker, or having a high-fat diet, is not enough on its own to account for the great majority of cancers. Even the cumulative and synergistic effects of the known physical factors do not explain them all. Also, we need to go beyond the "Why me?" question to "Why now?" Why has the cancer developed at this particular point in my life? Why now?

Now we need to go beyond the obvious physical risk factors and take account of the possible role of the psychological and even spiritual aspects of life. While it may be that some people do have a poor diet as a major precipitating factor, others may have a large psychological component; for others, conflict in their spiritual life may be a real issue. We need to consider other possibilities.

Do not despair! The more causes we identify, the more we can do to overcome them by taking appropriate action. Cancer is a dynamic process. When we replace destructive tendencies with constructive ones, we immediately begin to tip the scales back toward health.

THE CANCER-PRONE PERSONALITY

In my experience, psychological factors are important in the causation of most cancers. There is a typical psychological profile that occurs in more than 95 percent of the many thousands of people affected by cancer with whom I have discussed their disease. This profile, this cancer-prone personality, was first expounded by Dr. E. Evans in 1926! It has gained increasing attention over the last few years, especially through the work of Dr. Lawrence Le Shan,[25] as well as Dr. Ainslie Meares, Dr. Carl Simonton and Stephanie Matthews,[26] and Dr. Lydia Temoshok.[27]

This increase in attention is important for if the psychological factors are identified and treated appropriately, then a major driving force that has been keeping the cancer going is immediately removed.

Most people diagnosed with cancer recognize this psychological profile. For some it comes as a shock to hear their basic life history so accurately recounted.

HOW THE CANCER-PRONE PERSONALITY DEVELOPS

Childhood Stress

In childhood, a cluster of stresses build up over a period of time. The stresses often relate to the child's interaction with their parents or peers, the prime influences acting in their life at this time. The key component of this stress is that there is a sense of a lack of approval from the important people in their lives. They feel unappreciated, or more specifically, unloved for what they do, for who they are.

This stress may come from parents and others who are downright physically or emotionally violent, or more subtly from those who are actually quite loving but emotionally nonexpressive or even abusive in ways they do not realize. The end result is that the child begins to feel they have little worth because they are receiving little encouragement in their endeavors, or because they are not feeling adequately loved. Their self-esteem suffers and they become increasingly concerned by what they believe other people think of them.

Climactic Event

Next, usually around seven to nine years of age, there comes a major traumatic incident which, again, is like the final straw that breaks the camel's back—its psychological back. This event seems almost unbearable, and through it, the feelings of lack of self-worth, lack of self-respect, lack of self-love threaten to become overwhelming. They know that they cannot endure this type of stress anymore. The child cries, "Enough." Something has to give. They need to find a new way of relating to their world, a new way of coping. No longer can the child react in a free, uncomplicated manner.

Premeditated Pattern of Behavior

Now interestingly, the cancer-prone personality types do not become aggressive, rebellious or difficult at this point. Quite the opposite. They determine that the way out, the way back to feeling good about themselves, is to win back the love, to win back the approval. So while something does snap inside and the emotional shutters go down, they determine to become "nice," successful, likable people. They decide to adopt a rigid pattern of behavior in response to stress. They begin to actively focus on pleasing other people and winning their approval. By doing so their stress becomes manageable; life becomes tolerable again.

The key point here is that in the cancer-prone personality this rigid pattern of behavior revolves around attempting to be as other people want them to be, rather than as they personally feel they should be. This commonly leads to trying to please other people, to doing what others would want them to. There is often an overtone of passive subservience. The cancer-prone personality types are not the ones to become outwardly aggressive or antisocial. Maybe they become manipulative, but they want to be liked. They seek approval.

So cancer patients are frequently "nice people." When diagnosed, their friends often say, "Why her? She's so nice, always trying to help other people. How awful this has happened to her. Why her? Why not that old creep George down the road?"

The fact is, of course, that trying to please other people is a fine ideal. It is the motivation behind it, however, that creates problems for the people who develop cancer. For them, this begins as a conscious means of coping, a defense mechanism, not a pure motivation. It is taken up as a premeditated defense mechanism and means they become reliant on factors outside of themselves, outside of their control, for their fundamental happiness and their sense of self-worth. This personality type relies on external approval.

Rigid Response Becomes Automatic

This conscious effort as a child to be a particular type of person is soon repeated so often that it becomes an automatic response. Now all stress is handled in the same basic, rigid way.

As this involves putting other people first, this pattern works well and these people are liked and usually successful. They frequently seek out positions where they can gain their gratification through the approval of others. It is not easy for them to do things based simply on their merits and to be satisfied by them. They find it difficult to develop a good self-image, and frequently rely on the approval of others for their own self-esteem. This need for outside approval is very real, if not always consciously expressed. Outwardly, their rigid pattern of behavior can produce a confident and assured air, but all the time they are seeking to cover this lack of self-esteem. Deep down, there can lurk a marked lack of self-confidence with a tendency toward self-negation, almost self-destruction. Deeply bottled inside is the feeling that all is not well. True reactions, emotions especially, are often suppressed. There is a continual effort to block out basic feelings. It is like trying to push the truth from the conscious awareness, like trying to keep the lid on a constantly bubbling pressure cooker.

Inner tension is established and maintained. There is a limited range of responses possible when it comes to dealing with stress.

Another Major Climactic Stress

In later life, another cluster of stresses is followed by one major event that changes the person's whole life circumstances. For example, we see this happening with people who have put all their emotional security into one relationship. Then if that relationship fails through death or separation, the sense of loss can be profound indeed. This can involve relationships with parents, lovers, spouses—or even with a devoted mother whose children leave home. The same effect can occur when a "workaholic" retires or is put out of work. Suddenly there is no outlet. Their whole life pattern is upset.

Financial difficulties followed by a foreclosure may be enough to tip the balance for some people. Betrayal by a partner at work has been the precipitated factor for many in business.

Inability to Cope

This change in life circumstances threatens the person's very source of self-worth and purpose. There seems to be no way their rigid pattern of behavior can deal with it. Their very life has been undermined. The person feels to be a victim of circumstances beyond their control and they can see no answer to this new situation. They feel as if life has dealt them a bitter blow, often one they half expected to occur. Life no longer has any meaning for them. Because they do not feel they can change their way of coping, they can see no viable future.

Feelings of Hopelessness and Helplessness

Faced with an unsolvable problem, an underlying feeling of hopelessness develops. But there is even more to this. People with a cancer-prone personality have a strong need to be liked, to gain approval. So faced with what they perceive to be a hopeless situation, they are also helpless. They feel bound to appear well and cheery. Becoming angry, or even sad or grief-stricken has the perceived potential to upset the family or friends.

So on the outside, their rigid pattern of behavior keeps these people going. Often they carry on with their rigid, cheery, helpful front. They are often unable to express their loss, their feelings of hopelessness and helplessness and outsiders often remark how well they seem to be coping, how little they have changed, despite their adversity.

The Body Mirrors the Hopelessness

However, potentially, this style of coping comes with a high cost. The inner sense of hopelessness is soon mirrored by the body itself. It is as if the body, too, gives up. It is as if the body also loses the will to live, it loses the ability to defend itself. The effect is a significant drop in the effectiveness of the body's own physical defenses, the immune system.

Again, this concept ties in so well with the idea that cancer involves a basic fault in the body's own natural function. It is as if this stress is so major that the body is laid open to having a self-destructive disease like cancer to develop.

Another straw, another major cause, becomes apparent.

In my experience most people diagnosed with cancer can observe this scenario in their life. Most recognized a climactic stressful event three months to two years before their symptoms first appeared. The most common interval by far for the people that I have worked with has been around eighteen months. It is as if it takes this long for the body to produce the external symptoms of that internal state.

The key factor here, the key problem, is the long-held pattern of coping with major stress in a particular, rigid way. It is important to realize this fact because, as we know, most people during their lives will be confronted by events involving major stress. These stresses are an inevitable part of life. However, not everyone who experiences major stress has a cancer-prone personality. Clearly, not everyone who experiences major stress will develop cancer. Those who do develop cancer tend to respond to stress in a common but very particular way. So next we will review stress itself, then reexamine what we can do to reverse it.

QUANTIFYING STRESS

Dr. Richard Rahe has done interesting work quantifying the effects of life-changing stress on our lives. Initially with the help of his colleague, Thomas Holmes, Rahe developed a Social Readjustment Rating Scale that placed a relative figure on a range of potentially stressful events. First published in 1965, the scale has been reevaluated and updated in 1977 and 1995.[28]

Back in 1965, Holmes and Rahe identified loss of a spouse as being the event having the highest potential for stress. They rated it as 100 Life Change Units (LCU), and then identified a range of other events that might occur in our lives with potentially stressful consequences. Importantly, events we may perceive as "positive" such as marriage or retirement, figure prominently—as do the obvious "negatives."

When you study the Life Changes Scaling Across Time chart, you realize that the relative impact of some stresses has changed over time. However, overall, the general impact of stress using this assessment is calculated to have risen 43 percent in the years from 1965 to 1995. This validates what many people are feeling—life is becoming more stressful. Who is not in need of learning to cope more effectively so that stress affects us less? No wonder meditation has such wide appeal!

The chart can be used to assess the total amount of stressful events you may have experienced in a given year. Identify the events, add the 1995 LCU score (see the following table) and check your total! A score of more than 300 from the table in any one year produces a 40 percent change of developing illness, while a score of fewer than 200 produces less than 10 percent of risk. This demonstrates the direct link between stress and illness: the more stress, the more illness produced.

HOW WE REACT TO STRESS IS THE ISSUE

The emphasis with all these factors is the changes they produce in our life circumstances. What is at issue is the ability to adapt to change—and for people with cancer, the particular way they go about doing it.

The fact is that many of us do seek to preserve the status quo and do find change a hard thing to manage. However, when it is unavoidable, most people do manage to pass through challenging periods of change and while they may be stressed for a while, life goes on. While more significant or dramatic clusters of stress may produce more of a setback, even some level of related physical disease, most people still do manage to bounce back and do not develop cancer. Many people have their own ways of coping or find new ones, and are able to adapt to new circumstances. They do not feel hopeless for any lasting period.

For those who do go on to develop cancer, it would seem it is not so much the nature of the challenge that is the problem, but their rather rigid pattern of reacting to it. This is most important. Everyone is subjected to challenge. Everyone is likely to be faced with some major life-changing events during their lifetime. Whether it be the death of a loved one, the need to change jobs, a move to a new city, whatever, such events are inevitable. Certainly many of the lesser challenges in our lives actually give it zest and flavor. Many challenges work to extend and develop us, and life would be pretty dull without them.

Life Changes Scaling Across Time (1965–1995)

Life Events	1965		1977		1995	
	Rank	LCU	Rank	LCU	Rank	LCU
Death of spouse	1	100	1	103	1	119
Divorce	2	73	4	62	2	98
Marital separation	3	65	8	52	4	79
Jail term	4	63	6	57	7	73
Death of close family member	5	63	2	73	3	92
Major personal injury or illness	6	53	16	42	6	77
Marriage	7	50	10	50	19	50
Fired from work	8	47	3	64	5	79
Marital reconciliation	9	43	17	42	13	57
Retirement	10	43	11	49	16	54
Change in health/behavior of family member	11	44	9	52	14	36
Pregnancy	12	40	5	60	9	66
Sexual difficulties	13	39	12	49	21	45
Gain of new family member	14	39	14	47	12	57
Major business readjustment	15	39	21	38	10	62
Change in financial state	16	38	16	48	15	36
Death of close friend	17	37	15	46	8	70
Change to different line of work	18	36	22	38	17	31
Change in number of arguments with spouse	19	35	24	34	18	51
Mortgage or loan greater than $10,000	20	31	18	39	23	44
Foreclosure on a mortgage or loan	21	30	7	57	11	61
Change in responsibilities at work	22	29	32	30	24	43
Child leaving home	23	29	36	29	22	44
Trouble with in-laws	24	28	25	33	29	37
Outstanding personal achievement	25	28	25	33	29	37
Spouse begins or ends work	26	26	23	37	20	46
Begin or end school	27	26	28	32	27	38
Change in living conditions	28	25	19	39	25	42
Change in personal habits	29	24	30	31	36	27
Trouble with boss	30	23	20	39	33	29
Change in work hours or conditions	31	20	27	33	30	36
Change in residence	32	20	26	33	26	41

Life Events	1965		1977		1995	
	Rank	LCU	Rank	LCU	Rank	LCU
Change in schools	33	20	39	28	31	35
Change in recreation	34	19	33	30	34	29
Change in church activities	35	19	35	29	42	22
Chance in social activities	36	18	40	28	38	27
Mortgage or loan less than $10,000	37	17	42	26	35	28
Change in sleeping habits	38	16	31	31	40	26
Change in number of family get-togethers	39	13	41	26	39	26
Change in eating habits	40	15	38	29	37	27
Vacation	41	13	37	29	41	25
Christmas	42	12	*	*	32	30
Minor violations of the law	43	11	29	32	43	22
Mean LCU value for all events	–	34.5	–	42	–	49

Note: LCU—Life Change Unit

The problem for many people who develop cancer is this inability to cope with a major challenge, particularly when it involves a fundamental change in their life. The inability to react appropriately and find release from the situation produces the changes in body chemistry we know as stress. This in turn affects the body's metabolism and lowers the immune system, so adding a significant factor to the list of causes of cancer. The more I talk with individual patients and groups, the more I am convinced of the importance of this factor.

Being able to recognize this in their nature is a great asset for a cancer patient. By accepting that this did contribute to their situation, they can make a great deal more sense of it. It is then relatively simple, in principle at least, to learn to cope with these psychological aspects of stress. By dealing with it appropriately, patients can contribute greatly to their own well-being and return to health. We shall explore in more detail the means available to do this in the next chapter.

WHY ME? THE SPIRITUAL QUESTION

Finally, however, having considered the physical and psychological causes of cancer, we need to go one step further. We need to be brave enough to ask, "Why me?" once more.

Why do some people have this cancer profile, and not others? Why do only some people find themselves in those complex childhood situations that lead on to particular attitudes and a pattern of behavior that, in turn, predisposes them to cancer? Why are some people drawn to smoke, to eat potentially harmful foods, to work in dangerous environments and, as a consequence, be faced with disease?

Unless we can answer these harder questions, we will remain unsatisfied and still be tempted to wallow in victim consciousness. Again, is it just chance that these circumstances develop? Surely not! We are now faced with a basic philosophical question that must be tackled.

A PERSONAL ACCOUNT

I consider myself fortunate. Right from the time my cancer was first diagnosed, I recognized that there was a spiritual thread running through and connecting all the events in my life. Moreover, prior to the cancer, I felt that I had been living with disharmony between my inner spiritual attitudes and my outer physical actions. There was conflict between what I felt I should do and what I actually did.

Basically as a young and rather impecunious veterinarian, I had put my interest in spiritual matters on hold while I focused on making money and establishing myself in the material world. While I was not doing anything illegal or dishonest and while I was actually working very hard, I felt I was not being true to my own inner aspirations. I felt that this disharmony was another major factor in the development of my cancer.

Now, clearly I am not suggesting this existential problem I held inside by focusing on making money was the sole cause of my cancer. I did have a type C personality, I did have major issues courtesy of my diet and so on. However, I am confident this more deep-seated, more spiritual dilemma was a significant cause—for me. More important, recognizing this problem provided me with a basic stimulus and raison d'être for seeking harmony in my spiritual, psychological and physical nature. I saw the three as interwoven and interdependent. Because I could see the interrelatedness of my past actions and present circumstances, I felt confident that justice would prevail. If I could make the necessary changes and find the right techniques, health may well be reattainable.

Now it is relatively easy to talk of psychological and physical things. These issues are relatively straightforward and not too emotionally charged. It is not so easy with things spiritual. However, knowing the important stimulus it was to me and having seen so many others gain strength and direction from their own spiritual endeavor, I feel it appropriate to delve into these deeper areas.

I hesitate for one moment as I do not want to be simplistically and unhelpfully labeled, nor do I want to run the risk of having good, straightforward techniques like meditation labeled. All these techniques do stand independently in their own right and are quite free of spiritual bias. They can all be judged on their own merits.

At the same time, I feel that any life is rather facile without some spiritual loading. Most people diagnosed with cancer are interested—in fact, they are often preoccupied—with the quest for answers to spiritual questions. Many people do flavor their life with spiritual concerns and it is appropriate to recognize this. Being raised as a Christian in the Anglican Church, I grew up with an earnest desire to know the Truth. There was an ever-present feeling that behind the mysteries of life, beyond the basic teachings of religion, lay a profound, unshakable Truth. Truth with a capital T.

In searching for this Truth, I have been deeply blessed to read many great books and by meeting and studying with many great spiritual masters from all traditions, particularly the Tibetan Buddhist Lama Sogyal Rinpoche who for many years has been my main teacher.

So while I continue to value greatly my Christian heritage, the answers I found that helped me through my illness, the answers that helped me to find more meaning and purpose in my life, were not limited to the orthodox Christian ones.

It seems worthwhile to present these views as a means of provoking discussion in this vital area. It is for each of us to search out the meaning, to make sense of our own situations, our own lives.

So, why should any person be placed in that combination of conditions that eventually lead to cancer? While people do seem to learn best and develop most through adversity, is it really necessary to go through cancer? And why should young children get it? There must be some reason why.

There really is a clear-cut, basic choice to make at this point. There is either order or there is not. Either we have to say life is meaningless and harsh in the extreme as no loving God could allow such things, or we say there is some order, some reason for it, some logic behind it all. I confess to not being able to make sense of what I see happening around me just on face value. Why do some people get it easy, others apparently hard?

I have an undying faith in the basic structured order of the universe. There has to be an explanation. The only one that satisfies me is provided by the Eastern philosophy of karma and reincarnation, the spiritual laws of cause and effect. Karma is a concept that says every action we take produces consequences to match. As we sow, so we reap. Good action, good consequences and the opportunity to benefit by them; bad action, bad consequences and the need to face those consequences and learn to get it right.

We can certainly see this principle operating in current life circumstances. Most of our current situation is the product of events we can easily identify. But it is often difficult to see justice or order in all of our own life patterns and certainly it is easy to judge some others harshly. Some people seem to face impossibly difficult odds in life, while on the surface they appear blameless. Some appear to do terrible things and get away with them. I am drawn, therefore, to widen my frame of reference to include the concept of reincarnation, the notion that we have a series of lives, rather than just one. If we do pass from life to life and carry over basic traits and blemishes, it makes sense of many seemingly inexplicable events. The child genius, the congenital birth defects, the hopelessly poor, the uncaring rich, all assume explainable stations in life.

For me, these concepts provide a framework into which I can comfortably fit and feel confident working within. Regarding successive lifetimes as opportunities for spiritual evolution provides a reason to strive for ethical conduct in all situations. It also means that no effort is wasted. Every attempt we make to reach a greater degree of harmony in our lives will eventually bear fruit. Any effort, be it in the physical, psychological or spiritual realm, if made with a positive, harmonious motivation, will be to our benefit.

Recognizing this spiritual thread to life and its ongoing nature was a great comfort for me as I battled the odds. It helped me to understand my situation, even if I could not relate my present predicament to definite events of a previous lifetime. Also, it made me feel the efforts of attempting to get well were worthwhile. Death lost its sting as final arbitrator. If life went on and my attitudes and actions had effects on my future circumstances, it meant I would be sensible to give 100 percent in every situation. Anything more I could not do, but anything less would be totally inappropriate. Finally, I had to realize that I had to do my 100 percent and then be prepared to let the results take care of themselves. I had to learn the need to avoid being attached to the results of my actions and not to view them as win or lose situations.

Similarly, I came to recognize and accept that at the most fundamental level I was responsible for my own condition. It is relatively easy to accept our role in disease through our patterns of eating and thinking and the environment in which we live. I feel it even more satisfying to consider disease as an opportunity for spiritual growth through learning and endeavor. Our spirit has put us in this position to test our reactions and give us the opportunity to learn the lessons we need in a very intense way. We never get more than we have the potential to handle! Remember the people who say, "Cancer has taught me so much—much more than I could have learned without it."

THE CAUSE AND EFFECT OF RECOVERY

It is vital to recognize in all this that cancer is a dynamic situation. It is good to identify what causes you can in your own life, as then you can act, make changes and get well again. This thinking gives a rationale for a total approach for treatment.

On the physical level, the actual symptoms certainly need to be attended to. Appropriate, direct therapy must be considered for them. However, do not overlook the real possibility that the lumps and bumps are only symptoms. Do not forget to tackle the underlying causes. Again, on the physical level, it makes good sense at least to adopt the organic Wellness Diet or to be more thorough with the Healing Diet. It also makes sense to avoid any sources of pollution and to utilize any treatment that increases the body's natural defenses.

Psychologically, the big need is to change. If we recognize that a particular pattern has aided in creating the disease, then obviously a new pattern is required. Changing to that new pattern can be done through conscious action based on the desire to get better.

However, often it will just flow on as a result of the disease itself. The disease creates the excuse for change. It produces a new situation or insight that allows the patient the space to change their rigid patterns.

Hope is the key here. It may come from within with a change of attitude or be built by inspiration from without. Once that hope is revived, then the rebuilding process is under way. The attitude becomes positive and focused upon living well again. The sense of being a victim gives way to a feeling of being responsible and in control.

Many find that they no longer feel guilt about their past. Their new perspective sheds fresh light and allows them to seek forgiveness for errors of the past. Now they feel free to concentrate upon building a new future, to concentrate upon loving life and everything around them.

One step leads on to the next and the physical condition soon reflects this improvement. While there may be ups and downs, the healing process gathers momentum. Frequently, meditation takes the bumps out of this path. Having benefits on all levels of our being, it both smooths out and intensifies the healing.

For many people, the end result is a health that is described as "weller than well." Having recovered from such an illness, they have a new zest for life. Just getting well from cancer is cause enough for a boost in self-esteem. Add to this all that is learned along the way and people frequently portray a new confidence and a quiet but genuine regard for themselves and all around them. The joy they feel enhances their own lives and infuses joy into those with whom they come in contact. It is a process of self-discovery and self-fulfillment.

MOVING ON TO FIND SOLUTIONS

While considering the spiritual issues around disease and its causation may be somewhat esoteric for some, there can be no doubting the immediacy of the role played by our psychology and especially our emotions. Again to be clear, cancer is a chronic, multifactorial degenerative disease. So while I am not saying the psychological component is *the* cause of cancer, I am sure that it is another major contributing factor.

On the psychological level, the reality is that once the cancer is actually diagnosed, for many a seemingly hopeless situation will exist. However, what if the person diagnosed with cancer had previously lost the desire to live in the manner we discussed above, and now the diagnosis gives them the opportunity to not expect to live? A rather blunt friend, a fellow cancer patient, once described cancer as a socially acceptable form of suicide for people who found themselves in an intolerable position.

I can hear people yelling in protest, "It's not me! That's not me!" However, it is usually the families, not the patients, who protest most. Many patients recognize the sequence readily, are relieved to understand what is going on and are happy to set about correcting the situation.

To restate it, hope is the starting point. To re-create hope we need to bolster the desire to live and the expectation that a continuation of life is possible.

Now another curious fact. The desire or will to live can often be rekindled by the diagnosis itself! Having cancer can change a person's life dramatically and totally. Suddenly they become the center of attention. Friends and family rally, work may be avoided, a ready excuse is available for that long-put-off holiday, all manner of new possibilities present.

Some patients become very good at it—at being patients. While they may have a flourishing victim consciousness, under all the attention they rally. Life becomes enjoyable and worth living again, and the body responds to this new surge. Many then find new ways of coping and do get back to leading healthy lives again.

However, some do come to that difficult point where they are getting so well that their friends no longer call, the family returns to its own normal pursuits, and the need to work reemerges. A difficult choice: to be sick and happy, or well and miserable. This may well be funny if it was not real. It would be foolish to oversimplify the complexity of this problem, but very frequently psychological trauma is a major consideration for cancer patients.

A CRY FOR LOVE

The cry of anguish that creates disease is a cry for love. It is a genuine need that needs to be met. Love is the appropriate response and it works 100 percent every time.

In my experience, emotional factors do play a major role in cancer. People who are diagnosed with cancer are frequently emotionally tight. Many prefer to keep their emotions to themselves and they have difficulty in expressing them even if they want to. It has taken me years to feel comfortable telling people how I feel about them, particularly if I want to express my feelings of love.

When we recollect the stress response and the psychological profile involved in cancer, we see the challenge in that profile is frequently emotionally based. The fear that turns the challenge into a stress is usually one of not being loved, of being rejected, or of being emotionally hurt.

For cancer patients it is most frequently emotional challenges that produce the bodily reaction with its accompanying changes in body chemistry. For them, there often seems to be no adequate action they know of that can be taken to resolve their situation and so gain relief.

Emotional fear fixes them in a state of altered body chemistry. The contention is these biochemical changes can be so profound as to reduce their body's potential to heal and sustain itself in good health. Then, when a cancer begins—as might be prompted by a high-fat diet, cigarette smoking, some bodily malfunction, or whatever—the body no longer cares, it no longer recognizes it has a problem. It allows the cancer to develop and life-threatening symptoms can follow.

This being so, it is vital when we are seeking recovery from cancer to work on our emotions too—to "let go" emotionally, to heal the emotions as well as the body. Most people enjoy this part of it, once they get going! Everyone wants to feel love in their life and feel capable of giving it freely. So in the next chapter we consider the healing power of healthy emotions. How do we transform destructive emotions into healing emotions?

CHAPTER 16

Healthy Emotions 1

Feeling Well, Being Well

IT IS VERY USEFUL TO THINK ABOUT THE POWER OF THE MIND: TO ANALYZE, contemplate and plan how we train the mind; get the most out of its vast potential; use it as a key ally for healing.

By contrast, emotions need to be felt. And emotions have a powerful role in the healing process. So give yourself a moment or two to feel this.

If in the past you have felt resentment toward another person, or say you feel resentment for someone in current time, imagine you suddenly and unexpectedly meet that person.

Imagine they were in front of you now.

What happens in your body? Most people when face-to-face with resentment notice their muscles tighten up pretty quickly. Teeth clamp down harder; perhaps there is a grimace, the stomach contracts, maybe even fists clench and the arms draw close in to the body. Contact with the other person is avoided.

Now, maybe you have learned to mask all this, to sublimate the feelings and appear neutral from the outside. But if you go into the feeling, into the body, it is all about contracting, tightening, withdrawing. The feeling is of curling up or hunching over. The feeling is cold and hard and tight with a pervasive agitation.

What place has healing among that collection of feelings?

Now relax. Then bring to mind someone who delights you—maybe someone you have not seen for a while or someone whose company you really enjoy. Maybe you would say they love you, you love them. But now, just imagine meeting up with them again, suddenly and unexpectedly.

What happens in your body? Exuberance. Your arms probably go out and up. A smile breaks into happy laughter. If you were to check you would probably notice a feeling of gentle warmth and relaxation, maybe even a tingling in your body. Contact is welcomed. Maybe you hug, embrace, kiss.

What place has healing among that collection of feelings? Everything. While resentment almost feels like cancer itself, when it comes to the joy and delight of meeting an old friend, it is as if every cell in your body sings. That is a healthy emotion. That is a healing emotion.

THE STORY AND THE EMOTION

Now the crucial point. Emotions do not exist in their own right. You do not just feel angry, feel sad, feel joyful for no good reason. Emotions need to be produced by something and we can call that something "the story." So you feel angry because of the story relating to what he did. Or you feel sad because of the story relating to what happened in the past. Or you feel apprehensive based upon the story relating to what might happen in the future.

Simple is it not? There is "the story" and there is "the emotion." The emotion follows the story.

Of course, there is compelling logic in the way we link the emotion and the story. "Of course I am angry; let me tell you what he did." "Of course I am happy; let me tell you about my child's success." Etc., etc. But do you notice what it is like to be around someone who is miserable all the time? Complains all the time? Speaks badly of others all the time? Then remember what is it like to be around someone who recognizes the good in all they experience, who brings a sense of humor to all they do; a person who has warmth, compassion and love. Which person would you prefer to be with? If they were sick or needed help in any way, who would you be more likely to make time for?

So back to the crucial point. Just as we can decide how we will respond to our circumstances, we can decide to regulate our emotions. Now, if "regulating your emotions" sounds a little dry or calculating, or you have some other aversion to the notion, pause for a moment and consider the practical realities.

My old friend Jazzer comes to mind. Jazzer had a difficult form of leukemia many decades ago. He had chemotherapy off and on, actually more on than off, for over twelve years. These were in older times and Jazzer would vomit relentlessly and uncontrollably for hours and hours after each treatment. His reaction was so consistently bad he needed to be hospitalized for each treatment. Yet rather than develop an aversion, Jazzer welcomed the help he received. He would greet everyone in the hospital with genuine warmth, acknowledge even the smallest kindness, thank everyone for everything and, above all, use his natural humor to make light of his fairly extreme difficulties.

One of Jazzer's favorite ways of enduring the convulsive vomiting he was confronted with was to make his way to another ward in the hospital, get down on his hands and knees, and pretend he was a barking dog. Some probably thought he was barking mad, but we would crawl around on the floor, moving from bed to bed and alternating between making noises like a barking dog, making his involuntary noises associated with the dry retching, and pretending to lift his leg like a dog urinating on his fellow patients' beds. His smile and his manner was infectious and laughter accompanied his regular stunts.

Some will know of Dr. Patch Adams, another old friend who was portrayed by Robin Williams in the film *Patch*. Patch uses humor and clowning as a way to move past people's pain and into their hearts. A very skillful doctor and therapist, Patch is a living example of the healing power of laughter.

SCIENCE SUPPORTS HEALTHY EMOTIONS

In mentioning the medical profession again, let us consider another good reason why regulating our emotions makes good sense. There has been a great deal of research completed in recent years investigating how our emotions impact upon our health. The science is very clear. What commonly but perhaps unhelpfully are described as "negative" emotions generally weaken our health and well-being, they make us more prone to disease and adversely impact on our capacity to heal. Negative emotions are bad for us. No surprise there! Happily the converse is true—what we call "positive" emotions enhance our health and well-being, help to prevent disease and actively support our capacity to heal. Positive emotions are good for us, good for our recovery.

Now, what we do need to be very clear about is that our emotions are always valid. If you feel an emotion, it is real enough. So rather than describing our emotions as negative and positive, we will be kinder on ourselves and more accurate when we use the words destructive and constructive. Or life denying and life affirming. The real questions we need to address are: does a particular emotion harm or help you, and do you have the capacity to manage your emotions, particularly if you are intent on healing?

A quick answer comes with considering the scenario of living with yourself. Yes, if you were living with yourself, what would you be keen to change?

A more measured response comes by deliberately cultivating healthy emotions. Here is how:

FOUR TECHNIQUES THAT DEVELOP HEALTHY EMOTIONS

More good news. The answer to the last question, "Can I develop healthy emotions?" is a clear yes. Once you recognize the power of emotions and decide to cultivate healthy, healing emotions, there are four groups of potent yet straightforward techniques that will convert this intention into reality.

1. Meditation—has the natural power to release destructive emotions and foster the constructive ones.
2. General antidotes to destructive emotions—simple yet profound solutions for complex problems.
3. Specific antidotes to major destructive emotions—how to transform fear, shame, resentment, guilt and grief.
4. Techniques to cultivate constructive emotions—that are life affirming, healthy and healing.

We will consider the first two in this chapter; the other two in the next.

MEDITATION NATURALLY GENERATES HEALTHY, HEALING EMOTIONS

We have discussed this in some detail in the specific meditation chapters, but to recap:

When we meditate regularly and effectively, anger, resentment, depression, anxiety, fear, a whole range of unhelpful emotions simply falls away. At the same time, there is a natural rise in optimism, enthusiasm, joy and appreciation. It is natural for people who meditate to find themselves happier and more content, to be good humored and to smile more regularly and in a way that reflects a satisfaction that comes deep from within.

What meditation also does is to loosen up old habits, old states of mind. Therefore, against the background of regular meditation, the antidotes and the techniques to generate healthy, healing emotions become easier to work with.

GENERAL ANTIDOTES TO DESTRUCTIVE EMOTIONS

As with most things, there are a number of choices when it comes to managing emotions more effectively. None is better than the other per se; although the antidotes are a bit like treating the symptoms while the transformation gets at the cause. What makes sense is to consider the choices that follow and use whatever resonates with your own particular situation and needs.

The General Antidotes and the Transformation

CHANNELING THE ENERGY CONSTRUCTIVELY

Take anger as an example. There is a lot of energy in anger. The question is, how is that energy used? Many horrible things have resulted from uncontrolled and poorly directed anger. Many good things have been accomplished in the world when anger has motivated people to take strong, bold, decisive, and even prolonged action. Much that is good in social activism was inspired by anger.

Roger was caring for his wife, Beth, who had a series of difficulties associated with secondary bowel cancer. Their specialist seemed very despondent regarding Beth's case and was increasingly gruff and offhand in their meetings. Roger became increasingly agitated, increasingly angry.

Finally, with his wife complaining of pain and the doctor seeming intent on just getting them out of his office, Roger exploded.

"Look," he said, "we seem far more focused on trying to get my wife well than you are. How about you wake up to yourself and try to help us!"

Now the interesting thing is that this particular doctor had quite a good reputation for being caring, open-minded and a great communicator. To his credit, Roger's words had an electrifying effect upon him.

"I am so sorry," he said. "Please forgive me. I have been so busy, there is so much to do." Then he spent half an hour going over Beth's situation in detail and making sure her other needs, as well as her pain, were attended to.

What is important to note here is Roger channeled his anger wisely. He did not sit on it. He did not block it, he did not take it out on someone else. Also, he did not hit the doctor or abuse him! Very important. What he did was to use the energy of the anger to break through his natural reticence to speak up. He voiced the concerns he had for his wife and his dissatisfaction with the way she was being treated. And again, to his credit, the doctor took it in, realized his error, owned it, apologized and made good. As an addendum, Roger said they never had anything but the best of kind and attentive treatment throughout the time they saw that same doctor.

UNDERSTANDING HELPS

Part of what helps us to understand the difficulties people have with their emotions is to know where these difficulties come from. For example, in the cancer arena, we need to be aware that anger is a common reaction to grief. In Elisabeth Kübler Ross' classic description of the Five Stages of Grief,[29] denial comes first, anger second. Being aware that the diagnosis of cancer frequently triggers a grief reaction in patients, families and friends, we need to be on guard. Many unkind things have been said or done through anger, when actually grief was the real issue.

Jenny had six years cancer free after an initial diagnosis of breast cancer and a year of treatments. When it returned, her husband was dismayed by the way Jenny's attitude toward her teenage children changed. She began to find fault in every little thing they did or did not do. She withdrew from John, avoided contact, and yet several times John found her crying in their bedroom on her own. When asked what was wrong or if he could help, John was met with hostility and abruptly told to leave her alone.

Fortunately, John was helped to appreciate what Jenny was going through, to support her to express her anger with the relapse, and to begin to face her very natural fears of dying and leaving her family without a mother.

Supported by her husband's love and care Jenny began to be able to talk with others about her situation both in the support group where there was natural understanding, as well as with her closest friends where there was natural empathy, genuine care and love.

In my observation Jenny followed a common emotional path. Anger gave way to a lingering sadness that lay beneath a genuinely bright exterior. From time to time the sadness came out in tears or just the recognition of painful feelings. But the intensity, the heat of the early anger was gone and in the main, optimism, resolve and enjoyment of life filled Jenny's common experience. This seems natural and reasonable. Faced with a potentially life-threatening situation Jenny's disappointment and sadness makes sense. But if her emotions, coupled with fear, anger and resentment were to dominate her day, then she would both be having a miserable life and those emotions could well weaken her chances of recovery.

As it was, Jenny channeled a good deal of constructive energy into reinforcing her good nutritional and meditation habits. Given her relapse, she determined that her emotions were what needed the most attention, and focused on ways of resolving two significant, long-held resentments and becoming more loving with her family. Happily, she went into remission again and remains well.

RELEASING EMOTIONS SAFELY

People affected by cancer tend to bottle up their emotions. They feel them strongly enough, but they tend to keep them to themselves. We discussed some of the reasons for this when we addressed the cancer-prone personality type, and to repeat, blocked emotions are unhealthy emotions. For many of the people I have known who became long-term survivors, turning this around was pivotal to their success. They learned to be more open, more fluid, more authentic with their emotions.

Put simply, healthy emotions are authentic emotions. When emotions flow easily, comfortably, authentically, then health and well-being follow. Stifled emotions, repressed emotions and fabricated emotions all weaken the potential for healing as well as significantly reducing our sense of well-being. How then to change a deeply ingrained habit? How do we learn to release emotion safely?

The first thing is to recognize this is not so easy, but it can be done. This is an area where groups can play a particularly positive role. A good group leader creates what can be well described as a "safe place." Using a variety of techniques, it becomes increasingly obvious that the group is a place where people can express their emotions, be understood, be well "held"—as in supported and nurtured—and learn to be more at ease with being emotionally open.

Often it is among peers we learn best. So among other people going through similar experiences with cancer there is an inner knowing that binds the group. At first this goes unstated, but gently, as the more adventurous or "extroverted" speak up, what has been left silent, contained in silence, kept as secret, begins to be expressed.

CHANGING THE CHANNEL

This is a simple and effective technique for when a difficult emotion is really bugging you, but is not too strong. It is like turning the TV on and finding that what comes up first is unpleasant—maybe like a horror movie, and so you simply change the channels and watch something pleasant. This is a reliable method that aims to take your mind and your emotion away from something difficult and unpleasant to something comfortable and pleasant.

To change channels, all you need to do is choose to think of someone, something, or some event you enjoy. Or you could remember, reimagine your quiet place—that inner sanctuary which is reliably peaceful and calming (revisit chapter 10). This technique provides an easy short- to medium-term fix.

FEELING THE EMOTION AND DISSOLVING IT

For a longer-term solution this technique offers a wonderful possibility.

The theory is simple. The story resides in our head, the emotions are held in our body.

When we focus on the story, we continually rekindle old memories related to who said what, what happened when, and on and on. Focusing on the story can be like rerunning endless episodes of a classic soap opera where a few key players manage to recycle a never-ending list of problems. The more we dwell on the story, the more we fuel the emotions. When linked so directly to the thoughts in our head, emotions tend to become stuck, linked to their story and gone over again and again with no resolution. Left in our head, it is not surprising that emotions may well be painful and chronic and, as such, either suppressed or left uncontrolled and unpredictable.

Here then is the key point. Emotions are felt in the body. To work on our emotions, we need to turn our attention in to our body.

Often, before our awareness is brought to this and we train ourselves a little, we may well have felt our emotions as some vaguely pleasant or unpleasant feeling that we recognized as an emotion, but had difficulty really knowing what it was, or where it was. In this way, emotions remain rather abstract, vague and difficult to work with.

This antidote of dissolving emotions is based on the fact that when dealing with an emotion that is recurring, unpleasant or maybe quite painful, we can learn to use our willpower, to selectively drop any thinking about "the story," and instead go into "the emotion." By doing so, the remarkable outcome is that the emotion will actually dissolve. Here is how it works.

The solution is simple. If you have not done this before it is easy. It can be done in meditation posture, sitting casually or lying down—probably easier with the eyes closed. We simply bring to mind the emotion then notice where in the body we actually feel it. Most emotions register in our central core—abdomen, solar plexus region, chest; maybe up into the throat region, but mostly in the chest and abdomen. If you have a strong emotion, you can try this straight away. If not, and you want to experiment with this technique, you can recall one of your emotional stories for a moment, just long enough to generate the emotion, then drop the story, bring your attention into that central core area of your body, and go into the bodily felt sense of the emotion.

There are three crucial points with this technique:

Simply dwell on the feeling in your body

Avoid the temptation to think the feeling in your body needs to change or you need to fix something. Your awareness will take care of it automatically. By holding your awareness on the feeling, it will slowly, steadily and reliably dissolve.

Hold the physical feeling in your awareness nonjudgmentally

This is very important. Let go of any tendency to be critical or to analyze. Simply be interested to notice the feeling. That is all. Just notice it free of any judgment and free of any commentary or internal discussion.

To do this is the discipline, the personal kindness you need for the technique to be effective. So whenever you notice yourself becoming judgmental, simply drop the commentary and go back into the feeling. Be patient. Stay with the feeling.

Remain undistracted

Whenever you become aware that your mind has wandered or you have gone back to dwelling on the story, recognize this, be gentle with yourself (do not beat yourself up), and return to the bodily felt sense.

This technique is well described as mindfulness of emotions* and is a powerful way to actually become comfortable with, and then release, destructive and painful emotions.

DISSOLVING THE STORY

Any story that triggers an emotion lives in our mind. It is a complex construction, based on an event that actually did happen in the past, or we think may happen in the future. This event is then overlaid with our beliefs, habits, associated experiences, prejudices, knowledge, biases, preferences, hopes, fears, desires, dislikes, etc. We end up with a "story" made up of what we believed happened, or what we believe may happen. This becomes our version, our recollection of what actually did happen. The story.

However complex it may seem to be, once we have one, the story is the trigger for the emotion. So while we did learn in the last section how to dissolve the emotion, what about the story itself? There are three main techniques we can use to clear or dissolve the story:

Self-Analysis

This is possible but highly problematic. If our mind is deeply stable, then analysis of a past story may well be useful and effective; leading to perspective, clarity and resolution. However, for many of us, attempting to analyze the story tends to get us stuck in the unhelpful cycle of ongoing and unproductive thinking as described in the previous section.

---

* For more on the mindfulness of emotions, refer to the chapter of this name in my book *Meditation—An In-Depth Guide.*

Counseling or Psychotherapy

This is a real option, particularly if the emotions felt are distressingly painful and chronic.

There is a wide range of therapeutic techniques on offer, so where to go for the best help? The research is clear. When it comes to psychological change for the good, the quality of the relationship between you and your therapist is more important than the particular techniques or therapy style they use! It may be surprising, but constructive therapeutic change is most likely to occur when you have a good rapport with the health professional assisting you. So seek out a therapist you can develop confidence in and trust fairly quickly. It is always wise to regard the first visit to a potential counselor as a job interview. Is this person someone you can trust to help you with your life? If the answer is yes, make the next appointment and allow the real work to begin.

It is useful to mention that a well-run group also has the possibility to help in this regard. Sometimes I marvel at the shifts people experience in the group situation, so again, it is an option to seek out a well-led group in which you can feel confidence and trust.

Dissolve the Story Using Mindfulness and Meditation

This technique can be described as mindfulness of the story. Strange title, but great technique. This is a more advanced technique that requires some preexisting stability of the mind. Here is how mindfulness of the story works.

Preferably you take up your meditation posture, but you could do this sitting casually or lying down. Give yourself the time and space wherein you will not be interrupted. Then bring the story to mind. Being an old familiar story as the one you would work on will always be, it will only need a modest invitation. As you think over the story's details once more—who did what, what happened, what was said—allow the story to flow like a movie or a video clip in your head. And the key point again is to observe all that unfolds free of judgment. You need to avoid the running commentary of "That was good," "That was bad." You need to let go of attempting to manipulate the story, or attempting to reframe it in some way. Just let it run and remain aware, undistracted and nonjudgmental.

If you find emotion welling up to accompany the story, just observe that impartially as well. Even if tears flow or other emotions arise, simply observe them, stay with them, allow them their time, but in this technique, your focus stays with the story.

This exercise can be compared to allowing a bad movie to run through to completion, while you watch it as an impartial observer. When it is over, it is over. It is the emotion and the ongoing reflection and analysis that revives an old story. Simply letting it run under the light of full awareness allows it to reach completion and dissolve.

Now this is a powerful and effective technique but it is not without consequence. Often amidst the clarity of giving a story full awareness comes the realization that action is required. So maybe actively engaging in forgiveness is the next step. Maybe some restitution is required, some justice needs to be sought, or some personal change undertaken on your behalf.

Dissolve the Story in the View

The "view" is a word used to describe our philosophical understanding of life, coupled with the meaning and purpose we hold for it and our spiritual reality. So our view could be defined by our religious beliefs and our faith. We could hold a Christian view, Buddhist, Hindu, Islamic, Jewish view, etc. We could have our own personal philosophical view that has developed through our own experience, culture and learning. Our view may be abstract and vague, or well defined and precise. In simple terms, our view plays a major part in how we interpret and understand the world, its events and its people—and how we decide our part in all that goes on around us.

Many people find their view satisfactorily resolves past events. Things happen, you take them in, interpret them, make sense of them, act accordingly and life moves on. What we are discussing in this section is where our view fails and we are stuck with an unhelpful emotion. Maybe at such a time we can benefit from expanding our view.

Maybe resentment has been the issue. Maybe your view has accommodated holding on to resentment. You believe in your cause—"He did that atrocious thing," "She was so . . ." You believe in your right to be angry, to be chronically angry, to become angry over and over every time you recall the story. This is your view.

However, what if your view was expanded and you began to believe in forgiveness? If you did forgive, the story would dissolve!

Was Michael Leunig correct when he said:

"Love one another
And you will be happy.
It is as simple and as difficult as that.
There is no other way."

Reflecting upon this, we move on to examine specific antidotes to destructive states of mind and emotions.

CHAPTER 17

Healthy Emotions 2

Transforming the Negative, Accentuating the Positive

BACK AT THE END OF THE 1970S, WHEN I WAS BEGINNING TO FORMULATE the idea of starting a lifestyle-based cancer self-help group, it seemed clear that everyone was fully aware of the many problems associated with cancer. Virtually everyone I talked to at the time was beset with the difficulties they were facing; fear and despondency were commonplace. It was logical to conclude that a new approach was warranted.

Therefore, when the groups actually began in 1981, we concentrated on the positives. There was unspoken acknowledgment of the difficulties; we spoke of them very little, passed over them quickly and focused on the positives. So, positive thinking, positive emotions, meditation, exercise, diet. We talked about and put into practice the positive things that worked.

In the process hope was rekindled. Optimism soared, people felt rapidly better within themselves and many reported significant physical gains. Many doctors commented on the positive changes in the demeanor and the physical parameters of those attending the groups. The word spread, the numbers attending the groups increased rapidly, and all seemed wonderfully good.

OBSTACLES TO ONGOING PEACE OF MIND

Then came Barbara. Actually Barbara was there in the first group I ever ran, which started on September 16, 1981.

She had rung me the night before to tell me how difficult things were for her as a result of the advanced, medically untreatable brain tumor she was dealing with. She became more and more emotional and distressed as we talked, then she told me she was not sure if she would commit suicide or come to the group tomorrow. Then she hung up. Being new to all this, I had not yet taken her contact details so I could not get back to her. I could only spend a somewhat anxious time before experiencing considerable relief when she did turn up for the group.

Barbara was in her early forties and she came with her partner, Michael. Together they quickly warmed to the program, embracing all the recommendations, and Barbara experienced a swift, uneventful and complete recovery without any medical treatment. Barbara was a star patient—or so it seemed.

A little over a year later Michael called me. Barbara had been very well but recently was eating more and more things they both knew were not good for her. When Michael questioned her, he was told very curtly to mind his own business.

Michael and I discussed this a little but then a few weeks later he called again. Now Barbara had abandoned her meditation. Michael was increasingly worried. We discussed the situation some more. but a few weeks later he called again. Now the brain cancer was back and this time Barbara was completely opposed to meditating, eating for recovery or being positive. I went to see her in person.

Barbara was a very intelligent and articulate woman. She was reasonably open and frank with me. Barbara explained that before the cancer was diagnosed her life was in deep disarray. Problems abounded in every aspect of her life: a disturbing childhood, difficult past relationships, unhappy in work, conflict in her current relationship. The cancer diagnosis came as no surprise and she had related strongly to the group discussions regarding the cancer-prone personality. But the diagnosis changed everything.

Following the diagnosis of cancer, Michael had become more attentive and their relationship flourished. With the cancer, she was unable to go to work. With the cancer she had a ready-made, unarguable excuse to do whatever she liked. So she did. She came to know a new level of happiness.

Then she recovered. What now? She needed to face her life again. But she did not like it. The job seemed as unpleasant as ever. Now her friends were not so attentive. Her past felt as if it was crowding in on her.

Barbara put it to me quite simply: "Ian, I would rather die than go back to my old life." And despite everyone's best efforts at the time, she did die quite rapidly.

Often the stories that carry major insights or reveal key points are dramatic. Barbara's story, coupled with those of other people with similar dilemmas, affected me deeply and led to a new level of understanding. The so-called positive approach worked well as a starting point. It gave people hope and direction and nearly everyone who committed to the techniques involved improved dramatically in their health and well-being.

But over time, what we came to observe was that many people hit barriers to maintaining their peace of mind and when that was lost, the motivation to look after themselves was lost, and almost invariably, the health of the people involved suffered badly.

Now, with the benefit of many years of study and the cumulative experience of my colleagues and the many thousands of people from the groups, it is possible to categorize the barriers and to set out effective antidotes.

WHEN TO ADDRESS DESTRUCTIVE EMOTIONS?

There are five destructive emotions that people affected by cancer commonly encounter. But before we examine them, first a perspective and then the question of timing.

For any individual diagnosed with cancer the recommendation remains to focus on the way forward. By that I mean the positives—the food, the positive thinking, the healthy emotions, the meditation and so on. There is no need to go looking for destructive emotions. If they are an issue, they will find you. What is meant by this is that peace of mind is the thing to aim for. When it comes to states of mind and emotions, in broad terms it is peace of mind that will heal you. Experiencing more love, being happy, rekindling passion, experiencing joy, laughing—all these are powerful healers. So cultivate them in the manner we will discuss soon, but if you find a block emerges to your peace of mind, then that is the time to address the destructive emotions.

Some people do have fairly uneventful recoveries and experience peace of mind as an ongoing reality. Many more come up against one or more of the following destructive emotions and when the time is right, benefit from working through the problem.

How do you know when the time is right to address one of these issues? When the issue itself insists upon it. For example, an occasional fear is reasonable, rational and normal. There is no need to give attention to the occasional fear; just observe it, recognize it for what it is, a fear, and let it go.

However, if fear is with you all the time, if fear wakes you up regularly in the night, if fear takes up residence on your shoulder and whispers its message into your ear fairly constantly, then that is the time to address it.

FIVE BARRIERS TO PEACE OF MIND AND THEIR SPECIFIC ANTIDOTES

Now it is time to address fear, shame, resentment, guilt and grief. Something for everyone, really!

Fear and Its Four Antidotes

Fear is the most common emotion experienced by people when first diagnosed with cancer. Sometimes it is so strong it virtually paralyzes otherwise competent people. Curiously, in the groups' experience it is the easiest to deal with. For most people, a realistic hope and meditation combine in such a way that fear simply drops away without being addressed directly.

However, for those for whom it remains a problem, or for those who experience relapses and find fear rearing its head again, it is wise to address it on four levels.

PHYSICAL FEAR AND HOW TO FACE IT

This is the category in which we talk of the fears directly associated with the disease and the prospect of it advancing: fear of pain, fear of dying and fear of change. Each of these topics is discussed in other chapters of this book, but the actual fear is best overcome by facing it directly. If one attempts to ignore, minimize, suppress or even just take our attention off this group of fears, they simply return, commonly stronger than ever.

How to face these fears? First, some stability is needed. Denial is a common first response to grief because it puts the problem out of mind and helps to make things manageable.

Denial can be very useful short term—it just does not work well over the long term. It is helpful to understand this especially if you are supporting someone recently diagnosed. Denial can be a valid coping mechanism and people often need time to internally process their change in circumstances and support to regain the strength required to face their options with more awareness.

Rarely have I seen the benefit of dwelling on the issues of pain, death or change soon after diagnosis. However, when the time is right and if these early fears remain strong, the antidote is to "face the tiger."

Clive was a successful businessman who had lived on his own for many years. Diagnosed with advanced prostate cancer he began the program, reduced his pain, improved his health generally and stabilized his PSA. Then he found himself obsessing about his future. What would happen if the disease progressed? How would he cope? Could he manage at home? What to do? Clive became increasingly anxious, lost sleep and was heading into depression.

Acting on advice, Clive approached his GP, whom he valued for his skill and his capacity to communicate. Clive made a long appointment then explained that he was working hard toward his recovery and was essentially optimistic, but that fear for the future was really preoccupying him. He needed to understand his worst-case scenario—what might happen if all went badly and what he could he do about it.

The GP discussed the possibilities. He explained that pain was something he was very confident would be manageable medically if the need arose. He discussed how the cancer Clive had in his spine could progress and possibly interfere with his mobility, even lead to paraplegia if the possible treatment options he outlined were not successful. He pointed out that there may come a time when he would need home help or need to go into a nursing home or hospice. Then the GP described how in his experience many people die from cancer after first lapsing into a coma, and that again, in his experience, most die peacefully.

Clive recounted later how challenging this conversation had been. However, he stayed with it and at each point he and the GP made plans regarding Clive's options. He followed up by contacting the local visiting nurses' services, identifying home help options and visiting his local hospice, being pleasantly surprised by the quality of the facilities and the staff. Clive updated his will and did all he could to "put his affairs in order." Then he relaxed.

Having "faced the tiger," Clive now had a complete backup plan. Now, whenever fear for his future arose, he recognized the nature of that fear, reminded himself he had things well covered and was able to quickly dismiss the fear.

Facing death is a big enough issue to warrant its own chapter and that does come next, but the prompt here is to actually read and consider it when you come upon it.

EMOTIONAL FEAR AND ITS ANTIDOTE, LOVE

How will my relationships be affected by the disease? How will my friends react? My family? What about my work, should I tell people? Should I keep it to myself? How open and honest should I be?

First, there is no "should." Everyone is different. Every situation is unique. However, we can make some powerful general observations.

People who develop cancer tend to bottle up their emotions. They tend to "put on a happy face" and keep their distress inside. Many long-term survivors report that transforming this trait was integral to their recovery and one of the major benefits that came into their lives provoked by the harsh realities of their disease.

The simple antidote is to be more loving. Unconditionally loving. Many people these days, and many people with cancer particularly, love conditionally. I will love you on the condition that you are nice to me in return; if you look after me well, if you meet my needs. This is a neurotic form of love that is more like a deal, or a trade-off, than real love.

Real love heals. Real love is unconditional. Real love is cyclical. If you want it coming into your life, you need to be giving it out as well. The antidote to emotional fear therefore is to develop ways of becoming more loving.

The first step is to start working on reducing the conditional love. The two best ways to know this is working is when you can say no to requests, and when you can ask for help. Most people with cancer I ask—and I have asked thousands over several decades—have trouble saying no when asked to do just about anything, and similarly, most have trouble asking for help. These traits are powerfully linked to the cancer-prone personality. We can observe that these two habits are symptoms of an inner need to be liked, to be approved by those around us. The fear behind these habits is that if I do not say yes to all requests, people may not like me, may not approve of me, may not love me. If I ask for help, I may be a burden or create an inconvenience. To repeat, there is the fear people may not like me, may not approve of me, may not love me.

In my experience, revising these two ingrained habits is a very good indicator of long-term recovery. Of course, you do not want to spend the rest of your life saying no to everything and continually asking for help, but for a while, it is a very good idea! Once you have done both often enough to get over the usually acute awkwardness people feel when they first start this, once you have a free choice to unemotionally say yes or no, to ask for help or not as you really need it, then this job is done and you have taken a big step forward.

Regarding who to tell and how much to tell depends upon what type of relationships you have and what type of relationships you would choose to develop. This is a particularly important and obvious consideration for parents. What sort of model do you want to be?

Jacky had breast cancer, a difficult prognosis and was a single mother. Her two children were behaving differently. The fifteen-year-old boy was silent and sullen, the twelve-year-old girl argumentative, rebellious and obviously angry. Jacky's strategy had been to attempt to shield the children from what she regarded to be the harsh realities of her illness as well as the fears she held for the uncertain futures of herself and her children.

There is strong evidence that when children are left in the dark they "awfulize." So if important information is withheld, the truth is distorted, or worse still, if children are lied to, they tend to think the situation must be even worse than it is because why else would they not be given the accurate story?

The reality is that when given the truth, when included in a loving way, children are remarkably resilient. When this was discussed with Jacky, it brought to light another level of her difficulties. She had such a fear of what might happen to her children if she became incapacitated and then died, and struggled to face her own pain let alone share all of this with her children. She actually had a fear of the children seeing her cry.

Jacky was reassured that in her situation, tears were both reasonable and normal. She was helped to understand that how she chose to respond to her situation would provide powerful modeling for her children. Invited to consider what sort of model she preferred to provide, consciously she yearned to be open, honest and authentic. But underneath lay the habitual tendencies of nondisclosure and the emotional pain attached to all her doubts and fears.

Change begins with motivation and then comes intention. Jacky was highly motivated to do the best for her children. With the clarity that resulted from discussing and thinking through her choices, Jacky made a firm resolve, a strong intention to change her emotional habits, to share the truth of her situation with her children, along with the feelings that accompanied them.

A good intention needs a plan that results in action. Jacky realized what she proposed would take some doing. She needed help. Regular attendance at a group where other people were working on similar issues provided a good start. Then Jacky enlisted the support of school counselors for both her children as well as arranging several family therapy sessions. Finally she resolved quite simply to be more open and honest at home.

The outcome? At first Jacky was disappointed. She made a huge effort to consider how best to begin this new phase of communicating with her children. She was determined to explain to them the truth and how she was worried for them and for her; how she had thought so far it would be best to keep the details of her condition from them; and how she had been afraid of showing her emotion to them.

Jacky then made an even bigger effort to actually tell the children. Not surprisingly, it was not long before a few tears began to trickle down her face. She described how the children were riveted, paying full attention to her and what she was saying. However, they had little to say at the time, showed no real emotion themselves and once Jacky completed her spiel, they went off to their own activities.

But within weeks things were different. Regularly, each of the children came and asked her a question, one piece of the jigsaw puzzle they were trying to put together in their own heads. "What is chemo?" "What does this test mean?" "Will your hair grow back?" At school, behavioral challenges were seen and the counselor reported steady progress. Their grades improved and at home a new openness was felt. There were still times of acting out, still challenges, still issues, but a new level of ease and almost normality.

For Jacky the shift was life changing. In the groups she talked with a newfound ease and confidence. Whereas before her "atmosphere" was of tragedy and difficulty, now she had the quality of lightness and zest. Whereas before her physical situation seemed to involve one problem after another, now her reports were steadily improving, her energy up, her enthusiasm for the future buoyant.

Speaking personally, back in the eighties, a couple of years into running the cancer groups, I heard myself discussing all this with a group and it suddenly hit me. I had two children at that stage, one was four years old, the other two, and I had never told them I loved them. It occurred to me that I had never heard my own parents tell me they loved me—I did not doubt that they did, but they had never said it. I had adopted the same pattern. Simple, I thought. I will go home tonight and tell them.

Wow! It was so difficult! That was some habit to shift. Happily, what I do notice many years later is that my two children who have children of their own are very fluent with their love. They find it easy to express their love to their children and discuss the range of thoughts and feelings much more fully than I ever did in my younger days.

This is probably a good time to point out that making personal changes like these can take time. While some people become clear on what is needed and change rapidly, and while those in an effective therapeutic group may progress quickly, for many of us, changing habits takes months rather than days, sometimes even years. A helpful book to refer to is *How to Help Children Through a Parent's Serious Illness.*[30]

MENTAL FEAR

While it is true we could say that all fear is mental because fear essentially is in the mind, we have categorized it into physical, emotional, mental and spiritual to make it easy to understand and learn how to overcome fear on all levels.

There is an old maxim "knowledge dispels fear" and it holds an important truth. Just like the children who tend to "awfulize" when information is withheld, where anyone lacks knowledge there is ample room for doubt, uncertainty and fear.

The antidote, therefore, is simple—become informed.

What is needed is good information and a clear mind to assess it. This was well discussed in chapters 7–9 on positive thinking and mind training. Just one reminder: stress and anxiety also produce doubt, uncertainty and fear. Therefore, being free of mental fear is greatly assisted by our meditation. With meditation, fears dissolve.

SPIRITUAL FEAR

Why me? Why did I get this and not the person next door? Is there any rhyme and reason to my life and my illness? What is its meaning? What of its purpose? Where did I come from—before I was born? Where will I go to after I die? What is it all about?

These are the great philosophical questions. The questions that are at the heart of the spiritual quest as well as religious practice. We will go into them in some more detail in chapter 18, but for now the antidote is easy.

In the spiritual realm, when we seek answers to the big questions about life, we can begin by learning from other people's experience. It can be very helpful to read good books, to listen to authorities in this field, to discuss, reflect and contemplate these matters. However, other people's experiences or opinions can always be debated. Our own ruminations invariably have the quality of conjecture—maybe this is the answer, maybe that; maybe this is real, maybe not. No, the only satisfying conclusion to investigating the truth of major spiritual questions is direct experience. Hence the essence of meditation and its place at the heart of all the great philosophical and religious traditions.

Meditation provides a direct and reliable means to go beyond the speculation of the mind, beyond the ordinary thinking mind and to directly experience the truth of who we really are, what is in our heart's essence.

We live in a world where common, everyday truth is relative. I heard her say that, I think he did this. One authority claims this is true, but another argues the case. Is there an absolute truth? Meditation offers the way to explore that question and to experience the answer. Not to "think" we have the answer, but to "know." To know the truth of who we really are.

The value of experiencing this inner truth, this truth of who we really are, is that in doing so we find it is inherently good, fundamentally pure and absolutely inviolable. Just like the sky is never stained by the worst of stormy clouds, just as the sky is an ever-present, luminous, infinite presence, so too is this inner essence pure, whole, inviolable, unending.

To know this to be fact, to know this because we have experienced the truth of it directly in meditation, this experience leads to a deep confidence. We come to know there is a part of us that will be OK. Sure, our bodies may hurt, our emotions be fragile, our mind be troubled, but there is this inner core, this inner essence which is always pure, whole and OK. To reconnect with this essence is to find a place of inviolable refuge, a source of deep comfort and peace.

Meditation may well contribute to healing your body, emotions and mind, but even more, meditation can heal your spirit.

Shame—and Its Antidote, Self-Esteem or Self-Love

Shame is well described as the feeling of not being good enough and is commonly linked to low self-esteem.

Sally was in her late thirties, a single woman, diagnosed with leukemia. When asked why she was joining the cancer group, she replied in a very soft, fragile voice, "Oh, I was just hoping I could learn to cope a bit better."

When asked whether she could imagine any more positive, more forward-looking outcomes, it quickly became apparent that Sally was barely coping. She went on to express her deeper feelings. "I don't deserve anything more, this is the best I can imagine."

In later sessions, Sally confided the difficulties of her childhood and the troubled relationship she shared with her mother. For a variety of reasons, her mother had found it difficult to love Sally from her earliest days and gave her continual messages that she, Sally, was a nuisance and a burden. Everything she did was met with criticism. The feeling of not being good enough was deeply ingrained in Sally's psyche.

In an extraordinary, powerful moment, Sally revealed to her group that she even felt unworthy to be alive. For her, cancer made sense and on one level represented a way out. However, the group atmosphere encouraged her. She knew in her heart these really tough feelings were a product of her life experiences. They were not natural and, she reasoned, they could be changed. No doubt the warmth she felt from the group, the understanding, acceptance and encouragement helped her a good deal. In a real sense, attending the group was for Sally like attending a specific program to boost self-esteem.

Then the suggestion was made to choose an affirmation—a statement of intention to help change her way of thinking. It was suggested she consider using the word "worth," to counteract the shameful feelings of unworthiness.

Sally's first response? She came up with the affirmation "I am worthy of being here!" Quite a number in the group could not grasp its meaning and asked Sally to explain. She said she hoped that by using the affirmation she would reach a point where she felt OK to be alive, where she felt worthy to be here, as on the planet, as a living person. Several in the group were moved to tears.

Then Sally was encouraged to extend herself and to consider "I am worthy of being happy, I am worthy of being loved." Even to consider such a possibility was a real stretch of the imagination for her, but buoyed by the group and the possibilities, she embraced both and began repeating them regularly.

Sally remains clear in my mind as a woman whose life was transformed by affirmation. As she began to feel more worthy, she began to take better care of herself. She chose her company more wisely, she attended to her health more diligently, and she began to experience a new level of joy in her life.

What is of particular note is that as Sally began to feel better about herself, her meditation improved. She explained that early on when she began meditating, she often found excuses to avoid sitting quietly in her own company, finding that the meditation confronted her with her own inner feelings of inadequacy. As the feelings improved, so too did her comfort with herself. As she gradually came to experience the deeper stillness of meditation, Sally came to experience something of her inner essence. She realized the truth we talk of, that there is this pure, inviolable inner essence inside each one of us and as she reconnected with this more fundamental aspect of her nature, she felt deeply comforted, deeply at peace.

Although Sally's condition was expected to respond well to medical treatment, it was her life that was healed through her own awareness and efforts.

Resentment—and Its Antidote, Forgiveness

Resentment is well defined as chronic anger. Anger describes an immediate reaction to a person or circumstance that creates strong displeasure. Anger in the true sense of the word is a strong emotion that comes and goes fairly quickly. Resentment is when anger persists, lasts a long time, festers and stays with us. Resentment is always a destructive emotion.

Now we are all highly likely to have been involved in relationships in the past that have not turned out as we would have liked. This is quite normal, but often we get so enmeshed that the situation seems irretrievable and we can see no way around it. Such relationships can often be a constant sore point and a cause for chronic emotional stress. We need a way to let them go, a way to forgive. This can be done by using another meditation technique which, when combined with imagery and affirmations, can bring about profound and effective forgiveness.

The Forgiveness Exercise—Using Imagery and Affirmations

To begin, start as you would any meditation exercise and settle into your posture.

Relax. Take up a slightly uncomfortable position, preferably sitting in a chair or on the floor, and go through the standard relaxation.

Visualize the person you are considering. Aim to build up as clear an image of them in your mind as you can, as if they were sitting in front of you and you were looking directly at them. Some people find it helpful to begin by looking at a photograph, and in so doing, fixing the person in their mind.

Repeat the following four phrases, one at a time silently to yourself, over and over, as you would with an affirmation, until you can say each one with conviction, before going on to the next:

I forgive you.
Please forgive me.
I thank you.
I bless you.

As you begin this exercise, you will find that it takes an effort to concentrate on the person's image *and* the repetition of "I forgive you, I forgive you." Then, when you do begin to repeat the phrase, you will probably begin to think of all the good reasons why you should *not* forgive them!

"Forgive *them*? I have every reason to hate that person!" you may think. Every reason, except that the hate affects *you* more than anyone else. As you dwell on it more, a wider, healthier perspective will come.

As you keep repeating the phrase, you enter into meditating on why you would benefit from forgiving them. Think of all the reasons they are like they are, why they did what they did. You will find yourself slipping over into contemplation and a new insight developing. As you continue you *will* reach the point where, with conviction, you can say, "I forgive you!"

I found "Please forgive me" was the hard one. While at first I was beset by all the reasons why I should not forgive this person, how horrible they had been, how much they had hurt me, etc., I found that as I persevered I came to realize my role in all the problems. If I had behaved differently, the whole situation would have developed in a different, more harmonious way. This exercise led to remarkable insights and helped me to reframe my whole experience.

"I thank you" was sometimes something of a test too. Thanking someone for putting you through a hard time that finally taught you so much demands a fairly elevated perspective of forgiveness and acceptance. This exercise develops a great understanding of life and relationships in general.

"I bless you" is easy after the first three have reached the point of conviction. "I bless you" is a release, a letting go. At that point you recognized the worth in the other person. While you may agree to differ on points of view, you are now free to go your independent ways without any negative attachments.

I found it good to start this exercise with easy things, like the man who cut you off while driving home, the woman who stood on your toes, or the shop assistant who was so difficult. It is a great exercise to do regularly—choosing one person to work with each day for a while. I used to recall someone that I had met during each day and practice the exercise with them. Soon I found the whole thing happening automatically as any incident occurred. If a difficulty with a relationship looked like developing, it was as if those four little phrases whizzed around in my head, defusing the situation even before it developed. Then I worked on the hard relationships, the cluttered old ones from time gone by. The effect was considerable. I really felt freed of old attachments.

Alcoholics Anonymous takes this idea further and suggests that reformed alcoholics need to make restitution to people they have harmed. They recommend actually fronting such people, apologizing and doing all they can to physically make good any loss they caused. I do not think it is necessary to go that far unless you choose to. However, I know it works, for there was one particular person that I had been involved with in a difficult way and had not felt comfortable with since. I practiced the technique until I really could genuinely say those four statements. When I then called the person, the atmosphere between us was totally different to the usual tension. We fell easily into an extended talk, discussing our old problems in a way we had never done before. We both left feeling lighter and happier. It amazed me that the whole nature of that relationship was balanced by that exercise. Many of the people in our group have found it works for them and I recommend this exercise in forgiveness highly.

Guilt and Its Antidote, Self-Forgiveness

Guilt is when we dwell on the feeling of having done wrong in the past and feel badly about that. The obvious antidote to guilt is self-forgiveness, which can be helped greatly by developing more self-love.

So it is eminently possible to do the four-step forgiveness exercise with oneself. Doing so is easier for most people after having first used it to forgive others, and in the process becoming familiar with the four steps. Then when we come to do it with ourselves, the contemplations that result can be intriguing, insightful and freeing. What do I need to forgive myself for doing? What do I need to forgive myself for thinking about myself? For judging myself? What do I thank myself for? And then the fourth step, the blessing of self, the acceptance and the deep peace that follows.

But there is even more to this. With whom do you have the most important relationship—your wife, son, mother, or none of these? It is yourself! We all know that old maxim "Love thy neighbor as thyself." Yet we seem preoccupied with the first half of the saying. Everyone wants to be seen as loving and helping their fellows, but they overlook the ". . . as thyself" bit. This is the really vital part. If you do not have a good relationship with yourself, you can never relate openly or love honestly. You will be looking to other relationships to cover up your own seeming inadequacies, or seeking out people who show you in a good light. Only when you love yourself can you love another. This is not love in an egotistical sense, nor is it any other false emotion. It is a basic human right. You need to love yourself.

"Why should I?" you say. There is every reason. "But am I not fat? Haven't I got a crooked nose? My hair is not what I'd like and, besides, haven't I got cancer?"

You have a body that is so complex, so intricate, delicate and wonderful that if you consider it, really consider it, you cannot fail to be impressed. Your heart pumps one hundred thousand times each and every day. Can you imagine that? No mechanical pump could come close to doing it—especially without being taken out for regular overhauls and repairs, and yet yours does. No one else does it for you. Your body does it, regularly, automatically.

Think again. There was a time when you were just two cells: one from your mother, one from your father. They merged, became one, and then began dividing again. From those two cells, just two, your whole body has been created. In the process you have mirrored evolution. In the warmth of your mother you passed from being two cells through stages like a proto-plasm, fish, reptile, animal to man. You have this incredible, creative, inner force that has created the body that you are in at this particular moment. There were no genetic engineers standing by to direct the process—you pro-duced it all! You have the intelligence, the inner know-how to produce and to maintain a human body. Amazing!

Just as amazing, this same creative inner force maintains your health. It can heal broken bones with ease. Given the right conditions, it can heal or create anything. Those right conditions begin with love of self. That love is innate, a part of our natural being. Children show it perfectly. Adults often cloud it through fear. It grows, however, with reverent awe as the true won-der of the body and spirit are realized. If you have difficulty with this, I suggest you have another of those clear-cut choices. You either love yourself or you do not. It is a simple, basic choice.

If you want to reinforce that love, or come to feel it, meditate and con-template it. Think of yourself. Think of the workings of your body, emo-tions, mind and spirit. As you contemplate this, you may well become aware how your outer realities are temporary ones. Your body, your personality and your environment are all changing rapidly and frequently. But in the stillness you may become aware of something more permanent, more stable and more meaningful. This, your inner core, your true self, is what you need to recog-nize and love. Then you will be able to accept that you have limitations—everyone has those external limits. But also accept you have strengths. Think how you can put them to good use. Come to the point where you can accept totally that "Yes, I am worthy of my own love. I have strengths. I have weak-nesses and I have this inner core which is pure and true and inviolable."

Be prepared to admit your outer weaknesses in a nondefensive, nonag-gressive, open way. Be prepared to put your strengths forward and to make good with them. Know that you have that inner core which is perfect. Know that you are worthy of love!

Grief

This will be covered in the next chapter on death and dying.

CULTIVATING HEALTHY EMOTIONS AND HEALING STATES OF MIND

The big three states of mind that are powerfully constructive and healing are love, hope and faith and we have covered them well already. There are two more states of mind that, while they may be less recognized, can be equally powerful agents for healing and well-being.

Generosity

When we are sick, and especially when we are fearful for the future, we tend to contract, want to hang on to whatever we have and can verge on becoming stingy. Reversing that trend, transforming that state of mind and practicing generosity can be a powerful force for healing.

What to give? Start small—a few words of praise, a small gift, maybe then something larger. If you can give knowledge you give something of great value, and if that knowledge allays someone's fear and brings them peace and contentment, now there is a real gift.

I had a graphic lesson in this. Having been an athlete, I was always conscious of "style" in running. This has something to do with poise, with balance and flair, and, dare I say it, elegance. I enjoyed watching others who had it, and while I did not speak of it, I did try to develop it myself. It gave me joy to aim to learn to run with style and happily, the more I worked at it, the faster I went. Following my amputation, I then spent a lot of time trying to move on crutches with "style." It sounds funny, I suppose, but I tried to move fluidly and easily. I never told anyone about my "training." However, one day a young man quite unknown to me came up and said to me with clarity and conviction, "It is a pleasure to watch you move. You look as if you are just floating along," and left.

Nobody else before had ever commented. Most people simply ask me what happened, why I do not wear an artificial leg and what do I do with the other shoe! Having had an amputation through the hip, I continue to find crutches more convenient and comfortable than an artificial leg. As it happens, having one leg, a kaftan is more comfortable and in my view more esthetically pleasing than wearing trousers with one leg. And I have my one shoe personally made so as not to waste the other. While I have always felt comfortable with all of this, this young man's single remark, said with genuine feeling, sticks in my mind and warms my heart.

The old saying "A word of praise is worth a thousand of criticism" is so true. You can make someone else's day by seeking out what it is in them that deserves praise. A single, well-placed, genuinely felt word can have someone else smiling for a long time.

Of course, it would be no surprise to notice ourselves beginning the practice of generosity hoping that if we give someone something nice, we will receive something even better in return. This is understandable as a starting point, but the real power comes and the real benefits flow when we let go of the "trade" mentality and go unconditional. Experiment. Can you give even a small gift with no thought of being appreciated, let alone receiving a gift in return? The challenge with all the positive states of mind is to aim to develop them to the point of being unconditional. Now there is a real challenge!

Gratitude

Take a moment to go back to the feeling that goes with bitterness and resentment. Cold, hard, tight, contracted, withdrawn. Very antihealing, very pro-cancer! Now feel into gratitude: warm, positive, open, embracing—very anticancer, very much to do with healing!

Gratitude is another state of mind we can choose to develop very easily. We mentioned in the positive thinking section that one of the best ways to develop gratitude and to feel its benefits is to remember as you go to bed each night to list just three things from your day you can be grateful for. Maybe it is as simple as the fact that you did wake up again that morning. Maybe it was a sunny day, or a rainy day and it was good for the gardens. Maybe you were given something, achieved something. Maybe you had a good laugh or a moment of real peace. Just list three things. Some people actually keep a "gratitude diary," write them down, and marvel at the list as it grows.

This simple exercise is remarkably powerful and, as an aside, good research demonstrates it to be a powerful antidote against depression.

But then take gratitude further. Get into the habit of thanking people for what they do for you. You probably do a lot of this—however, it is all too easy to take someone who is helping you for granted and to think they know how helpful they are being and how grateful you are. Maybe they are psychic, but why not tell them! It reinforces their kindness and leaves them in no doubt. Express your gratitude.

WHAT TO DO? WHAT IS EMOTIONAL HEALING?

When you are focused on recovering from cancer, there is no need to go chasing problems. Sometimes you hear people saying, "Oh, she has cancer, she must be big on resentment, or have had a big childhood trauma, or . . ."

Maybe. Maybe not. Being judgmental of others is a risky business. What is very clear from my many years of helping people and getting to know their states of mind quite well is that there is far more healing to be gained from developing healthy, constructive states of mind than by going digging for the destructive ones.

The place to start is with valuing, generating, experiencing and giving as much of the following as possible: hope, love, faith, laughter, joy, gratitude. Be generous with your emotions!

Look over the list again. Almost certainly one, two, maybe even three of the above will speak directly to your heart. "Pick me. I am the one you need right now. Cultivate me; I will get you going. Together we can heal!" So focus on developing that emotion, that state of mind to begin with. As you progress, from time to time return to this chapter and the list. What next?

And if at some point it becomes obvious that resentment is an issue, then that will be the time to give some weeks, maybe even months, to focusing upon forgiveness. If fear raises its ugly head at some point and hangs about too long, consider how to alleviate it. Is it physical fear, emotional, mental or spiritual? Use your mind to train your mind; to identify the issues you face, to reason how to respond and to motivate you to follow through and transform any destructive emotions into the energy of healing.

Above all, meditate regularly. Meditation creates balance. Physical balance, emotional balance; balance in our mind and our spirit. For some, meditation has been enough on its own. For most, training the mind, using the power of the mind, transforming destructive emotions and cultivating constructive states of mind has transformed their health and their life.

These positive states of mind have an effect that is very similar to turning on a light in a darkened room. Turn the light on and the dark, which may have been in the room for just a few moments or for eons, is immediately transformed. Moreover, with the light on there is nowhere for the dark to hide. If illness is compared to the darkness, healthy emotions are like the light.

CHAPTER 18

Death and Dying

How to Live Well, and Die Well

YOU MAY WELL ASK, "WHY IS THERE A CHAPTER ON DEATH AND DYING? Isn't this all about conquering cancer, about being positive, and getting well?"

There are two compelling reasons why considering death and dying makes powerful, positive sense. First, and perhaps most obviously, many people have enough fear about dying to not only significantly inhibit their chances of recovery, but to adversely affect the very way they live. Learning how to transform the fear of dying leaves us free to heal.

Second, consideration of death can transform your life. During thirty years of working with people affected by cancer, it is truly remarkable how many of those people have told me how glad they are to have been diagnosed with cancer. This sense of gratitude, which sometimes not surprisingly can seem perverse to outsiders, can take a while to develop. However, months or years later, many people tell me that being diagnosed with cancer was the best thing that ever happened to them.

How remarkable is that? And the reason? Because by considering their death they addressed their life. Being aware of the real possibility of dying sooner rather than later, they had the impetus to prioritize, to make changes, to do what was important, to make time for the things they really valued, to transform their lives.

So be brave. This discussion definitely has the capacity to transform your life. Read on!

LIVING IN FEAR OF DEATH OR INFORMED BY DEATH?

All of us will die one day. However, we need to be careful not to glamorize death. When we die, everything changes. When we die, there is a great deal we will lose. We lose connection with this body and this life. We lose direct connection with our family and friends. We certainly lose the capacity to work and it appears fairly clear we can take nothing with us. Alexander the Great, who ruled over more of the world than just about any figure in history, insisted on being buried in a simple white shroud with his hands left exposed and empty—to show what he took with him.

When someone we love or care for dies, we lose that direct contact with them. Their qualities, their energy, their presence, their inspiration, strength and weaknesses may stay with us and continue to influence our lives, but everything changes. We need to acknowledge death can be tough and it has the potential to be fearful.

Everyone knows this. Everyone deals with this knowledge in one of two ways. People aim to live in denial of death, or they live informed by death. One of the key points here is the proposition that the latter, living informed by death, while not so common in our society and perhaps challenging when first considered, is a better way to live and can make a major contribution to recovery.

CANCER AND THOUGHTS OF DEATH

In my cancer work, many people have told me the only reason they gave consideration to death was due to the fact of their cancer diagnosis. That was because before the diagnosis they were in denial of death. On one level, denial makes good sense. By denying death, by pretending we will live forever or at least die at some convenient time way off in the future when we are ready, we can avoid dwelling on the immediate pain of the losses death may well bring.

But denial comes with a cost. With denial of death comes the optimistic hope that we will have time to do all the things that are important in life. Later. So with denial there is often a willingness to postpone, to procrastinate, to compromise. And there is also a tendency to take life for granted, to function on automatic and to just allow life to drift along.

A cancer diagnosis can cut right through that. That is its power. That is its positive potential. If life may end sooner rather than later, what is the priority? What is really important?

Of course many consider it is the cancer that provokes these thoughts. While this is often the truth of how life unfolds, everyone who is alive will die one day and no one knows when. Back in the mid-seventies, nearly everyone who knew me thought I would be dead in a few weeks. Decades later, I have been to quite a few of those people's funerals and I remain alive and well. The point is, if you are alive, you will die one day and you do not know when that day will be. If you take that fact into account, it will enhance your life.

When we live a life informed by death, we really appreciate how precious life is, as well as how fragile it can be. So we value life; we value each moment. Once we overcome the immediate fear of death and the shock that can often result when for the first time we do contemplate it deeply, then life becomes more vivid and more focused. There comes a freshness, a vitality that seeks to get the most out of life. Almost paradoxically, by considering death, we become truly alive.

This is where the thanks for the cancer diagnosis originates from.

IS A GOOD DEATH POSSIBLE? AND IF SO, HOW?

I have known people diagnosed with cancer who were deeply scared of dying and who thought that to speak of it, or heaven forbid, shed a tear over it, was a negative thing to do and as such was to be avoided at all costs. And the costs associated with this view are high: noncommunication, bottled-up emotions, deep-seated ongoing pain and anguish, and the capacity to heal significantly impaired. What then does being positive really mean? What do we do with the natural fears that most feel, especially in the early days after a diagnosis?

Most of us have experienced the death of some of the significant people in our lives. You may have noticed how some people seem to have what we could characterize as "a good death," while others we might describe as "a bad death." Having helped many people, including family and friends to approach death, I can honestly say that after many years nearly all who died having following the approach I advocate died well. Many confirmed this for me in the lead-up to their deaths. Many families tell me after someone they love has died how amazed they were at the extraordinarily high "quality of death" they all experienced.

Perhaps the greatest revelation, and to be open, the greatest surprise to me in my many years of working with people experiencing cancer, has been how consistently people died well with cancer. Sure, many do learn to live well with cancer and it has been wonderful to witness and be a part of people surviving against the odds, but that was expected. Transforming suffering, being with people who found happiness amidst what was real adversity, seeing people die well consistently, that has been a real blessing.

And do be clear: most of these people began the groups or picked up *You Can Conquer Cancer* in denial of death. Most had significant concerns, many suffered anxiety, and the majority were deeply fearful. The common fears are fear of the process of dying, fear for the moment of death and fear for what happens after death. These fears are held for the person themselves and for those they love and care for.

The question is simple. Given we all will die one day, is it possible to have a good death? And is it possible for those who survive us to go on to have a good life? Given some people seem to have "a good death" and others not, what can we do when our time comes? Do we approach death in denial and just hope for the best, or is it wiser to prepare?

Clearly, experience points to the great value that comes from being well prepared. There are four areas to consider:

1. How to prepare for your own death
2. How to help another approaching death
3. What to do at the moment of death
   1. For yourself
   2. For another
4. Coping with grief

HOW TO PREPARE FOR YOUR OWN DEATH

The type of death you experience will be most affected by how you have lived your life, the state of your mind at the time of death and how prepared you are. Before discussing these key points in detail, it may well be useful to revisit the highly recommended "What if . . ." exercise that puts life and death into perspective and is reproduced again here:

Now, some may have seen this exercise popularized in the film *The Bucket List*. It featured Jack Nicholson and Morgan Freeman playing two characters diagnosed with cancer who shared the completion of their "bucket list"—the things they wanted to do before they kicked the bucket. We have used this exercise for decades with those affected by cancer and those who

---

The Contemplation on "What If . . ."

- Take a piece of paper and a pen to a quiet place where you will not be disturbed for about half an hour.
- Imagine that for the next three months everything in your life will remain basically the same as it is now; but at the end of the three months you will die. So you have the same level of health, same finances, and the same capabilities. The fantasy is that only you die and the question is, what do you do in these last three months?
- Clearly, this is a fantasy. No one knows how long they will live. However, imagine you have three months to go, with everything else staying basically the same, and now write down the ten most important things you would choose to do in those three months.
- As the list forms, you may have a sense of priorities—some things may seem more immediate than others. If so, rank them in order of importance.
- Only write down the things that really warrant being on the list. If you do not reach a total of ten, just stay with the significant items.
- Once your list is complete, consider how much time you are giving currently to each item on the list. If there are items that are being postponed or unattended to, consider what it would take to get them done.
- Use this list. Refer to it regularly. Maybe you have been doing it somewhat already courtesy of a cancer diagnosis. Do it formally and continue to review your list. This list can transform your life. This list is particularly useful for people who are well. It is how they can obtain the benefit of a life-threatening illness—without needing to get sick!

---

are well. Do take time to review it regularly. It is one of the most useful techniques I know.

A Good Life Leads to a Good Death

This is a powerful generalization. The experience here is clear. The great majority of people who have lived to the fullest, done all they could, used their lives to help others wherever possible, minimized the regrets, forgiven others and themselves, developed a good heart with generosity and gratitude. People who have lived well invariably die well.

Now of course, unless we were fully enlightened from birth, there are things we will look back on with regret. So most of us will benefit from checking our guilt, shame, blame and resentment levels. Maybe this is a good time to be reminded that we can always change our mind, retrain our mind, reconcile the past and learn to be happy in this present moment.

Our State of Mind at the Time of Death

People who approach death in an unpremeditated way rely on their life experience to determine their state of mind. So for people who arrive at the end of their life full of fear, bitterness and resentment, it is easy to imagine things will not go so well.

This is where death can be like an ally to our life. In this sense, death can be a valuable friend, as it reminds us to live well, to develop what we call a positive state of mind, to address our fears, to forgive wherever necessary and to cultivate a sense of joy and gratitude throughout our life.

There is no doubt that a good state of mind is closely aligned with a good quality of death.

Be Prepared for Death, Be Free to Live Well

What follows is a fairly comprehensive list of the major items to consider when preparing for death. Many people find it useful to write this checklist out, complete it and then share and clarify it with the people they are closest to, so they understand the preferences.

This is a list that warrants regular review; maybe an update once a year is ideal.

End-of-Life Checklist

THE PRACTICAL MATTERS—GETTING YOUR AFFAIRS IN ORDER

- Prepare or update your will.
- Attend to your financial affairs and ensure your partner can access joint accounts and other key financial and legal matters if necessary.
- Create an enduring power of attorney (a simple power of attorney ceases if you become incapacitated).

- Consider establishing a living will or enduring power of attorney—medical treatment form. This will set out your preferences and directions for end-of-life treatment options. These directions would provide guidance to medical staff and family if you become incapacitated, are not likely to recover, and choices need to be made regarding being left to die naturally or to have major interventions. You can also mention the levels of pain medication desired (maximum or minimal) and whether you would elect to have CPR (cardiopulmonary resuscitation) if your heart were to stop in this end stage of life. You could also nominate who you might want present (or absent) at the end of life and indicate a preference for being at home, in hospital or a hospice.
- Consider your possessions. Do you prefer for some items to go to particular people? If so, make sure this is clear. Maybe consider giving some things away while you are alive.
- Designate who you wish to look after any children, parents or other dependants if you and/or your partner were to die. Make sure the designated people know and agree.
- Complete as many of the tasks in your life as possible. Give priority to your bucket list. Aim to die free of regret for things left undone—either do them or let them go.

COMMUNICATE. DO NOT DIE LEAVING PEOPLE WONDERING!

- Express your love. You may think they know, maybe they are psychic, but tell them anyway!
- Consider leaving messages for significant people to be read or viewed at significant times. This can be particularly useful and comforting if you have young children now. Ideally, write or record your messages and deliver them in person on the eighteenth birthday or at the wedding; but if you are not there, the message will have real meaning.
- Consider documenting your life. You could simply create a photo album from childhood on, or collate any old videos or DVDs. Or you could be more personal and specifically record your insights, reflections, regrets, passions, etc.
- Forgive. Forgive. Forgive. Resentment is like a cancer in itself. Forgiveness heals the heart and sets us free. Review the forgiveness section in the healthy emotions chapter and do it! Forgive others. Forgive yourself.

IMMEDIATELY AFTER DEATH

- What preferences do you have for your body? Should it be left undisturbed for a while, and if so, for how long? In hospitals especially, there is often a need to clear beds for the next person (a tough reality), but family and friends may find great value in being able to sit quietly with the body after death. Also, some spiritual traditions indicate there is real benefit for the person who has died if the body is left undisturbed for even up to three days after death. This length of time may not be practical, but you may choose to indicate your own preference.
- What procedures do you want carried out with your body? Have you registered for organ donation? Embalming is a highly invasive procedure and only legally required if the body is being transported internationally. Have you a preference for who should wash the body and what clothes it will be dressed in?
- Have you a preference for a particular type of coffin or casket?
- Burial or cremation? Where?

FUNERAL SERVICE

- Do you want one? If so, will it be closed to include only the immediate family, or open for everyone who wishes to attend? Be reminded a funeral can help those left behind a great deal and consider wherever possible what will help them.
- Where will the service be held and who will officiate—a civil celebrant or a member of your religious tradition?
- What style of service? Traditional according to your religion? Themed such as New Orleans jazz? What emphasis will there be on the celebration of life and the grief of loss?
- What music, poems, readings to include?
- Who will speak? Who gives the main eulogy? Will others reflect on your life, offer readings, etc.?
- Are there particular interest groups to include and feature, such as sporting or service clubs?
- What about after the funeral? Will there be a wake? If so where, who organizes it and how will it be financed and provided?

ANYTHING ELSE IMPORTANT?
If so, add it to your list.

A Healthy Lifestyle Makes for a Good Death

A surprising number of people make the mistake of approaching death in an unhealthy way. Some people tell me, "I tried the diet and the meditation. It helped for a while, but now I am approaching death I am going back to my old way." This is a crucial point. Eating well makes it easier to die well. Why? Because heavy foods and junk foods add a burden to your system. High-fat diets make for sticky blood and lead to higher risks of embolism, stroke and heart failure. Bad diets promote inflammation that is both uncomfortable and is likely to aggravate any health issues you have. Bad diets are degenerative, whereas our healthy diet is regenerative and anti-inflammatory. Meditation is also anti-inflammatory and regenerative, while it also clears the mind, reduces anxiety and pain and helps us connect with who we really are.

If I thought I was really closer to dying rather than just the fact of knowing I could die any day, I would be even more particular about what I ate and drank, and I would meditate even more than the average one hour per day I do currently.

Be gentle on yourself. Live well and die well.

HOW TO HELP ANOTHER APPROACHING DEATH

Be involved. Communicate. When a question occurs to you, such as "Do you still think you can recover or are you ready to die?" be brave and ask it. Ask it skillfully (we will discuss how to soon), but do communicate. Feel free to express your emotions. Be authentic. Be real. Do recognize your own needs. Look after yourself so you can be of most use to the one you love and care for. Here are some guidelines.

Clarify Your Role

Are you the key caregiver? Or are you a close member of the family or close friend, someone who supports both the person with the illness and their primary caregiver? Or are you a more casual friend who is intent on being as useful as possible, or a casual friend who has little time? It is wise for you and all involved if everyone is clear on your role as well as the roles others are contributing.

Is the Focus on Recovery or Dying?

Tricky question. Challenging to ask and often challenging to answer. In my experience, most people with cancer know the answer to this question within their own hearts. However, when someone reaches the point where they are ready to die, it is often difficult to express it. Close family and friends often attempt to dissuade them. "Don't talk like that. You'll be OK. Here, have another carrot juice."

Having the next carrot juice may make good sense, but so too does honoring the person you are helping. Many of the things that help people to recover, help them to die well. But if someone has accepted they are ready to let go of the intention to recover or even the possibility of recovery, they may well choose to focus their attention on different things.

The way to get the answer to this question is to do what is often quite difficult, to put your own preferences aside, to be open and nonjudgmental, and to ask. Sometimes these words help: "I can imagine that some people in the situation you are in at the moment would be focused on getting well. But maybe others might be at a stage where they would rather let go of that and accept they are ready to die. Where are you in that spectrum of aiming to recover and accepting death is becoming the more likely outcome?"

Adjust what you do and how you are to the intentions of the person you care for.

Be Aware of Intentions

Use the suggestions and checklists in the previous section, How to Prepare for Your Own Death, to clarify what your loved one has decided to do. Talk through the options. If you are the principle caregiver, it is highly recommended to work through the lists together. It may be emotional. Tears may flow from time to time. It may take a while, it may take several sessions, but then you have clarity.

Clarify What Sort of Friend You Are to Be

What happens if the person you are helping falls short on their intentions? For example, what if they say they will have seven juices a day and balk after three? Or they say they will meditate three times a day and only manage one?

It is wise to discuss this possibility in advance, when things are warm, friendly and rational. Does your person want you to remind them of their intention? Is it helpful and desirable for you to provide the proverbial "kick up the backside"? Or are you meant to be passive and watch quietly as they do their own thing. Plan for this, as many couples have suffered badly if the scenario unfolds where there is a disparity between good intentions and actual actions. Aim for peace of mind and accord. Work as a team.

Recognize Your Grief—Be Gentle on Yourself

For many caregivers, the diagnosis of cancer naturally triggers a strong grief reaction. Recognize this may affect you, and see the later section on coping with grief.

It is OK to express your grief as long as you do not get stuck in it. It is very normal for couples to share their grief at first diagnosis. Shock is common. Numbness, tears, even feelings of injustice or rage are common enough. There is a time for that. Then when the initial storm passes, there is a time to gather your energies, make plans and set about the task of recovery.

Balance Your Own Needs

Some people become so dedicated to providing full-time care they exhaust themselves. Illness can follow, as can a general level of grumpiness, resentment and disinterest.

There is a need to nurture yourself so you can best nurture the one you care for. It makes sense to take some time out. To give yourself permission to enjoy hanging out with friends, to go to a movie alone or with someone else, to play golf—to do something that provides a real break. Doing this is another form of kindness to the one you are looking after. Rather than the common feelings of guilt people initially feel taking time out, pat yourself on the back and be grateful you can balance things as best as possible.

Be Aware of Overconcern—Balancing Care and Trust

Just because someone has cancer does not mean they are completely incompetent. Obviously, I hope! But some caregivers do feel they need to do everything and go into full-on sympathy mode. This can be really counter-productive, really obnoxious.

While it can be a delicate balance to strike, the need is to communicate. Talk about what is easy, what is challenging, what requires help, what can be left to the person with cancer. Many patients clearly value their independence and struggle with the notion of being a burden on those they love, so they may well need to address this sensitive issue too and jointly develop a strategy you are both happy with. Talking is the key.

For the Immediate Caregivers

If you live with a person with cancer, there will be a cycle of routines with meals, treatments and other activities. Be on guard that life does not move into automatic. It is easy to get caught up in the routines and miss the moment. So do remember from time to time to be more intimate and to check on feelings, hopes, fears and aspirations. Do take time to go out of your way for fun, enjoyment and meaningful time together. You may need to put these events in the diary too—make sure you include time for life as well as healing (even though so much of healing is about living well).

If You Are an Occasional Visitor

Whether you are a family member or a friend, if you only visit occasionally, also be on guard. Occasional visitors often make a real effort to visit. They come from overseas or interstate, they give up time, and they feel the natural urge to have an impact.

Here is the caution: you do not have to fix everything in a visit of an hour or two, or a day or two. As an occasional visitor, the real job is to express your love and concern and to support the primary caregivers. Relax. Trust that those who are there the most are best placed to provide the active support.

Do feel free to enter into intimate conversations. Again it is fine for you to acknowledge and express your own feelings. When with someone who is close to dying, the two key areas of interest are entered into by saying something like, "Let's talk about your life and what you have come to know of love. Who did you really feel loved by? Who did you love? What did you love? What were you passionate about?" And second, "What did you learn in your life? If life was like going to school to learn lessons, what were the main lessons you learned?" These questions will take you directly into the heart of what most people are interested in toward the end of their lives—love and wisdom.

If You Get Frustrated

What about if you realize that you wish the person you care for was different, did things differently, and more fully agreed with you regarding what they should be doing?

For your own integrity and the one you love, it is wise to express your preferences rather than bottle them up for risk of confrontation or offense. The aim of course is to avoid discord, but if there are differences, you have a right to express an opinion, just as the person with cancer has an even stronger right to choose their own path.

Do your best to strike an accord. Use this book, use the lists, enlist professionals and friends; explore the options and aim for agreement. If conflict emerges, remember grief commonly produces anger and commonly people find it easier to express anger with people they are close to and trust. In an almost perverse sort of way, people can be angriest with those they love the most, so do what you can to be understanding and keep a perspective. Of course, unreasonable behavior is always unreasonable and so everyone needs to keep cool. If the atmosphere remains difficult, counseling, especially family counseling with an experienced therapist, can be very valuable.

The reality is there may be a need to accept the one you love is different to you, does make different choices, and through your love you need to acknowledge this, accept it and do what you can to support their choices.

By aiming to be attentive, present and nonjudgmental, at least you will know you are putting your compassion and love into action—you will do no harm and, who knows, maybe in that atmosphere a miracle may happen.

WHAT TO DO LEADING UP TO THE MOMENT OF DEATH

The moment of death is one of the most important moments in our life. Think of this. When we die we will get to find out the answers to the really big questions. If nothing happens, we simply die and that is the end of everything, well that will be OK. But if something does happen after we die, the chances are it will be really extraordinary. So while I am keen to live as long as possible, I look forward to dying and to finding out what happens. It should be truly amazing!

So how to die well? How to lead up to a good death? What to do at the very moment of death? And what about afterward?

Leading Up to Death—for Yourself

Ideally, all the issues raised so far in this chapter have been attended to. If not, there is a lot of homework to do! As well as using the "be prepared" guidelines, here are some other major issues to consider.

LOSS OF CONTROL

As people draw closer to death, particularly through an illness like cancer, it is common for their physical body to weaken. Weight loss is common, mobility can be reduced and, for some, there will be loss of control of bodily functions.

These changes deeply disturb some people, particularly those who are fiercely independent or proud. It is curious to me. No one balks at changing a baby's diaper or carrying them around. For many, these changes at the end of life are just as natural as the limitations we all experienced at the start of our lives. At the end of life, there is the challenge to let go, to accept things as they are and to be grateful for the people who love and care for us, or for those who are paid to look after us.

PERSONAL CHANGE

If we approach death gradually, rather than as an accident, we are bound to notice an array of personal changes. As well as loss of control, our body can change dramatically, our energy levels drop, and our range of interests narrow.

For some, the range of emotional expression also narrows and it is common that people's true nature emerges. Happy people emerge as basically happy, the grumpy ones grumpy. At the same time, intellectual capacity and interests can wane but then there is the good news. What we have talked about so far is all to do with our ego. As we approach death, our ego tends to dissolve somewhat. If we are aware of this we can free ourselves more from this aspect of our lives. We simply let it go. At the same time, almost invariably as the body and ego diminishes, our spiritual awareness and presence will strengthen and come to the forefront.

This is why many people choose to work in palliative care or hospices. Many people at the end of their lives come more fully into their spiritual nature. It is there for all to see. When someone is close to or at the point of dying, you will feel this presence, this spiritual quality. This goes beyond the intellect, even beyond emotion. It is the presence of the person's fundamental nature, their spiritual essence. It is real and it is tangible.

So when your time comes to die, it is a good time to consciously let go of the things to do with the mundane aspects of life and your ego. Focus your awareness on what you have learned, what you know, what you love and what you aspire to in the spiritual aspect of your life.

PAIN CONTROL

Refer to the chapter of that title but then think seriously about what pain, if any, is being felt and being addressed. Obviously, loss of control and personal change can be painful. No doubt some people appreciate being "bombed out" on heavy analgesics so these more emotional issues are dulled out of their awareness.

I recommend you to be as aware as possible at the moment of death. While the essential part of our nature is unaffected by pain medication, a conscious death is a real possibility and may have great value.

INCLUDE CHILDREN

Do not shut them out. Be prepared for their questions, which are often profound, often mundane; often come at odd and unexpected moments. Answer what you can, being confident and clear about what you do not know.

It is really helpful to offset children's main fears by repeatedly telling them two things. First, if you are coming to the end of your life and you have young children, assure them regularly that you really do love them, and that you have done and will continue to do all that you can to live as long as possible and to stay with them. Children, especially young children, can feel abandoned when a parent dies, so this needs regular repetition.

Children also commonly feel that they are at the center of the universe and as such are responsible for everything. While this may not be rational, they commonly feel responsible for their mom or dad's cancer. Therefore, the second thing to tell them regularly is that the illness is not their fault.

As with other crucial needs, if you are worried about how children are managing, seek professional advice. Judicious and skillful counseling can transform a lifetime of difficulties into a well-managed major life change.

CONFESSION, FORGIVENESS AND LETTING GO

As the prospect of death becomes real, what might help to clear the conscience if necessary, and allow us to die at peace? In the old melodramas, this was the time when people were advised to "make their peace" or to "make peace with their maker." It was good advice.

Maybe you have not been near a church or a temple for ages past. But anytime is a good time to return to your homeland or your spiritual roots. The Catholic Church has excellent rituals of confession and absolution and, when done meaningfully and authentically, these rituals can bring great peace. While other religious traditions have their own rituals, some people I have known developed their own personally meaningful rituals and techniques that enabled them to let go of guilt, shame and resentment. (Refer to the previous chapter on healthy emotions.)

Some leave it to their deathbed to forgive. Sure, you can make a case for doing it earlier, but it is never too late.

What would you benefit from letting go so that you are in a better state of mind to die?

Leading Up to Death—for the Caregivers and Friends

TRANSFORMING SUFFERING

As a caregiver, your first challenge is to maintain some stability—within yourself. Particularly if the person you care for feels that all is falling apart, stability provides an anchor, something to hold on to and something to be supported by.

If you find yourself overwhelmed by your own emotion, take it elsewhere— it will not help the one who is dying. Balance your own needs and, if necessary, seek counseling or share your emotions with others you are close to.

THE TWO GIFTS—FROM THE PRIMARY CAREGIVER

As a person draws near to the moment of death, there are two things that make dying much easier when they are heard to come from the person who is closest to them. Both usually take quite some preparation before that caregiver is able to say them in a heartfelt way.

First comes: "It is OK to die." This is like a permission. It is best said after explaining how much you love the person, how they know how much you would prefer them to live, and how you would do whatever possible to bring that about, but if it is their time to go, "It is OK to die."

Second: "We will be OK." Again, with the death of someone so close to you, and if families are involved, everything will change and clearly life will never be the same again. But life will go on for those left behind and while there may be difficult and challenging times to manage, if you can have the confidence to authentically say, "We will be OK," it can be deeply reassuring to the one who is close to death.

Preparing to say these two phrases can be deeply emotional. It may require some resolve to first contemplate and think them through, and then to be able to genuinely give voice to them. However, doing so can produce profound comfort for the dying person, allowing them to relax, be assured things will be OK and to let go into the process of dying. Also, for anyone who says these things authentically, there is immediately a very real and major step forward in resolving their own grief.

WHAT TO DO AT THE MOMENT OF DEATH

Ideally, all we have covered so far has been taken care of. What follows next is a sequence that in a conscious death you may remember to follow, or perhaps it could be spoken to you at the time of death by whoever is closer to you, as a reminder and as a guide.

Instructions for the Moment of Death

- Remember, it is OK to die. Dying is a natural process. We will all do it, and we will all do it successfully! When the time comes, all you need to do is breathe out and when you do not breathe in again, it is done. It is very easy. There is nothing to fear. Relax and go with it.
- While you can, remember the good things about your life, maybe dwell on what wisdom you learned, what love you experienced.
- Generate a sense of gratitude for this life and for the people who were a part of it. Know that they too will be OK.
- When you are ready, consciously bless those whom you are leaving behind, thank them again and let them go.

- Turn your mind away from the world you have known in this life and the people in it and bring your attention to your spiritual essence.
- Imagine whatever symbolizes or embodies your own spiritual truth as if they or it were in the sky above you. So it may be Christ, Mother Mary, a particular saint, the Buddha, Krishna or a beloved teacher. Or it may be a more abstract image—a ball of light like the sun that symbolizes the universal energy that runs through all of life. Even if you have a particular religious or spiritual view, this ball of light may be easiest, representing as it does all that is good and all that has your own best interests at heart.
- Generate whatever devotion you feel and direct it to that figure or ball of light. This is like the longing you might have felt as a small child to be with your parents. If you are comfortable with prayer, quietly repeat whatever prayer comes to mind.
- Imagine that this feeling is received by the focus of your attention and returned to you. There is an outpouring of love that streams toward you and that you imagine, that you see as a stream of luminous white or golden light. This light flows from the heart of the figure you see in the sky before you, or from the very center of the ball of light.
- As this luminous, loving light reaches down and touches you, you feel it drawing you magnetically toward its source.
- Consciously letting go of this life and being intent to remain undistracted by either pleasant or unpleasant diversions, allow the flow of light to carry you into the very heart of your spiritual figure or the center of the ball of light.
- When you do this, they say that dying is as easy as running into your mother's arms.

What to Do Following the Death of Someone You Love

- Hold the atmosphere of peace, love and reverence for as long as possible. Grief is natural. Tears may well flow. If necessary, move away from the body while emotions are really strong, then aim to sit quietly with it.
- It can be very helpful to repeat in your mind or speak out loud to the body the instructions for the moment of death.
- Most people have their own knowing of when it is time to leave the body, to move away and do whatever comes next.

- If possible, do not move the body for an hour or two—many prefer longer if it can be done.
- Ensure any specific religious or spiritual practices chosen by the deceased are carried out.
- It is really helpful if there is a designated "minder" who can protect the atmosphere, keep unthinking staff away if necessary, regulate visitors and monitor everyone's needs, especially those of the key people.

What if I Was Not There at the Moment of Death?

First understand this: I have been a part of family vigils that went on for days. Then, in the few moments when everyone left the room, dear old Grandpa died. Or other times where defying all expectations, someone held on to life for days, even weeks until a particular person arrived by their side, at which point they died almost immediately.

The reality is some people are very private, some really seek company. Whatever the fact of this, I know how some people find it deeply disturbing when they are unable to be there when someone close to them has died. What can you do?

- If you know someone is dying and you cannot be there, stop whatever else you are doing. Pray, meditate or just hold that person in your mind. Imagine the instructions for dying as if they are happening. Project with your mind as if you are with the person and guiding them. Take comfort that the mind can do this—the mind can transcend space and time.
- If you find out after someone has died, allow yourself to grieve. Once you are reasonably calm and clear, draw on prayer and meditation and project the earlier instructions even though the person has died—there is value in doing this hours, even days after the death.
- If there has been a long delay before you learn of a death, you can still be very helpful. What has been useful for many is to meditate and imagine in your own mind a place where you feel particularly peaceful and comfortable, just as you do when going to the inner sanctuary (see chapter 10). Then invite the person who has died to join you in that place. You imagine them joining you in that place, imagining all this to be as real as you can. Once you feel the connection with the person who has died, you can say what you need to, what you feel. Maybe they will say something

back to you or for you. Many people have found this exercise profoundly helpful in resolving the mixed feelings that commonly go with being apart from someone you love when they die.

COPING WITH GRIEF

For many people, a diagnosis of cancer triggers a major grief reaction. Some resolve this grief in such a way that the moment of death is experienced quite differently to the powerful grief reactions many feel at that time. What is normal? What is reasonable and OK? And what may require attention?

The Five Stages of Grief

Elisabeth Kübler-Ross identified five now-classic stages that dying people pass through. These are explained in her book *On Death and Dying*.[31] In my experience, it needs to be stressed that these stages overlap considerably and people can travel back and forth between them. Also, I see a secondary pattern emerging in people who are better prepared for death, and this pattern has some quite different elements. It is very useful to be aware of these stages as they help to make sense of our experiences.

DENIAL

"It's all a mistake. This cannot be true! The X-rays were mixed up in the lab." I remember thinking this one myself—for about two seconds! And then I accepted it was for real. Some people become stuck in denial and go from place to place seeking a new opinion. Others just refuse to believe that they have a potentially life-threatening illness.

ANGER

"Why me?" "Why did I get it, why not old George down the road?" Again, some people take this emotion to its extreme and go through a particularly difficult time.

BARGAINING

"If I go back to church regularly, then perhaps I will live another six months." The thing about bargaining is that it involves a fantasy. You may well go to church, find ingredients missing in your life, make changes and recover completely. No sense of bargaining there—just taking appropriate action. Any self-help techniques could be regarded as being bargaining unless the motivation was right.

The point about bargaining techniques is that they are not sustained. Because they are based on fantasy they are not carried through. Genuine self-help techniques are sustainable because they bring results, even if those results do not change the physical situation. It is important with cancer particularly not to view healing as a game of winners and losers with death the end point. Cancer is an intensification of the game of life. In one sense it is a game of winners and losers, but success is marked by wholeness, peace and harmony. This is not a cop-out or rationale to justify death.

I see people who accept their situation and work with it. Incredibly, they often feel death is of far lesser importance than what they are gaining through the process. For most in our groups, this third stage, then, is one of acceptance and commitment and it leads on to taking appropriate action. The acceptance is sustainable and it carries them through getting well or through dying. They can accept life and they commit to doing all they can to live well and to die well.

DEPRESSION

"I don't want to know anyone." People close to dying can go through periods of deep depression where everything is "wrong." In this state they can be very difficult to help and very insular. I feel depression happens when people are beset by the physical reality of their situation and preoccupied with thoughts and fears of their lack of immortality. Often, however, this can be interspersed with moments of great clarity when their spiritual realities appear more real and comforting.

ACCEPTANCE

"It's OK to die." People in this stage may be insular or not, but they are characterized as being at peace. Nearly everyone, it seems, unless they are absolutely overwhelmed by fear or anger, passes through this stage before dying. Physical pain often melts away and there is a great sense of calm. For people who work at it, this stage can be a wonderful peak experience. If shared, it can offer families and friends an experience they are unlikely to get in any other way.

It is as well to realize that friends and relatives can also be involved in this five-stage process. A little of them is dying too as they lose someone near and dear. They, too, can need help to get it right before death. People who exhibit love and faith have death marked by kindness and compassion. People who express bitterness and fear often find confusion and loneliness.

The art of dying well lies in the art of living well.

What Emotions Are Normal?

A wide range. It is common for people to fluctuate between the deep despair of loss and the exalted highs of the spiritual atmosphere that commonly surrounds death.

Most of us find it challenging to help another through a period of grief. It is always an emotionally charged time. What should we say or do? Faced with indecision it would be easy to do nothing. However, by using some simple principles we can be very helpful indeed. The aim is to communicate, to give the grieving person the opportunity to express their thoughts and particularly their feelings, and for you to communicate your care and empathy.

So if someone needs to talk about death do not try to change the subject. Do not make light of it but share in the difficulties it can produce. By being prepared to talk of the person who has died and the situation they face through the loss of that person, you give them the opportunity to express themselves. Often only emotions and feelings will come out and logic may not be a part of the conversation.

Quite often surprising negative emotions may come out. Guilt, anger, despair, even rage, are just as likely to appear as gratitude, acceptance and love. Do not develop an argument by trying to counter negative feelings with positive ones. What is being expressed is an emotional response and if it is not released in the early days after the death, it will remain. Repression of such emotions and feelings may cause bitterness and disillusionment. Frequently this means that your role is to say very little. It is certainly harder to be a listener than a talker and often the grieving person will say the same thing over and over. Often they will be expressing feelings, not logic. Given the opportunity to do this, the feelings will gradually settle, and at the next meeting a more logical discussion of the situation may well be possible. Sometimes the initial talks will lead to tears. Have the courage to let this happen if it is needed because it allows the person to "let go" of their inner tension, and that in turn leads to release.

Honoring the One You Love

There are many ways you can honor the life and memory of someone you love after they die.

- Prayer is common to all traditions and naturally is highly recommended.
- Planting a tree, particularly a deciduous one, both honors the person and reminds us of the cycles of life. Planting many trees is another option.
- In some traditions, freeing fish or animals that were destined to be eaten is valued.
- You can dedicate the merit of projects, or kind acts, or even simply the good thoughts you have to the benefit of the person who has died. You can make donations on their behalf, or simply meditate and wish whatever benefit comes from you doing something useful goes to them.
- If you come from a tradition that believes in reincarnation, these actions are considered to enhance the deceased person's chance of achieving full enlightenment after death, or of experiencing a better rebirth in their next life.

What Can I Do?

Action reinforces your own feelings, so find something to actually do for the grieving person. Whether it be taking around a prepared meal or accompanying them on a day's outing, the physical act shows you really do care. Remember that at the time of a funeral there is always a lot to do and a great deal of support comes forward. However, four to six weeks later, everyone is getting back to their own immediate concerns and it is at this later stage the loss will be most noticed by those closely affected. Make a note on your calendar to call on them and to help your friend to find new interest and directions. Helping them to do things for themselves is a start, but once they are helping others, life is well under way again.

Other Dimensions

One of the more fascinating aspects of dying is the work that has been done on the near-death experience. Raymond Moody in *Life After Life*[32] was one of the first to write of his experiences with people who had been revived after being clinically dead. Their experiences were remarkably similar. These near-death experiences are not only recalled by people with a yen for spiritualism, but by ordinary everyday people. A later study showed that 40 percent of all people who have been clinically dead recounted some or all of these experiences.

First, people who recount these experiences comment on how they were struck by their feelings of calmness and lack of fear. Even people who were involved in severe accidents and suffered serious physical injuries were aware at the time of the accident that they felt no pain. They felt like a calm observer—yes, an observer—standing to one side or, more commonly, looking down on the scene surrounding their physical body. People who have been on operating tables and lapsed into clinical death have often been able to recall the words spoken by the doctors and what was done to revive them. One of our group who experienced this recalled her exasperated doctor saying in the middle of intense efforts to revive her, "Don't give up on me now, you bitch—breathe!" It was a red-faced doctor who verified using those words.

Many have then experienced the sensation of leaving the vicinity of their body and passing down what seems to be a tunnel. It is often a tunnel of light, or there is a light at the end of this tunnel. Again, the feeling is one of comfort and security—not fear. Frequently, there is someone known and loved by the dying person at the other end as if to greet them. It is then, as if they reach a threshold—to pass over it would be irreversible and death would occur. Obviously, people telling these stories came back and usually they felt a compelling reason to do so. They either had unfinished business or a sense of mission. So one of our group, a devout Catholic, got to the end of her tunnel to be met by her deceased grandfather. "You're too early, lass. You have to go back for the children." She recovered from surgery and now has a profound knowing that death is OK.

This is the exciting thing. People who have this near-death experience are left with a feeling of comfort and peace. For them, death is transformed. It is no longer a thing to fear. In fact, it is described as a very pleasant process.

I had an experience like this following my amputation. It seemed to be triggered by an adverse drug reaction and it began with a weird feeling. It was as if my awareness became out of time with my body. I felt like I was outside of my body and that I was watching myself call for a nurse. Then it was as if I was watching someone else trying to explain what was happening, only that someone was me! Then I lost awareness of my surrounds altogether.

I recorded in my diary that I felt as if I was being propelled along a hose in a stream of water. If you have ever pointed a stream of water to the sky on a sunny day and seen the stream break into beads of sparkling light, you will know how I felt. It was as if I reached the end of the hose and had a glimpse of a glorious array of cascading beads of light in an infinite expanse of space. I felt strongly that if I kept going with those beads I would not return. It was a beautiful sight. I took one glimpse and said to myself, "No thanks, not yet," and I actively retreated. Soon my awareness returned to the hospital room.

At the time I wondered if I had hallucinated or had experienced something more. However, the experience having been so real, I felt sure I had been through a genuine experience. It left me knowing that death was OK. It is all very well to rationalize and talk about it, but after an experience like that, you have this inner knowing that death will be OK.

This positive view of death is backed by a philosophy that regards death as an integral part of life. Meditation has enhanced that feeling by adding to my appreciation of spiritual reality. So I would like to think that just as I can celebrate all the other life events, birth, marriage, child rearing, maturity, so I am able to celebrate death. While I accept that remorse, anguish and grief are real and need to be dealt with, I give thanks for life and wish people well in their new phase of it after death. I try not to cling to old memories and so bind people who have new directions to explore. I seek to avoid complications by communicating well with people before they die, seeking to explore the practical issues as well as feelings, thoughts and attitudes.

FINALLY • An Approach to Death

It is well to have the courage to develop a concept of what you think will happen when you die. You might like to meditate and contemplate it. This is not a ghoulish thing, but a useful prerequisite for approaching death in an open way. Again, you do not need a life-threatening illness to gain enormously from this. You will probably find fears well up and it is good to analyze them and use the techniques to let them go. Letting go of attachments is the key.

It is also good to discuss the practical details concerning any preferences you might have for when you do die, especially in case you die unexpectedly. What schools would you prefer the children to attend? Is it intended that outside help come into the family? What about remarriage? And so on. Remember the benefit of sharing the checklist.

Whatever else you do, talk about this vital area. It is probably one of the hardest conversations to get started, but everyone is amazed at how well it flows once it begins. Such sharing leads to increased bonding between families and friends, heightened peace of mind and does a great deal to enhance quality of life. Remember, if you are alive, one day you will die, and none of us know when that will be. So you do not need to have an illness for these conversations to be useful—you just need to be alive and to be interested in living well! In the words of the great impressionist painter Paul Gauguin:

How brief this life,
So little time to prepare for eternity.

Perhaps one of the most beautiful comments around death came from four-and-a-half-year-old Anna. When asked by her mother what she thought had happened when her grandmother died, Anna paused to reflect for a moment and then replied, "Well, Mommy, just the *living part* went out of her."

It occurred to me recently how many people dread the prospect of death. Yet so often the fear of dying inhibits both healing and life itself. To reconcile death, to face it, to integrate it; to be ready to die, is to be ready to live fully. Perhaps this is a feature of survivors—they have faced death, moved through its domain and reemerged to celebrate life. So we aim to become confident, confident to be able to live well and to die well, but not so confident with death that we become blasé and forget how precious this life is—instead we continue to do all we can to make the most of it.

On top of all this it may well be that the moment of death is a moment of delight, filled with mystery and magic—so here is what occurred to me:

The Clear Moment of Death
The moment of death may be the greatest moment of your life
It may be better than the best chocolate sundae you ever had
It may be better than the best orgasm you ever had
It may be better than the dearest, happiest moment you hold in your
*   memory*
For in that moment of death

The spirit separates from the body
And in that moment
It is free—totally free
If you can grasp that clear moment of death
Recognize it for what it is and experience it fully
Then you will experience fully who you really are
And unite with the mystery and essence of life itself
The only thing that scares me about the moment of death
Is that I may come to it unprepared
To be prepared for the moment of death
I would need to feel that I had lived fully
Loving and learning as much as I could during this lifetime
And feeling free of regrets
To be prepared
I would need to feel that those around me would be all right
That I could let go of my worldly attachments
And that they could release me
To be prepared
I would need to be free of fear
And to have had some glimpse of my own true nature—
Perhaps through the introduction of meditation
Being prepared for that clear moment of death
Then it may well be
That I would be able to recognize what I have been searching for always—
The heart and essence of who I really am.

CHAPTER 19

Your Healing Choices

Principles, Practicalities and Spirituality

HEALING IS ANOTHER INTEGRAL PART OF THE PROCESS OF LIFE ITSELF. IN seeking to understand the healing process we can compare it to a journey between two great cities—one called Disease, the other Health. Disease is known by suffering, separation and restriction; Health by joy, interconnectedness and authenticity. The journey between the two is that of healing.

It would be tempting to say the journey was on a purely physical level and that being free of physical symptoms assured a place in the city of Health. Experience tells us otherwise. We see people of sound body beset by emotional distress and mental anxiety. We see people of no purpose wandering the byways with no direction. We see others racked by physical disease whose inner light shines strong and pure. So, this is a metaphorical journey indeed—a journey of personal evolution.

The paths between any great cities are many and varied; the routes people take between Disease and Health are diverse indeed. It is as if we are born somewhere along that route with our own particular inborn level of health and our own range of talents with which to work. As we grow, we respond to the environment around us. Some of us, it would seem, pass our days being merely bumped along by the external events of life. In what appears to be a waste of a grand opportunity, these people make little progress as their life passes by. Others do move off in search of a better clime, but find no compass to guide them. Often they stumble deep into the city of Disease before realizing they are on the wrong track. Then comes the test—to change direction, to learn to read the map and to head back to the security of Health.

Those brave ones who do dare to tread the path to Health, unprovoked by such a stay in the compelling city of Disease, are the ones in life I admire most. Those who value life and its opportunities, who respect their deeper nature and their body, and work to better it have really grasped the purpose of their life. They are the ones who when you meet them along the path, exude the joy of the search and uplift all they encounter.

The paths between the two cities are as varied as the travelers. There are narrow, winding lanes for those who wish to dally, and wide, direct highways for those with purpose and perseverance. And for some, although few it seems, there are the airports where, spreading wings, it is possible to fly direct to the destination. All along these routes are towns and places of interest. Some are unrewarding, mere dalliances and distractions along the way, while other stops add quality and enrichment.

As the travelers move along the separate routes, their paths often cross. When they do, it may appear to the passing individuals as if they are heading in opposite directions. Without the benefit of a grander map they might be tempted to say the other was wrong in pursuing such a course, exclaiming, "You are going in the wrong direction. Follow me. My way is the right, my way is the best, my way is the only path to Health." However, those with a grander vision acknowledge their fellow seekers and bless them as they move on their way, for direction comes with discovering that this is more than a physical quest.

Disease: "dis-ease." The word says it all—lack of ease, lack of balance, lack of harmony. Health is harmony and the purpose of life is to seek harmony on all levels of our being—physical, emotional, mental and spiritual.

The further we journey, the more we realize that we are responsible for our own position on the map of life, and that we must accept this responsibility. We see that life has a pattern and we are an integral part of it. We are intimately involved with the complex pattern of events that has resulted in us being in our current situation. Maturity comes with finding our position on the map and accepting that position. Then, if we are strong enough not to indulge in looking back with guilt or regret, we can chart our own course and take the first steps toward Health.

Some of us find it hard to accept responsibility for being in our present position. Particularly if physical disease is evident, it is far easier to blame something or someone else for our own misfortune and so to feel a victim of circumstances. But some time, somewhere, the realization dawns and we appreciate that the pattern of the life we have been leading has determined our current circumstances. We *are* responsible, just as we can be in control.

If our past pattern has produced the symptoms of disease, and now we are seeking to reestablish health, we must be brave enough to look for a change in direction. Change is required to establish the pattern that leads to Health. Some can make that change almost instantaneously. With the speed of jet travel they can relocate themselves in new and happy surroundings. For most, however, the journey becomes a process, the healing process. It develops as a series of changes that gradually lead to the place of their dreams. Commonly, the first steps are superficial ones and there is a preoccupation with the obvious physical steps that need to be taken. So, people with illness journey to places of physical treatment, change their diet and begin to exercise. These outer things are easy to start with, easy to work on. As they come under control, the effort becomes more profound. The inner work begins. The need to change fundamental attitudes and direction becomes apparent. To change just one really basic trait for the better is a major accomplishment for any lifetime.

So, where is the map? Where is the compass? What can guide us through this maze? In essence it really is very simple. Once our basic course is realigned with harmony, once harmony is the prime motivation, then healing is under way. The more harmony in our actions, attitudes and spirit, the better our quality of life and the closer we move toward that wonderful city of Health.

Harmony comes with peace of mind, so as we seek peace of mind, we seek Health. If, at every step along the way, peace of mind is the basic criterion that must be satisfied, then each and every step will be a good one—one that takes us in the right direction. To begin with, the physical may lag behind, but in terms of inner development, once harmony is the aim and peace of mind the governing principle, then progress is surely under way.

In fact, once we are free of physical symptoms we often discover that the journey has only just begun. While many find that healing their physical ailments does bring great personal spiritual growth, they soon realize that the true aim of the process of healing is really synonymous with the aim of the process of life itself—to seek harmony on all levels. Their spirit leads the way and often aspires to journey beyond the place where their physical and psychological reality dwells and works.

So, often this journey takes us out of familiar territory, out of our comfort zone. This journey has the potential to produce tension, a tension of growth, as the spirit leads the personality toward its goal. If this tension is creative, the path runs smoothly. If the personality lags or resists, then bumps abound. When the prime motivation is peace of mind, the journey to Health is steady indeed.

The means to Health, the paths of healing, run on many levels and are extremely varied. To clarify the map a little we can summarize some of these many varied routes.

YOUR HEALING CHOICES

When we seek healing for ourselves or someone we love, what are our options? It must be obvious that a book like this can neither give specific advice, nor should it even attempt to do so. Sorting out your own particular needs requires specialized advice. What follows is merely an introductory overview of some of the possibilities. If you feel drawn to a particular area, then seek help from the appropriate qualified practitioner.

Let us review the choices systematically. There are three main areas of treatment and support we need to consider. Please note that it is important to use the right words to describe the specific area of treatment or support you are engaging with. Unfortunately, these descriptive words are often used loosely, with little attention to their real meaning. In my opinion there is a compelling need to use the words more accurately; particularly to know that what is advocated in this book is not "alternative" medicine, it is not even "complementary" medicine (although it does complement all other forms of therapy)—it is lifestyle medicine.

In the sections that follow, we will examine the three main avenues for healing, define our terms, clarify the concepts and discuss the options.

CONVENTIONAL MEDICINE

Conventional or orthodox medicine generally describes medical interventions that are taught at medical schools, are generally provided at hospitals, and that meet the requirement of peer-accepted mainstream medicine and standards of care. The main focus in the conventional treatment of cancer is on:

Surgery

Surgery is the first line of mainstream treatment for the majority of cancers and is associated with many people returning to their normal life expectancy. Surgery may well be crucial and directly lifesaving in some cases, as in the case where a bowel cancer may be causing an obstruction. But surgery also takes a load off the body, immediately reducing the burden of the cancer, freeing the body to regenerate and providing a better opportunity to prevent recurrences. Surgery is best used when tumors can be removed en masse, leaving nothing behind. When surgery is supported by a healthy lifestyle, it seems to have little significant adverse effect on the immune system. Surgery makes good sense for many cancers, especially where it is relatively straightforward.

Chemotherapy

The side effects need to be weighed against the benefits. In some situations chemotherapy can be effective, but quality of life can suffer and the balance needs to be watched. Many people these days have an inflated notion of how helpful chemotherapy actually is. There is good evidence that chemotherapy improves five-year survival rates for twenty-two of the major cancers by an average of less than 3 percent.[33] More detail of this is available on my website,[34] but this well-documented, evidence-based information comes with a word of caution. While chemotherapy can be quite useful for some childhood cancers and some of the less common adult cancers, and while there is more positive science regarding the potential benefits of what you can do for yourself, it is worth observing some people find some of the statistics relating to chemotherapy distressing and prefer not to know about them.

To my mind, if chemotherapy offers real benefit compared to any side effects, then it makes sense to consider it seriously. But the question should be "Why would I have chemotherapy?," rather than "Why wouldn't I have chemotherapy?" In other words, you need to be convinced it is in your best interests.

Radiation

This is often used to reduce pain and can do so, particularly when bone is involved. It is effective as a treatment in a limited number of situations, but personally, is my least favored form of treatment due to the potential long-term side effects. In recent years, radiation treatments have become more localized, more targeted, and so are relatively safer than they used to be.

Immunotherapy and Other "Biologically Elegant" Therapies

This is a rapidly developing area in conventional medicine. For example, monoclonal antibodies that aim to stimulate the immune system can be helpful in some cases. Angiostatins are new drugs that have the potential to halt the development of new blood vessels and starve the cancer.

Hormonal Therapy

Some tumors can be hormone responsive; for example, some breast cancers and prostate cancers.

NATURAL MEDICINE • Three Main Components

Complementary Medicine

In the United States, the National Center for Complementary and Alternative Medicine (NCCAM), defines complementary and alternative medicine (CAM) as a group of diverse medical and health care systems, practices and products that are not presently considered to be part of conventional medicine, as defined by medical peers.

The diversity of these therapies does make them difficult to categorize as a group, yet they are often collectively referred to as complementary, alternative, lifestyle, integrative, unorthodox, unconventional, unproven, natural, traditional and holistic medicine, and are contrasted with conventional, mainstream, allopathic, orthodox and scientific medicine. Hence the need to define our terms.

NCCAM classifies CAM into five categories or domains.

ALTERNATIVE MEDICAL SYSTEMS

Alternative medical systems are built upon complete systems of theory and practice such as homeopathic and naturopathic medicine, traditional Chinese medicine and Ayurveda.

MIND-BODY INTERVENTIONS

These interventions include patient support groups, cognitive-behavioral therapy, meditation, prayer, spiritual healing and therapies that use creative outlets such as art, music or dance.

BIOLOGICALLY BASED THERAPIES

These therapies include the use of herbs, foods, vitamins, minerals and dietary supplements.

MANIPULATIVE AND BODY-BASED METHODS

These methods include therapeutic massage, shiatsu, chiropractic and osteopathy.

ENERGY THERAPIES

These therapies involve the use of energy fields, They are of two types:

- Biofield therapies such as qigong, Reiki and therapeutic touch.
- Bioenergetic therapies involving the use of electromagnetic fields, such as pulsed fields, magnetic fields or alternating current and direct current fields.

You will notice how some of the above modalities such as nutrition and meditation are what we will define soon as lifestyle therapies. Also, unlike in America, where complementary medicine and alternative medicine are linked and the acronym CAM is used all the time, in Australia, the term "alternative medicine" is used by many in the medical profession in such a negative way that complementary medicine and alternative medicine tend to be spoken of quite separately.

Specifically then, complementary medicine has been defined as any therapeutic practice that does not satisfy the standards of the majority of the orthodox medical community, that is not taught widely at medical schools, and that is not generally available at hospitals.

However, even this definition creates some difficulty as these days many medical schools—both in Australia and overseas—offer courses in complementary medicine and many hospitals provide complementary therapies.

Although there is growing evidence that a number of complementary therapies can be safe and helpful in cancer management, particularly in the area of symptom control, there are a number of legitimate concerns regarding the use of CAM among cancer patients.

These concerns include:

- Heightened concerns for vulnerable cancer patients and families
- The suggestion of false hope
- The potential for monetary exploitation
- Delayed use of effective conventional treatments
- Little scientific evidence for some therapies
- Potential dangers, interactions and side effects
- Poor training and regulation of some practitioners

Of course, these issues are just as relevant for the conventional cancer care as they are for complementary therapies and lifestyle factors. When it comes to the evidence, it is clear that the side effects reported from complementary therapies are far less in number and far less serious in nature when compared to the side effects reported from conventional cancer therapies.

Traditional Medicine

Traditional medicine includes well-documented or otherwise established medicine or therapies that are based upon the accumulated experience of many traditional health care practitioners over an extended period of time.

The Therapeutic Goods Administration (TGA) in Australia provides a specific definition: "Traditional use refers to documentary evidence that a substance has been used over three or more generations of recorded use for a specific health related or medicinal purpose."

Traditional therapies include traditional Chinese medicine (TCM), Ayurvedic medicine (from India), Tibetan medicine, western herbal medicine, homeopathic medicine, indigenous medicines, and aromatherapy. These traditional medical systems represent a different paradigm of health care when compared to conventional Western medicine.

Alternative Medicine

This is the domain of what is sometimes described as unorthodox or unconventional or unproven medicine or therapies. Alternative medicine generally describes medical interventions that are not widely taught at medical schools, not generally provided at hospitals, and are outside peer-accepted mainstream medicine and standards of care. The strong implication, or even fact, is that these therapies are not supported by a significant Western medical research base.

Examples could include aromatherapy, intravenous chelation and vitamin C, ozone therapy and psychic surgery. There are many of these therapies, and they are often difficult to evaluate and they need to be considered with due caution.

Lifestyle Medicine

Lifestyle medicine is defined rather formally as the application of environmental, behavioral, medical and motivational principles to the management of lifestyle-related health problems in the clinical setting.

In practice, lifestyle medicine is concerned with what a person can do for themselves in the context of their daily life. By contrast, there are all the things that could be done to or for you under the banner of conventional, complementary, traditional or alternative medicine. Lifestyle medicine focuses on what you can do for yourself. The other approaches involve either a therapy provided by a therapist (whether that be surgery, acupuncture or a massage) or a compound you take (that could include antibiotics, chemotherapy, supplements or herbs).

Lifestyle factors or therapies include physical factors such as nutrition (food, fluids and juices), exercise, exposure to sunlight and creative activities. They also utilize mind-body interventions that can include psychosocial activities, group therapy, mind training (positive thinking, affirmation, imagery), meditation, yoga, qigong, tai chi, healthy emotions (relationships, communication, laughter, forgiveness, etc.), personal development and transformation. Lifestyle factors also encompass spiritual pursuits such as exploring meaning and purpose in life, prayer, spiritual healing, religious practice and spiritual development.

Lifestyle medicine forms the substance of this book and a summary of recommendations makes up chapter 21.

INTEGRATIVE MEDICINE • Healing in the Balance

Let us be clear now. Conventional medicine, traditional medicine and CAM focus on things that are done to you or for you. Lifestyle medicine focuses on the things you do for yourself. While some may choose to do only one or the other, it has always been my contention that it is wise to bring together, to integrate, the best of all that is available. I am committed to using what works best. Integrative medicine is the answer.

Integrative medicine is defined as the blending of conventional, natural and complementary medicines and/or therapies with the aim of using the most appropriate of either or both modalities to care for the patient as a whole. Integrative medicine considers the person's body, emotions, mind and spirit. Integrative medicine is open to integrating the services of a wide range of health practitioners and modalities in a way that is often described as holistic medicine.

Integrative medicine, therefore, is an umbrella term. In fact, integrative medicine is what good medicine always was. It takes account of the health, healing and well-being of the whole person and it works cooperatively within an interdisciplinary environment to draw on all means possible to achieve the best results possible.

THE TRUE NATURE OF HEALING • A Personal View

How wonderful it would be to fully recover physically from cancer. My wish is that everyone diagnosed with cancer has this experience. How then do we best set about healing a diseased body? If disharmony is the root cause, obviously anything that re-creates harmony will have a healing effect. However, if there is obvious physical disease, the symptoms may be so severe and so physical, it may not be possible for those involved to normalize the situation using only the energies available through subtler avenues. Often it is necessary to alleviate the immediate situation with surgery and purely physical medicine, just to ensure a continuation of life.

This is a fine balance to strike. Physical treatments are tried and proven and will have a place for a long time, a fact often overlooked by overzealous advocates of alternative medicine. But it is important to remember that it *is* physical medicine and frequently does not go beyond the treatment of the physical symptoms. Once the physical situation is stabilized, it becomes important to turn the attention to the underlying causes and their correction to effect a complete cure. Is being physically well enough?

Surely, we all know people in good physical health who are otherwise miserable—grumpy, bitter, angry, resentful, unhappy relationships all around. There are plenty of people for whom emotional healing seems like a distant dream. For them, to be emotionally well would be wonderful and there is no denying that, but would it be enough just to have good emotional health?

Leading health authorities claim over 20 percent of the population in countries like Australia and the United States suffer from a diagnosable mental illness in any one year. Twenty percent! That is one in five. For those people who are perhaps dealing with anxiety, confusion, mood or personality disorders, depression and so on, to be well in their mind would be marvelous, and that too is true. But is even that, even being mentally well, enough?

Clearly it would be wonderful to have a fit body, healthy emotions and a sound mind, but there is more to life—more to being really well, more to being fully happy. There is the spiritual dimension to consider.

One way to consider this is to contemplate what does bring happiness and contentment into our lives. Many people rely on things outside of themselves or the people around them for their happiness. If the kids are happy, I am happy. If people are speaking well of me, are being kind to me, I am happy. If work is going well, if the bank balance is OK, I am happy. If I have the right house, the right car, the right partner, then of course I am happy. Or am I?

What we can observe is that the people and the things around us can change; often at times and in ways that are both unexpected and seriously inconvenient as it may seem. So relationships change, finances change, status changes—everything around us has the clear potential to change.

So while it is true that having nice things around us and being in the company of nice people is pleasant and a cause for some happiness, if we are solely dependent on the things outside of us and the people around us for our happiness, we will always be vulnerable. Life changes; people change, move on or die; fortunes fluctuate. Many diagnosed with cancer know this to be all too true. However, take heart. There is a deeply comforting answer. Lasting happiness, enduring happiness, is a very real possibility. Clearly, lasting happiness is a state of mind. The answer to real happiness is not to be found outside of us. The answer to real happiness resides within us. The quest for real happiness leads to the spiritual path.

SPIRITUAL HEALING • The Quest for True Happiness and Good Values

Many people I have worked with found their cancer diagnosis profoundly challenged their spiritual view. Many with an established conviction found that conviction deeply disturbed, while others of little conviction found their thoughts turning to their church once again. The Bible is very clear on this. There is no need for guilt, no need to hesitate. The Prodigal Son story is definite. Any time is a good time to return home. If disease and difficulty does take someone back to their spirituality, that gives added meaning and benefit to the initial suffering.

However, while many people are passionately interested in their spiritual life, not everyone is interested in a formal religion. There is a significant difference between spirituality and religion. Religion is how we express our spirituality within the context of a particular system of faith and worship. Spirituality is to do with finding inner peace, finding meaning in our life and developing good human values. One would always hope that spirituality played a major part in religion, but clearly, spirituality can exist outside of religion.

While the primary motivation for entering the spiritual path may be to seek real happiness, the primary outcomes from following the spiritual path are to enhance our human values, to make ourselves into better human beings and to serve humanity.

All the great religious traditions have at their core this quest to find true happiness, to find meaning in life, and the desire to cultivate positive human values. All share the potential to fulfill that quest. However, because people are different, it is natural that different religions, different paths toward this same end will fit with some people more closely than with others. The best religion for any one of us will be whatever religion takes us most directly, most reliably to that inner happiness and helps us to become kinder, more useful people.

Unfortunately, in modern times many are disenchanted with the answers and the direction they receive on these matters from formal religions. Many are looking deeply in their own way. Seeking more than dogma, they want logical and compelling answers. They want practical and effective techniques and prefer to pursue their spirituality in a general sense rather than through a religion specifically.

What is clear is that the practice of a given religion is not essential to being a good, honest and sincere person. Indeed, there is plenty of evidence that tells us the practice of a given religion does not always ensure being a good, honest and sincere person. By contrast, it is almost impossible to consciously pursue the spiritual path and to not become a better, more honest and more sincere person.

When we are ready, the task for each of us is to find and to follow our own spiritual path. Of course, this may or may not be focused via a religious path. What is clear is that many I speak to say that cancer provoked their spiritual inquiry and practice. They report that doing so helped to make sense of their cancer, and that their spiritual development became a major reason why they express some gratitude for the cancer. Many feel that their most significant healing actually took place in their spiritual lives.

So, aspiring to inner peace, happiness and good human values is easy to understand. What of meaning?

There are three big philosophical questions that need to be satisfied on the spiritual path. Where did I come from? Who am I? and Where am I going? As in, what was I, or what was going on before I was born, what meaning and purpose is there in this life I am experiencing now, and what will happen after I die?

To explore these questions, one way to begin is that we could say spirituality addresses the gap between how things appear to be and how they really are. So I could be described as the son of my parents, father of my children, husband to my wife. In some of my various daily activities I could be described as teacher, a student, a health educator, an entrepreneur, a researcher. There are so many designations or names that can be assigned to the many and varied roles I fulfill and are all summed up in my name, Ian Gawler. You might like to take a lighthearted pause and consider all the "titles" that you function under from time to time. However, if all these are stripped away, who are you, really? What is in your heart's essence? What is your true nature?

These questions have been active in my own mind since I can remember. The answers I had already came to informed the way I managed my leg being amputated and my health descending into the depths before I recovered. Courtesy of the intensity of that recovery process and then courtesy of working with thousands of others exploring the meaning and purpose of life, more insights followed. In the spirit of sharing human experience and gently provoking your own spiritual inquiry and development, my biography *The Dragon's Blessing* authored by Guy Allenby,[35] documents some of those insights, along with the life events they were associated with and their observable consequences.

RECOMMENDATIONS FOR THE SPIRITUAL PATH

Making progress along the spiritual path is like learning or progressing in any field of endeavor. It requires study and practice. This is like the wings of a bird. If a bird only has one wing, it flaps around in circles in a pretty unhappy state. To fly, a bird needs two functional wings.

To develop our spirituality, first we need to study. Many gain great benefit from reading and from attending lectures, conferences or retreats. When the time comes, an authentic teacher will deepen all this. But clearly we then need to practice. This book is full of directions, and here is a specific summary for the spiritual path.

Value Your Spiritual Life

- Recognize the importance of your inner life. I have known people who died profoundly healed. Their bodies may have been weak, but the strength of their spirit was extraordinary.
- Give time for your spiritual life. Be gentle on yourself. Allow time for reading, for reflection, for daydreaming, for formal contemplation and meditation. Make time for this.
- Consider how you can be supported on the spiritual path. Who are your spiritual friends? Who do you discuss these matters with? Is there a group

to attend that nourishes you spiritually? What about professionals like a counselor with a spiritual focus, or even a spiritual teacher?

- Aim to be authentic. More and more, seek consistency between your inner and outer lives.
- Do be aware that often there are more questions than answers, particularly as we first turn our thoughts inward. Be comfortable with the mysteries, hold the questions—be patient.

Be Ethical, Avoid Harm

As much as possible, take your spiritual values into daily life and reflect these values in what you do, how you speak and how you think. It is a fact that a well-developed spiritual view will lead to a healthy, healing lifestyle. This is something to delight in—the fact that being motivated by good ethics leads to healthy eating and drinking takes us away from smoking, drugs and excesses in life, and takes us toward a healthy sex life and satisfying work.

Train the Mind

Everything in this arena makes sense. Consider what is helpful and most immediate to meet your needs. Consider:

- Affirmations and imagery—based upon understanding how the mind works and how we can use it intelligently to good effect.
- Psychotherapy, CBT and counseling—for when more personal help is wise.
- Practicing and developing:
  - **Generosity:** Learn how to give and let go.
  - **Discipline:** This is the discipline of kindness, doing what is kind to you and to others.
  - **Patience:** This is the quality of not being upset by others; it is the quality of spiritual endurance.
  - **Diligence:** This is like discipline but is better described as finding joy or delight, being enthusiastic about doing what is good for you.
  - **Meditation:** Recognize the difference between therapeutic and spiritual meditation. Do some regular meditation with a spiritual focus.
  - **Wisdom:** Develop your spiritual view. Aim to see things as they really are.

Deepen Your View

The way to take a spiritual theory into practice and embody it in your life involves three steps.

LISTEN AND LEARN

This is how we acquire new knowledge. Maybe we read, or we listen to teachers; we take things in with our intellect and develop some understanding.

CONTEMPLATE

To advance a theory, to deepen our understanding, we benefit from sitting quietly, relaxing and then focusing our mind on the topic at hand. This helps us to think things through thoroughly, but then it leads to deeper understanding, insight and even revelation.

INTEGRATION

Contemplation takes a theory down from our head into our body. We come to embody what we know.

So we repeat this process; we listen and learn, we contemplate and we integrate. The more we do this, the more we become authentic, the more consistency there will be between our spiritual view and our worldly life. One very good measure of profound healing and true health is this measure of our authenticity.

Coming back to our old friend death, when we die what will be most important is what sort of life we lived and the state of our mind. Authenticity is one of the best gauges of all this.

My wish is that you lead an authentic life. My wish is that you live a long and happy life!

Oh, and if all else fails, you might like to do what my old friend Barry the ophthalmologist recommends. Barry says when all else fails it is time to reach for the Viagra eye drops. You know them? They are really good for when you need to take a long, hard look at yourself!

And there is a moral to his recommendation—lighten up. While all of this is extremely important, do remember your sense of humor.

A FINAL WORD ON HEALING

So balance in all things. Start with the immediate things. Define your medical treatment plan. Attend to your lifestyle right at the start and then, once there is some stability, consider the other options. Chapter 21 provides a summary of all the options and a suggested pathway, but first, the more radical side of healing.

CHAPTER 20

The Sealed Section

The Special Case of Subtle-Energy Medicine

THERE MAY BE VALUE IN TAKING SOMETHING OF A RISK AND SHARING SOME of the experiences I had with subtle-energy medicine, with paranormal healing phenomena, and particularly psychic surgery in the Philippines. First, it is widely known that I have benefited from such treatments and I am sure this needs clarifying. Second, psychic phenomena are most intriguing. If they can be shown to be genuine in just one instance, the implications are vast indeed. I find it a fascinating area.

Warning: If this field of endeavor or this type of conjecture is not to your taste, please do not be put off by it. Having had remarkable experiences, I seek to explain them. If I do not do so adequately, that is my shortcoming. The other more concrete things covered in the book to this point stand in their own right, and in my experience are fully justifiable. What follows is the product of experience, reading, conjecture and contemplation. It may shed some light on what to me is a truly wonderful area—the mysterious area of subtle energy healing. But if this is of no interest, simply move on to the next chapter.

It is interesting to note how many types of paranormal phenomena are cropping up today, and the interest they are producing. Debate on psychic surgery has been intense for quite a few years. Reports of miraculous cures have been countered with claims of quackery, sleight of hand and the use of chicken's blood and tissues of nonhuman origin and in some countries practitioners have even been prosecuted. People like Uri Geller have bent spoons and started clocks. At the same time, the Russians experiment with psychokinesis, that is, moving objects using psychic energy alone without touching them. If these things are talked of openly, what experiments are going on in secret?

In the healing arena, Kirlian photography is being used to distinguish between healthy and diseased tissues. A sophisticated technique of photography, it reveals what is claimed to be the health aura. Clairvoyant healers now, and in ages gone by, have claimed to be able to see this subtle energy emanating from their patients. Acupuncture has been accepted into the conventional treatment repertoire despite there being no conventionally accepted explanation for its means of action.

We are getting a lot of hints, demonstrations of the possibilities. Frequently, patients in dire need are being drawn by such phenomena, sometimes turning their backs on conventional treatments. Patients can see that there are practical benefits to be gained. But there is a great need for balance—the ability to decide what to do and when.

So far we have been doing just this. We have been considering the patient's role in cancer and what they can do to help themselves back to health. While the principles of diet, positive thinking and nutrition break enough new ground for some, the area of psychic surgery introduces us to a whole new frontier.

A PERSONAL ACCOUNT

When my leg was amputated in 1975 with bone cancer (osteogenic sarcoma), there had been no other sign of the cancer. It reappeared, however, and secondary cancer was diagnosed later that year. I was told that the medical options of chemotherapy and radiation were not likely to improve my chances of living more than another three to six months and that they would have unpleasant side effects. No medical treatment was recommended, while at the same time I was told the cancers were likely to double in size every month.

Concentrating on meditation and diet, I saw no growth at all over the first three months. Then, through a combination of factors, mostly to do with my trying to do too much each day and so creating new stresses, I deteriorated rapidly. Initially the searing pain of sciatica running down my left side restricted my mobility. Then my weight fell away and I was confined to bed. Finally, it was confirmed that my right kidney was obstructed and severely swollen. I had reached my lowest point.

In desperation, my first wife, Grace, and I left for the Philippines in March 1976. I weighed a little more than 84 pounds, compared to my

normal 126 pounds (I was around 168 pounds before having my leg amputated). My color was likened to that of a jaundiced custard. Pain forced me
to lie down except when it was absolutely necessary to move.

We were motivated by the conviction I would still recover, but knew little
of what to expect. I had heard of the Filipino healers from several people,
notably an aunt and friends who had helped to introduce me to the dietary
regime some months earlier. They had provided the address of one healer,
one young Filipino boy whom they thought might be helpful, and one hotel.
While excited by the possibilities, and open to them, I was basically skeptical
and certainly critical in my approach to healers. The first thing I did in the
Philippines was to buy a movie camera. If I was to be tricked, I wanted to
record it.

Two days after arriving, I had my first operation performed by a small,
shy Filipino healer. Traveling to his house early in the morning, we were met
by his cousin who doubled as business manager. He told me that after the
treatment I was to return to my hotel and rest a few hours. For twenty-four
hours I was not to bathe or drink coffee, alcohol or carbonated drinks. He
also took twenty-two dollars from us, the amount this healer charged in
those days. It was the first and last time we were asked for money.

Most of the healers work on a donation-only system. Most are very simple people of peasant background with a strong Roman Catholic influence.
They are not used to handling large sums of money. They say they are using
a God-given power and accept what goods or money their patients can offer
in return. Those few who did charge large amounts seemed to have become
preoccupied with material things and found their healing powers had waned.
However, they were the exceptions, not the rule.

After the formalities, I was ushered into the operating theater. This was a
small bare room with a large wooden table to one side. The healer stood at its
center, flanked by two assistants. At his feet were two buckets. One was used
as a repository for the bits and pieces that were removed, the other contained
already bloodied water and was used for washing hands between operations.
There was no pretense of sterile technique. We later learned that the healers
have been shown to be able to destroy disease-causing organisms by merely
passing their hands over them.

This day, there was no preamble. I was asked to strip to my shorts, to lie
back down on the table, and to pray as best I knew. Under the circumstances,

it was easy! The healer moved forward and quickly entered my abdomen with his fingers. He held his hands together, with fingers outstretched and just overlapping a little. I felt a pop, as when you poke a finger through a stretched rubber balloon. Grace was called over for a better look. As the healer pulled his hands apart she could see the lining of my peritoneal cavity and the tumor inside my pelvis. He then continued by taking some fresh tissue, similar to loose connective tissue, from the area. Blood welled up from within the incision, while there did not seem to be any bleeding from the skin itself. He finished by withdrawing his fingers, leaving a small pool of blood on my skin. When this was wiped away there was no scar visible. The performance was repeated in several other places and then I was unceremoniously told to get dressed and to return the next day. It had all taken five minutes.

I was excitedly asking Grace what she had seen as we returned to our hotel where I reluctantly agreed to lie down for a short rest. I slept extremely heavily for the next three hours, and after lunch I had another unexpected reaction. All my joints began to ache, one after another. I felt nauseous and colicky, and my head began to spin. As these symptoms became more severe, I began thinking my surgeon's gloomy predictions about my death might prove correct after all.

However, the Filipino boy, who soon showed that he had wisdom far beyond his years, was familiar with the problem, and said this frequently occurred. He explained that the healers were able to mobilize the body's own defenses. Once this process was set in motion, it frequently produced a classic healing reaction with an intensification of some or all of the patient's symptoms. Chronic conditions are often brought to a head and after a short, acute episode, healing progresses.

After a very uncomfortable twelve hours and a good night's sleep, I did, in fact, feel a great deal better. Within two days I had flushed all my analgesics down the toilet. Pain relief is a common sequel to this type of treatment and I am sure this is due to both a physical and psychological benefit. The healers are very aware of the psychological impact of this visually dramatic procedure. They recognized that if a patient believes the disease they have is normally considered to be terminal, then it takes something quite out of the normal to change that belief system and replace it with positive healing thoughts. They happily admit that their healing relies on its psychological impact as well as its physical effects.

We stayed on for four weeks and visited five healers during our first trip. Some people seek help from just one healer—others, like me, go to more. There are no set rules and it is important for the patient to accept responsibility for their own decisions and be guided by their own thoughts and feelings. The effects must also be put into perspective.

I returned from the first trip about 13 pounds heavier in weight, with no pain and with good mobility. My surgeon was amazed by the improvement. While there was no decrease in the actual cancer, there was no doubt my general condition had improved dramatically. He said he could not understand it, and that there was no medical explanation to account for it.

I continued to meditate and develop my dietary program, as well as pursue any other avenue that might help keep this healing process going. Soon our movie films were back and they confirmed what we had seen with our own eyes. It appeared that I had been operated on without anesthetic or instrument. I had felt no pain, although I had bled and tissue had been removed. No scar remained as a visible sign of the procedures, but above all else, I had improved. *Something* had happened.

If just once a healer's hand, even a finger, had gone through my skin under these conditions, then my view of reality, my knowledge of physics and how surgery was possible, was quite inadequate to explain it.

SEEKING ANSWERS

There are three choices anyone faces when considering such an extraordinary phenomenon:

- It is a trick to be discounted.
- It is a miracle to be merely marveled at and thankful for.
- It is a genuine phenomenon that requires an explanation.

The history of physics is marked by the development of new theories that were required to justify previously unexplained phenomena. Whether it be Archimedes' "Eureka!" in his bath, or Einstein's theory of relativity, all of physics has been a product of our attempts to explain the world as we observe and experience it.

I feel sure that the current wave of interest in psychic phenomena is really prompting us to look again at the nature of the world around us. The real message of the Filipinos is to offer a psychic signpost to a new awareness. For, if it is genuine—as I have come to believe it is—then it forces us either to take the easy way out and dismiss it as a miracle, or be brave and reconsider the nature of matter and the power of the mind.

THE NATURE OF MATTER

Most of us accept matter as being solid and finite. We sit on a chair and it feels solid enough. It looks solid. We tap it and it reassures us further by sounding solid. No doubt it has a taste and smell to add to its claims to solidity. But is it? What is it made of, really?

For it is the evidence of our five senses that we are relying on to call the chair solid. These five senses of touch, sight, hearing, taste and smell are very helpful for us in day-to-day situations, but they have quite a limited range when compared to our modern precision instruments. If the wavelength of light our eyes registered was just a little wider, we would all have X-ray vision. Imagine the difference just that one small change would have. Our view of reality would be transformed! And how often do we "see" something, take it to be real, and only find out later we were mistaken?

So if we want to understand the nature of matter, we go to modern physics with all its marvelous technology. As the physicists analyze matter they look more closely at it, probing it with the aid of microscope, electron microscope and mathematical theory.

Most of us would be familiar with one of the results—the atomic concept of matter. The atom is a model for the ultimate building block. These building blocks are combined like pieces of a child's interlocking building game to form all the substances we know.

The atom is represented as having a central nucleus with electrons circling it in orbit, much like the planets as they orbit the sun. But, if we enlarge an atom to a size to which we can relate, we see just how "holey" matter really is. For, if we represent that central nucleus by a pea about one-quarter inch across, then, on that scale, the nearest electron would be the same pea-size; it would be 575 feet away and it would be going at the incredible speed of 1,242 miles per hour! Can there be all that space in what we consider to be solid? It has been calculated that if all the space was taken out of the atoms which make up the human body, the resulting mass would be smaller in size than a pin's head!

And it does not even stop there, for now the physicists have probed the atom still further. First they thought the nucleus and electrons were made of smaller and even smaller particles of solid matter. But now they say something even more startling. There is nothing solid there at all. The atom is merely the product of concentrated energy. *Matter is concentrated energy.*

We all know Einstein's famous equation, E=mc2. But we seem to fall short of grasping its implications. E stands for energy, m for mass, and c for the speed of light. The equation is saying that mass, or matter, is a product of energy and light—as esoteric a statement as formulated by any ancient sage.

This, to me, is the most remarkable thing of all. The modern physicists are becoming the New Age philosophers. For, as they probe deeper into the nature of matter, they are forced to investigate energy and so seek to understand it. For, if all matter is made of energy, what makes the difference? Why does one "block" of energy come together to build a rock, another a tree, and another me?

The brave few physicists in the vanguard, who once more are prepared to ask that most vital question, "Why?" Why does energy take the multitude of forms that it does? these physicists are forced to introduce another concept—that of consciousness. They say that it is consciousness that actually produces the energy we are talking of, and that it is then this energy which is interpreted by our five senses as the thing we call matter.

CONSCIOUSNESS, ENERGY AND MATTER

What a concept! Consciousness produces energy; energy produces matter. Thought precedes form. Thought produces form! It leaves me concluding that my physical form is the result of the sum total of my consciousness. I must presume, therefore, that I and all those around me are all essentially reflections of our overall consciousness. Further, given our highly ordered world, I must presume an all-pervading, interconnected consciousness to provide the basic framework in which it all happens.

Most humans have a similar view of reality—the world, as each one knows it, is basically similar. We interpret and respond to a basic universal energy pattern. Within this matrix we radiate our own sphere of influence—

project our own thoughts and energies and so adjust the picture. For those capable of generating novel thought and projecting it with power, the whole picture can change at will. Reality is limited by our ability to conceive its possibilities.

Can we then understand more of the true nature of man? How can we formulate a model that takes into account these ideas of matter being consciousness and which also accounts for the phenomenon of the familiar physical world?

Why does some vast, all-pervading consciousness create the energy patterns that combine to produce the things we call atoms, which in turn combine in varied ways to produce the many things we call matter? And what, then, sparks this matter to produce a living organism with consciousness in its own right? And given all that, why do we see so much disease? We are now getting to the basic questions to which healers and patients seek to find answers as they attempt to formulate a basic paradigm within which to approach disease and its treatment.

Presently, all forms of paranormal phenomena are coming under scrutiny in the West. Parapsychology is an emerging science wrestling with these questions, but as yet no unifying principles have been commonly accepted.

However, if we turn to Eastern thought and metaphysics, there is a recurring model that both makes sense of the phenomena and provides a framework in which to operate.

Most major civilizations have had a tradition of an esoteric science in their culture. Being esoteric, it was hidden from the mainstream of the people but used by those initiated into its secrets in a very practical way. Despite the diversity of cultures, there is a remarkable agreement on basic principles. Even more remarkably, these principles relate to the concepts now being put forward by the modern physicists.

In the esoteric lore of the Ancient Egyptians, Chinese and Greeks, the Indians of North America and the Incas of the South American continent, the Polynesian Kahunas and Filipino healers, the Vedic seers of India, the early Christians and, more recently, the medieval alchemists and mystics of Europe, we find this recurring vision of man. It is esoteric in nature but still it is used in a very practical way. All these people saw man's physical body as being the end result of a series of interrelated and interdependent subtle levels of consciousness.

LEVELS OF CONSCIOUSNESS

Basically, they saw man as being the sum total of seven levels of consciousness. To each level is assigned the form of an energy body. Only the energy of the physical body is dense enough to register immediately with the five senses and hence with the direct perception of another person. The other energy bodies can only be deduced by inference or perceived directly by clairvoyant or extrasensory perception. If we consider the emotional—or astral level, as it is frequently called—then I might think you are happy because I can see you smile and hear you laugh, but this does not mean I am appreciating your emotions directly or accurately. You may be putting on a front. A clairvoyant, however, might be able to see your emotional body directly, say in terms of subtle color emanations, and so have a better idea of how you really do feel. Similarly, healers often say they base their physical diagnosis on perception of the subtle energy of the health aura.

The seven levels of consciousness are given various names and I have used the following:

Divine or True Nature }	Spiritual Essence
Spirit mind Spiritual-intuitional mind } Higher intuitional mind	Higher self, soul or spirit
Mental-intellectual mind Emotional-astral mind } Physical-etheric mind	Lower self, personality or ego

The levels of consciousness are represented on an ascending scale purely for convenience as in actuality, each is interrelated with the other.

The different kingdoms are also related in this scheme. Each kingdom is said to be concentrated in a different area of consciousness. The mineral kingdom is right in the physical level. A rock is a very physical thing! The vegetable kingdom is primarily in the physical but peaks into the emotional. Experiments with lie detectors have confirmed this ancient esoteric view by registering the emotional reactions of plants. This is well explained in *The Secret Life of Plants* by Tompkins and Bird.[36]

The animal kingdom is strongly involved with the physical and emotional levels and also has activity in the mental sphere.

Bringing Ego and Spirit Together

Next comes man, who has the most exciting prospects. We human beings are active on the physical, emotional and mental levels, and for us there is the possibility of making direct contact with higher levels of consciousness. For human beings there is this exciting distinction between our egos and our spirits, and the even more exciting prospect of uniting the two.

The ego is very similar to what we call our personality, as it includes our physical form, our emotions and our thoughts. The ego is that part of our self we tend to be most familiar with as well as being the most obvious part of our self that other people tend to know us by. The ego is the vehicle through which we project ourselves out to the world at large. But also we have what is often described as our spirit, the higher self or inner core of our being. Our spirit is the more permanent, purer, less complicated part of our being.

Many of us are aware of the nature of our ego or personality and work on this level. Only in moments of contemplation or inspiration do we make contract with our higher self or soul. The gap that links our ego with our soul is "the eye of the needle" spoken of in the Bible, and the mind acts as the fulcrum between physical and spiritual man. Intellect must be transmuted into intuition to bridge that gap.

Our life purpose is to make that leap. Our goal is to be freed of the limitations of personality, and soar free as spiritual beings.

Death plays its part in this process by providing new beginnings. At death, all of us that is the ego—our body, emotions and thinking mind—drops off, and our consciousness persists in the other states. Usually, our new functional body is our astral body, or it may be a higher body, depending on our stage of development. In this altered state of consciousness, we develop further, before reincarnating into a new physical body for the purpose of advancing toward the state of perfection intended for all of us.

Reincarnation is governed by the Law of Karma, which is basically the spiritual law of cause and effect. Just as physically for every action there is an equal and opposite reaction, so also spiritually, as you sow you shall reap.

Hence, good actions have their rewards and bad ones need to be compensated. The aim of the game is to progress beyond the law of karma. Then, free of the bonds of past activity, actions can be performed for their intrinsic "correctness," without any thought as to the benefits they might produce. This leads to a state of enlightenment in Eastern terminology, or to reunion with the Divine in the Christian view.

This concept helps to explain the seeming disparities around us and provides an incentive toward ethical, moral conduct in all situations.

SUBTLE-ENERGY HEALING

But back to healing. The etheric body is vital to our considerations. It is the counterpart of our physical body. It is composed of a very subtle energy that is visible to sensitive people such as clairvoyants, and known as the health aura. It is this vehicle through which the other levels of consciousness impinge on the physical.

This subtle energy is centered on seven chakras. "Chakra" is a Sanskrit word used to describe the concentrations of this subtle energy that is said to be located in seven different regions located along the spine and up into the head. Each chakra is a reflection of one level of consciousness and in turn relates most directly to one particular endocrine gland.

Chakras can be thought of as energy transformers in an electricity grid. They relay energy to a network of power lines, that are called meridians or nadis and which radiate throughout the physical body. The meridians correlate with the nervous system that in turn regulates the secretions from the endocrine glands. The hormones, so released, travel throughout the body via the blood and are instrumental in maintaining the body in its natural state of balance; hence the link from consciousness to matter. From the realm of consciousness, energy streams forth to vitalize etheric energy in the individual chakras. This energy then passes via the meridians to influence the nervous system's regulation of the endocrine glands. The hormones that then flow via the blood are vital in maintaining the physical body.

In this view, then, the physical body is the end result of formative energies as mediated by the etheric body that is in a state of dynamic flux. The characteristics of our etheric body will vary with the quality of the energies coming from the various formative levels of consciousness and with how its physical counterpart, the body, interacts with its own immediate physical environment.

Disease can be due to purely physical causes such as diet and exercise or the rare case of a true accident. However, many current diseases relate to aberrations in our emotional world, while many others are centered in our mind. This fact is recognized by the growing attention being paid to psychosomatic disease and the role of tension and anxiety in the production of disease.

Accepting our basically spiritual nature, it is easy to see the spirit's overriding involvement and to consider disease in man as the end stage of disharmony between the spirit and the ego—or friction between the higher self's attitudes and the lower self's actions. When such disharmony is left unresolved, it manifests as a physical reality so that we are forced to confront it.

Disease then provides an opportunity to progress beyond our limitations. To gain the benefit of disease, to learn its real lessons, all aspects must be considered. Yet, in the immediate situation, it is often the physical condition that seems to be of prime importance. Most people living in the physical world do reject disease and death. They wish to continue here to experience and to progress as much as possible.

However, let us pause to reconsider the miracle of pure, physical surgery. Consider again the incredible trauma following a broken leg. It is easy to imagine the soft tissue damage, fragmented bones and then perhaps a steel pin inserted to hold things in place. Yet, after medical intervention and the passage of a relatively short period of time, function will return to normal and later X-rays will show little, if any, evidence of the damage. Just how can this be? What does initiate this truly wondrous healing that produces such magical effects?

We know quite a lot of the process, but what of the cause? We know a lot about how it happens. But why does it happen? I contend that a basic, relatively permanent blueprint of the body's form, as provided by the etheric body concept, does make sense of the situation. Although the physical form is traumatically altered in such accidents, the basic pattern, the etheric blueprint, remains. So, given the right conditions, healing will proceed so that the physical form once more matches the etheric, and normal function will return. It is a mistake to think that an outsider heals anything. A healer can be a most useful catalyst in the healing process, but the healer's role is to create the correct conditions whereby the patient's healing processes themselves can re-create the normal state.

Consideration of this subtle-energy model also accommodates the many other forms healing can take. Dietary considerations, for instance, act first on the physical level to purify the physical organism. But, as food has its own etheric energy, it can be a source of vitalization on this level also. This is one reason why many people advocate the use of pure foods raised in as natural a way as possible. The more natural, the fresher and more vital our food, the more subtle energy it has. Also, it is believed the subtle energy of food can be increased by being produced and prepared by a sensitive person, attuned to such ideas. On the other hand, the etheric value of much of the present-day mass-produced processed food must approach zero, or even have negative connotations.

Meditation acts to balance the higher and lower selves. In a state wherein the physical, emotional and mental levels are removed from one's direct awareness, the intrinsic purity of the higher self can operate to reharmonize the etheric blue print and so lead on to the re-creation of the normal physical situation. Dr. Ainslie Meares said that meditation produces a return to a state wherein the immune system is induced to function normally. This causes the body to recognize and reject the presence of cancerous cells. This, he said, is mediated via an influence on hormonal levels. You can see the similarities in concept, the explanations being to me a matter of degree.

The extraordinary Filipino healers are able to channel large amounts of direct healing energy. Sometimes they operate on a purely physical level. More often, however, they are operating on the precursive levels, notably the etheric and astral. Some are effective on the mental level, and a rare few heal on the spiritual level. Christ was a Divine Healer—capable of healing on any level.

This etheric energy of which we have been speaking has its global and universal counterpart, tied up with the all-pervading consciousness. It is on this energy that the psychic surgeons and other faith healers draw. Most of them merely accept their healing talents as God's gift of the Holy Spirit in action, and leave it at that. However, it is not too hard to use our model and to consider the possibility that what they are doing is drawing upon a universal energy, focusing it with their minds as a lens focuses the rays of the sun, and then emitting it through their fingers in a beam of energy that can be compared to a laser beam.

This beam of energy can then neutralize the positive and negative charges holding tissues together at the molecular level. In the absence of these forces, the tissues separate and can be entered. When the energy is withdrawn the body's etheric forces reassert their blueprint effect so that the physical structures resume their normal state, with no scarring.

Alternatively, some people believe psychic surgery is performed through the action of harmonics. They theorize that the healers are able to cause their hands to resonate in harmony with the tissue of their patients, so that the two can intersperse, much as two gases or two liquids can intersperse.

Regardless of how it is achieved, once the healers are inside the body, they utilize a magnetic faculty that enables them to draw together the diseased energies and remove them—a bit like a magnet can draw iron filings to itself. It is important to realize that such changes in phase do occur—a good example being how steam can be condensed to water. Maybe what the healers do is to concentrate the subtle, formative energies associated with a physical symptom of disease and actually precipitate them into physical form. Could this be a demonstration of energy giving rise to matter—a true materialization?

MY OWN INTEGRATION

In the Philippines I was told my bone tumors were too dense to be removed physically, but that the etheric energies associated with them could be taken away. My physical form would then return to match this normalized blueprint if I did not re-create the destructive etheric energies. So, after the initial boost, it became important to seek out the causes of disharmony within myself.

After the Philippines experience, I gained a remarkable and generalized healing boost. Yet the tumors kept growing, although slowly. It was obvious to me I had not made the necessary changes in myself. Only after many more efforts, culminating in meeting Sai Baba, a holy man of India, was I really able to get free of my cancer problems.

There still remains the ongoing process which faces each one of us—that of developing a system in which to maximize our potentials, correct our shortcomings, and live in accord with our principles.

These subtle energies we have been considering can be drawn upon and used in a positive, practical manner. All of us do radiate these subtle energies. They are colored by the quality of the "vehicle" through which they pass. Therefore, if we do want to use them more fully, it is vital that we seek to be as free as possible from complications within our own personalities or egos, and be open to allowing these subtle, but powerful, healing energies to flow freely.

SUBTLE-ENERGY MEDICINE • Recommendations

What to do? Times have changed. Few people I know these days go to the Philippines for healing. But many people continue to benefit from prayer, from Reiki, from visiting those who are regarded as having "healing gifts" and those who have some psychic awareness. There is no doubt in my experience some people have been helped greatly by subtle-energy medicine in one form or another.

This is another area where we need to be guided by our own sensibilities.

Maybe you regard all this as mumbo jumbo. No problem—just focus on what you find helpful. However, if you are curious, if you are interested, the best way to investigate is the way you would investigate anything. Find out what you can, check out the books, any references, the Internet; speak to your friends and seek word-of-mouth endorsements. Then if you do go to visit any practitioner of subtle-energy medicine, just like with a counselor, allow the first meeting to be like a job interview where the basic task is to decide whether or not you will go the second time. If you do decide to see a practitioner of this type, the best thing is to then commit. Do all you can to dispel any doubts, give yourself over to the treatment, and hope for a miracle. I know people who have been lucky!

Now it is time to pull all the pieces of the healing journey together, to summarize, and to formulate a plan.

CHAPTER 21

Recommendations

An Action Plan

SO OFTEN I HAVE MET PEOPLE WHO FEEL HOPELESS, AS IF THERE IS NOTHING they can do to help themselves. Then, presented with all the very real possibilities we have been discussing, they soon find themselves wondering where to begin, how to fit it all in, what to do. There is a great deal of information, a great many useful techniques, included in this book. The task now is to sort out the priorities and make a plan. While it is an obvious fact that individuals do vary, in general the following would be a reasonable order of priorities for those looking to help themselves toward maximizing their potential.

FOR PEOPLE RECENTLY DIAGNOSED AND BASICALLY WELL

Answer the four basic questions:

1. Do I really want to get well again?
2. Do I choose to accept responsibility for my situation? If taking responsibility, lifestyle medicine will always make sense; get started on that as soon as you can—meditation, positive thinking, diet and exercise being the immediate priorities.
3. How relevant is conventional medicine, traditional medicine and CAM?
4. Which particular external therapies shall I use?

(Details: The introduction and chapter 13.)

Assess each therapy according to the principles:

1. What are my expectations with no treatment?
2. What are the expectations for me if I have the proposed treatment?

3. Are there any side effects to the treatment and, if so, what might they be?

4. How will my own response to that treatment affect the outcome?

(Details: chapter 3.)

MEDICAL TREATMENT

If a specific therapy is suitable for you, and you decide to have it, commit yourself to it fully; work to minimize any potential side effects and maximize the benefits.

LIFESTYLE-BASED, SELF-HELP TECHNIQUES

Meditation

This is the ideal first step because it deals with stress, will help you to regain balance in body, mind and spirit, to think calmly and clearly, and to act appropriately.

If quality of life is your prime aim, begin with three sessions of ten to twenty minutes daily, and once it is working well, maintain one or two sessions of ten to twenty minutes daily.

If you want to gain maximum benefit from meditation, begin with three sessions daily of whatever period you feel comfortable with and build as rapidly as possible to three sessions of forty minutes, up to one hour each day.

(Details: chapters 4–6. Read *Meditation—An In-Depth Guide*. Consider using a CD to guide you or using my downloadable meditation program, Mind-Body Mastery.)

Dietary Considerations

Once the meditation is becoming integrated into your day, consider your dietary choices.

MAKE NO CHANGE

The average Western diet—high in fat, protein, salt, sugar, alcohol and refined foods, and low in fiber, vitamin and mineral intakes—may be inadequate. The "average" person would do well, therefore, to consider change. Recognize that change in this vital area has the potential to be stressful. Spend time to think the changes through, discuss them, and plan for them. Be clear on your aims and choices. Meditation makes change easier. Seek professional guidance. Get excited by the possibilities!

THE WELLNESS DIET (CHAPTER 13)

This is a good, sensible approach, as it avoids known risk factors and concentrates on foods that are known to carry preventative factors or actively promote health. Essentially, it is low in fat, protein and alcohol, avoids salt, sugar and refined foods, and has a high-fiber content. It is a plant-based, whole-food diet. Its primary constituents are the fruits, vegetables and grains. Ideally, the recommendations of the Wellness Diet then become a lifelong way of eating.

THE HEALING DIET (CHAPTER 14)

This is the more intense approach that is better suited to those who want to emphasize their dietary considerations. It includes consideration of an initial mono diet of three to ten days to provide an element of fasting, detoxification, transition and regeneration.

The recommendation is to continue with the Healing Diet until cancer-symptom free; or if you were symptom free when you started the Healing Diet, continue it for two months before gradually transferring to the ongoing Wellness Diet.

FOLLOW A SPECIFIC, FORMAL DIET

For example, the macrobiotic approach or the Gerson Therapy (see Appendix G). The last mentioned, particularly, is suited to a clinic situation and it is not recommended to be attempted at home without skilled guidance and the committed support of at least one permanent, full-time helper.

My personal experience, coupled with the feedback received from thousands of other people affected by cancers, leads me to believe that the suggestions summarized in (b) and (c) are the best way to proceed with your diet.

(Details: chapters 11–14.)

Positive Thinking

With meditation and dietary considerations, positive thinking completes the three basic ingredients of healing and well-being. Recognize the basic need to be positive, and to use the mind training techniques that you need in your particular situation.

If you do feel depressed or negative, start by working on exercise and a creative activity. By actually doing something physical and positive, you will set the whole process in motion. Gardening is my favorite activity. Exercise also warrants being a strong priority—aim for thirty minutes daily.

(Details: chapters 7–9.)

Spiritual Development

For most, this is another essential. Recognize that your endeavors in this area may be the most important of all.

RELIGION

Follow your own preferences here. Very few people change their religion through an experience with disease, but many find their convictions strengthened. This may well be a time to return to your religion.

REFLECTION, INTROSPECTION, CONTEMPLATION

Highly recommended as long as they are not associated with guilt or other negative emotions. Seek to understand your past, accept your present, and work "in the now" toward a happier, healthier tomorrow.

YOUR VIEW

Your view, or belief system, can limit your horizons or leave you free to soar above any situation with a smile on your face. Spend time reading, thinking, in contemplation, and in evolving your own theories. Open yourself to the possibilities.

SPIRITUAL HEALING

This may be catalyzed by others, but often comes with personal experience. Learning to love that part of your inner self, your spiritual essence, is an integral part of loving God, the universe, and your fellows. Once you can love yourself, you can recognize the inner truth in others. Then you can see that they too are seeking to be free of limitations and to express their inner perfection. Along with this, you will realize that it is not enough to dwell in spirit. The body is the temple of the soul and you need to give it due consideration.

Healing is complete when harmony is found in body, mind and spirit. (Details: chapters 19–20.)

Healthy Emotions

Relationships frequently require as much healing as the physical body.

Make peace with as many as you can. Use the imagery technique of forgiveness once your meditation is working well.

The immediate family may need all these principles just as much as you do. Often it is the patient whose physical symptoms reflect a malaise involving one or several other closely associated people. Encourage your family to support you and to join you in as much of your program as possible, particularly the big three: meditation, diet and positive thinking.

(Details: chapters 16–17.)

Pain Control

Another essential life skill for all to learn at some stage. Do the recommended pain control exercises and be aware of the other possibilities.

(Details: chapter 10.)

Consideration of Death and Dying

This is another vitally important issue that is best acknowledged, contemplated, discussed and then used as motivation to live well, to live fully in the present moment.

Formulate your will and an enduring power of attorney.

Discuss your choices for end-of-life care.

Principles: Be brave enough to reflect and contemplate upon what you anticipate to happen. Look at your fears if any. Actively seek the opportunity to discuss the whole area with a good listener and especially, if possible, with your closest relatives. With the fears confronted and allayed, and with the benefit of regular meditation and contemplation, death can be genuinely seen as another very natural and positive part of life.

(Details: chapter 18.)

Healing

Be convinced that true healing lies within and work toward your own health and well-being. However, healers who can act as catalysts in the process may be very useful and appropriate. Be aware of the possibilities and use your own judgment. I certainly *do not* routinely recommend that anyone should jump on a plane and dash off to the Philippines, India or wherever; nor would I say it is unwise to consider doing so. However, if you do seek healing help from an extraordinary source, find out as much as you can about it before you begin. Having made your choice, strive to be open to the best possible outcome and commit yourself to the requirements of the healing technique involved.

(Details: chapters 19–20.)

Imagery

Imagery can be an "optional extra" to add to the meditation once the latter is going well. It does utilize the active, more willful side of the mind, whereas meditation relies on the stillness.

You could use the gentle, abstract methods such as the white light imagery or the healing journey.

If you choose to use more active and personalized images, you are advised to read and study my book on this subject, *The Mind That Changes Everything*.[37] This will add extra clarity. Also, you may benefit from seeking qualified guidance. If you use imagery regularly, do it for a few minutes three times daily. Then aim to continue on from the imagery, to let go and to experience moments of stillness whenever possible. Seek to be as relaxed as you can be.

Whether you do use imagery or not, do persevere with the meditation, as almost all people who persevere do establish an effective practice, and it has special benefits.

(Details: chapters 8–9.)

Remember: A journey of a thousand miles begins with just one step.

FOR PEOPLE IN A CRITICAL CONDITION

The same basic approach applies. You may feel quality of life issues are more important than efforts to overcome your physical symptoms. In this case, some medical and self-help techniques may be counterproductive. Changes in diet may just cause anguish, whereas meditation always leads to peace of mind and remains the priority. Most people who use all the principles find they apply to any life situation and so make for a good life—and a good death.

Faced with a crisis, your attitudes and beliefs assume paramount importance and peace of mind should be the main aim. So do seek to avoid or resolve situations of conflict as the calm that follows is enduring. I would never abandon hope of conquering disease, as it is my firm belief that healing is possible in any situation.

I am confident the techniques we have discussed in this book can work. However, they only have a chance to work if you apply them. Of course it is important to gather the best support around you that you can, but then it is up to you. You can greatly improve your situation. You can be confident of that. It is not reasonable, however, to expect that everyone will be freed of their physical symptoms. Some still die as a result of their cancer, but success or failure is not marked by death. Success is marked by poise and equanimity. The greatest successes I have seen have been in people who have developed a strong, stable and life-affirming "I choose to live to the full" stance but at the same time have been able to accept what life had to offer in return, even if it is dying. However, a great many have become well, and virtually all who have applied themselves to these principles have felt a great deal of benefit. Any effort will be rewarded.

FOR THOSE INTERESTED IN PREVENTION
OR IN MAXIMUM HEALTH

Surprise! The same principles still apply. The degree to which you apply them depends on your priorities, beliefs and expectations.

As an ideal prevention program that would lead to maximum health, I confidently recommend:

1. **Meditation:** Ten to twenty minutes once or twice daily.
2. **Healthy Nutrition:** The basic Wellness Diet.
3. **Positive Thinking:** Keep developing this, using the techniques already summarized.

4. **Make time**—yes, *make* time—to dwell on and implement the recommendations for spiritual development, positive emotions, pain control, considerations of death and dying, and healing. Regular time for contemplation is highly recommended and imagery also may find a place in your life.

A SUMMARY

I am confident that these basic, self-help principles and techniques are worthy of application in virtually all conditions. They may be applied to other disease states besides those of cancer or merely used as aids to maximize health.

Make total health your goal. Make that elusive, ephemeral, wonderful, joyous state of harmony in body, mind and soul your life ambition. Seek to develop your potential to the full.

Be patient yet persevere, for the goal is real and within reach. Be gentle with yourself. Most have ups and downs along the way. Remember, it is your belief system that validates your actions. If your actions are not in line with your belief system, you are almost certain to produce disease. You may have pondered on boozing, smoking and shuffling old George, who probably thinks that his life is OK and so has no inner conflict. By doing so he accepts substandard health. But while he may have no obvious physical symptoms of disease, his version of health is a pale image of his potential.

Once you have a glimpse of *your* true potential you will realize that we all have the capacity, the potential to heal and to be really well. Accept that it can take time. Make a start. Just being on the path to true health in body, mind and spirit will transform your life and bring you peace. Life *was* meant to be good.

Happiness is to be found along the way, not just at the end of the path.

My wish for everyone is a long and happy life.

Appendices

How to Develop Effective Relationships with Your Doctors

FROM THE POINT OF VIEW OF A PERSON WITH CANCER, HAVING AT LEAST one doctor that you can trust and communicate with is a very important element in the healing process.

You need someone who can provide accurate and complete information, to the level it is known medically, and to the level you choose to know—someone who can be sensitive to the physical, psychological and spiritual state of both you and your family.

What is needed is a doctor who is focused on your welfare, who respects your thoughts and feelings, and who responds to them—a good communicator.

It is a sad fact, that with the thousands of people we have worked with over the years, it has been rare to find a patient who has not had at least one major medical complaint that had at its core poor communication. Many patients and partners are glowing in praise of the general care and attention they receive medically. Yet, it is unusual for these people not to have had at least one bad experience. Others are openly hostile about the way they have been treated and spoken to. Clearly, there is a need for good doctor/patient communications, better training for medical practitioners and more support for self-help techniques such as meditation and positive thinking.

Often it seems that the patient, the person with the illness, needs to take an active, gently assertive role in improving communication levels.

Communication is a two-way process. Your part as a patient/partner/ support person is to express yourself and listen objectively to the doctor. Here are some points that build good relations.

Practice Gentle Assertion

This means expressing yourself clearly and accurately, ideally free of emotion, with the intention of informing the doctor of your needs and preferences. Inform your doctor of:

- The level of information you want provided;
- Who you want involved in major decision making—which professionals, family members and/or friends;
- Which doctor is to take the central coordinating role and be the focus of your decision making and treatment;
- Who you regard as a technician, who a counselor, communicator, adviser. Ideally, doctors will fill many of these roles but some may need to be regarded as one only.

Ideally, Seek a Medical Partner

A key medical person that you can trust, a good communicator. Someone who will do their best to give you as accurate and complete information as you ask for, who can speak in a language you can understand, who is sensitive to and responds to your state of mind, who respects your choices and supports you. A general practitioner or family physician is highly likely to fill this role and so a warning. Often people go to their family doctor with their early symptoms and are then referred to specialists for detailed investigation and treatment. Many then become caught up in the ambit of the specialists and do not return to the family doctor. The point is the GPs are generalists. They often have a broad, holistic or integrated view. They are usually good communicators, are great problem solvers and excellent advocates for their patients. They can be ideally suited to be the head of your healing team.

At Consultations

- Take a second person, preferably a partner. They will provide good moral support, remember questions and answers and be more stable, especially if emotional issues arise.
- Write your questions down before consultations and take them with you.
- Request extra time (in advance) for questions and discussion if necessary.

- Take notes during consultations or even ask if you can use a voice recorder. The amount of important information that can be forgotten in a consultation is great and you do need to retain it!
- Feel free to ask for explanations, elaborations, options, opinions.
- Be prepared to explain and justify your preferences.
- Inform the doctor what self-help options you are using—for the sake of information, education and inclusion.

Consider a Second Opinion

For major decisions, always give strong consideration to obtaining a second opinion. Go to someone outside the medical group, hospital or circle of the first opinion, so that it is, in fact, an independent opinion. Cancer medicine, like any other complicated field, is subject to personal experiences and preferences. It may be that a second opinion could provide a very different treatment option that warrants your consideration.

Be Prepared to Change Your Doctor If You Are Not Satisfied

Always try first to resolve problems by communicating with the doctor. Explain your situation if you do experience any difficulties or dissatisfaction. Often this will lead to resolution and healing of another sort—the healing of an important relationship. If not, there is no need to feel guilty—ask for a referral to someone more suited to your needs or make your own enquiries. A good doctor-patient relationship is vital to your health and well-being.

Aim to Be Confident of All Your Choices

Keep enquiring, listening, questioning and talking until you feel you are clear on the options and what is the best approach for you to follow.

Remember, it is unlikely that you can know or appreciate all the facts, all the options, all the fine details. It is likely there will come a point where you will have to say, "In the light of all I know and feel at this point in time, this is my very best option."

Do aim to clarify that option as clearly as possible, so you can confidently commit yourself to it. This is the first essential in positive thinking and will set you on the path toward achieving the best possible results.

Further suggestions on decision making are in chapters 1–3.

Recognize, Value and Use Your Own Resources

Remember that whatever treatment is available medically, as a human being you have emotions, a mind and a spirit. That makes you an incredibly powerful being. Add to that the support and love of well-directed family and friends and you can achieve exceptional results—peace of mind and the best possible physical outcome.

Commit to Your Decisions and Follow Through

Once you have clarified your options and made definite decisions, commit to what you plan to do. Better still, embrace all you do. Be enthusiastic. Welcome any treatments you do commit to. Do all possible to support yourself, your good intentions and those around you, including your health professionals.

What to Do to Enhance Surgery, Chemotherapy or Radiotherapy

General Recommendations to Support Medical Treatment

Step 1. Mental Preparation

1. Collect a team

1. Decide who is on your team, who you consult, who you take advice from.
2. Decide who will be your key medical adviser—maybe a GP interested in integrative medicine is best for this, maybe a nurse-practitioner? Maybe your oncologist or your surgeon? Who will it be?

2. Decide and commit

1. The aim is to explore your options carefully, make an informed choice with a clear decision, then commit to it.
2. In some situations the logical choice regarding what to do will be obvious, and sometimes it will not be so obvious. To ensure good decision making, as well as using your intellect, meditate so that your mind becomes calm and clear, and you have more direct access to your intuition and your wisdom. Put all this together and you will make good choices.
3. Once you arrive at a decision, seek all the support you can and aim to embrace all that you do.

3. Prepare for the best

1. Once you do make a choice and commit to a particular treatment regime, be really conscious of preparing yourself and consider all you can do to:

2. minimize any potential side effects
3. maximize the benefits
4. make the whole experience meaningful.

4. Study and apply the healing principles set out in this book!
5. Work hard to be confident and have faith in your decisions and your plans. Aim to create a healing environment, physically, emotionally, mentally and even spiritually around yourself.

Step 2. The Immediate Practicalities

1. Eat well—at least follow the Wellness Diet, but ideally use the Healing Diet.

1. Include in your diet anticancer foods such as raspberries or pomegranate; fresh turmeric; broccoli sprouts; cabbage; etc.
2. Use the nutritional principles of the Healing Diet to create a cancer-unfriendly environment in your body and to turn the tables metabolically on the cancer.
3. Consider organizing healthy "meals on wheels" for hospitalization if the hospital food is inadequate. Friends or family might drop off juices, nutritious meals and snacks.

2. Keep the fluids up. Remember to keep drinking—at least 68 ounces in total per day.

1. Include seven juices per day—These are particularly good around chemotherapy treatment times, as they provide a good source of easy to absorb nutrients in a balanced package, are gentle on the bowel and their nutrients are easily absorbed. Green juice especially is particularly useful during radiation and chemotherapy.
2. Smoothies are excellent if eating is difficult, appetite is down, or weight loss is an issue. Use any nondairy milk as a base, add banana, soy yogurt, plus a little honey and/or carob or cocoa powder.

3. Exercise regularly—at least three to four times each week for around thirty minutes, but ideally daily.
4. Meditate—ideally, three long sessions daily (forty to sixty minutes per session).

5. **Imagery**—consider using the white light healing journey or specific personal healing imagery, especially while receiving treatments.
6. **Massage can be very helpful**—once a week or as it suits.
   1. Be mindful during the massage so you experience the greatest benefits for your state of mind.

7. **Supplements** may well be useful and ideally you clarify these possibilities with a doctor trained in nutrition, or another suitably qualified health professional. Particular supplements to discuss include:
   1. Multivitamin/mineral supplements
   2. Vitamin C
   3. Magnesium, iron and zinc
   4. Floradix as a supplement or eat liver (organic calves liver) to aid blood quality, especially if you know your blood cells or platelets have dropped down.
   5. Strath tonic has been shown to minimize potential side effects of radiotherapy and may be helpful with chemotherapy. Green tea, turmeric, seaweeds, rooibos tea and spirulina are all thought to offset potential side effects of chemotherapy and radiotherapy and are worth considering.
   6. Consider using slippery elm powder three times a day or aloe vera juice to protect from an unsettled stomach and bowel while undergoing chemotherapy.

8. **Support your bowel.** Take regular probiotics supplementation or eat yogurt daily (natural, organic soy yogurt is best) to maintain healthy bowel flora.
9. **Check your vitamin D levels regularly.** They need to be between 100 and 150nmol/l. Use supplements if necessary, especially if out of the sun for extended periods. Buy the 5,000 IU capsules that can be purchased over the Internet.

Step 3. Emotional Preparation
1. **Be authentic**. Healthy emotions are authentic emotions. Read the chapters on emotional health and find the people in your life you can share your emotions with safely and authentically. It is natural to have emotions

surface from time to time; express them authentically and then get on with what you need to do to recover.

2. **Communicate.** Think about who you need to say things to, and what you want to say—and do it!

   1. With children repeat two things regularly (as well as the obvious telling them that you do love them):
      - "It (as in the cancer) is not your fault" (offsets guilt).
      - A major reason why you are doing this treatment (including all you are doing for yourself) is because you want to survive and to continue to be with them (offsets feelings of abandonment).
   2. Read *How to Help Children Through a Parent's Serious Illness* by Kathleen McCue.
   3. Get professional help if you are stuck.

3. **Practice gratitude.** Develop a sense of gratitude for the skill of your medical team and for the effectiveness and accessibility of the medical system. Be grateful for all the support you generate.

Step 4. Spiritual Preparation

1. **Generate acceptance.** Accept what is happening now and what has happened to you in the past. Adopt a relaxed mode, but one that also has a resolve for a good outcome. Commit to making the best of the situation you are in (e.g., combine acceptance and commitment). This will provide the clarity to do whatever the circumstances require, which may be doing nothing in particular, or it may require action. The clearer you are, the clearer your choices will become—this is one of meditation's major benefits.

2. **Make time for the big questions.** Maybe this is time to be contemplating the meaning and purpose of life, to be questioning what it is all about.

   1. It is certainly a good time to be making peace with those around you, anyone outstanding from the past, and to be reconciling your own inner life. Consider your own spiritual tradition and how you relate to it now. Is it time to be going to church, or to be hearing a great spiritual teacher speak somewhere? Give attention to seeking out the organizations, the people, the books that can help you with this.

2. Take time to sit quietly and to also discuss these matters with a spiritual friend.

3. Many find that it is the time they spend on the big questions that enriches their lives for the better, and that this becomes a happy side effect of the illness.

Preparing for Surgery Specifically

Step 1. Consider Collecting Blood

Preoperation, organizing collecting your own blood via your doctor may well be possible and may make sense for a possible retransfusion.

Step 2. Practice Inner Rehearsal

This is a valuable technique you can start as soon as surgery is booked in, and you can do it daily right up to the time of the surgery. Many people find this exercise really useful even as they go into theater and are being anesthetized.

Imagine:

- The physical reality of the cancer shrinking in the time leading up to the surgery (particularly around its outer margins), and that when the surgery is performed the cancer will be easy to remove—a bit like shelling a pea out of its pod.

- The whole construct that goes with the cancer being contained within the physical mass of the cancer itself. What this means is that you imagine all the causes and all the physical, emotional and psychological dynamic of the cancer being contained within the cancer itself. You imagine everything and anything to do with the cancer is contained within its mass. Then you imagine that when the actual physical lump is removed surgically, everything associated with the cancer is removed at the one time. This is a bit like an exorcism, a purge, that takes more than just the physical lump—it takes the spirit, the energy, everything associated with the cancer out of your system.

- Imagine during the operation the surgeons being pleased with the surgery and saying things like, "This is easier than we expected," "It's all going really well," "The operation went well."

- Imagine that you will experience a rapid and complete recovery—you are pleasantly surprised by the lack of pain, and there or no postoperative infections or any other side effects.
- Imagine yourself in the future, fit and well, looking back at the surgery and being grateful for a full recovery. You could imagine visiting the doctor when you are well and you are looking back on the time of your illness and discussing all you did to become well again.

Regard the Postoperative Period as a New Beginning

Consider that you need a time of convalescence. Try not to go back to work for some time and rest your body regularly.

The Traditional 5-Step Process of Meditation

TRADITIONALLY, ONE COMMON WAY TO DESCRIBE AND TO TEACH MEDITATION was to consider it as just one step in a five-step process. This process began with:

Concentration

A beginner would take up a set position, relax physically and then attempt to concentrate upon just one thing. It should be emphasized that the relaxation and the concentration were complementary and some of the techniques actually did place emphasis on the means of becoming relaxed. The more you relax, the easier it is to concentrate.

The focus for the concentration may have been on just about anything, but these are the most common:

- An activity—Breathing, in particular, has been widely used, as has dance and meditative movement such as the Chinese art of tai chi.
- An object (such as a candle or a painting)—Icons have been used for this, as have mandalas or complex, symbolic paintings.
- A sound—Usually such a sound would be repeated over and over. This could be done out loud as with chanting, or silently as with a repetitive prayer or a mantra. A mantra is a word or group of words repeated continuously as in the practice of transcendental meditation (TM).
- A thought—Generally a particular quality would be concentrated upon; truth, honesty, love and compassion are typical examples used. This particular practice is often called contemplation or analytical meditation.

Whatever the nature of the focus for concentration, the aim was to think of that focus and nothing else. This took people's attention away from random, distracting thoughts and helped to focus their attention. Once this was achieved, meditation was under way.

Meditation

Meditation in this context was defined as the ability to concentrate on one thing to the exclusion of other thoughts. It was an active process of the mind that required some effort. In this traditional sense, meditation was really undistracted concentration. When practiced long enough it led on to:

Contemplation

Contemplation could begin once the act of concentration had become automatic and effortless. Then, it was as if the mind slipped into overdrive. When this occurred, instead of the logical, thinking part of the mind being at work, a heightened state of awareness developed and the intuitive, creative, wisdom aspect came into play.

It is important to recognize that the mind does have these two distinctive ways of functioning—one rational and conscious, the other more abstract, intuitive and wisdom based. Most of us are very familiar with the day-to-day rational processes of the brain. All day our brain is thinking, analyzing, evaluating. We have a steady flow of thoughts from the time we first arise to the time when we lapse into sleep at night. This rational, mental activity is normally associated with the left half of the brain.

Normally, we would associate times of nonthinking with sleep or unconsciousness. However, we may have experienced fleeting moments of nonthinking consciousness in the pleasant reverie that sometimes descends just before sleep. This peace is similar to those wonderful moments when a glorious sunset or a major work of art touches our inner core and leaves us in rapturous silence. We are then involved with that more abstract, less rational brain activity which is predominately associated with the right side of the brain. Often in those moments of reverie or silence, we can experience useful, even profound insights.

Many of us then, could be laughingly referred to as half-wits because, being overly rational creatures, we only use half our brain's potential! Contemplation complements our rational thinking and is a way to exercise the other half of our brain. By doing so, fresh insights can be gained and new levels of meaning obtained.

The mind, however, is still active during this contemplative phase of the process. In contemplation it is just being used in a way with which we are not so commonly familiar.

Prolonged contemplation leads on to the experience of unification.

Unification

This is a still more abstract state. To explain, during our normal daily experience, when we become aware of an object, we have a sense of duality. Look again at this book you are reading. There is the book in front of you, and there is that part of you that is aware of the book. It is natural to feel the two are separate. There is you, and there is the book. There is also the process of being aware of the book.

Now, here is the interesting and exciting bit! Through contemplation, you the contemplator, the object of whatever you are contemplating, and even the act of contemplation itself, merge so that there is no sense of separation, no sense of duality. Just an abiding sense of unity. A sense of oneness. In our example, you no longer feel separate from the book, you feel at one with it.

This union, this sense of oneness that can be catalyzed by concentrating on any particular object in the manner described; this union is what the mystics of all ages have sought so earnestly and waxed poetic about when they found it. It led on to a final state, illumination.

Illumination

This has been described as "the knowing that passes all understanding." In this state, a totally new experience of reality would be revealed. This experience was direct, immediate and totally satisfying. It was the experience of truth, absolute truth in a way that was clearly and unmistakably revealed. In some traditions this experience is called enlightenment.

We can understand how this five-step process works if we use the example of concentrating upon a candle. Initially, concentration is required to sit still and to focus our attention on a candle. To begin with, the mind will almost certainly tend to wander—What is for dinner? What am I doing tomorrow? Should I scratch my nose? Etc.

Eventually, with persistence and effort, we can concentrate on the candle without being restless or without being interrupted by other thoughts. This is meditation. This is undistracted awareness. Soon contemplation will follow and it is as if another thought process begins. Abstract thoughts of the candle become apparent. The symbolism of the candle, its shape, its light, its fire, may be reflected upon and these qualities provide a new level of understanding. For example, you may feel as if the light of the candle is a symbol of the spiritual essence within you and feel enriched by this awareness.

As time goes on such thoughts gently fade and all awareness of activity and time are lost. Only in retrospect can you be aware that you were in a state in which you felt at one with the candle. This is unification. This sense of oneness may extend beyond the candle and your immediate environment to give a direct appreciation of your oneness with everything around you. This type of mystical experience puts a smile on people's lips that does not readily fade!

Finally, a new clarity may dawn. From contemplating the candle you may have sensed something of the nature of your own inner essence; now, in illumination, you may experience the truth of that inner essence, and come to realize that it is within yourself and every one of your fellows. This knowing is irrefutable. It is not the knowing gained through reading or listening to others. It is the knowing of direct experience. It may not even be justifiable in rational terms; no worry, you know it as truth.

Prayer, Hope and Science

MANY PEOPLE HAVE A POSITIVE PERSONAL EXPERIENCE OF PRAYER SIGNIFI-cantly transforming some aspect of their own life or that of someone close to them.

Prayer is defined in the *Oxford Dictionary* as "a solemn request to God or an object of worship; a supplication, thanksgiving, or other mental act addressed to God" and as "a formula or form of words used in praying"—so in the literal English sense, God figures prominently in prayer.

Prayer in relation to healing falls into one of two categories: intercessory prayer, which involves praying for the benefit of another person; or personal prayer, which involves praying for oneself.

When it comes to scientifically validating the healing potential of prayer, nearly all the published research focuses upon intercessory prayer (IP).

Much excitement was created in the research and wider communities in 1988 when the cardiologist and committed Christian, Randolph Byrd published a landmark paper demonstrating the benefits of IP for people recovering in a coronary care unit (CCU). Working in the San Francisco General Hospital, Dr. Byrd used a prospective, randomized, double-blind protocol making the study quite sound from a scientific point of view.

Practicing "born again" Christians were assigned to pray for people they never met, and who did not know if they were being prayed for or not. They were instructed to pray daily for the rapid recovery of those assigned to them, and for the prevention of any complications and death, in addition to other areas of prayer they believed to be beneficial to the patient. The results demonstrated that those prayed for had significantly fewer complications and required less medication. Mortality was the same for those prayed for and the controls. Byrd's often-quoted study attracted a good deal of support and criticism.

The Harris study in 1999, was another similarly well designed and well-conducted study that showed positive benefits in reducing complications in a CCU. However, the most recent Cochrane Review (Roberts 2007) on IP is not favorable. The Cochrane Reviews, which are given a good deal of weight in medical circles, aim to provide the evidence base on a particular subject and commonly use a process that selects for high-quality research while filtering out observational and population based studies. Roberts concluded that the current evidence base for IP was so unequivocal as to not warrant further research of the subject. This view is not shared by many other researchers, clinicians and members of the wider public for whom the topic of IP remains of great interest.

Personal prayer involves a spectrum of inner practices that range from prayer in the traditional sense, through to the repetition of a particular prayer or the use of a mantra, and on into the use of contemplation and sitting quietly in silence. Techniques in this spectrum include praying for oneself by appealing for divine intervention or praying that the best outcome possible will flow from the present circumstances and trusting in that outcome. But this type of prayer can also cover a range of inner practices that may produce significant cognitive shifts such as from despair to acceptance, and can include the use of visualization and contemplation that leads to insight, clarity and the development of particular traits such as compassion and happiness. It even may be that simply sitting quietly in silence is the most powerful healing practice of all.

Personal prayer has had very little specific research published on it. However, this form of practice overlaps with that of contemplation and meditation which have attracted a great deal of recent study. It is relatively easy to make the theoretical connections between the practices of personal prayer, contemplation and meditation. As such, it is reasonable conjecture that many of the positive health benefits associated with the practice of meditation are likely to be reproduced via personal prayer. Here it is worth noting that there are currently more than six thousand studies in the medical literature around the world attesting to the positive benefits of meditation in a wide range of physical and psychological conditions.

In summary, the existing research on the healing benefits of prayer are scant and include both positive and negative findings. Research in this field is challenging but, due to the huge public interest, warrants more attention. There may be particular benefits in examining the linkages between the practices of personal prayer, visualization, contemplation and meditation and the wealth of research available and continuing in the latter fields.

Definition of the Mind

THE MIND IS AN EMBODIED AND RELATIONAL PROCESS THAT REGULATES the flow of energy and information.

To fully understand this definition you may find it helpful if we attempt to explain the terms a little first, and then you contemplate the words as a whole.

Let us start with the meaning of "regulates the flow of energy and information." Of course "regulate" means to control; but what is being controlled? "The flow of energy and information." The mind regulates how we use energy—what comes in and what goes out. In crude terms, it decides what we eat and drink, it decides what exercise and activities we pursue. It regulates how we use our energy. The mind also has the capacity to gather, to store and to control the way we use information. It decides what we read, what we learn, even how we learn—and then it uses that information as it sees fit. The mind has the potential to change everything.

What then of "the mind is an embodied and relational process"? Embodied first: the mind exists in a manner that is intimately connected to our physical body. While it is concentrated in the brain, it is widely accepted that the mind is not confined to the brain. In fact it even extends beyond the nervous system generally and is to be found actively functional in all parts of the body. Yet you can pull the body apart and you will not find "the mind." "The mind" is to do with the body, but it is far more than a piece of the body.

Next, we need to be aware of one of the most important qualities of the mind. You can change it. We used to laugh at the old, somewhat sexist maxim, "It is a woman's prerogative to change her mind." Good news! We all can do it. In fact, the exciting new field of neurobiology that focuses on neuroplasticity clearly establishes the brain and the mind are far more flexible and malleable than ever we thought.

It is not so long ago neurobiologists taught that the brain actively developed up until the age of around five to eight years. This theory dictated that all was set in proverbial concrete around that age and the brain only deteriorated as we became older.

The concepts, knowledge and clinical experiments connected with neuroplasticity have changed all that. Neuroplasticity refers to the brain's ability to change its structure and function according to how we use it. Norman Doidge's groundbreaking book, *The Brain That Changes Itself*,[38] has eloquently described the advances in the current understanding that likens the brain more to our muscles than our bones. Even our bones do change a little over time but our muscles respond rapidly to whether we use them or not. Importantly, when we choose to, we can train our muscles—and they respond.

Neuroplasticity tells us that we can learn how our mind works, train it, and have it function more effectively. When we train our mind, we can rely upon it to bring us better health, more effective healing and profound happiness.

But now, back to the definition. The mind is "a relational process"; it exists within the context of relationships. All that we do depends upon our relationships—those we have with our environment, other living things and ourselves. Because we have a relationship with our self, we look after it. Depending on the quality of that relationship we look after our body better or worse. Not many people self-harm by actually cutting their bodies; some do, but many self-harm by eating badly or not exercising. Many trash the environment and treat other creatures or people badly because they have a poor relationship with them. So the mind is a process that is affected by relationships.

That leaves "process" to consider.

Process: The *Oxford Dictionary*: "a continuous and regular action or succession of actions occurring or performed in a definite manner." Take a moment to consider this and be prepared to become a little excited. The mind being defined as a process means that it is an active "doing," not a sedentary object.

When all this is put together, these words define the mind not as a passive noun but as an active verb!

Viewed this way, the mind is well described as an emergent property. This means it is fluid, active, constantly changing. The mind exists in close relationship to our body, but is not our body, not even just the brain. The mind functions in relationship to all around us. It is affected by the environment we are in, the animals and the people we interact with. The mind regulates all our vital functions. It collects, stores, retrieves and uses information. It controls the energy that flows through us—the physical energy, emotional, mental and spiritual energy.

It is well worth taking the time to sit quietly and contemplate this definition. Sit quietly, learn the definition, close your eyes, and reflect on its meaning. Whenever your mind wanders onto other things or spaces out, notice you are off track as soon as you can, be gentle with yourself, and simply return to your contemplation. Practicing active reflection like this takes a thought from being nebulous and fleeting to something you anchor firmly in your understanding.

When you do this, you will have even more clarity regarding why we say, "It is all in the mind." It is the mind that regulates and changes everything.

Adapted from *The Mind that Changes Everything* by Ian Gawler, Brolga Publishing, Melbourne, 2011

Coffee or Caffeine Enemas

1. Use fresh ground coffee.
2. Add 2 tablespoons of ground coffee to 500mls (1 pint) of water, bring to the boil and simmer for ten minutes. Many people find half the quantity of coffee and half the quantity of water (250mls) has a very positive effect and is enough.
3. Cool to body temperature and pour through a fine filter into the enema bag. Use a gravity-fed type of bag.
4. Go to the toilet first if necessary. When first using enemas you may benefit from a washout enema of plain water to evacuate the bowel before the coffee enema is administered, but this is not necessary routinely.
5. If insecure, lie on a plastic sheet. Most people learn to retain an enema quite easily, especially if they relax.
6. Lie on your right side with your legs tucked up a little. Consciously relax.
7. Insert the enema tube's lubricated nozzle through the anus and gently allow the liquid to flow in.
8. Switch off the flow and remove the nozzle.
9. Relax for ten to fifteen minutes while retaining the enema. Reading is a good distraction if you need it.
10. Go to the toilet and evacuate the bowel.
11. Be sure to wash your enema equipment thoroughly after every use.

The Gerson Therapy and My Own Nutritional Path

MY INTEREST IN NUTRITIONAL THERAPY FOR PEOPLE AFFECTED BY CANCER was kindled when my own cancer reappeared after the initial surgery. At that time I was told that the conventional medical treatments offered no prospect of a cure. By a happy chain of events, I was taken to a lecture on the Gerson Therapy. I was amazed to find that Dr. Max Gerson had an exciting, comprehensive and novel theory on cancer and its nutritional treatment. Even better, he had documented cases of restoring terminal patients to health in his book, *A Cancer Therapy: Results of Fifty Cases.*

Gerson was a medical practitioner who as a young man used a dietary regime to relieve his own otherwise untreatable migraine attacks. He then developed this regime and documented good results treating tuberculosis patients. He treated his first cancer patient, reluctantly and with little optimism, in 1928. She had a complete remission.

Winston Churchill said, "Men occasionally stumble over the Truth, but most pick themselves up and hurry off as if nothing had happened."

No doubt Gerson did stumble across this treatment. However, he spent the next thirty years attempting to validate his results while modifying and improving the diet according to clinical experience.

My feeling from reading Gerson's work is that he had a great faith in nature. He believed that cancer was a multifactorial, degenerative disease. He regarded it as the product of our food and environment being too far removed from nature. He believed that we have exceeded the body's ability to cope with unnatural products. Like me, Gerson saw cancer as a disease of society, a disease of lifestyle. He listed the overuse of artificial fertilizers and chemicals in the soil, the overrefining and adulteration of food with toxic additives, the poor preparation of food and the pollution of our environment generally as being individual factors that combined to adversely affect the body's function as a whole. He postulated that over a period of time these factors weakened the body's resistance. Then, when one final trigger factor produced the localized symptoms, the depleted defenses of the body were unable to eliminate or even contain it. Cancer was the localized sign of a generalized condition—a multifactorial, chronic, degenerative condition.

Gerson had developed these views way back in the 1930s! He was one of the first to suggest that cancer involved the impairment of the body's natural defenses—the immune system—in this generalized way. He was stating way back then that cancer involved a problem of immune deficiency. It is only recently that the medical mainstream has begun to explore this avenue and to share this basic concept. Gerson was way ahead of his time. He recognized that once the symptoms of cancer appeared, there was a problem that included more than just the localized lumps and bumps. The whole body was diseased. Often, however, cancer is treated as a localized problem as if it is only the lumps and bumps that are the disease and the rest of the patient's body is fine. Gerson's hypothesis was that if the rest of the body can be returned to a healthy condition, then it would react to and eliminate any cancer, anywhere in the body.

This, then, was Gerson's aim—to restore the normal function of the body.

Gerson recognized the theory he worked with, the nutritional basis of his diet and the supplements he used, were subject to medical argument. He was very pragmatic, however. His saw results with his methods and so he preferred to work toward a fully acceptable medical explanation as he continued treating his patients. He claimed a high recovery rate, even of terminal cases. There is evidence that he did achieve remarkable results, made more remarkable by considering that most of his patients had been through the conventional treatments first and gained no success.

Gerson's is a very strict and involved regime to follow, and it certainly calls for professional guidance. I certainly recommend *against* anyone trying Gerson's diet on their own. It needs to be described as a therapy rather than a diet. As well as the need for supervision and monitoring, there is a need for at least one person to assist with preparation. My first wife was involved for about twelve hours each day helping me with it. Obviously, the level of commitment needs to be very high on everyone's part. It would not be possible to live a normal life, let alone go to work, while following the diet intensively. It is really a regime best conducted in a live-in clinic situation. Full details of the regime are best studied via the books he or his daughter, Charlotte Gerson, has written.

So, there are plenty of reservations regarding Gerson's therapy. However, it is well worth mentioning, as his ideas stand on their merits. Also, for those interested in intensive diets, Gerson's is the soundest and best to my knowledge. Most others are adaptations of his.

The main benefits I gained from the three months I did on the Gerson Therapy is that it certainly helped me to detoxify and to purify my system. As a consequence of this, along with the intense meditation I continued with, I found myself to be very sensitive to what new foods I could add and eat reliably, and those I continued to need to avoid. For example, for me, dairy products and eggs were two of the things I needed to avoid.

Using an ongoing process of experimentation, trying foods and observing their reactions, I steadily developed a new way of eating that stood me in good stead for the healing phase of my recovery—the Healing Diet. Once I was free of cancer, I continued to experiment and fairly soon arrived at what could be described as a maintenance diet—the Wellness Diet. Over the years, based on current research and particularly the feedback from thousands of people with cancer who have given serious attention their nutritional management and therapy, the Healing Diet and then the Wellness Diet have evolved to where they are today.

Fishing for Answers:
Sustainable, Healthy Fish

FOR NONVEGETARIANS, FISH HAVE HEALTH BENEFITS COURTESY MOSTLY OF their omega-3 fatty acids. Also, they are a good source of protein. However, most of us are alert to the vexed issue of contamination of our fish by pollution, as well as the sustainability and environmental problems of overfishing and damaging fishing practices.

It is claimed that currently 70 percent of the world's fish species are fully exploited, overexploited, depleted or recovering from depletion. It is a scary thought to know the best estimates are that if current trends of overfishing continue, stocks of all fish currently being commercially fished will have collapsed by 2048. The question, then, is what fish are best to eat? What to do?

Say No to Farmed Fish

The trend toward increasing aquaculture, the farming of fish, makes sense in theory but does not seem to have the right answers as yet in practice. Most people are unaware that commercially farmed salmon are genetically modified to become what are called tetraploids—that is, they have a double set of genes so they grow faster. Then they are fed on other fish, a practice that is very inefficient and damaging to other fish stocks. It takes 4½ to 9 pounds of wild fish to produce 2 pounds of farmed salmon. While increasingly vegetable proteins are being used for feed, these result in lower levels of the valuable omega-3 fatty acids in the salmon. Seaweed may be a more viable food source for fish farming, but that remains to be seen. Also, disease is emerging as a major issue among intensively reared fish. Increasingly, significant amounts of antibiotics are being used to manage infections (as happens continually in the intensive rearing of chicken).

So wild-caught fish are preferable, but which ones?

Know Where Your Fish Came From—The Further out to Sea and the Less Polluted the Waters, the Better

Fish that are caught in more remote areas away from built-up, polluted areas are obviously preferable. So choose fish that live further out to sea, that are the deeper sea varieties, and come from less-polluted areas and countries.

Choose the Smaller Species Rather Than the Big Predator Fish

Pollutants accumulate as you go up the food chain. For example, it is well known sharks accumulate heavy metals and the mercury levels in big fish can be very toxic.

Check Out What the Sustainable Fish Are in Your Area

This is a regional as well as international issue and the need is to check your local conditions. In Australia, a good guide is found on the Australian Marine Conservation Society's website: marineconservation.org.com.

The international Marine Stewardship Council has developed a certification system that mostly shows up on packaged seafood and features a distinctive blue MSC label. See their website: msc.org.

Goodfishbadfish.com.au has a very user-friendly list of sustainable seafoods, with reasons for the various listings and practical preparation tips.

Avoid the Unsustainable Fish That May Also Have Health Issues

Again, say no to farmed fish.

Say no to wild caught barramundi, blue grenadier, cods, garfish, gemfish (hake), groupers, Murray cod, orange roughy (deep-sea perch), shark, snapper, marlin, swordfish, toothfish and tuna (unless the tuna is troll, pole or line caught).

Fish That Are Best to Avoid, but Not So Bad

Blue-eye trevalla, coral trout, flathead, gunard, John Dory, kingfish, ling, mulloway, red emperor, red mullet, red snapper (redfish) and silver trevally.

Fish That Are OK to Consider

Wild-caught bonito, bream, eel, King George whiting, leatherjacket, mackerel, mahi mahi, mullet, tailor, trevally and whiting.

Imported canned salmon and sardines are usually acceptable.

Avoid Scallops from the Wild
Seafood That Is Best to Avoid, but Not So Bad

Lobster and prawns (farmed prawns are likely to be better environmentally).

Seafood That Is Acceptable to Consider

Farmed: abalone, oysters, scallops and blue mussels.
Wild: blue swimmer crabs, mud crabs, squid, calamari and octopus.

All this information may seem a little imposing at first, but it is like many things. Take your time to think it through. If you are planning to eat fish, find out what is available locally, where you can get healthy, sustainable seafood, develop a good relationship with your supplier, and then it is easy and satisfying.

Relative Levels of Caffeine

THE LEVEL OF CAFFEINE IN INDIVIDUAL DRINKS VARIES ACCORDING TO THE source and the method of preparation. What follows are general indications only.

Product	Approximate Levels of Caffeine per 100 ml—in mgs
Percolated coffee	38–65
Drip coffee	55–85
Espresso	170–225
Decaffeinated coffee	2–7
Black tea	28
Green tea	17
Coca-Cola	10
Red Bull	32

Dark chocolate tends to have around three times more caffeine than milk chocolate. The more cocoa in the chocolate, the more caffeine.

The average block of chocolate weighs around 100 grams (3.5 ounces) and 100 grams of dark chocolate contains around 70 milligrams of caffeine, compared to 21 milligrams in 100 grams of milk chocolate.

Approximate Alcohol Content in Various Drinks

THE LEVEL OF ALCOHOL IN INDIVIDUAL DRINKS VARIES ACCORDING TO THE manufacturer and other factors. What follows are general indications only.

Product	Approximate % of Alcohol in Various Drinks
Fruit juice	Less than .1%
"Nonalcoholic" beer	Around .5% or less
Light beer	Around 3%
Standard beer	4%–5%
Stout	5%–10%
Cider	4%–8%
Wine	10%–15%
Sparkling wines	8%–12%
Port	20%
Liquors	15%–55%
Spirits	Around 40%
Rum	35%–50%
Whisky	50%–60%

The Preparation of Sprouts

ADD A LITTLE LESS THAN ONE-QUARTER INCH OF ALFALFA SEEDS TO THE bottom of a 2-pound jar.

Cover well with water and leave soaking for eight hours.

Cover the jar with chicken wire or any screen, holding it on with a rubber band. Invert the jar, pouring off the water.

Rinse and drain twice.

Store upside down, ensuring good drainage and air circulation. You can obtain racks for the purpose. Sit them on the kitchen bench, away from direct sunlight.

Rinse the developing sprouts thoroughly with water twice daily, both morning and evening (three times in hot weather).

In four to five days the seeds will have sprouted and be nearly an inch long with little green heads. It is best to have four jars at various stages of development, as a family can easily devour the contents of one each day.

Sprouts are an ideal source of fresh, vital food, especially in winter. They are claimed to be one of the highest sources of vegetable protein and are packed with vitamins and minerals. Highly recommended and something young children often enjoy participating in producing. However, if you prefer, they are readily available for purchase.

Food Combining

THIS IS LIKE FINE-TUNING WHERE THE INTENTION IS TO EAT COMBINATIONS of foods that are most easily digested together.

To determine how well or how badly two groups of foods combine, refer to the following chart. Identify the first food in the left-hand column and follow it across until you reach the vertical column under the name of the second food. Where the two columns meet, provides the answer.

For example, starches (third down on the left-hand column) combined with fats (third from the left in the top column) equals a fair combination.

Acid fruits (bottom of the left-hand column) combined with sweet fruits (third from the right, top column) equals a poor combination.

Primary proteins: almonds, Brazil nuts, cashew nuts, hazelnuts, pine nuts, pistachios, walnuts, pepitas, sunflower seeds, sesame seeds, wheat germ, lecithin, soyabean.

Secondary proteins: peanuts, cheese, eggs, yogurt, poultry, meat, fish.

Fats: avocados, oils, macadamia nuts, pecans, coconut, olives.

Starches: oats, rice, wheat, corn, rye, millet, buckwheat, lima beans, red beans, navy beans, mung beans, broad beans, garbanzos, lentils, chestnuts, breadfruit, jackfruit, sweet potato, Jerusalem artichokes, pumpkin, taro yams.

Melons: cantaloupe, watermelon, honeydew.

Vegetables: globe artichokes, fresh sprouts, beetroot, carrot, peppers, rutabaga, parsley, Brussels sprouts, cauliflower, cabbage, celery, lettuce, turnips, fresh beans, fresh peas, zucchini, chayote, marrows, squash, broccoli, asparagus, eggplant, silver beet, spinach, tomatoes, onions (best cooked).

Sweet fruits: bananas, figs, custard apples, Monstera deliciosa, persimmon, all dried fruits.

Food Groups	Primary Proteins	Secondary Proteins	Fats	Starches	Melons	Vegetables	Sweet Fruits	Sub-Acid Fruits	Acid Fruits
PRIMARY PROTEINS	Good	Poor	Poor	Poor	Poor	Good	Poor	Fair	Good
SECONDARY PROTEINS	Poor	Fair	Poor	Poor	Poor	Good	Poor	Poor	Fair
FATS	Poor	Poor	Good	Fair	Poor	Good	Fair	Fair	Fair
STARCHES	Poor	Poor	Fair	Good	Poor	Good	Fair	Fair	Fair
MELONS	Poor	Poor	Poor	Poor	Good	Poor	Fair	Fair	Poor
VEGETABLES	Good	Good	Good	Good	Poor	Good	Poor	Poor	Poor
SWEET FRUITS	Poor	Poor	Fair	Fair	Fair	Poor	Good	Good	Poor
SUB-ACID FRUITS	Fair	Poor	Fair	Fair	Fair	Poor	Good	Good	Good
ACID FRUITS	Good	Fair	Fair	Poor	Poor	Poor	Poor	Good	Good

Sub-acid fruits: mulberry, raspberry, blackberry, blueberry, grapes, pears, apples, cherries, apricots, peaches, plums, nectarines, pawpaw (papaya), mangos, guava.

Acid fruits: grapefruit, lemon, orange, lime, mandarin, pineapple, strawberry, kiwifruit (gooseberry), passionfruit.

Prepare your food with love and joy. It is good stuff.

Dietary Analysis

THE NUTRIENT CONTENT OF THE DIETS SUGGESTED IN THIS BOOK WERE analyzed by Dietary Analysis (Australia). They used a computer model based on the Australian Food Exchange Tables. Where no Australian values were available, they used British tables. They then based comparisons on the recommended daily allowances set down for nutrients by the USDA. There were some problems. We found that there were some things that are normally used in this diet for which the computer did not have values. Also, the bread figures used were based on salted breads that, therefore, dramatically raised their sodium levels. But, overall, this was the best analysis available.

Samples were analyzed of the Wellness Diet as being used by:

1. A 110-pound female with light activity.
2. The same diet with the addition of six juices.
3. The Gerson Diet as applied to a 155-pound male with light activity.

The results are summarized and show a supplement of vitamins E, B_{12} and zinc may be useful. Perhaps this is another indication for a multivitamin formula that assures an adequate supply of all these vital nutrients.

The Wellness Diet came out low in energy. This was an expected finding based on our clinical experience. While we certainly see people lose excess weight in this diet, our experience is that people's weight very commonly stabilizes at a lean, fit level. If lack of energy was experienced or weight loss continued, it could be easily rectified by eating more carbohydrates. Also, you can see from the charts that follow, that adding six juices leads to a predicted weight gain. However, again in our experience, weight does again stabilize for most people at a lean, fit level.

It should be noted that the figures given are the result of examining a three-day sample diet.

Legend

PROT	= Protein
CHO	= Carbohydrate (sugars & starch)
ENGY	= Energy
Ca	= Calcium
P	= Phosphorus
Fe	= Iron
Na	= Sodium (constituent of ordinary salt)
K	= Potassium
B-CRT	= Beta-carotene (orange plant pigment)
RETIN*	= Retinal (vitamin A)
B_1	= Vitamin B_1 (thiamine)
gm	= gram weight
mg	= milligram weight
mcg	= microgram weight
B_2	= Vitamin B_2 (riboflavin)
NIACIN **	= Vitamin B_3 (niacin)
VIT-C	= Vitamin C
VIT-E	= Vitamin E
B_6	= Vitamin B_6 (pyridoxine)
B_{12}	= Vitamin B_{12}
Zn	= Zinc
FIBER	= Dietary fiber
CHOL	= Cholesterol
FOLIC	= Folic acid
Mg	= Magnesium
kJ	= kilojoules
CAL	= 1 calorie (4.2kj)
RDA	= Recommended daily allowance

  * Includes RETINAL produced in the body from B-CAROTENE
** Includes NIACIN produced in the body from TRYPTOPHAN

Wellness Diet—110-Pound Female

		Supplied by Diet	Recommended % of RDA (RDA)	
WATER	gm	1535.88	***	
PROT	gm	62.02	55.11	113
FAT	gm	52.36	***	
CHO	gm	325.71	***	
ENGY	kJ	8080.74	9184.80	88
ENGY	Cal	1930.42	2194.17	
Ca	mg	870.64	400.00	218
P	mg	1298.73	**	
Fe	mg	20.44	12.00	170
Na	mg	2418.24	***	
K	mg	5493.97	***	
B-CRT	mcg	21330.11	***	
RETIN	mcg	112.83		
RETIN*	mcg	3667.85	750.00	489
B1	mcg	1577.20	918.48	172
B2	mcg	1661.87	1102.18	151
NIACIN	mg	14.97		
NIACIN**	mg	24.90	14.70	169
VIT-C	mg	274.39	30.00	915
VIT-E	mg	11.33	12.00	94
VIT-B_6	mcg	2837.73	2000.00	142
VIT-$_{B12}$	mcg	.80	2.00	40
Zn	mg	10.51	15.00	70
FIBER	gm	62.88	20.00	314
CHOL	mg	123.00	300.00	41
FOLIC	mcg	627.67	200.00	314
Mg	mg	629.50	300.00	210

*** RDAs have not been set for these nutrients. However, dietary goals do exist for some of them.

% of Total Energy in the diet provided by:	
1. PROTEIN	= 12.3 (Recommended = 10%–12%)
2. FAT	= 23.3 (Recommended = 30%–35%)
3. CHO	= 64.4 (Recommended = 55%–60%)
Energy (DIET)	= 8,081 kJ (1,930 Cals)
Energy (RDA)	= 9185 kJ (2,194 Cals)
Difference (DIET—RDA):	= 1104 kJ (264 Cals)

If the diet record is accurate and is typical of the patient's diet for the rest of the week, then the above energy difference would result in the patient LOSING .2kg (.5 lbs) per week.

Wellness Diet and Juices—110-Pound Female

		Supplied by Diet	Recommended % of RDA (RDA)	
WATER	gm	2795.93	***	
PROT	gm	75.08	55.11	136
FAT	gm	54.98	***	
CHO	gm	499.33	***	
ENGY	kJ	11001.48	9184.80	120
ENGY	Cal	2628.16	2194.17	
Ca	mg	1387.75	400.00	347
P	mg	1745.93	***	
Fe	mg	30.94	12.00	258
Na	mg	3043.75	***	
K	mg	9475.91	***	
B-CRT	mcg	75950.76	***	
RETIN	mcg	52.83		
RETIN*	mcg	12911.29	750.00	1722
B1	mcg	2505.44	1100.15	228
B2	mcg	2467.31	1320.18	187
NIACIN	mg	21.97		
NIACIN**	mg	33.99	17.60	193
VITAMIN C	mg	561.56	30.00	1872
VITAMIN E	mg	12.63	12.00	105
VITAMIN B$_6$	mcg	3226.73	2000.00	161
VITAMIN B$_{12}$	mcg	80	2.00	40
Zn	mg	11.67	15.00	78
FIBER	gm	69.18	20.00	346
CHOL	mg	123.00	300.00	41
FOLIC	mcg	915.67	200.00	458
Mg	mg	792.00	300.00	264

*** RDAs have not been set for these nutrients. However, dietary goals do exist for some of them.

% of Total Energy in the diet provided by:	
1. PROTEIN	= 10.8 (Recommended = 10%–12%)
2. FAT	= 17.7 (Recommended = 30%–35%)
3. CHO	= 71.5 (Recommended = 55%–60%)
Energy (DIET)	= 11,001 kJ (2,628 Cals)
Energy (RDA)	= 9,185 kJ (2,194 Cals)
Difference (DIET—RDA):	= 1,817 kJ (434 Cals)

If the diet record is accurate and is typical of the patient's diet for the rest of the week, then the above energy difference would result in the patient GAINING .4kg (.9 lbs) per week.

Gerson Diet—155-Pound Male

		Supplied by Diet	Recommended	% of RDA (RDA)
WATER	gm	4,121.97	***	
PROT	gm	164.90	69.90	236
FAT	gm	95.00	***	
CHO	gm	642.35	***	
ENGY	kJ	16,312.35	11,650.00	140
ENGY	Cal	3,896.88	2,783.09	
Ca	mg	1,659.12	400.00	415
P	mg	3,743.34	***	
Fe	mg	86.09	10.00	861
Na	mg	4,091.26	***	
K	mg	15,108.84	***	
B-CRT	mcg	99,999 Plus		
RETIN	mcg	41,914.20		
RETIN*	mcg	69,373.41	750.00	9,250
B1	mcg	4,852.52	1,631.24	297
B2	mcg	1,7875.20	1,957.48	913
NIACIN	mg	105.20		
NIACIN**	mg	131.58	26.10	504
VITAMIN C	mg	927.28	30.00	3,091
VITAMIN E	mg	13.20	05.00	88
VITAMIN B_6	mcg	6,073.00	2,000.00	304
VITAMIN B_{12}	mcg	500.00	2.00	9,999 Plus
Zn	mg	50.27	15.00	335
FIBER	gm	62.14	20.00	311
CHOL	mg	1,850.00	300.00	617
FOLIC	mcg	2,268.37	200.00	1134
Mg	mg	969.68	350.00	277

*** RDAs have not been set for these nutrients. However, dietary goals do exist for some of them.

% of Total Energy in the diet provided by:	
1. PROTEIN	= 16.2 (Recommended = 10%–12%)
2. FAT	= 20.9 (Recommended = 30%–35%)
3. CHO	= 62.9 (Recommended = 55%–60%)
Energy (DIET)	= 16,312 kJ (3,897 Cals)
Energy (RDA)	= 11,650 kJ (2,783 Cals)
Difference (DIET—RDA):	= 4662 kJ (1,114 Cals)

If the diet record is accurate and is typical of the patient's diet for the rest of the week, then the above energy difference would result in the patient GAINING 1.0 kg (2.2 lbs) per week.

Dietary Regime for Small Animals with Cancer

THIS ARTICLE WAS FIRST PUBLISHED IN THE "CONTROL AND THERAPY" ARTI-
cles of the Post Graduate Committee in Veterinary Science *publication, University of Sydney, and has since been slightly revised.*

Does this sound familiar? "Your dog has cancer, there is nothing we can do. Shall we euthanase him now or later?"

This is a précis of an often repeated, if more gently expressed, diagnosis and sentence. It leaves the animal and owner without professional support, and likely to prematurely terminate a loved pet's life or to seek help from unqualified alternative sources. It leaves the practitioner missing out on an opportunity to follow through a stimulating and helpful exercise in disease management.

Having been through it myself with osteogenic sarcoma and having felt the benefits that dietary considerations offer, I have developed a dietary regime that I am confident offers help to animals with cancer. I present it on the basis of clinical experimentation with the knowledge that it does improve the quality of the animal's life. It has not cured anything as yet, although it has been instrumental in several remissions. I do feel, however, that it has prolonged life in many cases and am certain it has made the most of many difficult situations. It has also eased many people's minds when they want to do something constructive instead of just watching their animals die. Many owners comment on how fit and active their animals became on this nutritional package, despite the presence of tumors. Also, when the diet is followed, it is frequently noted that the animal's demise, when it comes, is rapid. Rather than the drawn-out, steady deterioration frequently associated with cancer, the animal remains well, often fitter than usual, until there is a sudden collapse. Then, if a decision regarding euthanasia is required, it is usually easily made.

Overall, the diet has many positive attributes. The principles are to detox-ify the body, correct mineral imbalances, restore the digestion, and feed a well-balanced diet. I have included several supplements including Vitamin C, as I believe there is good evidence to do so.

The diet recognizes that we are dealing with carnivores, but that protein intake is better restricted a little.

Here it is.

Basic Components

Meat 40% by volume—stewing steak type; lean is preferable.

Vegetables 40% volume—concentrate on yellow ones (e.g., pumpkin, carrot) and green ones cooked minimally.

Brown Rice 20% volume—well cooked.

Presented as a stew; meat and vegetables should be cooked as little as acceptance dictates (e.g., generally well cooked to begin with and less as the pet's palate adapts). It is useful if carrot and greens especially are given raw—just grate finely. If all except the grains will be eaten raw, so much the better.

Fed to appetite demands, once daily.

Fast one day per week.

Additives: for 33-pound dog (adjust according to the pet's weight.)

- 1 teaspoon cold-pressed flaxseed oil—added after cooking.
- ¼ teaspoon kelp powder or granules—presoaked or cooked with rice.
- 1 tablespoon brewer's yeast—not a bitter variety—add to stew.
- 3 drops Lugol's iodine (can be made up by a pharmacist on request)—add to stew or drinking water.
- 200mg Potassium Orotate—crumble onto stew.
- 2 pancreatic enzyme tables, give by mouth (dogs usually eat these like treats).
- ½ Oroxine (thyroxine sodium) 100 mcgm tablet Welcome Aust.—give by mouth.
- ½ teaspoon Sodium ascorbate powder—available in small packs from health food shops or chemists—sprinkle onto stew—generally well accepted. If not, use coated 1,000mg tablets and give 2 tablets.

Dogs generally accept the diet readily, cats more reluctantly. Implementation obviously requires the owner's participation and tends to lead to the veterinarian becoming intimately involved in the whole procedure. This diet can be used as an adjunct in the treatment of any chronic degenerative disease.

Ian Gawler's 1978 Case History

THE FOLLOWING REPORT IS REPRINTED FROM THE *MEDICAL JOURNAL OF Australia*, 1978, 2:433.

The patient, aged 25, underwent a mid-thigh amputation for osteogenic sarcoma 11 months before he first saw me two-and-a-half years ago. He had visible bony lumps of about 2cm in diameter growing from the ribs, sternum and the crest of the ilium, and was coughing up small quantities of blood in which, he said, he could feel small spicules of bone. There were gross opacities in the X-ray films of his lungs. The patient had been told by a specialist that he had only two or three weeks to live, but in virtue of his profession he was already well aware of the pathology and prognosis of his condition. Now two-and-a-half years later, he has moved to another state to resume his former occupation.

This young man has shown an extraordinary will to live and has sought help from all the alternatives to orthodox medicine which were available to him. These have included acupuncture, massage, several sessions with Philippine faith healers, laying on of hands and yoga in an Indian ashram. He had short sessions of radiation therapy, and chemotherapy, but declined to continue treatment. He has also persisted with the dietary and enema treatment prescribed by Max Gerson, the German physician, who gained some notoriety for this type of treatment in America in the 1940s. However, in addition to all these measures to gain relief, the patient has consistently maintained a rigorous discipline of intensive meditation as described previously. He has in fact, consistently meditated from one to three hours daily.

Two other factors seem to be important. He has had extraordinary help and support from his girlfriend, who more recently became his wife. She is extremely sensitive to his feelings and needs, and has spent hours in aiding his meditation and healing with massage and laying on of hands.

The other important factor would seem to be the patient's own state of mind. He has developed a degree of calm about him which I have rarely observed in anyone, even in oriental mystics with whom I have had some considerable experience. When asked to what he attributes the regression of metastases, he answers in some such terms as: "I really think it is our life, the way we experience our life." In other words, it would seem that the patient has let the effects of the intense and prolonged meditation enter into his whole experience of life. His extraordinarily low level of anxiety is obvious to the most casual observer. It is suggested that this has enhanced the activity of his immune system by reducing his level of cortisone.

Ainslie Meares, MD, DPM

[Since this report was written the patient has been declared free of active neoplastic disease. —AM]

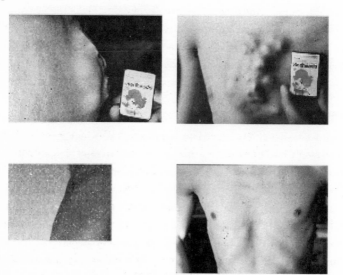

Important note. In the original article, the date for the top two photographs was incorrectly recorded. The photographs were taken in October 1976 (and have Kodak dates imprinted on their reverse), while the bottom two were taken on the April 25, 1978.

Ian Gawler—30-Year Follow-Up—2008 Case History

THIS ARTICLE APPEARED IN THE *MEDICAL JOURNAL OF AUSTRALIA*, 15 December 2008: 189 11/12663–665.

Thirty-year follow-up at pneumonectomy of a 58-year-old survivor of disseminated osteosarcoma

George A Jelinek and Ruth H Gawler

A 1978 case report in the Journal described a 25-year-old man with disseminated osteogenic sarcoma whose metastases regressed after treatment with diet and intensive meditation. Thirty years later, there has been no recurrence of his cancer, and a recent pneumonectomy for chronic bronchiectasis revealed mature cancellous bone in the resected lung. The man is otherwise well. (MJA 2008; 189: 663–665) MJA • Volume 189 Number 11/12 • 1/15 December 2008

Clinical Record

A man who is now 58 years old was diagnosed in 1974, at the age of 24, with histologically confirmed high-grade osteogenic sarcoma of the right femur (Figure, A). His right leg was amputated in January 1975. Histopathologically, the tumor was described (in a 1994 review of the case) as follows: "The tissue is replaced by a cellular malignant spindle cell tumor forming osteoid and bone and having a disorganized pattern of proliferation . . . confirming the diagnosis of a high grade endosteal osteosarcoma (osteogenic sarcoma)."

In December 1975, widespread bony and pulmonary metastases were diagnosed. Despite being told in March 1976 that he had only 2–3 weeks to live, the man survived until September that year, when he underwent three cycles of palliative chemotherapy with vincristine, adriamycin, cyclophosphamide and dacarbazine, as well as brief palliative radiation therapy. He elected to discontinue these therapies as his condition deteriorated further.

The patient then consulted prominent psychiatrist and hypnotherapist Dr. Ainslie Meares, who reported his case and his subsequent remarkable recovery in the Medical Journal of Australia in 1978.[1] When Meares first saw the patient, he had visible bony tumors protruding from his ribs, sternum (Figure B) and iliac crest, and was coughing up blood containing small spicules of bone (Figure C). Meares taught him how to meditate, and both he and the patient felt this was a key component in recovery, although he also adhered faithfully to a vegan diet and tried many alternative therapies, including massage, acupuncture, faith healing and others.

The patient recovered and returned to full time work, founding and running self-help groups for people with cancer, but had persistent reminders of the original illness. Presumably related to immune suppression from chemotherapy, he developed pulmonary tuberculosis in June 1978, and was treated for this condition for 12 months. This progressed to cavitation and severe bronchiectasis, causing repeated bouts of pneumonia and persistently elevated erythrocyte sedimentation rate (ESR).

Chest x-rays in November 1989, 15 years after the patient's diagnosis and subsequent recovery, showed evidence of previous tuberculosis and ongoing bronchiectasis, with a left hilar mass compressing the left upper lobe bronchus by 50%. Views of the lumbar spine and pelvis, taken at the same time to investigate ongoing back pain, showed abnormalities initially thought to represent progressive metastatic disease. The report noted "progressive metastatic disease with large osteoblastic deposit right ilium, sacrum, and invasion into L5." That report was amended 4 days later, after comparison with films from 1978, to state "The appearances in the body of L5 . . . are those of metastatic disease but this appearance is essentially unchanged." A thoracic computed tomography scan performed a few days later showed evidence of previous left lung tuberculosis.

With no further treatment, the patient's condition remained stable. X-ray images of the chest, pelvis and lumbar spine in 1993 were unchanged from 1989. Lung function testing in 1996 and 1999 showed satisfactory function, with an FEV1/FVC (forced expiratory volume in 1 second/forced vital capacity) ratio of 2.56 L/3.40 L. Indeed, the patient was well enough to go trekking in Nepal for three weeks in 1999 to a height of about 16,000 feet above sea level.

However, two episodes of left lower lobe pneumonia in 2004 and chronic bronchiectasis resulted in referral to a thoracic surgeon with a view to pneumonectomy. Noting the patient's chronically elevated ESR, indicating ongoing sepsis, and recurrent chest infections, the surgeon recommended left pneumonectomy while the patient was still young enough to tolerate the surgery.

In December 2004, pneumonectomy was performed. As the patient had relied on elbow crutches since the original leg amputation, it was hoped that a minimally invasive approach might preserve chest wall skeletal structure and musculature, but because of widespread adhesions and tuberculous scarring, this was not possible. A complicated 5-hour pleuropneumonectomy was performed, with the pericardium being opened to enable access to the pulmonary veins, precipitating a short period of intraoperative ventricular fibrillation.

Macroscopic pathological examination showed a small, collapsed, scarred left lung. The lung parenchyma was abnormal, and bronchiectasis, cavitation and scarring were widespread, but there was no obvious tumor. Microscopic examination showed severe bronchiectasis, but there was no evidence of mycobacterial infection. The report noted that "palpation of lung paren- chyma deep to the hilum reveals a rock-hard consistency, impossible to sec- tion with a knife. Using a saw, horizontal cuts . . . reveal a centrally located bony mass 35–30mm about, surrounding the bifurcation of the left main bronchus." Histopathological examination of decalcified sections showed "a bony mass surrounding and incorporating large central bronchi and neuro- vascular structures. Much of the bone has a mature cancellous appearance with normal appearing osteocytes, and mature fat within the intertrabecular spaces. In addition there are foci of coarse sclerotic and heavily calcified bone which are devoid of viable osteocytes. No viable tumor is present."

After steady postoperative recovery, the patient returned to fulltime work and remains well.

Discussion

Osteosarcomas are rare malignant tumors of the skeleton characterized by formation of immature bone by tumor cells. At the time of this patient's diagnosis, osteosarcoma was a devastating disease with very low survival rates.[2] Most patients died within a year of diagnosis. Management centered around limb amputation, with palliative chemotherapy and radiation ther- apy for recurrences. Over the past 30 years, management has improved dra- matically. With the use of limb-sparing surgery, induction and adjuvant chemotherapy, and surgical excision of metastases, survival rates of around 60% can now be expected for patients presenting with localized disease.[3–5]

There are limited data examining long-term outcomes among patients recovering from osteosarcoma. A few articles have reported long-term fol- low-up, including surveillance for recurrence,[6] the development of other can- cers,[7] and cardiac toxicity from chemotherapy agents.[8] Metastases have been known to develop as long as 14 years after diagnosis.[6] While there is a report of spontaneous regression of a pulmonary metastasis that developed 5 years after treatment for osteosarcoma,[9] the fate of regressed secondaries has not been well documented.

Today, pulmonary metastases are often resected, but this is while the tumor is active. In this patient's case, the lung was resected, for other rea- sons, 30 years after the original diagnosis, and incidentally, a large piece of mature cancellous bone was found surrounding the left main bronchus. This presumably represented bone formation by a long-since regressed secondary tumor, similar to the bone found in the primary tumor at the time of amputation.

It is clear from the 1978 report that large sections of the externally visible osteogenic secondaries were resorbed as the cancer regressed. This was most obvious on the patient's chest wall (Figure D). However, some spinal and pelvic bone formed by the secondaries appears to have remained intact after tumor disappearance, as illustrated by the fact that x-rays taken of the spine and pelvis 15 years after diagnosis and recovery were identical with films of 11 years earlier and by the presence of bone in the resected lung.

It is interesting to consider the possible factors involved in this man's remarkable recovery. Spontaneous remission is a possibility, although exceedingly unlikely at such an advanced stage of disease, and its coincident timing with a wide range of self-help measures adopted by the patient makes this explanation even more improbable. Certainly, the patient had widespread disease from which recovery, even today, would be very unlikely. Although the patient received a short course of palliative chemotherapy and radiotherapy to his lumbar spine, it is unlikely that this would have been curative with such widespread metastatic disease. Meares and the patient attributed the remarkable recovery to intensive meditation,[1] and it is true that the patient meditated from 3 to 5 hours daily after developing secondaries. He still regularly meditates and teaches others with cancer to do so. His fastidious adoption of the Gerson diet[10] for 3 months, followed by adherence to a plant-based wholefood vegan diet may also have played some part. Such a lifestyle approach, incorporating meditation and vegan diet, has recently been shown to cause significant modulation of gene expression and biological processes associated with tumor growth.[11]

Apart from illustrating the value of maintaining hope in the face of apparent hopelessness, this case shows that, long after tumor regression, metastatic lesions from osteosarcoma may contain significant amounts of residual bone. Even in the absence of tumor, these bony deposits may cause health problems in their own right, depending on their location. Our understanding of such unlikely survival continues to improve with the recent demonstration that modifiable lifestyle factors affect gene expression in patients with cancer.[11]

ACKNOWLEDGMENTS

We are grateful to Professor Peter Clarke, who performed the pneumonectomy, and Mr. John Doyle, who undertook the amputation, for their assistance with the provision of past records and review of the manuscript, and to Dr. Sandra Neate for her critical review and helpful suggestions.

Competing Interests

Professor Jelinek is a friend and colleague of the patient, and Dr. Ruth Gawler is related to the patient.

Author Details

George A. Jelinek, MD, FACEM, DipDHM, Professorial Fellow1,2

Ruth H. Gawler, MB BS, MGPPsych, FACPsyMed, General Practitioner and Therapist3

1 Department of Medicine, University of Melbourne, St. Vincent's Hospital, Melbourne, VIC.
2 Department of Emergency Medicine, St. Vincent's Hospital, Melbourne, VIC.
3 The Gawler Foundation, Yarra Junction, VIC.

Correspondence: George.Jelinek@svhm.org.au

References

1 Meares, A. Regression of osteogenic sarcoma metastases associated with intensive meditation. *Med J Aust*, 1978; 2:433.

2 Picci, P. Osteosarcoma (osteogenic sarcoma). Orphanet *J Rare Dis*, 2007; 2:6.

3 Jaffe, N., Carrasco, H., Raymond K., et al. Can cure in patients with osteosarcoma be achieved exclusively with chemotherapy and abrogation of surgery? *Cancer*, 2002; 95: 2,202–2,210.

4 Wittig, J. C., Bickels, J., Priebat, D., et al. Osteosarcoma: a multidisciplinary approach to diagnosis and treatment. *Am Fam Physician* 2002; 65: 1,123–1,132.

5 Tan, J. Z., Schlicht, S. M., Powell, G. J., et al. Multidisciplinary approach to diagnosis and management of osteosarcoma—a review of the St. Vincent's Hospital experience. *Int Semin Surg Oncol* 2006; 3:38.

6 Strauss, S. J., McTiernan, A., Whelan, J. S. Late relapse of osteosarcoma: implications for follow-up and screening. *Pediatr Blood Cancer* 2004; 43:692–697.

7 Kim, M. S., Sim, Y. S., Lee, S. Y., Jeon, D. G. Secondary thyroid papillary carcinoma in osteosarcoma patients: report of two cases. *J Korean Med Sci* 2008; 23:149–152.

8 Longhi, A., Ferrari, S., Bacci, G., Specchia, S. Long-term follow-up of patients with doxorubicin-induced cardiac toxicity after chemotherapy for osteosarcoma. *Anticancer Drugs* 2007; 18:737–744.

9 Bacci, G., Palmerini, E., Staals, E. L., et al. Spontaneous regression of lung metastasis from osteosarcoma: a case report. *J Pediatr Hematol Oncol* 2008; 30:90–92.

10 Gerson, M. *A Cancer Therapy: Results of Fifty Cases.* New York: Station Hill Press, 1995.

11 Ornish, D., Magbanua, M. J., Weidner, G., et al. Changes in prostate gene expression in men undergoing an intensive nutrition and lifestyle intervention. *Proc Natl Acad Sci USA* 2008; 105: 8,369–8,374.

Ian Gawler's History—A Summary

AS THIS HISTORY IS LONG AND COMPLEX, IT HAS OFTEN BEEN MISQUOTED. What follows is a chronology of key events in Ian's recovery from cancer and his ongoing life.

February 25, 1950: Born in Melbourne, Australia.

1972: Graduated in Veterinary Science—Melbourne University.

1973–1975: Leased veterinary practice at Bacchus Marsh, Victoria, at first in partnership, then as principal. Large practice with the focus on stud and performance horses and companion animals.

December 1974: Reported swelling in right thigh to local GP and referred to surgeon, Dr. John Doyle.

January 1975: Full anesthetic and open biopsy confirmed osteogenic sarcoma in right leg. Told prognosis was 5 percent chance of survival after five years. Five days later, on January 8, right leg was amputated through the hip. Postsurgical histology confirmed the diagnosis. Independent review of all pathology in 1994 confirmed the original diagnosis.

Found prosthesis less practical than crutches. Began to wear kaftans for comfort and esthetics. Began to meditate daily, improved the diet, and reflected deeply on the meaning and purpose of life.

November 1975: Rock-hard swelling detected inside right groin. Based upon the clinical picture, definitive X-rays and bone scans, Doyle diagnosed secondary osteogenic sarcoma in the right sacroiliac area and suspected more secondaries centrally in the chest. Advised medical treatment ineffective and not recommended. Advised prognosis was three to six months.

Ian reasoned that healing may be possible if the immune system could be activated. Began intensive meditation (initially three to five hours, then three) with Dr. Ainslie Meares (Melbourne psychiatrist and author of *Relief Without Drugs*). Began the Gerson Diet.

February 1976: No growth in cancer but complications began through weight loss and period of a couple weeks of severe back pain and sciatica. Confined to bed. Following more extensive investigations at Peter Mac-Callum Hospital, three palliative radiotherapy treatments to lower lumbar spine were administered, but were ineffective for pain relief. Chiropractic, megavitamin therapy and acupuncture gave slight relief but not persisted with. Medically directed injections of Plenisol, a mistletoe extract, relieved pain and increased mobility.

Married Gail Kerr (later Gail changed her name to Gayle, then Grace) who had been Ian's veterinary nurse and who continued to support him throughout his illness and recovery.

March 1976: Hydronephrosis developed, pain reintensified, severe night sweats, jaundiced, cachexia with marked weight loss.

March/April 1976: Travelled to Philippines. Over four weeks, psychic surgery received from five traditional Filipino shamanistic healers. Marked pain relief, weight gain and general health turn around, although cancer unchanged.

April–October 1976: Continued with meditation, diet, and explored wide range of natural therapies aimed at stimulating the immune system and healing. This was a period of intense reading, introspection and personal development. However, the cancer continued to progress, with large masses slowly enlarging inside pelvis, mediastinum and through left lung, plus large eruptions of cancer on the exterior of the sternum.

October 1976: Cancer progressed to its largest size (as seen in photos in this book. This photo has been regularly mislabelled as being taken in October 1977, but the original has the Kodak print date on its back and it forms one in a sequence of over a dozen photos that are dated by Kodak). Otherwise, health very good.

Concerned by cancer growth, consulted oncologist. After more investigations and confirmation of the diagnosis, advised of experimental chemotherapy that could be attempted with uncertain results and probably significant side effects (transient nausea, short-term hair loss, high probability of sterility, possible heart muscle and eyesight damage). Two-year course of treatment recommended with Adriamycin, vincristine, cyclophosphamide and dacarbazine. After two weeks deliberation, commenced treatment while intensifying the diet, the meditation and other supportive, self-help procedures.

After ten weeks treatment, felt whatever benefits the chemotherapy had to offer had been received. However, the cancer had only slightly diminished in size over the period of treatment (as confirmed by the regular photos taken and the oncologist's written reports); and warned of the very real possibilities of rapid rebound growth if the treatment was ceased. Against medical advice, elected to discontinue treatment.

January 1977: Returned to the Philippines seeking more healing for the cancer, any side effects from the treatment, and in an attempt to understand psychic surgery. Rented a flat in Baguio and spent three months being treated, filming, talking and studying with healers. After a visit to Manila that was very polluted, began coughing up blood for the first time. This may have marked the onset of the TB that would not be diagnosed until June 1978.

April 1977: Journeyed on to India. Met with Sai Baba, who is regarded as an avatar (a divine incarnation) in India. He said, "You are already healed, don't worry"—another turning point. Cancer began to recede markedly.

May/June 1977: Journeyed to Cairo; England—Glastonbury, Findhorn, Iona; Europe. Cancer continued to recede and began coughing up spicules of bone from the cancer breaking down in lungs.

June–December 1977: Back in Torquay, Victoria. Maintained the diet, meditation, positive attitude, natural therapies and personal development.

December 1977: Moved to Surfers Paradise, Queensland. Recommenced veterinary work.

December 1977–February 1978: Employed in companion animal practice, Surfers Paradise, Queensland.

April 1978: All visible cancer cleared. Returned to India for three weeks and then moved to Adelaide, South Australia, to take up companion animal veterinary practice at Morphett Vale, living at Old Noarlunga.

July 1978: Rosemary, first child born. Following extensive tests, cancer pronounced all clear, but tuberculosis diagnosed. Treatment commenced. Doctors advised given the medical history that recovery is likely to take around one year. Intensified the diet, meditation, etc. TB cleared in three weeks.

September 1978: Case reported by Dr. Ainslie Meares in *Medical Journal of Australia* (MJA) (see full report earlier). Media attention led to increased enquiries from other cancer patients and families.

1980: Moved to country property at Yarra Junction, Victoria, and established a mixed veterinary practice. Lived in small shed, while building own house over a four-year period. Three home births in shed: David, August 1980; Peter, March 1982; Alice, November 1983.

1981: Ian and Grace initiated the Melbourne Cancer Support Group (MCSG). This innovative twelve-week program had the specific aim of helping people to learn and put into practice those things they could do for themselves. The intention was to actively support people as they set about increasing their quality of life and their chances of experiencing long-term survival. The first meeting was held on September 16, 1981. The meetings lasted two and a half hours each week and on average over thirty people attended each program. Each session had a theme and time was provided for discussion and mutual support. This was the first group of its type in Australia, and one of the very first in the world; a lifestyle-based self-help program that focused upon therapeutic nutrition, attitudes, positive thinking and healthy emotions, meditation and peace of mind. This program continues to be presented and continues to evolve based upon clinical experience and research.

1983: In December, a nonprofit, nondenominational, registered charity was established to support and extend the MCSG. As the years progressed, the Gawler Foundation developed an additional emphasis on the prevention of disease, lifestyle counseling and the generation of well-being and peace of mind for symptom-free people. The programs, having been based upon Ian's recovery to begin with, continued to evolve in line with feedback from the participants and with the latest research findings.

1984: The veterinary practice was sold to focus on the newly established foundation. Ian has done very little formal veterinary work since.

1984: *You Can Conquer Cancer* was first published by Hill of Content (the book was based on MCSG program) and launched by Sir Edward "Weary" Dunlop, patron of the Anti-Cancer Council and long-term advocate for Ian's work.

ABC TV presented a landmark, mind-body medicine documentary featuring the work of Ian Gawler and Dr. Ainslie Meares called *Mind the Healer, Mind the Slayer.*

1985: The first residential program was conducted for cancer patients and their families in December 1985 at Monash University. These were the first residential programs for people with cancer in Australia.

1987: Australia Day Honors: Ian was awarded the Order of Australia Medal for services to the community.

1987: *Peace of Mind* published by Hill of Content (now published by Michelle Anderson Publishing Pty. Ltd.)

1991: First phase of the Gawler Foundation's (TGF) residential center at Yarra Junction opened.

1992: Second phase of TGF's residential center at Yarra Junction opened.

1995–99: Ian founded and convened Mind, Immunity and Health, the first Australian conference designed specifically for doctors and allied health professionals interested in mind-body medicine. This conference continues as the Holistic Health conference, the annual conference of the Australasian Integrative Medical Association.

1996: *Meditation—Pure and Simple* published by Hill of Content (now published by Michelle Anderson Publishing Pty Ltd.).

Grace ceased working at the Gawler Foundation.

1997: In November, Ian and Grace separated, then divorced in mid-1999.

The Creative Power of Imagery published by Hill of Content.

1999: Ian co-led a meditation-based trek for three weeks in the Himalayas to altitudes of 16,000.

2000: Ian remarried, to Dr. Ruth Berlin—now Dr. Ruth Gawler, a GP with a master's in general practice psychiatry.

2002: Dr. Ruth Gawler began working at the Gawler Foundation.

Ian and Ruth initiated lifestyle-based, self-help programs for people with MS—in collaboration with Professor George Jelinek, MS survivor, professor of emergency medicine, author of *Overcoming Multiple Sclerosis*.[39]

2004: Ian's left lung was removed following ongoing complications from bronchiectasis and scarring resultant from the TB. Histology confirmed there was a boney lesion removed with the lung that was consistent with osteogenic sarcoma treated with chemotherapy.

Health is now very good.

2005: Senate Inquiry into Cancer Services in Australia made a bipartisan recommendation that Gawler Foundation programs receive Medicare rebates. This is yet to happen.

2006: First endorsed training conducted for Cancer, Healing & Well-being—the twelve-week lifestyle-based cancer self-help group. (Ian first began annual trainings for people who wanted to lead cancer groups or teach meditation back in 1988). A network of the groups began across Australia, New Zealand and overseas.

2007: Endorsed training program commenced for teachers of meditation.

2008: Biography *The Dragon's Blessing* published by Allen & Unwin; author Guy Allenby.

Ian's medical case—a thirty-year follow-up of Dr. Ainslie Meares' report in 1978 written by Professor George Jelinek and Dr. Ruth Gawler—was published in the *MJA* in December (see full report earlier).

2009: Ian was featured on ABC TV in *Compass: A Good Life*.

Ian retired from the Gawler Foundation at the end of the year.

2010: *Meditation—An In-Depth Guide* is published by Allen & Unwin.

Grace Gawler challenged some of the timelines and reasons postulated for Ian's recovery in the *Medical Journal of Australia*. These claims were answered by George Jelinek and Ruth Gawler in the *MJA*.

2011: *The Mind That Changes Everything* was released by Brolga Publishing.

2012: Ian launched *Mind-Body Mastery*, a downloadable meditation program with an innovative support package to enhance learning and increase frequency of practice.

Haines and Lowenthal, writing in the *Internal Medicine Journal* (IMJ), disputed Ian's diagnosis of secondary cancer and hypothesized he only had TB. They did this without checking the facts with Ian or his treating doctors and without Ian's permission. These claims were refuted as being incorrect by Ian and Ruth Gawler in separate letters to the IMJ that were accompanied by details of the original medical reports from the time of his diagnosis along with statements from his original doctors.

You Can Conquer Cancer—a completely revised and rewritten version—was released by Michelle Anderson Publishing.

References

1. Meares, A. *Relief without Drugs,* 1968, Souvenir Press, London.

2. Sogyal, R. *The Tibetan Book of Living and Dying,* 1992, Ryder, London.

3. Gawler, I. J. ed. *Inspiring People,* 1995, The Gawler Foundation, Yarra Junction.

4. Kraus, P. *Surviving Cancer,* 2008, The Gawler Foundation, Yarra Junction.

5. Doll, R., and Peto, R. *The Causes of Cancer,* 1981, Oxford University Press, New York.

6. Kune, G. Edited Proceedings, The First Slezak Cancer Symposium, "*The Psyche and Cancer,*" 1992, Melbourne,

7. Gawler, I., and Bedson, P. *Meditation—an In-Depth Guide,* 2008, Allen & Unwin, Sydney.

8. Kraus, P. Op cit.

9. Kabat-Zinn, J. *Full Catastrophe Living,* 1990, Delta Books, Bantam Doubleday Dell Publishing Group, New York.

10. Frankl, V. *Man's Search for Meaning,* 1963, Pocket Books, New York.

11. Gawler, I. *The Mind that Changes Everything,* 2011, Brolga Publishing, Melbourne.

12. Coué, E. *Self-Mastery Through Conscious Auto-Suggestion,* First published 1922, this edition, 2007, Cosimo, New York.

13. Simonton, O. C., and Matthew, S. *Getting Well Again,* 1978, Bantam, New York.

14. Dossey, L. *Healing Words—The Power of Prayer and the Power of Medicine,* 1994, Harper Collins, New York.

15. Sackett, D.L.R., et al. "Evidence Based Medicine: what it is and what it isn't," *BMJ* 1996; 312: 71–2.

16. Yogananda. *Autobiography of a Yogi,* First published 1946, this edition, 2007, Sterling Publishers, New Delhi.

17. Gerson, M. *A Cancer Therapy: Results of Fifty Cases,* 1958, Totality Books, California, USA.

18. Ornish, D., et al. *Journal of Urology* 2005; 74: 1065–1070.

19. *The New Gawler Foundation Cookbook*, 2012, The Gawler Foundation, Yarra Junction.

20. Pauling, Dr. L., and Cameron, E. *Cancer and Vitamin C,* 1979, Linus Pauling Institute of Science and Medicine, New York.

21. Pert, C. *Molecules of Emotion,* 1998, Simon & Schuster, London.

22. Brandt, J. *The Grape Cure*, 1996, Health Research, Pomeroy, USA.

23. Kune, G. *The Home Health Guide to a Cancer-Free Family*, 2005, Michelle Anderson Publishing, Melbourne.

24. Doll, R., and Peto, R. Op cit.

25. Le Shan, L. *You Can Fight for Your Life,* 1978, Jove Publishing.

26. Simonton and Matthews. Op cit.

27. Temoshok, L. and Dreher, H. *The Type C Connection: The Behavioral Links to Cancer and Your Health,* 1999, Collingdale.

28. Miller, M. and Rahe, R. H. *Life Changes Scaling for the 1990s,* 1997, *Journal of Psychosomatic Research*: 43:279.

29. Kübler-Ross, E. *On Death and Dying,* 1969, Macmillan, New York.

30. McCue, K. *How to Help Children Through a Parent's Serious Illness,* 2011, St. Martin's Press, New York.

31. Kübler-Ross, E. Op cit.

32. Moody, R. *Life After Life,* 1979, Bantam, New York.

33. Morgan, G. et al. *Clin Oncol*, 2004; 16:549–60.

34. Gawler, I. *Cancer, Chemotherapy and Lifestyle*, available via the research section on the website www.iangawler.com.

35. Allenby, G. *The Dragon's Blessing*, 2008, Allen & Unwin, Sydney.

36. Tompkins, P. and Bird, C. *The Secret Life of Plants,* 1974, Penguin, Melbourne.

37. Gawler, I. *The Mind That Changes Everything*, 2011, Brolga Publishing, Melbourne.

38. Doidge, N. *The Brain That Changes Itself,* 2008, Scribe, Carlton North.

39. Jelinek, G. *Overcoming Multiple Sclerosis*, 2009, Allen & Unwin, Crow's Nest.
    The Australian Concise Oxford Dictionary, Melbourne, Oxford University Press, 1987.

The Holy Bible, Revised Standard Edition, New York, Thomas Nelson, 1972.

More Information on Ian Gawler

Book

Meditation: Pure and Simple

Downloadable Meditation Program

Mind-Body Mastery—with ongoing online support:
www.mindbodymastery.net

Ian's Website

www.iangawler.com

Ian's Blog

gawlerblog.com

To contact the Gawler Foundation:

PO Box 77, Yarra Junction, Victoria 3797, Australia
Phone: (03) 5967 1730, or Fax: (03) 5967 1715
International Dialing: +61 3 5967 1730
E-mail: info@gawler.org
Website: www.gawler.org

Index

Page numbers in *italics* refer to photos, illustrations, figures, and charts.

HANS KÜNG

Christianity

Its Essence and History

SCM PRESS LTD

Translated by John Bowden from the German
Christentum. Wesen und Geschichte,
published 1994 by Piper Verlag, Munich

ISBN 0 334 02571 0 (cased)
0 334 02584 2 (paper)

First published in English 1995 by
SCM Press Ltd,
9–17 St Albans Place, London N1 0NX

Second impression 1995

Typeset by The Spartan Press, Lymington,
and printed in Great Britain by
Mackays of Chatham, Kent

Contents

B. The Centre   21

The Aim of This Book

Now, of all times, a massive book on Christianity? Yes, now! For a massive crisis in Christianity makes a massive answer urgently necessary. The first thing to be said is that this answer is radical. It will not spare any Christian tradition and church from criticism, because it has a radical trust in the cause of the gospel. Without compromise or harmonization it will confront Catholicism, Orthodoxy, Protestantism and Anglicanism with the original message and in this way do them an ecumenical service. This book can and must be critical of the churches because it has been written in an unshakable faith in the person and cause of Jesus Christ, and because it wants the church of Jesus Christ still to be there in the third millennium.

But can one still have any confidence in the Christian cause? Confronted with the third millennium, mustn't one despair of Christianity? Hasn't Christianity become completely incredible and incomprehensible, at least in its European heartlands? Aren't today's trends more than ever away from Christianity: to Eastern religions, to all kinds of groups concerned with politics or experience, or simply into a convenient private world without any obligations? Don't many people even in our 'Christian' and especially Catholic countries associate Christianity with an institutional church greedy for power and lacking in insight, with authoritarianism and a doctrinaire dictatorship, which so often breeds anxiety, has complexes about sex, discriminates against women, refuses to engage in dialogue and treats with contempt those who think differently? Isn't the Catholic Church in particular identified with discrimination against women, when Rome wants 'once and for all' to forbid the ordination of women (along with the marriage of priests and contraception). And because of this inability to make any adjustments, in some countries hasn't the former more or less benevolent indifference towards Christianity turned into spite and indeed open enmity?

But what is 'Christianity'? Can one talk about 'Christianity' in the singular at all? Aren't there different **Christianities** – Eastern Orthodox, Roman Catholic, Reformation Protestant Christianity, not to mention the various Free Church Christianities and all the countless Christian sects and groups? It has to be conceded from the start that the mention of Christianity produces extremely contradictory feelings throughout the world. What isn't 'Christianity'? Even Christians feel a deep unease. Think of all the institutions, parties and movements, the dogmas, laws and ceremonies which bear the label 'Christian'. And how often in history Christianity has been neglected, squandered, indeed betrayed! How often it has been neglected, squandered, indeed betrayed by the churches themselves! Instead of Christianity there has been only ecclesiasticism. Instead of Christian substance and Christian spirit there has been the Roman system, Protestant fundamentalism or Orthodox traditionalism.

And yet, even more than Judaism, Christianity has remained a spiritual force present on all continents – despite all the threats posed by suppression in the former Communist East or by consumerism in the secular West. Christianity is by far the greatest of the world religions, which neither Fascism nor Nazism, neither Leninism, Stalinism nor Maoism, could exterminate. And although many Christians, too, can no longer tolerate their churches, they don't want to give up Christianity. Rather, they want to know what Christianity really means, could mean. They want courage, courage to be Christians even today. And it is help towards being a Christian today that this book seeks to give, for all its criticism, thus supporting the forces of reform in all the churches.

Christianity has remained my spiritual home, too, despite all my experiences of the lack of compassion in the Roman system. Perhaps an account of Christianity by a committed Christian may prove even more exciting than a 'neutral' approach from the perspective of religious studies or confessional apologetics, or even a cynical anti-Christian denunciation or caricature. No, I have not given up hope that it will still be possible to live out Christian faith credibly in the third millennium – with both devotion and criticism – a faith which has a convincing content without dogmatic rigidity and which gives ethical guidance without being moralistically paternalistic. **Christianity should become more Christian** – that is the only possible perspective for the third millennium, too. The Roman system, Orthodox traditionalism and Protestant fundamentalism are all historical manifestations of Christianity. They have not always been there, and one day they will disappear. Why? Because they are not of the essence of Christianity.

But if Christianity is again to become more Christian, conversion will be necessary: a **radical reform** which is more than the psychologizing or remythicizing of Christianity. A reform is radical, it 'goes to the roots', only if it brings something **essential** to light again. But what is this essence of Christianity? Here one cannot just appeal to religious experiences and dispense with all thought. Every possible means must be used to investigate the question: what holds together all these Christian churches, so varied and intrinsically different, all these Christian centuries which differ so much? Is there – despite all the abuses and violations – something like a recognizable **essence** of Christianity on which one can reflect in the different churches?

Many books have been written about this, and they contradict one another. The present book broadly takes up what I said about the essence of Christianity as early as 1974, in *On Being a Christian*, for it is impossible to answer the question of the essence of Christianity **without reflecting on the origins which give it direction.** These are the Bible, its foundation document, and its primal figure, Jesus Christ. Jesus as the Christ is the fundamental figure and primal motif of all that is Christian. Christianity gains its identity and relevance only from him as its central figure.

But at the same time this book is a continuation of *On Being a Christian*, into the history of theology and the church, for there can be no answer to the question of what is truly and authentically Christian in the divided two-thousand-year history of Christianity without a **critical survey of the church tradition** in its different confessional expressions. The criterion for what is Christian is not Christianity as it really exists at any time, but its nearness to or remoteness from its origin, its foundation and centre.

So in this way I shall attempt a **critical, historical account of twenty centuries of Christianity.** I know that this is a tremendously difficult undertaking. And not a few theologians and historians would regard it as simply impossible. But this difficult undertaking must be ventured on if we are not completely to lose sight of the whole of Christianity, if we are to understand the present and develop perspectives for the future. I should make it plain that this book is neither a neutral scholarly description of Christianity nor a systematic theological account of the doctrine of Christianity. It presents a synthesis of both dimensions, history and systematic theology, and it offers both a chronological narrative and an analytical argument about the substance of Christianity. It tells a story, a tremendously dramatic and complex story, but at the same time this story is constantly interrupted critically from the start to ask about the price paid by Christianity in a particular paradigmatic constellation. 'Questions for the future' are asked, of the kind that always arise when a church tradition has hardened and thus become incapable of true ecumenicity. The book is thus conceived on interdisciplinary lines, because it breaks out of 'disciplines' which have proved sterile and attempts **a multi-dimensional view of Christianity**. It sets out to be an ecumenical book in the best sense of the word, based on the conviction that the confessions of Christianity will survive in the third millennium only in the spirit and form of **true ecumenicity**. The four great church leaders to whom I have dedicated the book stand for these perspectives.

Such an attempt can be made only because paradigm analysis provides a theoretical approach and a conceptual tool. I have already reflected on its methodology in my books *Theology for the Third Millennium* (1987) and *Global Responsibility* (1990), and it has already proved its worth for the historical account in *Judaism* (1991). So I can dispense here with reconstructing in detail the two-thousand-year history of Christianity in the different periods and territories, with all the different trends and leading personalities; besides, any handbook of church history will offer more here.[1] Rather, thinking in paradigms means understanding the dominant structures of history with the figures who shaped them. Thinking in paradigms means analysing the different **entire constellations** of Christianity, their origins, the way in which they mature and (though here I can only be brief) the way in which they harden. Thinking in paradigms means describing the survival into the present of paradigms which have hardened into tradition.

And what is all this for? To understand the present more deeply. What I am interested in here is not the past as such but **how and why Christianity became what it is today – with a view to how it could be.** The specific character of this kind of historiography is not pure chronology, but an interlocking of periods and problems.

I have had to forego countless interesting details, attractive anecdotes and important aspects in order to achieve the sharp perspective that is needed with a constantly changing historical approach. I have had to concentrate on working out each of the great entire constellations or paradigms – the Jewish Christian apocalyptic (P I), Hellenistic Byzantine Russian (P II), mediaeval Roman Catholic (P III), Reformation Protestant (P IV) and finally Enlightenment modern paradigm (P V), against the background of a brief historical sketch of the development of the conditions, causes and pressures, the constants and variables, in order to survey and sound out the basic features of the contemporary paradigm. And as the older paradigms do not die out when a new one arrives, but develop in parallel to the new paradigm and then interlock in many ways, smaller overlaps are not only unavoidable, but very useful.

So this book is the second volume on 'The Religious Situation of Our Time', written within the framework of the project 'No World Peace without Religious Peace', which is promoted by the Bosch Jubilee

Foundation and the Daimler-Benz Fund. As with my account of Judaism, here too my starting point is that an investigation does justice to Christianity only if it seeks at the same time to provide two things. First, an **analysis** of the spiritual forces of a thousand-year-old history which are still effective in the present, i.e. a systematic historical diagnosis. This should, secondly, lead to **assessments of the prospects** of the different options for the future on the basis of the analysis of the present, with the **beginnings of** practical ecumenical **solutions**. However, work on this volume has made it clear that an account of the history of Christianity and the great Christian traditions alone is enough to fill it. So a description of the present and expectations for the future must follow in a further volume.

To understand this book it is equally important to see that the conception set down in it is the **end-product of a long process of thought**. This is not in fact the first time that I have written on the historical developments of Christianity. After four decades of theological research I can present a coherent overall account here. So I hope that it will not be taken amiss if in particular chapters I refer to earlier books in order to support and deepen the comments made here.

And one last thing is important to me. This book has been written in a German university, but by a 'world citizen' and as far as possible **against a universal horizon**. So I have tried, depending on the period, also to write from the perspective of another country if the forces which changed and shaped a particular historical constellation came from that country. Of course in this book the non-European continents could be discussed only on the periphery: not because they are less important, nor even because of limits on space, but because – at least as far as Christianity is concerned – it is only in recent decades that important stimuli have been emerging from these countries for the 'heartlands' of Christianity. For me this is a clear sign (among others) that after the Eurocentric constellation of modernity we have entered a polycentric constellation (both postcolonialist and postimperialist, taking shape after the First World War and establishing itself after the Second), a constellation of what goes under (among other terms) the name of 'postmodernity'. That is reason enough for describing the influence and special significance of the non-European continents (Africa, Asia, North and South America, Oceania) in the further volume I have mentioned. But first the project as announced, of a trilogy on the religious situation of our time, will be completed as planned, with a volume on Islam which will come next – God willing, and if I am still alive . . .

Tübingen, June 1994

Hans Küng

In grateful memory of
Pope John XXIII, Bishop of Rome,
Athenagoras, Ecumenical Patriarch of Constantinople,
Michael Ramsey, Archbishop of Canterbury,
Willem Visser't Hooft, First General Secretary of the World Council of
    Churches,
who embodied their paradigm of Christianity credibly,
yet opened it up to the wider Christian world.

A. The Question of Essence

Only the ignorant can claim that all religions are the same. On the contrary, it is extremely important for members of every religion and especially every prophetic religion, whether Christianity, Judaism or Islam, to ask, 'What is the difference between my religion and other religions? What is the special, the typical, the specific, the essential character, indeed the "essence" of this or that religion?'[1] I now want to raise this question for Christianity, as I have already raised it for Judaism – in an ecumenical spirit, without polemic against the other religions.

I. The Essence and Perversion of Christianity

It is clear that to talk of the typical, peculiar, essential element in a religion is not to focus on the abstract theoretical question of a systematic conception of unity: a single Christian system or regime. Rather it is to focus on the highly practical question what may be said to be the **permanently valid, constantly binding** and **quite indispensable** element in Christianity. I make no secret of my motive here: it is not the preservation of the status quo, which is so important to the conservatives; far less is it the restoration of the status quo ante, for which reactionaries from Roman Catholicism, Protestant fundamentalism and old Orthodoxy are fighting. My interest is in **change, reform, renewal of Christianity** with a view to a status quo post, the future. In that connection it is important to distinguish between an ideal picture of Christianity, a hostile picture of Christianity and a picture of how Christianity really is.

1. The ideal picture

There is not and there never was on this earth, a work of human policy so well deserving of investigation as the Roman Catholic Church. The history of that church joins together the two great ages of human civilization. No other institution is left standing which carries the mind back to the times when the smoke of sacrifice rose from the Pantheon, and when camelopards and tigers bounded in the Flavian amphitheatre. The proudest royal houses are but of yesterday when compared with the line of the Supreme Pontiffs. That line we trace back in an unbroken series, from the Pope who crowned Napoleon in the nineteenth century to the Pope who crowned Pepin in the eighth . . . The Republic of Venice was modern when compared with the papacy; and the Republic of Venice is gone, and the Papacy exists. The Papacy exists, not in decay, not a mere antique, but full of life and youthful vigour. The Catholic Church is still sending forth to the farthest ends of the world missionaries as zealous as those who landed in Kent with Augustine, and still confronting hostile kings with the same spirit with which she confronted Attila . . . The number of her children is greater than it was at any former time. The increase that she has experienced in the New World has more than compensated for what she has lost in the Old. Her spiritual rule extends over all the countries that lie between the plains of the Missouri and Cape Horn, and after another century these countries will perhaps contain a population equivalent in number to the present population of Europe. The Roman Catholic Church comprises certainly no fewer than 150 million souls; and it would be difficult to demonstrate that all the other Christian confessions number 120 million together. Nor do we see any sign which indicates that the term of her long dominion is approaching. She saw the commencement of all the governments and all the ecclesiastical establishments that now exist in the world; and we feel no assurance that she is not destined to see the end of them all. She was great and respected before the Saxon had set foot in Britain, before the Frank had passed the Rhine, when Grecian eloquence still flourished at Antioch, when idols were still worshipped in the temple of Mecca. And she may still exist in undiminished vigour when some traveller from New Zealand shall, in the middle of a vast solitude, take his stand on a broken arch of London Bridge to sketch the ruins of St Paul's.

That is how **Thomas B. Macaulay**, the statesman and famous representative of liberal English historiography,[2] described in grand style, in the last century – and I am quoting him word for word – the Catholic Church, the oldest, greatest and strongest representative of Christianity. And how many Catholics, non-Catholics and converts, like the Anglican Macaulay, have admired this Catholic Church in a similar way in our century also: its history maintained and shaped in a unique way, its venerable antiquity and at the same time its lively youth; its effective organization spread throughout the world and at the same time present locally, with hundreds of millions of members and a tightly organized hierarchy; the exalted ceremonial of its worship, rich in tradition; its well-thought-out system of theological doctrine; its epoch-making cultural achievements in the construction and formation of the Christian West; its modern social teachings. But, as is well known, men of power and criminals of all kind could also admire the Catholic Church – including Napoleon and the Austrian Catholic Adolf Hitler, who admired and imitated its organization, firm dogma and liturgical splendour.[3]

In the introduction to his work *The Essence of Catholicism*, which went through many editions and appeared in almost every European language, the well-known Tübingen theologian **Karl Adam**, one of my predecessors in Catholic dogmatics in Tübingen, quoted this passage from Macaulay and added: 'It is this that entrances our gaze in the wasteland of the present: this imperishability, this teeming life force, this eternal youth of the old, age-old church.'[4] And even after the experiences of Nazism and the Second World War, Adam, also once an admirer of Hitler ('he came from the Catholic south but we did not recognize him'), who had argued programmatically that 'nationalism and Catholicism' belong together 'like nature and supernature',[5] writes in the same way as ever. In the different chapters of his book he presents as the 'Catholic idea, untouched by space and time', the church as the body of Christ and the kingdom of God on earth, its marks, its claim to be the only source of salvation and the special forces through which it gives its blessing.

And the reality? Only in the last chapter does Adam the dogmatic theologian turn from 'Catholicism as an idea' to 'Catholicism in its manifestation' and state in feeble apologetic that, because of the institutionalization of Christianity and the all-too-human elements in the church, 'it is by no means surprising that historical Catholicism does not always coincide completely with ideal Catholicism, but rather that actual Catholicism falls considerably short of its idea; that never yet in history has it been finished and completed, but is always only coming into being, laboriously growing'.[6] Indeed, this is the way in which the history of Christianity has been thought of above all since German Idealism and Romanticism (Friedrich Schleiermacher in Protestantism, John Henry Newman in Anglicanism, Johann Adam Möhler in Catholicism): as a **reality growing organically** which, while it is certainly always also producing rotten fruit and dead branches, is in a process of permanent development, unfolding and growing to perfection: the history of Christianity is a process of maturing and penetration.

But how often a striking development has proved to be a false development; how often apparently grandiose progress has turned out to be what in the end was an extremely damaging regression. No, an optimistic idealistic view of history which seeks to detect organic growth everywhere – in doctrine, constitution, law, liturgy, piety – is untenable not only in the light of the New Testament but even more in the light of the reality of church history. There are utterly unorganic, abnormal, contrary, false developments in it – one only has to think, say, of the increasing splitting of Christianity into large churches and countless sects. Indeed, despite their occasional criticism (hardly ever of 'Rome' and the Pope), such idealistic and exalted descriptions of the church, whether those of Karl Adam or the distinguished French Jesuit theologian Henri de Lubac under the title *Méditation sur l'Église*[7] or of his pupil Hans Urs von Balthasar under the programmatic title *Sponsa Verbi* (Bride of the Word)[8] (it was not for nothing that both were made cardinals), not to mention the *Hymns to the Church* by the convert Gertrud von Le Fort, are utterly remote from the reality of Catholicism as it really exists.[9] But who still wants to sing hymns to the church today?

Be this as it may, the question 'What is Christianity?' can no longer be answered with such idealizations, mystifications and glorifications which, while not uncritical, have virtually no consequences for the Roman system. What is appropriate, rather, is unrestrained **truthfulness**. And I could not allow even Henri de Lubac, for whom I have great personal admiration, to forbid me this, despite his comment after my lecture in St Peter's on 'Truthfulness in the Church' at the time of the Second Vatican Council:[10] 'One doesn't talk like that about the church. *Elle est quand-même notre mère*: after all, she's our mother!' But in the meantime the mother-complex of many clergy has been thoroughly analysed, not least by Eugen Drewermann.[11] And three decades after the Council there has been a rude awakening from some beautiful 'church dreams'. Nevertheless, along with truthfulness, **justice and fairness** towards the church and Christianity are also called for. So now it is important to set a counterpoint.

2. The hostile picture

'**I condemn** Christianity, and confront it with the most terrible accusation that an accuser has ever had in his mouth. To my mind it is the greatest of all conceivable corruptions . . . it converted every value into its opposite, every truth into a lie and every honest impulse into an ignominy of the soul . . . I call Christianity the **one** great curse, the **one** enormous and innermost perversion, the **one** great instinct of revenge, for which no means are too venomous, too underhand, too underground and too **petty** – I call it the **one** immortal blemish of mankind.' This hate-filled 'curse on

Christianity' is the conclusion to *The Antichrist*, the last work which **Friedrich Nietzsche** personally wrote for publication, aimed directly at the annihilation of Christianity.[12]

A hymn instead of a curse! A curse only of its time? A curse which today has long been superseded by the further history of Christianity, which can easily be cursed but not so easily destroyed? Superseded? In no way! The same sentences have recently adorned a bestselling *Criminal History of Christianity* by **Karlheinz Deschner** as a motto. Unlike Nietzsche, the pastor's son, Deschner comes from a conservative Catholic background and was even briefly a theology student; he plans to continue the work in ten volumes in all.[13] And in such a critical history Deschner by no means intends only to give a history of the churches, 'an account of the different kinds of churches, church fathers, bishops, heresiarchs and heresiologists, the inquisitors and other rogues, holy and unholy, their purely clerical ambitions of power and violent undertakings, but far beyond that a history of Christianity, its dynasties and wars, its terrors and atrocities'. Thus the author himself in his publicity. His specific intention is to give a detailed report of the 'continuous interlocking of so-called secular and spiritual politics and the secularized consequences of this religion: criminality in foreign policy, in agricultural, trade and financial policy, in educational policy, in culture, censorship, in the ongoing dissemination of ignorance and superstition, the unscrupulous exploitation of sexual morality, the marriage laws, the criminal law.' And at the same time the 'history of clerical criminality' is to be brought out, in the 'private accumulation of wealth, in the jockeying for office, in the pious deception in the cult of miracle and relics, in the great variety of forgeries, etcetera etcetera.'[14]

There is considerable justification for a criticism of the church system, and it by no means needs to come from an ideological anti-clericalism. A great deal of acid criticism from former believers is the result of bitter disappointment. I am certainly the last person to take Nietzsche's accusation against Christianity lightly, since I not only quoted it fifteen years ago, but discussed it in detail with much empathy.[15] And I am also the last person to take Deschner's accusations lightly; after all, for some time now I have been discussing some of his critical questions from a historical perspective, for instance the attitude of the church to Jews, heretics and enthusiasts,[16] all the questions of reform within the church, and time and again the problem of the papacy.[17] And as in my *Judaism*, so now in this book on Christianity I shall have to investigate some errors and confusions. Deschner is quite right on many points, and he poses a challenge to the church ideologists in shaping knowledge and con-sciences. Now that the official church has felt able to ignore and suppress the serious criticism of well-disposed theologians, it must cope with the exaggerated criticism of malicious 'criminologists' (and some pamphleteers). These do not want to understand and make critical distinctions, but to accuse and utter sweeping condemnations.

But I hope that as one who has had much experience of church matters and who has been much tested by them, I may be allowed to observe that Deschner's 'criminal history' of Christianity (which already begins with Judaism!), often vulnerable in detail, does not contain much new material. In particular the scandal-mongering exploitation of the history of the Popes by this author, who became a historian as a result of bad experiences, is anything but original. Its only new feature, as the author openly concedes, is its hate-filled summarizing and amassing of all the mistakes and errors, crimes and blasphemies, false developments and signs of decadence in a spirit of 'hostility'[18] towards Christianity. All that is good and shines out in the two-thousand-year history of Christianity is simply passed over in silence. Why this great expenditure of irony, polemic, sarcasm and invective? To be able to maintain the thesis that Christianity is intrinsically criminal, a delusion, a lie and deception which must be destroyed 'scientifically'. But Deschner is not at all familiar with more recent theological literature, and instead quotes old apologetic tomes which have long been superseded.

It goes without saying that one can fill several volumes with scurrilous, pathological, criminal incidents from two thousand years of church history without ever coming face to face with the holy. That is the task of a lifetime. The author could easily write further 'criminal histories' in the same style and with similar motivation: the criminal history of Germany, France or America, or perhaps the criminal history of militant atheism and the criticism of religion. But in the long run will not such criminal histories, which merely gather shadows and walk through puddles, become as insipid as the emphatic 'hymns to the church'? Why insipid? Because those who passionately collect only shadows can offer only a shadow play. And those who deliberately tread in all the puddles wrongly make the way difficult for themselves.[19]

No, both genres of book – those written in bright triumphalist colours and stained-glass-window piety and those which are aggressively polemical and cynically condescending – are failed books of half-truths. For half-truths are at the same time half-errors, and neither is serious history. Hatred can certainly make one as clear-sighted as love can, but it can often also make one blind. One need only read the tirades of hatred by the former Bamberg theology student 'On the Need to Leave the Church' – for him the 'giant corpse of a monster of world history'.[20] But just as someone who was fundamentally anti-German would hardly be able to understand the authentic Germany, or someone aggressively anti-French would be unable to understand the authentic France, or someone fanatically anti-American the authentic America, so too someone who is militantly anti-Christian can hardly understand the real Christianity (for all his apt observations). Why do so many Germans, French, Americans want to remain German, French, American, despite all the criticism? Why do so many Christians not cease to be Christian?

No, a 'Chronique scandaleuse' is not yet historiography, but, to give a dictionary definition, is a 'collection of scandalous stories and gossip from a period or a particular milieu'. All that means that such a hostile picture cannot settle the question of what Christianity really is any more than a traditional ideal picture can. Instead of glorification or contempt, historical-critical understanding is asked in truthfulness and justice (which then, of course, have to be the foundation of a theological judgment) to use the origin, the foundation document of Christianity, as its criterion.

3. The real picture: a twofold dialectic

As long ago as the time of the Second Vatican Council, in the 1960s, it became clear to me that for a real picture of the church it is always necessary to distinguish and take into account two perspectives, which now in the context of the religious situation of our time and the great world religions will deliberately have to be extended to 'Christianity', understood as a sociological, political and theological entity:[21] these are the reciprocal relationship, i.e. the **dialectic**, between essence and form and essence and perversion.

Essence and form

The concept of Christianity is always shaped by the particular concrete form it takes at a period in history. Christianity can become the prisoner of the picture which it has made of itself at a particular time. Indeed, every age has its own picture of Christianity which has grown out of a particular situation, lived out and formed by particular social forces and church communities, conceptually shaped beforehand or afterwards by particularly influential figures and theologies.

However, anyone who is not blinkered can note that in all trends and counter-trends in social history, church history and the history of theology, in all the different, changing historical pictures of Christianity, an **abiding** element persists. It is to this that we shall have to devote all our attention: basic elements and basic perspectives deriving from an origin, which remains the valid norm. So in the history of Christianity and its self-understanding there is something which persists, indeed an '**essence**' (*essentia, natura, substantia*). I am well aware of the misunderstandings associated with this term. But against all rigid 'essentialism' I would immediately add that this essence shows itself only in what **changes**.

In other words, there is something identical, but only in variables; a continuum, but only in the event; persistence, but only in changing appearances. In short, the 'essence' of Christianity does not show itself in metaphysical immobility and aloofness but always in a constantly changeable historical '**form**'. And if we are to get a sight of this original abiding 'essence' – which is not static and rigid but takes place dynamically – we must take note of the historical 'form' which permanently changes.

Only when we see the 'essence' of Christianity in its changing historical form will we grasp the Christianity from which I want to begin in this account: not an ideal Christianity in the abstract spheres of a theological theory or poetry, but a **real** Christianity which really exists in the midst of the history of this world. The New Testament, too, does not begin with a **doctrine** of Christianity which is then subsequently realized, but with the **reality** of Christianity, on which there is subsequent reflection. Real Christianity is primarily a fact, an event, a historical movement. The real essence of real Christianity becomes event in different historical figures. Here we should note two things:

– **Essence and form** are **inseparable**: they may not be torn apart, but must be seen as a unity. The distinction between essence and form is not a real one but a conceptual one. In reality there never was nor is there anywhere an essence of Christianity 'in itself', separated, purely distilled from the flow of church figures. The changeable and the unchangeable cannot be neatly divided – this is important for praxis! Certainly there are abiding constants, but there are no spheres which are *a priori* irreformable. Essence and form are not related in the same way as kernel and shell. Essence without form is formless and thus unreal, just as a form without essence is inessential and thus equally unreal.

– **Essence and form** are **not identical**: they may not be identified, but must be seen in their difference. Though the distinction between essence and form is conceptual, it is necessary, with a foundation in reality. For how else are we to be able to define the abiding element in what takes shape? How else could we judge the concrete historical form? How else could we have a criterion, a norm, for defining the legitimate element in any particular historical empirical manifestation of Christianity?

How important this is becomes evident when we also note the second perspective:

Essence and perversion

In all the negative factors at which criticism of the church rightly takes offence and which an idealistic admiration happily disguises, we do not simply have the expression of a historical 'form' of Christianity. That would be to trivialize the evil in Christianity. Is the positive to be identified with the abiding 'essence' and the negative with the fleeting 'form'? No, inconvenient though this is, we also have to take seriously the negative element in the church, the perversion of Christianity. And this perversion of Christianity conflicts with its essence, although it is dependent on it. It is not the legitimate essence of Christianity but its illegitimate essence, not its authentic essence but its perverted essence. As a dark shadow this perversion runs alongside the essence of Christianity through all historical forms. In short, **the real essence of Christianity comes about in its perversion.**

So all the admirers and all the enemies of Christianity must be told that particularly those who are seriously concerned for the cause of Christianity and the church must reckon *a priori* with the dark perversion of Christianity. Like essence and form, the abiding and the changing, so too good and evil, salvation and disaster, essence and perversion, are interwoven and cannot be set off against each other without remainder by any human reckoning. The basic essentials also change. Even they can be perverted. Even the best is prone to evil. Sin is possible even with the holiest.

So we can see the history of Christianity from a negative as well as a positive perspective. If we do, we note that for all the shaping and mastery of history we can also recognize in Christianity a succumbing, a capitulation to history. In all the effective organization there is a powerful financial apparatus working with very secular means; in the imposing statistics of Christian multitudes there is an impoverished superficial traditional Christianity; in the well-ordered hierarchy there is a clerical officialdom which always has an eye on Rome, often servile and effeminate even in the way in which it dresses, remote from reality and vain; in the cultic ceremonial there is an externalized ritualism stuck in a mediaeval baroque tradition out of keeping with the gospel; in the clear dogmatic doctrinal system a rigidly authoritarian scholastic theology manipulating the husks of traditional concepts, unhistorical and unbiblical; in the achievements of Western culture secularization and a deviation from its real task. For many people that is the real church, the church which really exists. And that is why they have left it.

All this means that the basic object of our consideration must be not only historicity in general, but in particular the way in which Christianity has been infected by the anti-Christian. We must take this into account *a priori* and everywhere, without any false apologetic. Certainly some of those who are leaving the church in Germany (by no means poor people) are doing so for purely financial reasons (to avoid the church tax), and some charges levelled against the church are uncomprehending, arrogant, one-sided, unjust, indeed very often simply false and sometimes even malicious. All this can be answered; not, however, in a lazy apologetic but in an apologia, defence, justification, which accepts only justified, well-founded charges.[22]

So in this study I shall never simply take the present status quo of Christianity as a criterion, nor even justify it. Rather, I shall attempt a critical survey which is a presupposition for that renewal of Christianity which is constantly necessary, whenever it takes place. I already chose the same approach for **Judaism**, and I must also attempt it in my account of **Islam**. In the face of all the frustration and resignation which is always a threat to reformers in all religions, who sometime have the feeling that they are simply like dogs baying at the moon, and constantly coming up against brick walls, I want to offer help by means of an analytical account which is rather different from cheap unmasking, by providing a diagnosis of the present which attacks abuses, identifies those responsible, increases the pressure towards reform and encourages **structural changes**. We cannot be content with the status quo in any religion – whether in Judaism, Christianity or Islam (not to mention religions of Indian or Chinese origin). Everywhere parallel questions arise about future renewal.

Questions for the Future

In time, will a new consensus also perhaps develop in Judaism, a consensus which despite all the dialectic of essence and form, essence and perversion, which is also unavoidable here, will again make clear what is the abidingly valid, permanently binding and utterly indispensable element of Jewish belief?[23]

What possibilities does Islam have of distinguishing the essentials from the inessentials, in the face of all one-sided caricatures and despite often burdensome traditions, and of bringing out the essentials of Islamic faith more realistically, beyond all utopian ideals?

What needs to be done for the real essence of Christianity once again to appear clearly, despite all the changes of form and the distortions brought about by its perversion?

This aim must be made concrete in an approach which is not abstract and idealistic, but sober and realistic. Through the general question of the **essence** of Christianity (as opposed to its form and its perversion), we must answer the question of what is specifically, **authentically Christian.**

II. 'Christianity' in Dispute

1. The essence of Christianity – can it be identified by philosophers?

The Essence of Christianity – under this title there appeared in 1841 the work of a thirty-seven-year old philosopher, whose declared aim it was 'to turn theologians into anthropologists, theophiles into philanthropists, candidates for the next world into students of this world, religious and political servants of the heavenly and earthly monarchy and aristocracy into free, self-aware citizens of the earth'.[1] His name was Ludwig Feuerbach.

Religion – a human projection (Feuerbach)

This book made a powerful claim, since it sought to attack every religion once and for all by deriving the religious comprehensively from the human. And its influence was immense. After all, it converted not only Max Stirner and Bruno Bauer, the young Richard Wagner and Friedrich Nietzsche, but also Karl Marx and Friedrich Engels to atheism. For throughout the Communist system dialectical materialism presupposed the criticism of religion made by Ludwig Feuerbach, who thus became the 'church father' of modern atheism.[2] Ludwig Feuerbach's philosophy literally became a factor in world history.

Feuerbach's basic thesis was: 'The **secret of theology** is **anthropology**.'[3] That means that in belief in God human beings as it were extract their human nature and see it as something existing outside themselves, separate from them. So they project their nature as an independent form as it were on heaven, call it God and worship it. In short, the concept of God is nothing but a **human projection**: '**The Absolute nature**, man's God, is **his own nature**. The power of the **object** over him is therefore the power **of his own nature**.'[4] Thus the knowledge of God is a powerful searchlight: 'God' is nothing but a projected, hypostatized reflection of human beings, made by them, and splendidly confirmed by the properties of the divine being. What are the love, wisdom, justice of God? They are in reality human properties, the human genre! *Homo homini Deus est*, man is man's God: that is the whole secret of religion.

Chapter by chapter, in a way which is ultimately exhausting but very persistent, Feuerbach hammers home his new creed to the reader and in so doing applies his basic insight to all the Christian dogmas. One can soon almost think out the explanation of them for oneself. What is the secret of the **incarnation of God**? The incarnate God is now the manifestation of divinized man. What is the secret of the love of God for humankind? None other than the secret of the love of humankind for itself . . . In this way Feuerbach thought that he had seen through the essence of Christianity, indeed the essence of any religion, once and for all. And at the same time he was convinced that religion, and with it Christianity, would dissolve to the degree that human beings became aware of themselves.

Only a projection?

However, 150 years later the situation looks different. We can see that Feuerbach's expectations have remained unfulfilled. And that also has to do with the fact that Feuerbach's theory, which sounds so convincing, is ultimately not conclusive philosophically. So we can take it that Feuerbach's criticism of religion, repeated with variations in many quarters, has been seen through. It is fundamentally based on two arguments:

1. **The projection argument.** Time and again Feuerbach uses variants on the argument from individual or social psychology that religion is nothing but a human projection or, as Marx later described it pointedly in his critique of society, the 'opium of the people'. But does that conclusively prove that God is **only** a projection, that God is only a consolation conditioned by interests or only an 'infantile illusion', as Sigmund Freud was later to argue, along the same lines? 'Only' or 'nothing but' sentences must be treated with suspicion. They suggest a certainty for which there is no foundation.

We must certainly concede that belief in God can be explained psychologically. But whether or not belief in God is psychological is a false alternative. For from a psychological perspective, belief in God always displays the structures and contents of a projection; it is always suspect of being a projection. But the fact of projection in no way determines whether the object to which it relates does or does not exist. In other words, the wish for God can correspond to a real God. And why shouldn't I be allowed to want death not to be the end, to want a meaning in my life, in human history? In short, why shouldn't I want God to exist? So Ludwig Feuerbach is quite right: beyond doubt religion, like all faith, hope and love, contains an element of projection. But that does not prove that religion is only a projection. It can also be related to another reality.

2. The argument from **the extinction of religion**. The argument that

religion is at an end, with its constant variations in the philosophy of history and culture, is similiarly based on an extrapolation into the future for which ultimately no foundation can be given. 'Unbelief has taken the place of faith, reason the place of the Bible, politics the place of religion and the church, earth the place of heaven, work the place of prayer, material distress the place of hell, man the place of Christianity.'[5] Really? Today it is crystal clear that neither the 'abolition of religion' by atheistic humanism (Feuerbach), nor the 'extinction of religion' by atheistic socialism (Marx), nor the 'replacement of religion' by atheistic science (Freud) have proved to be true prognoses. Rather, on the contrary, faith (!) in the goodness of human nature (Feuerbach) has proved to be an understandable projection, faith in the future socialist society (Marx) to be a consolation governed by particular interests, and faith in rational science to be a dangerous illusion. And though we must take the problems of both theoretical and practical nihilism seriously, Nietzsche's prognosis of the death of God has proved to be a false prognosis. On the contrary, today – and this is one of the clearest signs of a new era after modernity – we face the fact of the return of religion even in the Soviet Union, which has been atheistic for so long, and in China, where atheism is official.

However, it may also be decisive for the future of religion in the postmodern period – whether Christianity, Judaism, Islam or an Indian or Chinese religion – whether the religion in question takes seriously the justified concern of these great critics of religion:
– whether religion in postmodernity is again (as so often in modernity) the expression of the intellectual, moral and emotional alienation and impoverishment of humankind – or its manifold enrichment and a true theoretical and practical humanism;
– whether it will again become 'opium', the means of social alleviation, consolation and repression – or the means of comprehensive enlightenment and social liberation;
– whether it is proved to be 'illusion', the expression of a psychological immaturity or even neurosis, regression – or an expression of personal identity and psychological maturity.

In respect of Christianity, at any rate, since the nineteenth century the question has become even more intense. What is Christianity? At that time, in the hey-day of historicism, this fundamental question increasingly began to occupy theology. And attempts were made to solve it by investigating once again the 'essence' of Christianity – no longer in a philosophical-speculative but a historical perspective.

2. The essence of Christianity – can it be reconstructed by historians?

'The Essence of Christianity': under this title, a good fifty years after Feuerbach, in 1900, lectures by the great Protestant church historian and historian of dogma, Adolf von Harnack, were published in book form.[6]

Back to the simple gospel (Harnack)

Like the lectures already given in Berlin to an audience drawn from all faculties, Harnack's book was a tremendous success – in contrast to another turn-of-century book published the same year, Sigmund Freud's *The Interpretation of Dreams*. Why? Because here someone who knew the whole complicated development of Christian dogmatics and had presented it in a multi-volume *History of Dogma*[7] took the trouble to enquire briefly and lucidly, and in a way which anyone could understand, into the original form of Christianity, the Christian message in its original simplicity, plainness and 'naivety': 'What is Christianity? What was it? What has it become?'[8] They were the leading questions.

It can in fact be said that Harnack's enterprise is a 'single bold attempt' to 'produce a historically responsible **reduction of the complexity** of theology, to achieve a kind of "disarmament" in matters which philosophically, speculatively and conceptually were excessively complex, so as to open up the nucleus of the Christian proclamation afresh for today'.[9] However, Harnack was still a typical modern man in the way in which his perspective of Christianity was restricted, was a Eurocentric one: 'The answer to this question may, we hope, also throw light by the way on the more comprehensive one, What is religion, and what ought it to be to us? In dealing with religion, is it not after all with the Christian religion alone that we have to do? Other religions no longer stir the depths of our hearts.'[10]

But among other things Harnack's thrust also provoked the question: for how long in the history of Christianity have people been seeking the 'essence' of Christianity? This question is not as novel as it sounds. In his great article 'What Does "Essence of Christianity" Mean?',[11] the Protestant theologian and historian Ernst Troeltsch – who had already previously called for the strict application of historical thought in theology as well[12] – put it in the period of Romanticism and Idealism, and others put it as early as Enlightenment theology.[13]

Only recently, the Protestant theologian Rolf Schäfer has been able to demonstrate that talk of 'Christianity' and its 'true essence' can be found as early as the father of Pietism, Philipp Jakob Spener, in a sermon of 1694; so talk of the 'essence of Christianity' does not come from academic terminology but from the language of edification and is 'a construction, not of the Enlightenment, but of Pietism'.[14] And the Catholic theologian Hans Wagenhammer[15] has been even more specific: the formula 'essence of Christianity' already occurs in a posthumous work of the Pietistic Lutheran pastor Joachim Betke in 1666 ('The Principal and Substantial Essence of Christianity'), while a first monograph with the title *Essentia religionis christianae* was written by the French Pietist (Labadist) Pierre Yvon.[16] What follows from this finding?

A question of the Reformation and the Enlightenment

If we take the formula 'essence of Christianity' together with similar or parallel forms like *Substantia christianismi* which already occur in the eirenic Strasbourg Reformer Martin Bucer, who was concerned to find the element in Christianity which bound together Lutherans and Reformed,[17] it seems to me that two conclusions necessarily follow.

First, in so far as talk of an 'essence' (or the *substantia*) of Christianity denotes a concentration involving a delimitation from what is not Christian, it presupposes the sixteenth-century **Reformation**. And that makes sense. Why? The Reformation would not put up with the decadence, the perversion of Christianity everywhere, but wanted to find its way back to the original gospel. However, the Reformers and after them the Pietists regarded the gospel set down in the Bible as the **unquestionable essence of Christianity**, quite apart from any specific definition one gave of it, whether justification, rebirth or blessing.

Secondly, in so far as the formula 'essence of Christianity' denotes a historical insight into the different formations, the 'forms' of Christianity, it presupposes the eighteenth-century **Enlightenment**. Why? This was primarily concerned with the reasonableness of Christianity, but at the same time recognized the fundamental historicity of all Christian forms and thus began to identify as a problematical question **the essence of Christianity** which was already given in the Bible.

Since then explicit questions have been asked – not for the sake of a reduction and a dissolution of Christianity, but in a quest for its most concentrated form – for what is important, decisive, characteristic, in other words for what is 'substantial', 'essential' about Christianity. However, today, as we have seen, this is no longer to be understood in idealistic but in realistic terms:

– as the abiding essence **in** changing historical forms of Christianity;

– as the authentic essence despite the constant virulent perversions of Christianity and – one can add after the split in faith and in acceptance of the reconciling tendencies of the Enlightenment:

– as the binding, common essence of all the different Christian confessions and churches.

Nowadays, on the basis of historical research, there may be agreement over the rejection of two standpoints which are diametrically opposed. The essence of Christianity **cannot** be identified:

– with a **religion of reason**, with a rational natural religion allegedly given to all times, as presented in pioneering form for the Enlightenment (still as a defence of the nucleus of Christianity) by the three English thinkers John Locke, in *The Reasonableness of Christianity*;[18] John Toland, in *Christianity not Mysterious*;[19] and Matthew Tindal in *Christianity as Old as the Creation*[20] (all three titles are significant);

– or with the essence of **Catholicism**, a line still taken even after the Second World War in a pre-conciliar spirit by two German Catholic theologians, Michael Schmaus[21] and Romano Guardini,[22] in their works on the essence of Christianity.

Where do we go from here? Or better, where do we find ground under our feet for a definition of the essence of Christianity not as a nature religion but as a historical religion? We can only look at the **origin** of Christianity. And here – historically speaking – there can be no doubt that right from its origins Christianity was not identical with a naturally given, reasonable religion for all human beings, far less with a particular Roman church system. Rather, from its origins Christianity has been inconceivable without a quite definite – **name.**

3. 'Christianity' – called by its name

I also want to avoid well-meaning over-extension, narrowing, twisting and confusion of Christianity by taking trouble to use clear language which calls things by their name and takes concepts at their word. The concept of Christianity has been diluted and randomly extended enough. Here I want to make it precise. For the Christianity of Christians should remain Christian; indeed, perhaps it should become Christian again.

No Christianity without Christ

If we stop focussing on the formula 'essence' or 'substance of Christianity' but keep in view **Christianity as it really is**, we can hardly deny that of course there was an 'essential' Christianity even before the questions of Pietism and the Enlightenment about the 'essence' of Christianity. The discovery that the word 'Christianity' was used relatively rarely in the early church and even less in the mediaeval church, and that people talked more of Christian 'faith' or of 'church' and the like, does not alter this fact. For example Justin, the second-century Christian apologist, philosopher and martyr, spoke of Christianity as the 'true philosophy'; however, by that he did not meant just a theory of religion but also a way of life.

It is not the history of the term which is decisive for us. If we move from conceptual history to real history, it is impossible to overlook the fact that, unlike Judaism, from its very beginning the two-thousand-year-old historical phenomenon of Christianity as a way of faith and life had to do quite essentially with a particular human name. However, when it comes to essentials, theologians are sometimes better at talking round the **substance** than calling it by its **name**. When we say in German 'the child needs a name', we mean that something needs a specific derivation, identification, basis. So if we ask quite basically why Christianity is Christianity, the answer can only be: because it does not have its **basis** in any principles, ideas or concepts, but in a **person**, who in ancient terminology is still called **Christ**. To be sure, that is an elementary answer. But as we shall see, this elementary answer proves extremely complex for theory and practice.

The name Christianity come from 'Christ' – which became the proper name of this person, the identification which distinguishes him from others. However, 'Christianity' is not a biblical term – perhaps one reason why Martin Luther rarely used the word. Yet it is almost as old as the phenomenon which it denotes. The word '**Christians**' already appears in the Acts of the Apostles, which reports that this name (perhaps as a nickname) appeared in Syrian Antioch, where the first Gentile Christians were living alongside the Jewish Christians who had fled from Jerusalem.[23] Possibly the word **Christianity** = *Christianismos* (like *Christos*, a Greek word) also first came into being in Antioch, in obvious analogy to the word Judaism = *Judaismos*,[24] which similarly denotes not only teaching and practice but also community. 'Christianity' appears for the first time around the year 110 in the letters of the bishop of this great Syrian metropolis, Ignatius, who, as he was being deported to Rome under the emperor Trajan's persecution, wrote to the Magnesians that they should live 'in accord with Christianity'.[25] In so doing he already differentiated Christianity extremely sharply from Judaism. He even thought that it was 'out of place to say Jesus Christ and to live as a Jew'.[26] By contrast, in Latin Christianity was simply called *Nomen christianum*, 'Christian name'.[27]

Concentration on Christ without christocentric narrowness

We may be amazed that already soon after the end of the first century a Gentile Christian bishop like Ignatius no longer wanted to have anything to do with a Jewish Christianity; however, we cannot mistake the fact that from the beginning the words 'Christ' and 'Christianity' are connected with this name Jesus Christ. Moreover he is constantly mentioned in the New Testament writings: as a historical person. This is also confirmed by the very first non-Christian witnesses from around the same time.

– **Flavius Josephus**, the Jewish historian. Around the year 90 in Rome, with clear reservations he reports the stoning of James, 'the brother of Jesus, the so-called Christ', which took place in 62.[28]

– **Gaius Plinius II**, the Roman governor in Bithynia, a province in Asia Minor. In 112 Pliny sent an enquiry to the emperor Trajan about the 'Christians', who were accused of many crimes. According to his interrogation, while they had refused to offer worship to the emperor, otherwise they seemed merely to have sung hymns to 'Christ as a god' and pledged to observe certain commandments (not to steal, rob, commit adultery, deceive).[29]

– **Cornelius Tacitus**, the great Roman historian and friend of Pliny. Somewhat later he reports the great fire of Rome: while in general the blame for this was put on the emperor Nero, Nero himself in turn had foisted it on the *Chrestiani. Chrestiani* (respectable citizens)? The word is said to stem from a 'Christus' who was executed in the time of Tiberius by the procurator Pontius Pilate, after whose death this 'pernicious superstition', like everything shameful and mean, had found its way to Rome, and after the fire had even gained a great host of followers.[30]

What this earliest Jewish and pagan evidence from the first and second centuries says about Christianity can be confirmed by countless witnesses from all twenty centuries, and indicates something that really should be taken for granted, yet is not. In essence, Christianity as '**religion**', i.e. as a **message and a way of salvation**, does not mean

- some eternal idea (whether of 'justice' or 'love')
- some dogma (however solemn)
- some world-view (even the best)
- but rather this all-determining significance of a concrete human figure, Jesus the Christ.

If first of all we leave aside everything that has been accumulated and piled up in the history of Christianity (in churches, theologies, legal ordinances, spiritualities, popular religion – we shall be talking about that at length later), at the **origin** of Christianity we find nothing but a person. With him alone we have the abiding **centre** of Christianity, and only in terms of him can the question of the **essence** of Christianity be answered.

So here I am primarily concerned with a **concentration on Christ**. But a concentration on Christ is **something different from christological narrowness**. So that we may avoid this from the start and keep the universal human horizon open on all sides, at this point I would like to formulate some interim questions.

Questions for the Future

Must a concentration on what is distinctively **Jewish** – Israel as God's own people and land – a priori exclude that one Jew from Nazareth in whose name Jewish belief in this one God was carried all over the world?

Must a concentration on what is distinctively **Islamic** – the Qur'an as the one God's word and book – not include authentic grappling with the history and message of that great prophet and messiah before Muhammad as he was described in Christian sources more than half a millennium earlier?

Must a concentration on what is distinctively **Christian** – this one person as God's Christ and Son – a priori lead to a sharp separation from the two other Abrahamic religions? Cannot essential connections be made with Judaism and Islam specifically from the Christian centre?

So let us attempt to define the essence of Christianity more precisely by coming to the centre of Christian faith. What forms the centre of Christianity? What is its basic form and original motive? What are its central structural elements?

B. The Centre

What could be said for Judaism applies even more to Christianity. Its 'centre' is not to be confused (in Hegelian fashion) with a 'basic concept', a 'basic idea' in comparison with which all other concepts and ideas of Christianity are only historical decisions and developments. Nor is its 'centre' (in dogmatic and orthodox fashion) to be confused with a 'basic principle' from which the whole of Christian faith can be constructed systematically. What, then, is the centre of Christianity?

I. Basic Form and Original Motif

We cannot deduce any unitary conceptual system or any coherent scholastic dogmatics from the New Testament any more than we can from the Hebrew Bible. Even if the New Testament writings, unlike those of the Hebrew Bible, in all span barely a century, historical criticism has shown how many different traditions, strata and theologies are to be distinguished even in the New Testament. But here too the question is no less urgent: given all the multiplicity, is there no connection between traditions and strata, persons and theologies?

1. What is common to the foundation documents of Christianity

Is the New Testament just a conglomerate of basically different writings which have no common denominator? Or is it more?[1]

Despite all the differences, a basic figure

There is no disputing one fact, which only a blind and dogmatically blinkered person could fail to perceive: the **different character**, the randomness, indeed partly also the contradictoriness of **the writings collected together in the New Testament**. There are Gospels which report above all discourses and miracles from the past, and prophetic letters which relate to the present and future. Extensive systematic doctrinal works stand along relatively unplanned answers to questions asked by those to whom they are addressed. The scope ranges from a brief occasional letter to the master of a runaway slave, barely two pages long, to a rather lengthy description of the acts of the first generation and its main figures. Some writings are stylish, others rough; in language and thought-world some come from Aramaic-speaking Jews, others from Greek-speaking Jewish or Gentile Christians; some really come from the author whose name they bear (authentic letters of Paul) and others are only attributed to the author concerned (pseudepigrapha); some were written very early (around 50), the last a long time after Jesus' death (around 100).

The **question** certainly arises: what really holds together the twenty-seven 'books' of the New Testament, which are so different – and the authors and communities behind them?

According to the evidence, the **answer** itself is astonishingly simple. It is the name of a Jew, **Jesus** of Nazareth, to whom his followers gave the loftiest honorific titles that Jews could give anyone. *Maschiach* (Hebrew), *Meschiach* (Aramaic), *Christos* (Greek) means the one anointed or sent by God. Jesus as God's Christ is the **basic figure** who holds together all the New Testament histories and parables, letters and missives, and also the Jewish Christian and Gentile Christian communities which are all so different. The abbreviated biblical formula is 'Jesus Christ'.

By contrast, there is absolutely nothing about Jesus of Nazareth in those famous scrolls which were found between 1947 and 1956 in the caves near the ruins of the destroyed settlement of **Qumran** by the Dead Sea.

A secret file on Jesus?

Since as early as 1974 serious scholarly literature has demonstrated in detail both the common features and the unbridgeable differences between Jesus and his community of disciples on the one hand and the Essenes and the Qumran community on the other (and already at that time virtually all the relevant texts were known).[2] One can only be amazed how some sensationalist authors who are not to be regarded as serious scholars have succeeded with the help of the media in leading millions astray with their claim that the Catholic Church and especially the Vatican have sought to suppress the truth about Jesus with repressive methods ('a secret file on Jesus'[3]). Although in this connection I myself am mentioned as a victim of Vatican repression, despite my battle with the

Roman Inquisition, in the face of these 'disclosures' I feel obliged to make the following **clarifications**:

– There has never been a Vatican conspiracy to suppress the truth of Qumran; but such widely accepted fantasies are indications of a crisis of confidence in the Catholic Church: people no longer believe the Vatican, which today is once again repressive and authoritarian, but think it capable of anything.

– The occasion for such rumours was provided by that self-seeking, narrow-minded and at the same time inefficient group of seven scholars of different confessions (but unfortunately, in what at that time was Jordanian East Jerusalem, without a single Jew) who wanted to publish absolutely all the fragments (around 100,000 of them, some only the size of a postage stamp) themselves, and thus did not make much headway.

– At the same time there is a manifestation here of the failure of an academic theology which constantly proves incapable or unwilling to make known the results of its research in understandable language to a wider public; but there is also a manifestation of the failure of church governments, who keep the results of criticial exegesis and history as far from the communities as possible (what people do not hear mentioned in the Sunday sermon they then pick up in a completely uninformed way on the television).

– None of this excuses those sharp publishers and media whose business is folly: allegedly scientific literature which does nothing but satisfy the desire of the masses for the religious, mysterious, occult and scandalous. But those looking for reasons for turning their backs on Christianity can in no way refer to this 'Dead Sea Scrolls deception' or to Jesus' (alleged) pseudo-death, the Turin Shroud (which is inauthentic),[4] Jesus' journey to India (which is a complete invention),[5] and similar fantasies or conspiracy theories.[6] They must give more solid reasons for their departure.

As for **questions of substance**, it is utterly beyond question that the Qumran writings offer an important insight into Jewish society and religion immediately before the appearance of Jesus and the rise of the first community of Christian disciples.[7] Serious Qumran research does not polarize Jews and Christians, but brings them together. For in many details, above all linguistic, the Qumran writings help us to understand the New Testament better (for example the phrase 'Son of God' appears both in the Psalms and in a Qumran fragment). Finally, they are related to the whole sphere of Jewish faith and culture, the seed-bed of Christianity.

Even if it is impossible to define clearly the function of the settlement which was presumably destroyed in 68 CE by the Romans, the majority of scholars still rightly assume that this was an Essene or sectarian settlement which cultivated its own radical observance of the Torah there in the wilderness by the Dead Sea. The following points are important in connection with the problems connected with earliest Christianity:

– The radio carbon tests carried out by the Israeli authorities in 1991 confirm that all the relevant Qumran writings were composed before the appearance of Jesus, in the second and first centuries BCE (at most, copies of earlier writings are of a later date).

– According to the sources known to us, neither John the Baptist nor Jesus himself nor his brother James nor the apostle Paul had anything to do with Qumran.

– In particular, Jesus' name is not mentioned once or hinted at, even in a cryptic form, in any of the writings which have been made known in the meantime; the identification of him with the 'Teacher of Righteousness', the unknown priest who founded the order and was active between 150 and 100 BCE, rests on blatant misdating and misinterpretation.

– So there are no traces of Christianity whatsoever in the Qumran writings (certainly not of a messiah who has come and indeed has been crucified and raised). On the contrary, the repeated baths, shared meals, shared possessions and hierarchy typical of Qumran are strikingly different from the practices of Jesus and his community of disciples.[8]

2. What holds Christian history together

Is the history of Christianity simply a quite arbitrary and contradictory sequence of contrasting ideas or events which are held together by nothing and nobody? Or is it more?

Despite all the contradictions, a basic motif

Similarly, all the rifts, jumps and breaks, contrasts and **contradictions** in church tradition and **in the history of Christianity generally** cannot be disputed, and only an ideological church historian could want to harmonize them and paper over the cracks. Thus developments took place almost in accordance with sociological 'laws': the small communities become a large organization, the minority becomes a majority, the underground church becomes a state church, the persecuted become rulers, and the rulers often in their turn become persecutors . . . Which century is the truly Christian century? That of the Neronian martyrs or that of the bishops of Constantine's court, that of the Irish and Scottish monks or that of the great mediaeval church politicians?

Think of all that Christianity has gone through! Centuries of barbarian converts in the rise of Europe and centuries of the Roman empire refounded by German emperors and Roman popes, to be ruined once again. Centuries of Crusades and persecution of the Jews, centuries of papal synods and of reform councils pressing the Pope. Christianity has experienced both the golden age of the humanists and Renaissance men and the great church revolution of the Reformers, who in turn were followed by the Counter-Reformation and the Inquisition: eras of baroque Catholic and also Lutheran-Calvinist orthodoxy, and then again eras of evangelical revival; periods of adaptation and periods of resistance, dark centuries and the *siècle des lumières*, phases of innovation and phases of restoration, times of despair and times of hope.

Indeed, here too the **question** becomes pressing: what really holds together the twenty centuries of Christian history and tradition, which are so tremendously contradictory?

The **answer**, here too an elementary one, can only be: it is the name of that **Jesus** who through the centuries has been called God's eschatological prophet and emissary, God's representative and son. The name of Jesus Christ is rather like a golden thread in the ever-renewed fabric of Christian history, which is so often torn and dirty: the binding **primal motif** in Christian tradition, liturgy, theology and piety which is never simply lost, for all the decadence.

That is still true today. One need only ask: what do such different figures of our century as the Jewish philosopher Edith Stein (died 1942) and the resistance fighter Dietrich Bonhoeffer (died 1945), the American civil rights fighter Martin Luther King (died 1968), the Salvadoran archbishop Oscar Romero (died 1980) and the Polish priest Jerzy Popieluszko (died 1984) have in common? They were Christians, and all fought non-violently under authoritarian regimes of violence for a more humane life for their contemporaries. They were all killed with brute force and thus came to resemble their model, the crucified Nazarene.

That brings us to a first answer to the question of the **centre** of Christianity; it may be general, but it is basic and definite:

- Without Jesus Christ there would have been no gathering of the New Testament writings and communities: he is the **basic figure** who holds together all the traditions (which are not, however, completely heterogeneous).
- Without Jesus Christ there would have been no history of Christianity and the Christian churches: he is the **basic motif** which holds them

together over and beyond all the breaks, which binds the historical eras together (though these are not totally different).

• The name of Jesus Christ, which had already become a proper name in New Testament times, is thus the **abidingly valid, constantly obligatory** and **simply indispensable** element in Christianity.

Instead of an abstract principle, a concrete person

So Christianity does not stand or fall by an impersonal idea, an abstract principle, a universal norm, a purely conceptual system. Unlike some other religions, Christianity stands and falls by a concrete person, who represents a cause, a whole way of life: Jesus of Nazareth. He himself is the embodiment of a new 'way of life'.

In fact Jesus does not proclaim any eternal ideas. So none of the 'eternal ideas' stands at the centre of Christianity, but a **tangible** person. Ideas, principles, norms and systems are characterized by clarity and particularity, simplicity and stability, and can be thought and expressed. But detached, abstracted from the particular and the individual, they appear monochrome and lacking in reality: abstraction almost necessarily leads to a lack of differentiation, to rigidity and a relative void in content, all sicklied over with the pale cast of thought. In short, by their very nature, ideas, principle, norms, systems, lack the mobility of life; they cannot be grasped in images, nor do they have the inexhaustible wealth of empirical concrete existence which cannot be comprehended in thought.

Jesus is different – a concrete person! So being a Christian must be different! And not only the New Testament, but the history of twenty centuries, shows this. As a concrete person Jesus has stimulated not only thought and critical, rational discussion but always also fantasy, imagination and emotions, spontaneity, creativity and innovation. As a person he made it possible for men and women to enter into a direct existential relationship with him in the Spirit: people could tell stories about him and not just reason, argue, discuss and theologize about him. And just as no history can be replaced by abstract ideas, so in the case of Jesus no narrative could be replaced by proclamation and appeals, no images could be replaced by concepts, no being grasped could be replaced by grasping.[9] The person could not be reduced to a particular definitive formula.

It is precisely this that constitutes the specific character of Christianity: **not a principle but a living figure**, who can be 'attractive' in the deepest and most comprehensive sense of the word: *verba docent, exempla trahunt* – words teach, examples attract. Indeed, Christians are not just to realize a general 'Christian' form of life but can attempt to trust in this

Christ Jesus whose spirit is still at work, and direct their lives in accordance with this criterion. So in all that he is and means for human beings Jesus himself proves – as the Gospel of John interprets it – to be 'the way, the truth and the life'.[10]

But what is special about this name, this person? **The history of his influence** gives us no answers, or at best **confusing answers**, since reformers and heretics, saints and villains, pious people and hypocrites, the moral and the immoral, the powerful and the helpless have all appealed to him. Only the **history of his origin** gives us a **clear answer**, and if we want to avoid any christocentric narrowness here we must investigate the New Testament foundation documents, indeed the basic message of the New Testament, to define what is special, typical, characteristic and specific about the Christian religion. So we shall attempt to find a concrete and at the same time brief answer to the question: in the different foundation documents of Christian faith, what is the

– constant presupposition (not a principle)?
– normative basic conception (not a dogma)?
– driving force (not a law)?

Here we are concerned with the central structural elements of Christian faith:
– in the one God as the constant presupposition,
– in Jesus the Christ as the normative basis,
– in the Holy Spirit as the driving force.

II. The Central Structural Elements

So many people are longing for an orientation in life. Where do we come from? Where are we going? That is answered by faith in the one God.

So many people are asking for directions. What should we go by? These are given quite specifically by faith in Jesus, the one Lord.

So many people are wanting courage and joy in life. Where do we get the power? This is given by faith in the one Spirit.

1. Belief in the one God

'There are varieties of gifts, but only the **one Spirit**.
There are varieties of service, but only the **one Lord**.
There are varieties of working, but only the **one God**,
who inspires them all in every one.'

Thus the apostle Paul in his first letter to the community of Corinth.[1]

What the three prophetic religions have in common

It is of fundamental importance for a present-day understanding between Jews and Christians that Christians, too, believe in the one God of Abraham, Isaac and Jacob, the God of Israel. The rejection of a Jewish God of creation, righteousness and the law in favour of a Christian God of the gospel, grace and love, such a repudiation of the Hebrew Bible for the sake of a radical concentration on and reduction to the gospel of Jesus Christ, which Marcion, the shipowner and bishop's son, had put forward as early as the first half of the second century, was rejected and excluded by the young Christianity of the time once and for all as arch-heresy. As we heard, Paul himself disavows Marcion, who allegedly appealed to him as the only one who really understood Jesus.

Thus from the beginning, Christianity along with Judaism and then Islam proves to be a typically **prophetic religion**, which is distinct both from the Indian mystical and the Chinese wisdom type of religion:[2] the decisive initiative in the event of salvation has been taken by **God**, with whom human beings are not one by nature and cannot be one by any human effort, but 'before' whom (before whose 'face') they act and in whom they may trust in faith.

That means that from the beginning, like Judaism, so too Christianity and then Islam are not governed by a unitive mysticism as in India or a world harmony as in China but – metaphorically speaking – by the **contrast** between God and human beings. Thus Christianity, like the other two prophetic religions, is a religion of the **confrontation** of God and human beings, the holy God and sinful human beings. But through God's **word** to human beings and through human **faith** in God it becomes a religion of **communication.**

So before working out in any way what is specifically Christian, it is important to stress just how much **Christianity has in common with Judaism and Islam**:

- **faith in one and the same God of Abraham,** the ancestor of all three religions,[3] who according to all the traditions is the great witness to this one true living God, who may be addressed in lamentation, praise and prayer. All three are religions of faith;
- a **view of history** which does not think in cosmic cycles but is **directed towards a goal**: it has its beginning in God's creation, is confirmed by God's action and saving signs in time, and is directed towards an end through God's consummation. These are religions which think historically;
- the ever new proclamation of the word and will of God by a whole series of **prophetic figures**. These are religions with a prophetic, not a mystical, stamp;
- the record of a revelation to human beings, given once and for all and remaining normative, in the form of a **revelatory writing**. These are religions of the word and the book;
- finally, a **basic ethic** of an elemental humanity grounded in the will of the one God: the Ten (or similar) Commandments of God (the Decalogue). These are religions with an ethical orientation.

A shared Jewish-Christian-Muslim basic ethic

Already in my study of Judaism it became clear that even the commandments and prohibitions contained in the Bible are mediated through human beings. Even the ethical demands of the Torah, the 'instruction', the 'five books of Moses', have not simply fallen from heaven, either in content or in form.[4] What is immediately evident in the case of the ethic of the prophets and wisdom literature is also true of the instructions of the Torah, the Five Books of Moses. We know today that the whole long Sinai history[5] consists of many levels of material containing divine ordinances which reflect different phases of time. And even the famous Ten Commandments – 'the Ten Words',[6] which we have in two versions[7]

The Common Basic Ethic

     †   ☾

The Jewish-Christian Decalogue	**The Islamic Code of Duties**
(Exodus 20.1-21)	(Surah 17.22-38)

I am the Lord your God.	In the Name of God, the merciful Lord of mercy.
You shall have no other gods besides me.	Set up no other deity alongside (the one) God.
You shall not make for yourselves any image of God. You shall not take the name of the Lord your God in vain.	Your Lord has commanded that you serve no one but Him.
Remember the sabbath day, to keep it holy.	
Honour your father and mother.	Show kindness to your parents. Give to the kinsman his due and to the needy and the wayfarer.
You shall not kill.	Do not kill your children for fear of poverty. Do not kill any man – a deed God forbids.
You shall not commit adultery.	Do not come near to adultery.
You shall not steal.	Handle the property of the orphan with integrity.
You shall not bear false witness against your neighbour.	Keep your bond. For you are accountable.
You shall not covet your neighbour's house.	Give full measure when you measure and weigh with just scales. Do not pursue things of which you have no knowledge.
You shall not covet your neighbour's wife, or his manservant or his maidservant, or his ox, or his ass, or anything that is your neighbour's.	Do not strut proudly on the earth.
(Revised Standard Version)	*(Translated by Kenneth Cragg)*

– have undergone a history, and instructions from the so-called 'second table' (duties towards fellow human beings) derive from the moral and legal traditions of the pre-Israelite semi-nomadic tribes. One can find numerous analogies to this in the Near East. Doubtless a long period of practice, polishing and testing was needed for the Decalogue to become sufficiently universal and brief in content and form to be capable of being regarded as an adequate expression of the will of Yahweh.

Whatever the historical background, this is the significance of the message of **Sinai**: what distinguish Israelites and Jews are not the individual commandments or prohibitions in themselves but **faith in Yahweh**, for which all these commandments and prohibitions express the will of Yahweh himself. So it is not these fundamental minimal demands, the origins of which preceded faith in Yahweh, that are specifically Israelite. What is specifically Israelite is that these commands were subjected to the authority of Yahweh, the covenant God, who is the 'object' of the 'first table' (duties towards God).

The new faith in Yahweh has **consequences for the previous ethics**: now these demands, like other series of commandments, in so far as they were compatible with faith in Yahweh, sketch out with the utmost possible brevity Yahweh's will for human beings. Now it is Yahweh himself who in the commandments watches over elementary humanity, and this is safeguarded in the 'second table' with reference to respect for parents, the protection of life, marriage, property and the honour of neighbours. So the distinctive feature of Old Testament morality does not consist in discovering new ethical norms but in rooting instructions which have been handed down in the authority of Yahweh and his covenant, in order to legitimate and protect them; it consists in incorporating a pre-existing ethic into the new relationship with God. This theonomy presupposes the autonomous development of ethical norms and at the same time also sets it in motion again: in the light of this God and his covenant there is further development and correction of the existing norms – not, however, consistently in all areas (marriage, the position of women).

So **God himself is the advocate of humanity**, of true humanity. Thus norms which came into being autonomously on the basis of human experiences, along with their evaluation, do not appear in the Torah as impersonal laws but as requirements of God himself. There is an unconditional 'You shall', backed up not by a human or state authority but by God's word and will: 'Thus says the Lord your God.' This is particularly true of the Decalogue, those 'Ten Words' which are indispensable for an ethic of humanity; they are elementary imperatives of humanity. Christianity appropriated these 'Ten Commandments' (apart from the one relating to the sabbath), and towards the end of the Mecca period the Qur'an, too, offers a summary of the most important ethical obligations (with many striking parallels to the Decalogue – again except that relating to the sabbath). Consequently, as I already remarked in the context of Judaism, we can speak of a **basic ethic common to the three prophetic religions**, grounded in God's word and will, which could be a highly significant contribution to the **global ethic** that needs to be formed.

What Christianity has in common particularly with Judaism

To the present day, belief in the one God of the Jewish 'fathers' also remains the **abiding presupposition** of Christian faith, which, like Jewish faith, knows no rival God of evil, and also rejects any female consort deity.[8] Moreover, this God is already addressed as **'Father'** in post-exilic Judaism.[9] But this is not meant to be a sexist emphasis on the masculinity of God and the inferiority of woman, who indeed according to the book of Genesis is created, like man, in God's image.[10] Rather, after the collapse of state structures God was to be invoked in his protective function as supreme head of the family. God's power, God's protection is meant, not God's 'masculinity'. To this degree, while this image of God excludes any polytheism, it does not exclude feminine traits.

But what Christianity has in common with **Judaism** in particular here goes very much further. On the basis of the traditions of the Hebrew Bible, Christian faith also recognizes the **three covenants of the one God**,[11] who indeed is the God of all human beings:
– the **Noah covenant** with the whole creation, the sign of which is the rainbow (Adam = man: all humankind);
– the **Abraham covenant** with Abrahamic humankind, the sign of which is circumcision (Abraham, the father of many peoples: Judaism – Christianity – Islam);
– the **Sinai covenant** with the people of Israel, the sign of whose covenant is the altar and the ark (Jacob = Israel, the father of the twelve tribes, the people of Israel).

Thus at the same time it has become clear that because Christianity believes in the one God of the Hebrew Bible, in principle it accepts the central structural elements and leading concepts of Israelite-Jewish faith:[12]
– **Exodus**: an election of the people of Israel, which the Jews understand not as a proud claim but as grace and obligation.
– **Sinai**: the making of the covenant and its obligation, as this is expressed in the lawgiving (Torah).

– **Canaan**: the promise of the land, which goes with the election of the people.

However, there is an unmistakable difference here: Christianity recognizes (at least again today) the reality of the elect people and the promised land in a concrete Judaism which is different from Christianity. But it has appropriated this to itself only in a complex **spiritualized** form: a people of God and a land of promise understood in spiritual terms. This spiritualization is connected with the history of that Jew whom Christians recognize as their one Messiah, Christ, Lord, but without ever giving up faith in the one God and Father or setting a second God alongside the one God. Let us look more closely at this.

2. Discipleship of Christ

It is fundamental to an understanding of the man from Nazareth[13] that the God of Israel is also his God. Like any devout Jew, he too stands over against this God, the 'Father in heaven'. He calls him 'greater',[14] indeed 'only good'.[15] And only in the Fourth Gospel, which is markedly interpretative, is a unity of will and revelation between Jesus and the Father stressed throughout, though here too this never does away with the contrast between God and Jesus.[16] But precisely in both the contrast and the unity with God his Father, Jesus is the central figure of Christianity.

The central figure

I can summarize here what I developed at length in *On Being a Christian* and demonstrated from the New Testament: Jesus made the **cause of the God of Israel** his own, governed by the typically apocalyptic expectation of living in an end-time, in which God himself will very soon appear on the scene and impose his will, establish his rule and realize his kingdom. Jesus wanted to announce in advance this kingdom, this rule, this will of God, **with a view to human salvation**. This alone he made the criteria. So he called not only for the renewed observance of God's commandments but for a **love** which in individual instances extends to unselfish service without hierarchy, to renunciation even without receiving anything in return, to boundless forgiving. It is a love which even includes the opponent, the enemy: love of God and love of neighbour in accordance with the criterion of self-love ('as yourself').

So Jesus **shows solidarity**, in a quite practical way which scandalizes the pious, with those of another religious faith, the politically compromised, the moral failures, the sexually exploited – especially with women,

**Jesus in the Cross of Co-ordinates
of Options within Judaism**

Establishment
(Sadducees)

Prophetic provocation

Not a priest

Against ascetism

Not a monk

of God

Love

Not a rabbi

Against legalism

Emigration   of neighbour   **Compromise**
(Qumran people)   (Pharisees)

Not a revolutionary

Against violence

Revolution
(Zealots)

God's will = human well-being = love

children and the sick, indeed with all those who had been forced to the periphery of society. He used his charismatic gift of healing for all of these – he did not just proclaim the word but healed the body – and did so even on the sabbath. By the criterion of love, particular precepts of the Law, particular regulations about food, cleanness and the sabbath were secondary for him – although in principle he himself observed the Law; he believed that the sabbath and the commandments were there for the sake of human beings.

Without doubt here was a man as provocative as a prophet, who in word and deed also showed that he was critical of the Temple and demonstrated against the commerce prevalent there. He was a man who exploded the usual schemes and would not be enlisted on any front. He was in conflict with the political-religious establishment (not a priest or theologian), yet no political revolutionary either (rather, a preacher of non-violence). He was no advocate of migration, either physical or

Jesus in the Cross of Co-ordinates of the World Religions

Moses
Prototype of the prophet

Moral mastery of the world
(Torah)

↑

not a lawgiver
and leader of the people

Buddha
Prototype of the enlightened

Monastic renunciation
of the world
(meditation)

not a mystic
and monk

Jesus Christ

Not a scholar
and teacher
of the virtues

Confucius
Prototype of the wise

Moral ordering of the world
(Harmony)

Not a military leader
and statesman

↓

Muhammad
'Seal' of the prophets

Religious conquest of the world
(theocracy)

spiritual (he was not an ascetic or a Qumran monk), nor was he a pious casuistic lawyer (not a Pharisee full of 'joy in the commandment'). To this extent Jesus of Nazareth differed not only from the great representatives of the Indian-mystic and Chinese-wisdom traditions (Buddha and Confucius) but also from the two other Near Eastern Semitic religions (Moses and Muhammad).

He was quite evidently a great enthusiastic-prophetic figure who, without any special office or special title, with his words and saving actions transcended the claim of a mere rabbi or prophet, so that some saw him as the Messiah. To justify himself in the great conflict into which he was increasingly drawn, he referred to none other than God himself, whom he used to address with unusual familiarity as 'Abba' ('Dear Father'). No wonder that he was drawn into a **conflict**:

– His criticism of traditional religion was too radical for many of the pious.

– His public protest against the Temple trading and those who guarded and exploited the Temple seemed too arrogant.

– His understanding of the Law, focussed as it was on human beings, was too provocative.

– His solidarity with the common people unversed in the Law and his dealing with notorious lawbreakers was too scandalous.

– His criticism of the ruling circles, to whom he was a problem because of his large following among the people, was too massive.

I have dealt at length in *Judaism* with this whole conflict of the man from Nazareth, not with the people but with the official authorities of the Judaism of the time, the hierarchy, which handed him over to the Roman governor Pontius Pilate (in a legal process which today is no longer clear); here too I want to recall some elements of the cross of co-ordinates given there.

The scandal of the cross

We now need to bring out more clearly a decisive point for determining what is specifically Christian, which hitherto has caused difficulties not only for Jews and Muslims and the adherents of other religions but also for many Christians: the significance of the **cross**[17] as a distinguishing mark of Christians. Already at this one point it becomes abundantly clear that the popular verdict that all religions and their 'founders' are the same is an untenable prejudice. If one merely compares the deaths of the founders, the differences are unmistakable: Moses, Buddha and Kung-Fu-Tse all died at a good old age, after rich success, amongst their disciples and followers, 'full of life' like the patriarchs of Israel; Muhammad even in the arms of his favourite wife after enjoying a good life in his harem. And Jesus of Nazareth? He died as a young man after an amazingly brief activity of at best three years, perhaps only a few months: betrayed and denied by his disciples and followers; mocked and scorned by his opponents; abandoned by God and his fellow human beings in the most abominable and thorough rite of dying, which according to Roman jurisprudence could not be inflicted on criminals who were Roman citizens, but only on slaves and political rebels: the cross.

It is understandable that even long after the abolition of this punishment by the emperor Constantine, down to the fifth century Christians avoided representations of Jesus suffering on the cross. This only became customary to any great extent in mediaeval Gothic – and then unfortunately all too much. And it is even more understandable that neither a Jew nor a Greek nor a Roman could have arrived at the idea of attaching a positive, even religious, sense to these gallows of the ostracized. The **cross of Jesus** must have seemed a barbaric folly to an educated Greek, a scandal to a Roman citizen, a divine curse to a believing Jew. So why for Christians was it a **sign of salvation?**

We have simply to note that just as the cross is a harsh, cruel and undeniable historical fact, so it is an equally undeniable fact that the very first generation of Christians already saw the cross of Jesus in quite a different light. Why? In short, because on the basis of particular charismatic experiences ('appearances', visions, auditions) and at the same time a biblical pattern of interpretation, they had come to the conclusion that the crucified Jesus had not remained dead but had been **raised** by God **to eternal life,**[18] **exalted** to God's glory. However the details of this are to be understood, he had not died into nothingness but into the most real reality, at any rate into God himself.

Soon people began to sing the songs of the psalter, understood messianically, in honour of the one who had been raised from the dead, especially the enthronment psalms. A Jew of the time could easily understand the exaltation to God in analogy to the enthronement of the Israelite king. Just as the king was **appointed 'son of God'** at the moment of his accession, probably taking up the kingship ideology of the ancient Near East, so now the crucified Jesus was appointed 'son of God' through his resurrection and exaltation.

In particular it may have been Psalm 110, in which King David celebrated his future 'son', who at the same time was his 'Lord', which was sung and quoted time and again: 'The Lord said to my lord, "Sit at my right hand!"'. For this verse answered the burning question of the Jewish followers of Jesus as to the 'place' and function of the risen Christ.[19] Where is the Risen Christ now? The answer could be given: with the Father, 'at the right hand of the Father', not in a communion of being but in a 'throne communion' with the Father, so that the kingdom of God and the kingdom of the Messiah were in fact identical: 'Thus the appointment of the crucified Messiah Jesus as the "Son" to the Father "through the resurrection of the dead" is probably the earliest message common to all preachers, with which the "heralds of the Messiah" called on their own people to repent and believe in the "Messiah of Israel" who had been crucified and raised by God and exalted to his right hand.'[20]

So faith in the one who was crucified and yet is alive through and with God made an inconceivable claim for that time: this man who had suffered a shameful execution was the one confirmed by God with power, so that this **sign of shame** was a sign **of victory.** Indeed, this dishonourable death of a slave and rebel could finally be understood as a saving death bringing redemption and liberation. The cross of Jesus, this bloody seal on a life of sacrifice, thus became a summons to the renunciation of a life shaped by selfishness, a call to an unpretentious life for others.

This was no more and no less than a **revaluation of all values** – as Nietzsche rightly detected in his invectives against Christianity. But what is meant by this is not a way of narrowness and weak self-abasement, of the kind evidently communicated to the pastor's son Nietzsche as a child, a 'creeping to the cross'. What is meant, rather, is bold everyday life without anxiety, even in the face of deadly risks, through the battle which is now unavoidable, through all suffering and even through death. Everything is to be done in unshakable trust ('faith') and in hope of the goal of true freedom, love, humanity and finally eternal life. The scandal *par excellence* had become an astonishing experience of salvation, the way of the cross a possible way of life for those who accepted it, who became Christians.

Of course the young Christian community could not cope all at once with the tremendous scandal of a crucified Messiah – indeed the legitimation of Jesus was the question of the spiritual survival of the community. The confusion of Jesus' disciples was not simply removed by the Easter experience. At every level the various New Testament writings are steeped in this **grappling with the cross**, and it is no coincidence that the earliest consecutive narrative about Jesus is the story of his passion. Only with time was the cross recognized as the sum of Christian faith and life. For both the controversies within the communities and their justification of themselves to outsiders compelled a deep reflection which soon made it clear how much the Christian community on the one hand and Jews, Greeks and Romans on the other, indeed faith and unbelief, part company at the cross.

In the light of the Easter experience the initial disconsolateness and speechlessness was first replaced by the simple conviction that everything that had happened to Jesus must have taken place in accordance with God's counsels, that Jesus 'had' to go his way according to God's will. There were **models for this from the Hebrew Bible:**
– the prophet commissioned by God but persecuted by men;
– the servant suffering innocently and vicariously for the sins of many;
– the sacrifical animal which symbolically takes away the sins of humankind.

All these notions helped slowly to give significance to the cruel, meaningless event of the cross. They were not meant to propagate the archaic idea of a bloodthirsty and sadistic god who could only be satisfied by a human sacrifice, or the mythical ritual event of a god torn into fragments and restored to life again (like Dionysus). It was to become clear that what had happened with Jesus was not simply arbitrary or meaningless. Everything happened 'according to the scriptures', as people said, by which initially they meant the Hebrew Bible as a whole, which, if Jesus was Messiah, must necessarily refer to him everywhere.

However, to discover this they needed a kind of exegesis of their own which found the 'type' of the new throughout the 'Old Testament'. Was not for example the righteous man, depicted in the prophet Isaiah[21] in the Servant Songs, such a clear pointer to Christ? And could not the Hebrew Bible, thus understood, increasingly be interpreted in terms of the cross and, conversely, the cross increasingly be interpreted in terms of the Hebrew Bible, so that it proved more and more clearly that in Jesus, too, and particularly in him, God, the God of Israel, had in fact acted in person? On a large scale we have such a developed 'theology of the cross' on the one hand in narrative form in the earliest of the four Gospels, in Mark, and on the other in the thorough discussion in the letters of the apostle Paul. The word of the cross became the great Christian answer to the age-old question of the incomprehensibility of suffering and above all of innocent suffering.

Christianity as radical humanism

Now we have a clear definition of what is **distinctively Christian** – in contrast not only to Judaism but also to all religions and humanisms: **what is distinctively Christian is this Christ himself, who was crucified and yet is alive.** And faith in this Christ is truly no empty formula, nor merely a doctrinal formula. For:

- Faith in Christ relates to a very concrete historical person, Jesus of Nazareth. So it has behind it the beginnings of Christianity, and also the whole great tradition of 2000 years: what can refer to this Christ is Christian.
- Faith in Christ is expressed not only in a message but also in tangible rituals: in baptism in his name and in the meal celebrated in his memory.
- At the same time faith in Christ offers a fundamental pointer to the present and the future: Jesus Christ does not bring a new law, but love as the normative basic notion for Christian life and action, suffering and dying.

As New Testament research shows,[22] the ethical demands of the New Testament, too, did not drop from heaven either in form or in content. This applies to the ethics of the whole of the New Testament, but can be demonstrated particularly clearly from the ethical demands of the apostle

Paul. We should not speak a priori of a Pauline 'ethic', since Paul did not develop any system or casuistry of morality. Rather, he draws his admonition (paraenesis) largely from Hellenistic and especially Jewish tradition.

The household tables current in the Graeco-Roman ethics of the time (Epictetus, Seneca) with their admonitions to those in different positions do not appear in Paul himself, but only in the Letter to the Colossians[23] and the Letter to the Ephesians which is dependent on it, and in the Pastoral Letters and the Apostolic Fathers. However, Paul himself also already uses concepts and notions from the Hellenistic popular philosophy of his time. Clearly a **universal human ethic** and a **specifically Christian ethic** are not **mutually exclusive**. And while Paul only once uses the term 'virtue', which was central to philosophical ethics, at this one point in the Letter to the Philippians he so surrounds it with Greek and especially Stoic ethical conceptuality that we can see the result as something like a summary of customary Greek ethics: 'Whatever is true, whatever is honourable, whatever is just, whatever is pure, whatever is lovely, whatever is gracious, if there is any excellence, if there is anything worthy of praise, think on these things.'[24] However, in the other catalogues of virtues and vices[25] Paul then keeps more to the Jewish than to the Hellenistic tradition.

So what is specifically Christian[26] is not the making of some particular, intrinsically incomparable, ethical demand. There can also be other foundations for the ethical demands which Paul takes over from Jewish or Hellenistic tradition. Nor does Paul have any particular principle of synthesis or selection; rather, he uses different motives as the foundation for his ethical demands: kingdom of God, discipleship of Christ, eschatological kerygma, body of Christ, Holy Spirit, love, freedom, being in Christ. Even if he uses key words like obedience or freedom, these do not denote any systematic leading ideas, but simply the totality and indivisibility of the obligation of the believer and the believing community to its Lord.

So what is specifically Christian is that all ethical demands are understood in the light of Jesus Christ, crucified and risen. Jesus, to whom Christians **are** subject once for all in baptism, through faith, **should** remain their Lord. All this means that just as belief in Yahweh is the distinctive feature of Jewish ethics, so **belief in Christ** is **the distinctive feature** of **Christian ethics**. All the individual commandments or prohibitions are to be understood and observed in the light of Jesus Christ and his spirit. So we now have confirmation in the other direction, from ethics, that the starting point in defining what is Christian is not an abstract principle but this concrete Jesus Christ.

Now in this perspective, being a Christian can be understood as a truly radical humanism: as a **humanism**, because being a Christian comprises being human to the full. Christians are no less humanists than those humanists who give their humanity an un-Christian, anti-Christian, indeed anti-religious foundation or no foundation at all. No Christian need be afraid of using the term humanism. But Christians advocate a **radical** humanism. In this human life which is so divided, in this society which is so full of conflict, they not only affirm all that is true, good, beautiful and human, as an idealistic neo-humanism said, but also confront the untrue, the ungood, the unbeautiful and indeed the inhuman, which are no less real. Certainly, even Christians cannot do away with all these negative features of human life and society (that would be another pernicious illusion leading to a contemptuous compulsive back-slapping and mass slavery), but they can endure, fight against and assimilate the negative.

In this way and only in this way it is also possible to attain true **happiness** in this life (though it will by no means be free of suffering): not through peak experiences produced artificially by every possible means; not through a constant lofty mood of happiness which has to be striven for; but through a basic mood of happiness in realistic contentment with life which is maintained even in distress, and in the depths of the soul. All this means that being a Christian is an attempt to achieve a humanism which can cope not only with all that is positive but also with all that is negative, like suffering, guilt, meaninglessness and death, in an unshakable trust in God which in the end does not rely on its own achievements and successes but on God's grace and mercy.

But what help is this great leading figure of the past, if today he no longer has a present or a future? How is Christ continually to become present, to have a future? How can Christians gain courage and joy in life from this faith in Christ? For this, the third central structural element of Christian faith is of essential significance: belief in God's Spirit, in and through which Jesus lives and works.

3. The activity of the Holy Spirit

It is belief in the God of Abraham which unites Jews and Christians; however, it is belief in Jesus as God's Christ which distinguishes Christians from other believers and non-believers. Alongside these two central structural elements there is a third, which gives the faith of Christians its profile and at the same time can combine with other traditions: the power of the Spirit. For – on the basis of the New

Testament witnesses – Christians do not just believe in an isolated event of the resurrection of the dead, brought about in Jesus the crucified one; they also believe that this risen Christ now continues to live, rule and work in the Spirit of God. How is that to be understood?

What is the Spirit?

Here too we do best to approach from the **Jewish tradition**. According to the Hebrew Bible and then also the New Testament, God is spirit, Hebrew feminine *ruach*, which originally means breath, breeze, wind. Tangible yet intangible, invisible yet powerful, as important to life as the air that one breathes, laden with energy like the wind, the storm – that is the spirit. What is meant is none other than the **living force and power** emanating from God, which works invisibly in both the individual and the people of Israel, in the church and in the world generally. This spirit is **holy** in so far as it is distinguished from the unholy spirit of human beings and their world: as the spirit of **God**. The understanding of Christian faith is that it is the driving force (*dynamis*, not law) in Christianity.[27]

But we should beware of misunderstandings: in the light of the New Testament the Holy Spirit is not – as often in the history of religions – some third element distinct from God which is between God and human beings; it is not a magical, substantial, mysterious-supernatural fluid of a dynamic kind (no spiritual 'something'), nor is it a magic being of an animistic kind (some spiritual being or ghost). Rather, the **Holy Spirit is none other than God himself.** God himself, in so far as he is near to human beings and the world, indeed works inwardly as the power which grasps but cannot be grasped, as a life-giving but also judging force, as a grace which gives but is not under our control. So as God's Spirit, the Spirit can no more be separated from God than the sunbeam from the sun. Thus if we ask how the invisible, intangible, incomprehensible God is near and present to believers, the answer of the New Testament is unanimous. **God is near** to us human beings **in the Spirit**: present in the Spirit, through the Spirit, indeed as Spirit. And Christ?

In connection with the person of the crucified and risen Christ this means:
– Jesus Christ taken up to God and exalted now also lives in God's mode of existence and activity. Therefore Paul can quite consistently call the risen Christ 'the life-giving Spirit',[28] indeed can speak of him as 'Spirit',[29] and conversely speak of the Spirit of God as the 'Spirit of Jesus Christ'.[30] Specifically, this means that through the Spirit, in the Spirit and as Spirit, Jesus can be near to his community – whether in worship or in service of one's neighbour, whether in the community or in the

heart of the individual – helping, encouraging, comforting, judging.
– But this christological perspective must not lead to neglect of another
perspective which is also attested in the Bible: the **Spirit of Jesus Christ is
and remains God's Spirit**. And this Spirit of the incomprehensible,
infinite, immeasurable is at work not only in Christianity but – as we
already read on the first page of the Hebrew Bible at the very beginning[31]
– throughout creation, everywhere. According to the New Testament,
too, God's Spirit is at work '**where** he wills',[32] and his activity cannot be
limited by any church. In other words, God's Spirit works not only in
Christianity but throughout the world. What does that mean?

Prophets even after Christ

Certainly the free Spirit of God is not a spirit of arbitrariness, of pseudo-
freedom, but a spirit of true freedom; it is not a spirit of chaos but a spirit
of just order. But it works **when** it wills, and no church order in teaching
and praxis can compel it to act or not act now. No, the Spirit of God
works when and where it wills, as on that **feast of Pentecost** on which,
according to the tradition of the evangelist Luke, the first 'assembly' took
place in Jerusalem of the followers of Jesus who had returned (above all)
from Galilee and among whom **the birth of the 'church'** (Hebrew *kahal*,
Greek *ekklesia* = assembly) took place in enthusiastic charismatic
circumstances. So the Spirit is also at work in the later history of
Christianity, and is, again, according to a saying of the Gospel of John, to
'lead into all truth'.[33]

And because the Spirit of God continues to work, according to what the
New Testament says there will be **authentic prophets even after the death
of Jesus**, people who, inspired by God's Spirit, confirm, interpret and
express him and his message for a new time and situation. Thus for
example in the Pauline communities (as emerges from the First Letter to
the Corinthians[34]) prophets, men and women, occupy the second place
after the apostles. The early church is built not only on the apostles but
also on the prophets.[35]

However, soon after the end of the Pauline mission and with the decline
of Jewish Christianity, prophecy disappeared from the phenomena found
in most Christian communities. But in the light of the New Testament we
cannot a priori and dogmatically object if even *after* Jesus new prophets
emerge who claim to stand in fundamental accord with his proclamation
of the will of God. The most prominent example in world history is
Muhammad – for Islam **the** Prophet, whose revelation in the Qur'an is
attributed to the 'Spirit' (however this is understood)[36] – and who is to be

taken with the utmost seriousness, say, in the face of an exaggerated christology.

Anyone who puts the Bible, especially the Hebrew Bible, and the Qur'an side by side will ask: Don't the **three religions of revelation** of Semitic origin, Judaism, Christianity and Islam, and don't especially the Hebrew Bible and the Qur'an, have the **same basis**? Doesn't one and the same God speak abundantly clearly in both? Doesn't the 'Thus says the Lord' of the Hebrew Bible correspond to the 'Say' of the Qur'an, the biblical 'Go and proclaim' to the Qur'anic 'Stand up and warn'? Indeed, the millions of Arabic-speaking Christians, too, know no other word for 'God' than 'Allah'! So isn't it perhaps merely a dogmatic prejudice if we recognize Amos and Hosea, Isaiah and Jeremiah and many others, as prophets who have been called, and not Muhammad?

The relationship between Christianity and Islam

For centuries the Qur'an was despised in the history of Christianity and the prophet Muhammad calumniated; the philosopher Karl Jaspers, whose thought was otherwise so universal, did not even want to include him in his book about 'normative people'.[37] Only today is a self-critical ecumenical theology recognizing the world-historical significance of this man for the history of **belief in one God** – which binds together Jews, Christians and Muslims. And without smoothing over the differences, a Christian theology can also concede today that:

– The people of seventh-century Arabia were right in listening to the voice of Muhammad;
– By the standard of their very this-worldly polytheism, the old Arabian tribal religions were elevated by the preaching of Muhammad to a quite different religious level, that of a monotheistic high religion;
– Hundreds of millions of people between Morocco and Bangladesh, between the steppes of Central Asia and the Indonesian archipelago, have received infinite inspiration, courage and power to make a new religious start from Muhammad – or better, from the Qur'an: a breakthrough to greater truth and deeper knowledge, a breakthrough which brings their traditional religion alive and renews it.

So it could basically be said of the **relationship between Christianity and Islam**:[38]

● Christians and Muslims believe in a single God and therefore in a single salvation history: just as Christians already regard Adam, Noah, Abraham and all the patriarchs of Israel as 'Christians' before Christ, so Muslims recognize the same patriarchs (whatever may be the historical position over the descent of Ishmael, which cannot be verified) and also Jesus as a 'Muslim' before Muhammad;

- For Christians this Muhammad (who bore witness to Jesus) is not a matter of indifference, nor can he any longer be dismissed as a pseudo-prophet, as though there were no more prophets after Christ;
- For Muslims this Jesus (to whom Muhammad also bore witness) has something of abiding importance to say with his gospel.
- So Christianity and Islam cannot be separated from each other as two totally different religions, but are interwoven as religious movements in the same way as Judaism and Christianity. Together they form a great religious river system of Near Eastern Semitic origin with a prophetic stamp, which differs from the two other great river systems – Indian mysticism and Chinese wisdom (not to mention the nature religions). In so far as Islam seeks again to inculcate the fundamental message of the one God, it has proved to be a great help, inspired by the Spirit of God, for countless people in living in accordance with the will of God.

The view of the Spirit in particular thus makes it possible for Christians to combine the preservation of Christian **identity** with the affirmation of religious **plurality**, a concentration on Christ with a **universal** humanity. In such an open attitude Christians can recognize humanity, fellowship and religion **wherever they appear,** not only in Judaism and Islam, but also in high religions of Indian or Chinese origin, in the nature religions and in religious and ethical groups of all kinds. Christians can recognize them **without commandeering them** a priori for Christianity (say as 'anonymous Christianity'), but also without appropriating them un-critically.

But – and this is the question of Christian identity in practice, against a universal horizon – what makes a person a Christian?

4. What makes a person a Christian?

So now we sum up and bring matters to a head. What is the ultimate distinguishing mark of Christianity? Here the circle is closed for our extremely brief introduction to the centre of Christian faith.

The ultimate distinguishing mark of Christianity

- *What distinguishes Christianity from the old world religions and modern humanisms is this* **Christ himself.** But what preserves our faith from any confusion of this Christ with other religious or political Christ figures?

- What distinguishes Christianity from the old religions and modern humanisms is the Christ who is identical with the real, historical Jesus of Nazareth; in other words it is specifically this **Christ Jesus**. But what preserves our faith from any confusion of this historical Jesus Christ with false images of Jesus?

- What distinguishes Christianity from the old world religions and modern humanisms, the ultimate distinguishing mark of Christianity, is quite literally, according to Paul, 'Jesus Christ and **him crucified**'.[39] He is the content of the gospel; believers are baptized in his name, and they commemorate his passion, death and new life in the eucharist. The cross – in a very different way from the seven- branched lampstand (Menorah) for Judaism and the crescent for Islam – is the real and central symbol for Christianity.

Therefore the evangelist John sees the distinguishing mark of Christianity in just the same way as Paul when, as we heard, though in very different conceptuality, he calls Jesus the way, the truth and the life[40] and illustrates this with the following images: he is the bread of life,[41] the light of the world,[42] the gate,[43] the true vine,[44] the true shepherd who gives his life for the sheep.[45] Here Jesus is evidently not a name which needs constantly to be uttered (saying 'Lord, Lord'). He is the way of the truth of life which is to be done. Indeed Christianity is throughout concerned with the **truth**. However, here 'truth' does not mean purely theoretical truths of reason but practical truths of faith, which are grounded in experience, decision and action. Indeed, the truth of Christianity is not to be 'seen', 'theorized', but to be 'done', '**practised**'. The Christian concept of truth is not contemplative and theoretical, like the Greek concept, but operative and practical. It is a truth which is not just to be sought and found, but to be followed and made true, guaranteed and preserved in truthfulness. It is a truth focussed on praxis, which calls people to a way which gives new life and makes new life possible.

So what makes a person a Christian? Not simply being human, social or religious, but attempting to live out one's humanity, social life and religion **by the criterion and in the spirit of this Christ** – for better or worse, as is the case with human nature. We shall be occupied later with what this means. But first of all we must ask: isn't the creed fundamental to becoming a Christian?

Shared short formulae of faith

Christian faith is not dumb faith. It knows what it believes and confesses what it knows. There can be no act of faith (*fides qua creditur*) without a

First Christian Confessions of Faith

One member:

'**Jesus** is Lord.'

(I Cor.12.3; cf. Rom.10.9)

Two members:

'For us there is **one God**, the Father,
from whom are all things and for whom we exist,
and one Lord, **Jesus Christ**,
through whom are all things and through whom we exist.'

(I Cor.8.6)

Three members:

'The grace of the Lord **Jesus Christ**
and the love of **God**
and the fellowship of the Holy **Spirit**.'

(II Cor.13.13)

'Baptize them in the name of the **Father**
and of the **Son**
and of the Holy **Spirit**.'

(Matt.28.19)

More extended:

'What I received,
that **Christ** died for our sins
in accordance with the scriptures,
that he was buried,
that he was raised on the third day
in accordance with the scriptures.'

(I Cor.15.3f.)

'The Gospel of **God**... concerning his **Son**,
who was descended from David according to the flesh
and designated Son of God in power
according to the **Spirit** of holiness
by his resurrection from the dead,
Jesus Christ our Lord.'

(Rom.1.3f.)

content of faith, however that is defined (*fides quae creditur*). In so far as this knowing and confessing faith expresses itself, it is dependent on words and statements of faith. And in so far as Christian faith is never just the faith of abstract individuals, never individualistic and solipsistic, but faith in or in relation to a **faith community**, for communication within the faith community it is dependent on language which takes place in words and statements, in **statements of faith** in the broadest sense of the word.

So at a very early stage the community of those who believed in Christ formulated **shared** statements of faith. These are summary confessions of belief in Christ, not yet statements which polemically lay down dividing lines or defensively make definitions, nor yet definitions or dogmas of faith of the kind the later church was to know, but statements which **abbreviate and recapitulate**, statements which briefly and tersely sum up the decisive points and seek to impress them on the memory: confessions of faith, symbols or creeds.

It is not so important for our enquiry whether here we have more the word of proclamation or the response of the confession; whether worship, catechesis or church order is the concrete setting for such statements. It is not always easy to decide whether in individual instances statements are more liturgical, kerygmatic, catechetical, juridical or edifying; whether more precisely we have shared shouts (acclamations) like 'Amen', 'Hallelujah', '*Iesous Kyrios* = Lord Jesus', or words of praise and thanksgiving (doxologies) mentioning the name of God, and then also of Christ, and later elaborated as hymns; whether we have blessings (like Jewish greetings and beatitudes) or sacramental formulae (liturgical formularies for baptism and eucharist with a fixed terminology) or confessional formulae or homologies in the strict sense. The transitions between the individual forms and formulae are a priori fluid: especially the transition from acclamation to doxology and to the confessional formula proper, which is presumably often used in a special context with baptismal instruction and the baptismal liturgy.[46]

At all events, there is no disputing the fact that already in the New Testament communities there are such **shared short formulae of faith**, all of which centre on the Christ event:

– The briefest of these formulae of faith are the numerous **one-member** ones which combine the proper name Jesus with a particular honorific title taken from the Jewish or Hellenistic world: 'Jesus is Messiah', 'Jesus is Lord', 'Jesus is God's Son'.[47]

– But at the same time, in the New Testament we also find **two-member** confessional formulae about God and Christ,[48] or already developed short confessions of faith, especially referring to the death and resurrection of Christ.[49]

– Finally, in liturgical passages there are quite isolated confessions in **triadic** form (faith in Father, Son and Holy Spirit).[50] Such short formulae of faith, early, from the New Testament and later, have been preserved in the churches to the present day.

No laws of faith

If we keep these earliest Christian confessions in view, we are immediately struck by a difference from the creed in the present Christian liturgy. At the centre of the early confessions stand the cross and resurrection of Jesus, not his **virgin birth, descent into hell and ascension,** which are mentioned only very occasionally in the New Testament (the virgin birth only in the infancy narratives of Matthew and Luke, the ascension only in Luke, the descent into hell at most in an extremely disputed passage in the non-authentic First Letter of Peter[51]). Cross and resurrection form the **centre** of Christian faith. Moreover, the Apostles' Creed, for a long time attributed to the apostles, demonstrably existed in this form only from the fourth century (I have shown how one can understand this creed, which is still used today in many churches, in the light of both scripture and our contemporary world, in a separate short book, so as not to burden the present book excessively[52]).

So there should be no disputing that such short formulae, old or new, can make sense even today, perhaps as from the beginning in connection with baptism, catechesis or other aspects of the life of the church community. Here, however, we should reflect that the original formulae of faith and confessional formulae were never fragments of a single creed. They are too different for that, with all their concentration on the Christ event, the significance of Jesus for the community of believers: different in content and form, with this or that honorific title, this or that series of motifs.

It is even more important that the original confessions of faith were in no way concerned with dogmas in the present-day sense. They were not doctrinal laws: spontaneous, variable, varied as they were, they were not meant to be fixed statements of a definitive and binding character, not to be gone beyond and not open to discussion, excluding new and other formations, nor could they be. No, faith is not based on such formulae, but expresses itself in them: statements of faith not as a legal foundation but as a free expression of the faith of the community. This insight is important for making possible the formation of new confessions of faith which may perhaps be more comprehensible to a new time – for 'edifying' the community and perhaps also for ecumenical understanding between the separated churches.[53]

But in the face of creeds which have now got more and more complicated, mightn't critical questions occur not only to Jews and Muslims but also to Christians: couldn't these confessions of faith in Jesus Christ, his God and Father, and the Holy Spirit endanger what is common to the three Abrahamic religions from the beginning? So:

Questions for the Future

In Christianity, in the long run will not **belief in the one God of Israel** be endangered if in the course of history a second article of belief in Jesus Christ is to gain increasing weight and prominence in the course of history?

In Christianity, in the long run will not also **belief in the world-encompassing activity of the Spirit** be all too limited to the church, so that prophets outside the church, even the Prophet Muhammad, a priori find no recognition?

In Christianity, in the long run will not also trusting **faith in Jesus Christ** be replaced all too much by a propositional belief which interrogates, makes demands and can be enforced with sanctions, so that, compared with a correct creed, life according to the criterion and spirit of Jesus Christ becomes secondary: orthodoxy instead of orthopraxy?

Certainly, all the Christian confessions of faith – both old and new – must be held in honour, but something else is more important for being a Christian. Jesus nowhere said, '**Say after me**', but rather '**Follow me.**'[54] That means that Jesus did not first require a confession of faith from his disciples, men or women, but rather called them to utterly practical discipleship. The important thing is not to say 'Lord, Lord' but to 'do the will of the Father who is in heaven'.[55] That is why in all his words and activity, his suffering and dying, Jesus is the great central figure from the beginning, through the centuries, to our day.

Jesus Christ as leading figure: the specifically Christian ethic

What is the decisive factor for Christian action, for Christian ethics? What is the **criterion of the Christian**, the distinguishing mark of the Christian in practice, the much-discussed *proprium* of Christian ethics?[56] The answer is: Jesus as the **normative concrete person**, as we saw, as a tangible figure, with all the possibilities of perceiving him and realizing him. I also developed this in the context of my book *On Being a Christian*: for Christianity of all ages Jesus Christ represents a **basic model** of a view of life and a way of life which can be realized in many ways. He is in person, both positively and negatively, the invitation (You may), the call (You shall) and the challenge (You can) for the individual and society. Specifically, he makes possible:

- a new basic orientation and basic attitude,
- new motivations, dispositions and actions,
- a new horizon of meaning and the identification of a new goal.

The key New Testament concept of Christian ethics is discipleship of Christ.

Discipleship distinguishes Christians from other disciples and adherents of great teachers of humankind, in so far as Christians are ultimately directed to this person, not only to his teaching but also to his life, death and new life. A Platonist or an Aristotelian, a Marxist or a Freudian, would hardly claim that for their teachers. Although Plato and Aristotle, Marx and Freud, composed their works in person, these works can also be studied and followed without a special tie to their persons. Their works, their theories are in principle separable from their persons. But we only understand the real significance of the Gospels, the teaching (message) of Jesus, who as we know did not write a single word, when we see them in the light of his life and passion, death and new life: throughout the New Testament his 'teaching' cannot be detached from his person. So, for Christians, Jesus is certainly teacher and model, but also at the same time decidely more than teacher and model; he is in **person the living and normative embodiment of his cause**, Jesus as God's Christ, which is why those who believe in him are not called Jesuans, but Christians.

However, in so far as Jesus in person remains the living embodiment of his cause, he may never – like, say, Marx and Engels earlier in totalitarian systems – become an empty, unemotional portrait, a lifeless mask, the domesticated object of a personality cult. This living Christ is and remains Jesus of Nazareth, as he lived and preached, fought and suffered. This living Christ calls

- neither to inconsequential adoration nor even to mystical union,
- nor to literal imitation,
- but to practical, personal discipleship.

And what does such discipleship mean? '**Following**' – significantly, the New Testament has only the verb[57] – means 'going round after', though now no longer outwardly through the land, as in the time of Jesus, but by entering into relationship with him in token of the same discipleship, attaching oneself to him permanently and making decisions about one's life in accordance with him. That is the meaning of discipleship: trusting **oneself to Jesus** and his way and going one's own way – we each have our own way! – in accordance with his directions. This possibility was seen from the beginning as the great opportunity: not as a 'must' but as a 'may'. So it was a real call to such a way of life, a true grace, which presupposes only one thing, that one takes it on trust and **guides one's life** by it.

Thus Christian faith is the foundation of that great religion whose strength it is to be able to point to a quite particular normative historical figure for a detailed justification and basis of an attitude to life, a way and life-style. For a person's basic attitude and orientation, **form of life, life-style and way of life**, can be described both comprehensively and concretely in terms of Jesus Christ – with the same justification, as we saw. Indeed, beyond question the whole Christian message is not just aimed at particular decisions, actions, motivations and dispositions but at a completely new **attitude to life**, a fundamentally changed consciousness, a new basic attitude, another scale of values, radical rethinking and conversion of the whole person (*metanoia*[58]). This is the significance of the Sermon on the Mount, the core of Christian ethics.

The significance of the Sermon on the Mount

'The message of Jesus as I understand it, is contained in His Sermon on the Mount. The spirit of the Sermon on the Mount competes almost on the same terms as the *Bhagavadgita* for the rule of my heart. It is that sermon which has endeared Jesus to me.'[59] This was the confession of no less a figure than Mahatma Gandhi. The Sermon on the Mount,[60] in which Matthew and Luke have collected the ethical demands of Jesus – short sayings and groups of sayings mainly from the Logia source Q – has continually challenged Christians and non-Christians, Jacobins of the Revolution and the Socialist Kautsky, Leo Tolstoy and Albert Schweitzer. What is its purpose?

Certainly not one thing: it is not meant to be an **accentuated ethic of obedience to the law**. Sometimes it has erroneously been described as the 'law of Christ' – as a substitute for the Jewish law. But the 'Sermon on the Mount' addresses something which cannot be the object of a legal regulation. The love commandment, of all things, should not be a new law. Rather, in a quite concrete approach, remote from all casuistry and legalism, unconventionally and with a sure eye, Jesus calls individuals to an **obedience to God** which is to embrace their whole lives. Here are simple, clear, liberating calls which dispense with arguments from authority and tradition but give examples, signs, symptoms of the changed life. Great, helpful instructions, often deliberately formulated in

The Decalogue
and the Sermon on the Mount

                         †

'I am the Lord your God, you shall have no other gods besides me.

'No one can serve two masters... You cannot serve God and mammon.' (Matt.6.24)

You shall not make for yourself a graven image. You shall not take the name of the Lord your God in vain.

'But I say to you, Do not swear at all, either by heaven or by the earth... or by Jerusalem.' (Matt.5.34f.)

Remember the sabbath day, to keep it holy.

'What man of you, if he has one sheep and it falls into a pit on the sabbath, will not lay hold of it and lift it out? Of how much more value is a man than a sheep? So it is lawful to do good on the sabbath.' (Matt.12.11f.)

Honour your father and mother.

'He who loves father or mother more than me is not worthy of me.' (Matt.10.37)

You shall not kill.

'But I say to you that every one who is angry with his brother shall be liable to judgment.' (Matt.5.22)

You shall not commit adultery.

'But I say to you that every one who looks at a woman lustfully has already committed adultery with her in his heart.' (Matt.5.28)

You shall not steal.

'If any one strikes you on the right cheek, turn to him the other also.' (Matt.5.39)

You shall not bear false witness against your neighbour.

'Let what you say be simply "Yes" or "No"; anything more than this comes from evil.' (Matt.5.37)

You shall not covet your neighbour's house.

'So whatever you wish that men would do to you, do so to them; for this is the law and the prophets.' (Matt.7.12)

You shall not covet your neighbour's wife, or his manservant, or his maid-servant, or his ox, or his ass, or any-thing that is your neighbour's.' (Ex.20.1-21)

'But I say to you that every one who divorces his wife, except on the ground of unchastity, makes her an adulteress.' (Matt.5.32)

(Revised Standard Version)

an exaggerated way without any ifs and buts: If your eye offends you, pluck it out! Just say yes and no! First be reconciled with your brother! All have to apply these instructions specifically to their lives.

At all events the 'better righteousness' or 'perfection' does not mean a quantitative heightening of the demands. As the antitheses of the Sermon on the Mount[61] indicate, Jesus does not put into practice that obedience to the jot and tittle of the letter of the Law which is required by a Jewish Christian logion quoted by Matthew.[62] That would blunt obedience, in this case not in a liberal but in an ultra-conservative way.[63] Jesus' message is not at all a sum of commandments. To follow him does not mean observing a number of commands. It is no coincidence that promises of happiness for the unfortunate stand at the head of the Sermon on the Mount. The gift, the present, grace precede the norm, the requirement, the instruction: everyone is called, everyone is offered salvation without having to do anything first, and the instructions themselves are consequences of Jesus' message of the kingdom of God. He adopts a standpoint only by way of example, symbolically.

The general heading of the Sermon on the Mount is '**God's will be done!**' God's demand undermines, transcends and breaks through the limitations and legal ordinances of this world. The challenging examples of the Sermon on the Mount[64] are specifically not meant to indicate a legal limit: only the left cheek, two miles, the coat – in that case the attractiveness ceases. God's demand calls for human generosity, tends towards a 'more'. Indeed, it ends up in the unconditional, the boundless, the whole. Can God be content with a limited, conditional, formal obedience – simply because something is required or forbidden? In that case a last something would be missed out which all the regulations of justice and the Law, however detailed, cannot embrace, and yet which is decisive for human behaviour. God wants more: God does not claim just half the will, but all of it. God does not call just for externals, which can be controlled, but also for what happens inside, which cannot – the human heart. God does not want simply good fruits, but the good tree;[65] not simply action, but being; not something, but myself, all of me.

That is the meaning of the amazing antitheses of the Sermon on the Mount, in which the Law is contrasted with the will of God: it is not just adultery, perjury, murder, but also what cannot be embraced by the Law, an adulterous disposition, lack of truthfulness in thought and speech, a hostile attitude, that are against God's will. Any 'only' in the interpretation of the Sermon on the Mount curtails and dilutes the unconditional will of God: 'only' a better fulfilment of the law, 'only' a new disposition, 'only' a list of sins in the light of the one righteous Jesus, 'only' for those called to perfection, 'only' for that time, 'only' for a short period . . . In the face of what is last and final, the kingdom of God, a fundamental change is expected of people. The Sermon on the Mount is primarily addressed to the individual and does not aim at a new state order or a new law. But anyone who complacently thinks that 'no state can be made' with the Sermon on the Mount overlooks its implications and consequences for state and society, as we already saw in the discussion of Judaism.[66]

Jesus' demands are **radical**. Here are three examples which can easily be applied not only to individuals but to social (and indeed ethnic, national and religous) groups:

– Renounce your rights in favour of the other: go two miles with the one who has forced you to go one mile with him.[67]

– Renounce power at your own expense: give your cloak to the one who has taken your shirt.[68]

– Renounce violent retaliation: offer the left cheek to the one who has struck you on the right.[69]

These last examples in particular show even more clearly than anything that has gone before that Jesus' commands must **not** be understood as **absolute laws** to be followed literally. They are and remain **ethical appeals**. Jesus does not express the view that retribution is not allowed for a blow on the left cheek but is for a punch in the stomach. Certainly these examples are not just meant symbolically: they are very significant limit situations (often formulated with typically oriental exaggeration) which can become reality at any time. But they are not meant legalistically, as though only this and always this were commanded. Renunciation of violent retaliation does not a priori mean renunciation of all resistance. According to the accounts, when Jesus himself was struck on the cheek before the court he by no means offered the other cheek, but protested. Renunciation must not be confused with weakness. Jesus' demands are not for ethical or even ascetic achievements which would make sense in themselves. They are vivid appeals for a radical fulfilment of the will of God from case to case in favour of one's fellow human being. All renunciation is merely the negative side of a new positive practice.

Here is an expression of the degree to which not only a universal ethic of humanity but also the **Jewish ethic is radicalized**. In the light of Jesus' message of the 'better righteousness', even the Ten Commandments of the Decalogue[70] appear 'sublated' in the threefold sense of the word: dropped and yet preserved, because raised to a higher level.[71]

Not many words are needed to demonstrate what a tremendous **challenge** the Sermon on the Mount is **for Christianity itself**. Any of its statements becomes a question to Christianity as a whole, to the different churches and groups and the individual Christian.

Questions for the Future

✝ What challenge would be posed to politics, economics, culture and private life if it were the rule:

– not only to have no other gods than the one God, but to love God 'with all one's heart' and one's neighbour, even one's enemy, as oneself;

– not only not to speak the name of God casually, but not to swear by God at all;

– not only to hallow the sabbath by rest, but to do active good on the sabbath;

– not only to honour father and mother in order to live long on earth, but if necessary to turn one's back on natural human relationships, if that was necessary for authentic life;

– not only not to kill, but even to dispense with killing thoughts and words;

– not only not to commit adultery, but even to avoid adulterous intent;

– not only not to steal, but even to renounce the right to retribution for injustice suffered;

– not only not to bear false witness, but in unconditional truthfulness to let one's Yes be Yes and No be No;

– not only not to covet one's neighbour's house, but even to endure evil;

– not only not to covet one's neighbour's wife, but to avoid intrinsically legal divorce?

Love as fulfilment of the law

So we can understand why the apostle Paul – here too in striking accord with the Jesus of history – was right when he expressed the conviction that someone who loves has fulfilled the law![72] And after Augustine, it has been put in even more pointed form, '*Ama, et fac quo vis*', 'Love, and do what you will.' Here is no new law, but a new freedom of love. Here love is not understood as a primarily sentimental and emotional inclination (which it fact it is impossible to have for everyone), but as a being there for others which shows good will and a readiness to help. Jesus embodied this love in all his teaching and behaviour, conflicts and suffering. And had he not had this extraordinary fate – living and dying for his 'good news', his 'gospel' – we would hardly have had anything like the Sermon on the Mount handed down to us.

Is this message of love perhaps all too abstract? Is the great love song which Paul strikes up in his letter to the community of Corinth, very much in the spirit of Jesus, all too remote? Some simple antitheses by an author unknown to me may make it clear how much a different basic attitude can change life in a very concrete way:

Duty without love breeds weariness;
duty with love breeds constancy.

Responsibility without love breeds unconcern;
responsibility with love breeds concern.

Righteousness without love breeds hardness;
righteousness with love breeds reliability.

Education without love breeds contrariness;
education with love breeds patience.

Wisdom without love breeds rifts;
wisdom with love breeds understanding.

Friendliness without love breeds hypocrisy;
friendliness with love breeds grace.

Order without love breeds pettiness;
order with love breeds generosity.

Knowledge without love breeds dogmatism;
knowledge with love breeds trustworthiness.

Power without love breeds violence;
power with love breeds readiness to help.

Honour without love breeds arrogance;
honour with love breeds modesty.

Possessions without love breed avarice;
possessions with love breed generosity.

Faith without love breeds fanaticism;
Faith with love breeds peacemaking.

But wait a minute; here at the latest someone will object with deep horror: How noble the ideal and how sorry the reality! What has Christianity made over the past two thousand years of this invitation, this call, this challenge of its Christ? No, now that we have dealt so thoroughly with the essence and the centre, the central structural elements and the central figure of Christianity, we must tackle its **history**, its extremely ambivalent and often broken history, as concretely as is possible within the framework of this book.

But first of all here is a concluding and transitional reflection. If we look back at the previous remarks, it is no longer difficult to define what in all the changing historical constellations was and is the abiding substance of Christianity.

Abiding substance of faith and changing paradigms

What, after our reflections thus far, are the **centre and foundation**, in other words, what is the abiding **substance of faith** of the Christian religion, the New Testament, Christian belief? Regardless of all the interpretations and reductions of historical, literary or sociological criticism of the Bible, from the perspective of the foundation documents of the Christian faith which have become normative and influential in history the central content of faith is **Jesus Christ**: as Messiah and Son of the one **God** of Abraham, also active today through the same **Spirit** of God. There can be no Christian faith, no Christian religion, without the confession '**Jesus is the Messiah, Lord, Son of God**.' The name of Jesus Christ denotes the 'centre of the New Testament' (which is in no way to be understood in static terms).

Of course it can be argued that the one God of Abraham himself constitutes the centre of the New Testament, its '**theocentricity**'. But the 'new' element in the 'New Testament' is precisely the fact that this one God is never seen alone, but always together with the one who proclaimed him 'anew'. The New Testament writings do not centre on the innermost 'mysteries of the Godhead' but on the history of Jesus Christ, which has consequences for our understanding of God. For these Jews of that time, the Jewish people (which in any case was soon dispersed) and the Jewish land (which in any case was soon lost) no longer had a central place as an expression of God's covenant. The centre was this Jesus, who now for his part was regarded as the guarantor of the ongoing covenant, who was expected as the 'Messiah' or Lord' ('Son of man', 'Son of David', or whatever other title).

So while faith in the one God is unchanged, the **centre of faith is defined afresh**: Jesus' name stands for the kingdom of God, the coming of which he preached. Faith in God thus becomes specifically christological, indeed is personified. Here Christians have not put a second God alongside the one God; they do not honour any bitheism in place of monotheism. But the one God of Israel is seen afresh through this his last prophet and Messiah, and this prophet and Messiah is himself constantly understood anew, as God's image, word and son. To this degree the 'theocentricity' is determined by a '**christocentricity**' and the description of the centre of

Christianity in terms of Jesus Christ is natural, faithful to the original confession of faith in earliest Christianity.

If we describe the distinctive structural elements and abiding guidelines of Christian faith more precisely, according to all that we have heard, they are as follows:

- faith in Jesus, the Lord who was crucified and raised to life;
- faith in the God of Abraham who is shared with the Jews, whom Jesus called his Father;
- faith in the power of the Spirit of God who has become powerful in and through Jesus.

This special relationship of Jesus Christ to his God is the germ from which Christianity begins and the nucleus around which it crystallizes. And despite all the failure and reluctance of Christian people right from the beginning, and all the developments and confusions of the history of Christianity, this will nevertheless remain the basic conception of the Christian religion, which is never abandoned. Even as a Christian, one may interpret this constant centre which is the prime motive force in different ways, but here alone is the foundation of Christianity's

- **originality** from earliest times,
- **continuity** in its long history down the centuries,
- **identity** despite all the difference of languages, cultures and nations.

And even if Christianity (together with Islam) has also taken over the historical legacy of Judaism – belief in the one God – it issues a new challenge which in its way Islam also recognizes in principle: Jesus as the Messiah of the one God.

However, this centre, this foundation, this substance of faith – in my schematic description the paradigm shift is always indicated by a bisected circle – was never abstract and isolated but has been constantly interpreted anew and realized in practice in the changing demands of the time. To this degree, in the following long main section C, 'History', the **systematic theological account will be combined with a historical chronological account**, without which the former cannot be convincingly justified. This was already the approach in my account of Judaism – with the regular insertion of explanatory diagrams and topical interim reflections.

Now it can be said that this faith in Jesus Christ is an 'object' of faith, and as the by no means obvious revelation of God is visible only to the eyes of believers. That is true. But as a concept, notion, historically relevant entity it is there in the biblical writings for historians to recognize, describe and test – whether they are believers or unbelievers. And that is also the case in the subsequent history of Christianity.

Again and again, **new epoch-making constellations** of the time – society in general, the community of faith, the proclamation of faith and reflection on faith – interpret this one and the same centre and make it concrete once more. That is what I understand by paradigm, following Thomas S.Kuhn: 'an entire constellation of beliefs, values, techniques and so forth shared by the members of a given community.'[73] I have explained at length in earlier publications,[74] and already demonstrated clearly in the previous volume on *Judaism*, that it is possible, important and urgent to transfer the paradigm theory (in the sense of a 'macroparadigm') from the sphere of the natural sciences to that of religion and theology, and how far this can be done.

As we shall see, this history of Christianity now becomes unusually dramatic. First of all a small faith community, which then grows extraordinarily rapidly, will undergo a whole series of fundamental religious changes, indeed, in the longer term will undergo revolutionary paradigm shifts, in response to great new challenges which keep arising in world history. I shall end this section by sketching out my interest in this paradigm shift, once again, in the words of Søren Kierkegaard: 'Christendom has done away with Christianity, without being quite aware of it. The consequence is that, if anything is to be done, one must try again to introduce Christianity into Christendom.'[75]

C. History

How can an individual today survey two thousand years of the history of Christianity? It would be madness, on the next pages, to want to write even an approximation of a history of Christianity. But how are we to be able to understand Christianity without surveying its two-thousand-year-old history, which is still ever present? A historical understanding of earliest Christianity first of all calls for some basic reflections on history and history-writing.

I. The Jewish Apocalyptic Paradigm of Earliest Christianity

The specialist knows more and more about less and less. Many hundreds of secular and church historians, working in every possible corner of the history of Christianity, sigh over the complexity of the detail. In history, too, the flood of information has swollen to such a degree that even the specialist can hardly cope with all the articles, reports, dissertations and books. In addition there is the explosive increase in the assimilation of information with the help of novel computer technology: more than 300,000 pages of typescript text will fit on a compact disc the size of a hand! Individuals with their own limited ability to assimilate feel completely overwhelmed when confronted with this highly technological capacity for assimilating information.

1. The need for a basic orientation

In the face of excessive information – now already, unconsciously, at every moment – our brains cope by selection. And anyone who wants to achieve any survey at all of the history of Christianity has only this means of selection. It is certainly always dependent on the perspective of the onlooker, but it has to be done, not arbitrarily, but through clear rules which are related to the subject-matter.

Survey of the entire constellations

A distinction has to be made between information which is necessary and useful and information which is useless, between pure information and the necessary knowledge for orientation. What use is any information without a basic orientation?

Already in my *Global Responsibility* I showed why the **paradigm theory** seemed to me to be a very suitable instrument for this basic orientation. I can presuppose it here. In fact the idealistic way of thinking about history in the forced system of thesis, antithesis and synthesis (Hegel) is inappropriate for a global description and analysis of the high religions, and so too is the deterministic-pessimistic morphology of the great cultures (Spengler) or the more empirical and optimistic synopsis of cultural cycles (Toynbee). However, the strictly historical analysis of the paradigms of a religion, those **macroparadigms or epoch-making entire constellations**, is a possible way of making a selection for an overall view of the history of Christianity which is as comprehensive as possible, yet also precise.

Paradigm analysis makes it possible to work out the great historical structures and transformations by concentrating on both the fundamental constants and the decisive variables at the same time. At any rate, in this way it is possible to describe those breaks in world history and the epoch-making basic models of Christianity which have arisen from them, and determine the situation of Christianity to the present day.

But the history of earliest Christianity in particular shows that history is by no means concerned only with the ideas and acts of heroes and the powerful, peoples and states, the great policies or the decisive battles which are characteristic of the historiography of the Greeks Herodotus and Thucydides or the Romans Sallust, Livy and Tacitus. For in the first phase of Christianity there are few 'great figures' and 'great events' from the perspective of world politics – which were still the object of historical accounts in the nineteenth century for the modern historiography of historians like Ranke. Other things are more important.

The 'new historiography'

Present-day, postmodern historical research is concerned to be more comprehensive: ' . . .the history of people, all people, not exclusively of kings and great lords. The history of structures and not just of events; history in movement, the history of developments and transformations, not static history; no book-keeping and stocktaking, but rather explanations instead of narratives or descriptions, interpretations instead of dogmas . . .' That is how the programme of the French 'new historio-graphy', the *'nouvelle histoire'*,[1] describes itself. This approach took shape, with reference to Voltaire, Chateaubriand, Guizot and Michelet, as early as the crisis year of 1929, and was disseminated through the journal *Annales d'histoire économique et sociale*, edited in Strasbourg by Lucien Febvre[2] and Marc Bloch,[3] and inspired above all by Fernand Braudel and his pioneering work *La Méditerranée* (1949). Although they concentrated primarily on France and the Mediterranean world, and chronologically on the Middle Ages and the early modern period, these scholars led historical research as a whole along new paths, as the leading representative of this school today, Jacques Le Goff, points out: their concern was to achieve 'new (thematic and methodological) insights into economic and social history, into the history of structures, into the *longue durée*, into the history of outsiders, the body, sexuality, the imaginary and, above all, the history of mentalities'.[4]

These new thematic and methodological insights need to be drawn on by Christian historiography in particular. For it would be foolish to construct a national opposition between, say, French and German historiography. Indeed, the representatives of the *Nouvelle histoire* themselves point out that the German *Vierteljahresschrift für Sozial- und Wirtschaftsgeschichte* was the 'model' for the formative stage of the *Annales*;[5] and of course Max Weber, who thought historically as a sociologist, and as early as 1901 pointed out the connection between religion and social morality, should be mentioned as a forerunner.[6]

Yet there is no overlooking the fact that German historiography in particular is primarily the history of institutions, and that it displayed anxiety about the impact of newer methods and theories. Until the 1960s it was somewhat hesitant in accepting the stimuli of economic and social history, though for example in the ten-volume *History of the Church*[7] edited by Hubert Jedin and John Dolan along the lines of a particular Catholic ecclesiology one can also find some information about the social, economic and existential conditions of religious life, as one also can in the twenty-one volume *Histoire de l'Église* edited by Augustin Fliche and Victor Martin.[8] Only the most recent *Histoire du christianisme des origines à nos jours*, edited by Michel Mollat du Jourdin and André Vauchez, begun in 1990, which will eventually comprise 14 volumes and 16,000 pages, may be said to come closer to the programme of a multi-level *histoire totale*, which in ecumenical fashion aims at a comprehensive account of the life of Christianity.[9] A good supplement from the German-speaking world will be the series *Christentum und Gesellschaft*,[10] edited by Henneke Gülzow and Hartmut Lehmann, in which authors like Arnold Angenendt ('Early Middle Ages'), Hartmut

Lehmann ('The Age of Absolutism') or Martin Greschat ('The Age of the Industrial Revolution') achieve a comparable level to that of French research.[11]

Of course even the professional church and secular historians will not be able to assimilate with the same intensity all these volumes, with their excessive wealth of information. But there is no disputing that such works (together with the specialist literature) are of inestimable value in bringing into our paradigm analysis as many aspects and facets as possible of what has taken place over twenty centuries under the label 'Christian'. And even if it is completely impossible to reflect in the various paradigms the **'histoire totale'**[12] which the *nouvelle histoire* strives for, basic frameworks can be indicated which are significant for a history of Christianity in postmodernity – supplementing the traditional ('modern') church history which above all has an institutional and political orientation.

The return of suppressed aspects

Present-day history should strive to be what can only be hinted at here:
– not just a history of events with an accumulation of mere facts, but a history of structures, modes of thought and mentalities, in other words a history of ideas and mentalities, a social history;
– not just a political history of powers and institutions, of church and state, but a problem-orientated history of piety, theology and culture;
– not just a history of the great and powerful, the elites, but also a history of the social groups which hitherto have been neglected by history, the powerless, the underprivileged, the little people, the men and the women;
– not just a history of public life but also a history of private life, of the everyday world;
– not just a history of European Christianity, but also a history of American, African and Asian Christianity, a universal history;
– not just a history of the Roman Catholic world church but also a history of Eastern Orthodoxy, of Reformation Christianity and the more recent churches, as far as possible in the context of the other world religions: an ecumenical history.

Of course a paradigm analysis can only bring all these different aspects to bear to a very limited degree. But it is particularly concerned with the long-term perspective, 'the notion that the impulses of history work in long stretches and can only be grasped in them . . . systems which lasted for centuries'.[13] However, with this more recent view of history it is necessary to guard against all exaggerated views of what Fernand Braudel called an 'almost unmoved history'; the decisive results of modern historiography must be maintained.

Already in the history of Judaism the one example of King David showed that 'great men' are not just supernumeraries, and events like the conquest of Jerusalem or later its destruction are not marginal events. So there can be no contempt for the 'event', for biography, narrative and political historiography, no separation between the history of events and the history of structures or mentalities. Even the French *nouvelle histoire* is now conceding that the epistemological process of historians is continuing and that today a return of **suppressed aspects of historiography** – which is quite ambivalent – can be noted: 'the return of the "event" is the most spectacular; the return of biography the most familiar; the return of narrative historiography the most polemical; the return of political historiography the most significant'.[14]

But once again: this book is not meant to be a history of Christianity but a historical and systematic **analysis of its epoch-making overall constellations** – against the background of history. Even the *'nouvelle histoire'* emphasizes that a positive (and fundamentally illusory) description of 'how it really was' is not enough, that even historiography without dogmatic partisanship has to derive its criteria from the present. With Henri Fefbvre, Marc Bloch 'bequeathed a twofold step to the historian as a method: understanding the past through the present'.[15] It will emerge how far it has been possible to work out the very different structures, forms and figures of Christianity up to the present in a way which is both sufficiently comprehensive and sufficiently concrete. The tasks at any rate are clear:

- what must be offered is not a confessionalist but an interconfessional-ecumenical view of Christianity;
- what must be striven for is not a Eurocentric but a universal historical view of the great intellectual and world-historical connections;
- what must be pursued is not a historical approach which is in love with the past but one which is critically related to the present, and in such a way that the present can be understood from the past and the past from the present.

2. The earliest community

Now it might be very difficult to discover anything about the everyday life of the first generations of Christians after almost 2000 years. After all, we know hardly anything about the normal, usual course of their lives, their everyday cares, anxieties and joys. For who was the subject of this history?

Jews from lower classes

Three perspectives are important if we are to understand the history of the earliest community:[16]

- This is not a history of Romans and Greeks but of **Jews born** in the sphere of Hellenistic Palestinian culture. Though some may have spoken Aramaic and others Greek, they communicated to the whole church that was coming into being Jewish language, a Jewish world of ideas and Jewish theology and thus left an indelible stamp on the whole of Christianity in the subsequent period – including the Gentile Christianity which was to come – down to the present day.
- But at the beginning it was not on the history of an upper class that historiography was usually orientated, but on the history of the **lower classes**: fishermen, peasants, craftsmen, little people who normally have no chronicler. The first generation of Christians did not have the least political power and did not strive for positions in the religious and political establishment. They formed a small, weak marginal group of the society of their time, under attack and discredited.
- In the end this was initially not only a male movement but also a history of **women** who followed Jesus, who gave financial support to him and his followers and who followed him to Jerusalem (one of these women, Mary Magdalene, was a witness to the resurrection). The practice of also calling women disciples was unconventional and undermined existing patriarchal structures.

But there was no ideal beginning period of Christianity. The reports that we have of the early Christians are usually stylized, with 'ideological' colouring, selected with the specific aim of proclamation. When we read, for example, in the Acts of the Apostles that 'the community of believers was of one heart and one soul', that 'none of them called what he had his property', but that 'they had everything in common',[17] we may have here an idealized description by Luke two generations after the events described.

Certainly **Jesus** himself, who came from an artisan family and spoke Aramaic, had addressed his message provocatively to the 'poor', whom he called blessed, along with those who wept, were hungry and downtrodden.[18] Sociologically, the renewal movement sparked off by Jesus must have been one of those typical religious movements from the **country population** (and the small towns) which, like that of John the Baptist and Qumran, had a mistrustful or even hostile attitude to the great Hellenistic cities and especially the conservative and rich capital. Moreover, Jesus' opponents belonged above all to the narrow petty-bourgeois urban middle class (mostly Pharisees), who maintained the primacy of the law, and the thin layer of the upper class, also urban (above all the Sadducees), who occupied remunerative positions around the temple. Jesus' message certainly disturbed not only their religious but also their social consciences.

But already the prophet Isaiah, whom Jesus quotes in his answer to John the Baptist, understands the word *anawim* (the **poor**) in a comprehensive sense, denoting all the oppressed, the afflicted, the failures, the despairing, the wretched. And despite all the polemic against the rich, Jesus, who did not want to be a public benefactor by force, did not preach the dispossession of the rich or a 'goulash Communism', or even a 'dictatorship of the proletariat'. There was no primacy of the economic for him: 'Food is the first thing. Morals follow oñ', as Bert Brecht remarks in *The Threepenny Opera*.[19] But in the Sermon on the Mount we hear Jesus saying precisely the opposite: 'First the kingdom of God . . . and all these things shall be yours as well.'[20] Jesus required from everyone contentment and no desire to make claims, a trusting lack of care, inner freedom from possessions; and anyone who wanted to lead a free itinerant life with him necessarily had to leave everything behind. But Jesus was not like the Essene comunity of Qumran by the Dead Sea in requiring possesions to be given to the community. He allowed Zacchaeus to distribute just half his possessions; he laid down no law and no regulations. Various of his followers, including Peter, who was later to be so important for the earliest comunity, had houses to call their own.

Even in the **earliest community** – in Jerusalem and probably also in parallel, in Galilee – individual followers of Jesus who probably came from various Jewish groups (Pharisees, Essenes, Zealots, priests are mentioned) had houses which they made available for house meetings. Scholars can agree today that 'the poor' (*anawim* or *ebionim*) is not a proper name for the earliest community; Paul's collection for the poor is not for the Jerusalem community as such but for those in it who really were poor or needy.[21] Certainly there were cases of voluntary unselfish renunciation of possessions, possibly especially among Essene Christians,[22] and the earliest Christian itinerant missionaries were to devote themselves exclusively to proclaiming Jesus' message, with a disregard of personal possessions, which is probably what Peter and the Twelve also did.[23]

But Luke – unlike Paul – subsequently idealizes conditions in the earliest community: 'No one said that any of the things which he possessed was his own, but they had everything in common.'[24] He bases this on a saying of Jesus against all possessions to which he himself adds a rigoristic emphasis (as comparison with Mark and Matthew shows). In reality even the earliest community did not know any general renunciation of possessions, despite all the brotherliness and sisterliness that it practised. Luke himself lets the difference between the needy and those not in need show through in his Acts of the Apostles (for example in the care of widows).[25] Help for the needy and sharing, not abandoning property, was evidently the aim. An ideal social utopia was not realized, but a 'community of social solidarity'.[26] But what was the spiritual horizon of this community, in the light of which we must also understand its social attitude?

The expectation of an end of time

The spiritual horizon, the spiritual 'climate' of the Aramaic-speaking earliest community in Jerusalem (and possibly also elsewhere in Palestine), can be described in a word: it was **apocalyptic**, eschatological; in other words, the early Christians were expecting that the world would end soon. Thus this first generation of Christians was influenced by the 'apocalyptic' (= 'unveiling', 'revelation') movement which had become increasingly strong since the time of the Maccabees in the second century BCE among the pious Jews, the 'hasidim', and which in the form of prophecies, testaments, dreams and visions claimed to be able to 'unveil' the divine mysteries and above all the future.[27]

For these people in the Palestine of that time were not interested, like some in Greece, in physics, in knowledge of phenomena on earth and in heaven, or in metaphysics, knowledge of the primal principles of all that is. They were interested in **the future**: not just what would develop from 'below', from human beings and the world, but what was dawning, coming from God, from 'above'. And in view of the great disappointment over the decadence and the downfall of the Maccabees, already in the second century BCE people had arrived at the conclusion that deliverance could not come from an earthly Davidic 'Messiah' ('anointed'), but only from one sent by God direct from God's heaven, the heavenly Messiah, the pre-existent and transcendent saviour and judge figure of the 'Son of Man'.

What about **Jesus**? Although there is disagreement over whether Jesus specifically claimed the title Son of Man, and if so, how far he did, it is certain that he worked in this apocalyptic climate, hardly noticed by the wider world and not listed in its chronicles.[28] His thought and preaching were governed by a typically apocalyptic expectation of the end-time: I have already indicated this in the previous section.[29] There are several extremely inconvenient texts[30] which attest that Jesus, too, expected the kingdom of God in the **imminent future**. The end time had already begun with his activity. In his unassuming words and actions, in his message proclaimed to the poor and the unhappy, those who wept and were trampled on, and in his charismatic actions which helped the sick and those who had fallen into debt, he proclaimed the expected kingdom where debt, suffering and death would have an end.

However, Jesus constantly refused to put a precise date to the end of the world.[31] He was not at all interested in satisfying human curiosity, in giving a precise date and place to the kingdom of God, in unveiling sensational apocalyptic events and mysteries, in forecasting the precise course of the eschatological drama. But the fact remains that even if apocalyptic was not the centre of Jesus' preaching and attitude – that centre is, of course, the kingdom of God – it was his horizon, the framework to all his understanding and imagining. Present-day exegesis has established that beyond all doubt.

It is also indisputable that the **earliest community**, all its thought and activity, its whole mentality, is stamped by apocalyptic notions.[32] And not just its theology but also its understanding of sexuality and marriage, prayer and asceticism, life and death is to be seen against this spiritual horizon. It took over traditional apocalyptic material in particular to depict the end events – as already in the Markan apocalypse[33] – and in this way interpreted its own experiences around the time of the fall of Jerusalem. But to the first generation of disciples this apocalyptic expectation seemed already to have been filled in two ways: by the resurrection (exaltation) of Jesus and by the experience of the Spirit.

Pneumatic-ecstatic experiences

For the followers of Jesus, however, this apocalyptic expectation had a specific focus. Hadn't they experienced how the one who had proclaimed and initiated the coming of the kingdom of God had been executed as one forsaken by God? But had they therefore really given up all belief and hope in the kingdom of God? After the shock of Jesus' arrest and execution, at any rate Jewish women (in Jerusalem?) and men (in Galilee?) had various kinds of pneumatic-ecstatic experiences, a series of visions and auditions which made them certain that Jesus was alive. However present-day exegesis and religious study attempt to explain these phenomena in historical and psychological terms,[34] Jewish disciples, men and women – doubtless against the horizon of Jewish hopes of resurrection and models of interpretation (e.g. the transportation of Enoch and Elijah, the raising of martyrs, legends of ascensions like those of Moses and Isaiah) – saw these experiences not as interpretations which they had produced themselves, but as revelations granted by God: he, the one who had been humiliated and put to shame, had not been left in death by God but **raised to life**. And where was he now? Their conviction was that the one who had been condemned and executed in a collaboration between the Jewish authorities and the Roman procurator Pontius Pilate had been exalted to God, now dwells with God in heavenly glory and – as was announced in Psalm 110 – rules over the world in a place of honour 'at the right hand of God' until he comes again in judgment. Indeed, he is now the one who bears the hope of the coming kingdom of God: the pioneer, bringer of salvation and judge of the world. Here lies the origin of all christology: God has made Jesus, who had proclaimed his kingdom with authority, 'Lord and Messiah',[35] despite his death on the cross, by raising him from the dead.

At any rate there was a new gathering of the disciples who had fled on Jesus' arrest, under the leadership of Peter – again in Jerusalem. Whatever historical events lie behind the manifestly ecstatic phenomena of glossolalia and rapture in the **account of** the pouring out of the Spirit of God at **Pentecost** in the Acts of the Apostles,[36] it bears witness to the eschatological-enthusiastic spirit in which the first **messianic community** formed – on the Jewish harvest festival and pilgrimage festival, the 'Feast of Weeks' (seven weeks and a day after the Passover), which Christians call Pentecost (from the Greek *pentekoste* = fiftieth day). The spirit of God, which according to traditional Jewish notions had been quenched in the present, was experienced in the young community, and not a few of those possessed with the Spirit expressed themselves in prophetic discourse.

Early Christianity was not just a child of apocalyptic, any more than apocalyptic was a fruit of earliest Christianity. Rather, the phenomena were interdependent. People fortified themselves in the faith that the one who had been raised to life by God would come again as judge of the world to complete the rule of God which had already dawned and set up the definitive kingdom of God. In the meantime the message about him had to be proclaimed: his name was the signet and the banner for the coming kingdom, which could be experienced 'already now' in the Spirit, but had 'not yet' been manifested, not yet been realized. Now already it was important to decide for him. But did this decision for Jesus – a question of topical and at the same time abiding significance then and now – mean bidding farewell to the Jewish community? By no means.

3. The Christian centre – with an abiding Jewish stamp

No long explanations are needed to describe how the first generation of those who believed in Jesus of Nazareth as the Messiah still remained completely **integrated within Judaism** – like Jesus himself, his family and his first disciples, men and women.[37]

What are Jewish Christians?

The group of disciples who had fled after the execution of Jesus and who reassembled under the impact of the resurrection experience consisted of Aramaic-speaking Jews who understood themselves to be a group within Judaism which preserved its external connections with the Jewish world and indeed initially was also regarded as a Jewish sect. Today we call them '**Jewish Christians**' (in the strict sense). The first Christian community:

- shared with all Jews the belief in the one God of the fathers ('Shema Israel'),
- held fast to the holy scriptures (Tenach),
- observed the Law (Torah): circumcision,[38] sabbath,[39] festivals,[40] and regulations about purity and food,[41]
- visited the temple,[42] sacrificed, and prayed the same psalms and hymns as other Jews.

The young messianic community which had accepted Jesus of Nazareth in faith as the true Messiah hoped that finally the whole people of Israel would accept him. It felt called to continue the proclamation of Jesus in his name. Initially its mission, too, was limited to its Jewish fellow countrymen. However, here it continually clashed with official Judaism, which strictly repudiated Jesus as a lawbreaker and false Messiah. Indeed, this dispute over Jesus of Nazareth, his provocative message, his unconventional behaviour and cruel fate, bore within it the germ of a split.

For there is no overlooking the fact that the **whole life of the earliest community**, not only its thought but also its practice, its liturgical commemoration and celebration, **centred primarily on him, Jesus, the one who was crucified and yet raised by God.** He embodied both continuity and discontinuity (because of his rejection by the religious and political establishment) with the official Judaism of the time. They had known him personally; he it was whom they confessed, but in the subsequent period they endowed him with various Jewish honorific names like 'Son of David', 'Son of Man', 'Messiah', 'Christ', 'Son of God'.

The Jesus Movement

Believed in
Jesus Christ

Jews
(='Jewish Christians')

Aramaic-speaking, from Palestine:
'Hebrews' with the 'Twelve'; **faithful to** the Temple and **the Law**

Greek-speaking, from the Diaspora:
'Hellenists' with the 'Seven'; **critical of** the Temple and **the Law**

**The apocalyptic paradigm
of primitive Christianity (P I):**

**Saul/Paul
apostle of the Gentiles**

Non-Jews
(='Gentile Christians'): Greek / Latin-speaking; **free of the Law**

World religion:

**The Hellenistic paradigm
of the early church (P II)**

These individual titles and the different notions they imply are not the decisive thing. What is decisive is that already in this first apocalyptic paradigm, still wholly stamped by Judaism, none other than Jesus himself is the basic figure who from the beginning stands at the centre of all the different traditions; indeed, he is the central figure who binds together the various traditions and indeed literally is their centre. To this degree **Jesus' theocentric proclamation of the kingdom of God** quite naturally turned into the **christocentric proclamation of Jesus as the Christ**: the gospel of Jesus became the gospel about Jesus Christ. The whole earlier history of God with his 'elect people' was increasingly read as coming to a new definitive climax in Jesus: in Jesus there was a new criterion by which even God's relationship to **all** peoples (the non-Jewish pagan peoples) could be judged anew. Here we have not just the faith of individuals but the faith of a community.

The new faith community

Truly it was not just with Paul but from the beginning that in this first Jewish Christian apocalyptic paradigm the one who had been crucified and raised showed himself to be the element that distinguished Christians from the Judaism of the time: **Jesus Christ** as the **constant centre and abiding substance** of Christian faith and life. Without him even the beginnings of Christianity cannot be understood, nor can its later eras. Ignored and betrayed though he may have been in the course of church history, Jesus Christ is indisputably the element in Christianity which is abidingly valid and represents a constant obligation. It is to him that the faith of the community is directed and he is the one whom its tangible signs of faith recall.

Faith – here understood in the light of the Hebrew Bible as unconditional, unshakable **trust** in God as Jesus had modelled him in his life – was also the foundation of earliest Christianity. That did not yet distinguish these Christians from other Jewish brothers and sisters. 'Your will be done', this prayer of the Jew Jesus, is the Jewish foundation stone of faith, a reason why to the present day Jews and Christians can pray the 'Our Father' together without difficulty.

But Jews who recognized Jesus as the Messiah were soon to form their own **community of believers**. For their confession in faith of the crucified Jesus as Messiah distinguished them from all previous messianic expectations in Judaism and inevitably had to lead to a separate community of believers, a community of those who **believed in Christ**. This and nothing else is the original description of what was later to be called with another word, 'church'. **Faith in Christ** – as the human response to the message of

Christ – was already the **basis for the new community** in the framework of the earliest Christian paradigm: this community was borne up by the conviction that the Risen One was as it were God's agent[43] – in post-exilic Judaism this was already believed of God's wisdom, of significant patriarchs and high angels! – to whom the community of Christians had a living relationship on the basis of deep spiritual experiences. The common expression of this faith was the **confession** of Jesus as the Christ, **hymns** in praise of the exalted one, **prayers** to Christ as the 'Lord', **prophecies** which were now regarded as words of the exalted one, and calling on his **name**.

Calling on his name? In this connection the question arises: but how does one become a member of this faith community? From what point does one belong visibly to it? And what did Jesus have to do with this new sign of faith? There are two **basic symbols** of the faith community: baptism and the celebration of a meal.

What distinguishes the community: baptism

One belongs to this community when one has publicly demonstrated one's faith through a distinctive **rite of initiation**: that of **baptism**.[44] This is the **first basic symbol** of the new faith community. Even this sign need not at first have cut off the followers of Jesus from their Jewish past. For forms of baptism had long also been in use within Judaism. Jews baptized their proselytes – at least this is attested for a later period, and here legal and ritual considerations were in the foreground. There was also 'baptism' in the Qumran monastery, though this was self-baptism, immersions for expiation which were repeated daily. Certainly according to the Synoptic Gospels Jesus himself did not practise baptism,[45] nor did he explicitly require it of his followers in his lifetime.[46] But like others he had himself baptized, as we know, by John the 'Baptist',[47] for whom the single rite of baptism already symbolized repentance for sins and a readiness to be renewed before God.[48] So the baptism of John may have been the model for Christian baptism, in so far as it was already given as baptism of repentance of the forgiveness of sins in the light of the end-time. The definitive conversion of men and women was to be manifested and sealed by immersion in purifying water by the person baptizing (not by the person being baptized), once for all, so that no repetition was allowed. This unique baptism of repentance in the eschatological sense was probably John's original creation, so that it is not for nothing that he was named 'the Baptist'.

Even if Jesus' post-Easter 'baptismal command' is not historical, the community felt **empowered to baptize by Jesus and his message**. Granted, there was no formal 'institution' of a baptismal rite, but equally there was no initial period of a Christianity without baptism: the first evidence goes back to the time immediately after the death of Jesus.[49] The noun 'baptism' (*to baptisma*) – in contrast to the verb 'immerse', 'baptize' (*baptizein*) – is limited to Christian terminology. The community now baptized in remembrance not only of the baptism of John but of Jesus' own baptism, indeed it baptized '**in the name of Jesus**', as Acts[50] and Paul[51] report. And what does 'in the name of Jesus' mean? In the Hebrew context 'name' is a legal term which is meant to express authority and legal status. Believers are to entrust themselves wholly to him, the exalted Lord, putting themselves under his lordship and protection. In this way, those baptized are to receive forgiveness of sins, a share in his life, his Spirit, his filial relationship with God.

In this sense the formula '**in the name of the Father, the Son and the Holy Spirit**', attested only in the Gospel of Matthew,[52] is the further development of the content of the christological formula 'in the name of Jesus', which expresses the structural elements of Christian faith. Baptism takes place in the name of the one (= the Son) in whom the one God himself (= the Father) is present with us through his Spirit (= the Holy Spirit). However, nothing is said here of a unity of these three extremely different entities at the same level.

What holds the community together: the celebration of a meal

A further question arises: what holds the Christian community together? The celebration of a communal meal may have been a central element.[53] People gathered regularly in private houses for prayer and the '**breaking of the bread**' and 'partook of food with glad and generous hearts'.[54] That Jesus himself 'instituted' a supper as it were legally is as questionable as that he formally 'instituted' baptism; an invitation to repeat the meal is missing in particular in the earliest Gospel according to Mark. But on the basis of the sources we cannot doubt that Jesus celebrated a kind of **farewell meal**, a last meal before his death, with his disciples. The tradition of this event is unusually rich and comparatively constant in the different writings of the New Testament. Four variants have been handed down,[55] of which the First Letter to the Corinthians, written about 55, is particularly important. It is the earliest, and contains a reference to a tradition which goes back to Jesus himself and could have been checked by eye-witnesses who were still alive.[56]

However, this last meal of Jesus' may not be isolated from the concrete situation and stylized as the institution of a sacramental meal. It must be seen against the background of a long series of meals which Jesus celebrated with his disciples. For whereas penitential baptism as a symbolic act was characteristic of John the Baptist, for Jesus the characteristic act was a meal held in a joyful mood, which celebrated sharing together in the coming kingdom. And as a sign of the grace and forgiveness offered in advance, those who were discriminated against and rejected, the 'publicans' and 'sinners', were not excluded. Now, in expectation of the coming kingdom and his departure, Jesus wanted to hold one more such meal with his followers: possibly (according to Mark but not John) this was a ritual Passover meal, or at any rate was in the shadow of the Jewish idea of passover, if it was celebrated one night earlier.

The special **words of Jesus** spoken on this occasion did not drop as it were from heaven as sacred words of institution. They fitted easily into the course of a festal Jewish meal regulated by ritual, of the kind that is partly still customary in Jewish families today:

– The **word over the bread** takes up grace before the main meal, where the father of the house says words of praise over the bread, breaks or tears it, and shares pieces of it with the others at table.

– The **word over the wine** takes up the prayer of thanksgiving after the meal, where the father of the house circulates the cup of wine and has everyone drink from it.[57]

So Jesus did not invent a new rite, but dared to give a new interpretation to the old rite at a dramatic moment. He combined a **new symbolic word** with the **old symbolic action**. Referring to the threat of his violent death he interpreted the broken bread and blood-red wine as so to speak **prophetic signs** which at this moment most deeply symbolized what he was, what he had done and wanted: the sacrifice, the surrender of his life. Like this bread, so would his body be broken; like this red wine, so would his blood be shed: 'This – my body; this – my blood!' The 'is' which later was so hotly disputed between the Christian churches was in all probability not spoken at all in Aramaic (and Jesus spoke the Aramaic vernacular). Both times he meant his whole person and its sacrifice. And just as the father of the household makes those who are eating and drinking share in the table blessing under the sign of bread and wine, so Jesus gives his followers a share of his body given in death (in Hebrew or Aramaic 'body' or 'flesh' always mean the whole person) and his blood shed for 'many' (an inclusive term meaning 'all').

Their master's farewell had been announced to the group of disciples, and yet there was a new foundation for their communion both among themselves and with him on the basis of their experiences of his death and resurrection. So in great simplicity and in a very natural way, in homes whether in Jerusalem or outside, a **memorial celebration** (Greek *anamnesis*, Latin *memoria*), a thanksgiving (Greek *eucharistia*), was observed: in grateful, believing remembrance a participation in the effect of this unique abiding sacrifice of Jesus' life. At a very early stage this meal was called '**Lord's Supper**'[58] or '**eucharist**'.[59] Alongside baptism this was the **second basic symbol** of the new faith community. It was a meal of commemoration and thanksgiving which at the same time was to be a covenant and community meal, indeed a sign and image of the meal of consummation in the kingdom of God. The Aramaic acclamation 'Marana tha', 'Our Lord, come', was later to be preserved even in Greek worship.[60]

We should remember that on the presupposition of the faith in the one and only God (and his Spirit) attested in the Hebrew Bible, this **Jesus Christ** – faith in him and, as a tangible expression of this faith, baptism in his name and the meal in his memory – from the beginning formed the **constant centre** and the abiding substance of Christianity. Here lay the foundation of the tremendous dynamic of original Christianity.

In retrospect, we can now already define some characteristics of the **entire Jewish Christian constellation** which remained important even after the destruction of the temple in the year 70:

- the eschatological horizon which the Jews who followed Jesus had in common with many Jews;
- also the Jewish attitude to life, by continuing to observe the Mosaic ritual law, above all circumcision, sabbath and festivals, regulations about cleanness and food;
- finally, Jewish theology: apocalyptic motives, wisdom speculations.

However, the expectation of an imminent end was to be disappointed, and here already it is clear that a simple restoration of earliest Christianity would inevitably lead one astray. The 'end time' of the expectation of the immediate coming of the kingdom of God was followed by the 'interim time' of the church. The church? Did Jesus want a church at all? This is not a rhetorical question but a very serious one, especially for those who are serious about the church.

4. The foundation of a church?

The man from Nazareth, without any office and dignities, had proclaimed the kingdom of God, but he had not wanted to create a special community distinct from Israel with its own creed and cult, its own constitution and ministries. In other words, Jesus had sparked off a great **eschatological collective movement,** and for him the Twelve with Peter were a sign of the full number of the tribes of Israel that was to be restored. However, Jesus had no thought of founding a great religious structure; there are no words of Jesus addressed to the public which programmatically summon a community of the elect or call for the founding of a church. Indeed according to the Gospels he almost never used the word 'church'.

What is church?

'Church' in the sense of a religious community distinct from Israel is clearly already something to do with the Jewish Christian communities **after Jesus' death**: they were not founded by Jesus but came into being with reference to him, the crucified one who was alive. For it is only after Easter, under the impact of the experience of resurrection and the Spirit, that there is a community with an eschatological orientation. Its foundation is not initially its own cult, its own constitution, its own organization with particular offices, but, as we saw, simply and solely the confession in faith of this Jesus as the Messiah, as it is sealed with baptism and celebrated by the meal in his memory.

A **community of those who believe in Christ** – that is my short definition of '**church**',[61] Congregatio or Communio Christifidelium: the community of those who have committed themselves to the person and cause of Jesus Christ and who bear witness to it as hope for all men and women. So where the church distorts the cause of Jesus Christ instead of serving it and bringing it to fruition, it sins against its own being and perverts itself. The degree to which the church is committed to the cause of its Lord is already clear from its name. The usual word 'church' in English, 'Kirche' in German, 'kyrka' in Swedish (cf. the Slavonic 'cerkoc') does not come from curia, as Luther thought. It probably comes via the Gothic from the Byzantine vernacular form Kyrike and means 'belonging to the Lord ('kyrios'), viz. 'house or community of the Lord'. But with 'ecclesia', 'iglesia', 'chiesa', 'église', the Romance languages have even preserved a direct linguistic connection with the word used in the New Testament: in secular Greek, ekklesia means the assembly, the political popular assembly. However, in the New Testament this is a translation for the term kahal used in the Hebrew Bible, and found in the Greek translation of it known as the Septuagint, where it is the solemn designation of the 'assembly of God (Yahweh)'.

So when the earliest Jewish-Christian community took over this particular designation, it was making a great claim (within Judaism): that it was the **true** divine assembly, the **true** eschatological community of God which was now assembling in the name and in the spirit of the Messiah confirmed by God. In other words, it was the '*kahal* of Jesus'. In the New Testament *kahal-ekklesia* means both the **process of assembling** and the **assembled community** itself. That means that without assembling there is no community, no church. Already in the Jewish Christian paradigm the concrete gathering for worship was regarded as the manifestation, representation, indeed realization of the newly formed Jesus community.

That provides the norm once and for all: *ekklesia* originally in no way meant an abstract and remote hyper-organization of functionaries set above the concrete assembly, but in origin a community gathered at a particular place at a particular time engaged in a particular action. However, this is no isolated, self-satisfied religious association, but a community which forms a comprehensive community with others. Each **local church** fully represents the **whole church**. To it is given all that it needs in its place for human salvation: the proclamation of the gospel, baptism, the Lord's Supper, the different charisms and services. Each individual community, all its members, may understand itself as the people of God, the body of Christ, a spiritual building.

The significance of women

That Jesus himself relativized the 'fathers' and their traditions, also called women to his group of disciples,[62] and even expressed his high esteem for children shows that patriarchal hierarchies cannot appeal to him. Nor did he make, for example, celibacy a condition of discipleship. A law of celibacy cannot appeal to Jesus for legitimation either; moreover the Hebrew Bible nowhere thought celibacy praiseworthy. The apostles were and remained married (Paul regarded himself as an exception[63]). The church of the Jewish Christian paradigm could have called itself **democratic** in the best sense of the word (at any rate not aristocratic or monarchical): **a community in freedom, equality and brotherhood and sisterhood**. For this church was:

– not an institution of power, not a Grand Inquisition, but a community of free people;

– not a church of classes, races, castes or ministries, but a community of those who in principle were equal;

– not an empire under patriarchal rule with a cult of persons but a community of brothers and sisters. Sisters? This in particular needs to be explained.

According to present-day research there can no longer be any question that women played a considerably more important role, not only among the disciples of Jesus, but also in earliest Christianity, than is directly indicated in the New Testament sources. We are above all indebted to the

German American New Testament scholar Elisabeth Schüssler Fiorenza for having investigated the New Testament material from a 'feminist theological perspective'. Her investigation confirms that in the early Jewish Christian Jesus movement there was a 'praxis of equality and the involvement of all, both male and female disciples': 'The majority of them were not rich, like the Cynic philosophers who could reject property and cultural positions in order "to become free from possessions". Rather, they were called from the impoverished, starving and "heavy laden" countrypeople. They were tax collectors, sinners, women, children, fishers, housewives, those who had been healed from their infirmities or set free from bondage to their evil spirits. What they offered was not an alternative lifestyle but an alternative ethos: they were those without a future, but now they had hope again; they were the "outcast" and marginal people in their society, but now they had community again.'[64]

How far, however, women were active as charismatic itinerant preachers in the early Jewish Christian community can only be conjectured. Historically this can no more be verified than the thesis that 'women were decisive for the extension of the Jesus movement to gentiles'.[65] So we should be very restrained in concluding 'historical leadership'[66] or even 'leading positions for women[67] from individual texts (e.g. that about the Syro-Phoenician woman in Mark 7.24-30). That also applies to the role of Mary Magdalene, who may have been the most significant female figure from Jesus' immediate circle.

All this, however, does not detract from the important recognition that the activity of Jesus called to life a community of disciples who were equals, and this also has a critical message for the present situation. And if explicit criticism of patriarchy was also no essential part of the Jesus movement, Elisabeth Schüssler Fiorenza is still right: 'No one is exempted. Everyone is invited. Women as well as men, prostitutes as well as Pharisees. The parable of the "Great Supper" jolts the hearer into recognizing that the *basileia* includes everyone. It warns that only those who were "first invited" and who then rejected the invitation will be excluded. Not the holiness of the elect but the wholeness of **all** is the central vision of Jesus. Therefore, his parables also take their images from the world of women. His healings and exorcisms make women whole. His announcement of "eschatological reversal" – many who are first will be last and those last will be first – applies also to women and to their impairment by patriarchal structures.'[68]

However, we should note here that although all members in this early church in principle have equal rights, in principle the same rights and duties, this did not mean a uniform egalitarianism, a co-ordination and uniformity which levelled out the multiplicity of gifts and ministries. On the contrary: the earliest Jerusalem community in which, according to Luke, people were 'of one heart and one soul',[69] showed opposed persons, a variety of positions, differentiated functions.

Provisional structures: no 'hierarchy'

On the basis of the texts we cannot ignore the fact that from the beginning – despite the apocalyptic expectation of an imminent end – there were **provisional structures** in the community: above all the group of **Twelve**, but also the group of **Seven** whom the Acts of the Apostles calls 'Hellenists'. From this we can conclude that the community which followed Jesus will by no means have consisted only of Aramaic-speaking Jews, but also to no small degree of Greek-speaking Hellenistic Jews.

At any rate the conflict over the daily care of widows reported in Acts 6.1 seems to reflect a marked division in the earliest community between 'Hellenists' on the one hand and 'Hebrews' on the other. It is further underlined by the fact that to all appearances other Jewish Christian groups had their own synagogues and their own house communities in which scripture was read at worship in their own language – Hebrew or Greek. These Jewish Christians who had Greek as their mother tongue – deriving socially and culturally from the urban milieu of Hellenistic Diaspora Judaism and, because they were educated, probably also spiritually more active – may have been led by the Stephen group ('the Seven', all of whom have purely Greek names); they were probably relatively independent from the group of apostles representing the 'Hebrews' ('the Twelve', who represented the twelve tribes of Israel). At the same time that means that 'the Seven' may well have been much more than simply welfare officers subordinate to the 'Twelve', as Luke's Acts of the Apostles reports a generation later. We should see them more as the 'leading group of an independent community' which was already engaged in active mission in Jerusalem at that time.

Apostles? Not just the Twelve, nor even the Seven, were apostles, but all those who were regarded as the primal witnesses and messengers: those who proclaimed the message of Christ and founded and led communities as the first witnesses. We cannot tell whether the title apostle was also given to women in Jewish Christianity; it would be otherwise in the Gentile Christian sphere. But it is certain that right from the beginning in Jewish Christianity – and this is easily overlooked – there were not only prophets but also prophetesses: in addition to Agabus, Judas and Silas mention is explicitly made in Acts of the four daughters of Philip; in addition there were evangelists and helpers of very different kinds, here too men and women.

Offices? These various church ministries and callings were not given that name at this time. In fact in the New Testament secular terms for 'office' were avoided, and with good reason. Why? They express relationships of domination which the Christian community did not want to take over. Instead of this another general term was used, a quite ordinary unreligious word with a rather inferior tone, which could in no way conjure up associations with any authority, rule, or position of dignity and power: '*diakonia*', service – originally serving at table. Here it was evidently Jesus himself, serving his disciples at table, who set the irrevocable standard. That is the only explanation of the frequency of the saying which has been handed down in six different variants: 'The highest shall be the servant of all (at table).'

And **hierarchy** = '**holy rule**'? From the beginning of Christianity this would have been the last term of all which people would have used for serving in the church, which aimed to avoid any style and allure of domination: it was only introduced five hundred years later, by an alleged disciple of the apostle Paul, Dionysius the Areopagite (Pseudo-Dionysius). Certainly, there is also authority and power in the church, but in the spirit of Jesus it is never to become domination (and the preservation of privileges), but is to be used for the service and the well-being of all. In the light of the New Testament only '**church ministry**' is allowed, a phrase which must never be veiled with the pseudo-humility of clerical domination.

Moreover, it is striking that in the New Testament the word '**priest**' in the religious sense of sacrificial priest (*hiereus, sacerdos*), like all sacral cultic titles, is avoided in connection with functions of the community – in favour of designations of function drawn from the secular sphere. Certainly the word 'priest' is used as a matter of course for Jewish and pagan dignitaries, but strikingly never for those serving in the Christian communities. For this reason it is usually avoided in Protestant churches.

Though the English word 'priest' (like '*Priester*', '*prêtre*', '*prete*', '*presbitero*') traditionally denotes the cultic and sacral *sacerdotium*, it originally derives from the uncultic title of the elder of the community, so that as is usual in some churches it can appropriately be replaced by '**presbyter**' or '**elder**', or *presbyter parochianus*. There had been *zekenim*, presbyters, elders, at the head of each Jewish community from time immemorial. Probably from the 40s on, the earliest Jewish community had its own elders, though we have no report of their being appointed. Presumably already at the same time there was the laying on of hands or ordination, similarly deriving from Jewish tradition, which in the Christian community meant the authoritative sending of particular members for special service. Luke first reports this in Acts in connection with the Hellenists' 'Seven' mentioned above.

Historically speaking, we cannot discover whether there was a distinctive constitution of elders in Jerusalem who claimed local authority and then authority over the whole church before Peter left and the leadership of the earliest Jerusalem community was taken over by James. Possibly the college of presbyters came into being as the community became increasingly distanced from its origins and the Twelve disappeared. The community was growing, and this group of older, well-tried members could govern it and perhaps also guard against an increasing danger of heresy. But we need to investigate one question: what was the precise position of Peter and James, of John and finally also Paul, with whose names the first conflicts in earliest Christianity are associated?

5. The first great conflicts

According to the New Testament, there is no disputing the fact that that Simon whom perhaps Jesus himself nicknamed the 'rock' (Aramaic *Cepha*, Greek *Petros*[70]), the fisherman who came from Bethsaida and was married in Capernaum – was already **spokesman of the disciples** during Jesus' public activity,[71] even if his role was subsequently stylized, so that his name also appears at the head of the group of the Twelve.[72]

Peter: a move to the Gentiles

However, Peter was *primus inter pares*: the **first among equals**. And he was a man – evidently passionately committed to Jesus, but changeable and wavering – whom the first two Gospels in no way idealize. He is errant and fallible; he is no hero or genius. His failure to understand, his lack of courage, his unreliability and finally his flight are unsparingly reported, as is the flight of the other disciples. Only Luke, who also idealizes the earliest community as a model, tones down or removes some offensive features: he passes over Jesus' 'Get behind me, Satan' to Peter after his messianic confession,[73] abbreviates the Gethsemane scene in favour of the disciples, then suppresses the note of their flight and makes amazingly positive statements about Peter and the disciples.[74]

It is also historically certain that – if we leave aside Mary Magdalene and the women – Peter was also the **first witness to the resurrection of Jesus**,[75] and consequently could be regarded as the rock of the church. But we can assume with the same certainty – today even according to Catholic exegesis[76] — that the famous saying about **Peter as the rock** on which Jesus will build his church,[77] which has an Aramaic character but strikingly has no parallels in the other Gospels, is not a saying of the earthly Jesus but a post-Easter construction of the Palestinian community or Matthew. The details of what the historical Peter believed and preached cannot be developed either from the speeches in Acts, which have been edited by Luke, or from the New Testament letters of Peter, which are not authentic.

Certainly, already in the New Testament Peter became increasingly important as a type for Christian faith and for the unity of the church made up of Jews and Gentiles ('Peter typology').[78] According to the first chapters of the Acts of the Apostles he remained unassailably the spokesman of the disciples. But Peter by no means had exclusive authority, or even a monarchical legal power of leadership (jurisdiction). Historically, we cannot get round the statement that up to the Apostolic Council in Jerusalem (around 48) Peter was only **leader of the earliest Jerusalem community**[79] **together with** the group of Twelve and later in the college of the three 'pillars'[80] — James (now in first place!), Peter and John.

In Jerusalem Peter showed himself to be a representative of that tolerant Jewish Christianity which was well disposed towards the Pauline mission to the Gentiles — in contrast to those Jewish Christians in Galatia who were causing confusion, who required full observance of the Law from Gentile Christians and promptly provoked the anger of the apostle Paul. Moreover at the Apostolic Council there was an official agreement over the division of mission between the Jerusalem people (the three pillars mentioned) and Paul: Peter was now regarded as the one destined by God to 'serve as apostle among the circumcised',[81] Paul was the one chosen by God 'for service among the Gentiles'.[82] So Peter carried on **a mission among Jews bound by the Law,** in the wake of which Jewish Christian communities came into being in different parts of the empire.

And **Rome?** Had not Peter been in the then capital of the world — with such well-known consequences for church history? Here, too, historical caution is appropriate. Certainly it is clear that Peter is the only one of the Twelve who carried on a mission outside Jerusalem, although there is no itinerary for his journeys nor any precise chronology. A stay of Peter in Antioch (probably 49/50) is attested by Paul,[83] and a visit to Corinth, where there was possibly a Jewish-Christian group, is quite likely.[84] But as far as Rome is concerned we read nothing anywhere in the New Testament in connection with Peter. And above all, there is not even a hint of a specific 'successor' to Peter (and also in Rome). That would also be quite improbable, simply because of the logic of the image of the rock:[85] Peter's faith is to remain the constant foundation of the whole church!

And yet the tradition which connects Peter with Rome (initially free of any church-political tendency) – the so-called First Letter of Clement[86] (around 96) and Ignatius of Antioch[87] (c.110) – is so old, so clear and above all unrivalled that our historical starting point must be that Peter was in Rome at the end of his life and probably died as a martyr in the Neronian persecution. Even if it is impossible to identify his tomb under the Vatican basilica by archaeological means, 'Today there is increasing agreement that Peter went to Rome and suffered martyrdom there.' That statement appears in the Joint Lutheran-Catholic declaration made in the USA in 1974, though there is a significant 'but': 'but there is no reliable evidence that Peter was ever at the head of the local church of Rome as supreme head or bishop. We learn nothing from the New Testament about a successor to Peter in Rome.'[88]

We shall have to look closely at the consequences for theology and church history of the tradition about Peter in Rome. However, already at this point we need to take note of what the Catholic New Testament scholar Paul Hoffmann said about the 'formation of a monepiscopal community constitution as the foundation of the later hierocratic church structure': 'Personal charisma is replaced with the charisma of office, the institution itself becomes its vehicle and guarantor, the "grace-giving institution" – a process which in the further course of church history leads to the first rational bureaucracy in the history of the world in the form of the mediaeval church and finally in the nineteenth century to the ecclesial formation of a dictatorial bureaucracy – legalized by making the Pope's primacy of jurisdiction a dogma – of the kind that shapes the real existence of Catholicism today.'[89]

James: in favour of the link with the synagogue

However, not Rome (the inscription on the Latern basilica *caput et mater omnium ecclesiarum urbis et orbis* is triumphalistic but wrong) but **Jerusalem** was **the centre and mother community of the first Christianity.** And at the latest from the 'Apostolic Council' on, and especially after the departure of Peter, another man increasingly became the central figure in Jerusalem: **James**, the 'brother of the Lord', so called because he was presumably the oldest of the four physical brothers of Jesus[90] – not to be confused with James the son of Zebedee, the brother of John, who was one of the Twelve and had been executed around 43 by Herod Agrippa.[91] James, the brother of Jesus, who like his other brothers was at first ashamed of the outsider[92] and did not take his side in the confrontation in his home town of Nazareth,[93] had evidently only come to faith in Jesus after Easter; it is said that he had a personal experience of a christophany.[94] In the 'Apostolic Council' he had generously contributed to the compromise with Paul: the liberation of pagan believers in Jesus from the Jewish ritual law, but the unconditional continuation of strict observance of the Law for Jewish believers in Jesus.[95] Jewish Christians and Gentile Christians were to live together in a single church community, and the Jewish Christians could remain in their ancestral synagogues – in hope of a conversion of all Israel to the Messiah Jesus.

So after Peter's departure this brother of Jesus, a strict observer of the Law yet at the same time accommodating, and personally blameless, along with like-minded 'elders', became **supreme head of the earliest community** during the persecution under Agrippa I in the 40s; as such he had an authority which went beyond the region, and in the succeeding period he remained the normative figure who provided the guidelines for Jewish Christianity. While Simon Peter was revered as 'the rock', James was revered as 'the just'.

According to the report by the Jewish historian, priest and eyewitness Josephus,[96] he, the 'brother of Jesus who is called Christ, James by name, along with some others (Jewish Christians)', was condemned between the death of the procurator Festus and the arrival of his successor Albinus. This was presumably in 62, and the charge of the supreme Jewish court (the 'Sanhedrin') under the Sadducean high priest Annas II may have been one of 'transgression of the Law', carrying the penalty of **death by stoning**, the punishment for serious religious offences. Pharisees in particular ('those in the city who had a particular concern for the Law and were committed to a strict observance of the Law') protested against this judicial murder. Possibly James, as the leader of a messianic movement, seemed politically destabilizing, and was burdened not only with his affinity to Jesus but also by his acceptance and toleration of Paul, the representative of a mission to the Gentiles outside the Law. Be this as it may, a little later Paul too was arrested in Jerusalem as a 'lawbreaker' (and because of his 'desecration' of the sanctuary[97]), and after a two-year trial in Caesarea was executed in Rome in 64, two years after James.

For the earliest community the execution of its leader James and those close to him represented 'a catastrophe . . . from which it was never to recover': 'Evidently the supporters of the party of the priestly nobility saw in James and his friends the same kind of religious and political danger for the people that they had seen thirty-two years earlier in Jesus.'[98] For many Jewish Christians James later became a legend, a figure who was increasingly transfigured and absolutized; the letter attributed to him corrects Paul at various points; in the non-canonical Gospel of the Hebrews (not to be confused with the canonical Letter to the Hebrews) James – in contradiction to all the other sources – not only takes part in the Last Supper, but is also promised the first appearance of the risen Christ.

But this persecution had fatal consequences for the relationship of the early Christian community to the Jewish authorities: after the executions of, first, the Hellenistic Jewish Christian Stephen (with the flight of the Hellenistic Jewish Christians from Jerusalem) and then James the son of Zebedee, this stoning certainly made a major contribution to the break between Jews and Jewish Christians. The persecution and then – after the catastrophic year 70 – the expulsion from the synagogue resulted in a definitive separation from the synagogue. The **excommunication of Christians** by the now Pharisaic establishment preceded all the persecution of Jews by Christians.[99] It is here that the early anti-Judaism even of the Jewish Christians which has been recorded in the Gospel of Matthew and then especially in the Gospel of John – lamentable as it is – has its historical roots. Hence the question: what about John?

Excommunication by the synagogue: John's community

According to the most recent scholarship the author of the Gospel of John, which was written in Greek, was also a Jew: a **Hellenistic Jew** who was deeply rooted in the Hebrew Bible and the Jewish wisdom tradition and who wrote for a predominantly Jewish-Christian community with Gentile Christian members, for whom he explained the Jewish terms and customs which frequently occurred.[100] And at this point it is striking that unlike the name of Peter, the name of the third leading man in Jerusalem, that of James, who was well known and highly respected in all the communities, is deliberately passed over in silence; indeed, in a striking scene the brothers of Jesus are even all presented as unbelievers.[101]

However, we must bear in mind that at the time of the composition of the Gospel of John around 100, i.e. more than three decades after the judicial murder of the brother of the Lord, James' way – confession of the Messiah Jesus and participation in synagogue life and worship – had failed. For now the **formal excommunication of Christians** was already **in force**: that pernicious 'cursing of the heretics' which had been pronounced after the Jewish-Roman war and the destruction of the Second Temple by a 'council' in Jamnia (near Jaffa), dominated by Pharisees, and which was repeated at the beginning of every act of worship in the synagogue.[102] Granted, it also related to other heretics, but it had particularly fatal consequences for the Jewish followers of Jesus of

Nazareth, who were specifically named. From now on they were excluded from the worship and the whole life of the synagogue, and for them this had not only religious but also far-reaching social and economic consequences: 'Old ties were totally cut, all personal and social converse was interrupted and all help was excluded.'[103]

So why is there constant **silence** about **James** the brother of the Lord **in the Gospel of John,** indeed why is he indirectly disqualified? The Tübingen exegete Christian Dietzfelbinger has investigated this question and has offered a convincing solution.[104] His answer is that the exclusion of the brothers of Jesus, who were accused of unbelief, did not apply to the historical brothers of Jesus, who were already dead, but to those Jewish Christian groups which still appealed to James and his way. For the author of the Gospel of John was living in a community in which the exclusion from the synagogue had become a reality.[105] This community no longer wanted to have anything to do with the synagogue, as it no longer allowed the message of Jesus to be proclaimed, was hostile towards the Christian community, and thus proved to be part of the evil and dark 'world' hostile to Jesus. An atmosphere of anxiety must have prevailed in John's community: a 'fear of the Jews'.[106] The synagogue critical of Jesus had become a synagogue hostile to Jesus.

So for the author of the Fourth Gospel an understanding between the Christian community and the synagogue was no longer possible: 'Belief in Jesus and membership of the synagogue were now no longer compatible, and if they had formerly been compatible, such compatibility had now come to an end through the continued "no" of the synagogue to Jesus and the Jesus community.'[107] Thus the Johannine community set its own **'no'** **against the 'no' of the synagogue to the Messiah Jesus.** Confronted with the synagogue, it saw itself as the new internalized, spiritualized community of the new age, exclusively focussed on Jesus as the Light of the World and the Good Shepherd. The manna of the Exodus, the pouring out of water at the Feast of Tabernacles and the spirit of the end-time – all these were now related to Jesus, who also stood for the Temple and the Law. Instead of the Torah, it was Jesus who was 'the way, the truth and the life'; only through him did one come to the Father.[108] Moreover, according to John Jesus was not condemned to death by the Romans as a political rebel but by the Jewish authorities for the religious crime of blasphemy.

We can no longer discover how far the Johannine community's very **high christology** (Jesus as the heavenly Son of God already existing before Abraham) – as compared with the Synoptic tradition, which was evidently regarded as inadequate – and the equally very high understanding of the eucharist (Jesus as the bread of life) was the presupposition or the consequence of excommunication by the synagogue. But it is certain that such high christological statements must have seemed sheer blasphemy to orthodox Judaism. Moreover this charge is clearly reflected in the Gospel, where there is no longer a conflict with the Law (over the sabbath) but over the identification of Jesus with God: 'This was why the Jews sought all the more to kill him, because he not only broke the sabbath but also called God his Father, thus making himself equal with God.'[109] What appears in the Gospel as a charge against Jesus is a reflection of the repudiation of the community by 'the Jews': 'We stone you for no good work but for blasphemy; because you, being a man, make yourself God.'[110]

But what really was blasphemous? It will be said that the basis for the pre-existence of Jesus seems already to be laid in the famous prologue to the Gospel. But what kind of pre-existence was this? The answer is that at least in the prologue, what is spoken of is not the pre-existence of the Son but that of the Logos, the Word.

Pre-existence of the Logos in the Gospel of John

The view has largely become established in exegesis that the author of the prologue has used an older, probably **Jewish-Hellenistic hymn** which in good Jewish fashion is not about a pre-existent divine being 'Son', but about God and his Logos, his Word, his Wisdom in creation and revelation. The Christian author of the prologue did not change this text about the Word which was from the beginning with God, but only gave it a Christian **focus** at the end: 'and the Word was made flesh and dwelt among us'.[111] For the Christian author this is the 'climax of the prologue',[112] which in this way has lost nothing of its universality: God's Word remains the life and light of human beings;[113] God's Word was and already is there at creation, is at work everywhere. But now it has become visible and tangible among us in a human being.

So this Christian 'focus' simply seeks to provide a concrete location for the universal Word of God in history: Jesus of Nazareth is the Word made flesh, God's Logos in person, **God's Wisdom in human form**. The Jew Philo of Alexandria, Jesus' contemporary, had already described the world-embracing Stoic Logos as 'God' and 'Son of God', but for the sake of strict monotheism he subordinated him as 'second God' to **the** God (*ho theos*). The evangelist John, though, was the first to identify the titles Logos and Son of God with a concrete person, the earthly Jesus, and thus give the title Son of God a personal content which it did not have for Philo and which was unacceptable to Jews.[114]

But at the same time it must be noted that God's wisdom is active not only in Jesus but everywhere among human beings. The New Testament scholar Leonhardt Goppelt has identified this difficult problem: 'The Logos of the prologue **became** Jesus: Jesus was the Logos become flesh, but not the Logos as such.'[115] And Hans Conzelmann emphasizes that here John does not have a pre-existence christology but a christology of mission and revelation: 'There are no pictures either of the pre-existence (John does not relate any heavenly conversations of the Son with the Father before his incarnation) or of the course of the incarnation (there is no virgin birth). Both come under the radical reduction made by John. There is only a portrayal of what happens after the incarnation, the appearance of Jesus in the world. Pre-existence and incarnation form the **foil** to this description: they designate the indescribable origin of Jesus.'[116]

Only recently have we had a comprehensive account of the **problems of pre-existence** which considers both the problem in the New Testament and contemporary attempts at a solution in systematic theology (from Harnack and Barth to Rahner and Moltmann). In his *magnum opus Born Before All Time?*,[117] the Tübingen theologian Karl-Josef Kuschel has emphasized the essential point:[118] one cannot talk of a self-divinization of Jesus in the Gospel of John any more than one can talk of a divinization by his disciples. Indeed the few statements that are made about a pre-existence of the Son of God do not mythologize or engage in conceptual speculation, but describe his mission, which has a soteriological orientation of a kind familiar to Jews for centuries: the Redeemer comes from God. John's christology is not pre-existence christology but a revelation and sending christology in which the statements about pre-existence have the function of emphasizing the significance of the Redeemer and Messiah Jesus of Nazareth.[119] That means: 'The Johannine writings are not interested in protology in isolation and for its own sake, whether in speculation about divine beings before all time, or in the assumption that the man Jesus is pre-existent in the temporal sense. Rather, they state in trust that the existence of Jesus Christ "in the world" owes itself to the initiative of God.'[120]

But how are we then to understand the **unity of Father and Son** which is so emphatically emphasized by the Gospel of John in particular? The answer is: as with similar Johannine sayings, the statement that the Father and Jesus are 'one'[121] is not meant as a 'metaphysical statement about the unity of the Father and the Son'.[122] This is not about a unity in categories of Hellenistic ontology but about a 'unity in activity',[123] a 'unity of action'[124] – understood not in metaphysical but in personal terms – a unity of revelation: 'Whoever sees me (the human being) sees (God) the Father.'[125] So Kuschel rightly says against any theology of metaphysical speculation (in the style of Karl Barth): 'In defining the unity, John is not concerned with either mythological speculations or metaphysical conceptualizations of Jesus' Godhead, divine being or divine nature.'[126] More recent exegesis, both Catholic and Protestant, is largely agreed: 'John does not investigate the metaphysical nature and being of the pre-existent Christ; he is not concerned to know that before the incarnation there were two pre-existent divine persons who were bound together in the one divine nature. This way of conceiving things is alien to John. So too is the conception of a "begetting within the Godhead".'[127]

So what is John's positive concern? It is 'the confession that the Word of God which is with God from eternity, God's Word and thus God himself, has become man in Jesus of Nazareth. Jesus is the eternal word of God in person, not because people believe in him or because he asserts it of himself, but because this is what he is from God. Jesus is the eternal Son of God, not because human beings have understood this to be the case or because he has made it plausible, but because this is what he is and always was, from God.'[128] This explanation does not yet explode the structure of the conceptual framework of what Jews and Jewish Christians can believe. On the contrary: the christology of the Jewish Christian John still remains fully within the Jewish horizon of understanding of the time. It is part of the original Jewish Christian paradigm.

But what then about the apostle Paul, whose high christology is often made responsible for the alienation of Christians from their Jewish roots?

In continuity with Jesus: the faith of the Jew Paul

Whatever will need to be said later about the attitude of the former Pharisee from the tribe of Benjamin to the Jewish law, Paul can only be understood from his origin in Judaism. His theology remains completely in continuity with the preaching of Jesus and so utterly tied to its Jewish roots.

The great themes of Pauline theology cannot be understood without this continuity. Paul shares with Jesus:
– the expectation of the imminent coming of the kingdom of God;
– knowledge of the actual sinfulness of human beings;
– a summons to faith and conversion;
– belief in God's activity in history;
– belief that the God of Israel is also the God of all peoples;
– an understanding of faith as unconditional trust in God and the conviction that sinners are justified on the basis of this trust in God without having merited it by their own achievements or earning it through works of the Law;

– love of God and love of neighbour as actual fulfilling of the Law: unconditional obedience to God and unselfish dedication to fellow human beings.

In his sympathetic transformation of the proclamation of Jesus – now interpreted by him in the light of Jesus' death and resurrection – Paul did not create a new system, a new '**substance of faith**'. As a Jew he built on that foundation which in his own words has been laid once for all by God: **Jesus Christ**.[129] This is also the origin, content and critical norm of his, Paul's, proclamation. So in the light of a totally different situation after the death and resurrection of Jesus he did not advocate another cause, but the same one: the **cause of Jesus** which is none other than God's cause and the cause of human beings – but now, sealed by death and resurrection, understood summarily as the **cause of Jesus Christ**.[130] This living experience of Jesus Christ was for Paul the origin and criterion of the new freedom, the irrevocable centre and norm of what is Christian.

So in the **substance of faith** Paul does not differ from the Jewish Christians who wanted to maintain the Mosaic ritual law. Central for him, too, are:

● faith in Jesus as the Messiah/Christ of God and practical discipleship;
● baptism in his name;
● a ceremonial meal in his memory.

The question is, though: didn't Paul remove himself far from Judaism, particularly in his christology? Isn't there in Paul in particular the notion of a personal pre-existence of Jesus as the Son of God which is unprecedented within Judaism and in conflict with Jewish monotheism?

Pre-existence of the Son in Paul?

Karl-Josef Kuschel has also investigated and set out the alleged 'pre-existence christology' of the apostle Paul step by step on the basis of the most recent scholarly exegesis:[131]

– Surprisingly, Paul did not make fruitful use for his christology of the statements about pre-existence already 'lying ready' in Jewish apocalyptic and wisdom theology.

– In adopting a text like the Philippians hymn,[132] which probably for the first time in the New Testament contains a christological statement about pre-existence, he put the emphasis not on the heavenly origin but completely on the humiliation and the cross.

– But even in his further christology Paul showed no interest in shaping the heavenly 'form of existence' of Christ in God.

– Rather, from the beginning of his theology to the end, against an apocalyptic horizon (an expectation of an imminent end), the apostle presents a theology which is concentrated on the crucified one who is risen.

Kuschel's final conclusion on Paul is: '**Paul's authentic christology does not recognize any independent statements about a being of Jesus Christ before the world or before time** (in direct statements either about "being with God" before appearing on earth or about his own mediation at creation, or even identifying him with God), though Paul also has no difficulties in taking over a statement about pre-existence from the Hellenistic community. Protology has no independent significance for him. In the strict sense, the word "pre-existence" is open to misunderstanding in Pauline christology; it is unusable and should be avoided in the future. Paul's confessions are about the **origin, derivation and presence** of Christ, from God and in God, but not about a temporally isolated 'existence' before the creation of the world. **For Paul, Christ is the crucified wisdom of God in person, not personified pre-existent wisdom.**'[133]

On this point Paul remained within the framework of the rest of Jewish Christian christology. When he says that God has 'sent' his Son,[134] there is no underlying mythological scheme of pre-existence and existence but a prophetic scheme familiar to Jews for centuries: just as God sent the prophets, now in the end time he is sending the definitive saviour, the Messiah Jesus Christ. The Dutch exegete Bas von Iersel rightly states: 'It is more likely that the sending of the Son must be seen against the background of the prophets whom God sent before him. The idea is then that God is no longer satisfied with a prophet, but that he sends his own Son who is greater than the prophets. Does he send him from heaven? This is not mentioned even once, in contrast to what Wisdom 9.10 says about wisdom. There is no mention either of this Son having previously been with God – as is the case with wisdom in Wisdom 9.9. On the contrary, the Son who is sent was born under the law, i.e. at a moment when the Torah was already in force, and he was born from a woman (Gal.4.4); and he is sent when the fullness of time comes. What Paul writes about the sending of the Son can in no way be understood of a situation preceding the beginning of history, but rather of an event following Jesus' birth and preceding his resurrection. Sent by God, Jesus, as God's own Son, revealed more of God and realized more of God's intentions than any prophet before him, and more, too, than all his predecessors together.'[135]

So there is no trace of a real pre-existence christology, far less of a 'triune God' in either Paul or John. Paul's **christocentricity** remains grounded and comes to a climax again in a strict **theocentricity**: his intellectual model was **not** the **co-ordination** of Father, Son and Spirit **but** the **concern** of God for human beings, 'from God through Jesus Christ in the Spirit', and the concern of human beings for God, 'through Jesus Christ in the Spirit to God'. We need to remember that although Paul already introduced the paradigm shift to Gentile Christianity through his mission to the Gentiles outside the Law, in his christology he did not for a moment shake Jewish monotheism. For him in particular the very different 'roles' and functions of Father, Son and Spirit are often characterized by three different prepositions (for example: from God – through Christ – in the Spirit) or through different properties and activities. However, Paul calls God himself '**Lord**' very much less, since this name is usually used for the 'Lord' Jesus Christ – displacing the many lords and gods. But conversely, Jesus is hardly ever called 'God'.

God? Why is there never talk of the 'triune God'? Should there not be mention of this 'triune' or 'threefold' God, of the Trinity, particularly in the New Testament, if here, as some theologians say, the 'central mystery' of Christianity is to be dicussed? But where is there mention of the Trinity in the New Testament?

6. What Jewish Christians believe

In the **earliest Jewish Christian community**, belief in the one God was so much taken for granted that the idea of rivalry from another being who was equal to God a priori could not arise. That the one who had been executed had been exalted by God to God and now (wholly in accordance with Psalm 110) occupied the place of honour 'at the right hand of God', that he had now been made 'Lord and Messiah'[136] through the resurrection and now is the pioneer, bringer of salvation and coming judge of the world – all this was regarded in the Jewish Christian paradigm – and also in Paul and John – **not as rivalry to faith in the one God but as its consequence**. Jesus Christ was the embodiment of the rule and kingdom of God, which could now be experienced in the Spirit. Baptism was a tangible sign of faith, first 'in the name of Jesus' and finally also 'in the name of the Father, the Son and the Holy Spirit' – a liturgical development of the christological formula in Matthew's community. Baptism took place in the name of the one (the 'Son') in whom the one God himself (the 'Father') is with us through his Spirit (the 'Holy Spirit'). And yet:

No doctrine of the Trinity in the New Testament

Although there are so many triadic formulas in the New Testament, there is not a word anywhere in the New Testament about the 'unity' of these three highly different entities, a unity on the same divine level. In I John there was once a sentence (the *comma Johanneum*) connected with the saying about the Spirit, the water and the blood, which went on to speak of the Father, the Word and the Spirit, which, it said, are 'one'.[137] However, historical-critical research has unmasked this sentence as a forgery which came into being in North Africa or Spain in the third or fourth century, though the Roman Inquisition was still vainly attempting to defend its authenticity at the beginning of our century.[138]

In short, in Judaism, indeed throughout the New Testament, while there is **belief in God the Father, in Jesus the Son and in God's Holy Spirit**, there is **no doctrine of one God in three persons (modes of being)**, no doctrine of a 'triune God', a 'Trinity'. But how does the New Testament understand the relationship between Father, Son and Spirit?

There is probably no better story in the New Testament to show us the relationship of Father, Son and Spirit than that of the speech made by the protomartyr Stephen in his own defence, which has been handed down to us by Luke in his Acts of the Apostles. During this speech Stephen has a vision: 'But he, full of the Holy Spirit, gazed into heaven and saw the glory of God, and Jesus standing at the right hand of God; and he said, "Behold, I see the heavens opened and the Son of man standing on the right hand of God."'[139] So here we have God, Jesus the Son of Man, and the Holy Spirit. But Stephen does not see, say, a God with three faces, far less three men in the same form, nor any triangular symbol of the kind that was to be used centuries later in Western Christian art. Rather:

– The **Holy Spirit** is at Stephen's side, is in Stephen himself. The Spirit, the invisible power and might issuing from God, fills him fully and thus opens his eyes: 'in the Spirit' heaven opens to him.

– **God** himself (*ho theos* = **the** God)) remains hidden, is not in human form; only his 'glory' (Hebrew *kabod*, Greek *doxa*) is visible: God's splendour and power, the brilliance of light which issues fully from him.

– Finally **Jesus**, visible as the Son of Man, stands (and we already know the significance of this formula) 'at the right hand of God': that means in throne communion with God, in the same power and glory. Exalted as Son of God and taken up into God's eternal life, he is God's representative for us and at the same time, as a human being, the human representative before God.

What is the meaning of belief in Father, Son and Spirit?

In accordance with scripture, the relationship between Father, Son and Spirit could be described like this:
– God, the invisible Father **above** us,
– Jesus, the Son of man, as God's Word and Son **with** us,
– The Holy Spirit, as God's power and love, **in** us.

The apostle **Paul** sees this in a very similar way: God himself creates salvation **through** Jesus Christ **in** the Spirit. Just as we should also pray to God **in** the Spirit **through** Jesus Christ: prayers are directed *per Dominum nostrum Jesum Christum* to God the Father himself. Jesus as the Lord exalted to God has so made God's power, might, spirit his own that he is not only seized by the Spirit and powerful in the Spirit, but on the basis of the resurrection is even himself in the mode of existence and activity of the Spirit. And in the Spirit he can be present to believers: present not physically and materially, nor in an unreal way, but rather as a spiritual reality in the life of the individual and the faith community. There he is present above all in worship, in the celebration of a meal with the breaking of the bread and drinking of the cup in grateful memory of him. Therefore the encounter of 'God', 'Lord' and 'Spirit' is for believers ultimately one and the same encounter, God's own action, as Paul expresses it, say, in the greeting: 'The grace of the Lord Jesus Christ and the love of God and the fellowship of the Holy Spirit be with you all.'[140]

It was also possible to speak of Father, Son and Spirit in this way in the farewell discourses in **John**, where the Spirit has the personal features of a 'supporter' and 'helper' (this is what 'the other paraclete'[141] means – not, say, 'comforter'). The Spirit is as it were the representative of the exalted Christ on earth. He is sent by the Father in the name of Jesus. So he does not speak for himself, but only recalls what Jesus himself said.

All this should have made it clear that according to the New Testament **the key question in the doctrine of the Trinity** is not the question which is declared an impenetrable 'mystery' (*mysterium stricte dictum*), how three such different entities can be ontologically one, but the **christological question** how the relationship of Jesus (and consequently also of the Spirit) to God is to be expressed. Here the belief in the one God which Christianity has in common with Judaism and Islam may not be put in question for a moment. There is no other God than God! But what is decisive for the dialogue with Jews and Christians in particular is the insight that according to the New Testament the **principle of unity** is clearly not the one divine 'nature' (*physis*) common to several entities, as people were to think after the neo-Nicene theology of the fourth century. For the New Testament, as for the Hebrew Bible, the principle of unity is clearly **the one God** (*ho theos*: **the** God = the Father), from whom are all things and to whom are all things.

So according to the New Testament, Father, Son and Spirit are not metaphysical and ontological statements about God in himself and his innermost nature, about a static being of the triune God resting in itself and not at all open to us. Rather, these are soteriological and christological statements about how **God reveals himself** through Jesus Christ in this world; about God's dynamic and universal activity in history, his relationship to human beings and their relationship to him. So for all the difference in 'roles' there is a unity of Father, Son and Spirit, namely as an **event of revelation** and a **unity of revelation**: God himself is revealed through Jesus Christ in the Spirit. This is a thought-structure shaped in the framework of the Jewish-Christian paradigm which, as a structure – unlike that of a 'triune God' – need not have been absolutely alien to a Jew even down to the present day.

Thus it is not surprising that in the subsequent period, too, Jewish Christianity always insisted on the historical fact that the Messiah and Lord Jesus of Nazareth was not a divine being, a second God, but a human being from among human beings. It is not surprising that during the doctrinal development from the second century onwards, Jewish Christianity imposed restraint on the notion of the pre-existence of Jesus Christ. Nor is it a coincidence that though the Gentile Christian church historian Eusebius had no understanding of Jewish Christianity, as late as the third/fourth centuries he was still reporting about Jewish Christian circles which would not concede that Jesus Christ 'pre-existed as God, Logos and Wisdom'.[142] Therefore the momentous question arises: since the Jesus of history (who presented only an implicit christology) did not proclaim his own pre-existence, and the Jewish Christian community (which did have an explicit christology) did not allow a doctrine of the Trinity to arise, where does this doctrine of the Trinity really come from? The answer is that it was a product of the great paradigm shift from the early Christian apocalyptic paradigm to the early church Hellenistic paradigm. We shall hear more of this later.

In conclusion, we must ask: what was the later history of Jewish Christianity? What was the fate of the Jerusalem community and the other Jewish-Christian communities which – can we ever forget it? – made up original Christianity?

7. The fate of Jewish Christianity

In his *Church History*,[143] Eusebius reports that the **earliest Jerusalem community emigrated** from Jerusalem after the execution of James and before the outbreak of the Jewish-Roman war in 66 and settled in **Pella**, east of the Jordan. Attempts have been made to dispute this.[144]

The end of the earliest Jerusalem community

But why should an emigration be a priori excluded when one thinks that Jesus himself resolutely refused to be chosen as 'king', i.e. leader of an anti-Jewish rebellion? What has been handed down to us in summary form in the Sermon on the Mount is the opposite to an ideology of national revolt against the Roman empire; it is a message of non-violence. It is in line with the attitude of the prophets Isaiah and Jeremiah, who had expressly warned against war, indeed against resistance to very much stronger foreign powers. And since now the supreme head of the earliest church, James, and others had been executed by the Jewish authorities – were they still to take part in a revolt against Rome contrary to their religious conviction?

At any rate the most recent investigations[145] have shown that it is credible that at least important parts of the earliest community emigrated from Jerusalem into Transjordan before the Jewish War against the Romans, which had no prospect of success: 'The danger and deep uncertainty which had arisen for the Jerusalem community as a result of the execution of James the brother of the Lord (and other Christians) during the interregnum between procurators in 62, and especially for its "respected members", strengthened their resolve (sanctioned by a divine revelation to precisely these *dokimoi*) to turn their back on the city and emigrate to the nearest foreign land, the Decapolis. Therefore a large number of Jerusalem (and other Judaean?) Christians left the sphere of Jewish rule, possibly as early as 62, and – perhaps by way of Jericho and the Jordan valley – reached the city of Pella, belonging to the Decapolis, where they (or the majority of them) settled.'[146]

We can no longer establish how far members of the earliest community remained in Jerusalem or returned there after the war. At any rate, according to the list of bishops in Eusebius,[147] no less than fifteen Jewish Christian 'bishops' could be counted in Jerusalem – all circumcised (perhaps presbyters and relatives of Jesus were also included in the count) – up to the fatal year 135. This year, after a renewed Jewish rebellion, brought the complete destruction of Jerusalem, the expulsion of all Jews, the renaming of the city Aelia Capitolina and thus also the **end of the**

Jewish Christian community of Jerusalem and its dominant position in early Christianity. Its aura had now disappeared, for the Gentile Christians in particular. And modern church historians are not afraid to call Jewish Christianity, in derogatory fashion, the 'palaeontological period' of church history. Are they right?

The dark history of Jewish Christianity

Granted, the history of Jewish Christianity in the next century is one of the **darkest chapters** of church history. But why?[148] The most important reasons are:

– Whereas European 'classical antiquity' was at first exclusively orientated on Graeco-Roman antiquity, Christian patristics for a long time understood Jewish Christianity uncritically (following the heresiological remarks of the church fathers) as a single heretical entity.

– The Greek– and Latin-speaking theologians of the first centuries already showed little interest in manuscripts in Semitic languages; but now in addition to Aramaic and Hebrew there was also Syriac, Arabic and later Ethiopian.

– The Jewish Christian communities bordering on the Roman empire were a priori suspected of heresy, since they were in contact with Jewish Baptist and Gnostic sects.

– A large part of the writings were lost, since the Jewish Christian communities on the Euphrates and Tigris did not have the good fortune of the people of Qumran on the Dead Sea or the Gnostics in Egyptian Nag Hammadi, whose writings were preserved from destruction by the dry climate of the wilderness.

So for the Jewish communities of the Near East, where – to exaggerate somewhat – we often have only a couple of documents for a century of history, we depend far more on conjectures than we do in the church of the West, where we can often evaluate thousands of pages of source material for a decade. And whereas Simon Peter is mentioned by name around 190 times in the New Testament and Saul/Paul around 170, James is mentioned only eleven times (in Acts only three times), which according to some present-day exegetes indicates a suppression of Jewish Christianity (and the brothers of Jesus) in the Gentile Christian church.

So did Jewish Christianity, as traditional church history similarly asserts, soon become a **heretical sect** because it persisted at its earlier stage? Today scholars at least no longer dispute that there continued to be a Jewish Christianity even after the destruction of Jerusalem in 70, and many scholars are devoting themselves to the exciting task of finding **early traces** of the many branches of Jewish Christianity.[149]

It is generally recognized that the **Sayings Source** (abbreviated by scholars to Q, from the German *Quelle* = source, translated from Aramaic into Greek by a lucky coincidence and integrated into the Gospels of Matthew and Luke) is of Jewish Christian origin and dates to the first century. It has preserved definite sayings of Jesus from the earliest time.[150] The **Gospel of Matthew** (possibly written around 80 in Antioch), the **Letter of James** and the **Gospel of John** (written about 100) – where the controversy with 'the Jews' is sharper than that in Matthew – also come from a Jewish-Christian milieu. But are there traces of Jewish Christianity outside the New Testament as well?

On the trail

In addition to the New Testament there are **three non-canonical Jewish-Christian Gospels**: the Gospel of the Hebrews; the Gospel of the Nazoreans; and the Gospel of the Ebionites, which may be related to the Gospel of Matthew, but like the earliest canonical Gospel (Mark) has no infancy narrative and understands the divine Sonship of Jesus in terms of the descent of the Holy Spirit at his baptism.[151] If one may believe the hypothesis of the American New Testament scholar J.Louis Martyn, Jewish Christians even seem still to have been engaged in a mission to the Gentiles requiring observance of the Law in the second century.[152] They may already lie behind **Paul's opponents in Galatia** (and also in Philippi), who evidently see Christ in the light of God's Law – instead of, like Paul, seeing the Law in the light of Christ.[153] Moreover, because they obeyed the law (circumcision, festivals, precepts of purity), they saw themselves as the real children of Abraham.[154] The Jewish Christian work **The Ascension of Isaiah** (c.100-130), in which against an apocalyptic background a group of prophets put revelations in the mouth of the prophet Isaiah and precisely in so doing expressed faith in Jesus as the Messiah, is also illuminating.[155]

The **ongoing existence of Jewish Christians** who appealed to Peter or James instead of to Paul, and who were still in no way infected by Gnosticism, may also be attested by further pieces of tradition which were worked into a **Christian romance about a recognition** (attributed to Clement of Rome and therefore called the Pseudo-Clementines) which describes the conversion of the Roman Clement, Peter's companion in Palestine and Syria, and the rediscovery of his family, who were believed dead; along with the Kerygmata Petrou ('Proclamations of Peter') these include above all the 'Ascension (*Anabathmoi*) of James'.[156]

The background to this is probably the existence of Greek-speaking

Jewish Christians in Transjordan in the second half of the second century, who practised baptism in the name of Jesus but at the same time observed the law of Moses (probably including circumcision). They venerated James as the leader of the Jerusalem community and attacked Paul for preventing the possible conversion of the whole of the Jewish people to the Messiah Jesus through his mission outside the Law. Insistence on observance of the Law separated this Jewish Christian community from the new Gentile Christian mainstream church, but belief in Jesus who was a prophet like Moses and identical with the Messiah whom so many Jews had expected separated it from mainstream Judaism.[157]

Furthermore, the existence of Jewish Christian communities in Syria loyal to the Law is attested by the **Didaskalia** ('Instruction') of the apostles. In the Jordan valley and the upper reaches of the Euphrates there were followers of Elkesai, who represented a sect which was Jewish Christian but at the same time syncretistic and Gnostic.

Christian synods had to take action against Jewish Christian customs which were evidently still widespread even in the time of the shift under Constantine: in Spain the Synod of Elvira (in 305) and in Asia Minor the Synod of Laodicea (between 343 and 381). And even at the end of the fourth century Jerome tells us of the existence of a small Jewish Christian community of **Nazaraei** (Nazarenes) known to him in Beroea (Aleppo, Syria) which, while recognizing Paul as apostle of the Gentiles, evidently used a Hebrew Gospel of Matthew.[158]

But we still know infinitely more about the Near Eastern Gentile Christians, although from an orthodox Chalcedonian standpoint for the most part these were later also regarded as 'heretics' (Monophysites or Nestorians), than we do about that Jewish Christianity which after the fall of Jerusalem preserved the earliest views of faith and practice. It probably still had its focal point in Palestine and adjacent territories, but had adherents as far away as Rome and Egypt, Mesopotamia and southern Arabia. According to the sources in the church fathers, which need to be read critically, at any rate we need to distinguish **different groupings** in different areas and with different names, though it is very hard to make a historical reconstruction of what really lay behind the names.[159] Whereas 'Nazorean' (following the 'Nazorean' Jesus) stems from the Hebrew-Aramaic term used by Jews of Christians (probably to be distinguished from the 'Nazarenes', a pre-Christian sect), 'Ebionites' (God's 'poor') is the self-designation of a particular Jewish Christian group (there was no such person as Ebion). 'Cerinthians', 'Symmachians' and 'Elkesaites' derive from persons (Cerinthus, Symmachus, Elkesai or Elchasai).

Heretical or legitimate heirs of early Christianity?

In the chapter on the Jewish context and the Christian centre I have already described what qualifies all these groups as 'Jewish Christians' in the strict sense: to put it briefly once again, Jewish Christians embody **that form of Christianity** whose members (mostly of Jewish origin) **combined their faith in Jesus as the Messiah with observance of the Mosaic ritual law.** These Jewish Christians wanted to practise discipleship of Jesus specifically by observing the Law. These Christians, these Jews, who often also remained in contact with the mainstream church that was coming into being and sometimes celebrated the Sabbath and Sunday one after the other, wanted to retain their own way of life and theology with its Jewish stamp.

However, it was the fate of these Jewish Christian communities from a very early stage to be ignored, despised and finally **branded heretics** – because they could not go along with the complications of a Hellenistic christology which was growing increasingly higher and more intricate. They were branded heretics by bishops first like Ignatius of Antioch, who already around 110 had categorically ruled out any combination of belief in Christ with Jewish practice,[160] and then in 180-185 by Irenaeus of Lyons, who similarly wrote in Greek and listed all Jewish Christians without distinction among the 'heretics' as Ebionites (it is in his work that this name first appears).[161]

But before him a church father who himself came from Palestine (Nablus) proved to be well informed about Judaism, and around the middle of the second century reported on these Jewish Christians. This was **Justin Martyr**, who (like Hegesippus) had a more differentiated picture of the many forms of Jewish Christianity. He avoided the word heresy and made a precise distinction between the majority of **Jewish Christians**, whose beliefs were quite **orthodox** and who, while observing the Jewish ritual Law and circumcision as Christians, did not want to impose it on the Gentiles any more than did Paul or the Apostolic Council, and the **legalistic Jewish Christians** who wanted to impose the Law also on Gentile Christians as being necessary for salvation. Justin thought the latter line inadmissible. In his view, Jewish Christians accepted Jesus as Messiah/Christ, but claimed that he was 'a man from among men' and was 'elected' Messiah/Christ.[162] But was that in itself heretical? In the East at any rate, as we can see, say, from Origen and Eusebius, people were less dismissive of Jewish Christianity, which in part they still knew at first hand. It was Epiphanius of Salamis, that specialist on heretics, who first included in his famous account of eighty heresies dating from 374-7 (the *Panarion*) a number of Jewish Christian groups which he knew either from writings which have been lost or personally. However, it is very difficult to identify the historical reality behind the individual names of heretics. At any rate, all that Epiphanius says about the 'Nazoreans' is: 'While the Nazoreans confessed Jesus as the Son of God, in other respects they lived wholly in accordance with the Jewish laws.'[163]

And indeed this statement cannot be heretical, simply because Jesus' first disciples, the majority of the earliest community and all the Christian missionaries known to us were Jews, or more precisely – as we heard – 'Jewish Christians' (what else could they be?). In principle they observed the Law and circumcision, and had a **christology with a Jewish stamp** which represented an illuminating combination of belief in the Messiah and observance of the Law and was only later branded as heretical (because it was allegedly 'natural' or 'adoptianist'). Seven types of Jewish Christian christology have been distinguished, but they are by no means mutually exclusive.[164] There are three christologies 'from below': the royal (Jesus as 'Son of David'), the prophetic (Jesus as the 'new Moses') and the priestly (Jesus as 'high priest'); and four christologies 'from above': the 'Son of Man', the one above all the angels, the 'Son of God' and the 'Word of God' – all notions with a clearly Jewish background.

In fact, as is well known, christology began quite modestly 'from below', from the perspective of the Jewish disciples of Jesus: not with lofty metaphysical speculations but with the questions 'Who is this?'[165] and 'Can any good come out of Nazareth?'[166] If we wanted to judge Christians of the pre-Nicene period after the event, in the light of the Council of Nicaea, then not only the Jewish Christians would be heretics but also almost all the Greek church fathers (at least in essence), since as a matter of course they taught a **subordination** of the 'Son' to the 'Father' which according to the later criterion of the definition of a 'sameness of substance' (*homoousia*) was regarded by the Council of Nicaea as heretical. In the light of this we can hardly avoid the question: if one wants to make just the Council of Nicaea the criterion instead of the New Testament, was anyone at all orthodox in the early church of the first centuries?

Whatever their detailed assessment of the Jewish Christian sources, present-day scholars see more the **continuity** of Jewish Christianity with the beginnings of early Christianity and less its heretical distortion. For them, Jewish Christians are the **legitimate heirs of early Christianity,** whereas the rest of the New Testament for the most part reflects the view of Gentile Christianity as this was defended by Paul and his followers.

The Göttingen exegete Georg Strecker, distinguished for his research into Jewish Christianity, clearly brings out the present-day theological significance of Jewish Christianity for relations between Christians and Jews: 'In the universality of its appearance, which has taken concrete form in many ways not only in the early Christian period but down to the present day, Jewish Christianity shows itself to be a connecting link between synagogue and church. To the synagogue it witnesses that the promises to the Fathers were disclosed by the Christ event and that the will of God revealed in the Old Testament is being realized. To the church it provides a reminder of its Jewish heritage and represents the abiding claim of Israel. While Jewish Christianity is hardly to be identified with a "natural" Ebionite christology (the idea of pre-existence also occurs), it can help to limit the tendency within the mainstream church and outside it towards docetism and spiritualization, by returning to the historical foundations of the Christian faith.'[167] So Jewish Christian theology is a critical corrective to an all-too-remote christology which is exposed to the dangers of docetism and spiritualization!

However, since Epiphanius Jewish Christianity had now also permanently been branded a 'heresy' in the East, and in 386/7 John Chrystostom felt obliged to give eight anti-Jewish sermons[168] in Antioch in which he attacked Christians who proved to be attracted by synagogue worship and Jewish festivals and customs (including circumcision). After the first half of the fifth century, traces of Jewish Christianity seem increasingly to be lost. Syncretistic tendencies become stronger. But what happened to the Jewish-Christian groups? Neither Judaism nor the mainstream church can have absorbed them all fully.

Two traces – which cannot be pursued in detail here – point to present-day Africa and India:

– In **Ethiopia**, a former Jewish-Christian paradigm seems to have laid the foundation for official Monophysite Christianity, as I was able to observe at an Epiphany celebration in Addis Ababa: veneration of the ark of Moses (Tabot), Semitic liturgical language; priests who sing psalms and dance to the accompaniment of drums and trumpets; circumcision as well as baptism, the Sabbath as well as Sunday, and finally special regulations for fasting and food (prohibition of pork).[169]

– In **South India** there is an ethnically different group of around 70,000 people, called Tekkumbagam Christians or Southists, who according to their local tradition of a Thomas of Cana (Canaan?) came to Kerala in 345 with seventy-two Christian families from Syria or Mesopotamia. These were Jewish Christians who believed in Jesus as the Messiah for the Jews, whereas the Christians already living in Kerala were disciples of the apostle Paul.[170]

But a third trace had even more consequences at the time. It relates to that prominent Persian **Mani** (Greek *Manes, Manichaios*, 216-76) who, following Zarathustra, Buddha and above all Christ understood in Gnostic terms, wanted to found a new kind of 'Christian' world religion. During the third and fourth centuries it spread, as a serious rival to Christianity, from the Atlantic to China, from the Caucasus to the Indian Ocean. This was dualistic and ascetic **Manichaeism**. But the new discovery in our day is that according to the tradition of the Arab bibliographer Ibn an-Nadim and the newly discovered Greek Mani Codex in Cologne,[171] **in his youth** Mani had **belonged to the Jewish Christian sect of the Elkesaites**: 'Jewish influences like legalism and apocalyptic thought came to him (Mani) via Jewish Christianity', remarked the Tübingen Mani specialist Alexander Böhlig at his own congress on the Cologne Codex: 'The Baptists among whom Mani grew up were indeed Elkesaites. They saw Elkesai as the founder of their law . . . The legal character of Jewish Christianity forms the foundation for the legalistic character of Manichaeism.'[172] So the Elkesaites are the connecting link between Palestinian Baptist sects and Jewish Christianity on the one hand and Manichaeism on the other. But there is yet another, far more important, trace, which takes us further.

8. Jewish Christianity and the Qur'an

Another, surprising, influence from Jewish Christianity must occupy us further precisely because of its ecumenical interest. If we can trust those researching in this area, although the Jewish Christian communities were branded as heretics, became syncretistic and were finally exterminated, with their theology they may have exercised an influence which was even to have world-historical significance: in Arabia, through the monotheistic reform movement which the Arab **prophet Muhammad** sparked off six hundred years after Jesus' death and three hundred years after the Council of Nicaea.

Jewish Christianity on the Arabian peninsula?

Moreover underground relations between Jewish Christianity and the message of the Qur'an have long been discussed by Christian scholars.[173] As early as 1926, in his *History of the First Christianity*, the distinguished Protestant exegete **Adolf Schlatter** had written: 'However, the Jewish church had died out only in Palestine west of the Jordan. Christian communities with Jewish customs continued to exist in the eastern regions, in the Decapolis, in Batanaea, among the Nabataeans, on the edge of the Syrian desert and into Arabia, completely detached from the rest of Christianity and out of communion with it . . . For Christians the Jew was just an enemy, and the Greek mood which overlooked the murders carried out by generals Trajan and Hadrian as the well-deserved fate of the evil and despicable Jews was also carried over into the church. Even its leading men who lived and taught in Caesarea, like Origen and Eusebius, remained amazingly ignorant about the end of Jerusalem and its church. Similarly, their reports about the ongoing existence of Jewish Christianity are sparse. They (sic!) were heretics, because they did not submit to the law which held elsewhere in Christianity, and were therefore set apart from that Christianity.' But he adds: 'None of the leaders of the imperial church guessed that the day would come for this Christianity which they despised on which it would shake the world and destroy a great deal of the church which they had built up. It came when Muhammad took over the prize possession of the Jewish Christians, their consciousness of God, their eschatology proclaiming the day of judgment, their morality and their legends, and established a new apostolate as "the one sent by God".'[174]

Monotheism instead of the doctrine of the Trinity, servant christology instead of a two-nature christology: the thesis of the influence of Jewish Christianity on the Qur'an had already been discussed and consolidated earlier by Adolf von Harnack,[175] and by Hans-Joachim Schoeps.[176] Present-day scholars like Christopher Buck also come to the same conclusion: 'In the course of time the Ebionites along with the Sabaean Baptists seem to have established themselves in Arabia. This fertilization invites the hypothesis that the Qur'an reflects Ebionite prophetology.'[177] Indeed, Georg Strecker says that it is 'indisputable that **Islam** was open not only to Jewish and Christian but also to Jewish-Christian influences, even if this is a field of research which is still largely unworked'.[178] So the original **Jewish Christian paradigm** may have been handed on in some form or another. But is there really any connection with the Qur'an? At all events, there is more than a century between the Jewish Christianity of the fourth/fifth century and the Qur'an.

We should probably not think of the early Christian Nazoraeans as possible direct **links between Jewish Christianity and the Qur'an**. Rather, since Harnack, scholars have thought in terms of Jewish Christians of a Gnostic stamp like the Elkesaites, who according to the most recent research may have been identical with the Sabaeans mentioned in the Qur'an.[179] At any rate, today the existence of a Jewish Christian scripture in Arabic can hardly be disputed any longer. Julius Wellhausen[180] already mentioned by name the Ibadians of Hira and Ambar and some poetic personalities. And as the Berlin scholar of religion Carsten Colpe points out in a summary,[181] plenty of references have been found to liturgical books for an Arab-Christian liturgy, which indicates the presence of Christian communities on the Arab peninsula; there seem to have been Arabic translations of the Psalter and the Gospels.

But Colpe has made another surprising discovery. The famous designation of the prophet Muhammad, the '**seal of the prophets**',[182] already appears in one of the earliest works of the earliest Latin church father, in Tertullian's *Adversus Judaeos* (before 200)[183] – of course as a designation of Jesus Christ.[184] Was the title 'seal of the prophets' claimed by the prophet Muhammad in a controversy with Jewish Christians or Manichaeans? 'We need not go so far as to claim that the Jewish tribes with which Muhammad had hostile clashes in Medina were all Jewish-Christian,' says Colpe. 'But there is no doubt that Judaism was established on the Arabian peninsula by a variant which we call both Jewish and Christian. It may have been this Jewish Christianity which the title "seal of the prophets" reached, and the title may have been used there and in principle throughout Jewish Christianity to guarantee a particular confessional identity.'[185]

Possibly there may also be some other traces. Colpe himself pursues a **first trace** in applying a text from the Byzantine Sozomen's church history, composed between 439 and 450, to Jewish Christians who legitimated themselves by descent from Ishmael and his mother (Hagar), in other words through the Ishmaelites or Hagarenes: 'Here an Eastern Jewish Christian "confession" emerges which is older than the Nestorians and Jacobites and continued to exist alongside the latter, especially among the Arabs. By type they could have been Jews, from whom Muhammad got his Jewish traditions – Jews with midrashim but without Talmuds, who at the same time were Christians venerating Jesus and Mary, but without dyophysite or monophysite christology. Such Jewish Christianity is also conceivable on the Arabian peninsula, above all in Medina. It may have been a vehicle for biblical traditions and traditions of biblical exegesis of the kind that we find in the Qur'an.'[186]

The Jewish scholars S.M.Stern and S.Pines found **a second trace** in an Arab manuscript of 'Abd-al Javar (Gabbar), who was active in Baghdad in the tenth century, or even of an earlier Muslim scholar who worked over a Jewish Christian text, probably from the fifth and sixth centuries. This contains an early history of the Christian community, laments the split between Judaism and Christianity, criticizes the 'Romanization' of Christianity, and at the same time claims to continue the original tradition of the Jerusalem community before it was corrupted. This tradition, it was held, had its foundation in the first disciples of Jesus, who believed that he was a man and not a divine being, and observed the Mosaic commandments.[187] Here there is evidence of a Jewish Christianity both in Palestine-Syria and Arabia and Babylonia – one which continued at any rate into the seventh century.[188]

Are the Jewish Christian and the Qur'anic pictures of Jesus related?

What historical genetic references in the Qur'an point with what intensity to which Christian group is a question which perhaps must ultimately be left open. However, one thing cannot be disputed: the **analogies in content between the Qur'anic picture of Jesus and a christology stamped by Jewish Christianity** remain perplexing: the parallels are indisputable and await a historical explanation.

Claus Schedl has ventured a first attempt in his comprehensive study of the picture of Jesus in the Qur'an. His findings: 'The sketch of a servant of God christology, fragments of which are preserved in the Acts of the Apostles, was not developed further by the Hellenistic church of the West; the designation of Jesus as servant (*'abd*) seems to have been the dominant christological confessional formula. So when Muhammad puts the title "servant" at the centre of his preaching about 'Isa (Jesus), he is adopting a scheme from earliest Christianity, purging it of contemporary misinterpretations, but avoiding ontological precision – of the kind one would expect from Hellenistic Eastern thought . . . So it should no longer be said that Muhammad had only a defective knowledge of Christianity. Certainly in the Qur'an he does not argue with the doctrinal decisions of the councils of the Western church; however, the overall picture which we have gained from our investigations may demonstrate that he knew the basic structure of Syrian Semitic christology very well and developed it further on his own. If a Muslim-Christian dialogue is to bear fruit, then it needs to start from these basic facts.'[189]

And indeed these historical references open up surprising possibilities for dialogue between Jews and Muslims. However, the Muslim dialogue partner needs to be assured from the start that with this perspective on history there will be no revival of the old apologetic by means of which Christians tended to reduce the Qur'an to Jewish or Jewish Christian sources and a 'heretical' redaction of them. After all, since the days of the last church father, John of Damascus, Christians have been fond of disqualifying Islam as a 'Christian heresy'. No, the **authenticity of the Qur'anic revelation**[190] is not being put in question if we establish links with the Christian tradition, any more than the Christian revelation is diluted if we reconstruct all the possible Jewish sources. So parallels and analogies will not be cited here to prove the superiority of Christianity or to cast doubt on the authenticity of the Qur'anic revelation, but to indicate the affinity between Christianity and Islam, which represents a challenge and an opportunity for all those engaged in dialogue.

Let us be clear just for a moment what it would mean for a dialogue between Jews, Christians and Muslims if Muhammad could be understood as the 'Jewish Christian apostle' of the one true God in Arabian garb, whose day came when he 'took over the prize possession of the Jewish Christians, their consciousness of God, their eschatology proclaiming the day of judgment, their morality and their legends, and established a new apostolate as "the one sent by God"', to quote Adolf Schlatter once again.[191]

Opportunities for an inter-religious dialogue

Unless the signs of the times are deceptive, despite all the tremendous political difficulties and all the ethnic and religious tensions, indeed wars, we are at the beginnings of new theological dialogues which could shed new light on the differences between the three great monotheistic religions, sufficiently known and not to be denied here.

Jewish-Christian dialogue made decisive progress (after centuries of reciprocal anathemas) when Jews and Christians together began to take seriously for their faith the abiding basic features of Judaism to be found in the figure and message of Jesus. The implications of the insights into the **affinity between earliest Christianity and earliest Islam** should be made fruitful for Christian-Muslim dialogue – the earlier the better: the Qur'anic understanding of Jesus no longer as a Muslim heresy but as a christology on Arabic soil coloured by earliest Christianity! We must be clear that these insights would at first be highly inconvenient for all three prophetic religions. But if an understanding is to be reached, the questions which arise must receive an answer:

Questions for the Future

✝ May Christians still go on appealing unthinkingly to the high christology of the Hellenistic councils and make them the sole norm of belief in Jesus as the one sent by God for all 'children of Abraham'? What significance do they attach to the **Jewishness** of **Jesus of Nazareth**? What status do they give him for their faith? How far are they prepared to take seriously the much more original christology of the Jewish disciples of Jesus and the early Jewish Christian communities as these are also reflected in the Qur'an?

May Jews today still simply exclude the figure of Jesus in polemi-cal fashion and ignore his significance for Jewish faith and life? What significance does Jesus also have for the faith of Jews today if he is taken seriously as the **last great prophet of the Jewish people with abiding Jewish features**, as also happens in the Qur'an?

May Muslims today still be content with criticism of Hellenistic christology (which is alleged to be a danger to monotheism)? How prepared are they also to consider the religious significance of Jesus from the **perspective of the New Testament**, so as to understand the authentic figure of Jesus more comprehensively and avoid narrowness and one-sidedness?

There is no doubt that much will be asked of all three Abrahamic religions. But the same inconvenient insight into the affinity between Jewish Christian and Qur'anic christology could prove highly fruitful. We should also be clear that **all three prophetic religions are given an opportunity** here:

- An opportunity for the **Jews**: they could maintain their faith in the one God of the fathers, Abraham, Isaac and Jacob. And they could recognize Jesus of Nazareth as a great son of Israel and acknowledge this last of the great prophets, who solely for the sake of God and human beings relativized the absolutes of descent, sabbath and law and with his message and his fate proved to be a successor of Moses yet 'more than Moses'.
- An opportunity for **Christians**: they would not need to delete anything from their belief in Jesus as the one Messiah or Christ of God. Yet they could explain their understanding of 'sonship' in a way which was more comprehensible to Jews and Muslims: in so far as the Hebrew Bible and the Jewish Christian community could not have conceived of this divine sonship in terms of any kind of sexual, physical or even metaphysical ontic begetting, but rather in the 'appointment' and enthronement of Jesus on the basis of his resurrection through God himself as 'Messiah' (king) 'in power'.[192]
- An opportunity for **Muslims**: they could firmly maintain their belief in the one and only God and the impossibility of giving God associates or envisaging any earthly being in partnership with God. Yet they could attempt a more comprehensive understanding, in the light of the New Testament, of Jesus, the one sent by God, God's Word, Messiah, who according to the Qur'an was exalted to God.

II. The Ecumenical Hellenistic Paradigm of Christian Antiquity

A **paradigm** is – to repeat the definition given by Thomas S.Kuhn – 'an entire constellation of beliefs, values, techniques and so on shared by the members of a given community.'[1] A **paradigm shift** is the replacement of a paradigm previously held to be valid by a new one.[2]

Now if, as I am attempting in my analysis of 'The Religious Situation of Our Time', one wants to apply paradigm theory to the history and present situation of the world religions, it is natural to distinguish between:

– **Microparadigms**: paradigm shifts on individual questions, as for example the transition from the celebration of the sabbath (or the sabbath and Sunday) to the celebration only of Sunday;

– **Mesoparadigms**: paradigm shifts in partial areas, as for example the transition from an apocalyptic christology (Christ the end of time) to an early Catholic christology (Christ the centre of time);

– **Macroparadigms**: paradigm shifts in theology, church, society generally, like the transition from Jewish Christianity to Gentile Christianity.

Now there is no doubt that the paradigm shift from Jewish Christianity to Gentile Christianity which was already becoming evident in the New Testament period is the replacement of a macroparadigm which includes countless meso– and microparadigms. The conflict and dispute thus caused was throughout an expression of creativity and vitality. Such fundamental paradigm shifts never, of course, simply involve individual persons, individual events and individual symptoms; they are never just about individual theologians, theologies and theological schools. Nevertheless, individuals (individual theologians or church members) can play an almost revolutionary role as catalysts. And the first theologian – who was not to be the last – to play a fundamental role in a paradigm shift was without doubt that persecutor of Christians and preacher of Christ who at the same time stood in both continuity and discontinuity to Jewish Christianity: Saul/Paul.

1. Paul: the initiator of the paradigm shift

Paradigm shifts in the religious sphere in particular do not normally take place suddenly. A macro-paradigm needs a long time to mature before it establishes itself historically. And the **ecumenical Hellenistic paradigm (P II)** which replaced the apocalyptic paradigm (P I) of the earliest church almost throughout the Roman empire did not simply 'appear' in the third and fourth centuries, but was already initiated by persons and circumstances in the first century.

Here beyond question the person of the apostle Paul plays a key role. But the way was prepared for Paul by Hellenistic Jewish Christians (especially the apostle Barnabas from Cyprus), who after the martyrdom of Stephen had fled from Jerusalem and settled in **Antioch** (present-day Antakye), the capital of the then Roman twin province of Syria and Cilicia, the third most important city in the Roman empire after Rome and Alexandria. Antioch was an international trade centre and at the same time controlled the land routes which linked Asia Minor, Mesopotamia and Egypt.[3] Here Hellenistic Jewish Christians addressed their preaching directly to the Gentiles. Here the **first mixed community** made up of born Jews and born Gentiles was founded.[4] Here those who believed in Christ were for the first time given the name 'Christians' (Greek *christianoi* = 'Christ-people'[5]).

So it is no coincidence that the great city of Antioch became the centre of the Christian mission to the Gentiles. Here already, both sociologically and culturally, in milieu and language, a paradigm shift began to take shape to which Gerd Theissen[6] above all has drawn attention:

– Whereas the Palestinian Jesus movement was at home in a rural milieu, Christianity now became an **urban phenomenon** (at the end of antiquity the term *pagani* = 'village dwellers' became a synonym for the last to retain the old ways).

– Whereas Jewish Christianity could retain the old vernaculars spoken in the country (Aramaic in Syria-Palestine), in the cities Gentile Christianity had to speak the language of universal communication, namely *koine* Greek.

Once a Pharisee – now an apostle

The **theology and mission of Paul,** by far the most successful of the earliest Christian apostles, came to be of fundamental significance for the paradigm shift in Christianity which was now taking shape. As we saw in connection with the Jewish Christian paradigm, his roots were Jewish through and through, though they were steeped in the Hellenistic spirit. And on the basis of his restless intellectual, theological and missionary church political activity, Paul the apostle to the Gentiles introduced the first great change in early Christianity: the transition from Jewish Christianity (speaking partly Aramaic, partly Greek) to an exclusively Greek- (or later Latin-)speaking Gentile Christianity. This is the background to the well-known conflict between Paul and Peter in Antioch.[7]

Here we may presuppose what was said in my *Judaism* about the theological profile of the apostle Paul (above all about his attitude to the Torah) and his conflict with the Jewish establishment of his time:[8] that the Jew Paul – who had had a strict Pharisaic upbringing – had originally raged against the Christian communities with great zeal for God and God's law; but that after a radical shift, caused by a revelation of Christ, he felt called to be the authoritative missionary to the Gentiles. Today Jewish scholars, too, take the 'authenticity of Paul's conversion experience'[9] as seriously as that of the prophets of Israel: the **conversion of Saul, the Pharisee loyal to the Law, from Pharisaism to belief in Jesus Christ**, whom he had experienced as being alive in a vision, a christophany which he regarded as being equivalent to the original apostles' experiences of the resurrection. And for Paul this conversion was to prove much more than just a paradigm shift within Judaism.

For the decisive consequence of Paul's conversion experience was that he saw himself called to proclaim Jesus, the **Messiah of Israel, as Messiah of the whole world made up of Jews and Gentiles**. And although he himself was a Jewish Christian, he saw that for him the observance of the Jewish ritual law, the halakhah, was no longer obligatory in any respect: human beings are not 'righteous' before God by painstakingly fulfilling all the particular 'works of the law'. What is decisive is unconditional trust ('faith' = *pistis*) in God, trusting acceptance of God's will – and this can be given regardless of whether one fulfils the specifically Jewish commands of the ritual law, the halakhah, or not. Here Paul did no more and no less than undermine the exclusive saving function of the comprehensive halakhic system – referring to the God who raised the crucified Jesus in the name of the Law and thus confirmed him as Messiah and Lord.

No wonder that wherever Paul went he was suspected of apostasy and given a hostile reception by the Jewish establishment. Paul did not dream of simply abolishing the halakhah. Indeed, he himself observed it when he moved among Jews: for the sake of this message he wanted to be 'all things to all men'; 'to the Jews a Jew, to those outside the law one outside the law', always bound to 'the law of Christ' (the law of love).[10] Nor did Paul want to replace Jewish belief in one God with a Christian belief in two Gods. Rather, he always regarded the Jesus who had been exalted by God's Spirit to God as subordinate to this one God and Father: as the Messiah, Christ, image, Son, of the one God. So his christocentricity remains grounded in and culminates in a theocentricity: 'from God through Jesus Christ' – 'through Jesus Christ to God'.[11] To this degree Paul's christology is directly compatible with Jewish monotheism. But there was another decisive factor.

On the way to a world religion

Paul wanted the Gentiles, who did not belong to God's elect people, also to have unconditional access to belief in the universal God of Israel without first having to submit to circumcision and thus to the Jewish commands relating to cleanness, the halakhic regulations about food and the sabbath. In other words, a Gentile was to be able to become a Christian without first having to become a Jew and then having to fulfil the specific 'works of the Law'.[12] And at a very early stage this theological insight and missionary practice of Paul's meant a **revolution in world history** with long-term **consequences for world history**:

– Through Paul the Christian mission to the Gentiles (which already existed before Paul and alongside him), in contrast to the Jewish Hellenistic mission, became a decisive **success** throughout the empire (as far as Spain?).

– Through Paul there was an authentic **inculturation** of the Christian message in the world of Hellenistic culture.

– Through Paul the small Jewish 'sect' finally developed into a **world religion** in which East and West were more closely bound together than even by Alexander the Great.

The fact remains that without Paul there would have been no Catholic church, no Greek or Latin patristic theology, no Christian-Hellenistic culture, no shift under Constantine. But at the same time the fact remains that Paul was not the real 'founder of Christianity', as is unfortunately still maintained to the present day, though without any new arguments, by some people who just will not be taught.[13] No, according to the whole of the New Testament, including Paul, Jesus Christ who was crucified and rose again is the founding figure, and his message is the foundation of Christianity. But Paul is certainly responsible for the fact that despite its universal monotheism, Judaism, which at that time was similarly engaged in an intensive mission to the Gentiles, particularly in Antioch, did not become **a universal religion of humankind**, whereas Christianity did.

The new Gentile Christian Hellenistic paradigm

That does not make Paul the founder of Christianity, but it does make him the **first Christian theologian**, who gave a brilliant theological explanation of what Jesus had in fact said and done only implicitly, and put it into practice. Here Paul, a Roman citizen of Tarsus (in Asia Minor) with a Hellenistic education, made use not only of his rabbinic training and exegesis but also of concepts and notions from his **Hellenistic environment**. This environment was certainly not just unsettled and suffering an internal crisis, as historical research long assumed; in many respects it was enjoying its hey-day: a colourful world of cults, sects, religions. We have seen that Paul's theology maintains continuity with the preaching of Jesus. But in his letters – unfortunately we do not possess his original catechesis – it at first appears in a somewhat off-putting light. Why? Because it has been remoulded into quite different perspectives, categories and notions: it has been transferred into a quite different overall constellation, into another, **Hellenistic paradigm!**

However, for Paul it is quite clear that the decisive feature, the **'essence' of Christianity** as compared with Judaism and all the religions of the world, is and remains this **Christ Jesus himself.** For it is as the crucified one in particular that he differs fron the many risen, exalted, living deities and divinized founders of religion, Caesars, geniuses, lords and heroes of world history. And at the same time belief in the concrete Jesus as God's Christ makes possible a universal openness, so that all human beings can come to God through Christ. This is the new element. No longer is membership of a particular (elect) people decisive, but only faith. This alone explains why **Christianity is not just another paradigm within Judaism but** is in the end really a **different religion (though it cannot give up its roots in Judaism)**, since Jesus as the Messiah of Israel was repudiated by the majority of the people of Israel and was accepted by many Gentiles.

So Paul does not differ from the Jewish Christians in the substance of faith but he does so in having a completely different paradigm. And at a very early stage the consequences of this first paradigm-shift within Christianity, from Jewish Christianity to a Gentile Christianity with a Hellenistic stamp, become abundantly clear. This is a new macroparadigm which includes several paradigm shifts in the meso-sphere, a paradigm shift in the understanding of the Bible, the Law and the people of God.

1. A new **understanding of the Bible:**

– The Jewish Christians had already begun to read the Hebrew Bible in retrospect in order to interpret it in terms of the Messiah Jesus. Good Jewish honorific titles like 'Messiah', 'Lord', 'Son of David', 'Son of Man' (used in the Hebrew scriptures only occasionally for Israel's king and the whole people) were transferred to him to express his significance for God and humankind.

– The Gentile Christians now understandably read the 'Old Testament' wholly against a background stamped by Hellenism. Like his older contemporary Philo of Alexandria, similarly a Hellenistic Jew from the Diaspora, Paul had already interpreted the Hebrew Bible allegorically and symbolically, and conceded the primacy of the 'spirit' over the 'letter'. Gentile Christians could make nothing of Jewish notions and honorific titles like 'Son of David' or 'Son of Man'. So they concentrated on a title like 'Son of God' which was popular among them (it was used for emperors and other heroes), and after the New Testament period, under the influence of Greek Hellenistic ontology, this title was understood in an increasingly naturalistic way.

2. A new **understanding of the Law**:
– The Jewish Christians (especially the Hellenists) had already begun to take the ceremonial and ritual commandments less seriously than the ethical commandments, in accordance with Jesus' attitude to the sabbath, attaching special importance to works of love.
– But the Gentile Christians no longer felt that bound to the Jewish ceremonial law: there was no compulsion towards circumcision and the ritual halakhah.

3. A new **understanding of the people of God**:
– Although the Jewish Christians felt themselves by nature and on the basis of circumcision to be members of the people of Israel, they were already more distanced from the Temple and the Law, especially to the degree that they spoke Greek.
– However, for the Gentile Christians who did not belong a priori to the elect people, the decisive factor for membership was not so much descent as faith in Jesus Christ, sealed in the initiation rite of baptism in the name of Jesus.

Now as we know, Paul was not only a perceptive theologian but also an uncommonly effective organizer; not only a theoretician in the church, but a practical man, a founder and leader of churches. And as we know, already at that time Christians did not just live for themselves as individuals, but in fellowship, in communities which required a concrete structure or constitution. Here, too – in the question of church order – we can recognize a meso-paradigm shift (similarly initiated by Paul).

2. The origin of the hierarchical church

In communities, as a rule people have tasks, ministries, functions, and already in the New Testament a whole series of functions can be distinguished: preaching, and the functions of apostle, prophet, teacher, evangelist and admonisher; then as auxiliary ministries the functions of deacons and deaconesses, distributing alms and caring for the sick, widows serving the community; and finally for leading the community the functions of the first converts, overseers, *episkopoi*, pastors and so on.

A *charismatic church in Paul*

All these functions in the community (and not just specific 'offices') were understood by Paul, about whose communities we have by far the best information, as gifts of the Spirit of God and the exalted Christ. Those who exercised such functions might feel themselves to be **called by God to a particular ministry in the community**. In Paul, such a gift of the Spirit is called briefly, in Greek, **charisma**. The Protestant exegete Ernst Käsemann[14] has strongly emphasized the charismatic dimension of the church in Paul: according to Paul, not only the extraordinary phenomena highly prized in present-day charismatic communities (like speaking in tongues and healing the sick) are charisms, gifts of the Spirit, but also quite everyday and as it were 'private' gifts and ministries like the gift of consolation, of admonition, of knowledge, of speaking wisdom, of discerning the spirits. They are not limited to a particular circle of persons. One cannot talk of either clericalism or enthusiasm in Paul. On the contrary, **any** ministry which in fact contributes to the building up of the community (permanent or temporary, private or public) is **church ministry**; and as a concrete ministry it deserves recognition and subordination. **Any** ministry, whether official or not, thus has authority in its own way if it is established for the benefit of the community in love.

But how was it possible to preserve **unity and order** in the Pauline communities, which in fact were often enough endangered – through rival groups, chaotic administration, dubious moral practices? Paul's correspondence with his communities is clear on this point: Paul did not want to restore unity and order by levelling out the differences, by introducing uniformity, hierarchy, centralization. Rather, he saw unity and order guaranteed through the working of the one Spirit, though this does not give all charisms to every person but gives each person his or her own charism (the rule is: 'to each his own'); this charism is not to be used egocentrically, but for the benefit of others (the rule is: 'with one another for one another') and in submission to the one Lord (the rule is: 'obedience to the Lord'). Anyone who does not confess Jesus and does not use his or her gift for the benefit of the community – this is how the spirits are to be discerned – does not have the Spirit of God. Action in solidarity, collegial harmony, conversation, communication and dialogue in partnership – in the life of the community these are signs of the Spirit of God which is identical with the Spirit of Jesus Christ.

Apostolic Church Order

The Jewish Christian Community of Jerusalem around 48

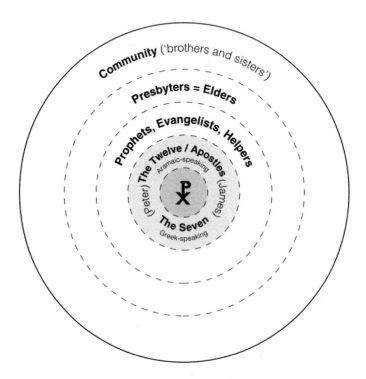

'When they came to Jerusalem, they (Paul and Barnabas) were welcomed by the church and the apostles and the elders, and they declared all that God had done with them.' (Acts 15.4)

'I (Paul) went up (to Jerusalem) by revelation; and I laid before them (but privately before those who were of repute) the gospel which I preach among the Gentiles...' (Gal.2.2)

'And when they perceived the grace that was given to me, James and Cephas and John, who were reputed to be pillars, gave to me and Barnabas the right hand of fellowship.' (Gal.2.9)

'Now in these days prophets came down from Jerusalem to Antioch.' (Acts 11.27)

Charismatic Church Order

The Gentile Christian Community of Corinth
according to Paul around 55

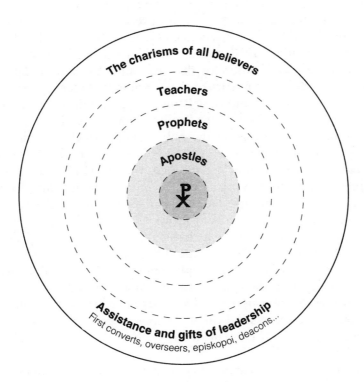

'In every way you were enriched in him (Christ) with all things... so that you are not lacking in any charisma...' (I Cor.1.5,7)

'To each is given the manifestation of the Spirit for the common good.' (I Cor.12.7)

'And God has appointed in the church first apostles, second prophets, third teachers...' (I Cor.12.28)

'And God is able to provide you with every blessing in abundance, so that you may always have enough of everything...' (II Cor.9.8)

As we have heard, in the **Jewish Christian** paradigm, given the apocalyptic end which was expected soon, there were provisional structures in the community: the Twelve, the Seven, the apostles, prophets, elders, evangelists. **Paul**, too — also in expectation of the imminent advent of Christ — knows ministries of order and leadership in his communities.[15] But in his list of charisms the 'helps' and 'gifts of leadership' stand far behind apostles, prophets and teachers — in penultimate (!) place, immediately before glossolalia or enthusiastic speaking with tongues, which is the most relativized.[16] As far as we can still establish, at first the **ministries** of order and **leadership** became **established autonomously** in the communities founded by Paul. We hear no word of a legal institution (on the basis of an 'apostolic authority' of Paul) to the different ministries of the community. Indeed, an examination of the undisputedly authentic Pauline letters produces the following significant characteristics.[17] In the Pauline communities there was:

– **no monarchical episcopate**: the only passage which is evidence for 'episkopos', the formula of greeting in Philippians, speaks of *episkopoi* (and *diakonoi*) in the plural[18] (so too Acts; the Pastoral Epistles differ);

– **no presbyterate**: there is not a single mention in the authentic letters of Paul of presbyter or presbyterate (Acts and the Pastorals differ);

– **no ordination**: there is never any mention of a prior laying on of hands in the case of those who have a charism (again Acts and the Pastorals differ). Nevertheless Paul is convinced that his Gentile Christian communities, too, are in their way complete and fully equipped churches. He writes specifically to the conflict-ridden community of Corinth, where evidently there are no *episkopoi, diakonoi* or presbyters at all (otherwise Paul would have addressed them on the topic of particular abuses): 'You were enriched in him (Christ) in all things . . . so that you are not lacking in any charisma . . .'[19]

Now not only is a monarchical episcopate nowhere to be found in the Pauline communities and in the Didache, but in the first period it is not to be found anywhere else either, even in the Acts of the Apostles.[20] According to the Didache ('Teaching' of the Apostles), the oldest early Christian community order (*c.*100), above all prophets and teachers, and only secondarily elected bishops and deacons, celebrated the eucharist.[21] The community of Antioch was evidently led not by *episkopoi* and *presbyteroi* but by prophets and teachers, and this statement may be historically reliable.[22] In Rome, too, at the time of Paul's Letter to the Romans there was evidently as yet no community order of presbyters and *episkopoi*. The fact remains that Paul does not yet know any office which was to be institutionalized throughout the communities in the same way, to which one was appointed and which alone gave one the right to celebrate the eucharist. Certainly 'overseers' are mentioned in his First Letter to the Thessalonians,[23] but not in the two important letters to the Corinthians; Stephanas and his family had made themselves available voluntarily.[24] That means that the Pauline communities are largely still fellowships of free charismatic ministries, though that does not mean that such ministries had no authority. On the contrary, these voluntary charismatic community ministries, especially of rich women who made their houses available to the community, had authority; submission could be called for. For Paul, authentic service does not depend simply on the possession of a particular function but on the way in which this function is exercised.

Conflicts over the place of women

There is no question that if the church of the Jewish Christian paradigm can be called democratic in the best sense of the word, a community in freedom and equality, a community of brothers and sisters, that is probably even more the case with the **Pauline communities**. Nowhere is this made more impressively clear than in the sentence which Paul writes to his community in Galatia: 'For as many of you as were baptized into Christ have put on Christ (as a garment). There is neither Jew nor Greek, there is neither slave nor free, there is neither male nor female; for you are all one in Christ Jesus.'[25] Indeed there can be no doubt; in his letters Paul addresses women as his *synergoi*, which literally means 'fellow workers', i.e. colleagues.

We have only to read the **greetings at the end of the Letter to the Romans** to see how many women were actively involved in the proclamation of the gospel: ten of the twenty-nine prominent people addressed here are female.[26] First we have **Phoebe**, who was on an official mission for the church of Cenchreae. She is called *diakonos*, which suggests that she was the leader of a house community.[27] **Junia** is of special significance; Paul even describes her with Andronicus as 'distinguished among the **apostles**' who had already 'confessed Christ' before him.[28] Apostle (in Greek there is no feminine form) is the highest predicate Paul can bestow. Moroever, as Ulrich Wilckens has rightly pointed out, Junia may have been one of the 'numerically limited group of those leading missionaries who had extraordinary authority as "apostles" and to whom Paul himself was only added later. This is a wider circle than the group of the Twelve.'[29]

At all events the general evidence is unambiguous: many of the women mentioned by Paul are called 'hard workers' for the gospel – a favourite word of Paul's for apostolic dedication.[30] According to the Letter to the

Philippians women like Eudonia and Syntyche – with exactly the same status as Paul and his other male fellow-workers – 'fought for the gospel'.[31] The fight to which Paul alludes was evidently so important to him that he entreats them to come to an agreement. A woman like **Prisca**, who with her husband Aquila is mentioned several times in Paul's correspondence, also has a special status.[32] The couple may have had a house in Ephesus in which they gathered a house community,[33] and we may also assume that later they led a group in their house in Rome. That Prisca is usually mentioned before her husband Aquila shows the special significance of this woman as a missionary and founder of a church.

We have heard that the activity of **women prophets** is also attested, with no objections to them, even if the New Testament no longer identifies any individual in the Gentile Christian sphere. Paul also knows such prophetesses. Certainly he wants to oblige women uttering prophecies to wear a veil in worship, but at the same time he confirms their right to free speech in the community assembly: 'Any woman who prays or prophesies with her head unveiled dishonours her head . . .'[34] So there can be no doubt that the community as Paul sees it, and as according to the Letter to the Ephesians it 'is built upon the foundation of the apostles and prophets',[35] was also a **church of women apostles and women prophets**. Therefore in summary we may say with Elisabeth Schüssler Fiorenza: 'The Pauline literature and Acts still allow us to recognize that women were among the most prominent missionaries and leaders in the early Christian movement. They were apostles and ministers like Paul, and some were his co-workers. They were teachers, preachers, and competitors in the race for the gospel. They founded house churches and, as prominent patrons, used their influence for other missionaries and Christians.'[36]

But already in Corinth the first **conflicts** were brewing over the public preaching of women, and even Paul is ambivalent here: although he defends the right of women to speak, by insisting on the **veil** he takes over arguments from an anti-feminist polemic of early Judaism[37] which he reinforces with christology: the man is the head of the woman, and Christ is the head of the man.[38] A few decades later in some texts women are then totally prohibited from **speaking** in the community: the notorious saying 'Women are to keep silent in church' has even been manipulated into the selfsame letter to the Corinthians,[39] although three chapters earlier Paul had expressly confirmed the right to prophetic utterances. The prohibition against speaking then finds its sharpest expression in the so-called Pastoral Epistles, which, while claiming the authority of the apostle to the Gentiles, come from a later time: 'Let a woman learn in silence with all submissiveness. I permit no woman to teach or to have authority over men; she is to keep silent.'[40]

All this shows that the early Christian baptismal confession of the unity of man and woman 'in Christ' which Paul quotes in Galatians was not really put into practice everywhere. There were always also **forces at work which sought to limit the equal treatment of** Jews and Greeks, freemen and slaves, **men and women.** This tendency finally gained the upper hand, so that gradually even the women mentioned in the New Testament came to be forgotten, or their significance was played down. Thus over the centuries in the Latin-speaking West the **Junia** in Romans who is distinguished with the title apostle was turned into a man, 'Junias'.[41] Thus, too, later the apostle's disciple Thecla of Iconium who preached and baptized (though she is not mentioned in the New Testament) was transformed into an ascetic recluse.[42] And already in the Gospel of John, **Mary Magdalene,** who in the Synoptic Gospels is still depicted as a leading figure among the women from Galilee, is no longer mentioned as the first of the women under the cross but is displaced by Mary the mother of Jesus,[43] who, according to the Synoptic Gospels, was strikingly not to be found under the cross. Granted, in the Gospel of John in particular Mary Magdalene then becomes the 'first witness to the resurrection',[44] and consequently is later even honoured with the title 'apostle of the apostles'.[45] But as time went on, people no longer wanted to draw conclusions from this for the right of women to preach the gospel as men did. Indeed, the question of the status of women shows an increasing repression of the original 'democratic' and 'charismatic' structures at the beginning of Christianity and a process of institutionalization which now ran its course increasingly in favour of men.

Institutionalization: apostolic succession?

However, in the long run an **institutionalization** was unavoidable even in Paul's communities, indeed, a degree of **institutionalization** had already set in at a very early stage even in the Palestinian tradition – as we heard: **by the adoption of the college of elders and the rite of laying on of hands from Judaism.** Moreover Luke's Acts of the Apostles in the 80s and even more the still later Pastoral Epistles – the most important link with the later monarchical episcopate – show an advanced stage of institutionalization in the Pauline communities as well (ordination by the laying on of hands, but still no distinction between bishops and presbyters by office and title[46]). That even applies to the community of Corinth which had so charismatic a structure; here – presumably not without resistance (I Clement) – the system of *presbyteroi* and *episkopoi* similarly began to be established. However, towards the end of the first century other communities (around Matthew or John) still show marked 'brotherly' structures, so that at the end of the New Testament period there was a great **multiplicity of community structures and forms of ministry** (partly charismatic and partly already institutionalized), which could not be harmonized without disturbing the unity between the communities.

The complex historical evidence had to be worked out on the basis of the biblical texts. Only now can the more systematic theological questions be answered. For a series of problems now seems even more insoluble: after such results from historical criticism can one still speak of an 'apostolic succession', that series of apostles to which Orthodox, Catholic and in part even Protestant clergy refer in order to legitimate the authority of their office and its demands? Here different partial aspects need to be distinguished:

1. **Apostolate.** As we already saw in connection with the Jewish Christian paradigm, among the regular public ministries the **apostolate** had the function and significance of **founding the church**, for all times. The apostles (first reduced by the evangelist Luke to the Twelve = 'twelve apostles') are the original witnesses and messengers who predate all church ministries, and to whom therefore the whole church and each individual member remain obligated. They were the first witnesses to preach the message of Christ; they founded and led the first churches and at the same time saw to the unity of the churches. So on them – together with the prophets – the church is built.

2. **The 'apostolic succession' of the church.** In principle the succession is not a matter simply of particular officials but of the whole faith community and each individual Christian. What is meant is that the church as such, and each Christian, has constantly to strive afresh to maintain a substantial unity with the apostles, specifically to maintain agreement with the **apostolic testimony** (which has come down to us in the New Testament) and constantly to perform an **apostolic ministry** (the building up of the community and missionary witness in the world). So apostolic succession is primarily succession in apostolic faith and confession, and in apostolic ministry and life.

3. **The 'apostolic succession' of bishops.** Given these basic reflections, how can a special 'apostolic succession' for bishops be maintained? At first sight the historical response seems a sobering one: it is **not** possible to verify that **the bishops are in a direct and exclusive sense the successors of the apostles** (and even of the college of the Twelve). As the immediate first witnesses and first emissaries of Jesus Christ, the apostles a priori could not be replaced and represented by any successors. An uninterrupted

sequence of 'laying on of hands' from the apostles to the bishops of today, an unbroken chain of succession (of the kind cited in later lists of succession) cannot be demonstrated historically.

Nevertheless we can rightly speak of an **apostolic succession** of the manifold ministries of leadership in the church if this is **understood functionally**. Why? Because the ministries of leadership in particular – both bishops and presbyters/priests, which can be distinguished in terms of law and discipline but not of theology and dogma, because they were identical in the early period – take further in a special way **the apostolic task of leading and founding the church**. To this degree a call to church ministry by the community leaders (bishops) – though with the participation of the community – rightly became the norm (though not exclusively).

That means that the **special** 'apostolic succession' of the bishops (and pastors) consists in leading and founding communities and churches, but it was to be rooted wholly in the proclamation of the gospel. The bishops were not to 'quench'[47] the other charisms, but support them. **Prophets** and **teachers** have their own original authority.[48] Ordination with laying on of hands, which eventually became established, is not a rite which works automatically or mechanically; it presupposes and requires faith, which is to be active in the apostolic spirit. This in no way excludes the possibility of mistakes and errors among the church leaders; so they need to be constantly examined by the community of believers. But how did the development continue?

Concentration on the one bishop

The **presbyteral-episcopal church order** which has been retained to the present day not only by the Eastern Orthodox churches but also by the Catholic, the Anglican and Methodist and individual Lutheran churches is neither an accident nor a lapse, but part of the paradigm shift towards the Hellenistic paradigm initiated by Paul and thus the consequence of a historical development. Important and generally successful though this structure of office was, it would be unhistorical today still to insist on the traditional dogmatic explanation that the episcopal church order rests on 'divine institution' or on 'institution by Jesus Christ', i.e. on divine right (*ius divinum*).

Historical research clearly indicates that church order centred on the bishop is to be derived from a long and not unproblematical **historical development**[49] which took very different courses in different regions.

Phase 1: The local **presbyter-bishops** prevailed over the prophets (who were often itinerant), teachers and other charismatic ministries as the

The Order of Three Ministries

The Gentile Christian Community of Antioch
according to Ignatius around 110

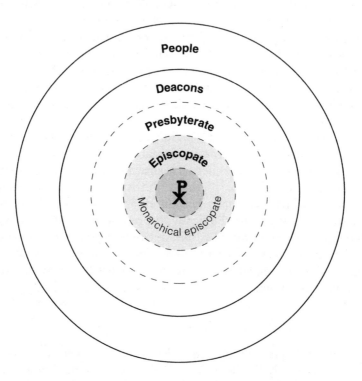

'Follow your bishop, every one of you, as obediently as Jesus Christ followed the Father. Obey your presbyters, too, as you would the apostles; give your deacons the same reverence that you would to a command from God. Make sure that no step affecting the church is ever taken by anyone without the bishop's sanction. The sole eucharist you should consider valid is one that is celebrated by the bishop himself, or by some person authorized by him. Where the bishop is to be seen, there let all his people be; just as wherever Jesus Christ is present, we have the catholic church. Nor is it permitted to conduct baptisms or love-feasts without the bishop. On the other hand, whatever does have his sanction can be sure of God's approval too. This is the way to make certain of the soundness and validity of anything you do. You have only to acknowledge God and the bishop, and all is well; for a man who honours his bishop is himself honoured by God, but to go behind the bishop's back is to be a servant of the devil.'   (Smyrnaeans, 8.If., 9.1)

principal and eventually **the sole leaders of the community** (at the eucharist as well). What is problematical here is that the 'collegiality' (*communio*) of **all** believers increasingly became a collegiality (*collegium*) of particular ministerial groups **over against** the community, so that a division of 'clergy' and laity began at a very early stage.

Phase 2: The **monarchical episcopate of an individual bishop** in a city as opposed to a number of fellow presbyters in the communities spread increasingly: first in Syrian Antioch with Ignatius, in whose letters for the first time we find the order of three ministries – bishop, presbyter, deacon. Certainly what Ignatius wrote about the bishop was probably in some respects still wishful thinking at the time: evidently the eucharist was still often celebrated without a bishop. But this development was already problematical by then: the collegiality of the different bishops or presbyters now became the collegiality of the **one** bishop with his presbyterate and his deacons, so that the division between 'clergy' and 'people' finally came about.

Phase 3: With the spread of the church from the cities to the country the bishop changed from being the head of a city community to now being the **head of a whole church region,** a diocese and so on. He was the bishop in the present-day sense, for whom the 'apostolic succession' was now historicized, formalized and also externalized by indicating the succession in lists of names. The problem here is that alongside the collegiality of bishops and presbyterate, increasing importance was attached to the collegiality not only of the individual monarchical bishops among themselves (the college of bishops) but also, though only in the West, in connection with the Bishop of Rome.

The slow rise of the Bishop of Rome

We already saw in connection with the Jewish Christian paradigm (P I) that there is no mention of a **Bishop of Rome** (or of Peter in Rome) anywhere in the New Testament.[50] It is still more striking that **there is no mention of a Bishop of Rome even in the earliest post-New Testament sources:**
– **Ignatius** of Antioch[51] (c.110), who shows such concern for the church (he uses the phrase 'catholic church' for the first time), the unity of the community and its eucharist, and for the rejection of 'heresies' (Jewish Christian or docetic?), already addresses monarchical bishops emphatically in his letters to communities in Asia Minor and defends the monarchical episcopate (after the model of James?) with theological and ideological arguments. However, in his letter to the Roman community, which according to him 'has the primacy of love', like the apostle Paul before him, strikingly enough he does not address a bishop.

– And even in the earliest letter from the Roman community itself (to the community of Corinth around 96), the authorship of which is to be attributed to a **Clement** (according to a statement by Dionysius of Corinth around 170, preserved by Eusebius), no single author appears anywhere; no monarchical bishop is mentioned either for Rome or for Corinth.

– As the communities in the West continue not to know a monarchical episcopate (according to the letter of **Polycarp**, for example, in Philippi in Macedonia), contrary to Antioch and Asia Minor, some historians conjecture that 'this institution, coming from the East, was able to establish itself only gradually in the West'.[52]

So when did a **monarchical bishop** first emerge from the host of *episkopoi* and *presbyteroi* **in Rome**, that metropolis with its many house churches? We can no longer discover this. The reports of Peter's successors – for example the earliest list of bishops of Rome in Irenaeus, though this does not mention Peter as the first Bishop of Rome, but rather Linus, to whom both Peter **and** Paul are said to have transferred the episcopal ministry – are second-century reconstructions, which in some cases have made use of Roman names which were still known. A monarchical episcopate can only be demonstrated at a late stage – say from the middle of the second century (Bishop Anicetus). Our information about the Roman church and its bishops is very fragmentary down to the middle of the third century; the first precise chronological dating of a Roman pontificate is the resignation of Pontian on 28 September 235.

Nevertheless, there is no question that from the beginning the Roman community understandably had a very **high self-esteem**[53] and rightly enjoyed **great respect**.[54] Why?

– It was the community in the capital of the empire,

– it was old, large and prosperous,

– it was the site of the tombs of the two chief apostles Peter and Paul,[55]

– it was famous for its charitable activity ('primacy of love'),[56]

– it had proved to be a guardian of apostolic tradition in the fight against Gnosticism, as Irenaeus of Lyons confirms.[57]

And if even in Rome neither the community nor an individual claimed primacy for many centuries, now – after the fall of Jerusalem and its Jewish-Christian community in 135 – Rome had in fact become the leading church of Christianity. The **paradigm shift** from the Jewish Christian (P I) to the Gentile Christian (P II) constellation can hardly be described more symbolically: **instead of Jerusalem, Rome** (along with other cities of the pagan empire) had become the main vehicle of Christianity. And in the newly built Aelia Capitolina (Jerusalem) there was now only a Gentile Christian community.

Structural characteristics of the early church paradigm

If we look back on the complex development of young Gentile Christianity in its first century the following **dominant structural characteristics** of the new paradigm initiated by Paul emerge – while the substance of faith remains the same:

- instead of a church community made up of Jews there is now one made up of Jews and Gentiles and finally of **Gentiles** alone;
- instead of Hebrew and Aramaic, **Greek** is now the dominant language, and all the New Testament writings have been handed down to us in Greek;
- instead of having a rural breeding ground in Palestine and the Near East, Christianity is now inculturated in **Hellenistic Roman culture**;
- instead of Jerusalem, **Rome** is now the centre and leading church of Christianity;
- instead of a community with presbyters as leaders there is now an increasingly institutionalized presbyteral and episcopal church order.

Indeed, the three-level presbyteral-episcopal church order (bishop – presbyter – deacon) finally established itself in a slow and complex history in post-apostolic Christianity, for reasons which can still be followed and accepted today. However, it cannot claim universal validity, as our paradigm analysis has demonstrated. Measured by the intentions of Jesus himself (mutual service) and the impulses of the first Jewish Christian community (no hierarchy but mutual diakonia) and also the charismatic Pauline community (each has his or her charisma), it has no absolute significance, unpopular though this may be for bishops.

The New Testament scholar Paul Hoffmann has rightly described the negative consequences of this development: 'The price for the "overwhelming persistence" of a church of males and patriarchs was not least the discrediting of women, the degeneration of any responsible community, the far-reaching repression of charismatic gifts in favour of an office of leadership which attracted all authority to itself, the division of the church into clergy and laity, the replacement of prophetic preaching with a tradition which became increasingly fossilized – not to mention the many who were sacrificed in the name of the "unity of the church" or the "purity of doctrine" in order to preserve the system. And this ends in the loss of church unity.'[58]

The ecumenical explosiveness of such a statement can easily be seen by those who know the centuries-old strategies of legitimation and argumentation used by the churches to maintain their own doctrinal positions and their power. So already at this point we must raise some self-critical questions which show what ecumenical significance this historical evidence also has for the future, even if we do not strive in any way for an anachronistic repristination of New Testament community structures:

Questions for the Future

• Are the **Orthodox Churches of the East** well advised for the future to continue to treat the clearly post-biblical church order of three ministries (bishop – presbyter – deacon) as though it were unchangeable in every respect? In the future, is it not necessary to go more by the gospel itself than by the 'fathers' (most of whom were bishops), that gospel which gives freedom in so many questions of church order and church discipline (marriage of bishops, ordination of women)?

• Can the **Catholic Church of the West** continue to exist in the future if it retains its absolutist and centralist system, which in practice in the Middle Ages did away with a presbyteral-episcopal church order that had been functioning well for a thousand years in the West, too? Can it still attempt to regulate all questions of dogma, morals and church discipline by a Pope who in effect exercises absolute rule from the centre, in Rome?

• In the future must the **Churches of the Reformation**, too, rigidly and unconditionally maintain the present status quo of their church order? Wasn't the old presbyteral-episcopal order replaced by a 'church governed by local rulers', first as an emergency (rulers as 'emergency bishops'), and then as a matter of principle (rulers as 'summepiscopi'), and then by systems of local, regional and national autonomy – all often at the cost of a church provincialism without links to the universal church?

• Can the **Churches of the Orthodox and Catholic tradition** continue in the future to deny that the ministries and eucharists of the Churches of the Reformation tradition are valid by appealing to an apostolic succession which seems not to exist? Didn't the church order of the Pauline or Gentile Christian communities from the start also leave open other modes of leadership and apostolic succession of church leaders? And according to the New Testament, couldn't someone also become a church leader on the basis of a call by other members of the community, or on the basis of a free charism which led to leadership or the foundation of a community?

So in the comments which follow we shall always have to be keenly aware of the historical relativity of particular developments, and the forms of church order which emerge from them. Since according to the New

Testament itself other possibilities exist, or at any rate cannot be excluded, **every church must be open to other options.** And churches are not allowed to brand other church structures as un-Christian, or out of keeping with the gospel or the church. The gospel itself has to be the only criterion for the truth or falsehood of a development in the church, and here we must look carefully to see whether there is an *evolutio contra evangelium* (a development contrary to the gospel), an *evolutio secundum evangelium* (a development in keeping with the gospel), or an *evolutio praeter evangelium* (a development outside the gospel). The paradigm analysis in particular makes it possible to relativize developments regarded as absolute in the church in the light of the 'Absolute' itself, to put in question what are alleged to be ordinances with divine sanction in the light of God's original will (as attested in the gospel), in order to introduce the dynamic of development and loyalty to origins into the ecumenical dialogue between the Christian churches.

But after this brief critical interlude we must turn to the further history of the young Gentile Christian church. Of course it cannot be related in detail here, but it does have to be analysed in respect of the further development of this paradigm of the early church.

3. Persecution of Christians and dispute over faith

Who in the Roman empire, a century after the execution of Jesus of Nazareth under Pontius Pilate, would have given Christianity a chance of establishing itself in the Graeco-Roman world with its numerous religions and philosophies, its thousands of temples and theatres, arena and gymnasia?[59]

A persecuted minority

'In the second century of the Christian era,' wrote the Enlightenment British historian **Edward Gibbon** about the period after Nero and Domitian in the introduction to his famous seven-volume *History of the Decline and Fall of the Roman Empire* (albeit somewhat too optimistically), 'In the second century of the Christian era the Roman empire comprehended the fairest part of earth and the most civilized portion of mankind. The frontiers of that extended monarchy were guarded by ancient renown and disciplined valour. The gentle but powerful influence of laws and manners had gradually cemented the union of the provinces. Their peaceful inhabitants enjoyed and abused the advantages of wealth and luxury. The image of a free constitution was preserved with decent reverence. The Roman senate appeared to possess the sovereign authority and had devolved on the emperors all the executive powers of government. During a happy period of more than fourscore years the public administration was conducted by the virtue and capability of Nerva, Trajan, Hadrian and the two Antonines.'[60]

The first official Roman report on the Christians, the letter of **Pliny** the Younger which has already been cited, comes from this time (to be precise, from 112). Pliny was governor of the province of Bithynia on the Black Sea, where there were already many Christians even in the country, and he was writing to the Emperor Trajan: some temples were standing empty, and it was almost impossible to sell meat for sacrifices. In fact Christians were refusing to worship the state gods and the emperor. Now a **refusal to respect the cult of the state** was a **state crime** (*crimen laesae Romanae religionis*); here no Christian was safe from accusation and punishment. Moreover, Pliny writes unmoved that he had had some Christians who were not Roman citizens executed, but had sent others to Rome for trial. Otherwise, he had not been able to establish any crime with which they could be charged: hence his question. At that time numerous rumours were going the rounds about atheism and treachery, indeed incest (in connection with the agape?) and cannibalism (in connection with the eucharist?) at their nocturnal meetings. These people would merely sing alternately a hymn (psalm?) to 'Christ as a god' on a particular day (certainly Sunday) before daybreak, and had sworn an oath (baptismal vows?) to refrain from theft, robbery, adultery, falsehood and deceit.[61]

The Emperor **Trajan**'s famous reply ('rescript') is the first constitutional regulation for the trial of Christians known to us, and in principle it remained the policy of subsequent emperors down to the middle of the third century. No anonymous denunciations should be entertained, nor should Christians be hunted down and investigated, but orderly individual accusations should be acted upon; those who then recanted and offered prayers to the gods would be acquitted, and only the stubborn would be punished. At first the emperors did not regard the Christians – still few in number – as such a danger to the state that they felt that they had to order a general persecution.

Persecutions of Christians[62] – the first under Nero in 64 (numerous Christians cruelly executed as scapegoats for the great fire which Nero had himself staged in Rome) and the second under Domitian (81-96: he had made an 'oath' on the genius of the emperor compulsory) – were not systematic and uninterrupted down to 250, but were local, limited, sudden and sporadic. So the church was not driven into the catacombs everywhere; that is a later 'Romantic' notion. In any case, the eucharist was celebrated in private houses. But the Neronian persecution was a fatal precedent: one could be condemned – man or woman, slave or free – simply for being a Christian. Indeed, to become a Christian was now always a risk, because the Christian faith called for a decision. In some circumstances, being a Christian meant a readiness to *martyrein*, to 'bear witness' to the Christian faith: through suffering, through torture (and for women, being made prostitutes) and finally death. But here too we should guard against idealizing. Beyond doubt numerous Christians were tried, but the number of 'martyrs' like Ignatius, Polycarp and Justin, Blandina, Perpetua and Felicitas – the word 'martyr' was now increasingly used in the strict sense of 'those who bear witness with their blood' – remained quite limited. Moreover, martyrs brought Christianity great publicity everywhere. Those 'confessors' who survived persecution also enjoyed great respect. The Christian was to endure martyrdom in an emergency, but not provoke it – and that is in fact what happened.

The earliest Christian theologians

The so-called 'Apologies', the first Christian literature, came into being in this precarious situation.[63] We must note that the few Christian '**Apologists**' like Quadratus, Aristides, Justin and others felt in a quite impossible position in writing their defences, in part presented to the emperor, against pagan misunderstandings, attacks and calumniations. Their public and political effect on the society of the time was at first small. But their influence in the church was all the greater. These authors, all of whom wrote in Greek, were after all **the first Christian men of letters**, who for the first time produced Christian 'literature', because unlike the New Testament authors and the 'apostolic fathers' who followed them (Ignatius, Polycarp and a few others[64]) they did not merely compose works (mostly 'letters') for use within the church but wrote for the public. Their purpose was to present Christianity by means of generally understandable Hellenistic concepts, views and methods. Here not only was scripture quoted, but there was philosophical argument. In this way these defenders of Christianity became **the first Christian theologians** – after Paul – who provided a hitherto unprecedented spiritual and intellectual **impetus towards Hellenization** within the church community.

However, at a very early stage a different attitude to Greek **philosophy** made itself felt within Christianity, which was continually to recur down the centuries: whereas Theophilus and Tatian and then the Latin North African Tertullian repudiated philosophy, Athenagoras and Justin, like the Alexandrians Clement and Origen later, proved well-disposed to it. **Justin** above all (we have already met him) was to become important for the future.[65] He came from Palestine and then worked publicly as a philosopher in Rome as well (he was executed around 165). He was the only one of the apologists to have had a philosophical education. He argued intelligently and emphatically in four directions at the same time: against the mockery of the intellectuals, the oppression of the state, the enmity of the Jews and the disputations of the heretics. Justin was able to make use of Platonic metaphysics, Stoic ethics and the Hellenistic criticism of myths, on the one hand to unmask pagan polytheism and pagan myth (the immoral stories about the gods) and cult (bloody sacrifice, the worship of animals) as superstition and the work of demons, and on the other to claim the great philosophers like Heraclitus and Socrates as 'Christians before Christ'[66] – all for a Christianity which he now wanted to proclaim as the universal, only **true philosophy**. For him Christianity had become a reasonable wisdom which fulfilled the age-old prophecies of the prophets, which produced brave martyrs and fearless confessors: it was not by chance that it had spread throughout the ecumene so rapidly (in fact already from the Caspian and Black Sea to Spain and Britain).

However, the fact that this Justin, who, as we heard, had not broken off relations with the Jewish Christians, and thought of the God of the philosophers and the creator God of the Bible together, was to be of special significance. At the same time he took up a popular key term of Hellenistic spirituality, the **Logos**,[67] which already occurs in Jewish form as 'Word' (= 'wisdom') in the hymn that is the prologue to the Gospel of John: the Logos which 'was in the beginning with God'.[68] Now Logos is understood as the divine reason, which as the 'seed-giving Logos' (*logos spermatikos*)[69] implants the seed of truth in all human beings, and as 'the true light lights everyone'.[70] And this Logos revealed itself not only through the prophets of Israel but also through the sages of Greece, and then truly 'became flesh'[71] in Jesus Christ and assumed a human form. While in other human beings it can only be known weakly and unclearly, now it is clear and plain in Jesus.

This is beyond doubt a grandiose conception with much promise for the future. It preserved Christ, the bodily revelation of the divine Logos, as the centre of Christianity and yet also attempted to do justice to other philosophers, poets and historians, all of whom had a share in the divine Logos: 'Whatever is well said among them belongs to us Christians.'[72] However, one thing cannot be ignored from the beginning in this Hellenization of the gospel: now Christianity was understood less and less as existential discipleship of Jesus Christ and more – in an intellectual narrowing – as the acceptance of a revealed doctrine about God and Jesus Christ, the world and human beings. And it was above all to be the Logos

christology which increasingly forced back the Jesus of history in favour
of a doctrine and finally a church dogma of the 'incarnate God'.

Mixed or segregated?

But even in the face of such Christian apologetic, educated Romans and
also well-known critics of Christianity like Galen and Celsus in the
second century, or Porphyry in the third and even later Julian, the
'apostate', in the fourth century were asking:[73] did such a religion have a
chance of establishing itself in the Roman empire? At best, this could
happen:
if Christianity, too, adapted itself to the existing order of Roman society;
if – since it was 'unfortunately' an offspring of Judaism, though without
having retained the Jewish law – it adopted the splendid Hellenistic
culture fully and completely;
if, since it was after all a new religion, it finally came to terms with the old
Roman state religion, was tolerant to other religions, did not encourage
any rebellion or undermine morality;
if it thus observed the same morals and customs which had time and again
been handed down from generation to generation;
if, finally, it confessed the gods to whom the empire now owed its
greatness and strength.

Now for better or worse Christianity was in fact compelled to establish
itself in this world: turning away from the Jewish Christian apocalyptic
paradigm was the answer to the new cultural, social and political
situation. Theologians who still argue today in a very anachronistic way
for 'apocalyptic' ought to note that the **apocalyptic expectation of an
imminent end**, which was cherished by many Jews in the earliest
community and also by Paul, was not fulfilled (and even later was
disappointed time and again). After the death of Paul and the destruction
of Jerusalem – the time during which the Gospels and other New
Testament writings were produced – what alternative did the Christian
communities have but to settle down for the long term in the world of the
Roman empire?

Already in the New Testament, towards the end of the first and the
beginning of the second centuries, above all Luke's works, the Pastoral
Epistles and finally II Peter, and in another way also the Gospel of John,
bear witness that the eschatological and apocalyptic view of Christianity
had been quietly overcome – apart from the very earthly 'chiliastic' hopes,
widespread among the people, for a 'thousand-year' messianic kingdom
on earth before the judgment of the world. Instead of this there was now a
salvation-historical perspective: Jesus Christ was not just the end of time

but the 'middle of time'.[74] An evidently lengthy intermediate period was put between him and the coming of the kingdom of God: the **time of the church**.[75] In the meantime, as we saw, a church of Jews had become a church of Gentiles. It now began, quite unconcerned about its Jewish origins, increasingly to become Hellenized, institutionalized and established.[76]

But this departure from Judaism and the increasing immersion of the church and theology in the Hellenistic-Roman world raises a **question of principle** which is still significant today:

– Should not Christianity, like Roman state religion, simply accept everything religious and thus **mix** with other religions of the Hellenistic world: 'syncretism' as a 'fusion' of religions?

– Or should Christianity totally **dissociate** itself in decisive matters from these religions, fascinating though they are in many ways, with their mysterious cults ('mysteries') and doctrines, and which in Syria and in Egypt were strongly influenced by Eastern thought (and which ultimately might perhaps even have Indian roots)?

Gnosticism: redemption through knowledge

Syncretism was the trend of the time and was in the interest of the Roman state, and a current catchword – already in Paul's Corinth – was '**Gnosis**', '**knowledge**'. But 'Gnosis' was more than a slogan. 'Gnosis' (which is also known as Gnosticism) was one of the great religious movements of late antiquity which promised redemptive knowledge about the mysteries of human beings, the world and God.

Already from the first Christian century, extremely different Gnostic groups, trends, schools and systems had formed in the Eastern provinces of the Roman empire.[77] Today we no longer know about them only from the reports and refutations of the church fathers, primarily Irenaeus (c.140-200).[78] Between 1945 and 1948 in the desert of Upper Egypt near the present small town of **Nag Hammadi**, the sensational discovery was made of a collection of Gnostic and non-Gnostic manuscripts in Coptic, written in the first half of the fourth century but originally composed in Greek in the second/third centuries. Since then, for the first time we have had a small library of thirteen volumes with fifty-one different works (1153 pages) which give the 'world-view' of Gnostics themselves, whether these were non-Christian or Christian, Christian-Gnostic or Gnostic-Christian.[79] At any rate the majority were Christian, since Nag Hammadi is the territory of the ancient Chenoboskion, where, also in the fourth century, Pachomius (mentioned in the fragment of a letter) founded the first monastery for Christian monks, some of whom had presumably taken their scrolls into the wilderness. Possibly such scrolls were buried after an anti-heretical Easter letter from the Alexandrian patriarch Athanasius, which was translated into Coptic in 367 and communicated to the Egyptian monks.

Many **historical questions** about Gnosticism had long been disputed, for example whether there was already a Gnosticism before or outside Christianity (which is demonstrated at the latest after the Nag Hammadi finds by writings which are not influenced by Christianity), whether the Simon called a magician in Acts was the first Gnostic (which is claimed by Irenaeus but not proven), or whether Marcion should be reckoned a Gnostic (a matter of definition), indeed, whether the New Testament is already influenced by Gnosticism (which cannot be ruled out in the case of the letters of Paul, the Pauline school and the Johannine writings).[80] There is no dispute that with Basilides from Alexandria and above all with the Egyptian Valentinus teaching in Rome around the middle of the second century Gnosticism experienced its heyday, and in the third century as it were reached its culmination with the syncretistic world religion of Mani.[81]

Where does Gnosticism come from? Presumably it has Jewish roots: first from the sphere of Jewish apocalyptic, which had already adopted elements of Iranian dualism and eschatological thinking, and secondly from Jewish wisdom teaching, which in time had shifted in the direction of scepticism. But it had also allied itself with enlightened Greek thought and, philosophically, especially with Middle Platonism, whose dualism and thought in terms of ascent and descent it took over. So the language, vocabulary, conceptuality, indeed the whole garb of Gnosticism was Greek and Hellenistic. Gnostic dualism differed from Iranian-Jewish and Greek-Platonic dualism by its marked **hostility to the world, matter and the body.**

From the perspective of the Gnostics themselves, their eirenic and polemic writings, the character of Gnosticism of course became clearer than it had been through the often tendentious reports and quotations of the church fathers who were fighting against it. Here it is important to see that for some Christians the **boundaries between the mainstream church and Gnosticism** were for a long time **fluid.** Gnosticism was not a priori heresy; after all, there were even already traditions in the New Testament itself (above all the Johannine prologue, the Philippians hymn) which Christians with a Gnostic orientation could take up.[82] In the third century many Gnostics were still living and working within the framework of the mainstream church. Gnosticism is primarily a **religious form of thought, attitude and mood** characterized by striving for 'knowledge', which is widespread and not limited to Christianity. Gnostics are those who want to interpret the shared Christian traditions in their own highly distinctive way. Klaus Koschorke has pointed out that the Christian Gnostics, who could not be recognized as such outwardly, but rather attempted to influence the mass of mainstream Christians from within, understood themselves as the 'inner circle, the spiritual centre of the mainstream church': thus Gnostic Christianity did not construct itself 'as **opposition to** but as a higher stage **above** ordinary Christianity, presupposing this and building on it'.[83] So the belief of mainstream Christians was not rejected a priori but relativized. It might not be made absolute and exclusive: it was the lower, provisional way of salvation for the *simplices*, for ordinary people.

Thus 'already in early Christianity there were **interactions between Christian and Gnostic ideas**'.[84] In very different ways the Gnostic theologians who had penetrated the Christian communities attempted to integrate material from the Greek, Jewish and Iranian spheres into Christianity. Christianity was not to remain a popular religion with a cultic orientation and a hierarchical stamp, but rather was to raise itself to become an intellectually reflective and highly spiritual elite religion of 'those who know': a Hellenistic 'mystery religion' which could be lived out, experienced and thought through in a wholly personal way. Thus 'Gnosticism' was an esoteric tradition of 'the few' (probably mostly intellectuals, above all in the great Hellenistic cities of the East and in Rome with a following from the lower classes) with a philosophical and theological orientation. Moreover today we should not disparage mainstream Christianity and say that Gnosticism was a broad current, as though the mainstream church tradition had only made a 'small selection of specialist sources'.[85] This unnecessarily reinforces the views of those who in any case believe the slogan used by researchers that 'everything is Gnosticism'.

Why did Gnosticism make more impression on some people of the time than the biblical message? The answer can only be that Gnosticism claimed above all to give a comprehensive answer to the constantly oppressive question of the human condition: the **origin of evil** and the whole process of God and the world. According to Gnosticism, the origin of evil does not simply have to do, as in the Bible, with human beings who have a proneness to evil, but with the fall, stage by stage, from the supreme deity itself (a fall for which there were different explanations). The inferior creator God, the ignorant demiurge, who emerged from this had created the evil world, remote from God, through his self-glorifying actions; however, sparks of the original divine world of light imprisoned in the human body have still been preserved. Certainly the Christian Gnostic systems of the second and third centuries differed widely, but their 'central idea' was the **descent and ascent of the divine 'spark'**.[86] The Gnostic thought-models and explanations of the world are thus defined by a pessimistic-dualistic view of the unknown, incomprehensible transcendent God (with a 'fullness' of angels, heavenly beings and hypostases) and the visible world dominated by evil powers, evil matter, the body, which is the prison of the soul, the spark of light.

This was a dualism hostile to the world on both the cosmological and the anthropological level, though it had a quite hopeful outlook. For at the same time Gnosticism promised a **way of redemption**, and offered **knowledge** (and other means) to liberate human beings from the constraints of earthly living and entanglement with the world powers. So was this self-redemption? No, for only on the basis of a call to resurrection by a redeemer, mission preaching or esoteric instruction does the soul, which has been put to sleep and bewitched by evil demons, succeed in breaking the darkness of ignorance and achieving self-knowledge. And this self-knowledge consists specifically in the knowledge of the divine spark of light ('spirit', 'soul') which is the authentic essence of human beings. So the aim is to make it possible for the divine spark to return from the evil world of matter to its divine home of light. Thus begins an 'ascent of the soul' or a '**journey of the soul**', constantly put in the utmost danger by the powers which rule the world, through the spheres above the earth back to that divine unity which right at the beginning a lowly arrogant creator god had broken by creating the world.

Here an important role is played in many Gnostic writings by a **redeemer figure** (sometimes even several redeemer figures) who possibly already existed before or outside Christianity, or who may only have been produced through Christianity: a redeemer who as a light form shares the fate of the sparks of light which are akin to him and brings them back with him into the world of light. Here Gnosticism knows no unitary 'redeemer myth' of the kind still assumed by Rudolf Bultmann (following Wilhelm Bousset and Richard Reitzenstein). The Nag Hammadi writings compel us to abandon this position, since here there are very different conceptions of a redeemer, liberator, revealer, messenger.

For the Gnostic it is decisive that redemption can already be experienced and introduced here and now, though the final breakthrough only comes about in the separation of the spark of light from the body in death. Thus a monistic vision of unity forms the background to Gnostic dualism. Redemption is understood as a return of the soul from the world and the body to its pre-existent, purely spiritual, primal state, and not as in the New Testament writings as a historical new human beginning through Jesus Christ, as liberation from sin and guilt.

Furthermore, remarkably enough the highly spiritual Gnostics, who were certainly effective in their recruitment, also offered very material help as a **means against the dangers of the journey of the soul**: tokens of recognition and protection ('seals'), magical sayings, amulets and ceremonies of the dead (with the communication of passwords). Without doubt, what was fascinating for many people was that in the Gnostic system the world was often described with the help of polar opposites, in which human bisexuality appeared through couples (syzygies) in a quite different way from a God envisaged in masculine terms. Here masculine and feminine appeared to be taken up into the Godhead on equal terms. This has led individual feminist interpreters today to see a better foundation for the idea of a priesthood of women in Gnosticism than in orthodox Christianity. Indeed, even today we can easily imagine that it must have been extremely attractive at the time for many people, women and men, educated and uneducated, to entrust themselves to particular 'revelations', myths, secret traditions and world systems with mysterious rituals and magical practices instead of to the simple Gospels, commandments and rites of the church.

Be this as it may: Gnosticism was concerned to answer the question of the origin of evil and the way to redemption from a life of anxiety and confusion, suffering and death. It was by no means just a primarily theoretical 'philosophy of religion', as the founder of research into Gnosticism, the Tübingen church historian Ferdinand Christian Baur, thought: in essence it was concerned with **existential questions** – though of course these first had to be dealt with intellectually, as Hans Jonas and Rudolf Bultmann already emphasized.[87] In the face of so much cultural stagnation and political apathy, especially in the Eastern part of the Roman empire, Gnosticism, with the help of Eastern religiosity, which had also streamed into Hellenistic culture, offered a way of achieving a particular attitude to life which made it possible to overcome alienation and find a way out of political and social constraints. To this degree Gnosticism also expressed a social protest.

Here the Gnostics – unlike 'the many' in the mainstream church – did not simply want to hold to particular rules of faith and a selection of sacred scriptures, particular church rituals and the clerical hierarchy. They turned against the church's doctrine of God and creation, christology, ecclesiology and the sacraments. They wanted to take a way of solitude and inwardness which led them to accept only what was confirmed by their own religious experience. Here they did not advocate a 'physical theology' of salvation, a distortion so often presented by the church fathers, as though the Gnostics were physically connected with the light world, 'redeemed by nature', and dependent neither on grace nor on perseverance. No, the way of life of a Gnostic had to correspond to his or her enlightened state; Gnostics had to prove themselves ethically until their entry into the *pleroma*, the 'fullness'.

And some in fact asked themselves whether the simple '**faith**' (Greek *pistis*) of the Christian community was not perhaps just a simplistic, superficial form of this higher, radically spiritual '**knowledge**'. In the face of bishops, priests and deacons of the institutional church, who often seemed authoritative, wasn't a reaction and appeal to one's own religious insights, spiritual experiences and an ethic of freedom justified?[88] More recent research has indeed made us realize that we must not see the Gnostic speculations, practices and systems just as special, abstruse and un-Christian! From a present-day perspective we can understand all too well why some Gnostics rejected as naive faith notions of a biological virgin birth of Jesus or a bodily resurrection understood literally.

The danger of Gnosticism: mythologizing and syncretism

But even the most benevolent interpreters of Gnosticism cannot overlook its **danger for Christianity**: quite untroubled by the unmythological and historical origin of Christianity, indeed despising the simple church faith of the mere 'believers', the 'pistics', Christian 'Gnostics', 'knowers' – all the Valentinians Basilidians, Ophites (snake worshippers) and rival subordinate and parallel groups – attempted with the help of every possible myth, image, metaphor, symbol and ritual to transform the message of Christ rooted in history into a **mythical theology**. They promised a radical spiritualization and liberation from earthly fetters and displayed a tendency which was usually hostile to the world and ascetic (sometimes even libertine, though there is no evidence of that at Nag Hammadi). Was there not thus a danger that the original Jewish Christian faith would disappear in the undertow of a Hellenistic syncretism which swallowed up everything?

Of course there was no objection to a constantly new description of what Christianity was, nor can we deny the originality of anti-Gnostic theologians from Irenaeus to Origen, who doubtless learned from Gnosticism. But unlimited theological speculation? Was Christ, say, the reborn great Seth, son of Adam? Was just any allegory, any arbitrary symbolism and any conceptual acrobatics to be allowed? Was it legitimate, contrary to what is said in the book of Genesis, to make God the creator a hostile inferior being who grudges human beings redemptive 'knowledge'? In the face of this allegedly envious God, was one even to say that the serpent in paradise who seduced human beings into having 'knowledge' was right and the bearer of a redemptive primal revelation which had constantly to be regained down to the present day? Didn't this make the whole of Jewish history ridiculous, because it was a work of this creator God?

The **danger of syncretism** was real; was the young Christianity in some circumstances to accept more than one God and redeemer? Was it also to accept true gods and redeemers from other religions? God the Mother as well as God the Father? And instead of faith in Father, Son and Spirit, a Trinity of Father, Mother (or Wife) and Son? A mythicization of the couple, so that the heavenly Wisdom as universal mother also had to stand as consort alongside the heavenly Christ? For example, might one assume, against what was to be read in the Gospels (read aloud in the liturgy of the mainstream church) that as a spirit-man Christ (who was probably only inserted into some Gnostic texts at a later stage) could not suffer at all and was not even crucified?

Certainly we must not judge Gnostic notions by the later christology of the church; we shall see that in earliest and early Christianity there was a very varied understanding of the relationship of Jesus to God. Nevertheless, even now we can understand the negative reaction of the church fathers to **Gnostic christology** if we reflect with the Gnostic specialist Kurt Rudolph:[89]

1. Gnostic christology undertook a de-historicization of the Gnostic redeemer figure which at the same time resulted in a **mythologization** of the Christ figure: a ' "mythologizing" of the Christ figure to an unprecendented degree'. In fact, 'it was this side of the development above all which prevented Gnosis from obtaining permanent right of domicile in Christian thought, even if there were again and again – even in the present day – movements in that direction'.[90]

2. To bring the historical and mythical aspects under the same heading the Gnostic theologians undertook a '**division** of the Christian redeemer into two completely separate beings': whereas the earthly and corruptible Jesus of Nazareth 'as a temporary earthly manifestation of Christ takes over the above-mentioned task as revealer of Gnostic teaching', the heavenly eternal Christ is 'a higher being of light who from the very beginning dwells in the *pleroma* with the "Father", and is usually described as his "image", as the "self-originate", "son", "first born" (or identified with these). In this capacity he plays a role in the world of light . . .'[91]

3. The anti-worldly dualism of Gnosticism which completely devalued the earthly and bodily went so far in some systems that Jesus could only be

credited with a **phantom body**. Certainly there are Nag Hammadi writings which can put forward a view of Christ akin to the Gospel of John, and which cannot be suspected of docetism. But there are also Nag Hammadi texts in which Jesus himself takes on the form of Simon of Cyrene and looks on at the crucifixion, laughing: 'It was not I whom they struck with the reed. It was another, Simon, who bore the cross on his shoulder. It was another upon whom they placed the crown of thorns. But I was rejoicing in the height over all the wealth of the archons and the offspring of their error, of their empty glory. And I was laughing at their ignorance.'[92]

4. On the basis of this view of the crucifixion, which is not the crucifixion of Jesus, we can also understand that for Gnostics the **resurrection** of Christ took place already before or at the same time as the crucifixion – the liberation of the spirit and annihilation of the flesh together. So there is no question of Gnosticism having aimed at a **dissolution of the substance of Christianity**: '"Redemption", "crucifixion" and "resurrection" are for Gnosis largely understood as symbolic incidents of cosmic significance and accordingly were subjected to entirely new interpretations which often become visible only on a closer inspection. This was one of the facts which demonstrated the danger of the gnostic teachings for an orthodox Christian understanding.'[93]

Was there then to be a **double truth** in the church: a truth that people generally could understand and an esoteric truth for those in the know? Right from the very beginning, the serious criticism of Gnosticism was that in many cases the text of the New Testament and Gnostic 'knowledge' were diametrically opposed. 'They speak like believers, but in so doing understand not only dissimilar but even opposed and quite blasphemous things,' remarks Irenaeus.[94] No, there is nothing against faith with knowledge and knowledge with faith; Paul often speaks of the knowledge of faith, and the Gospel of John largely identifies believing and knowing. **Faith** can be the presupposition of knowledge and **knowledge** the presupposition of faith. But according to the New Testament, knowledge may never reach out above faith and dialectically sublate faith into knowledge, the attempt that Hegel was later to make in his philosphy of religion.[95]

In these circumstances, the existence of the Gnostics within the communities of the mainstream church proved increasingly difficult. No wonder that these people who understood themselves as the 'elect', 'children of light', the 'spiritual', the 'free', indeed as God's 'unchangeable family', as 'seeds' from the world of light and therefore the 'family of Seth', also formed their own **communities**. We can only guess what these might have been like, made up of an educated elite (the 'knowers' and leaders) on the one hand and a relatively uneducated community on the other: they were evidently more 'cultic associations' with arcane discipline than hierarchically organized churches.

It is certain that **women**[96] could have functions among the Gnostics which were forbidden them in the official church: not only as prophetesses, teachers and missionaries, but also as liturgists in prayers, hymns and sermons, and also in baptism and the eucharist – to the degree that these rites were celebrated at all among the Gnostics, who were hostile to the cult in principle. At any rate baptism and the eucharist are attested in a Nag Hammadi fragment, as similarly are washings, anointings with oil, meals and rites for the dying. The notion that the redeemed are brothers and sisters may have served as the ethical basis of communal life: brotherhood and sisterhood in terms not of the shaping of worldly society, but of redemption from worldly existence.

However, a warning must be issued here against any **idealization of Gnosticism** – at the expense of the community church. Alongside the equal status for woman in practice and in the cult, in some texts there is also a marked devaluation of women, indeed a castigation of the feminine and a rejection of marriage. In view of the ideal of bisexuality which in part is attributed even to the supreme being, blame for the separation of the sexes is often foisted on the woman (Eve). Indeed, according to individual texts the woman has to be made man in order to be able to enter the 'pleroma'.

So – despite all the long overdue rehabilitation of Gnosticism by most recent scholarship – the question remains: was not young Christianity forced to **dissociate** itself from the Gnostic speculations, compositions and compilations? Or in the name of higher knowledge should it have admitted into the community every possible mythological or religious idea from the most varied spheres of religion and culture? Wouldn't the monotheistic legacy of Judaism have been changed into a syncretistic paganism by the Gnostic mixing and transformation? Wouldn't mainstream Christianity have split up into numerous Gnostic groups and small groups? This is not to dispute that every religion is also a syncretistic construction; there are no 'pure' religions as concrete instances, any more than there are 'pure' races. But there is an essential difference between a paradigm shift in which the substance of this religion is preserved inviolate and a growing together and fusing of religions in which not only the paradigm but the substance changes: this is **syncretism** in the real sense.

The **church fathers** – bishops, theologians and theologian-bishops – of the late second and third centuries gave the decisive answer to this challenge from a fundamentally 'parasitical' form of religion which was now endangering the existence of the church: in Greek, first Irenaeus of Lyons and then his 'disciple' Hippolytus of Rome (c.160/170-238), and in Latin first of all Tertullian of Carthage (c.160-220). For all their partisan approach and construction of a 'succession of heretics' we should not regard them as having been completely intolerant and simply accuse them of clericalism. In scholarship there is sometimes a tendency to go from one extreme to the other. Instead of following the church fathers' picture of the Gnostics uncritically, as once happened, we should not now condemn it in principle – again uncritically. Church teachers from Irenaeus to Clement and Origen, who still had personal experience of Gnosticism, often dealt with the legacy of ancient education and Gnostic theology in quite a sophisticated way, and extracted from the Gnostic world-view those notions which were usable in the light of the original Christian message. So the Gnostic doctrines provided quite positive stimuli for the development of the teaching of the church fathers. Thus for example Irenaeus already supplemented the Pauline Adam-Christ typology with an Eve-Mary typology, and we shall be hearing more in detail about Clement and Origen. On the whole, however, the church fathers spoke out against any undifferentiated mixing or crossing with any alien cult; they rightly argued for an independent theological, ethical and spiritual Christian profile.

Theologically and politically this meant that **Christianity was not to fit into the existing syncretistic system of state religion** with the help of Gnostic speculations. Christians maintained the Jewish legacy in two respects, and opposed any compromise between Christianity and any other religion or philosophy:

– In the face of the many gods Christians held fast to the **one God** who tolerates no other gods beside him, not even the emperor-god, or Isis (for women) or Mithras (for men). And the Christ Jesus who stood for the one God, and who was therefore praised in hymns, was in no way to be brought down to the level of the pagan pantheon or taken up into the heights of uncontrolled speculation and rampant fantasy.

– In view of the moral collapse in the later empire, particularly in the great cities, the **ethics**, the strict commandments of the God of Israel, were maintained and Christians never tired of hammering them home. In addition there was a call not primarily for philosophical 'knowledge' but for resolute devotion to those in need: feeding the poor, looking after the sick, burying the dead. The church did not know any magical passwords for entrance into the many levels of heaven. Because Gnosticism had turned away from the world and was orientated on the beyond, it was uninterested in society and had no desire to shape it; it was more intent on inner detachment from existing conditions of power than on reforming society. Both ascetic and libertine consequences were drawn in Gnosticism from its hostility to the world. In the community church people generally maintained a middle way between succumbing to the world and hostility to the world, between libertinism and asceticism. This was the only way in which Christianity could become a broad mass movement, whereas Gnosticism finally stagnated and perished, by the sixth century, at the latest.

However, in this development in the mainstream church we should not overlook the fact that the emphasis on monotheism and morality led to intellectualism and moralism, and both had their price: the specifically Christian was all too much repressed. And something else was lost with the rejection of Gnosticism, which was offered here as an authentic alternative: for example in respect of the origin of authority, equal rights for women, relations with other religions. Some things were suppressed all too quickly and took centuries to surface again. Some **Gnostic ideas continued to have an influence for a long time**, even in Christian dogmatics (say in the two-natures doctrine in christology), but especially through Manichaeism in Islam, and finally through the mediaeval Cathars in southern France and the Bogomils in Bulgaria. However, only one old Gnostic sect has managed to survive to the present day: the baptist sect of the Mandaeans (whom the Muslims call Sabians, Baptists) with about 15,000 adherents in the southern reaches of the Euphrates and the Tigris.

Was there an alternative to the exclusion of syncretistic Gnostics? Elaine Pagels strongly idealizes Gnosticism, by tendentious selection stylizing it as the prefiguration of an alternative, democratic-feminist-ecological Christianity. But even she has to concede: 'Had Christianity remained multiform, it might well have disappeared from history, along with dozens of rival religious cults of antiquity. I believe that we owe the survival of Christian tradition to the organizational and theological structure that the emerging church developed.'[97] But it is certain that first of all there was greater simplicity, and only with time a more structured order. The question is, what kind of organizational and theological structure do we have here?

Three regulators: rule of faith – canon – episcopate

How did early Christianity cope with the flood of Gnostic wisdom? At first, at any rate, not by force but by clear **criteria** (Greek *kanon* = measure, guideline, rule). These **regulators** were basically already in existence, and they are known to us. But in the second half of the second century they were formally set up as the **boundary line** of the 'Catholic Church', now also expressly called the 'great church', **against heresy,** and with reference to the apostles (who were now already highly idealized) they were termed 'apostolic'. Those who pointed the way for the great church of the third century were Irenaeus, Bishop of Lyons, who wrote in Greek, and Tertullian of Carthage, the orator, lawyer and creator of the language of the Latin church. The drawing of this boundary involved three parallel processes:

- The **confession of faith** – made by Christians on the occasion of their baptism – now became the **rule of faith** (*kanon pisteos, regula fidei*) = '**rule of truth**' (*kanon aletheias, regula veritatis*), which summed up the main events of salvation history: this was a first regulator.

The confession of Christ at baptism had become a tripartite confession of Father, Son and Spirit at a very early stage, particularly in Rome; it was increasingly developed and in the fourth/fifth century finally became a present-day 'apostolic confession of faith'.[98] The rule of faith increasingly also became the norm for the exposition of the Bible, although in turn it could only be grounded in and interpreted in the light of the Bible. From here developed the dogmas of the early church, above all around christology and the Trinity; other spheres were not 'de-fined', 'marked off', doctrinally.

- The **Old Testament** (the Hebrew Bible in the Greek translation, the Septuagint) was retained, but now a **canon of the New Testament** was laid down: a 'canonical', i.e. official, corpus of sacred scriptures set apart by the criterion of apostolic origin: this was a second regulator.

So the young Christian community did not allow the rejection of the Old Testament (= 'law' of the evil creator god) in favour of the New Testament (= 'gospel' of the good redeemer God). This had been proposed by a convinced admirer of Paul by the name of Marcion, from Asia Minor, who at the same time rejected any symbolic or allegorical explanation of the Hebrew Bible. Marcion, who wanted to limit the Christian canon to the Gospel of Luke and some letters of Paul, was excommunicated in Rome around 144 – with the consequence that at that time a powerful Marcionite anti-church came into being. But at a very early stage the three or four Gospels and the letters of Paul were read out in worship. The Gospels and letters stemming (really or supposedly!) from the apostles or disciples of the apostles were regarded as apostolic writings, as were the Acts of the Apostles and the Apocalypse of John.[99] But to the rule of faith and the biblical canon was added a third regulator: in cases of dispute, Irenaeus above all argued,[100] one went by the earliest churches in which the apostles had already been at work.

- The monarchical **episcopate**, for a long time already the focal point of the unity of the church, now became a **teaching office** which increasingly set itself apart even from fellow presbyters. It now became more and more important because it was responsible for administering the church's income and on the basis of an allegedly uninterrupted **chain of succession** from the apostles it was also entrusted with decisions on the correct apostolic teaching: this was a third regulator.

I have clearly indicated the historical problems of the development towards the monarchical episcopate. The three-level system of offices, which only developed over time, with now increasingly professional office-bearers, had eventually established itself everywhere. This now led to a system of provinces (a metropolitan constitution) which gave the bishops of the main cities of the imperial provinces a special dignity, and those of the three greatest cities of the empire (Rome, Alexandria and Antioch) the highest dignity. First of all extraordinary and then regular provincial synods were in fact synods dominated by the bishops. Lists of bishops were made to establish the most certain tradition – Rome as the imperial capital with the tombs of the two main apostles was particularly important here. 'Tradition', Greek **paradosis**, Latin **traditio**, now became an important word. With the charismatic teachers the prophets also vanished: the last flickers of prophecy in the earliest church, to which we shall return, emerged in so-called Montanism.

There is no question that this development inevitably led to a **tremendous increase of power for the bishop**. From being a servant of the community the bishop increasingly became the lord of the community with authority to bind and loose, and claimed to be the teacher, high priest and mystagogue who alone made the decisions. Now the opposition between 'clergy' and 'laity' which had already begun at an early stage became institutionally established; apart from assent to the election of the bishop, the laity lost almost all their original rights as a 'holy priesthood'.[101] But at first this was welcomed, as the bishop increasingly developed into a 'patron' or guardian in the social system of late antiquity. His support was increasingly sought by his clientele not only for heaven but also on earth; in the period after Constantine, moreover, one of the main occupations of bishops (which was often a burden to Augustine) was the writing of letters of commendation and petitions and presiding as arbiters.

Be this as it may, by means of the normative rule of faith, the biblical canon and the episcopal teaching office, at any time the mainstream Catholic Church, now firm and cohesive, could define where the true, apostolic doctrine was to be found. With the introduction of the **rule of**

faith, canon and episcopate, the **ecumenical paradigm of the undivided church** had gained its **three classic criteria**. The apocalyptic paradigm of Jewish Christianity was thus finally replaced. And these regulators were also maintained by the mediaeval Roman Catholic Church which was to develop later – though transformed in a papalistic direction. It was only at the Reformation that the third regulator (the episcopate) was put in question, after which the Enlightenment put in question the second (the canon) and finally also the first (the rule of faith). However, for most churches these regulators preserved and still retain great significance down to the present, though in many ways they have been revised.

Still, for our argument the question arises: what is the relationship of this church, secure within, to the outside world, to the problems of Hellenistic Roman society? For the pagans around them, how Christians lived was more important than what they believed. 'Christianity is also antiquity,' as Jacques Fontaine remarked, and is certainly bound up with the environment of late antiquity. But Christianity is not just antiquity but also an 'experience of novelty' (Karl Prümm) and manifested innovative power to change society.

4. Are Christians different?

Over specific social questions, the position of Christians varied quite considerably:

– Even if they rejected emperor worship, Christians were loyal to the **state**: in accordance with Jesus' slogan 'Render to Caesar what is Caesar's'[102] and the view of the apostle Paul that the state authorities had a divinely-willed function in fighting against evil, with the result that he called for obedience to state authority and the payment of taxes.[103]

– The institution of **slavery**, which had such deep social roots – the whole of Roman society was not structured so much by classes as by a system of patronage – was also not put in question by Christians (or by the slaves themselves) in the first centuries. Because differences of race, nation, gender and class were not to count before God, and all human beings had the same status before God, only a brotherly treatment of slaves was called for; slaves could even become priests and deacons (and the freeman Callistus even became a Roman bishop). However, the treatment of slaves as equals in the communities, which was largely the practice initially, could not be maintained in the long run.

– At first Christians had reservations about **military service**: the predominant view was that the soldier need not leave the army after conversion and baptism, but those who were already baptized should not embark on a career in the army. Clergy above all were to refrain from military service and other offensive professions. In general the professions rejected were those associated with idolatry, sexual permissiveness, superstition, astrology and magical practices, and above all those of gladiator, actor and artist.

– Christians were also strict about **morality in marriage**: they were known for their faithfulness in marriage, their rejection of divorce and above all of remarriage. But celibacy was voluntary, if only for ascetical reasons; initially there was no law of celibacy for bishops and priests.

The gentle revolution

There can be no doubt that through the communities Christianity displayed a **moral power** which changed society. **Peter Brown**, the Princeton patristic scholar who in his researches into 'private life' does not want to make any kind of distinction between 'private' and 'public' life, sees the social change beginning with Christianity primarily in a new ethical ideal: action not just in accordance with law, custom and class morality but from a personal centre which constantly needs to be examined anew. It comes from an unfalsified, undivided, **simple heart** – directed to Christ and one's fellow human beings. This was not, as in paganism, the morality of the pagan upper classes, who used to spend a large sum on 'their' city, in its and their honour, so to speak as a one-day firework celebration (*panem et circenses*). Rather, it was the everyday morality of all those with more means than others who dedicated themselves in continuing, regular solidarity to the suffering and poor: 'The eventual replacement of this model of urban society, which stresses the duty of prominent people to promote **their** city, with a model based on the implicit solidarity of the rich with the poor in misfortune: this remains one of the clearest examples of the change of the classical world into a post-classical, Christianized world.'[104]

So **Christians** – in this world, but not of it – could not by any means join in all aspects of ancient society: they maintained a profile of their own. And for a long time the **social cohesion** of Christians, who regarded themselves as 'brothers' and 'sisters' on the basis of their common faith in Christ, was still astonishing, and attractive to quite a few, for all the differences of race, class and education. For the Christian communities in many respects not only developed their own structures but also acted on stimuli deriving from Jesus: organized care for the poor, the sick, orphans, widows, travellers, prisoners, those in need and the old – made possible through unusually high voluntary gifts (usually presented at the eucharist) which were administered and distributed by the bishop.

The shared eucharistic celebration, which did not discriminate against anyone, strengthened community consciousness, as did the hospitality practised towards Christian strangers. Right living (ortho-praxy) was still always more important than right teaching (ortho-doxy) at this time, and was certainly one of the main causes of the unexpected success of Christianity. Despite all the verbal polemic, tolerance over questions of doctrine was still relatively great. Indeed Christianity slowly established itself in the Roman empire by a **gentle revolution**. Or, as the Oxford patristic scholar Henry Chadwick describes the '**paradox of the church**' at this time: 'it was a religious revolutionary movement, yet without a conscious political ideology; it aimed at the capture of society in throughout its strata, but at the same time was characterized by indifference to the possession of power in this world.'[105] Chadwick sees the humanizing influence of Christianity above all in the following points:
– Emphasis on the conscience and the value of the individual;
– A striving for a juster society with a higher degree of equality for human beings as children of God;
– The creation of welfare organizations for the needy, orphans, widows and others to a large degree declassed;
– belief in a divine plan in history and the possibility of real change in individuals and society.[106]
Let us look rather more closely.

What changed

However, much also changed in the institutional church in the first Christian centuries, producing features which today are often still felt to be 'original Christianity' but which in fact are of later and partially even of pagan origin:
– For **baptism**, which was still mostly adult baptism and not infant baptism, a lengthy period of preparation (catechumenate) began to be introduced, though because baptism was the occasion for the forgiveness of sins, this led to the postponement of baptism until as soon as possible before death. Baptism now had an increasingly rich ceremonial: exorcisms above all, and **anointing** with oil after baptism, which was later to develop into a separate sacrament of **confirmation**.
– The **ceremonial meal**, now celebrated in the morning and allowed only to the baptized (the arcane discipline, silence in the presence of those who were not baptized), was supplemented by a public **liturgy of the word** on the Jewish model (the reading of scripture, psalms, hymns, prayers and sermon). Whereas the worship of Christianity was not sacrificial, the celebration of the eucharist was now increasingly understood as a

sacrifice. Here not only the gifts brought and put on the altar (for the celebration itself and the poor) but also the pronouncing of the eucharistic prayer with the offering of the bread and wine or body and blood of Christ by the bishop or priest were understood as a sacrifice. The agapes (love meals) which were originally combined with the evening ceremonial meals disappeared in time or were abolished because of abuses.

– Whereas originally liturgical gatherings took place in **private houses,** already in the third century special **buildings for worship** (= churches) were in use. **Basilicas** – previously used for every possible public purpose – were to become the characteristic Christian sacral buildings. The eucharistic **table** increasingly became a **sacrificial altar** which was regarded as 'holy' even outside the ceremonial meal.

– There are already the beginnings of markedly symbolic early Christian **painting** and also sarcophagus decorations in the often subterranean ancient cemeteries ('catacombs'). This not only adopted Jewish or Graeco-Roman motifs but also developed its own Christian types: the *orantes* (praying figures), the fish, Jesus as the good shepherd (as an unbearded young man), various scenes from Old and New Testaments, but no depictions of the passion.

– There is already **veneration of martyrs and relics** in the second/third centuries: a cult of tombs, many chapels for martyrs, apostles, patriarchs, archangels and an increasingly crude belief in wonders (holy bones, amulets). Christian saints increasingly suppress pagan heroes and gods.

It follows from this that despite all the **detachment** of Christianity from the culture of Hellenism, the more time went on, the less Christianity could avoid a practical adaptation to existing conditions. This applied particularly to questions of church discipline. In earliest Christianity as a rule there was only **one chance for repentance**: before baptism, which forgave all sins. And from the beginning excommunication, exclusion from communion, was the punishment for serious moral crimes; at this time it was increasingly imposed for doctrinal deviations.

Now in the long run it was inevitable that a '**second repentance**' should be granted in the case of serious faults – existence as a penitent, first for life and then for a limited period. After a long, very strict period of penance involving exclusion from the eucharist, penitents were finally received back into full church communion: initially the three deadly sins of murder, adultery (fornication) and apostasy from the faith were not forgiven. But pastoral wisdom as represented in the third century above all by the church of Rome counselled first that those committing the sin of fornication and then – after the large number of lapsed in the persecution under the emperor Decius – apostates, too, should be taken back into full church communion. In North Africa, Bishop Cyprian at a synod of

Carthage in 251 established that the re-reception of the lapsed should be controlled solely by the bishop – in the face of martyrs and confessors who were all too ready to forgive, and a revolt of presbyters. This was beyond doubt a considerable increase in power for the bishop! Similarly, at the same time Cornelius, Bishop of Rome, opposed the rigorism of the highly intelligent, morally strict presbyter Novatian, leading to the foundation of a heretical church of the 'pure' (*katharoi*) scattered throughout the empire, which existed in the West until the fifth and in the East until the seventh century.

The losers in history: women

There is no doubt that the Gentile Christian church stood up to the first great external threat (persecutions) as it did to the first great internal crisis (Gnosticism). But since the fundamental work of **Walter Bauer** on orthodoxy and heresy in early Christianity[107] we know that the early Christian authors cannot so easily be divided into winners and losers, 'orthodox' and 'heretics' – if we adopt a strictly historical perspective. For today we know that the history of theology and the church, too, was predominantly written by the victors at the expense of the losers – along dogmatic or church-political lines. The losers in this kind of traditional church history are not just individual 'heretics' who have been rehabilitated by more recent historiography.[108] Whole areas of Christianity were the losers, like the Jewish Christians who, as we saw, for the most part were already being regarded as heretical in the second and third centuries. And the whole of the other half of Christianity, **women**, were losers, as we shall now see more closely.

Truly, for all too long traditional historiography has neglected the question of women as subjects of history – a key field for the kind of 'new history' which I mentioned at the beginning of Part C. However, while the **sources** for the situation of women in earliest Christianity were already **scanty** enough, the situation is almost hopeless when we come to the Christianity of the early church. Certainly there are numerous statements by numerous church fathers 'about' women, but there are very few testimonies from women themselves – all in all only four works certainly written by women, all extremely different.[109] Or there are scattered and fragmentary references in texts composed by men, most of which are about other questions.

It has constantly been pointed out how many statements there are, particularly in the Greek church fathers, about the **equal status of men and women before God**: both are created in the image of God; both have the same ethical and spiritual capacities and duties; women are the first witnesses to the resurrection of Jesus. But on the other hand it cannot be denied that at a very early stage in Christianity – and not just in monasticism, though it was especially encouraged there – there were **tendencies** hostile to the body which **devalued women**. Even a theologian as open to the world as Clement of Alexandria, who defended the equality of man and woman in the spirit of the Stoa, who had reservations about lifelong sexual continence, and who in no way wanted to regard celibacy as the higher ideal for Christians, argues for the subordination of the woman to the man. And with him there were countless bishops and theologians who constantly argued that women are inferior and should be excluded from church offices.

The history of the interpretation of the New Testament and the writings of the early church speak their own language here. And in the 'women's question' in particular it becomes clear how much the interpretation of the facts is dependent on the particular ideological interest of a time. For a long time it was taken for granted that the subordination of women desired by the church was legitimated by divine revelation and sacred tradition, and this is still the position of some clergy in Rome, England and elsewhere, for ever yesterday's men. Today in the Christian world the tendency is, rather, to emphasize the positive statements about women in the church fathers and credit Christianity with a special contribution to the emancipation of women. Who is right?

Here at a very early stage the historian **Klaus Thraede** surveyed the material concisely and drew attention to the decisive point: while the number of women in the communities in the second and third centuries seems to have been high, the church's equal treatment of women did not take account of this; rather, orthodox theologians attempted to stem the emancipation of women: 'Here, the more ascetical ideals became established in orthodox Christianity, the more it thought in a markedly old-fashioned way, which included a stereotyped criticism of cosmetics, hygiene and fashion . . . Contrary to a view widespread today, that Christianity furthered the emancipation of women, in its basic ethical attitude the mainstream church lagged far behind the real conditions of the period of the empire (in part even behind philosophical doctrines: the legacy of the pre-Christian moral preaching which was hostile to women predominates).'[110]

However, in order to have some understanding not only of the testimonies of the church fathers 'about' women, but of the world in which women of the time lived and the way in which they understood themselves, we need to read the whole of **'patristic' literature** in part 'against the grain' – a difficult business. For even if we limit ourselves to early church canons and church orders, ascetical treatises and hagiographical narrative writings, here too historical **detection requires laborious and detailed work to reconstruct how women really lived and how they understood themselves.** The Catholic theologian and historian **Anne Jensen** has done pioneer work here in the context of the Tübingen research project 'Women and Christianity', and I can now use her main findings as a basis.[111] She has rightly been concerned to overcome a traditional way of writing church history in which the 'view of the victors' dominates, in other words, which uncritically takes over the boundaries which later centuries drew between the mainstream church and the 'heretics'.[112]

A comparison of the four normative **histories** of the early church, by Eusebius, Socrates, Sozomen and Theodoret, which Anne Jensen has undertaken for the first time,[113] produces a clear result: in the account of the first three centuries by Eusebius, Bishop of Caesarea, around 325, we learn essentially more about the active participation of women in church life than in the three later authors, who report on the fourth and fifth centuries; in them we can note a clear tendency to **marginalize women and make them anonymous.** Strikingly, there are no reports in these church histories of autonomous women ascetics, whose great spiritual authority is described in other sources; by contrast, in Eusebius and the witnesses mentioned by him there are no deaconesses or their predecessors, no 'widows' recognized by the church in the service of the communities. But the fact that in later centuries one increasingly comes upon these ordained women office-holders in no way indicates a revaluation of active community work by women. Rather, a critical comparison with other sources shows that the establishment of the diaconate is to be seen as a tendency towards restrictive measures, even if it allows women some freedom of action in the church sphere. The same applies to the communities of 'virgins' which were formed by ascetics living a determinedly autonomous life, who increasingly came under episcopal supervision.

To be rediscovered: women martyrs, prophets, teachers

After this general panorama, which was produced from histories of the early church, Anne Jensen has also investigated individual groups of women who were particularly important in the early period of Christianity. The evaluation of reports of women martyrs[114] leads to the conclusion that while here, too, men predominate numerically, where women are mentioned they are depicted as their equals and put on the same level. Special attention should be paid to the martyr acts of the trial in Lyons in 177 in which the slave girl Blandina has the central role, and the trial in Carthage (203) of Perpetua and Felicitas, on which Perpetua herself made notes during her imprisonment – one of the few testimonies to come from a woman at this time. The theological analysis of these documents demonstrates that women confessors, who risked their life in bearing witness to Christ no less than male confessors, were recognized as witnesses empowered by the Spirit. Many members of the community acknowledge their right in times of persecution to receive lapsed Christians back into church communion. However, here we must be careful not to generalize: the egalitarian practice of individual groups of this 'confessing church' was only partially representative of the Christianity of the time.

In the early period of Christianity, **prophetesses** above all were regarded as witnesses empowered by the Spirit.[115] Here once again we encounter 'Montanism', which has already been mentioned, a prophetic movement in second-century Phrygia which is associated with the names of the prophetesses Prisca and Maximilla. Virtually no trend in early Christianity has been so vilified and contested by an uncritical reading of later polemical texts than this 'new prophecy' – the name chosen by this movement which developed into an independent church. However, thorough investigation of the early sources to discover the facts which underlie the polemic, and investigation of the few prophetic sayings which have been handed down, demonstrate that the modern designation 'Montanism' is wrong in two respects: first, because it puts Montanus, the 'advocate' of the prophetesses, who gave them organizational support, at its centre rather than the spiritual women leaders of this movement; and above all because it suggests a 'supreme head' for the movement which did not exist, since this movement in particular had a charismatic ethos with an egalitarian orientation. According to the extant sources, **Prisca** must have been the most significant personality of the 'new prophecy'. So here again we discover **traces of a real practice of putting men and women on the same level** in second-century communities. It is particularly striking here that the activity of women as such becomes the object of criticism only in later polemic.

How fruitful it is if we get beyond the 'perspective of the victors' in historiography is particularly evident from the investigation of those women who were active in public in the community as **teachers**.[116] These must be understood against the background of movements especially connected with Gnosticism. Then it is possible to rediscover and evaluate **Philoumene**, a woman theologian almost forgotten today, but a significant one. She was head of a school in Rome in the second century and was a rival to no less a figure than Marcion. Occupying a moderate position between Gnosticism and the mainstream church, this teacher and prophet argued for a radically spiritual understanding of resurrection (not bodily) but without falling victim to a christological docetism. The notion that creation was the work of a demiurge certainly puts the good creator God at a distance from evil in the world, but does not lead to a radical dualism in which the world and matter are rejected as evil. So Philoumene was an important pioneer of the new synthesis between Jewish-biblical and Hellenistic philosophical thought in late antiquity. But already in the fourth century, though far more in modern church history, the intiator of this school came under the shadow of her disciple Apelles, who preserved her preaching in writing and disseminated her teaching.

If we look at the results of research into women so far, the picture proves to be more complex than was perhaps expected. As with the work of Elisabeth Schüssler Fiorenza on the New Testament period, Anne Jensen's investigation also brings out contradictions:

• Women were more intensively involved in the dissemination of Christianity than the sources with their androcentric colouring at first give us to understand.

• At the same time, forces are at work everywhere which seek to prevent putting the sexes on an equal footing. Resistance to the consistent realization of an egalitarian ethos increases.

Alternative forms of life for women – and the shadow sides

Now Anne Jensen has been able to show that many measures which repressed the activity of women in the church at first had little success, since the Hellenistic Roman women who became Christians were not going to submit to discipline lightly. Though they had no access to political office, they were nevertheless 'e-mancipated' in the literal sense: they were no longer under the *manus* (= 'hand', in the sense of power and protection) of a spouse, but were free partners and economically independent to the degree that they had personal resources. So it was quite possible for women of the upper class to lead their own lives even within marriage. And this explains why there are no indications in the sources that women hoped for an improvement of their feminine condition by going over to Christianity.

Nevertheless, many women who were still single or had again become single decided against a traditional family life. So **widows** now play a significant role in the communities, as soon also do **virgins**, young women who a priori do not want to get married. Certainly a preference for continence was a universal phenomenon of the time, and thus specific neither to women nor to Christians. Yet these voluntarily celibate

Christian women created organizations within the churches which are unique in contemporary Hellenism on this scale. In Christianity, **alternative forms of life** were now possible for a large group of women, forms of life which were not defined by biological determination. This institutionalization guaranteed women both material provisions and a high degree of social recognition. Thus the association of women with a particular social role was broken through and transcended. Doubtless the Christian women themselves created the foundations for these new forms of female life, and even now the alternative to marriage provided by convents, communities and associations of very different kinds was chosen essentially more by women than men. This new understanding of femininity which freed itself from the exclusively biological determination of women was an **essential contribution to the history of emancipation.**

However, this relativizing of the old role of the sexes had problems of its own. For only through radical **renunciation of sex** was it possible for women to escape their biological determination. And the woman who was not a spouse and not a mother found social recognition in Christianity only if there was a **religious and ascetic foundation** to this renunciation of sex. Now at this point **conflicts** arose. Why? Evidently women who decided against the usual family life had different motives. For some, renunciation of sex at the same time meant a radical rejection of a worldly life, which was accepted and indeed finally praised on the church side. However, for others, sex was renounced simply to make it possible to take on other tasks free from biological constraints. But this was regarded by many as grasping at 'male' roles and the claim to leadership associated with them. While it could be tolerated in exceptional cases, as a mass phenomenon it was evidently thought increasingly more threatening on the church side. So there are ambivalent reactions:

– The **'positive' solution** was the theological construct of the **'sexless'** *parthenos* (the virgin woman or man), in other words the radical transcending of sex, which in theory was to lead to completely equal rights for women and men and in practice to an open brotherly and sisterly pattern of behaviour. For this model, a hierarchy of the sexes was inconceivable. So here the effort to overcome the sexual is not a priori to be identified with hostility to sex, though this could easily develop.

– The **'negative' solution** consisted in a specific form of contempt for women which was soon to become dominant in part of the ascetic movement. Anxiety about a drive which might possibly get out of control produces the hostile image of the seductress. This tendency begins increasingly to become established in the early church and leads to the principle of the separation of the sexes.

Thus a fatal interplay begins: in the imperial church hierarchical thought increasingly suppresses the original Christian efforts at egalitarianism and leads to asceticism; conversely, increasing sexual pessimism even outside the monastery has an effect on church and society. Even unmarried women who wanted to play an active part in church life were finally almost completely eliminated from the clerical state. In defining the relationship between the sexes, hierarchical thought finally proved victorious – and only in the free churches of modern times did the egalitarian ethos again gain ground within Christianity. So can we speak of an emancipation of women through Christianity in the time of the early church?

Were women emancipated by Christianity?

According to Anne Jensen, two current theses which fundamentally represent only apologetic feminist or conservative anti-feminist variants of the same false conclusion now prove to be wrong: 1. the heresies were better disposed towards women than the mainstream church; 2. because women were more prone to heretical trends, the church had to forbid women to teach. Rather, a precise investigation of the sources leads to the conclusion that even in the contested 'heretical' churches a consistent egalitarian ethos could not maintain itself for long. That means that in late antiquity the **demarcation line between hostility to women and openness towards them was identical neither with the frontiers of religion nor with the confessional frontiers.**

It is also important to note that in traditional Christian apologetic the charge of hostility to sexuality is readily blamed on the pagans, with reference to the biblical heritage. But that of course makes things too easy. For early Christianity did not just take over a tendency to shun the world from Hellenism. With its original expectation of an imminent end of the world and the judgment of the world, Christianity considerably accentuated any aversion to the world. This becomes particularly clear in the **ideal of continence**: whereas in late antiquity outside Christianity the decision for an ascetic life could ultimately remain a matter of individual preference, in the **teaching of the church, celibacy** in time took on a **pre-eminence** grounded in salvation history. This led directly to a devaluation of sexuality and indirectly to a devaluation of women, who, in so far as they did not live continent lives, were increasingly defined in a one-sided biological way as sexual beings.

Certainly there is no disputing the fact that the ideal of humanity in antiquity already emphasized that all human beings, men and women, slaves and masters, poor and rich, had the same dignity. So an alliance between the Christian and the ancient egalitarian ethos might have been expected. Why did historical developments turn out differently? Further factors must have been in play. For the expansion of Christianity **alone** cannot explain the increasing discrimination against the female sex in the history of Western Christianity.

So it seems more appropriate first of all to ask a neutral question: **what prevented a true emancipation of women in the early church?** Among the different factors involved here, three seem especially important, and unfortunately they now came increasingly to determine the Hellenistic paradigm of the early church.

– The establishment of **hierarchical structures**: as in the Roman empire, so too in the churches there was rivalry between an egalitarian ethos and political power-interests; the principle of equality primarily asserted itself only in the private sphere, whereas male domination became established especially in the sacramental sphere.

– **Hostility to sexuality**: this does not derive from Christianity, but is a general phenomenon in late antiquity; however, it became particularly developed in Christianity.

– **Devaluation of education**: education was a Hellenistic ideal which, though initially not neglected in Christianity, was later in part openly despised – especially for women. This made a major contribution towards perceiving women exclusively as 'body'.

Is tradition an argument today?

So how are we to evaluate this tradition of hostility to women, compared with the basic attitude of Jesus, the Jewish Christian communities in Palestine and also the Gentile Christian communities with a Pauline stamp? The evidence is clear: vertical hierarchies increasingly began to get in the way of the brotherliness and sisterliness which was the stamp of Jesus and the early Christians. Hostility to sex was taken over from ancient tradition and propagated at the expense of women, although nothing of the kind can be discerned in the preaching of Jesus, which at most shows a marked relativization of marriage and family in favour of the kingdom of God. Education as a positive value hardly appears in the preaching of Jesus: one can enter into the kingdom of God without being educated. But Paul is already an educated Jewish Christian, as are the (anonymous) authors of such highly theological and highly educated letters as the letters to the Ephesians and the Hebrews. But equally, those concerned to devalue education cannot appeal to Jesus either, not to mention Paul and other authors. In particular, any devaluation of education which results in a 'ban on teaching' for women or serves as an excuse to define women exclusively in terms of their sexual role is completely ruled out.

So what significance did Christianity have for the emancipation of women in the early church? The answer is that Christianity did not produce women's liberation, but it could have encouraged it and should have done more to do so than just through alternative forms of life. Instead of this, in the second and third centuries a shift took place towards increasing hostility to women in the church teaching and practice of the following centuries. Since in the society of late antiquity women had largely already achieved their emancipation, 'the abundant prohibitions against women participating in church office after the third century attest contrary practices which become all the clearer, the more they are repeated': 'So the political and dogmatic growth of orthodoxy goes hand in hand with the battle against the emancipation of women in both church and society.'[117]

Things need not have turned out like this, since both the heritage of ancient humanity and the message of the gospel could have pointed in another direction. But in respect of the present day it must be said that what may still have been 'understandable' for the Christianity of the Hellenistic paradigm of the early church becomes completely incomprehensible if open or latent discrimination against women in Christian churches is still grounded in and maintained with the support of 'church tradition'. So here too questions arise for the future.[118] These questions must be put above all to the Orthodox and Roman Catholic churches.

Questions for the Future

• By what right do the Orthodox and Roman Catholic Churches deny women equal treatment, including church office? Shouldn't the traditional structures of theological legitimation, like the view that a woman cannot be a 'symbol of Christ', be put in question in the light of the original ethos of Jesus and the early Christian community?[119] Since women exercised leading functions in the earliest church (Phoebe, Prisca), and the place of women in business, science, culture, state and society has now completely changed, can the admission of women to the priesthood be delayed any longer? Weren't Jesus and the early church ahead of their time in their evaluation of women, so that churches which maintain the prohibition of the ordination of women are lagging far behind the gospel and the practice of other churches?

- The Methodist Church was the first to consecrate a woman bishop in 1980; the Anglican Church in the USA followed in 1989 and the Evangelical Lutheran Church in Germany in 1992. What right do representatives of the Catholic and the Orthodox Churches have to threaten serious problems and difficulties for ecumenical 'dialogue'? May ecumenical 'dialogue' between the churches go on at the cost of the equality of women? Rather, should not churches which reject women bishops and priests self-critically examine their practice in the light of the gospel and the tradition of the early church?

- Isn't it time for the Orthodox and the Catholic Churches to concede that the Protestant and the Anglican Churches are nearer to the gospel than they are in the question of women's ministries? Isn't the appeal to conservative 'sister churches' an excuse for stopping the reforms in one's own church? Isn't it time, in the spirit of the gospel, to end the practice of discrediting, defaming and discriminating against women? Isn't it time to grant them, too, their due dignity and appropriate legal and social position in the church?

But there is one thing that women, too, should never forget. The male domination which imperceptibly became established in the church of the early church Hellenistic and then even more in the mediaeval Roman Catholic paradigms would hardly have been conceivable in this form without a prohibition which does not appear anywhere in the New Testament: the **prohibition against the marriage of the clergy** (the law of celibacy) – though in the Eastern churches this applies only to bishops; in the Roman Catholic Church it was also imposed on all priests and deacons. As Peter Brown rightly says: 'At this point Christianity chose the "great refusal". In the very centuries when the rabbinate was achieving its paramount position because it accepted marriage as a quasi-obligatory criterion of wisdom, the leaders of the Christian community orientated themselves in a diametrically opposed direction. Access to leading positions in the Christian community is identified with a quasi-obligatory celibacy. Seldom has a power structure been built up with such speed and such a sharp drawing of boundaries, on the basis of so intimate an act as sexual renunciation.'[120]

5. Paradigm shift in christology

According to Henry Chadwick, the Alexandrian philosopher Celsus in the third century was the first to recognize the strength of earliest Christianity: 'that this non-political, quietist, and pacifist community had it in its power to transform the social and political order of the empire'.[121] It took the most capable brain in the Christian church of the third century to provide a convincing answer to Celsus and his comprehensive philosophical and theological argument for traditional polytheistic religion. This was none other than the highly praised and highly controversial **Origen**[122] from Alexandria in Egypt, the city of learning. I have written a long chapter about Origen in my recent book *Great Christian Thinkers*, so here I can limit myself to giving some basic information.

Origen: the first model of a scientific theology

It is important here for us to see that Origen, the only real genius among the church fathers, a man with an insatiable thirst for knowledge, a wide-ranging education and tremendous creative power (the list of his writings made by Eusebius is said to have contained 2000 'books'), did theology with a great passion. He aimed at a definitive reconciliation between Christianity and the Greek world, or, better, at a **sublation of the Greek world into Christianity.** But this Christianizing of Hellenism inevitably resulted in a Hellenization of Christianity. So while Origen's theology does not represent a paradigm shift, it does represent the theological **completion of the Gentile Christian Hellenistic paradigm initiated by Paul.**

Completion here means that Origen, a deeply committed Christian who remained a Greek (as Porphyry, Plotinus' biographer, attests in admiration and bitterness), a pacifist who argued that Christians should not serve in the army and yet loyally supported state authority (except in matters of faith), created, indeed embodied, what in effect was the **first model of a scientific theology** – which had a tremendous effect on the whole of ancient Christianity. Both critical and constructive, this universal spirit, who found things of value everywhere, attempted to bring together all previous theological approaches and materials, including those of Gnosticism. Thus this pious thinker proved to be a cultural mediator *par excellence*, indeed to be the greatest scholar of Christian antiquity. According to the unanimous view of patristic scholars, he can be regarded as the inventor of theology as a science. So the French patrologist Charles Kannengiesser rightly says: 'Origen invented the appropriate **praxis** for this kind of theology, and the methodological **theory** which it needed. One wonders only if inventing a new paradigm need always entail as much innovation as Origen's creativity required.'[123]

Be this as it may, Origen, completely at home in the church community and yet at the same time in constant dialogue with the pagan and Jewish scholars of his time, was able to open up various new ways in comprehensible language: not only for Christian apologetics (in his work *Contra Celsum* he refuted the pagan philosphers sentence by sentence) and biblical exegesis (commentaries and homilies on every possible book of scripture) but also for the systematic and theological penetration of the biblical message. And we can be even more specific about what the completion of the Gentile Christian Hellenistic paradigm meant:

Origen opened up new ways in the **systematic presentation of Christianity.** Presumably as an answer to criticism which had been voiced, Origen, the greatest philologist of Christian antiquity, broke off work on his *Hexapla* (his text-critical Hebrew and Greek edition of the Bible in six columns) to sum up his theological views in a major systematic sketch. This is inspired in its idealism by Plato and in its evolutionary character by the Stoa. *On the Principles* (Greek *Peri archon*, Latin *De principiis*) is the name of this work, and it deals with the basic principles of being, knowledge and Christian doctrine. Because of some excessively bold theses (especially on the pre-existence of souls and the reconciliation of all things at the end) it made Origen a controversial theologian and led to accusations of heresy lasting long after his death and finally to his condemnation – with devastating consquences for his work, which has come down to us only in fragments (his *Peri archon* above all in Rufinus' Latin translation). Here Origen made a precise distinction between the *dogmata* of the church tradition which had to be maintained and the *problemata* which needed to be discussed. In answering these open questions he already claimed freedom of thought for theologians from the bishops, and put this into practice.[124]

Christianity as the most perfect of all religions

Origen attempted to combine Christian faith and Hellenistic education in such a way that **Christianity** appeared **as the most perfect of all religions.** He presented it in a first theological doctrinal system which sought to build on Holy Scripture, albeit measured by the tradition of the faith of the apostles and the church: less a first 'dogmatics' than a first account of Christian faith.[125] For this deeply reflective thinker, coherence in the discussions of different topics was a sign of truth. Moreover in the four parts ('books') of his work *On the Principles* Origen presents the whole of Christianity, in three great arguments: God and his unfoldings; the fall of the creaturely spirits; redemption and restoration (Part 4 deals with the allegorical understanding of scripture). From the central 'element and foundations' of Christianity Origen thus works out a 'coherent and organic whole',[126] a great synthesis. It corresponds throughout to Greek philosophical thinking, to the degree that here everything is presented in the Platonic Gnostic scheme of fall and ascent and the thoroughgoing division of eternal idea and temporal manifestation.

So – very much in line with his predecessor Clement of Alexandria – he can understand the history of humankind as a great **educational progress** continually leading upwards: as **God's pedagogy** (*paideia*) with human beings. That means that the image of God in human beings, obscured through guilt and sin, is restored through the providence and educational skill of God himself in Christ. Thus human beings are brought to perfection according to a quite definite plan of salvation. In Christ 'the union of the divine nature with the human took its beginning so that the human might itself become divine through close association with the divine'.[127] According to this '*oikonomia*' the **incarnation of God** is itself the **presupposition of the divinization of the human being**.

The **allegorical understanding** of scripture is the instrument for carrying through this systematic conception. As Greek philosophers before him explained the myths (especially the Homeric myths), and around the beginning of our era in Alexandria the Jew Philo explained the five Books of Moses, so now Origen explains the Old and New Testaments in essentials not historically but '**allegorically**', in other words symbolically, metaphorically, spiritually. He does not do this simply because the content of scripture, taken literally, is unworthy, immoral and contradictory, a fact which the Gnostics and Marcion already advanced at an early stage as criticism of the Hebrew Bible. Rather, he believes that only in this way is it possible to sound out the whole depth and mystery of the Bible as the inspired word of God, as the place of the presence of the Logos. For Origen, everything in Holy Scripture has a 'spiritual' sense, but by no means everything has a historical sense. Indeed, just as cosmos and human beings consist of body, soul and spirit, so too scripture has a **threefold sense**:[128]

– the somatic-literal-historical (the somatic can only see Christ as a human being);

– the psychic moral sense (the psychic sees Jesus only as the historical redeemer of his world age);

– the pneumatic-allegorical-theological (the pneumatic sees in Christ the eternal Logos who is already at the beginning with God).

If we attempt a historical evaluation of the work of Origen, this cultural mediator *par excellence*, we note how different everything is here from what we heard about Jewish Christianity – which was still very much alive at this time. Here we have a great new **Hellenistic** formulation of an 'entire constellation of beliefs, values, techniques' which is quite different from that of Jewish apocalyptic, what we would now say was the modern paradigm for this age of Hellenism: 'Exemplifying as an individual the unfettered access of Christian faith to the universal culture to which he belonged,' says Kannegiesser, 'Origen experienced, with the unique capacities of his genius, what was to become a paradigm for the whole church of the future generation: **the acceptance of modernity in Christian theology.**'[129]

The characteristics of the new constellation – biblical canon, church tradition of faith, episcopate, and in addition Middle and Neo-Platonic philosophical thought – all this also forms the hermeneutical framework for Origen's allegorical interpretation of scripture, which superelevates the biblical words and without doubt often reinterprets them. But his spiritual pneumatic interpretation of scripture in the long run largely became established in the theology of both East and West – even in the face of the more soberly literal and historical interpretation of the Antiochene school, which went back to Lucian of Samosata. And in place of that model of apocalyptic expectation of an imminent end taken over from Judaism, now for the first time the Hellenistic conception (already prepared for in Luke-Acts) of Jesus Christ as the middle of time was complete. The incarnation of God in Christ was the hinge of world history, understood as a drama of God and the world. Yet all in all this was:

A problematical shifting of the centre

For there is no overlooking the fact that Origen's thought represents a **shifting of the focal point** of Christian thought under the influence of a Hellenism with a Neo-Platonic stamp. It had been in the making for a long time, but now it was abundantly clear. Even if we do not want to go as far as Adolf von Harnack, who sought to see the 'establishment of the Logos christology in the **faith** of the church – as a fundamental article' – as 'the transformation of faith into a **doctrine** of faith with a Greek philosophical stamp',[130] we cannot avoid putting some critical questions to Origen:

– What, for Origen, is the basic problem with which human beings find themselves confronted? It is the radical dualism of the spiritual and the material cosmos, of God and humankind, which neither the Old nor the New Testament knows.

– And what therefore is the central saving event of this salvation history for Origen's systematic thought? The overcoming of this infinite difference between God and man, spirit and matter, Logos and flesh, through the God-man Christ in a way which is alien to the New Testament.

And the price? The centre of Christian theology is now no longer, as in Paul, Mark and the New Testament generally, the cross and resurrection of Jesus. Now largely speculative questions stand in the centre: how the

Shifts of Accent
in the Proclamation of Christ

three hypostases in the one Godhead are related; how the incarnation of the divine Logos and thus the bridging of the Platonic gulf between the true, ideal, heavenly world and the untrue, material, earthly world is to be envisaged; how Jesus can be described as the 'God-man' (*theanthropos*), son of the virgin and 'mother of God' (*theotokos*), who as a human being had to be able to eat and drink, but as God could suffer no need or feel no sexual drive. How difficult and distorted the picture of Christ had become – measured by the original message!

There is no mistaking the fact that already among the early Greek fathers the main theological interest shifted from the concrete salvation history of the people of Israel and the rabbi from Nazareth to the great soteriological system, and here from Good Friday – though of course that never failed to be mentioned – (and Easter) to Christmas (Epiphany), indeed the pre-existence of the Son of God (his divine life before all time) and thus the three 'hypostases' (in the West called 'persons') in the Godhead.

Questions for the Future

About Judaism: do Christian theologians do justice to the Hebrew Bible when they heighten the divine inspiration of the Bible and regard it as a book of deep Christian mysteries which they attempt to unveil with the help of the allegorical, symbolic method, so that they even think that they can discover a Trinity of Father, Son and Spirit in the 'Old Testament'?

About Christianity itself: don't Christian theology, literature and piety distort the original message of Jesus and the New Testament proclamation of Jesus as the Christ of God who was crucified, raised and is present in the Spirit, when they shift the main interest from the cross and resurrection to the birth and 'appearance', indeed to the pre-existence, of the Son of God and his divine life before all time? Doesn't that make the gospel, the 'word of the cross', a priori a triumphalistic doctrine, a 'theology of glory'?

About Islam: is it in keeping with the Hebrew Bible and the New Testament for the salvation history narrated in the books of the Bible increasingly to be forced into a more and more complicated dogmatic system, which already split the church in the century after Origen and became entangled in more and more tortuous disputes, so that Islam with its simple message of the one God, the prophet and Messiah Jesus and the 'seal' of the prophets, Muhammad – close to Jewish Christianity – could have such a decisive success?

Origen was firmly convinced that throughout his theology – in exegesis, apologetics and systematic theology – he had simply deciphered and decoded his dearly beloved Holy Scripture. But he was not aware how far he himself remained imprisoned in a quite specific philosophical world-view. And down to the present day the all too natural conviction has remained in Eastern Orthodoxy that the orthodox teaching of the church fathers is simply identical with the message of the New Testament, and that the Eastern churches thus stand in unbroken continuity with the earliest church – as though no paradigm shift at all had taken place!

Now if we look more closely at the development of Hellenistic christology in particular and the formation of a speculative doctrine of the Trinity, of the kind that is beginning to emerge in Origen, the need inevitably arises to make a more detailed investigation into whether it was really only the biblical message that was being interpreted for the centre of Christian faith in this Hellenistic paradigm or whether the message of the New Testament had not been swamped by Hellenistic conceptualities and ideas. But we should not forget the difficult situation of young Christianity at that time.

The empire-wide persecutions

When Origen – after arrest, torture and release from prison in the midst of a new persecution of Christians – died, Christianity, which hitherto had spread above all in the Eastern part of the empire and even in Rome was so far Greek-speaking – was still the religion of a relatively small minority. What had spread most widely in the third century was the cult of Mithras, deriving from the Indo-Iranian sphere, a sun cult which was compatible with the emperor cult but not with Hellenism. Christianity was quite different. Since Origen, hadn't it had at its disposal the power and intellectual methods of Hellenistic philosophy? Hadn't it also adopted many stimuli from syncretistic Hellenistic piety – for example in its understanding of baptism (now increasingly disseminated as infant baptism) and the eucharist (understood as a sacrifice)? Hadn't it at the same time increasingly developed a strict discipline and compact organization borrowed from the empire?

For many people the question now arose: wasn't Christianity, as the religion increasingly penetrating the empire, perhaps the religion of the future? There is no doubt that with his combination of faith and science, theology and philosophy, Origen had achieved a **theological shift** which made a **cultural** shift (the combination of Christianity and culture) possible and in turn prepared for a **political** shift (the combination of church and state). It is amazing that this was to come about only fifty years after Origen's death – despite all the reactions of the pagan state which now became increasingly vigorous.

The persecutions of the emperors Decius (249-251) and Valerian (253-260), who recognized the danger for the pagan state and attempted to exterminate Christianity with empire-wide measures, were the first persecutions of Christians which were not only sporadic and regional but universal and brought Christianity a whole decade of terror. In particular Valerian's edict of 258 intensified former edicts for all provinces of the empire: the summary death penalty for bishops, presbyters and deacons; the death penalty also for Christian senators and *equites* if loss of rank and confiscation of goods did not make them see the light; confiscation of possessions and possible exile for prominent women; confiscation of possessions and forced labour on imperial estates for high imperial officials; confiscation of all church buildings and cemeteries. There were numerous victims of the bloody slaughter in those years, including figures like Bishop Cyprian of Carthage, the great defender of episcopal rights against the Bishop of Rome, who was claiming more and more power.

But despite all the compulsory measures, the persecutions were a fiasco. Moreover in 260/1 Valerian's son Gallienus found himself compelled to withdraw the anti-Christian decrees. There followed a period of peace for around forty years, so that Christianity, which in fact was tolerated, if not legally, at least *de facto*, could spread increasingly also in Mesopotamia, Persia and Armenia, in North Africa and Gaul, and even in Germany and Britain. And increasingly it also found acceptance among the educated and well-to-do (even in the imperial court and in the army) as a more philosophical and spiritual form of worship of God without bloody sacrifices, statues of gods, incense and temples.

This time of relative peace was one of the presuppositions for the heyday of church theology which was to come, and without it a wide discussion and a structured theology could hardly have developed. At the centre of christology, in particular, it was to bring the momentous paradigm shift to an end.

The shift towards Hellenistic metaphysics

Let us remind ourselves: from the beginning the Christian communities believed:
– that the man Jesus, who was crucified, had been raised by God to new life and appointed Messiah, and ruled as exalted Lord over the earth;
– that God, the God of Abraham, Isaac and Jacob, was also that God whom Jesus called his Father;
– that the power of the Spirit, which had become powerful in and through

Jesus, was God's Spirit, which not only permeated all creation but also gave power and comfort to all those who believed in Jesus as the Christ.

So we spoke of three essential structural elements and permanent guidelines of Christian faith which had already been expressed in the New Testament in creeds with one (in Jesus Christ), two (in God and Jesus Christ) or three (in God, Jesus Christ, and the Spirit) members.[131] But nowhere does the significance of the **paradigm shift also for the centre of Christian faith** become clearer than in this belief given from the beginning in – as the triadic baptismal formula of the Matthaean community tradition puts it – 'Father, Son and Spirit'. This centre in particular was already seen in the Gentile church of the first centuries, in an epoch-making, different constellation. And only if we understand this paradigm shift in christology can we understand,

– why belief in the Messiah not only among Christians and Jews but also among Gentile and Jewish Christians drifted so far apart;

– why belief in Christ led to divisions in the church even within the Hellenistic Gentile Christian churches of the East, and

– why finally already in the first millennium a deep gulf developed between the Eastern and Western churches, which then led to a definitive schism in the second millennium.

So the development was that after the fall of Jerusalem, that christology of Jewish Christianity which mostly knew no pre-existence of the Son of God was increasingly brushed aside, while conversely the prologue of the Gospel of John with its statement about the pre-existence of the Word proved a powerful force which literally made history: the history of dogma. The **paradigm shift** becomes unmistakable the moment when already in the second century Justin and the early Christian apologists connected the Johannnine concept of the Logos, which had a Jewish Hellenistic stamp, with the Greek metaphysics of the Logos, and at the same time sought to emphasize belief in one God and the universal significance of Jesus Christ. Why? Because the starting point of Christianity had been shifted: from the earthly and exalted Christ to the pre-existent Christ. The great historian of dogma, Frierich Loofs, rightly makes a critical comment on this process: 'The Apologists, taking for granted the transference of the concept of Son to the **pre-existent** Christ, made possible the rise of the christological problem of the fourth century; they shifted the starting point of christological thought (from the historical Christ to his pre-existence) and put Jesus' incarnate life in the shade; they combined christology with cosmology, but they were unable to link it with soteriology.'[132]

Precisely what characterizes this paradigm shift in christology which comes about with the apologists and reaches its first climax with Origen?

The historians of dogma have emphasized features which dogmatic theologians in general have not taken very seriously. Here are three of them:

– Instead of an apocalyptic temporal scheme of salvation directed forwards (earthly life – the suffering, death and resurrection of Jesus – return), theologians now think principally from above downwards in a **cosmic-spatial** scheme: pre-existence – descent – ascent of the Son of God and Redeemer.

– Instead of being explained in concrete biblical language (logia of Jesus, narratives, hymns, baptismal confessions) the relationship of Jesus to God is now explained in the **essential-ontological concepts** of contemporary Hellenistic metaphysics. Greek terms like *hypostasis, ousia, physis, prosopon* or Latin terms like *substantia, essentia, persona* dominate the discussion.

– Instead of continuing reflection on God's dynamic activity of revelation through his Son in the Spirit in the history of this world, the focal point of reflection is shifted to a more static **consideration of God in himself in his eternity and his innermost, 'immanent' nature** and thus to the problem of the pre-existence of three divine figures. The decisive theological problem is no longer, as in the New Testament, 'What is the relationship of Jesus the Messiah to God?', but increasingly, 'What is the relationship of Father, Son and Spirit to one another already before all time?'

Here is just one example of the shift in perspective: the difference between the old (probably already pre-Pauline) confession of faith from the introduction to the Letter to the Romans and the famous christological formula of Ignatius of Antioch, about two generations later. Both speak of Christ as **Son of God**, but in clearly different ways:

The **Pauline** confession, like the well-known passage from Peter's speech in Acts,[133] briefly gives a sketch of the story of Jesus, beginning from below with the man Jesus from the tribe of David, who since the resurrection has been appointed Son of God: 'The gospel concerning his Son, who was descended from David according to the flesh and designated Son of God in power according to the Spirit of holiness by his resurrection from the dead, Jesus Christ our Lord.'[134]

– By contrast, **Ignatius** already says quite naturally that Jesus Christ 'was from eternity with the Father and will appear at the end of time'.[135] Indeed he unhesitatingly brings God and Jesus together and speaks of Jesus as a 'God come in the flesh', which then leads to paradoxical formulations like this: 'There is one physician, who is both flesh and spirit, born and yet not born, who is God in man, true life in death, both of Mary and of God, first passible and then impassible, Jesus Christ our Lord.'[136]

We cannot overlook the fact that in the subsequent period the **exaltation christology** with an original Jewish Christian stamp, beginning from below and centred in the death and resurrection (exaltation of the human Messiah to be Son of God, two-stage christology), was in fact increasingly **suppressed**. It was suppressed **by an incarnation christology beginning above** (Logos christology), which ontologically intensified the lines of the Gospel of John or the individual statements about pre-existence and mediation at creation in the hymns in Colossians and Hebrews: the pre-existence and incarnation of the Son of God whose emptying and humiliation are the presupposition for his later exaltation to God. We can also say that in Old Testament terms, for the 'ascending' christology, divine Sonship means an election and assumption as Son (in exaltation, baptism, birth). It is now supplemented or even replaced by a **'descending'** christology. For this christology, divine Sonship means an **essential begetting** of a higher kind – always to be described more precisely in Hellenistic terms and notions. Indeed, think of all that has been read into the New Testament and legitimated as 'apostolic'!

In fact, in the future the concern is less with Jesus Christ's position of power as judge, understood along the lines of the Hebrew Bible, than with his descent understood in Hellenistic terms. The concern in future is less with the function of the redeemer and more with his being. Terms like being, nature, substance, hypostasis, person, union take on increasing significance. But how is the relationship between Father and Son (and finally also Spirit) to be described on these new presuppositions? What increasingly emerged as the central theological problem as a result of this was that on the one hand Christians called Christ God and prayed to him, but on the other, on the basis of the Jewish tradition, they unconditionally wanted to maintain the unity and uniqueness (*monarchia*) of God. The only solution seemed to lie in the sharp subordination of the Logos (Son) to God and the Spirit to the Logos, though both were to participate in the divine *substantia*. But could all this be? A long dispute now began.

The battle over orthodoxy

Had people kept to the New Testament, they would have spared themselves the notorious difficulties which now arose over the relationship of the three persons 'in' God, all the speculations over the numbers one and three. But something like a **speculation with the number three** was in the air at the time. The Greek word *trias* already appears in the apologist Theophilus of Antioch in the second century (but for God, the Logos and Wisdom[137]); the Latin *trinitas* first appears in the African Tertullian in the third century. The formula of three *personae* in one *substantia* also occurs in him for the first time,[138] but this had hardly any influence on Greek theology, which was intellectually in the ascendant. In many religions and philosophical systems of the time there was a fascination with the number three, so that the notion of a Trinity within the Godhead also emerged for the Christian theology of the time:

– because of the attraction already exercised by the prime number three in the numerical symbolism of the Pythagoreans (a multiplicity in a closed and ordered unity);

– because of the significance (evidently almost magical) of this 'most holy number' in myth, art, music, literature and also in everyday life ('three times');

– because of the threefold deities not only in ancient Babylonia and Egypt, in India and China, but above all in the Hellenistic sphere: in Delphi, in the cult of Dionysius, in the religion of Asclepius, in the emperor cult;

– because of the metaphysical triads in Gnosticism (Father-Mother-Son; God-Counsel-Reason) or in Neo-Platonism (the One-the Spirit-the World Soul).

This last was particularly important; contemporary philosophy with its Neo-Platonic stamp regarded three hypostases in God as necessary, and here again **Origen** was particularly important for the development of a doctrine of the Trinity – now a 'scientific' one. He laid the foundation for the intellectually demanding trinitarian speculation which in time led to an increasingly complex conceptual apparatus. For it was Origen who took over the Middle-Platonic/Neo-Platonic doctrine of the **hypostasis** (Latin *substantia*)[139] in order to give an intellectual definition of the relationship between Father, Son and Spirit. He boldly interpreted the three 'entities' as three hypostases, that is, as three essentially independent beings, though at different levels from one another, indeed clearly subordinated to one another.

– Only the Father is 'God in the strict sense' (written with the article, *ho theos*) or, as Origen says, *autotheos*, God himself.

– The Son (like the Logos in the Johannine prologue) is only *theos* ('God', written without the article), who is not God the Father but participates in God. The Son is not created, far less merely adopted, but is begotten by God, as the splendour of light is constantly begotten from the light itself.[140]

– In this understanding of Father and Son (and Spirit), God's eternal being, resting in itself, stands in the foreground, and Jesus' humanity and history are largely left out of account. The concern is with the mystery of God in itself and not primarily with God's activity in the world, God's revelation for us.

Something that originally stood on the periphery of faith and knowledge now came into the centre and thus became exposed to controversy. Now Christianity was increasingly driven into a **crisis of orthodoxy** on the basis of different philosophical speculative systems, and this was to have devastating consequences. For it was by no means the case that Origen at that time dominated the theological scene alone. However, the second half of the third century after Origen, in particular, is extraordinarily sparsely attested in the sources, and is quite a dark period for historians. This is not only because we often have only very fragmentary evidence and do not know how far communities (larger of smaller) stand behind particular names, but because,

1. Many independent theologians (like Paul of Samosata) were condemned as heretics although, as their rehabilitation by twentieth-century historians attests, they were quite orthodox in their way;

2. Most of the books of the 'heretics' (including some by Origen after his condemnation) were destroyed, so that we are dependent on often tendentious and selective quotations by their opponents;

3. The Hellenistic terms of that time were ambiguous and were often used in contradictory ways: for example *hypostasis* (in any case identical with the Latin *substantia* only in etymology) could be used for God alone (i.e only one divine hypostasis); for God, Father and Son (two hypostases); or even also for the Holy Spirit (three divine hypostases).

Indeed, who can count the names which were entangled in the battles over the correct 'right faith', 'orthodoxy' – this unbiblical word increasingly entered church terminology at the end of the third century. There is little point in enumerating all the persons and schools, defining their positions and sketching out their developments. One can read long chapters about this in any history of dogma.[141] However, it should not be forgotten that in the third century there was still stubborn opposition to all Hellenistic Logos-hypostasis doctrines – above all in the name of the Jewish heritage. Here the concern was for belief in one God, which even Greek theologians resolutely defended in the name of the **monarchia**, the 'sole rule' or 'oneness' of God. So there is often talk of 'monarchianism', though this is confusing, because monarchianism has two completely opposed variants, both of which also caused considerable turbulence in church politics in Rome, and remained virulent at a popular level even longer:

– **Adoptionist christology** (that of Theodorus of Byzantium and, in the view of his opponents, later also Paul of Samosata, Bishop of Antioch), which regarded Jesus as an ordinary human being, though distinguished by a unique fear of God, who had been 'adopted' as Son of God at his baptism (or earlier: Paul combines with this doctrine the doctrine of an impersonal divine Logos coming from outside, which provoked special criticism).

– **Modalistic christology** (that of Noetus and Sabellius), for which Christ and the Father are identical: they are just different modes, energies, names, faces, roles, manifestations of the one God. Now if Christ was understood as the mode of appearance (even mask) of the Father, already at that time the critical objection had to be made that here the Father himself had become flesh and suffered (patripassianism); this completely contradicted the Gospels, according to which Jesus prayed to the Father and commended his Spirit into the Father's hands when dying.

However, most of the theologians from the second half of the this century whom we know by name maintain the line of Origen's Logos theology and doctrine of three hypostases, understood in sub-ordinationist terms: the Logos is subordinate to and put after the Father. Both the unbiblical modalist ('Sabellian') christology and the adoptionist christology, which was better grounded in scripture, though incompatible with the rule of faith, were condemned as heretical.

6. The shift under Constantine and the christological dispute

Every persecution which had aimed at exterminating Christianity – including the last great persecution under the emperor Diocletian at the beginning of the fourth century – had failed; so all that was left for the Roman state was the course of toleration and recognition. The Gentile Christian Hellenistic paradigm of the early church, which had been constructed theologically, ecclesiastically and culturally over so many long decades, now also succeeded in making a political breakthrough within a few years. The combination of faith and science, theology and philosophy, church and culture, was now followed quite consistently with the combination of Christianity and empire.

From persecution to toleration: Constantine

Toleration and recognition were prepared for by an edict of the emperor Galerius before his death in 311; it was implemented by the new Augustus who went by the name of **Constantine**. Though not himself a Christian but a hard man of power, Constantine attributed his victory over the Roman usurper Maxentius at the Milvian Bridge near Rome, not without the superstition characteristic of late antiquity, to the God of the Christians and the sign of the cross. The next year, 313, he promulgated a constitution in Milan – together with Licinius, co-regent in the East – which now granted **unlimited freedom of religion** to the whole empire. Here Constantine was neither a pious Christian nor a hypocrite. Rather, he was a statesman who coolly took Christianity into the calculations of his power politics, which, as we saw, were not free from superstition. From then on he always took around with him in his camp a precious standard with the Christ monogram (and there was a replica of it in every division of the army). He soon favoured Christianity in a variety of ways. Thus in 315 crucifixion (so hated by Christians) was abolished, in 321 Sunday was introduced as a legal festival and the churches were allowed to receive legacies; in 324 he won a victory over his fellow-emperor Licinius, who was more inclined towards paganism. Constantine was already sole ruler in 325. And in practical terms this meant that with him Christianity could develop throughout the empire, although as a skilful politician Constantine always tolerated the other cults.

So the **universal empire** very soon again had a **universal religion**, one which offered charitable help to many in distress and a hope of immortality to every individual. In any case it would be wrong to attribute the **'victory' of Christianity** only to its comprehensive charitable church organizations with their solid local roots or solely to its adaptation to the society of late antiquity. There was no mistaking the fact that Christian monotheism commended itself as a more progressive, enlightened position than polytheism, which was rich in myths, and that the lofty ethos of Christians, ascetics and martyrs to the death, proved superior to that of paganism. Here were clear answers to problems like those of guilt and death. Here the Christian religion, quite unlike paganism, appeared grounded in a holy book, the Bible, which as a book of deep mysteries sketched out the history of salvation from the beginning of creation to the end of time with more moral earnestness than the divine myths. The new religion seemed to have a magnificent centre in the idea of the incarnation of the Son of God in this corrupt world. And in practice it was guaranteed not only by preaching and catechesis, but by holy mysteries like baptism and eucharist, which promised liberation from the tremendous anxieties about demons and eternal salvation.

The relief and joy at the revolution in world history was tremendous in a Christianity which shortly beforehand had been persecuted and oppressed (events comparable with those in Eastern Europe in 1989). But unfortunately, at the same time (and here again we may compare events after 1989), when the longed-for freedom of religion had finally been granted, the religious tensions within Christianity which had been present for so long clearly came to light, tensions which above all derived from Hellenistic christology and not least from Origen's doctrine of three hypostases.

The **great crisis** broke out soon after the shift, when a pious Alexandrian presbyter and popular preacher with great self-confidence, **Arius** (Greek *Areios*), opposed his bishop Alexander, a prominent pupil of Origen's, by whom he had been accused of innovation. The dogmatic issue here was the question of Christ and the nature of his pre-existence as the presupposition for a particular understanding of redemption. Here we must go more precisely into this momentous controversy.

Christ – God or demigod?

Arius' basic concern was the one God who, for him, steeped as he was in the spirit of Middle Platonism, dwelt in absolute transcendence: un-created and unbegotten, eternal, without a beginning and unchange-able.[142] Here Arius, too, in good Origenist fashion, assumed three hypostases in God which were subordinate to one another. But on the basis of his strict monotheistic presuppositions, for him only the first hypostasis, God himself, was uncreated; the second, the **Son**, was **created**, though Arius made the correction that he was not simply created in time but 'before all time'. So using a very formal argument, he attacked the doctrine, put forward by Origen and Bishop Alexander, of the 'contem-poraneity' of the pre-existent Logos with the Father.[143] What caused most offence was his much-quoted statement (though we have no direct evidence of the original) 'There was once (a time), when he (the Son) was not.'[144] For Arius, the Son is certainly there 'before all time' (and here he differs fundamentally from all other creatures created 'in time'), but he is not uncreated, he is not eternal, since he has been created by the eternal God as God's foremost and most important creature.

Thus for Arius, while the Son is the great divine intermediate being and instrument for the creation of the world, precisely in this capacity he is essentially different from the Father: he is **not of one substance with the Father** (*homoousios*, 'consubstantial'[145]); rather, he is different in being from the Father. In this way Arius wanted to provide a vigorous defence of monotheism. As transcendent, untouchable, unbegotten substance without a beginning, eternal and not subject to change, his God could not have a Son in the real sense. The Son could be called 'God' only by analogy, thanks to the grace of the Father who gives him only part of his Godhead, as he does to all creatures. That explains why according to Arius the 'Father' is ultimately unknowable by this Son, so that the Son does not know the Father at the deepest level. The Logos is not God (*ho* *theos*) in the strict sense, but the first creature, though as such he is creator of the world.[146] That also explains why the Son is changeable, why he can 'become', and why incarnation and humiliation in the flesh are to be attributed only to him. In the human being, for Arius this Logos even takes the place of the human soul and unites itself directly with the flesh (*sarx*): here we have an explicit Logos-sarx christology. Thus the incarnate Logos is the redeemer and the exalted model for all human beings.

It would certainly be wrong to blame Arius – he has been called the most cursed heretic of the century – for all the subsequent confusions. Here something had broken through in the Hellenistic paradigm which had already been a basic problem for a long time: the more Jesus as the Son was put on the same **level of being** as the Father – in contrast to the Jewish Christian paradigm – and the more theologians described this relationship with **natural categories**, the more difficulties they had in envisaging monotheism and Christ's divine Sonship together convincingly.

Arius' main opponent was the deacon **Athanasius**,[147] Bishop Alexander's right-hand man, who was soon himself to become Bishop of Alexandria: he was a theologian with a strong faith and a pastoral disposition and a militant church politician. He was concerned with more than just philosophical theology; he was concerned with piety, church practice, monasticism, asceticism, redemption. Indeed, he too was concerned with the unity of God, but even more with **redemption through God** and therefore with the **unity of Father and Son**. He was convinced that anyone who like Arius added a second hypostasis or substance to God to be worshipped as divine – to some degree as *deuteros theos*, a second God – was bringing back Hellenistic polytheism through the back door. For what else was that created intermediate being between God and the world for the purpose of creating the world if not a mythological being as useless as it was senseless? And shouldn't God really be Father from eternity? Was he only to become Father through the creation of the Son? For Athanasius, that was no longer the Christian God!

Indeed, how was the redemption of human beings for divine life and the certainty of salvation in Jesus to be guaranteed if Jesus was only a creature and not the **God-man**? The Son cannot be redeemer if he is not one with God and God has not entered our humanity. And the notion of redemption understood in physically real terms – that man is divinized by God himself, adopted as son and made incorruptible – was quite decisive for Athanasius, as we can see from his famous dictum (which takes up a saying of Irenaeus): 'He (God) became man that we might become God' (Greek *theopoiethomen*).[148] By the incarnation of God and the divinization of human beings, for Athanasius Christianity differed both from Judaism and from paganism. By concentrating on incarnation and divinization he provided the strongest motivation for monasticism, which had meanwhile been growing stronger and stronger in Egypt. It is clear that Athanasius had formulated a clear counter-position to Arius, and the dispute called for a decision.

The establishment of orthodoxy: the councils of the early church

Not only theologians and bishops passionately took part in this controversy, but also every level of the population; Christians, Jews and Gentiles; the educated and the uneducated. The **Emperor Constantine** himself found the church dispute which had seized the whole of the East highly inopportune; indeed in the last resort it threatened to split spiritually the empire which he had again united politically. After vain attempts at mediation in Alexandria, having experienced a synod of bishops in Arles at close quarters a few years before, in 325 he gathered the bishops of the empire – who, having been persecuted not long before, could now use the imperial post! – to an imperial synod: an '**ecumenical council**' for which he put his splendid palace hall **in Nicaea** near the imperial residence of Nicomedia at their disposal.[149] In addition to the Bishop of Rome's adviser Bishop Ossius of Cordoba, only two Roman presbyters were present from the West as his representatives, along with a representative of the Bishop of Carthage; one bishop each represented Calabria, Gaul and Pannonia.

So right from the beginning it was clear **who had the say at the ecumenical council** – at this one and then at the next. It was not, say, the Bishop of Rome, as later ideologues of an absolutist papacy might like to have it, but simply and solely **the emperor**: he not only convened the ecumenical council but directed it through a bishop whom he had commissioned, with the assistance of imperial commissioners; he adjourned it and concluded it; by his decision the resolutions of the council became imperial laws. Constantine used this first council not least to **adapt the church organization to the state organization**. The church provinces were to correspond to the imperial provinces, each with a metropolitan and a provincial synod (especially for the election of bishops). A patriarchal constitution was already taking shape from the first council on, by the elevation of the patriarchates of Rome, Alexandria, Antioch and, with the same honorific status, Jerusalem (now no longer Jewish Christian but Hellenistic). In other words, the empire now had its **imperial church**!

It was now clear to Constantine the political strategist that the imperial church needed more than just the more or less varied confessions of faith of the individual local or provincial churches. It needed a uniform **'ecumenical creed'**, and this was to be the **church law and imperial law** for all the churches. He believed that only in this way could he ensure the unity of the empire under the slogan 'one God – one emperor – one kingdom – one church – one faith'. The imperial court theologian and church historian Eusebius presented a draft. But the council itself wanted to insist more clearly than he did on the ontological equality of God the Father and Jesus Christ, following the line of Athanasius (and some Westerners). It was not permissible either to degrade Christ to a pure creature or to have a concept of God which was not specifically Christian (God for ever Father of this Son). This meant that God is not the dark incomprehensible primal ground of the Neo-Platonists; God has not just revealed part of himself but has revealed himself without restraint in Christ. Christ knows the Father wholly, so in him the eternal living God and Father, inoriginate and uncreated, is present in him with no reduction. Christ is certainly not a second God or demigod alongside the true God, but the true God is himself present through him: '**God from God, Light from Light, Very God from Very God, begotten, not created,** being of one substance (Greek *ousia*) with the Father.'[150] Only because in Christ is there the God who is really God, is the redemption of human beings, their share in the Godhead and their eternal life, a reality through Christ. To make that clear, various statements by Arius were explicitly condemned and Arius himself was excommunicated.

The unity of Christ with God was to be emphasized by the inserted word **homo-ousios** = '**of the same being**' or 'of the same substance' (with the Father), which replaced any subordination along the lines of Origen and earlier theologians by giving the Son equal rank with the Father and strict unity with him: the Son has one and the same being in common with the Father (the council did not reflect on the Holy Spirit, which was soon to provoke great discussions). Beyond question *homoousios* is an unbiblical word which had been condemned by an earlier important synod and finally, for theological or political grounds, was imposed on the council by the emperor in person, who otherwise avoided a one-sidedly partisan position (perhaps he took this action at the suggestion of the Westerner Ossius). It was a scientific term with materialistic overtones (*ousia* = 'substance', 'matter') which could be quite incomprehensible and misleading. Athanasius himself (who was Bishop of Alexandria from 328) relativized the word after the council and hardly used it for many years: later he also accepted the counter-term *homoiousios* = 'of similar being', provided that there was the addition *kata panta* = 'in all things'. His concern was not this word as the shibboleth of orthodoxy but the matter of redemption. However, for us the question of the consequences of the council now arises.

The Hellenization of christology

Had the council solved the problem? If the quest was only for a formula, then certainly. But a solution of the substantive theological question and church unity? The confusion continued, as is evident from Athanasius' changing fortunes. At all events we must not overlook the fact that the **Hellenization of the Christian message** (which already begins in the New Testament) reached a first climax, which was also an official one, at the Council of Nicaea, as Adolf von Harnack has clearly emphasized. And the attempts by Catholic historians of dogma (like Alois Grillmeier) to make a *de facto* distinction between two kinds of Hellenization, good and orthodox and bad and heretical, are not convincing. According to such a scheme the Council of Nicaea in fact de-Hellenized, because it did not engage in Neoplatonic speculations about the deity and its emanations, about these descending developments of the divine, and thus opposed the Hellenistic Neo-Platonic thought of Arius with its hypostases. In that case only Arius and the heretics would have 'Hellenized', for opposite reasons. No, such an apologetic scheme is far too clearly dogmatic to correspond to historical reality.

If we take the New Testament as a criterion, we cannot deny that the Council of Nicaea certainly maintained the New Testament message and did not Hellenize it totally. But it is equally beyond dispute that the council remained utterly imprisoned in Hellenistic concepts, notions and thought-models which would have been completely alien to the Jew Jesus of Nazareth and the earliest community. Here in particular the shift from the Jewish Christian apocalyptic paradigm to the early church Hellenistic paradigm had a massive effect.

There is a tremendous difference between an eschatological '**throne community**' of God with his Christ after the latter's earthly life through resurrection and exaltation, as proclaimed in the New Testament, and a '**community of being**' between God the Father and God the Son that is to be thought of in protological, pre-temporal terms, i.e. that has always existed from eternity and is understood ontologically. In this perspective even the Johannine concept of the Logos, the Word of God, seemed dangerous to some council fathers – because it could be misused by Arians. So the word 'Logos', which was very much less open to misunderstanding, was deleted from the creed presented to the council by Bishop Eusebius of Caesarea (who was in any case suspected of Arianism) and replaced by 'Son of God'. But this confirmed that the more the Son was put on the same level of being with the Father and this relationship was described with natural categories, the more difficult it became to think of Jesus' distinction from God and his unity with God conceptually at the same time. In that case, all that was left was an appeal to a conceptual mystery which had neither been preached by Jesus nor witnessed to by the apostles, but which the theologians themselves had produced by transposing the biblical statements to another level.

So once again, had the council solved the problems? At least it has looked like that after the event. But in fact the consequence was first of all a tremendous confusion of different groups and trends and fifty years of dispute – carried on not only with theological but also with political means. Constantine himself, until his death in 337 (perhaps he had received baptism shortly beforehand), pursued a 'peace policy' which was tolerant of the Gentiles and integrated the orthodox and the Arians in the church. However, his sons, who divided the empire, and above all Constantius (who was master of the East), pursued a fanatical and intolerant policy against the pagans: the threat of the death penalty for superstition and sacrifices, the cessation of sacrifices and the closing of temples – for the Christian mob a call to storm the temples (the attempt to restore paganism by Julian, the 'Apostate', 361-3, with the help of a Neoplatonic state church on the Christian model, remained an episode). Within the church the sons of Constantine for the most part supported the Arian position; in the meantime this had attracted majority support in the Eastern episcopate, which called the tune. This dispute now extended to the question of the consubstantiality of the Holy Spirit, which was energetically disputed by numerous bishops, known as 'fighters against the Spirit' (Pneumatomachoi).

State religion and state power against heretics and Jews

The definitive church-political settlement in the Arian dispute took place under Emperor **Theodosius the Great** (379-395), who was a Westerner and a convinced Nicene. However, his religious edict *Cunctos populos* ('All peoples') was not concerned generally with legislative measures against Jews and pagans, but with the Arians. Only towards the end of his reign in 392 did he decree 'the general prohibition, never to be revoked, of all pagan cults and sacrificial rites, threatening those who acted to the contrary with punishment for *laesae maiestatis*'.[151] Thus in fact he made Christianity a **state religion**, the Catholic church a **state church** and heresy a **state crime**.

How short even the memory of the church can be! It took less than a century for the **persecuted church** to become a **persecuting church**. The enemy of the church was now also the enemy of the empire, and was punished accordingly. In 385 the Spanish ascetic and enthusiastic lay preacher Priscillian, with six companions, was executed in Trier for heresy – a bad sign for the Christian centuries to come. For the first time Christians killed other Christians over a difference in faith. Despite objections from different sides people soon got used to this. Leo the Great already expressed his satisfaction with the procedure.

Indeed, the church began to go along with all the compulsory state measures against Arians and Gentiles, and even to intensify them with new attacks on temples. Bishops, too (prominent ones like John Chrysostom), were active in this. The **Christianization of public life** was carried forward consistently: now the Roman senate solemnly abjured the old faith (even if individual members of senatorial families were long to remain pagans), removed the altar of *Victoria adveniens* from the hall in which it met and abolished all privileges for pagan priests and Vestal Virgins. The Olympic Games were banned, and Gratian, co-emperor with Theodosius for the latter's first years, declined the title of the Roman high priest, Pontifex Maximus, so that from the fifth century on it could be claimed by the Bishop of Rome without much opposition.

Now Christianity penetrated not only political institutions and religious convictions, but also philosophical thought and artistic culture. This was an **inculturation** of a depth and breadth that Christianity hardly achieved again in later paradigms. Paganism increasingly disappeared from the public life of the cities and could sustain itself only among individual learned philosophers in the great cities and in the country, among the village-dwellers (*pagani*).

However, the establishment of the Christian church as an imperial church was a particularly hard blow to **Judaism**, which had survived the catastrophes of the years 70 and 135 (the destruction of the temple and the city of Jerusalem) and existed dispersed over the Roman empire. It was now no longer remembered that the Christian church had once lived by the power of its roots, as Paul said: perceptibly and imperceptibly a specifically **Christian ecclesiastical anti-Judaism** began to develop from the anti-Judaism which already existed in the pagan state.[152] This too – regrettably – was also a hallmark of the early church Hellenistic paradigm. And it would be no service to inter-religious understanding for us to suppress the fact.

Some **church fathers** had learned Hebrew and biblical exegesis from Jewish teachers, and the first Christian theologian to work in a scientific way, the brilliant **Origen**, lived among Jews as head of the Catechetical School of Alexandria, maintained friendly relations with them and defended them against pagans, even if he vigorously censures them in his homilies for their rejection of the Messiah Jesus. So how did it come about that the hostility between Jews and Christians now became increasingly shrill, and as early as the second century an *Adversus Judaeos* literature (Barnabas, Melito of Sardes, Tertullian, Hippolytus), explicitly hostile to Jews, developed?[153]

Libraries have been written about this, and in the volume on Judaism I discussed at length the origins of the completely separate lives of Jews and Christians.[154] Here, without comment, I shall mention just a few important **factors** (which in practice often overlapped) that were responsible for **specifically ecclesistical anti-Judaism**:

1. Growing alienation of the church from its Old Testament roots as a result of the Hellenization and doctrinalization of the Christian message.

2. Increasingly more exclusive claims to the Hebrew Bible (albeit only in the form of the Greek Septuagint) by a church which no longer valued it in itself but used it almost exclusively to legitimate its own existence with the help of typological and allegorical interpretation.

3. The breaking off of the reciprocal dialogues between church and synagogue and mutual isolation, in which dialogue was usually replaced by apologetic monologue.

4. Blaming Jews for the crucifixion of Jesus, which was now generally attributed to 'the Jews', indeed to all Jews. The expulsion and dispersion of the Jews was now regarded as God's just curse on a condemned people.

Already in the second half of the second century we find in Bishop **Melito** of Sardes in Asia Minor a pernicious remark (governed by an un-Jewish anti-Jewish christology) which was to prove particularly disastrous historically: 'Hear, all you families of mankind and see the strange murder that has been committed in the midst of Jerusalem . . . God has been murdered, the King of Israel has been slain by an Israelitish hand.'[155] The charge that the Jews were 'God's murderers' was thus born. Here already the intent was no longer the conversion of Jews but a fight against them.

However, the shift under Constantine in 312/313 had not made the status of Judaism any worse. Certainly Constantine was extremely unfriendly (perhaps under the influence of his Christian advisers?) in his choice of vocabulary about the Jews (particularly when he was addressing the church). Yet it would be a mistake, as G.Stemberger points out against sweeping verdicts which speak of the end of tolerance of the Jews, 'to describe Constantine as an outspoken opponent of the Jews', especially as 'the laws which Constantine decreed did not really make the situation of the Jews worse, and in some respects rather strengthened their privileges under the law'.[156]

The real shift in imperial policy towards the Jews came almost exactly a century after the death of Constantine. Theodosius the Great had already forbidden conversion to pagan cults. Now under the emperor **Theodosius II** (401-450), direct action was also taken against Judaism. By **exceptional laws of the state church** (the Codex Theodosianus of 438) it was excluded from the sacral realm, to which access could be had only through the church sacraments. And as after the formation of an **imperial church** the Jews now consistently rejected the imperial ideology with its Christian colouring (the Christian emperor as the image of the heavenly ruler!), the specifically pagan anti-Judaism was formally adopted by the imperial church and powerfully reinforced by Christian motifs.

Now the church no longer remembered that it had once been persecuted. On the contrary, with the help of the state this same Christian church which not too long beforehand had been a persecuted minority with no rights, with the help of the state reduced Judaism (in the Roman empire so far still a *religio licita*, a permitted religion) to an entity with lesser rights. Granted, Judaism was not to be exterminated, like the heresies, but it was to be segregated from the spheres of Christian life and isolated socially. The **first repressive measures** were implemented for this purpose: prohibition of mixed marriages with proselytes (converts to Judaism); Jews barred from holding official positions; a ban on building or extending synagogues: prohibition of any proselytizing. It was this ban on recruitment which compelled Judaism, formerly a successful missionary religion on the offensive, to concentrate fatefully on itself and reproduce itself, so that it was later possible to speak of it as a separate 'Jewish race'. To this degree, in this period rabbinic efforts at segregation (for halakhic reasons) and the Christian practice of discrimination (for political and theological reasons) conditioned one another, and towards the end of the Roman empire led to a complete isolation of the Jews.

Thus the Jews now lived in the imperial sphere, in practice outside the empire; this made many of them feel their situation more than before to be that of a 'gola', a real exile, and again led them to hope that the Messiah would soon come to redeem them. And while theologians and bishops like Augustine still felt that they had a missionary task towards the Jews (contrary to the current thesis that the Jews were God's murderers, **Augustine** believed that despite their guilt the Jews had a hope of conversion), others, like **Ambrose**, prevented the rebuilding of synagogues, and indeed bishops like **Chrysostom** already preached against the Jews in the style of the later anti-Jewish firebrands:[157] the synagogue – a place of hostility to the Law, a quarter of the evil one, a bulwark of the devil; the Jews – gluttons who delighted in feasting and greedy rich people who, unfit to work, were suitable only for slaughter (!). But despite all counter-measures Judaism remained present as a living religion throughout the empire. Indeed, at the time of Chrysostom there were still Christians (*Ioudaizantes* = Judaizing Christians or Jewish Christians?) who went to the synagogue on sabbaths and feast days and also took delight in Jewish ceremonies.

The coronation of the state religion: the dogmas of the Trinity and of Christ

Fixed to its creed of Nicaea, the Christian church now had to advance the formation of its doctrine. This was required simply by imperial policy, for in the religious edict *Cunctos populos* of 380 the orthodox Spaniard Theodosius the Great invited 'all peoples' of his kingdom to accept belief in the one Godhead of the Father, the Son and the Holy Spirit in equal majesty and holy Trinity, as presented in the churches of Rome and Alexandria. And precisely this faith was now also to be established definitively at a further council, to end the Arian dispute, against those who saw the Holy Spirit as only a 'servant' or a 'creature'.

As early as 381 the emperor convened an Eastern council in the capital, which was then later called the **Second Ecumenical Council of Constantinople.**[158] This council condemned Arians, semi-Arians (Pneumatomachoi), Apollinarians and other heresies and spoke of the **identity of being of the Holy Spirit with God** (without using the word *homoousios*). Belief 'in the Holy Spirit, the Lord and Giver of life, who proceeds from the Father and with the Father and the Son is worshipped and glorified' was inserted into the Creed.[159] Presumably this expansion was taken over from a *Symbolum Romano-Nicaenum*, composed by a Roman synod.[160] At any rate, this creed, which is still used in the liturgy today, was only later called the 'Niceno-Constantinopolitan Creed'. And what about Arianism? It lived on for centuries, above all because the West Goths, accepted into the empire a year after the council and converted by Ulfilas, were and remained Arians and handed on their Arian faith to the other Germanic tribes.

We should note that whereas the Council of Nicaea in 325 spoke of a single substance or hypostasis in God, the starting point in the 381 Council of Constantinople was three hypostases: Father, Son and Spirit. There has been much discussion in the history of dogma as to whether the transition from a one-hypostasis theology to a three-hypostasis theology is only a terminological change or – more probably (as the temporary schism in Antioch between old and new orthodox shows) – also involved an actual change in the conceptual model. At all events it is certain that we can speak of a **dogma of the Trinity** only after the Second Ecumenical Council in Constantinople.

The Creed of the Councils

We believe in **one God**,
the Father, the Almighty,
maker of heaven and earth,
of all that is, seen and unseen.

We believe in one Lord, **Jesus Christ**,
the only Son of God,
eternally begotten of the Father,
God from God, Light from Light,
true God from true God,
begotten, not made,
of one Being with the Father.
Through him all things were made.
For us men and for our salvation
he came down from heaven;
by the power of the Holy Spirit
he became incarnate from the Virgin Mary,
and was made man.
For our sake he was crucified under Pontius Pilate,
he suffered death and was buried.
On the third day he rose again
in accordance with the scriptures;
he ascended into heaven
and is seated at the right hand of the Father.
He will come again in glory to judge the living and the dead,
and his kingdom will have no end.

We believe in the **Holy Spirit**,
the Lord, the giver of life,
who proceeds from the Father and the Son.
With the Father and the Son he is worshipped and glorified.
He has spoken through the prophets.
And the one holy catholic and apostolic church.*
We acknowledge one baptism for the forgiveness of sins.
We look for the resurrection of the dead,
and the life of the world to come. Amen.

* Some Protestant churches use the formula 'Christian church'
or 'universal Christian church' here.

The Niceno-Constantinopolitan Creed

At the Council itself there were also marked tensions between the Egyptians (allied with Rome) and the Christians from Asia Minor, rooted in the Origenistic tradition, who were now intellectually in the lead. The classical doctrine of the Trinity was developed in the second half of the fourth century by three famous theologians and bishops from Cappadocia in Asia Minor: Basil the Great, after the death of Athanasius in 373 the most prominent churchman in the East; his friend Gregory of Nazianzus; and Gregory's younger brother, Gregory of Nyssa. These **three Cappadocians** were able to combine Athanasius' faith with Origen's theory. On the basis of their new interpretation of Nicaea they were called 'Neo-Orthodox'. Following an extremely complex and often contradictory process of christological thought after Nicaea, which in any case was a tedious one, they were finally able to establish a new linguistic rule: God – **one divine being** (one substance, *ousia*, *physis*), but **in three hypostases** (three persons, subsistences, *prosopa*).

The foundations for this formula, which has become classic, had already been laid by Origen and in Latin by Tertullian with 'one substance, three persons' (but only in the event of revelation and strictly subordinated to one another); so it also met with the approval of the Latins. But whereas for the **Latins** the substantial unity was the clear starting point and the multiplicity was the mystery, conversely for the **Orientals** the Trinity of divine hypostases was the assured starting point and the unity the mystery. Like Origen, the three Cappadocians a priori included the **Holy Spirit** in the Godhead by combining the confession of the *homoousios* with the statement of three hypostases which were not subordinate to one another (as in Origen), but completely of the same order in the one *ousia*, in the one being of God. However, each of the hypostases preserved its peculiarity, its own mode of existence, its characteristic: the Father was 'not begotten', the Son was 'begotten', and the Holy Spirit 'proceeded' (no more specific word was found). From now on we can speak quite formally of the **triune God** in Christianity. Here the principle of unity, the *arche*, was again more clearly than in Nicaea the monarchy of the Father. From this alone the Spirit, too, proceeded as from the heart of the deity.

But the theological conflicts were by no means ended with the decisions of Nicaea and Constantinople; they continued. And now the direct concern had to be the person of Jesus Christ. For the great Cappadocian 'solution', set down in the Niceno-Constantinopolitan creed, had basically already pre-programmed a new church dispute. Its consequence was to be a whole series of further councils, and it was finally to split the Eastern church definitively. What was the problem? It had really already been posed by the formula of Nicaea: if the Son is of one being with the

Father, what is the relationship **between the divine and the human being in the one Jesus Christ**? Here of course there were very different models. A well-known contemporary and teacher of the three great Cappadocians, the anti-Arian Apollinaris of Laodicea, had asserted that while in Christ the divine Logos took human 'flesh' and a human psyche, he did not assume a human 'spirit'. The divine Logos simply replaced the human spirit. This view was very attractive to many religious people of the time: Jesus was fully God in human garb. But in the view of most theologians, for the Logos to take the place of the human spirit was to deny the full humanity, the whole human nature, of Christ. So this doctrine was condemned at several synods in both East and West. But the problem raised by Apollinaris persisted: how was it possible for there to be a 'two = one' in Christ? Was this a further 'mystery' like the 'three = one' in the Trinity?

At the beginning of the fifth century the christological question got caught up in the vigorous power struggles between the patriarchates of Constantinople and Alexandria over the ecclesiastical primacy in the East and the rivalry between the schools of Antioch and Alexandria which lay behind this. The dispute once again took on dramatic dimensions, and its confusions and complexities need not be described in detail here. It is enough to mark the basic fronts which emerged in 428 as a result of the polemic of Nestorius, Patriarch of Constantinople, against Cyril, Patriarch of Alexandria:

– The Alexandrian patriarch Cyril and the **Alexandrian school** in fact defended a complete **unity** and divinity of the person of Christ: the Logos had assumed the human nature like a garment, indeed the human nature was submerged in the divine, so that only a 'single nature' (hence 'monophysitism'), the divine-human, remained. So Mary was called *theo-tokos*, the 'Mother of God'. This seemed to be the more 'pious' solution and the one that was nearer to popular opinion.

– Nestorius, the Patriarch of Constantinople, and the **Antiochene school** did not want any substantial unity but unconditionally held firm to a **distinction** between the divine and human natures in Jesus Christ; this seemed to them to be the only way of guaranteeing the complete humanity of Christ. It seemed to be 'scientifically' the clearer solution. Moreover, by using the name 'Mother of God' (instead of 'Mother of Christ') for Mary one laid oneself open to ridicule in preaching.

However, Cyril was an unscrupulous power politician who had no inhibitions about forcing through his position at a new council, even manipulating it to achieve his aim. In 433 at the Council of Ephesus,[161] which was completely under his influence, he had his rival from Constantinople condemned, and with him Antiochene theology, without even waiting for Nestorius to arrive. Moreover the council, wholly following the line of Cyril's Monophysite christology, rejected the title 'Mother of Christ' for Mary and instead of this defined Mary as '**Mother of God**', which is still the dogma of the church today. Nestorius and his followers – understandably – retorted with a counter-condemnation (and deposition) of Cyril; once again Christianity was threatened with a deep split, so that Emperor Theodosius II had to force both sides to a union at a further Council of Ephesus (433). However, this could not settle the dispute. There was another council in Ephesus in 449, where Dioscurus, Cyril's no less power-hungry successor, terrorized the council fathers with his gangs of monks and deposed the most significant Antiochene theologians (which is why Pope Leo called this not a *concilium* but a *latrocinium* = Robber Synod).

However, a political revolution in Constantinople was soon to alter the situation. The Empress Pulcheria and her husband Marcian ascended the throne and were resolved to reimpose the traditional imperial rule over the church in the face of the church's claims to power. With the agreement of Pope Leo I, they resolved on the downfall of the Alexandrian Dioscurus, who was behaving in all too 'papal' a fashion, and summoned a new council for 451, at **Chalcedon**.[162] This council recognized only the councils of 325 (Nicaea), 381 (Constantinople) and 431 (Ephesus) as ecumenical and no others, and is therefore counted as the **Fourth Ecumenical Council**. Dioscurus was deposed in a shameful trial. This opened up the way for the emperor to dictate to the council the christological statements which he found illuminating, from a letter of Pope Leo. In this way neither Cyril's nor Nestorius' position came to the fore, but largely the Western, Latin christology of Tertullian, Novatian and Augustine. It is to them that Christianity is essentially indebted for the christological formula of the Council of Chalcedon which later became classic: 'one and the same' Lord Jesus Christ is 'perfect in Godhead and perfect in manhood, truly God and truly man'. One and the same is 'consubstantial with the Father as to the Godhead and consubstantial with us as to the manhood'. Thus 'one and the same Christ . . . exists in two natures unconfusedly, unchangeably, indivisibly, inseparably'.[163] The famous four adverbs were directed against both the Alexandrian extremists (unconfusedly, unchangeably) and Nestorius (indivisibly, inseparably).

But the council's acceptance of these formulae governed by Latin christology did not prevent it, once again at the instigation of the emperor, from inflicting a notable defeat in the political sphere on the Bishop of Rome, who had already become all too powerful and who now had an endorsement of his theology. In fact canon 3 of the Second

Ecumenical Council of Constantinople had already laid the foundation stone for the power base of the Bishop of New Rome: 'The Bishop of Constantinople shall have the place of honour after the Bishop of Rome, because this city is the new Rome.'[164] So the famous canon 28 (though, as we shall see, it was never recognized by the old Rome) assigns to 'the holy church of Constantinople', **the younger Rome, the same primacy** as the old Rome – a primacy which for both sees is not based on Peter, but politically on the status of the imperial capital. Thus between 381 and 451 the **five classical patriarchates** developed, in the following sequence: Rome, new Rome (Constantinople), Alexandria, Antioch and – lastly – Jerusalem! This, too, is a clear indication of the paradigm shift which had taken place. Even now the Bishop of Constantinople (now Istanbul) is called the 'ecumenical patriarch'.

Questions in the interest of ecumenical understanding

However, it may be asked today, did the Council of Chalcedon **achieve its aim**? Adolf von Harnack described the Chalcedonian formula as a purely external compromise, working with negations: 'The four bald negative definitions (unconfusedly, etc.) with which all is meant to be said . . . lack any warm, concrete content; they make the bridge which is the believer's faith, the bridge from earth to heaven, a line which is slimmer than the hair on which the confessors of Islam one day hope to enter paradise.'[165] But did the Council of Chalcedon want, say, to replace the New Testament? No, for this council, too, the New Testament remained the basis. Conversely, however, we may have inhibitions about taking over the triumphalist Roman Catholic apologetics which regards the dogma of 451 'as the mature result and to some degree the conclusion of all the efforts which had been made in previous centuries to give right expression to the content of revelation about the person of Christ'.[166] Even a dogmatic theologian like Karl Rahner, whose thought deliberately remained within the system, was prompted by the 1500th anniversary of Chalcedon to raise the provocative question 'Chalcedon – End or Beginning?'[167]

In the meantime discussion of Rahner's compromise theology has been extended, and the results are no longer evaluated from a purely dogmatic perspective, but from perspectives which are far more comprehensive. Certainly the christological formula found at Chalcedon (*vere homo – vere deus*) gave a lasting dogmatic foundation to both the Byzantine and the Western church, which was also to be significant for the liturgy. As already in the doctrine of the Trinity, so now again in christology there was a formula which could be accepted only as a 'mystery' inaccessible to reason. But this formula by no means ended the struggles. On the contrary:

– The **christological disputes** over Chalcedon still **continued** for centuries in both the Byzantine and the Western spheres; for the dispute over one or two natures in Christ, combined with much politics and diplomacy, now turned into a dispute over one or two energies, and then over one or two wills in the one Christ (the monenergetic and monotheletic disputes). Increasing tensions and disputes between Byzantium and Rome were also mixed in with this. Indeed, an imperial 'Formula of Union' (*Henotikon*, 482) to which Acacius, Patriarch of Constantinople, contributed, and his recognition of the Monophysite Patriarch of Alexandria, led to the first formal schism between East and West Rome, which lasted for thirty-five years (the Acacian Schism, 484-519).

– The christological disputes were increasingly mixed up with aspects of church politics. For they expressed not only the antagonism between the Eastern and the Western church but also all nationalistic resentment, especially that of the Egyptians and Syrians towards the domination of Byzantium. In the end even the emperors could no longer compel unity. On the contrary, **the imperial church split up.**

Down to the present day, several old and important Christian churches have not recognized the Council of Chalcedon, which was governed all too much by Western theology. So these **non-Chalcedonian churches**[168] have split both from the Orthodox Byzantine church of the East and the Roman church of the West. They are:

1. The Monophysite Coptic Church in Egypt;

2. The Nestorian Syrian Church, which then spread above all in Persia, but also in India (the 'Thomas Christians') and in East Asia as far as Peking;

3. The Armenian and Georgian Churches, which later went over to Monophysitism.

Let us once again survey this whole development. Certainly the Christian churches had to come to decisions about their formulations of dogma. But at the same time can we overlook the cost of this process? Let us reflect:

– The theology which became manifest at the councils led to a considerable **alienation from the New Testament.** In four centuries the simple and easily understandable baptismal formula in Matthew had become a highly complex trinitarian speculation which could only 'solve' the problem how three 'entities' could be one in a logical formal way through verbal distinctions. In essence there can be no doubt that the **'triadic'** is **not the distinctive feature of Christianity.** The distinctive Christian feature is christological. It is not a doctrine of Christ to be speculated on, not a dogma of Christ which one 'must believe', but, as we saw in the basic reflections on the essence and centre of Christianity,[169] Jesus Christ whom one must follow, on the way to God his Father, moved by the Holy Spirit. Theologically, everything depends on the scriptural relationship between Son, Father and Spirit. The norm for the interpretation of the councils of Nicaea, Ephesus, Constantinople and Chalcedon, too, cannot be a Hellenistic ontology but only the New Testament. And the council fathers also wanted unconditionally to retain monotheism (but combining with it the divinity of Jesus); they would have turned in their graves if in the style of modern theologians their trinitarian theology had been assigned a middle position (which for them was already logically impossible) between monotheism and polytheism.

Theology similarly alienated itself from a **preaching which was near to the people**. The doctrine of the Trinity became a highly demanding intellectual exercise, a kind of higher 'trinitarian mathematics' in which even theologians and preachers take little interest, but which can still be presented to reasonable people simply as a 'true mystery' which they have to accept by sacrificing their understanding.[170] At least in the Latin liturgy, down to the present day prayers are never addressed to the 'Trinity', but to 'God the almighty Father', 'through Jesus Christ in the Holy Spirit'. Traditionalist Orthodox, Catholic and Protestant theologians immunize themselves against any reasonable questions about the dogma of the Trinity with the irrational verdict, 'That is rationalism.' However, Christians are increasingly asking whether such Greek speculation, which boldly attempted to spy out the dizzy heights of the mystery of God, is not perhaps like the attempt of Icarus, the son of Daedalus, ancestor of Athenian craftsmanship, who with his wings made of feathers and wax flew all too near to the sun – and fell.

– The conciliar decisions plunged Christianity into undreamed-of theological confusions with constant entanglements in church politics. They produced **splits** and sparked off a **persecution of heretics** unique in the history of religion. This is what Christianity became as it changed its nature from a persecuted minority to a majority persecuting others. In the name of Jesus Christ, the preacher of non-violence and peacableness, those of other faiths were persecuted and indeed executed; cultural objects beyond price (books!) and art treasures were not only destroyed and discriminated against but eradicated. And even today, Christianity itself is split into the different churches. This split began with the first councils, when the Arians were forced out of the church and eventually persecuted, and when even after the Council of Chalcedon a whole series of churches were excluded from the fellowship of the church.

If Jesus of Nazareth is still to remain the criterion, this development must lead the Christian churches to criticism, to conversion and to renewal. So questions arise for the future:

Questions for the Future

✝ The concepts, governed by philosophy, became more and more specific; the distinctions between the schools became more and more sophisticated; the explanations became more and more complex; the safeguards to orthodoxy through dogmas which became state laws became more and more numerous. But so too did the misunderstandings, the parties, indeed the splits, the synods directed against one another and the bishops who excommunicated one another. Would it not be appropriate in a new world era, instead of simply repeating the old Hellenistic dogmas, to concentrate again on the message of the New Testament and interpret it afresh for contemporary Christians, as the Hellenistic theologians once rightly did for their time?

✡ Hellenistic Christianity seems largely alienated from its Jewish roots – despite its retention of the 'Old Testament'. And even today Jews can only interpret the distinction between the unity of God ('one being') and a real threeness in God ('three persons'), as in practice putting monotheism in question. So can one ever expect a Jew to assent to the Hellenistic councils between Nicaea and Chalcedon, to a two-natures christology or a theology of three persons? Isn't it therefore necessary in connection with terms like 'Son of God' and Jesus' relationship to God, once again to reflect on the original Hebrew context of Christianity and its roots in the Hebrew Bible?

☪ The divine element in Jesus was emphasized so strongly and so exclusively at Nicaea that all the human characteristics of Jesus receded into the background. And the problem of the differentiation in the personality of the Son was solved in all too formal and inadequate a way in terms of a being begotten (as distinct from begetting). The Christ of history retreated behind the Christ of dogma, and the Gospels behind the doctrines of the church; discipleship of Christ behind the orthodoxy of doctrine and the liturgy. Down to the present day Islam, which accepts Jesus completely as prophet and even Messiah but rejects Hellenistic christology, has not been able to understand that here we have a historical person and a personal human life. So isn't it necessary to begin to understand Jesus Christ once again 'from below', and to attach as much importance to his humanity as the Qur'an does, going on from there to understand how in him God's wisdom has taken human form?

In the previous section I have dealt at length – for some, perhaps at all too much length – with theological and christological problems. This has been for two reasons:

1. Over the centuries the dogmatic structure which was created in the Hellenistic paradigm in the fourth and fifth centuries continued to be of decisive significance not only for the church of the East but also for that of the West.

2. After the crisis over the legitimation of the authority of the emperor in the third century, the christology of the only begotten Son of the Father developed at this time was to provide the new basis of legitimation for him in the fourth century: the imperial autocrator as friend and representative of Christ.

So christological dogma becomes a constitutive element not only for theology and church but also for emperor and state in this old and yet new Byzantine world which was coming into being.

7. Byzantium – birthplace of Orthodoxy

The **Hellenistic** paradigm is the **ecumenical paradigm of the early church**, the whole of the early church, East and West. However, despite all the significance of the old imperial capital, Rome, its focal points – 'apostolic' churches, i.e. churches founded by the apostles, later patriarchates, councils, centres of learning and monasteries – lay above all in the East. And after the transfer of the imperial capital to the Bosphorus, the paradigm was still handed down for around another thousand years by this **empire of the East** – until the Rome of the East and thus the Roman empire generally fell in 1453.

The second Rome: Byzantium as a norm

For a long time the early church Hellenistic paradigm was handed down above all in the **Rome of the East,** whereas, as we shall see, in the West ancient culture generally sank with the Roman state and at the same time the Bishops of Rome, now called Popes, purposefully developed and extended their indepedence from the Rome of the East and their autocracy over the Western church. And in the West this pre-eminence of the Popes – together with the specifically Latin theology of Augustine and finally the political predominance of the Germans – was to form the essential presuppostion for the rise of a new constellation in world history: the new, Latin, specifically Roman Catholic paradigm (P III); it was to break through in the eleventh century with the Gregorian reform and at the same time lead to a definitive split between the Eastern and Western churches.

But before we go into this history of the West, we must first of all continue our analysis of the early church Hellenistic paradigm (P II) which was handed down in the East and boldly defended both externally and internally, as it has unfolded to the present day. Perhaps because of the difficult political and academic situation, more recent Eastern Orthodoxy has shown relatively little interest in the Rome of the East, and apart from specialist problems has left research into it largely to secular historians.[171]

On 11 May 330 the Emperor Constantine had inaugurated his new capital, **Constantinople,** on the Bosphorus on the site of the ancient Greek city **Byzantium,** which was to become the modern scholarly name for the Eastern Roman empire. The new centre had been carefully chosen: it was nearer to the Danube and the Euphrates and thus nearer to the imperial frontiers under attack from the Germans and the Persians; it was also nearer to the regions which were now economically prosperous; nearer, finally, to the religious centres of the East. It was still in Europe, yet the gateway to Asia, at the crossroads of great trade routes: the new representation and demonstration of Roman power and a strong support for Christianity in the East. With similar forethought the street plan of the new capital Constantinople had been assimilated to ancient Rome: it was given its own Senate, and both the most important senatorial families and also the imperial administration had moved to the Bosphorus. Constantine now proudly called it the '**second Rome**'; later it was also called the '**new Rome**', which essentially meant 'the continuation of Rome', and this was to be solemnly confirmed by the ecumenical council of Constantinople in 381, as we heard.

In 395, after the death of Theodosius, the **empire was finally divided into a Western Roman and an Eastern Roman empire.** Its frontiers ran through a country which in our century has called itself Yugoslavia, and in which in most recent times the old antagonism between Western Rome and Eastern Rome, Roman Catholicism and Byzantine Orthodoxy, has been aggressively intensified, although formerly a fruitful cultural exchange (for example with Western monks from the Adriatic as master builders for Byzantine churches) had taken place. At that time the institutions in the Byzantine empire remained Roman, and at first the constitutional and legal language remained Latin. But the population, the vernacular, the culture and even more the religion were Greek – apart from some Latin provinces in the West. Whereas in the West over the course of the centuries the Roman empire was to become a **Germanic** empire by association with the Franks, in the East as a result of Byzantium it became a **Greek** empire, whose primary orientation was less and less on Rome and the West, and more on the East, Asia, from which constantly new threats arose for the empire.

The inhabitants of the Eastern Roman empire simply called themselves *Romaioi*, Romans. For they regarded their Eastern empire as the direct development of the Roman empire, while the Western empire increasingly disintegrated under the waves of Germanic migrations which now rolled in, and in 476 finally collapsed. The **Hellenistic paradigm (P II) of the early church was preserved**; initially it was simply that the old pagan capital had been replaced by a new Christian one. And had not this replacement come about wholly in accordance with the plan of divine providence? So soon the official ideology was that the new Rome had been chosen to take over the world rule of the old Rome and now to exercise this world rule in the sign of Christ. This was a true **saving state**: for this new, Christian Rome, liberated from the demons of pagan Rome, not only had the best possible political administration for ruling the world but in addition also had the only true faith.

So what constitutes 'Byzantium' as a city and empire? The life, culture and the whole development of Byzantium draw on three very different 'primary sources': 'Without all three the Byzantine way of life would have been inconceivable,' says Georg Ostrogorsky, the great scholar of the history of the Byzantine state, who was born in St Petersburg.[172] What elements are they? They are three elements which clearly attest the permanence of the early church Hellenistic paradigm:

- the Roman state,
- Greek culture,
- Christian faith.

To take the third element, which is central to Christianity: **faith** is now no longer understood, as it is in the New Testament, as primarily believing trust (in God, Jesus Christ) but above all as **right belief**, as **orthodoxy**, as a conviction of the correctness of particular doctrinal statements of the church sanctioned by the state. Significantly, the words 'orthodoxy' and 'orthodox' do not appear in the New Testament, but became popular in the fourth century. It is 'orthodoxy' which distinguishes the Byzantine church from earliest Christianity (P I) and finally also from other churches. It was to become the proper name of this church.

Present-day Eastern Orthodoxy cannot in any case be understood without Orthodox Byzantium. Alexander Schmemann, a Russian theologian who died prematurely, to whom I owe much of my understanding of Orthodoxy, has put it more clearly than others: 'In a sense the Byzantine period must be acknowledged as the decisive period in the history of Orthodoxy, as the age of the crystallization of church life. The modern Orthodox Church is from the viewpoint of history the church of Byzantium, which has survived the Byzantine empire by five hundred years.'[173] Of course individual developments of liturgy, theology, iconography, piety and law, with some changes, can also be established in the sphere of Eastern Orthodoxy. But we cannot overlook the fact that just as the concrete form of the Catholic Church of the West down to the present day remains determined by mediaeval Rome, so the concrete **form of the Orthodox Church of the East has been shaped to the present day by Byzantium**. If we leave aside the special developments in the non-Chalcedonian churches, we can see something that will become clear in what follows:

• The liturgy continues to have a Byzantine shape.
• Theology has a Byzantine form.
• Iconography appears to have a Byzantine norm.
• Piety continues to have a Byzantine inspiration.
• Law and constitution have a Byzantine basis.

This last point needs special attention.

Co-existence of paganism and Christianity

Of course we should not succumb to the illusion that with Constantine the world of the Roman empire became Christian overnight. In the time of Constantine the majority of the population of the empire was still pagan. All the more recent researches into late antiquity – and nowadays private life is increasingly being investigated alongside public life[174] – show that particularly in the East, quite apart from the many heretical groups and sects, **Christianity and paganism by no means** confronted each other as **rigid blocks**, but largely existed contemporaneously and grew together.[175] Didn't Constantine exercise a wise tolerance towards the pagan cult and allow the building of new pagan temples even in Constantinople? And much as the directly political influence of paganism declined in the subsequent period, down to the sixth century it remained the foundation of culture. The main reason for this is simply that even the church fathers with their 'classical' education in no way wanted to dispense with 'classical' education in the framework of the church, and classical education, still continually the aim of all the elite, was connected with pagan literature, art, rhetoric, science and philosophy. One could not have all this without taking note of the Graeco-Roman world of the gods.

So it is no wonder that initially the pagan system of **schooling and**

education remained intact. Indeed, it even proved an attraction for Christians once again after the emperor Julian the Apostate in his short-lived pagan restoration had wanted to exclude Christians from it. Although Christian philosophy, along with poetry and historiography, was orientated purely within the church, the spiritual leaders of the church were able to 'democratize' pagan philosophy, which had previously been destined only for a certain elite, and use it for the completely new structure of Christian faith. So this education was also important for Christians, at least as a propaedeutic, despite the abiding normative significance of the Bible and church tradition. Thus the majority of Christian children went to pagan schools and Christians also thronged the ancient places of education: above all Athens, Antioch (until the great earthquake of 526 and its conquest and depopulation by the Persians in 540), and especially Alexandria, where Christians joined pagans in hearing, among others, the famous Neo-Platonic philosopher Hypatia, until she was stoned by a Christian mob in 415/416.

Thus many pagan social structures and external forms of life remained relatively unchanged, particularly in the East in the fourth and fifth centuries. In the upper classes of society, work was still regarded as undignified. And while even the Christian elite dedicated themselves to a life of luxury and enjoyment, in the lower classes, whether pagan or Christian, people all too often became parasites, work-shy and eager for pleasure. In the East the culture of 'late antiquity' was far less threatened by the 'barbarians'.

What about **the church**? The privileges granted to the church, the bishops and the clergy by the emperor at first made little difference to the situation of the elite, and even in popular culture, to the scandal of the clergy, many pagan customs (the theatre, the circus, gladiator fights, chariot races) and superstitious practices (amulets, soothsaying) continued. As one of the greatest experts of late antiquity, the British historian and patristic scholar Peter Brown, can write: 'Imposing as the church of the fourth century appeared, for this *saeculum* it remains marginal for a world the many structures of which are developing under the strong pressures of power and the need for security and hierarchy. Christianity is peripheral to this *saeculum*, even if it is now the nominal faith of the powerful.'[176] But what united Christian society? To quote Brown once again: 'a quite special pretence: that of a solidarity which can now express itself in the clear light of day during the ceremonies in the bishop's basilica'.[177] So in worship, where all were equal before the bishop and clergy, the hierarchy and structure of the world were now no longer present; here all without distinction were confronted with three new themes for which the church and no one else was responsible, themes which it also preached to the powerful, and with the help of which it was finally to 'Christianize' the society of late antiquity: the themes of sin (all are sinners), poverty (all have a duty to give) and death (all constantly face death). These were obligations all of which were of basic significance for attaining the soul's everlasting salvation.[178]

As R. A. Markus has shown,[179] 'a Christianizing of time and space' gradually developed. Thus gradually some pagan festivals, marriage and funeral customs became filled with a Christian spirit. A Christian calendar with many feasts of martyrs and confessors replaced the pagan calendar, and through relics the churches became Christian sanctuaries which were soon linked together by a network of pilgrimage routes, overlaying the topography of the pagan sanctuaries. So increasingly it was not life in the assimilated secular culture but aversion from the world, **asceticism**, which became the characteristic of authentic Christianity. However, **public penance** was now practised less and less. A public confession of sins? That could no longer be made before a small community but had to take place before a large public – with possibly fatal social consequences. So in the East **private confession** first of all quietly developed in place of public confession: initially by monks to one another and then also by laity voluntarily to a monk (not a priest). This was not an obligation but an opportunity. But for many people, by far the most important of all the new things that the church brought was the **social network** which was built up by a church now becoming increasingly rich, to help the masses impoverished by an economy dominated by large estates and the pressure of high taxation. There were numerous places for the poor, widows and foundlings, for refugees, the sick, lepers and the old, especially in the East.

However, we must not conceal the other side of the coin, that the church now itself became one of the greatest **land-owners**. It thus condoned that prime evil of the economy of late antiquity, and instead of fighting against the mass distress increased it and made a by no mean insignificant contribution to it. And as an land-owner, it was also quite naturally a large-scale **slave-owner**. It was now very much less interested in the legal improvement or even liberation of slaves than many pagans, influenced by Stoic ethics, had been even before the shift under Constantine. Indeed, whereas formerly a slave (like the freeman Callixtus) could even become a Roman bishop, Leo the Great now forbade the election of a slave as bishop. And whereas the situation of slaves in the West improved under the Germans, in Byzantium slavery continued until the fall of the empire: in the framework of a 'Christian' state and a 'Christian' church, both now under a 'Christian' emperor.

Theocracy: political theology

Constantine the Great remained the model for all Christian caesars, emperors, czars. That meant that at the centre of the Christian empire, which combined state and church, there was not a bishop or pope, but the Imperator Romanus. Athough a 'lay person' (and Constantine was not even baptized until shortly before his death), he had more say than any member of the clergy, and in the church the last say, even if he did not constantly intervene 'papally' in the everyday affairs of the church. Constantine was convinced that the emperor was nearer to God than any bishop. Very much in the succession of the old Roman pagan god-emperor, the Christian emperor saw himself as **God's representative on earth**. He had been given rule by God and no one else. Indeed the emperor now saw himself as the **friend of Christ, the consubstantial Son of God** (Nicaea!). He had the power and the duty to subject all men and women to the true law of God and Christ. Thus the emperor had virtually a kind of apostolate and was recognized as confessor of the true faith (though not infallible).[180]

No one gave an earlier foundation to the Christian imperial ideology, propagated it better and ultimately stamped it more deeply on the historical consciousness, on the ideas of state and church in Eastern Orthodoxy (of the Byzantines and then also of the southern and eastern Slavs), than **Eusebius of Caesarea** (who died in 339). It is no coincidence that he was a pupil of the great pioneer Origen, was able to use Origen's important library in Caesarea, and after initial sympathies for Arianism was promoted to be Constantine's court theologian with access also to the state archives.

If we are to do justice to Eusebius,[181] we must not forget what it meant for a generation which, like him, had still experienced the ranks of martyrs in his home city, for Christianity now to become a *religio licita*, a permitted religion, in the empire. So it was understandable that in his church history (which was written around 324/5, on the eve of the Council of Nicaea, just as work on building the basilica of St Peter's in Rome was beginning) Eusebius made the whole history of Christianity hitherto culminate under God's gracious providence in the Christian emperor. Moreover Eusebius cannot praise him enough elsewhere in writings and panegyrics. Like other contemporaries, he knew nothing of a special status for the Bishop of Rome, far less of a transfer of the city of Rome and the Western half of the empire to the Pope (the Donation of Constantine, now recognized as an eighth/ninth-century forgery).

Thus Eusebius, the father of church history and court theology, also became the **father of political theology**, though this has now been unmasked as the veneer to an ideology of the ruling class, indeed of **the** ruler. Eusebius' defence of the embellishment of the Church of the Holy Sepulchre in Jerusalem against the criticism of contemporaries in his *Basilikon* ('Address to the Emperor', 335), with a reference to the divinity of the Logos, is one of the more harmless forms of his mystifications; now pomp was put on show everywhere in the church of the poor Nazarene and the rich emperor. What was far worse was that in his *Life of the Blessed Emperor Constantine* (written after Constantine's death), Eusebius described the religious traits of the emperor (a 'new Moses' leading the church into freedom) while simply suppressing all that was negative about his person and politics; this created a fatal trend for Christian court theologians and historians in the Eastern and Western churches. It had not been the way of the classical Greek and Roman historians.

However, what was most important for world history was that already in his church history Eusebius so emphasized the **function of the emperor as the providential guardian and protector of the church** (the *episkopos* over 'external' church affairs) that it was easy to draw every possible consequence for church law and theology from it. Here the position of the absolute Roman ruler was in any event excessively powerful. Constantine now also exploited it in the direction of the church which he had liberated, to convene the first ecumenical council of the church on his own authority in his residence at Nicaea and to direct it largely in accordance with his will through his officials, even down to formulations of the Creed. Constantine and then his successors exercised a *potestas suprema*, a **primacy of jurisdiction** over the church, even if John Chrysostom and many Byzantine theologians denied them power over the church. Now they possessed a threefold imperial authority:

– supreme legislative authority: the appointment, direction and endorsement of ecumenical councils; council decisions became state laws;

– supreme judicial authority: a court of appeal for bishops who had been deposed by provincial synods;

– administrative oversight: nomination of patriarchs, often confirmation of the election of bishops and intervention in the affairs of individual communities.

Nevertheless, what Anton Michel thought he had proved, citing hundreds of sources of all kinds, and what Franz Dölger (who laid the foundation for research into Byzantine archives)[182] summed up as follows, can hardly be maintained, 'that in Byzantium from the beginning the emperor – as the successor of the divine Constantine the Great, as "Christ's representative" – was the sole master of the church in all areas, in church organization and administration, in church legislation and the judiciary, down to the innermost spiritual concerns of the church'.[183] That is far too much a Roman Catholic interpretation. It is more in keeping with Greek Byzantine thought to speak of the emperor as the copy of the divine original. But of course it remains beyond dispute that the **lordship of the emperor**, which could already be felt throughout the church in the period before Constantine, characterized the **Hellenistic Byzantine paradigm** in which, after Constantine, Hellenism and the state church appeared bound together by the **theocracy of the emperor of the Romans**: humanity united in Christian faith, united in a political body under the emperor.

The development of the state church: Justinian

The **end of paganism** came irrevocably with the sixth century, when Christian culture imposed itself totally, not without compulsion. In the sixth century, the Eastern Roman Christian empire which initially reached from the Balkans and the Danube through Greece and Asia Minor to Syria, Egypt and Libya but then during the Germanic migrations had lost many areas to the barbarians, was formally 'restored' by the most significant of Constantine's successors, the Macedonian **Justinian I** (527-565), who had a marked Latin stamp: in foreign policy by the reconquest of lost areas and domestically by a reform of administration and the law. Indeed Justinian again extended the *Imperium Romanum* – though this was to prove only transitory – right across the Mediterranean area, by wars against the Vandals (in North Africa), the East Goths (in Italy) and the West Goths (in Spain).

In addition Justinian, who was a resolute supporter of orthodoxy, also completed the internal, **Greek orthodox transformation of the empire**. Here are just a few dates:

527: All heretics and pagans ('Hellenes') lose state offices, honorific titles, permission to teach and public support.

528: Justinian first commissions a comprehensive collection of the law which in a Greek translation was to become the new basis for justice (later called the *Corpus iuris civilis*).

529: Closure of the philosophical school in Athens, the last support of pagan cultural independence, and forced baptism for the pagans in Constantinople and Asia Minor, who were still numerous.

535: With the publication of Justinian's legal *novellae*, Greek becomes the official language (this Graecizing was probably also a political strategy).

537: In Constantinople, now with around 300,000 inhabitants the symbolic centre of the empire, Hagia Sophia, the largest church in

Christianity, is built. In future it was to be the church in which emperors were crowned. (From then on in Eastern architecture the triumphal feature was the cupola, with its mosaics the focus of prayer for believers, the image and gateway to heaven.)

553: The Fifth Ecumenical Council in Constantinople, convened because of further christological disputes (the theopaschite dispute, then the dispute over the Three Chapters). This elevated the Cyrillian Monophysite interpretation of Chalcedon as the only legitimate one, though despite all the favours granted them the Monophysites could not win assent to their position.

With Justinian (on whom history bestowed the title 'the Great'), the **Byzantine state church** was fully established and shaped politically, legally and culturally – down to the financial starvation of the pagan educational system, the regulation of curricula and a takeover of the schools by Christians. Particularly since the Justinian restoration, in Byzantium people had been convinced that the second Rome was now not just equal to the old Rome: **the new Rome was politically superior to the old**. For in contrast to the Rome of the West, which had grown old and died out, shattered by the barbarian storms, plundered and largely destroyed, wasn't Byzantium clearly the renewed, lively, abiding Rome? There is no doubt that with Justinian the idea of a Roman empire in Christian garb reached a climax.

This ideology of a renewal was by no means just the conviction of the rulers; it was also that of the people, who could not think of a better form of government than the monarchy, now in Christian form. Indeed, people were so fixed on their own state-church ideology that they could not conceive that the bishop in old Rome – still an imperial subject, though in fact without an imperial master – could in time develop his own ideology of church and state. For the emperor still appeared the largely un-challenged master of the state and guardian of the church.

Symphony of empire and church

It is understandable that in the East a pope could not emerge as the political adversary of the emperor. Moreover in his functions the **Patriarch of Constantinople** remained almost completely limited to the spiritual sphere: to the preservation of the purity of doctrine and liturgical order in the narrower sense. Still, the patriarch might examine the orthodoxy of a future ruler before he was crowned emperor. Thus – quite apart from his independent administrative role in the church – developed at least the beginnings of a counter-force, which could be brought into play by significant patriarchs like Photius and Cerularius.

Imperial territory before Justinian

Justinian's conquests

The Empire of Justinian I around 565

The Empire of Basil II around 1025

Maps based on G.Ostrogorsky, *Geschichte des byzantinischen Staates*, Munich ³1963.

Asia Minor and the Balkans around 1214

The Collapse of the Byzantine Empire in the 14th/15th Century

A 'symphony' ('harmony') of empire and imperial church was the
demand of the time and became the watchword for Byzantium. However,
the emperor largely wrote the score of the 'symphony' and conducted it
himself. In succession to the Roman god-emperor and at the same time in
keeping with the Christian model provided by Eusebius of the direct
imparting of divine grace, the Christian 'autocrats' saw themselves as
copying God's sole rule over the whole 'inhabited earth', the 'ecumene'.
Justinian, as earthly governor for the heavenly 'pantocrator', proudly
called himself 'cosmocrator'. The earthly kingdom was thus a copy of the
heavenly kingdom. For a long time Greek Platonic thought in the
categories of 'above' (invisible) and 'below' (visible) had replaced Jewish
apocalyptic thought with its scheme of 'now' and 'then'.

So all in all, what developed in the East was **not** a **church state**, as this
was to develop in the West, **but** a **state church**.

– Since Ambrose, who regarded the emperor as a Christian **under** the
bishops in matters of faith and the possessions of the church, for a long
time Byzantium had not been taken seriously into account in the West.
Through the expansionism of the Roman Popes, in time a marked
antagonism developed between church and state ('city of God' and 'city
of this world'), and finally a system of **papalism** in which the church was
wholly orientated on the 'Papa', the 'Pope'.

– By contrast, in the East a unity of state authority and supreme
jurisdiction over the churches was established and then a unity of church,
state and people generally of a kind which in the West is termed
'**Caesaropapism**', though this label is better avoided. The emperor at the
same time pope? The emperor is not a priest and does not possess
infallibility like a modern pope. Rather than a system of one-sided
dependence, an **interdependence** of church and state prevailed. Unlike the
Pope today, the emperor had no absolute authority in questions of church
teaching, and more than once he was to come to grief in attempting to
impose dogmatic positions (for example in favour of Monophysitism or
union with Rome). Indeed, an emperor who became unfaithful to
Orthodoxy was to be regarded as a tyrant.

Despite everything, in practice the emperors had few inhibitions about
behaving 'more papally than the Pope', not only ordering popes to
Constantinople but even deposing rebellious patriarchs. For them, what
counted was not just the New Testament 'one God, one faith, one
baptism', but also the '**one empire, one law, one church**' of Constantine
and Justinian. In the narrow, 'harmonious', 'symphonic' combination of
church and state the state and its supreme representative, raised above all
others by a ceremonial and highly sacral symbolism which had been
refined for centuries, had the pre-eminence. This remained a **character-**

istic of the Hellenistic Byzantine paradigm – from Byzantium to Moscow, where the Czar was even to have absolute power. However, the state church is only as it were the outside of Orthodoxy. What governs it from within?

The liturgy – the living backbone of the Orthodox Church

The **ecumenical church of the first centuries** remains a church which understands itself not primarily as a great hierarchical organization with a centralist direction but as the great community of those who believe in 'Christ', spread throughout the 'ecumene', the whole inhabited earth. This community is concretely alive in the individual local and episcopal churches, and here above all in worship.

For the excessive power of the state should not lead us to forget that through all the changing epochs the **liturgy** was to remain the **greatest strength of the Orthodox church**, as it were its living backbone, which supported it even in difficult times and at the same time made it capable of adaptation to the different nations. It is a liturgy at the centre of which stands not the 'bloodless repetition' of Jesus' sacrifice on the cross (as later in the Latin Middle Ages) but the messianic banquet of the exalted Lord with his community. It is a liturgy the basic tenor of which is not repentance and forgiveness for sins but Easter joy and jubilation at the presence of the Lord. It is a liturgy which consequently is not celebrated kneeling, as in the West, with folded (Old German 'fettered') hands or with hands pressed together (the symbol of the 'flame'), but in principle standing upright with arms hanging down or stretched out above, and sometimes also crossed (accompanied – another Byzantine feature – by countless crossings, genuflections, prostrations and kissing of sacral objects).

Here the notion of the personal encounter of believers with the risen Lord in the first centuries turned into a whole wealth of spontaneous and very different liturgical forms (often improvised eucharistic prayers). This original freedom and variety was then, however, increasingly restricted. After the shift under Constantine, **families of liturgies** formed around the great cities:[184]

– from Alexandria the Greek Liturgy of Mark and the Coptic and Ethiopian liturgies;

– from Antioch the Greek 'Liturgy of James', the Western and Eastern Syrian liturgies;

– from Constantinople the Byzantine and also the Armenian liturgy.

These Eastern liturgies were as different as their churches, but despite their regional languages and characteristics they all developed within the framework of the Hellenistic paradigm (P II). They came to differ increasingly clearly from the Roman liturgy which spread from Rome, and which was above all to put its stamp on the empire of the Franks and produce a separate liturgical paradigm (P III).

Later, like Rome in the West, in the East Constantinople insisted on liturgical uniformity – of course not least for political reasons. And as the Roman city liturgy became established throughout the whole Western Roman and then the Frankish empire, so the Byzantine city liturgy came to be established throughout the Eastern Roman empire and most of the Slavonic kingdoms. Down to the tenth century the Liturgy of Basil the Great seems to have been most in use, and then more the Liturgy of John Chrysostom, which came from Antioch.

It is important for us to remember the liturgy, because it says something about the inner life of the church in the state church system. For it is true particularly of the churches of the first centuries that if after the shift under Constantine they became increasingly institutionalized and, at the wish of Constantine, adapted themselves to the organization of the one empire, they were by no means a uniform church organized strictly from above under a supreme bishop. They still formed a *koinonia, communio*, fellowship of churches whose unity and cohesion was not understood in legal and institutional but in sacramental and spiritual terms. They were a **federation** of churches in which the many city bishops felt bound together collegially, subordinate to the metropolitan and the patriarch, and certainly linked to the Bishop of Rome. They regarded him as the bishop of the old imperial capital and recognized him as the first of the patriarchs (*primus inter pares*); not, however, because of a special 'promise' or 'authority' but because of the tombs of the two chief apostles Peter and Paul. Many of these Eastern churches were, after all, themselves apostolic foundations and in this sense *sedes apostolicae*, apostolic sees: Jerusalem, Antioch and Alexandria along with Ephesus, Thessaloniki or Athens. They had received the faith directly from the apostles and not, say, from Rome (like most of the later Germanic churches) or Byzantium (like most of the later Slavonic churches).

However, for all the praise of Orthodoxy it would be a great delusion to fail to see that already the then **liturgy and constitution of the Orthodox Church** were **no longer simply the original apostolic ones** (P I). Why? One need only think of the position of the clergy – alongside the over-powerful position of the bishops. As we saw, in the Jewish Christian apocalyptic paradigm there was complete freedom in the specific shaping of church ministries, as long as they represented service and not power. To exercise a special church ministry was for a long time no small burden and a great risk; so many people paid a high price, in times of persecution even with their blood. All this changed as the office of bishop accrued power, as also indirectly did the clergy even in the century before Constantine.

After the shift under Constantine, however, a development took place which now made the clergy increasingly a separate social class.

The clergy – now a separate class

The Jewish-Hellenistic term **'layman'** (*laikos*) in the Greek sense means the uninstructed mass, in the Jewish sense the man who is neither priest nor levite. It does not appear at all in the New Testament, but in the so-called Letter of Clement[185] at the beginning of the second century. Here it means the simple believer in contrast to the high priests, priests and levites. The term is frequently found throughout the church after the third century.

By contrast, the Greek word *kleros* originally meant 'lot', 'portion', and was already used in the pre-Constantinian church for a share in the presbyterate and then also for other officials. Already in Origen *kleros* is a fixed **designation for church officers as distinct from the people.**[186] In the period after Constantine the biblical division between (priestly!) 'people' (*laos*) and 'non-people' (*ou laos*[187]) increasingly became the division between 'people' (*laici*) and 'priests' (*clerus*).[188]

After Constantine there was an amazing **return to the Old Testament** – even down to liturgical texts which now became increasingly fixed, ceremonial, priestly clothing and the shaping of the house of God.[189] Everywhere people resorted to the symbolism of a Temple and a Temple liturgy which Jesus himself had relativized and early Gentile Christinaity had ignored; post-Constantinian Christianity had never seen this Temple with its own eyes, but now took it as its transfigured model. It was as if, as Justin had already supposed, the Temple and Temple worship had been taken from the Jewish people as God's punishment and had now been given to the church as the 'new people of God' and the 'true Israel'. 'Solomon, I have surpassed you,' the emperor Justinian is said to have exclaimed on seeing the completed Hagia Sophia. And some churches in Syria and Georgia were called 'Zion'. Did Christianity, now that its liturgy was now largely fixed, as a recognized religion in competition with other religions perhaps also want to characterize itself, as Fairy von Lilienfeld conjectures, with a concrete '*nomos*' ('law' or 'religious practice', meaning both rite and church law), in other words with a strict liturgical order?

Be this as it may, the tension between church and world (which now itself became increasingly a 'Christian' world) had been transferred more and more into the church: it had become a tension betwen 'clergy' and laity. Here the clergy were increasingly given a special social status and developed into a distinctive social class. Three interconnected processes can be observed, which complete the **paradigm shift in the status of the church's ministry**: the development towards professionalization, towards privilege and towards celibacy. I shall indicate the differences briefly.

(a) In the Jewish Christian apocalyptic paradigm most of the church ministries were **part-time** occupations: even the apostle Paul earned his own living – according to tradition – by tentmaking. But now the higher church ministries increasingly became **full time**. Being a bishop or a presbyter or a deacon became a **profession**. The result of this was that gifts had to be given not only for the poor but also increasingly for the support of the clergy; it was advantageous to elect a well-to-do bishop who could then make over his possessions to the church. So the churches now became rich, and while this encouraged new generations of clergy, it did less to encourage a clerical life, as many abuses were soon to show.

The clergy was now 'essentially' different from the laity: through ordination, which was performed by the laying on of hands (see the Pastoral Epistles) and anointing. Now a presbyter could only be ordained by a bishop, a bishop only by the metropolitan (along with neighbouring bishops). There were also increasing gradations within the clergy following from the type of consecration (lower or higher). And alongside the clergy, especially in the larger communities, there was a whole series of administrative officials and sometimes hundreds of church musicians, people to carry the sick and bury the dead – a power which could also be used politically.

(b) In the Jewish Christian apocalyptic paradigm most church ministries had **no privileged position** in society; on the contrary, because of their belief in Christ those holding them were also the underprivileged, who often had to reckon with denunciations, discrimination and worse. But in the period after Constantine the clergy increasingly developed their own **privileged rank**. This meant:
– **Privileges of status**: that already began under Constantine with freedom from personal burdens; in part the clergy were granted their own jurisdiction (arbitration, the right of intercession and asylum).
– **Status symbols**: thus from the fifth century the tonsure, that way of cutting the hair which had been taken over by the monks (originally from the priests of Isis?); and then also special clothing (still strictly rejected by Pope Celestine I in 428).

– **Cultic ceremonial**: this included splendid liturgical garments and valuable church vessels; a ceremonial enriched in many ways with usages taken over from the Old Testament and paganism (despite original repudiation): lighted candles, the burning of incense (against the demons), penitential processions, and finally church singing (a separate *schola*) in the splendid basilicas adorned with precious mosaics.

All this must in fact have considerably distanced the clergy, who now celebrated worship with high ceremonial 'for' the people, from the people themselves, who became bystanders and were increasingly passive. Instead, the people were generously allowed a 'lower cult' of the kind formerly customary only in polytheistic paganism: saints, angels and especially Mary as 'patrons' or mediators of salvation, to whom one prayed; relics and a trade in relics, the veneration of images, and pilgrimages to Palestine, Rome and Tours.

(c) In the Jewish Christian apocalyptic paradigm most church ministers were **married**; celibacy in the service of fellow human beings, lived out in exemplary fashion by Jesus and Paul, was not a law but a charism, i.e. a calling freely undertaken. But now **celibacy** slowly became established for the more senior clergy. This was a phenomenon which must be seen against the background of the widespread development towards asceticism in late antiquity. For at that time there were ascetic forms of life in both Judaism and Hellenism. The Stoa in particular had pleaded for discipline and restraint in sexual intercourse; the view was that if a man gave too much of his power he would risk losing his virility – a principal virtue of the ancient Romans – and become soft.

Already in the third century the custom developed that bishops, presbyters and deacons who hitherto were normally married (also, of course, in Rome) might not marry **after their ordination**: if they did, they had to leave office. If we want to know why they had to have married before their first ordination (as deacons) we must read the regulations for cleanness in the book of Leviticus and the instructions for priests in the book of Chronicles: certain Old Testament precepts about what was clean and what unclean form the background for many procedures of the Orthodox churches, their bishops and priests.

After the fourth century things became more strict. Attempts increased to impose sexual abstinence on married clergy as well. Whereas Western synods (first of all the rigorist Synod of Elvira in Spain in 306/12) took up these demands, the Council of Nicaea rejected them. And it is significant for the different developments in East and West that here, too, the original church order was maintained more in the East. To the present day, the East goes by the Second Trullan Synod of 691 or 692, held in the Byzantine imperial palace ('Hullos') under Justinian II. It has always allowed married men to be ordained priest and also allows them to continue to have marital intercourse as clergy; that is the situation today, in contrast to the West, where since the eleventh century all the secular clergy have been obligated by rigoristic Popes to fundamental celibacy (in the real sense). In the East a separation from one's wife (who had to agree to this) was required only for candidates for the episcopate; this was theologically inconsistent and had fatal practical consquences. For in the long run this regulation meant that in the East bishops could be elected almost only from the monks. Otherwise to the present day celibacy in the East remains limited to monks, who freely chose this form of life. However, widowed priests might not marry again.

Thus the paradigm shift in the status of church ministry had considerable consequences for the spirit and structure of the church. Here there was more than the necessary cultural assimilation. There were substantive shifts in the understanding of the church's ministry: alongside the formation of a social class a **sacralization of the church's ministry** which can also be found in the Old Testament with its demarcation of 'clean' and 'unclean', but which is alien to the New Testament. Where in the New Testament is the office-holder a sacred person, set apart from other people, exalted above ordinary Christians as a mediator towards God, so that ordination often appears more important than baptism? Not even in the Pastoral Epistles. But in Orthodoxy baptism appears only as a kind of 'beginning', 'germ' of Christian life; only dedication as monk or ordination as clergy produces a really 'new creation'.

But a so-called 'christological foundation' for the church's ministry, which, falsely appealing to statements by Paul and jumping over the community of Christians, isolates the church leaders from the community as a 'second Christ' and 'mediator', does not correspond to the New Testament view of the uniqueness of the mediatorship of Christ and the universal priesthood of believers. On the contrary, according to the New Testament all believers have a share in the priesthood of Christ, all have a special position in the world through faith and baptism, in order to live in accordance with the gospel for the world, for fellow human beings. Questions arise, and not only for Orthodoxy, where 'the royal priesthood' of all believers, while certainly affirmed, hardly plays a great role in the life of the church. Questions arise which have to be put from both a Jewish and an Islamic perspective.

Questions about the Future of the Clergy

✝ If the **church's ministry** was not initially full time and did not necessarily have to be a profession, is it not conceivable that in the future it could again become a part-time activity, which in some circumstances need not be lifelong but could be engaged in for a particular period?

If initially the church's ministry did not necessarily have to have any special social status, is it not conceivable that in the future it could again be the ministry of one human being among others, without special privileges and status symbols?

If initially the church's ministry was not bound up with celibacy for bishops and priests, and if in the Eastern churches it still does not involve celibacy, at least for priests, in the future could not celibacy for priests and bishops also be a voluntary calling in the Western church as well? A ministry which in our time can also be open to women, as is already the custom in many Western churches?

If the church's ministry was not initially sacralized and those in office were not singled out from others as 'holy persons' and elevated as mediators to God, could not the unbiblical clericalism which now prevails once again be overcome?

✡ Since the destruction of the Second Temple, Judaism no longer has priests, but something like religious scholars. However, these **rabbis** are not sacral persons, but experts in the Bible (Torah) and tradition (Mishnah, Talmud), especially the all-embracing religious law (halakhah). They can also exercise this ministry part-time, and in any case are not cut off from the people by a celibate life. But does that of itself banish the danger of 'clericalism' in Judaism? Don't many of these experts and interpreters of religious law impose an all-embracing legal system on people: not an orthodoxy, but certainly an orthopraxy, which can similarly become a burden?

☪ Unlike Judaism, Islam had no priests from the start, but something like the religious scholars in Judaism: in Sunni Islam they are called **Ulama** and in Shi'ite Islam **Mullas**. They too are experts in scripture (Qur'an) and – except among the Shi'ites – in tradition (Sunna), and again especially in religious law (Shari'a). They too can exercise this ministry part-time and are normally married. But does that of itself banish the danger of a 'clericalism' in Islam, when in Islam, too, in some circumstances experts in religion impose on a whole people a comprehensive order of life thought out to the smallest detail, and in some circumstances even want to impose this Islamic 'system' universally in the political sphere with all the means of the state?

A point needs to be made about the clergy generally. Orthodoxy is often said to be rigorist about the 'laity' and their morality in matters of eroticism and sexuality. However, a close examination indicates that: 'The gulf between public and private morality on the one hand and the norms of church authority on the other is as deep in Byzantium as almost anywhere . . . Orthodoxy was by no means hasty with verdicts on erotic literature. We know enough cases from the church history of Byzantium where books were put on the index and burned, or at any rate expressly banned. But these were almost exclusively works which were at war with Orthodox dogmatics. It seems that they did not include a single text which could have been counted light reading and which was too erotic or too close to eroticism.'[190]

However, things were different with **monasticism**. First of all, monks were not clergy, but on the other hand not only wanted to be set apart in the world through faith and baptism but specifically sought to depart from the world. Monasticism – like the cult of icons which is connected with it – clearly came into being in the East and has been of crucial significance there to the present day. And as monasticism and the cult of icons are an indispensable element of Eastern Orthodoxy, we must now briefly turn our attention to them.

8. The mark of the Eastern church: monastic rule and the cult of icons

Monasticism[191] is not a Christian nor even a Jewish invention (Qumran!), but an old **Indian institution**. The Upanishads already give a reason why renunciation can be one of the supreme virtues. Monasticism is central to Buddhism, which in its origin and nucleus is a monastic religion, since those who followed the Buddha and accepted his teaching as normative were mostly hermits and itinerant monks, and then also cenobites (monks living together) in monasteries. Moreover it is monks who are addressed everywhere in the Sutras of Buddha Gautama, though the message also applies indirectly to the laity.

What monasticism originally was and sought to be

If we now move from Indian and Buddhist monasticism to the history of Christian monasticism, we can see striking **similarities between Buddhist and Christian spirituality**, despite the very different backgrounds.[192] And since with the downfall of the militant monks in the second Jewish-Roman War in 135, **Jewish** monasticism in Qumran had come to an end and nothing is reported to us of a **Jewish Christian** monasticism, the question has long been asked whether the origin of monasticism in Egypt (but at the same time also in Syria and Asia Minor) perhaps goes back to **Indian** influences. From the time of Alexander the Great there was in fact a commercial and cultural exchange between India and Egypt. So it is not surprising that the first mention of Buddha in Christian sources is as early as 200, in the *Carpets* (*Stromata*) of Clement of Alexandria, whom we have already met. He seeks to demonstrate that Christian gnosis is an ideal superior to any other gnosis: 'Some, too, of the Indians obey the precepts of Buddha; whom on account of his extraordinary sanctity, they have raised to divine honour.'[193] But it is difficult to demonstrate in detail how far Indian influence extended in the Nile Valley and the Hellenistic world. Influence from Gnosticism and especially pessimistic Manichaeanism, from Hellenistic philosophy and ascetic theology and Origen's mysticism of the soul, are more evident. So we must leave the question of historical dependence open, though it should be mentioned that the life of Buddha was widely disseminated in Eastern Christianity as the legend of Barlaam and Josaphat.[194]

But didn't the beginnings of Christian monasticism already lie in the earliest community? Weren't the sharing of goods, poverty and the unmarried state the ideals of earliest Christianity, apostolic ideals? Quite apart from the question whether here we have generalizing and idealizing accounts, we should reflect that neither the sharing of possessions nor poverty nor the unmarried state alone are characteristics of monasticism. There were already tendencies towards solitude and self-sufficiency in classical antiquity: there were pagan ascetics (for example, the self-sufficient Cynics) and Jewish ascetics (according to Philo, the Egyptian Therapeutae).[195] So it is not surprising that already in the second and to a greater extent in the third century there were also Christian ascetics in cities and villages. They renounced marriage, contented themselves with a minimum of possessions and devoted themselves to prayer and 'works of mercy'. But this asceticism – still completely without any rule, any special clothing and any common purse – did not yet have the form of monasticism.

For what is characteristic of the monk is a **retreat from the world** into solitude – which was not the attitude of the earliest community. The monk, from the Greek *monachos* = living alone, is someone who lives alone in the world; he can also be an 'anchorite', one who has 'escaped', 'withdrawn' (from the world into the wilderness), or – since the Greek for wilderness is *eremos*, a 'hermit', 'dweller in the wilderness'. So the eremitic-anchoritic-monastic tradition aims at a critical distancing and withdrawal from the world, in the name of Jesus Christ. This withdrawal (even from the regular community of Christians) first took place around the villages or even the cities, and finally was made into the complete solitude of the wilderness, though often in groups which gathered around 'father' figures. Here, at least according to Athanasius, a battle against the demons played an extraordinary role,[196] since the wilderness was often regarded as the place to which the pagan demons, who had to be fought against, had withdrawn.

On the other hand, the withdrawal into the wilderness was a sign that these drop-outs had a special, new relationship to heaven.[197] The wilderness was a place not only of exodus, of demons, but also of inwardness, of nearness to God. Here an **alternative form of life** was shown to the people of the society of the time: a person could be solitary, self-sufficient, truly free. The aim was not just to mortify the body, to overcome hunger and triumph over sexual needs, but above all to distance oneself completely from one's former settled community. 'Social death' was the alternative, in order to gain a new life through self-examination and self-mortification, to become a 'new Adam'. For the pagan world of antiquity, a completely new access to the divine appeared here in the Christianity of the fourth and fifth centuries. Here was no longer that quite natural, convenient approach which for example the pagan priests thought they had, needing only to call on a deity who was ever near. Rather, this was an access to a heaven which was no longer by any means near, to the hidden God, an access laboriously wrested from the demons and above all from one's own sinfulness. So the Christian monk represents something like a 'holy man' of a new kind who, precisely because he has rejected secular power, receives spiritual power, which does not, as in the case of pagan 'friends of God', derive from trances, dreams and visions but is achieved by constant and extremely ascetic efforts. Not only transitory visions of other-wordly things are communicated, but the constant gift of searching the hearts of human beings here and now. A **new spiritual elite** of Christian 'friends of God' was coming into being here which was finally to develop its own organization and legislation, literature, art and architecture.

What was the **origin of the Christian eremitic movement?** Historically it can be traced back to before 300 – and to Egypt. In rural Egypt, so different from the highly-cultivated Hellenistic city of Alexandria, where because of the growing pressure of taxation, distress, poverty and legal uncertainty had increased in the villages, there lived a man called **Antony**. Formerly a well-to-do landowner, but illiterate, for a long time he lived outside the village in a tomb, then in an abandoned citadel and finally on a wild rocky hill, where he fought his battle with the 'demons of sensuality' and where people came to him in search of consolation, advice and help.

After the death of Antony (around 356), who is said to have lived for over one hundred years, Athanasius wrote an idealized life of this desert father, interwoven with legends (*The Life of Antony*), which has come down to us. Most of it is taken up with Antony's battle against the demons, his miracles and his rejection of the Arian (and perhaps also the Gnostic?) heresy. The Gospel story of the rich young man[198] is said to have prompted Antony to give his possessions to the poor and go into solitude.

Others imitated Antony, and the sayings (the *Apophthegmata Patrum*) of these greatly venerated fathers were to form the beginning of monastic literature, all the spiritual letters, biographies and moral treatises. It emerges from them that the desert fathers saw themselves very much as successors to the prophets of the wilderness (in addition to Amos, especially Elijah and John the Baptist, patrons of many desert churches). The monks often protested later against the rich and elaborate liturgies of the city churches, but otherwise did not address the people as such, but individuals.

Athanasius' work quickly made **eremitism popular** in the Greek East but only very much later also in the West. Thousands went into the wilderness, often heeding social distress (and at the same time robbing the unpopular Roman state of financial, administrative and productive resources). Moreover settlements of hermits and monasteries soon extended in Palestine and Syria, where strange special forms developed: some spent their time on pillars (Stylites), kept awake in rotation to offer eternal worship (Akoimetes), or performed miracles (Thaumaturgoi[199]). Such monks were not normally clergy; often they were originally illiterate peasants who did not understand Greek. Many were authentically in search of God, but some were financially ruined and avoiding taxation, psychopaths and criminals on the run.

Even more popular, however, was **cenobiticism**, the 'common life', the organized **monastic community**. With its disciplined, humane and social character, this was to shape Christian monasticism more than the hermits, not least because the life could be lived by both men and women. It was the former recruit **Pachomius** (292-346), from a Coptic peasant family, a contemporary of Antony, who – because of the numerous dubious itinerant monks – for the first time organized a tightly regulated monastic life with Roman military discipline by the Nile in Southern Egypt (in Tabennisi): its foundation was unconditional obedience to one's superior; commitment to poverty and chastity; silence (an ancient Egyptian ideal); and heavy manual labour. In the end Pachomius had nine male monasteries under him, and two women's convents supervised by his sister Mary; with several thousand members this represented the most significant monastic organization in early Christianity. Athanasius' *Life* *of Antony*, the *Sayings of the Fathers*, the monastic rules of Pachomius and the lives of Abbot Shenute and his disciples are today the main works of the **Copts**, that age-old indigenous group of Egyptian Christians, so different from the Greek incomers (who were often felt to be arrogant). They have handed down Coptic, the last stage of the Egyptian language.[200]

But it was the great **Basil**, Bishop of Caesarea, who was first to help monasticism towards a theological foundation in the face of the pious individualism, separatism and often even exhibitionism of the monks: an orientation on the gospel and practical love of neighbour. He was also the one who gave the monks a **fixed rule**: novitiate, vows, strict obedience towards superiors with punishments and control of extreme asceticism. His rule was spiritual reading in all Orthodox monasteries and thus became universally authoritative throughout the East, so that here there were and are no different religious orders. The Council of Chalcedon in 451 finally integrated monasticism, which was often unorganized, into the organization of the church and put it under the supervision of the bishop.

The golden age of monastic foundations then came in the reign of Justinian in the sixth century; here, however, a culture supported by the laity was preserved in the East – in contrast to the West. John Cassian, a wise and moderate monk of Scythian origin, mediated monasticism to the Latin West (above all in Marseilles) with his *Institutions*, and in the same century **Benedict of Nursia** with his Benedictine rule (using the anonymous *Regula magistri*) also gave shape to Western monasticism. The decisive **elements of monastic life** are and remain:
– **communal living space** in abodes, places of work and places of worship;
– **uniformity** in clothing, food and ascetic attitude;
– a **written rule** to safeguard the community; and therefore
– **obedience** to the superior.[201]

We can easily imagine how from the beginning there were constant **tensions between monks and bishops**: because of their separation from the local church and its worship, because of exaggerated asceticism or demands of the monks which were hostile to the hierarchy. The separation weakened the communities, but quite often hordes of boorish monks formed the storm troopers of the bishop (e.g. Cyril of Alexandria) in the destruction of pagan temples and in conflicts with 'heretics'. However, what proved even more suspicious for the future was the view that monasticism embodies the higher form of Christian life, which the married cannot achieve in their active life in the world. But what theological evaluation is to be made of monasticism? This question arises within the framework of this paradigm analysis.

Certainly the monks were intent on a literal discipleship of Jesus. But in many things would they not have been more justified in appealing to John the Baptist? If we look at the **New Testament**, we find no invitation of Jesus like 'Go into solitude'. Jesus' call is 'Follow me', and this did not mean 'Separate yourself from everyone', 'Die the "social death"'. Certainly, according to the Gospels, after his baptism by John Jesus had himself been driven by the Spirit of God into the wilderness, where he is said to have lived for forty days (here already we have the symbolic number) among the animals, ministered to by angels, and to have experienced temptation from Satan.[202] But however much or however little of this narrative, which possibly sought to present Jesus as a 'new Adam', is historical, the fact remains that Jesus did not stay in the wilderness; he did not become a 'desert father'. Certainly he was unmarried, but he did not perform any public penance, nor was he the advocate of a pessimistic dualism and a Gnostic hostility to the body. He called women to be his disciples, and in contrast to the later hermits we hear nothing of his having had constant, tremendous fights with demons, who appeared as fearful wild beasts, as satyrs or as seductive women (repression phenomena?). We hear nothing of a command to be silent or obedient to a superior, no efforts to find access to God through works of ascetic mortification and to achieve a new identity.

But what about 'perfection'? It is even more striking that when asked this famous question, Jesus did not send the questioner (the rich young man) to the Jewish monastery of Qumran by the Dead Sea which was known at the time, where he could have practised the 'common life' in the strictest observance of the Torah. No, from Jesus' perspective, **monasticism** is to be understood **only as a charism**, only as a special personal calling focussed on the kingdom of heaven.[203] So it has to be regarded as only **one** form of discipleship of Jesus, as Paul rightly interpreted it in the cases of the married Peter, the brothers of the Lord and the other apostles.[204] It is not a higher form of discipleship for all Christians. Jesus himself did not advocate a spirituality turned away from the world, which is what the spirituality of Orthodoxy was increasingly to become under the influence of the monks. However, nowhere does the classical spiritual literature which Orthodox and ancient Eastern monasticism has used for edifying reading to the present day[205] teach that human beings can be justified before God by works of piety or asceticism, which were radically rejected after Jesus by a man like Paul. This only came about in modern Orthodox theology (under Roman Catholic influence?).

The triumphal progress of monasticism was unstoppable, and Palestine now became the promised land for the monks (St Sabas, who died in 532, led seven groups of anchorites there). At first the monks still lived in considerable isolation on the periphery of the church and society, and the monasteries were mostly poor, with no commercial and economic ambitions. However, in the reign of Justinian in particular many monasteries were founded, with the result that these now also began to play a certain political role in the imperial church and at court. The most important monasteries in Egypt, Palestine and Syria were overwhelmed by Islam in the seventh century, but in Byzantium itself the position of the monks became increasingly unassailable.

The great political hour of monasticism then came in the eighth and ninth centuries. For it was monks who played a historical role in that great dispute which was to shake both the Orthodox Church and the state to the foundations: the so-called iconoclastic dispute. A dispute over images? 'How can one have a dispute over images?', people kept asking in the West.

May images be venerated?

Anyone coming from the West who enters an Eastern Orthodox church today will immediately be struck by the many images of saints which are greeted and kissed by believers in hieratical sequence. Often, especially in Russia, a whole wall of images (iconostasis) separates the sanctuary from the body of the church. And in fact whereas the 'Constantinian' basilicas and mosaics were still common to both the Western and the Eastern churches, **icons** (Greek *eikon* = image) are a specifically Eastern development. It took place above all in the sixth and seventh centuries, when **images for pious remembrance became images for cultic veneration**, which, it was believed, would bring the help of the saint concerned.[206]

Here we should note that at the time of the pagan empire, any veneration of images was still tabu in the church. Even in the period after Constantine, at first this was seen as a continued influence of pagan thought. Reference was made here above all to the Old Testament prohibition of divine images. Early images of Christ (say of the Good Shepherd on sarcophagi) and of saints and saving events therefore had a purely symbolic character. They did not seek to represent or even portray the Son of God, but to indicate the means of salvation: Christ, the shepherd, baptism or the eucharist. So one participates in grace not through images but through the living Christ, his word and his sacrament. Eusebius, for example, had rejected any form of pictorial representation, even of the earthly humanity of Christ. In any case Christ's spiritual, divine nature could not be depicted, and a depiction of the man Jesus alone was not a depiction of the true Son of God. Even at the end of the fourth century Epiphanius of Salamis had attacked the veneration of images out of hand as a new form of idolatry.

By contrast, images were defended by the great Cappadocians, Basil and the two Gregories, and by Chrystostom. Finally, the portrait of each new emperor had formerly been taken to all the provinces to make it possible to experience his presence even in the farthest corners of the empire. The honour shown to the **image** was directed towards the **original**, in reality represented Christ, Mary or the saints. This was now explained Platonically, as 'participation' of the man-made image in its divine original. At all events, as early as the fifth and sixth centuries, in Eastern Christianity people no longer had any inhibitions about putting lighted candles or lamps in front of images in church or at home, burning incense, kissing the images, washing them or clothing them liturgically or kneeling before them – practices which were formerly quite usual among non-Christians. Now it was said that anyone who kissed the icons kissed Christ and the saints themselves, whose power and grace was present in the image. As in paganism, now too among Christian people, the Christian image was thought to have a prophylactic and miraculous effect.

This new kind of Christian veneration of images was markedly a movement from below. Theology with its theories of the 'incarnation' of God in Christ, which allowed the divine (in the form of Christ) to be painted, attempted to justify the veneration of images after the event, and sometimes to correct it. Anyone who denied that Christ could be painted, also denied the real incarnation of God in Christ. And it was above all the monks who acceded to the age-old **longing of the people for something to look at and for help**, for experiences of **grace and wonder**. All this was powerfully encouraged especially at the places of pilgrimage. The Monophysite view of 'Christ our God', widespread not only among monks, for which the earthly is only the garb of the divine, doubtless further strengthened these tendencies. The veneration of images was also encouraged, as archaeological evidence demonstrates, by pilgrimages to Simeon, the pillar saint. And soon the belief was widespread that some images of Christ (and later also of Mary) had come into being in a miraculous way and therefore had miraculous effects. Icons could work miracles of all kinds, could heal the sick, raise the dead, drive out devils, even intervene in war, make arrows rebound and destroy hostile siege machines, just as they could also take revenge on those who shamed them (for example by bleeding). And beyond question there are also models for all these miracles before and outside Christianity.

So finally **images** became **omnipresent** in the world of Byzantium; they were not only displayed in the church, in houses, businesses and monks' cells but also carried around in processions and taken on journeys, or to war. Finally, in 626 in a highly personal way the Patriarch of Constantinople confirmed the miraculous effect of icons and in the face of the onslaught of the Avars had prophylactic images of Mary attached to the western gates of the city. It is not always easy to establish how far all this was just 'veneration' and not also 'worship' (due only to God 'in himself'), how far a distinction was made between the image and the person depicted, or how far authentic piety was at work and how far superstition and magic. All too often popular religion goes beyond theological distinctions. Be this as it may, now some lovers of icons in the seventh and eighth centuries seem to have interpreted the images virtually as a new form of incarnation: Christ incarnated himself here and now in wood and oil, as he incarnated himself then and there in flesh and blood, though this view was not elevated to become Orthodox doctrine.[207]

What did the criticism of icons have to say to this? Of course, as we heard, the scepticism about and criticism of this novel veneration of images, expressed at a very early stage, never fell silent. We have evidence of this not only from Armenia and Asia Minor. Often material and physical contact with the icons (for example, kissing) was more important than the liturgy itself, and reports of crude superstition cannot be overlooked. There was a great gulf between the more restrained theological theory of icons and the exorbitant pious practices here. And the treatises of the theologians could not compete with the highly popular legendary literature which gave colourful reports of the miraculous behaviour and effect of icons. Nevertheless, a large number of Christians must have felt that this novel, materialized piety centred on icons was idolatry in Christian garb. That is the only explanation for the outbreak of a great dispute over these images. It came in the eighth century.

A fanatical dispute over images

This dispute, which was carried on with the help of theology, discipline and the police, was to plunge the empire into strife for more than a century, strife worse than that before and after the Council of Chalcedon. Strikingly, it was sparked off by the emperor **Leo III**, a soldier from the Eastern frontier states, who had already fought off the second siege of Constantinople by the Arabs in 717/18 and ended both the immediate threat and the inner disorder in the Byzantine empire. Historians have discussed widely what specific motives Leo may have had in supporting a movement which was not only critical of images but also **destructive of** images (**icono-clastic**). Was he concerned to fortify the troops fighting in the East against the armies of the Caliphate – a geo-political explanation? Was he concerned to oppose a movement among the middle-class farmers and their bishops in the Eastern frontier states – a socio-political explanation? Or was this the sole decision of a man who in 725/6 gave the first iconoclastic addresses and had the beloved image of Christ over the Bronze Gate between his palace and the city destroyed – a psychological explanation?[208] Be this as it may, in view of the strong tradition which already existed in the church that was either opposed to images or critical of them, it is inappropriate simply to attribute the dispute over the images to 'innovators' and to explain it in terms of direct influence from Islam and Judaism. Those who venerated images had already attempted in the eighth century to force their critics into an un-Christian corner. But as the Tübingen Byzantine scholar Stephen Gerö points out after a thorough investigation of the sources: 'There is little concrete support in the sources for direct Jewish or Muslim influence.'[209] Rather, the opponents of images saw themselves as the guardians of the old Christian tradition against 'pagan innovations'.

However, perhaps too little notice has been taken of the fact that Leo III, the founder of the Syrian dynasty in Constantinople, was a religious reformer who came from that Christian Semitic tradition[210] which a priori had reservations about Greek culture and its enthusiasm for images; like the Armenians, the Syrians too had accepted pictures as illustrations of the biblical writings, but they did not want to incur the suspicion of a neo-pagan idolatry with the veneration of images.[211] To speak here of Hellenistic 'spiritualism', of 'Asian qualities' (in contrast to the Greek character)[212] or even of 'a kind of secularization of art'[213] is foolish, in view of the biblical prohibition of images.[214] Hans-Georg Beck, one of the greatest experts in Byzantine church history, rightly points out that 'those in favour of images did all that they could to divert attention from the real causes, namely the excesses in the veneration of images', and therefore thinks it probable that 'the excesses of the cult of images also seemed to the emperor to be contrary to Christianity, whether he came to this view of his own accord or others convinced him of it'.[215] In other words, the movement against images did not arise outside, but **inside the imperial church**. It is clear that the state authorities intervened only after the event. And when the emperor put a total ban on the images in 730, he had not only a majority of the army but also many people in the population behind him.

However, he had the monks and thus the monasteries against him. They often owed all their reputation and indeed their existence to icons, their manufacture and their cult. And he also had the people dominated by the monks against him; with his direct prohibition of images he also had the Western Latin territories and the Pope against him, though demonstrably only from Gregory III (731-41) on. Finally, he had an important theologian against him (in this case more important than the Pope): this was **John of Damascus** (*c.* 700-753), who is regarded as the last of the great church fathers. He is held to be the most important systematic theologian of the Orthodox Church, and his dogmatic theology, entitled *Fount of Wisdom*, has remained normative throughout Orthodoxy to the present day. John, previously for a time the Caliph's treasurer, paradoxically wrote his **Three Discourses against the Iconoclasts** under Arab protection as a monk in the monastery of St Sabas in Jerusalem. In them he develops a comprehensive theology of icons: the making and veneration of images of Christ (and even more of the saints) are justified at length in terms of the incarnation of God, which has given a new meaning to everything in the world and has also prepared matter for sanctification. Therefore seeing is more than hearing, and the image of God (in human form) is clearer than the Word of God. So the cult of icons is a duty.

However, under Leo's important son and successor Constantine V, who continued the military, economic and administrative reform of the state, at the great council in Hiereia near Chalcedon in 754, which wanted to see itself as the seventh ecumenical council, **iconoclasm** was declared the **church doctrine** of the whole of the Eastern hierarchy, regardless of the fact that it had been explicitly condemned beforehand by the Pope. The iconoclastic theology of this council now no longer insisted just on the essential incomprehensibility of God and the impossibility of depicting him in images but also on the fundamental impossibility of depicting Christ. This must either tear apart Christ's human and divine natures or curtail his divine person, as this could not be depicted.

What was now a dogma of the imperial church (John of Damascus had been declared a heretic!) at first did not lead to persecutions. However, many public images (not private ones!) were destroyed or painted over. It was only years later that those in favour of icons were persecuted, monasteries were destroyed or secularized, and some monks who often opposed the emperor's supremacy over the church anyway were driven out, banished, forced to marry, tortured or in individual cases even killed. One hardly finds bishops and other clergy at that time among those who were to be venerated as 'martyrs' (but in 766 the emperor also had nineteen senior officials and officers executed).

A first change came only after the death of Leo IV (Constantine's son), under the Dowager Empress Irene (780-802). She came from the Greek heartlands and was under the influence of the monks; she appointed her

Secretary of State patriarch and by arrangement with the Pope (who, however, allowed only the veneration of images like those in the illustrated 'Bible of the Poor') summoned an ecumenical council in **Nicaea in 787** which is still counted as the seventh ecumenical council. It again **allowed the veneration of images.** This was the decision of this Second Nicene Council, which was unwilling to separate image and word, regarding them as two sides of the one thing: 'The veneration of the image passes over to the original (*prototypos*)' (Basil). True 'worship' (*latreia*, adoratio) here remains reserved for God, but relative veneration (*timetike proskynesis, veneratio*) of images is allowed: through genuflection, kissing, incense and candles.[216] All this is a plea for 'church traditions' and a condemnation of all 'innovations'. In the future bishops and clergy are to decide what may be depicted; the artists are simply to do the painting. This was a momentous decision for Byzantine art: 'For the first time in the history of Christianity, a control of graphic art by the church' was resolved on here which tacitly presupposed 'that the freedom of the Christian painter should be limited'.[217] The foundations had been laid for the theological control of Byzantine art, even if initially this control was only of subject-matter.

Today the Orthodox Church sees the **official formation of its doctrine** as being **closed** with the Seventh Ecumenical Council (Nicaea II). Indeed, all its important dogmatic conciliar definitions centre on the two themes of Trinity and incarnation, and the decision for icons in particular was already seen at the time as an ultimate consequence of the doctrine of the incarnation. Since then **tradition** has been the **criterion of truth** for Eastern Orthodoxy; to be specific, not so much the Bible as
– the faith of the seven ecumenical councils;
– the consensus of the early fathers.

However, the Second Nicene Council had by no means ended the dispute. On the contrary, after the death of Irene, in the ninth century, under the iconoclast Leo V and his successors – he was again not of Greek but of Armenian descent! – , there was a thirty-year **second phase of the iconoclastic dispute** (814-843), characterized by palace intrigue and changes of patriarch. Here the church hierarchy proved (with exceptions) to be tools of the emperor and fanatical monks who were greedy for privileges. In this phase, after the deposition and banishment of Nicephorus, the patriarch, who was in favour of icons and abbot of the Studios monastery in the capital, which he had restored, a major supporter of those in favour of icons was Theodore of Studios, who was backed by a well-organized monastic community utterly obedient to their abbot.

But it was once again under a woman, the Dowager Empress Theodora, a supporter of the monks and of icons, that the dispute was settled. She appointed Methodius, the monk, the new patriarch, and at a Synod of Constantinople in 843 the dispute was **finally settled in favour of icons**; bishops hostile to icons (as previously those in favour of them) were deposed. To commemorate this victory over this last of the great 'heresies', every year on the first Sunday in Lent the Orthodox Church still celebrates the **'Feast of Orthodoxy'**. Everything now seemed to have been achieved: the orthodoxy of faith and that of icons. But here too today we have to inquire into the cost of the dispute over icons – aesthetic, theological and political.

The theology of icons – critical questions

Since this time, **Orthodox icons** have certainly changed further, but have they changed very much more than the official Orthodox **theology**, which has been established as dogma since John of Damascus? Of course time and place of origin have their influence on the technique and motives of the icons and on the method and themes of theology. And just as historians of theology can distinguish different phases in the history of Eastern theology, so too art historians can distinguish different periods of Byzantine painting and mosaic art; finally, the Western Renaissance or Baroque have also influenced icon painting in Russia and in the Balkans. Nevertheless, apart from non-representational images, the **Byzantine style**, to which moreover present-day Orthodox works on the theology of icons refer, remains. Because of this continuing aesthetic influence of Byzantium and its successor churches, these images from the ancient Eastern church, governed though many of them are by the word of Holy Scripture, still seem very strange to some Westerners today: all too strict, all too archaic. But in the meantime – not least because of some exhibitions and publications – many Western prejudices against icons have disappeared. We now know that the icon painters – unlike Western artists since the Renaissance – were not concerned with the wealth of artistic inspiration in an artistic personality. Their art is not to be understood in the light of a Western principle of originality and individuality, of the kind that also became established in the nineteenth century in Russia, in the religious (often anti-church) art of a land which was already largely de-churched.

In Orthodoxy today not only dogmatic theology but also aesthetic composition is largely governed by canons, though this was not the case for many centuries. The doctrine of the church is defined once and for all by the seven ecumenical councils and the consensus of the early fathers, though later there were important further developments in theology and piety like Hesychasm, to which we shall be returning. The new – as in theology, so too in art – is usually suspect as *neoterismos*: novelty = heresy. Creative fantasies are tabu in both areas. Rather, standardized norms handed down over centuries without legal regulations are to be observed. Moreover, like theology, icons are to correspond precisely with the texts of the liturgy, where, for example, the birth of Jesus is said to have taken place in a cave (and not in a manger). Ideal types are to be preserved everywhere; this can happen in icon painting even if one painter paints, say, only the eyes and another only the hands of a figure.

Furthermore, icons are meant to **reproduce the heavenly archetypes, the divine originals**. They are to let the eternal significance of earthly figures shine through, like colourful mediaeval windows; twentieth-century Russian philosophers of religion have further reinforced the theory of images with its former Platonic stamp. This understanding explains the relatively constant symbolism of the colours and forms, the clothing and gestures, and above all the symbolic gold (yellow, ochre) as a constant background.[218] It explains the limitation to a two-dimensional depiction in which the original can be reflected, and conversely the ban on statuary which is strictly observed in Byzantine art, since originally this was probably too reminiscent of pagan divine images. It explains how painting icons becomes a religious art: not only does the artist pray and fast before beginning work, not only are colours and instruments blessed, but the finished painting is dedicated in a special liturgy and the identity of the image painted with the original is confirmed by the church. An icon is 'valid' only if it bears the name of the subject depicted or pictures a biblical scene.

It should now have become clear that icons are more than merely aesthetic exercises, and also more than pedagogical instruments for educating simple people. Rather, for the Orthodox, icons, along with proclamation of the word and celebration of the eucharist, are something like 'sacramentalia': a special form of the **communication of the believer with God**. That should also be understood in the West and not condemned. Nevertheless, questions arise over the traditionalism in art and theology, which should not be excluded from the ecumenical dialogue of the church.

First of all neo-Byzantine **aesthetics**: in the West, too, works of art from earlier periods in no way lose their value after a paradigm shift; in principle the old works retain their validity, for all authentic art has an abiding value which transcends time. But however much one treasures the 'old masters' in art, isn't an art which has remained in a particular period and is only more or less copied (like a theology which is handed down only more or less formally) perhaps an indication that a particular church and theology and thus a particular art has remained behind in a former era, in a former paradigm? This former paradigm need not totally be 'superseded'; no one today simply wants to abolish icons (or a traditional theology). But isn't there a danger that the old images and thinkers may lose their old content in a new time? The spirit of life and the life of the spirit cannot simply be borrowed from an earlier period.

So a question must be asked, not of the Eastern artist or theologian, to whom no one should a priori deny creative power (the great initiators of abstract modern art were the Russians Kandinsky and Malevič!), but of the church: doesn't this church reduce its great artists (and theologians) to superior copyists by its normative aesthetics and dogmatics? In a new entire constellation, 'old masters' can certainly preserve their artistic value for piety. But an 'old style' can be maintained in the production of art, whether neo-Gothic or neo-Byzantine, only at the price of fossilization. For in art (and theology) a crisis in time sooner or later leads to a crisis in style and this in turn to a change of style, though without excluding the adoption of old stylistic elements in a new time.

Then there are also direct questions to theology: as I indicated, there is the general question of the historicity of theology and its need for constant renewal. With the decisions in the iconoclastic dispute the development of the dogmatic structure of Eastern Orthodoxy came to an end and the form of liturgy and theology was given its essential stamp. Of course there are also interesting developments later, for example 'Hesychasm' in the realm of monasticism (especially on Athos).[219] This represents a form of mediaeval mysticism in the Eastern church demonstrable from the twelfth century on, which through a particular technique of breathing and incessant appeal to Jesus is meant to lead to *hesychia*, tranquil silence and the vision of the uncreated divine light. It was psychotechnically refined under Gregory Palamas in the fourteenth century and, with a technique of ecstatic vision which had also been thought through theologically, strove for the immediate vision of the divine energies of the threefold God. The writings of Palamas were condemned by two synods, but recognized as Orthodox from the time of the emperor John VI Cantacuzenus (middle of the fourteenth century). Both the Old Believers in their resistance against liturgical reform and the Startsy in the nineteenth century were inspired by Hesychasm. It was able to revive the **paradigm of Eastern Orthodoxy which was already established**, but hardly to change it in any decisive way.

The special question of **communio** also arises. Theologically the Orthodox Church attaches great importance to *koinonia*, fellowship. And in practice, in the community the Orthodox presbyter in fact often lives closer to his people than the Catholic cleric with his celibate life. But the iconostasis, the wall of images which arose in the Orthodox churches in the centuries after Nicaea II, like the Gothic screen in Western churches replacing a simple lower barrier, now introduced an unbiblical **separation of the community from the eucharistic table of the Lord,** a separation of priests and people, clergy and laity in the liturgy. Now the emperor was regarded as '*isapostolos*' ('like the apostles'), and was the only lay person to receive communion in both kinds behind the iconostasis – although the Trullan Synod in its sixty-ninth decree had maintained that the laity generally had this right.

Now is it not more of an Old Testament idea – however much Orthodox believers may have got used to particular theological justifications of this state of affairs – to separate the 'holy of holies' (interpreted as the image of heaven on earth) from the nave and the church people (the pilgrim church on earth)? As if the New Testament did not relate how the curtain before the Holy of Holies had been torn down, and by his offering Jesus Christ had opened free access to the Holy of Holies to all believers![220] The *koinonia*, the *communio* of believers with their Lord and with one another, should be celebrated in the eucharist. Therefore questions press in here about reforms which would be worth discussion at a pan-Orthodox synod.[221]

Questions for the Future

– A precisely regulated hierarchy of saints on the iconostasis separates the people from the clergy; shouldn't the question of a **liturgical reform**, of the kind that the Reformation Churches carried out with good reason in the sixteenth century and the Catholic Church – 400 years too late – then carried out in the twentieth century, also be discussed in the Orthodox Churches? The eucharistic table again close to the people in accordance with ancient tradition; the eucharist again celebrated in the sight of the whole congregation; the presbyter turned towards the people; Jesus' supper (and not the Jerusalem temple) as a model.

– Shouldn't the practice of the **veneration of icons** also be examined? Certainly it will be said that the iconostasis makes heaven appear on earth. But isn't a work made by human hands (even the holiest of works) still a human work? And in the view of theologians, doesn't even a holy image which has an ecclesiastical, indeed a liturgical, function, still remain a depiction, just as the finest mosaic or stained-glass window is only a reflection, since human hands cannot make the Holy itself appear? And isn't even the eucharist, where in the Orthodox Church the appearance of Christ with all his angels and saints is celebrated with particular solemnity, merely a representation and not an incarnation? So would a change to the earthly copy really be a change to the heavenly original itself?

– Even if in the West art and theology have undergone several epoch-making paradigm shifts, the Latin Christianity of the West since the Middle Ages has increasingly developed from a religion of hearing and following to a religion of seeing and touching. Isn't there a need in the Roman Catholic sphere, too, to subject phenomena of unenlightened religiosity like the cult of relics and supposedly miraculous images to a theological and pastoral examination?

The aim here is not an enlightened rationalism: of course the **notion of the icon** in Orthodox theology should **not be abandoned.**
– Orthodox theology and the church rightly attach importance to the biblical statement that human beings were created in God's image and likeness, and that they therefore carry God's icon within them.
– Rightly, no doctrine of original sin developed in the Byzantine world as it did in the West, where it leads to the view that the image of God in human beings was completely sullied and distorted because of sexual implications.
– Christ is rightly regarded not only as the Logos but also as the original likeness of God in which the original image of human beings is again to be renewed. So this belief in the divine pantocrator has rightly outlasted belief in the imperial autocrator – as will be demonstrated. But this also raises the question of the political cost of the iconoclastic dispute.

The victory of the monks

Is there one **victor** in the great dispute over icons? The victor was doubtless **monasticism**. It could increasingly evade the authority of patriarch and bishops, or monks could find their way to such leading offices. First, many of the monasteries which were ruined in the iconoclastic dispute were given to well-to-do clergy or laity to restore ('the coming ones'), though what was thought of as help in many cases all to easily became the exploitation of a benefice by the proprietor. But in the ninth and tenth centuries new monasteries were increasingly founded by the emperor and other well-to-do people, above all in Constantinople and then on Mount Athos. On this 'holy mountain' at that time a more or less independent 'monastic republic' developed whch now became the spiritual and church-political centre of Byzantine monasticism. This of course posed special problems.

For in the subsequent period the number of monks in Byzantium rose to around 100,000. This was an enormous proportion of the total population and was of course – because of the monks' privileged position (exemption from taxes) – a burden on the Byzantine state, which could hardly proceed against the monks by legal means. The monasteries became rich and increasingly extended their lands; abuses set in. Now monks were present all over Byzantine society as advisers, mentors and confessors.

Once again we should be clear that monasticism began as a charismatic, individual, private, lay movement on the periphery of the church. But now it regarded itself virtually as the inner core of the church (and thus also of the state). A **new monastic ideology** came into being, propagated above all by the perceptive and energetic abbot Theodore of the Studios monastery. Those who had formerly described themselves as the 'escapers' and the 'sons of the desert' now became the 'nerves of the church', indeed regarded themselves as the 'salt of the earth' or the 'light of the world'. For Theodore, the decisive feature of the gospel lies in renunciation and withdrawal from the world. And who can practise this with more perfection than the monks, while other people make compromises with the world and are marked by minimalism and often laxity? And although in principle there is also salvation outside monasticism, monasticism is now, according to this monastic view, utterly the norm of what is Christian.

No wonder that the monks now also felt that they were the guardians of true doctrine and the guides of the souls of the people, and that for Byzantium the Studios monastery functioned rather as a controlling authority for Orthodox faith and a place for forging bishops. Theodore of Studios, like some other monks, is venerated as a saint, while laity hardly ever achieve this honour. Monastic hagiographies in which the iconoclastic dispute was hardly mentioned came into fashion rather than theology; again, there are hardly any hagiographical lives of laity. Opposition groups like the Paulicians and the Bogomils, who though pious were hostile to the hierarchy and social revolutionaries, find no mention in them. But on the other hand it cannot be denied that monasticism in the East increasingly proved markedly critical of the state, or at least showed detachment from it.

Church and state – a real symphony?

Of course the victory of monasticism did not mean a revolution in the Byzantine state church. The **emperor** retained his strong position – particularly even over against the patriarch: he saw himself confirmed as the one who did the will of God. The **patriarch** and all his hierarchy remained dependent on the emperor – although in the context of his 'standing synod' in Constantinople he determined all the affairs of the church. Thus after the dispute over icons (847), the affectedly pious

Empress Theodora dared to nominate the zealous monk Ignatius as patriarch uncanonically (by-passing the synod); this led to endless disputes in Byzantium and with Rome and finally to a coup against Theodora (who was banished to a convent), the deportation of Ignatius and the election of the highly-educated Photius. Then Ignatius was appointed again (and later deposed again). Even so pre-eminently spiritual a patriarch as Photius twice suffered banishment in this complicated and difficult situation. Given this development it almost goes without saying that in the future the monks took the place of the intellectuals, just as they had taken over many sees and also the patriarchate. Indeed, alongside this 'pan-monasticism' the dispute over icons had a further consequence: the fact of 'heretical' emperors. So at a stroke the whole problem of the link established by Constantine, the 'symphony' of church and state, defined precisely by Justinian, became manifest.

But how must we evaluate this development? Did the Byzantine church perhaps prove victor over the state in the fight for its character, but succumb in the fight for its freedom? Did a complete fusion of state and church finally crown the process introduced by Justinian? This is the view of the Protestant church historian and historian of dogma, Adolf von Harnack,[222] and it is shared by many Western scholars. Or didn't the empire rather than the church prove victorious in this struggle? That is the view of the Orthodox theologian Alexander Schmemann,[223] who like Georg Ostrogorsky[224] before him put forward the opposite theory: late Byzantine theology was governed by that definition of the relationship between state and church which came into effect when Basil I the Macedonian presented it at the end of the tenth century in the *Epanagoge* (thought of as the introduction to a legal handbook): the positions of emperor and patriarch are parallel. The patriarch is the guardian of Orthodoxy and interprets doctrine; the emperor is required to be loyal to the Orthodox faith. Church and state did not need a legal demarcation of their spheres of action, since both were bound by the Orthodox faith. However, Anton Michel has pointed out that this scheme (an ideal one, evidently drafted by Photius) never became law,[225] and Schmemann, too, knows that in practice little was left of the theory of the dual rule (dyarchy) of emperor and patriarch: 'The completely arbitrary nature of state authority always still remained an incurable sore in the life of the church; even worse was the equally almost complete aceptance of this arbitrariness by the Church hierarchy.'[226]

It is evident that once church doctrine had completely become state doctrine, the church in fact no longer needed to set any limits to imperial authority. And once the emperor had become totally Orthodox, he himself needed to observe even fewer limits over against the church. The more clericalized the Byzantine state became (and everything took place in the name of the 'Christus Pantocrator', down to court ceremonial and the army), the more efficiently the emperor could also make definitions in church matters – where everything had not already been laid down in dogma. Whereas there were still important patriarchs in the iconoclastic dispute in the eighth and ninth centuries and the dispute with Rome in the eleventh century, the patriarchs of the subsequent period – with few exceptions – increasingly disappeared behind the splendour of the emperor. Moreover in this late period the frontiers of church and empire in any case largely coincided, since all non-Orthodox territories had been lost and all non-Orthodox dissidents had been excluded.

Here at the latest, **critical questions** arise about this Orthodox state-church system with its unity in duality which people sometimes described with the christological formula of Chalcedon 'unconfused and undivided'. They are put not in a confessionalist but in an ecumenical spirit, but they have another ecumenical side. For we shall see later – self-critically in connection with the Roman Catholic tradition – that the problems of the Western theocracy of the Popes, who wanted to subject the state to the church, were as serious as those of the Eastern theocracy of the emperors, who subjected the church to the state. Moreover these questions are not about anachronistic verdicts on a past system which in many respects was unavoidable and had performed a service, but questions for the future. They relate not only to the Byzantine church system but also to the Russian church system, and indeed any church system which presupposes a harmony with the state concerned.

Questions for the Future

– Doesn't a combination of church and state – Byzantine, Muscovite or whatever – almost of necessity lead to a supremacy of the state over the church and in the last resort to a capitulation of the church to the state?

– Don't a church and theology which are integrated into the state lose their prophetic function, which they need to have in society if they are to remain true to the gospel?

– Doesn't a state which is concerned less and less with the truth of faith than with the unity and peace of the empire tend towards a preservation of the status quo and the avoidance of any unrest? Isn't an orthodoxy of the church and the state a cradle of traditionalism?

But the history of the Hellenistic early church paradigm is not limited to Byzantium and the Greek world. We have to mention the mission of the Byzantine church in world history.

9. The Slavs between Byzantium and Rome

The migrations of the Germans from Eastern Europe and the expansion of the **Slavs** from their previous tribal territories between the Carpathians and the Dnieper took place early, between the fourth and the seventh centuries. In the West they penetrated as far as the Baltic and in the south to the Adriatic, the Balkans and Greece, where they destroyed the church organization. But they were slowly Christianized and in the process wooed by both Byzantium and Rome. That in itself shows that Christianization was always both a religious and a political matter.

Christianity as inculturation: the Slavonic liturgy

There is no doubt that the Christianization of the southern and eastern Slavonic peoples is the **epoch-making achievement of Byzantium.** Some of these peoples, who had been thrown back further and further beyond the Danube by Byzantium, but as early as 580 had flooded Greece with great hordes, had finally settled in the Roman provinces of Illyria, Mosia, Dacia, Thrace and Macedonia in the seventh century. And after the iconoclastic dispute, Byzantium was again so strong that in the ninth and tenth centuries it was able to develop a great mission among the Slavs, who were still an agricultural, farming people.

Byzantium, the new Rome: it appeared to all these 'barbarians' the queen of cities and centre of the world, embodying all possible wealth, art and culture. Its hospitality was famous, its diplomacy proven, its history and prehistory unique. It was here and not in ancient Rome that Graeco-Roman culture had survived down the centuries: Greek poetry, philosophy and science, and Roman law. No wonder that Byzantium in particular proved attractive to many pagan princes, above all its sacral monarchical state principle; some of the more lowly court titles were popular at a very early stage. For princes and for their subjects who were baptized at the same time, conversion to Christianity meant a transition from 'barbarianism' into world culture and the one ecumenical church, at whose head was the emperor as God's representative.

It was from **Byzantium**[227] that the Christianization took place of those **southern Slavs** who in the eighth century had invaded Greece, ravaged by the plague. There they were Hellenized and in the ninth century converted to Christianity. The Christianization of the **Bulgars** was particularly important. They received Christianity in 864 with the baptism of Khan Boris, who worked to have his own patriarchate and a church which was as autonomous as possible by means of a policy of steering between Rome and Byzantium; however, neither Rome nor Byzantium would allow this. In 870 Bulgaria was promised to the patriarchate of Constantinople, against the vigorous objections of the papal legates, by a conference of representatives of the Eastern patriarchates convened by the emperor in connection with the Council of Constantinople.

The two brothers **Methodius and Constantine** from Thessaloniki, which was surrounded by the Slavs, had already been working in Moravia since 863. As children they had learned Slavonic and were among the intellectual elite of Byzantium. Sent as missionaries by Patriarch Photius to Moravia, they were very successful because they used Slavonic – at the time only a peasants' language with no literature – in the liturgy and not Latin like the Franks or Greek like the other Byzantines. In deliberate contrast to current Byzantine practice, Greek linguistic arrogance and imperial demands, the brothers stood for the fundamental equality of all peoples before God and for free lands and monarchs bound together only by the spiritual affinity of the rulers of Europe.

It was Constantine, a scholar, philosopher and linguist, who, after the model of the Armenian Mashtotz-Mesrop, in a highly creative way invented the Old Slavonic (Glagolitic) alphabet, **the first Slavonic script**, with a view to what we would now call the 'inculturation of Christianity'. Both Gospels and liturgical texts were translated into Slavonic. Thus in Moravia and Pannonia the two brothers founded a mission independently of the East Franks with a **Slavonic liturgy**, which initially was given Roman approval for this territory which was still under Roman control.[228]

For Pope Hadrian II invited Constantine and Methodius to Rome during their interim stay in Venice *en route* to seek help in Constantinople, and against the opposition of the Bavarian and East Frankish bishops and the representatives of the 'three-language tradition', who recognized only the 'three sacred languages' Hebrew, Greek and Latin for the liturgy, took them under his protection. Constantine, seriously ill, entered a religious order in Rome, was given the name **Cyril** and died soon afterwards. Methodius, now ordained priest and consecrated Archbishop of Moravia and Pannonia in Rome, could not return to Moravia because of a change of rule and so worked in Pannonia, where he came up against vigorous resistance, especially from the Latinist Archbishop of Salzburg, who claimed this territory for himself. In 870 Methodius was even arrested, condemned and imprisoned until three years later Pope John VIII ordered his release. The Slavonic liturgy was at first banned, then allowed again with restrictions, and then wholly banned by Pope Stephen after Methodius' death in 885.

The immediate successors to Methodius and Cyril were driven out of Moravia, which remained in the kingdom of the East Franks under Frankish-Roman influence. But they found acceptance in newly converted Bulgaria, where the Glagolitic alphabet was now changed into the simpler Cyrillic and from there rapidly spread among the southern Slavs. Methodius and Cyril are therefore rightly called 'apostles and teachers of the Slavs'. Their efforts towards a Slavonic Christianity, which not least were also to benefit Russia, were to have world-historical significance. The foundations for a distinctive Byzantine Slavonic ecumene had been laid.

The Byzantine-Slavonic ecumene

Despite everything, the **Bulgars** achieved the autonomy that they wished under Czar Symeon (893-927), a grandson of Khan Boris. He had had a Greek education, and created a splendid Slavonic-Byzantine culture – Slavonic in language and Byzantine in spirit. He was the first Slavonic ruler to strive with all his might to become Emperor of Byzantium, and this was to result in the first great civil war in the Orthodox world. The rivalry between Bulgars and Greeks continued until after another cruel thirty years war. Bulgaria was reconquered by Emperor Basil II, the 'Bulgar-killer', and again wholly incorporated as a province into the Byzantine empire; however, it achieved new strength at the end of the twelfth century and even entered into a provisional coalition with Rome, until finally at the end of the fourteenth century the Bulgarian empire, too, fell under Turkish Islamic rule.

The Christianizing of the Bulgars also led to the Christianizing of the **Serbs** by Byzantium. These had already long been under the political and cultural influence of Bulgaria, but then they managed to gain their independence in 1077 under Prince Mikhail Voyislav. For political reasons they turned – provisionally – to Rome and even had a royal crown sent by Pope Gregory VII. But the Serbian rulers, too, sought the Byzantine crown in the subsequent period and after the Fourth Crusade in 1204 were granted autonomy for the Serbian church and ultimately also for the state by the Byzantine emperor.

The Christianizing of the **Rumanians** took place at the same time. The Rumanians not only derived from Romanized Dacians (thus the Ceaucescu ideology), but by language and the history of their settlement are related to the Wallachians and Aromuns, and probably for the most part immigrated only between the thirteenth and fifteenth centuries into the Danube delta, where they were under Bulgarian rule; so despite their romance language they adopted Church Slavonic as the language of their church, liturgy and diplomacy.

The one Slavonic world – but two paradigms

The fate of the Hungarians, the Western Slavs (Bohemia and Poland) and the western Southern Slavs (Croatia and Slovenia) was different. They were orientated, not on Byzantium but on the old **Rome**. They include:

– The **Hungarians**, originally Ugro-Finnish nomads from the steppes, from the region betwen the Don and the Dnieper, who sometimes penetrated as far as Central Greece. After their settlement and Christianization (Hungarian emissaries were baptized in Constantinople in 948) they remained incorporated into Western Roman Christianity. This position was sealed by St Stephen I (997-1038), who had himself crowned king with a crown sent by the Pope in 1001.

– The Western Slavonic **Bohemians**. In the ninth century they were Christianized under the Przemyslids of Regensburg and in 973/76 were given Prague as their bishopric. They adopted the Latin alphabet and Latin as a liturgical language.

– The **Poles**, also Western Slavonic, between the Vistula and the Oder, united under the Piast dynasty. In the tenth century, under Count Miezko, they joined the Catholic Christianity of the West; this was marked by the baptism of the Count and the establishment of the mission see of Poznan in 966. Under Boleslav I Chrobry, Poland became a member of the Roman empire of Otto III and dominated the Christianized Slavonic world (for a time as far as Kiev). At a very early stage it had its own national church, the Archbishopric of Gniezno, which was founded in 999/100. The Poles also remained orientated on the Latin West in alphabet and liturgical language.

– Finally the Southern Slavonic **Croats** (and **Slovenes**). Their territory, the Roman province of Illyria, had already been assigned ecclesiastically by Emperor Heracleius in the seventh century to the Pope as the patriarch of the West; but Illyricum remained a constant bone of contention between Rome, Byzantium and the Frankish imperial church (the bishops of Salzburg and Passau also claimed jurisdiction over Pannonia and Illyria). Croats and Slovenes had now been Christianized and also Latinized from the West above all since Frankish rule in the ninth century. Under Prince Tomislav (910-928), who took the title king, they definitively detached themselves from Byzantine supremacy and thus – unlike the Serbs – remained in the sphere of influence of Romano-Germanic culture.

Of course in subsequent centuries there were many further shifts in frontiers and spheres of influence, which need not concern us here. But the fate of later southern Slavia = Yugoslavia was fundamentally decided as early as the ninth century by a permanent bisection, and unfortunately not just a *laissez-faire* one. On the contrary, the arrival of Greek missionaries in Bulgaria and Moravia led to a battle between the Latin and the Greek churches over the mission to the Slavs, which was finally to be accompanied by a vigorous dispute between the Pope (Nicolas I) and the Byzantine patriarch (Photius), which we shall be discussing later.

The consequence is that from that time we are confronted with the **division of the Slavonic world between the Byzantine and the Roman church**, between cultures with a Greek Byzantine and a Germanic Roman stamp, in which **two completely different paradigms** are now emerging: the early church Hellenistic and the mediaeval Roman Catholic. Here the mission area of Moravia and Hungary was under Rome – despite some links with Byzantium – but the great Bulgarian church with its own patriarch remained bound to Byzantium, as in the long run did also the Serbian church. The effects of this polarization between Rome and Byzantium can be traced to the present day, and indeed have become especially virulent in the post-Communist era. For the different church developments – different alphabets, different liturgical and literary languages, and thus also different cultures – have had an effect to the present day on the ethnic, political and cultural identities and antagonisms of the southern Slavs. The current conflicts over nationality cannot be understood without taking note of this frontier between Eastern Rome and Western Rome which has existed for almost a millennium.

But the development of the **eastern Slavonic tribes** who had penetrated as far as the Black Sea coast, who even attacked Constantinople in 860 and then built up the **Russian empire**, were to be very much more significant for world history.

Kiev: the first phase of Russian history

In the ninth century, under the Rurikids – the first Russian ruling family of which there is evidence in history, who derive from the Norman-Swedish Varingians – the eastern Slavonic tribes of Rus had gained their independence from the eastern people of the steppes in the **kingdom of Kiev**.[229] A legend which came into being at the end of the tenth century describes how the apostle Andrew went through Russia on his way to Rome, but no direct claims to church rights were derived from it (as they were in Byzantium in reaction to Rome).[230] Like a first conversion of leading nobility around the middle of the ninth century, the baptism of Princess Olga of Kiev at first remained an episode. But in 988 her grandson Prince Vladimir, who sought a lasting ideological foundation for his country after victory in a bloody civil war, brought Russia into the community of Christian peoples. He was baptized and married a Byzantine princess ('born to the purple') and there was a mass baptism of the population of Kiev in the waters of the Dnieper.[231]

Like the baptism of the Bulgars previously, that of the Russians was thus also a well-considered affair of state aimed at the **entry of Russia into the Christian tradition of the civilized world.** So in Russia, too, Christianity not only grew from below but was finally imposed from above; immediately after his baptism Vladimir set to work building hospitals and houses for the poor, and establishing a juster state system. But for a long time Christianity remained something more for the political and religious elite; the people often kept to their own pagan views and practices. Given this situation we can understand how some Russian historians have adopted a critical attitude to Kiev Christianity, for which more recent scholars like G.Fedotov[232] have then attempted to compensate by describing the Kiev period as the 'golden days of childhood', as 'a model, a golden mean, a royal road of Russian Christianity'.

Russia, too, had connections with Rome at the latest from the eleventh century and had to choose between the Hellenistic Byzantine and the Latin Roman paradigm. It chose the Byzantine paradigm in its Slavonic form. This meant two things:

– On the one hand Russia adopted **Slavonic in its liturgy and as a literary language,** though contrary to legend Methodius and Cyril were never in Russia: doubtless Bulgaria in particular exerted a strong influence here.

– On the other hand, Russia fitted into the **Byzantine church organization** under the Patriarch of Constantinople. The Patriarch nominated the Metropolitan of Kiev and all Russia, whose church extended from the northern forests to the Carpathians and from the Baltic to the lower Volga. In the first 250 years of Russian church history up to the beginning of Tatar rule he had a defining influence on the Russian metropolis, though this was not without its tensions. For only twice down the centuries were the Metropolitans of Kiev Russian;[233] otherwise they were always Greeks, who usually brought their own clergy, artists and diplomats with them. But unlike the Bulgars and Serbs, the Russians were never formally members of the Byzantine empire, so no political struggles for autonomy disturbed the relgous, emotional and cultural ties between Russia and Byzantium. Vladimir's embassy to Constantinople in 987 had already brought back a fascinating report about Byzantium: about the beauty of Hagia Sophia and the Byzantine liturgy with its intimations of God's presence. Vladimir himself even experienced the superiority of

Byzantine 'philosophy' by hearing the address of a Greek philosopher or theologian in Kiev. And this admiration was to continue in the future.

There is no doubt that the Kiev period is not, as was sometimes thought, just a prelude, but the first significant phase of the history of Russia and its Christianity. Moreover – as we heard – historians have attempted to present it as a 'golden age': a period of the saints (above all Boris and Gleb, the two sons of Vladimir murdered by their brother) and the famous Crypt Monastery in Kiev. This was founded by St Antony and organized by the holy abbot Feodosy (Theodosius, died 1074) in accordance with the rules of the Byzantine Studios monastery. It became the school for Russian clergy (more than fifty bishops) and the spiritual centre of the kingdom of Kiev. At the least we can say that in Russia from the beginning Christianity had a strong **monastic** stamp (what was asked for was Byzantine saintly life rather than Byzantine theology), and in the spirit of the Byzantium of the time it also had a markedly **traditionalist** orientation. But here at the same time there was evidence of a 'symphony' between church and state in which the church with its Christian ideas at first exercised leadership, although the pagan Slavs (like the Germans) already had a sacral kingdom.

There is also no doubt that this epoch-making development also led to a powerful extension of the cultural sphere of Byzantium itself. Now Greek architects were building countless churches like the cathedral of St Sophia in Kiev, adorned with mosaics. Byzantines established schools and founded cities in Russia, resulting in a time of marked cultural expansion immediately before the West-East schism under Vladimir's son, the educated Jaroslav the Wise (1019-1054). Jaroslav had numerous Byzantine books translated by a whole team, so that his reign is identical with the beginnings of Russian historiography and literature. At the time of the Mongol invasion (1240) Russia already had sixteen dioceses.

Our **conclusion** must be that at the end of the first millennium the process of Europeanizing and Christianizing the peoples and states of the Southern and Eastern Slavonic peoples had essentially been completed by Byzantium, even if the history of these states – sometimes independent, sometimes not – remained extraordinarily varied. Thus the cultural cohesion of Slavonic Christianity was to be severely shaken by the Mongol onslaught of the thirteenth century, which extended from Asia right to the edge of Central Europe, while the Byzantine empire itself was only marginally affected.

Now in the context of our paradigm analysis it would make little sense to give a detailed account of the many vicissitudes in the fate of the Slavonic peoples and the Byzantine empire: all the developments from the early Byzantine through the middle Byzantine to the late Byzantine phase.

Here was an empire which time and again experienced a political and cultural hey-day (the blossoming of Byzantine art and literature under the Macedonian dynasty in 867-1056 and especially under the Paleologi, 1259-1453), but was entangled in constant controversies along its long frontiers and from the eleventh century was increasingly to be forced on the defensive by the advance of the Muslim Turks in the East and the Normans in the West, by the revolts of the Slavs and finally the 'Crusades' of the Latins.

However, what is indispensable for an understanding of present-day confrontations is a more precise analysis of that conflict in world history into which the old and the new Rome, the Rome of the Popes and the Rome of the emperors, were to be drawn. For none of the political antagonisms between Byzantium and the Slavonic realms (above all the Bulgarians and the Serbs) ever destroyed the unity of Orthodoxy with its Byzantine stamp, which also remained the paradigm of the Slavonic churches. But the conflict between Byzantium and Rome with all its political implications was finally grounded in the shaping of two very different paradigms of Christanity. It went correspondingly deep, burst apart the unity of the church and thus led to a schism between East and West which has still not been mended. We need to understand this.

10. How the split between the Eastern and Western churches came about

If we want to understand the almost ineradicable aversion of countless Eastern Christians to Rome, which is grounded in a long history and again became virulent in 1989, we must know the various factors which led to the East-West schism. For the Catholic and Orthodox churches, coping with the past is not just a theological and dogmatic but primarily a historical and psychological problem. A historical survey – of events which will be more than familiar to Slavonic and Byzantine scholars – is necessary.[234]

The gradual alienation

It may sound surprising, but the schism between the Eastern and Western churches cannot really be dated. There is no individual date of separation, but there is a long history of separation. So the Russian Orthodox theologian John Meyendorff, Professor of Church History and Patristics at St Vladimir's Orthodox Seminary in New York, who died all too prematurely, was right when he stated: 'All historians today are agreed that East and West separated on the basis of a **progressive** alienation which coincided with the equally **progressive** growth of papal authority.'[235] And Francis Dvornik, the Catholic historian from Washington, who is probably the greatest expert on the genesis of the East-West schism, remarked: 'In considering the development of the relationship between Byzantium and the papacy and its position in the church, we must recognize that for the Byzantine mentality the extension of the absolute and direct authority of the Pope over all bishops and faithful, as preached by the reformers (of the eleventh century), went against the tradition which was familiar to Byzantium.'[236]

The description of the varied history of the Slavonic peoples has already indicated that their split is the product of a paradigm shift in the West. And in fact the more time went on, the more clearly everything led to the formation of **two different paradigms of Christianity** in Rome and Byzantium: a new, Latin, Roman Catholic paradigm (P III, which we shall have to investigate separately) alongside the existing early church paradigm (P II) of which Byzantium is to be regarded as the heir.

It is certainly undeniable that the East, too, by becoming increasingly Graecized since Justinian, in its way contributed to the special formation of the two earlier shared paradigms and thus to the alienation between them. Thus the Greek elites – in contrast to Cyril and Methodius, the apostles to the Slavs – constantly refused to speak Latin or even, in Syria or Egypt, Eastern (and now also 'heretical') vernaculars. Consequently resentment against Byzantium was nurtured everywhere. The following are to be noted as important factors of alienation:

- the different **languages** in the Western and Eastern churches: they often led to mutual spiritual and cultural encapsulation and to numerous misunderstandings, even extending to theological terminology. Even a highly educated Pope like Gregory the Great (590-604), formerly ambassador in Constantinople, could not speak Greek, while the Byzantine patriarchs had no command of Latin. In communication they were constantly dependent on translators, secretaries and experts;
- the different **cultures** with different spiritual values and attitudes: the Greeks seemed to the Latins arrogant, pernickety and deceitful, while to the Greeks the Latins seemed uneducated and barbaric; there was either misinformation or no information at all about new developments on the other side;
- the different 'rites': for the Easterners they did not represent just a different liturgical ceremonial but a whole independent form of church life and faith with equal rights, embracing theology, worship, piety, church law, constitution and organization. Despite a shared dogma,

these liturgical 'rites', including the liturgical calendar, the cult of the saints and forms of piety and that religious feeling which is so important generally, had a divergent development from the fifth century on. In the Eastern church the sacrament of penance remained reserved for the monks. To the Latins the bearded married Orthodox clergy were alien, while the Easterners regarded with abhorrence the clean-shaven celibate Latin priests.

But did these cultural, religious and then also social and psychological factors necessitate a division? By no means. Rather, certain **church-political factors** were **decisive** here. Granted, in the often extremely confusing church controversies both Rome and Byzantium offered numerous provocations and engaged in diplomatic manoeuvres which could have been avoided. But what was decisive was probably what Meyendorff has called the 'progressive growth of papal authority', which has been felt threatening by the church in the East down to our day, despite its recognition of Rome as the first patriarchate in Christianity. This is confirmed from a present-day perspective by Francis Dvornik, who has dispelled many Western prejudices against the Constantinopolitan patriarch Photius: 'One may with full justification claim that today the only serious hindrance to a wider convergence between the Orthodox Churches and the Catholic Church lies in the question of the Roman primate. The other obstacles, above all the difference in rites and liturgical formulae, which played so large a role in the Greek and Latin polemical literature from the eleventh to the fifteenth centuries, can be said to have been overcome.'[237]

Certainly the East, too (as we saw), transformed its ecclesiology under the influence of Hellenistic thought more than it was aware of doing, and thus increasingly became independent. But a monarchical absolutistic centralized uniform church of the kind that was slowly forming in the West had been rejected in the East from the beginning as an innovation. The Eastern (and African!) understanding of the church never began from a universal bishop but from the *koinonia*, the communion of believers, from the local churches and their bishops. They did not have such a fixation on the legal aspect as the Romans. It was not canon law but sacraments, liturgy, symbols of faith that stood at the centre of a church which understood itself as a collegially ordered, federal communion of churches.

Certainly the Patriarch of Constantinople was now increasingly active as his own canonical authority, since after the seventh ecumenical council the East recognized no further ecumenical councils. A Byzantine law of decretals had begun to develop, and it was then followed, as in the West, by a science of church law (canonistics) which in part was highly developed. But we must always concede that the church of the East, which also understood itself as the **church of the 'seven councils'** (from Nicaea I in 325 to Nicaea II in 787), preserved the original church order far more strongly than the Western church. In matters of church order the Christianity of the East has the New Testament far more on its side than does the Roman church of the West. And the Reformation churches of the West also returned later to some basic elements of this church order.

However, the more time went on, the less people wanted to know anything about this earlier church order. The concern there was to establish the Roman primacy over all churches with all the means of canon law, politics and theology, and thus to establish a centralistic church system in the East as well, tailored to Rome and the Pope. The signals between the Eastern and Western churches began increasingly to be set for alienation, tension and division. And it is part of the psychological and historical process of coping with the past so needed today between Rome and Byzantium that we should remember **three phases of alienation** and address them in all historical honesty and fairness. So first of all let us look back – in the interest of a future ecumenical understanding – and then forward:

Phase 1: New Rome against Old Rome (fourth-fifth centuries)

Had the Roman emperors remained by the Tiber, the Bishops of Rome would not have been able to develop their political power in such an imperialistic way. But now the emperor had gone to the 'new Rome', and 'old Rome', for so long unconquerable, was to become the victim of that new political world constellation connected with the migrations of the Germans. In 410, for the first time since its early history, Rome was seized and plundered for three whole days – by the armies of the Germanic leader of the West Goths, Alaric. What a tremendous, almost apocalyptic event! Rome wiped out as a state and administrative centre! Many pagans said that this was the gods' punishment of a Rome which had become Christian. Many Christians said that it was God's punishment of the ancient Rome which was pagan or had still remained pagan. Who was right?

But hadn't what 'Rome' meant long been replaced according to the wise plan of providence by the new, second, now Christian Rome? That is how things looked above all in Byzantium. But in the West people saw this differently, as we shall discover in a later context (P III). Byzantium and its claims were increasingly ignored by Rome, quite deliberately. And the Bishops of Rome did all they could to fill the power vacuum which had come about through the confusions of the migrations in the West with their own power.

Increasingly with reference to a 'primacy' of Peter, the concern was to legitimate and perceive Rome's claim to leadershp in church and politics – to the point of levying taxes. In the eyes of Byzantium, which was usually preoccupied in other directions, this naturally looked like obstruction – of the one legitimate imperial authority. At any rate, East and West understood each other less and less and **began mutually to dispute the claim of the church to political leadership.**

– Attempts were made from **old Rome** to carry through the **principle of the papal church** which had already led to a first rupture between East and West at the Synod of Sardica in 342. But only at the end of the fifth century did a Pope like Gelasius I claim supreme and unconditional priestly authority over the whole church, completely independent of imperial power.

– By contrast **new Rome** – often also with means which were not particularly choosy – uncompromisingly defended the **principle of the imperial church.** This was further strengthened in the sixth and seventh centuries in the West, where attempts were made to impose it uncompromisingly. Thus because of their traditional understanding of their office the emperors Justinian (in the 'Three Chapters Dispute' in the sixth century) and Constans II (in the Monotheletic dispute of the seventh century) simply imprisoned recalcitrant Popes and transported them to Constantinople, where they compelled them to obey the imperial will in both political and dogmatic matters. There is no trace anywhere here of an infallibility of the Roman Pope. The conflict led to a first climax.

Phase 2: A German as emperor and the Photian schism (eighth-ninth centuries)

Imperial treason, betrayal of state and church – that is what many people were exclaiming in the East in the eighth century. What had happened? Pope Stephen II had travelled to the court of **Pepin, king of the Franks,** to have himself guaranteed a church state at the expense of former Byzantine territories ('The Donation of Pepin', 754). But that was a blatant offence against the political unity of Christianity, which had hitherto been maintained as sacrosanct. For the Pope was now also acting as a political ruler over a territory which previously had been simply and solely that of the emperor. Moreover, for purely political ends the Pope had turned to the barbarians, the enemies of the empire.

The political break became definitive when, on his own authority, a good fifty years later Pope Leo III also took a decisive step further: he autocratically bestowed the **title emperor** – hitherto reserved for the Emperor of Byzantium (and his representatives) on a barbarian ruler, Charles King of the Franks, in St Peter's in Rome on Christmas Eve, 800, a date which later became famous. We can see here with Byzantine eyes (P II) what we shall later see with Latin eyes (P III): a barbarian ruler had now been crowned Emperor of Rome by the Bishop of Rome as though there were no longer a Roman emperor. The consequence was that by the Pope's grace a new, Western, Germanic emperor stood alongside and confronted the sole legitimate Roman emperor in the East. A Germanic sacral state sanctioned by the papacy now rivalled the Byzantine saving state. In Byzantine eyes, Rome had thus finally become heretical, a view which many Eastern Christians, including theologians, maintain to the present day.

The political break was to follow the church break a few decades later, in the middle of the ninth century. The extremely complicated events after the iconoclastic dispute, involving the two patriarchs Ignatius and Photius, who have already been mentioned, need not be described here.[238] Be this as it may, after the dismissal of the monk Ignatius (successor to Methodius), who had similarly been nominated patriarch in uncanonical fashion by the Empress Theodora, in the end a scholar who was the head of the imperial chancellery, **Photius**, had been elected patriarch. He was a layman who had to be consecrated to all the ministries within five days. This gave Pope **Nicholas I** (whose understanding of his office was probably inspired by the Pseudo-Isidorian forgeries) the pretext of advancing the papal claim to rule over Illyricum (which Emperor Leo III had handed to Byzantium in the eighth century because of the weakness of Rome) and the Eastern church generally. He had a Roman synod declare the Byzantine patriarch deposed out of hand in 867, and a synod in Byzantium responded to this by deposing the Pope: this was the **Photian Schism**.

More recent Western research into Photius by V.Grumel, F.Dvornik, H.-G.Beck and many others has brought to light the spiritual stature of someone who was much vilified in the West: Photius was an excellent philologist, with a good knowledge of patristics and exegesis, the author of a great many biblical commentaries, theological writings and a lexicon of ancient authors and biblical writings. He was not a deliberate schismatic but a theologian and churchman who was also recognized by his opponents. In addition he was a bishop who thought pastorally and was not afraid of others; he played a decisive part in the dissemination of Christian faith among the Chasars, Bulgarians, Moravians and Russians, and moreover is still venerated in the East as a saint. Photius recognized the traditional Roman primacy (without rights of jurisdiction in the other patriarchates), sought reunion with the Armenians and was also behind the mission of his friend Cyril and Cyril's brother Methodius and the Bulgarian mission. He must not in any way be presented as an illegitimate counterpart to the Pope. Basically he was simply making a resolute defence of the traditional patriarchal Eastern Roman autonomy against the Western Roman patriarch's completely centralized jurisdictional understanding of primacy which had developed in the meantime and which was manifest in the excesses of the Frankish mission in Bulgaria and Pope Nicolas I's contempt for Greek customs. What was happening here?

In an encyclical issuing an invitation to a synod in Constantinople, Photius had summed up the points of dispute with Rome. In addition to the celibate priesthood there was also mention for the first time of a dogmatic dispute. Photius showed himself alarmed at an **addition to the Creed** by Roman missionaries in Bulgaria: in the article on the Holy Spirit, in fact first in Spain (above all at the Synod of Toledo, in 675, which countered Arianizing tendencies among upper-class Western Goths[239]), the formulation '**and** the Son' (*filioque*) had begun to be added, contrary to the original text of the Niceno-Constantinopolitan Creed: 'the Spirit who proceeds from the Father **and the Son**'. Charlemagne had already forced Pope Leo II to accept this expansion, and it had spread throughout the West after the Synod of Aix in 809. But it was Henry II who at his coronation in Rome (*c*.1013) first caused *filioque* also to be used there. What lay behind this Latin doctrine of two principles? We shall see this more closely in the framework of the Latin paradigm (P III): no more and no less than a different view of the Trinity. For the **East** it was a principle of unity, the one God and **Father**; for the **West**, however, it was the one divine **nature** common to the three persons.[240]

But shortly after the council of 867 dramatic events began to accumulate: Pope Nicholas I died without hearing of his condemnation by Byzantium. Emperor Michael III was murdered, and the usurper Basil I the Macedonian overthrew Photius in order to win over the conservative circles in Byzantium and the new Pope Hadrian II, reappointing Ignatius. A further Council of Constantinople in 869/70 with only 12 bishops at the beginning and only 103 at the end – completely under the control of papal legates – excommunicated and banished Photius. But he retained the support of the great majority of bishops, was finally recalled from exile, appointed the prince's tutor and reconciled with Ignatius – in the face of all the difficulties with Rome. Hardly had Ignatius died in 877 than

Photius again became patriarch, and at the **Council of Constantinople in 879/80** was splendidly rehabilitated with the participation of 373 bishops. The anti-Photian council of 869/70 was repealed, so that even in the West, up to the end of the eleventh century this was not counted as one of the ecumenical councils. The Pope, now John VIII, explicitly recognized the pro-Photian council of 879/80 as did subsequent popes for more than 200 years – down to the Gregorian reform in the eleventh century. At that time Gregorian canon lawyers in the investiture dispute unearthed and evaluated canon 22 of the anti-Photian council of 869/70 against the German emperors, so that the West had an interest in counting this particular council as the eighth ecumenical council, though of course no one in the East went along with that. However, at the council of 879/80 a wise compromise was resolved on: the traditional Roman primacy was recognized for the West, but all papal jurisdiction was repudiated for the East. At the same time the original text of the Creed (without the *filioque*) was endorsed.

However, the Byzantine church's confidence in Rome, which had previously been always treated with respect, was persistently shaken. And ingratitude was the world's reward in Constantinople as well: during his second patriarchate Photius had generously tried to achieve reconciliation with all his opponents, but was forced to resign by the next emperor, Leo V – his pupil, who then made his own sixteen-year-old brother patriarch. Photius died in exile in Armenia in 891. This was a sign that not only in the church of the old Rome but also in that of the new Rome imperial power politics and intrigue continued uninhibitedly. However, anyone in the West who criticizes the system of political Orthodoxy in the East should at the same time criticize that system of theologized Roman policy which – after the complete downfall of the papacy in the tenth century (the *saeculum obscurum*) – was to break through fully in the eleventh century.

Phase 3: Excommunication, scholasticism and the Crusades (eleventh-twelfth centuries)

Around the middle of the eleventh century a papacy reformed by the German emperors and thus reinforced could embark on a new trial of strength with Constantinople. In view of the threat to southern Italy from the Normans, which had been sparked off by the Arabs, both the Roman Pope and the Byzantine emperor were at that time very interested in a military alliance and a theological understanding. But new tensions were developing. The Norman campaign of the German reform Pope Leo IX and the Roman interventions in the Byzantine provinces in southern Italy (the replacement of the Greek liturgy with the Latin liturgy) were followed by heated reactions from the patriarch **Cerularius** of Constantinople (1043-1058), which sparked off a new dispute. A sharp letter from Archbishop Basil of Ochris went the rounds attacking the liturgical customs of the Franks (Latins), above all the use of unleavened bread (*azymes*) at the eucharist, Saturday fasting in Lent and similar ritual differences. The *filioque* was not mentioned. At the same time Cerularius threatened with closure those Latin churches in Constantinople which did not adopt the Greek rite.

As ill fortune would have it, this theologically uneducated and immoderate patriarch found an equally immoderate and theologically prejudiced counterpart in the leader of the Roman delegation to Constantinople, Cardinal **Humbert** of Silva Candida. He had already replied with cutting sharpness to the letter against the 'Franks' in a 'Dialogue between a Roman and a Constantinopolitan'. For this papal legate was a passionate advocate of the Cluniac reform movement and the leading theoretician of an absolutist papal rule, the doubtful foundations of which we shall hear about later.

On arrival Humbert challenged the right of the ecumenical patriarch to his title, even doubted the validity of his consecration and indeed agitated against him publicly. He insulted a Studite monk who defended Eastern customs by saying that he had not come from his monastery but from a brothel, and also introduced the *filioque* into the conversation as if the Byzantines and not the Latins had changed something in the Creed. And when he understandably got nowhere with the negotiations, although in the meantime he had heard of the death of the Pope, Humbert himself composed a **bull of excommunication** against 'Bishop' Cerularius and his helpers. He put this on the altar of Hagia Sophia on 16 July 1054 and departed with his delegation. The bull simply teemed with false and incorrect assertions (for example about the ordination of priests and the wearing of beards) and of course in return provoked a ban in return from the patriarch against the cardinal and his entourage (not against the Pope).

So instead of an alliance between Rome and Byzantium there was a **breach.** Today attempts are made to play down this fatal event as far as possible, not least for ecumenical reasons; it was not really the churches which excommunicated each other but individuals. But from now on the name of the Pope was no longer mentioned in the Byzantine liturgy, and in Constantinople the churches for those who spoke Latin remained closed. There is no mistaking the fact that although later the two parties constantly had dealings with each other and could have achieved peace, the break between the Eastern and Western churches was beyond repair.

The old Byzantine and the new papal ideas of rule over the world were now mutually exclusive. After that the Popes regarded the Greek church as separated from Rome, schismatic and also heretical.

As early as the end of the Byzantine exarchate of Ravenna (751), and after the 'Donation of Pepin' (754), the Pope ceased to see himself as the emperor's subject. The Gregorian reform, which already began before Leo IX with the German popes in the old Rome (Hildebrand, later to become Gregory VII, had been appointed with Humbert to the Roman Curia by Leo IX), on the one hand and the completely different Latin scholastic theology on the other cemented the split. In the West, although here too a Christian theocracy prevailed, a paradigm which was completely different from that of the early (and not just the Byzantine) church had broken through, a specifically Roman Catholic paradigm (P III). 'The Roman church recognized a new political ideology which was very different from that which was increasingly coming to prevail in the East. There was hardly any chance that a compromise could be arrived at between the two ideologies.'[241] But there was still hope of an understanding on both sides.

However, the nadir of mutual relations was still to come: the **Crusades**, which began towards the end of the eleventh century. They offered Rome the opportunity not only of forcing back Islam, which meanwhile had begun to pose a threat, but also of bringing Illyricum (the greater part of the Balkans!) and the insubordinate church of Byzantium under papal supremacy. Previously there had been acts of violence on both sides. But now there was a favourable opportunity of compelling unity, if need be by military means, since all appeals and negotiations had been useless. For the Byzantine emperor, threatened simultaneously by the Normans in southern Italy and the Turkish Seljuks in Asia Minor, was dependent on the Pope's help, but at the same time wanted to maintain the autonomy of the Orthodox Church in matters of dogma, rite and church organization. Thus his problem was 'how to find the right balance between military help from the West mediated through the Pope and the return of the Byzantine church to obedience to the Roman see which was asked for in exchange'.[242]

So Emperor Alexius I Comnenus co-operated with Pope Urban II in organizing the First Crusade (which assembled in Constantinople!), without suspecting that this would soon threaten the system of political Orthodoxy from within. For very soon Emperor and Pope lost control of the course of events, and under the influence of Norman politics the Crusades against Islam soon also became Crusades against Byzantium, which in the West, because of a good deal of disinformation, was customarily but wrongly accused of 'treachery'. So we should have no illusions: up to the present day it is a trauma for Eastern Christianity that the Pope accepted leadership of a 'holy war' with countless cruel atrocities, a war against Islam which then also became a war against its Eastern sister church. Rome achieved a mighty triumph – but at the price of a nadir in its relationship with the Western and Eastern churches. In 1204, on the **Fourth Crusade, Constantinople was conquered and plundered by the troops of the Latin West**. If we look at this once again with Byzantine eyes:

– The emperor (who alone was legitimate for Byzantium) and the Patriarch of Constantinople (who had equal rights with the Pope, the patriarch of the West) were expelled from the city to Nicaea in the territory of Asia Minor ('the Nicene empire').

– Against all justice a Latin emperor (Count Baldwin of Flanders was crowned emperor of Byzantium!) was installed in Byzantium, along with a Latin patriarchate and a Latin hierarchy with a parallel structure.

– All Greek clergy were forced to take an oath of obedience to Rome, and thus the conquered territories were largely Latinized.

– Through a Roman cardinal the crusading Pope Innocent III had Ivan Kalojan crowned 'emperor of the Bulgars and the Wallachians (Rumanians)'.

The Byzantine emperor, hard pressed in his search for allies, gave **autonomy** to the **Serbian church** at that time, and made Sava, a monk from Mount Athos and brother of the first king of Serbia, its archbishop. Moreover to the present day St Sava is venerated as the father of Serbian Orthodoxy and the Serbian state. It was only in 1261 that the Byzantine rump state of Nicaea, which was completely disorganized both militarily and economically, was able to reoccupy Constantinople.

Is reunion possible?

Only in 1204 did the split between Rome and Byzantium become irrevocable, so that any notion of a long-term reunion of the Christian church was ruined. Rome itself had decisively undermined its own bulwark in the East. The later attempts at union, made by Popes and weak Byzantine emperors – the Second Council of Lyons in 1274 and the Council of Ferrara-Florence in 1438/39[243] – did not have religious but political motivation: because of the danger from the Turks and the financial crisis they had been striven for above all by the emperor in the face of the church people of Byzantium and the majority of the hierarchy. In the East they were felt to be total capitulation to Rome, and that was also the view from Rome. They accentuated the schism instead of doing away with it, plunged Byzantium into internal conflict, and because of the compromises agreed on shook its credibility throughout Slavonic Christianity. In the subsequent period people grew so accustomed to the schism that it was no longer really felt to be a split in the church but the natural status quo; this allowed each side to perceive the other only as a caricature of itself.

However, after the 'Council of Union' in Florence no one could have guessed that it would be more than 500 years before another serious attempt would be made at an understanding between Rome and the Eastern churches. In fact the Christianity of our century – after the tireless and indefatigable preliminary work of ecumenical theologians on both the Catholic and the Orthodox side – is indebted first of all to Pope John XXIII and the Second Vatican Council (1962-65), and then to Pope Paul VI and Patriarch Athenagoras of Constantinople, for coming to terms with the passionate history of the centuries of alienation and the 900-year old separation and at least in part arriving at an understanding and a *modus vivendi*. And precisely because the present Polish Pope has again irresponsibly rekindled the differences after the collapse of Soviet power through his short-sighted Roman 'missionary policy' in Russia, Bulgaria and the Ukraine, here, in an ecumenical spirit of understanding, some critical but hopeful questions need to be formulated for a better future:

Questions for the Future

– If according to Vatican II

the difference between churches does not weaken, but strengthens, unity;

the churches of the East have the same rights as those of the West;

the churches of the East have the right and the duty to cultivate their own independent liturgy, legal order and spirituality:

couldn't this in principle be a basis for a new church fellowship between West and East?

– If according to Vatican II

the old rights and privileges of the patriarchs of the Eastern churches are to be restored and in particular they are to nominate bishops:

couldn't the problem of Roman primacy, so long an issue between West and East, also at last be discussed, and an ecumenical solution be put forward on the basis of the seven ecumenical councils accepted by both sides and the consensus of the early fathers?

- If the compromise of the Council of Constantinople in 879/80 was accepted even by Rome for many centuries, couldn't this also point the way forward for today: the Roman legal primacy could be accepted for the West, but for the East any papal jurisdiction could be rejected as it always as been, and the original text of the creed (without the later addition of the *filioque*) could be endorsed.

- If at the end of the Second Vatican Council, on 7 December 1965, the mutual excommunication was 'blotted out of the memory of the church' and the schism was regretted by Pope Paul VI and Patriarch Athenagoras, wouldn't it have been logical long ago to follow up the lifting of the sentences of excommunication with the restoration of communion?

But at that time Byzantium was condemned to a slow death. And in retrospect we may ask: wasn't the Byzantine ideal of a neo-Roman universal rule of the world, given by God himself, exaggerated from the start? Didn't it have to come to grief on the limited possibilities for action in this empire?

Byzantium at an end, but not Orthodoxy

Alain Ducellier, one of the greatest experts in Byzantine history and culture, sees the basis for the 'dull dissatisfaction which runs through the history of the Eastern empire like a scarlet thread' grounded in this tension between **boundless ideal and inadequate political possibilities.** But he also states, perhaps not wholly without admiration: 'Orthodoxy as a Christian commonwealth sees its ideal of earthly perfection almost always compromised by a refractory reality, but nevertheless never puts in question its goal of a world rule which is given by God himself. Not even in the blackest moments of its history can Orthodoxy concede that in the meantime this or that claim has become completely untenable, that this or that territory has been lost for ever.'[244]

At all events, the state-church transformation of the early church Hellenistic paradigm of Christianity has been able to sustain itself over more than a thousand years, although Byzantium constantly had to adapt itself to changed political situations and thus continually seek a new centre and new limits to its power.[245] Whereas Byzantium under Justinian had been a Mediterranean power, in its hey-day it became a Eurasian power, and then an Aegean power. In its final phase it was concentrated on a kingdom limited to Constantinople and the Peloponnese.

In this final phase Byzantium was utterly dependent on the help of the West. But this help did not come – despite the church union proclaimed in

Florence. The West was too disunited, Rome was too uncommitted, Byzantium itself was too exhausted, paralysed and burdened with resentment of the Latins. It was no help to anyone that in the face of the manifest preparations for war by the energetic young Sultan Muhammad II, the Pope sent to Constantinople Cardinal Isidore, who, five months before its fall, proclaimed union with Rome and celebrated a Latin mass in Hagia Sophia, to the indignation of the Byzantine clergy and people. At best this appealed to the circles which preferred a union to Rome to an understanding with the Turks. The siege by an army almost ten times stronger, with artillery of improved range (thanks to Western engineers), lasted seven weeks. One needs to read the history of the **capture of Byzantium** and the death of the Byzantine emperor in battle, which is still unexplained today, as described in detail by an expert like the British Byzantine scholar Steven Runciman, to get a concrete impression of the drama of this world-historical event.[246] 29 May 1453 saw the fall of the Second Rome, protected by its unique situation and fortifications. After about 1100 years, the work of Constantine the Great found its sorry end with Constantine XI. Tremendous wealth and art treasures, church vessels, icons and manuscripts beyond price fell victim to the plundering, which lasted three days and three nights before the sultan himself made his triumphant entry.

A natural centre, now called Istanbul, held together the European and Asian possessions of the Ottoman empire, a Turkish empire which reached from Mesopotamia to the Adriatic, and to which the rest of the Balkan lands were soon to be subjected. However, for Christianity, after its early loss of the Christian heartlands in Near East and Africa, now the great Eastern bulwark of Byzantium had fallen victim to Islam. The anti-Byzantine policy of the Roman see over centuries bears a substantial part of the blame for this fall. The mistrust and antipathy of the Easterners to Rome and the Latins was total after the fall of Constantinople. Against all the Latin proselytism, throughout the following centuries people constantly repeated the slogan of the time. 'Better death than Rome!' 'Better the turban than the mitre!'

Now comes the amazing thing: the end of Byzantium was by no means the end of the Hellenistic early church paradigm. For this paradigm (P II) in no way perished, as the Jewish Christian paradigm (P I) had before it. On the contrary: Orthodox faith and Eastern Christianity, so different from Latin Christianity, held Greeks, southern and eastern Slavs together in the 'dark centuries' which now followed and preserved them from being dissolved into Islam (remember the Christian communities of the Near East and North Africa). No, the Hellenistic early church paradigm, first of all fully supported by ancient Rome, with its political and religious traditions, was now taken over by a new empire – of course with considerable changes and adaptations: this was the Russian empire, based on Moscow, which slowly but steadily developed into the great guardian of Orthodoxy, above all in the Balkans. There – in the second, Muscovite period of Russian history – it was again to show its vitality.

11. The Third Rome: Moscow

A similar hatred of Rome spread later from Byzantium into **Russia**.[247] Here the role of the **Latin Order of Teutonic Knights** is often underestimated. During the Tatar period this offered military protection on the flanks to the mission among the Baltic tribes, which led to territorial frontier battles with the Orthodox principalities of Novgorod and Pskov. The invasions of the **Catholic Poles** were already more serious; in the time of the 'troubles' (*smuta*) in 1605 these even occupied Moscow. The Poles tried to take over leadership of the Moscow empire and subject the Russian Orthodox Church to the rule of Poland and thus of Rome. It is tragic to see how John Paul II's re-evangelization campaign has rekindled the controversies over the church in the Ukraine, and the appointment of Latin bishops in Russia has again revived such memories, so that the Slavonic Pope in particular (like some aggressive American missionary sects) is proving a serious hindrance to any understanding with Slavonic Orthodoxy.

In the view of the East, over the centuries Rome did all that it could to undermine and weaken the two great bulwarks of Christianity against the non-Christian Arabs, Turks and Mongols: first the Byzantine empire, the Second Rome, and then the Moscow empire, the Third Rome. But what were the developments in Russia? We must not – like some modern historians – look at Russian history only from predominantly economic, social and political perspectives. Whatever may be retained of the significance of the idea of a Third Rome for the beginnings of the Russian state ideology – which certainly also had an increasingly nationalist inspiration – we must not forget how great the religious and cultural influence of Byzantium was. At any rate for almost five hundred years (988-1448) Russia was a church province of the Patriarchate of Constantinople. And there were far fewer changes in the church of Russia with its Byzantine stamp than in the Russian state (which was also increasingly influenced by the West).

Moscow: the second phase of Russian history

For more than two hundred years, from 1240 to 1447, Russia, which had already been Christianized for so long – we might recall the Kiev empire –

was under the **rule of the Mongol Tatars.**[248] It began with Batu, the grandson of the Genghis Khan who in 1206 united all the Mongol tribes including the Tatars under his rule and founded a world empire of 'the Golden Family' extending as far as the Black Sea. Batu was a nephew of the new Great Khan Ugudei, and as ruler of the Western empire had taken it upon himself to implement the resolution of the Mongol imperial assembly of 1236. This was that Russia, Poland, Hungary and the whole of Europe were to be conquered. Batu and his hordes of cavalry succeeded first in destroying the Volga Bulgars and seizing some minor Russian principalities (including Moscow). Then in 1240 Russia's nominal capital Kiev fell, so that breakthroughs into Poland, Silesia and Hungary could follow. Only the sudden death of the Great Khan led Batu to withdraw, so the rest of Europe was spared the Mongol assault – unlike the proud Islamic empire of the Caliph of Baghdad, which was to fall in 1258.

But Russia itself remained for two centuries under the rule of the Tatars. Granted, the unity of Old Russia no longer existed, but the church was still there. And beyond doubt in the thirteenth and fourteenth centuries it was above all the Orthodox **Church** which at this time of political dissolution, economic decline and cultural collapse kept alive the awareness of the **national unity of Russia.** Since then, being Russian has meant being Orthodox – and this has had an effect right down to the present day. Be this as it may, the Mongol rule of force was at first mainly limited to the demands for tokens of obedience, the payment of tribute and contingents of troops. So the church at least could continue its activity and develop its spiritual and theological tradition. Indeed, later it would even start missionary activity along the lines of Methodius and Cyril; this was done above all by **Stephan,** Bishop of Perm (*c*.1340-1396), the most significant missionary of the Russian church, among the East-Finnish Syrjans, after careful preparation, with the help of a runic script. Here the church of Russia still regarded itself as part of the Byzantine ecumene, and the admiration of the Russians for Byzantium, already very weakened, was unbroken. Not only the Grand Princes of Kiev, as before, but now also the Russian princelings among the barbarian army in fact regarded themselves as younger members (nephews) of the imperial family.

But why in this emergency didn't Russia turn to the West, with which it had connections above all through Novgorod and the Hanseatic cities on the Baltic? The answer is that the Grand Prince of Novgorod, **Alexander Nevsky** (1252–1263), the ancestor of the Moscow dynasty, preferred the pagan rule of the Tatars to an orientation on the Latin West – for religious reasons. For Alexander feared that Rome would exploit the opportunity to force the allegedly 'schismatic' Russia under its authority. And we need only read the letter of the lawyer Pope Innocent IV addressed to him[249] to see that this fear was no idle fancy. Alexander, who was on diplomatic visits to pay homage to the Khans of the Golden Horde, turned against the Western invaders from the beginning and inflicted heavy defeats on the Swedes, the order of Teutonic Knights and the Lithuanians. So to the present day he is honoured as a national saint and as a symbol of the defence of Russia against the West. He resolutely secured the demarcation of the Russian Orthodox world from the Western world, although of course Russia always wanted to belong to Europe and not to Asia. Alexander was one of the first Old Russian princes to have himself consecrated monk before his death.

Kiev was far from having recovered from the Tatar onslaught, and the focal point of Russia shifted to the north-east, where – after an intermediate phase in Vladimir – the princes of **Moscow** in the fourteenth century, not without bloodshed, formed a new political power centre. The second, Muscovite phase of Russian history had thus begun, and now the church leadership, after disputes among the metropolitans, moved from Kiev to Moscow. Here an important role was played by Russia's greatest saint, **Sergei** of Radonezh (1314–1392). Originally a recluse, he attracted companions, and finally at a due distance from Moscow, in the Russian 'wilderness' he founded the Monastery of the Trinity (near the later Sergei Pasad, renamed Zagorsk in 1920 by the Communists but now Sergei Pasad again). This was soon to become Russia's largest monastery. With its ascetic spirituality, it also became a model for many other monasteries (around 180 of them), which in the next 150 years also began to take care of those farmers who were very slowly starting to cut down the Russian forests. Sergei, a friend of the Grand Princes of Moscow, dedicated himself to a new union of the country under the leadership of Moscow and in 1380 – through a letter of blessing to Grand Duke Dimitri – he made a decisive contribution to the very first victory of the Russians over the Tatars at the battle of Schnepfenfeld. This victory shattered the Tatar rule, which had seemed so unconquerable, and considerably raised the prestige of Moscow and the Russian national consciousness. But Sergei rejected the dignity of metropolitan. He was not a politician by nature, but remained a man of the spirit and faith, who even as abbot lived in poverty and continued to engage in physical work. So he proved to be an authentic starets (= elder), a spiritual leader who was an exemplary embodiment of the ideals of Russian holiness: simplicity, humility, compassion, social and national commitment.

And such ideals were desperately needed, for Russian history had its dark side, which, also according to Russian experts, is all too often concealed by Orthodox and non-Orthodox admirers of Russian

Orthodoxy. From earliest times an underground **'second culture' of old Slavonic paganism** had persisted among the Russian people beneath the Byzantine Christian culture and liturgy; as one of the most important Russian theologians of our day, George Florovsky, put it: beneath the 'Christian "day" culture' of the spirit and the intellect lay a '"night" culture which concealed itself too long and too stubbornly, which evaded examination, verification and purification through "thought"' and was mainly responsible for the 'unhealthiness of the development of the old Russia'.[250]

In addition there were then the two centuries of **Tatar enslavement**, during which the Russian princes gave tokens of Slavonic submission to the Tatar Khans and every Russian had to bow as a Tatar rode by. As A. Schmemann explains, the consequence for Russian society was a "Tatarism" – a lack of principle and a repulsive combination of prostration before the strong with oppression of everything weak' which 'unfortunately marked the growth of Moscow and the Muscovite culture right from the very beginning'.[251] And he adds that in the face of this dark world of superstition, alcoholism, dissipation, barbarism and violence, the monasteries above all (where now great libraries had also been built up) embodied a counter-reality, a counter-reality of absolute, holy values with the possibility of repentance, purification and renewal: 'The monastery is not the crown of the Christian world, but on the contrary, its inner judgment seat and accuser, the light shining in the darkness.'[252]

The new stronghold of Orthodoxy

So in the fifteenth century Moscow was the undisputed centre of the great Russian kingdom, and now also the centre of a Russian art stamped by Italian architects in church building (the Uspenski Cathedral in the Kremlin), painting (Theophanus the Greek) and iconography (Rublev's icon of the Trinity). Byzantine forms and norms were adapted to the Russian character. But above all Moscow now became the new stronghold of Orthodoxy, which was soon to free itself from the domination of Constantinople.

The time for that came in 1438–39 when at the **Council of Ferrara – Florence** Byzantium accepted a union with its old rival Rome. This was short-lived (Constantinople fell fourteen years later), and as we heard, it was a measure never really accepted in the Byzantine church. However, in Russia, where people had been brought up by Byzantium to hate Rome, in deep disillusionment the event was seen as a sheer betrayal of the cause of Orthodoxy.[253] And when Metropolitan Isidore of Kiev and all Russia, a Greek and a prominent member of the union party, who had gone to the council against the wishes of the Grand Prince (Eugene IV[254]), returned and made a solemn entry into Moscow with a Latin cross in order to read out the documents of the union at the liturgy, Grand Prince Vassily had him summarily arrested and thrown into prison. In any case, people in Moscow would have nothing of an 'eighth council' after the seven ecumenical councils. Isidore was later able to escape, was made cardinal in Rome and died as Latin Patriarch of Constantinople – in Rome. But in 1448, probably at the desire of the Grand Prince, Bishop Iona of Rayazan was elected Metropolitan of Kiev and all Russia without any permission from the Patriarch of Constantinople, who remained in union with Rome; from now on Russia chose its own metropolitan.

But the separation from Byzantium, which had now become 'heretical', and which in the Russian view had forfeited the right to leadership of Eastern Orthodoxy by its 'betrayal' of the true faith, did not become a schism. As soon as orderly conditions returned in Constantinople/Istanbul after 1453, the Russian church made efforts to normalize relationships. But it left no doubt that from now on it regarded itself as an '**autocephalous church**', that is, it claimed its 'own head'. That was understandable in church-political terms. But at the same time the Russian church paid a high price for this step: the definitive subjection of the church to the Russian state, which did not remain uninfluenced by Western nationalistic thought. In contrast to earlier times under Byzantine, supra-national authority, the church was now subject to every kind of political manipulation by the rulers in its own country.

All this explains why after the fall of Constantinople in 1453 Moscow (although for another 140 years it was a metropolis and not a patriarchate) not only had an interest in entering into the heritage of Byzantium as far as possible, in time **taking over the leadership of Eastern Orthodoxy** (though making no universalistic claim), but was also politically prepared for this in both church and state. For in Russian eyes it could be no coincidence that Byzantium fell at the precise moment when Russia freed itself from the last traces of Tatar rule. And no one could fail to overlook the fact that after the subjection of yet further 'Orthodox' countries (Bulgaria, Serbia and Rumania) by the Islamic Turks, in the second half of the fifteenth century Russia was now left as the last politically independent power of the Christian East. Had not the fall of Byzantium to be seen as divine punishment for the union with Rome? Moscow began to understand and then to take up its historical 'mission'.[255]

It was then Grand Duke **Ivan III** (1462–1505) who took the decisive step here: by marrying Zoe (Sophia), the niece of the last Roman emperor, who had fallen at the capture of Byzantium. She had fled to Rome and the plan was hatched in the Vatican, in order to win over Russia for the Union.[256] However, it had precisely the opposite effect. Granted, historians argue over how far Ivan, who was already under the influence of the Western European states, formally entered into **the heritage of Constantinople** in 1472. At all events he now came before the Byzantine (or Habsburg) imperial nobility in Russian state heraldry. And now he proudly called himself 'self-ruler' (= *autocrator*), as the lords of Byzantium had once proudly done. For Ivan, the title 'Czar (= Emperor, Caesar) of all Russia' became particularly important and was confirmed by the Patriarch of Constantinople – although Czar had been used very much earlier for king/emperor (*basileus*).

There is no doubt that in all this Ivan, the one who united Russia, had no thought of union with Rome, although Russia always understood itself as part of Europe. Italian Renaissance artists made their way to Moscow (Italian architects rebuilt the Moscow Kremlin), but not Catholic prelates. On the contrary, Moscow now increasingly saw itself as the new Byzantium or – as it was then called for the first time by the monk Philotheus of Pskov (around 1510) – the **third Rome**. Philotheus, who applied the apocalyptic Daniel prophecy of the last of the great world empires to Moscow, saw history through Russian eyes like this: 'All Christian czardoms have come to an end and according to the prophetic books entered into the Czardom of our ruler, the Russian Czardom. For two Romes have fallen and the third stands fast. A fourth there cannot be.'[257] The first Rome? That had fallen into the hands of the barbarians and become heretical. The second Rome? That had succumbed to heresy through the Council of Florence and was now in the possession of the pagans. Moscow was now the last centre of Orthodoxy and thus the only right-believing Christianity. This idea became popular much later. Then it was the nineteenth-century Slavophiles and above all their political 'sons', the pan-Slavists, who activated the idea of the third Rome. Here was the foundation for no small part of the Russian messianism which kept breaking through later, and of course could also be all too easily secularized.

And what about Constantinople? Moscow was soon able to secure the recognition of its independence from Constantinople. In 1589 the Russian Metropolitan Job was appointed '**patriarch** of Moscow and all Russia' – by Patriarch Jeremias II of Constantinople, who made a special journey to Moscow for the purpose. But there was one thing that Moscow did not achieve, a change in the hierarchy of patriarchates. It did not become, as it wished, the third patriarchate (after Rome and Constantinople), but for ever remains the last of the six patriarchates. This did not prevent Moscow from not only taking over but also accentuating the

Byzantium ideology.[258] For on the one hand the Byzantine state and imperial ideology linked Moscow with Byzantium, and on the other the Muscovite ideology attributed to the **Czars** as God's representatives not only a wealth of uncontrolled power over the state but also (in contrast to Byzantium) a wealth of in practice uncontrollable **power over the church**.

We should note that in Constantinople the patriarch had still been able to reprove the emperor for deviating from church teaching and the moral law; and in the Kiev period the Metropolitan of Kiev and All Russia still had considerable independence from the local rulers by virtue of his nomination by the Patriarch of Constantinople. But from the beginning the Metropolitan of Moscow and All Russia, who since 1448 had been elected by the local Moscow synod, was under the direct control of the Grand Princes and then the Czars. At the same time criticism of the church increased. Even in the time of Ivan III the close connection between state and church, including the execution and torture of 'heretics', was affirmed in the great controversy between the strict abbot Joseph (Sanin) of Volotsk, administrator of the monastic lands (the leader of the party of the 'possessors') and Nil Sorsky (the representative of the party of 'those without possessions'). However, the limits of the obedience of subjects to the Czars were also emphasized.[259] Sometimes Asiatic Mongolian traits as well as Byzantine traits emerged in the rule of the Czars, who had taken over some brutal customs of the Tatars (for example flogging); at the same time, everyday life was markedly ritualized by the constant repetition of religious formulae, gestures, prostrations and so on.

But in the face of the mass murder and mass transportations, the confiscation of goods and plundering under Ivan IV the Terrible – equalled only by Stalin – in 1568, had not the Metropolitan of Moscow, Philip, finally dared to protest publicly during the liturgy? Certainly. But what were the consequences? The Czar removed him from office, indeed had him arrested and finally murdered by his own henchmen, so that to the present day Metropolitan Philip is venerated as a martyr. Indeed, when his relics were ceremonially brought to Moscow, the Czar asked for forgiveness for the sin of his predecessor. Even later there were still public protests against the ruler in this now largely totalitarian system, to which everything and everyone was subjected, virtually ruling out any self-criticism. The **church** was now **part of the state**, which did all it could to centralize the church, too, even its liturgical texts, chronicles and administration, in Moscow, and even to collect the most famous icons from all over Russia in the Kremlin church.[260]

The question arises: doesn't the transition from Byzantine to Russian Christianity represent a large-scale paradigm shift? Historians say that aspects of legitimacy and renewal were bound up with the transference of imperial rule (**translatio imperii**). But can one speak of renewal in respect of Russian Christianity?

Even through Russia – no paradigm shift

There is no doubt that the political and cultural changes connected with the rise of Russia and its Orthodox Church were considerable. But in the religious, church dimension – and we are dealing with Christianity here – amazing continuities are evident. If we again use as a basis the three components of Byzantine society worked out by Ostrogorsky, the following complex picture emerges:

- The **Roman political tradition** was not taken over in Russia. Russia was never part of the Roman–Byzantine empire. Granted, Ivan III already adopted the title 'Caesar', acted in a centralistic and absolutist way, and also behaved as if he were lord over the church. But as 'Czar of all Russia' he did not make any universal, ecumenical claim. To this degree there was no question of a Third Rome. Here **discontinuity** becomes evident: a **Roman–Byzantine universal state** became a **Russian national state**.

- **Greek language and education** were not introduced in Russia (as say, Latin was in France). Certainly numerous translations of church texts were made from Greek into Slavonic, but Hellenistic-'pagan' educational material (apart from collections of sayings) and especially classical Greek philosophy were not accepted. Indeed in Russia, up to the early Enlightenment, which came from the West (second half of the seventeenth century), Greek and Latin were virtually unknown. Here too **discontinuity** is evident; Russia took over only **Byzantine Christian religion** without **Greek-Hellenistic** civilization.

- By contrast, in Russia **Orthodox Christian faith** was taken over from Byzantium. Granted, here, too, there were certain changes of detail, above all conditioned by the Slavonic language. But on the whole in Russia **dogma, liturgy, theology, discipline and piety continued to have a Byzantine stamp**. Thus in the understanding of Christian faith and life a fundamental **continuity** between Byzantium and Moscow was evident. There was:

- the same Orthodox tradition of the church;
- the same theology of the seven ecumenical councils and the early fathers;
- the same world of monks and icons.

That means that on the way from Byzantium to Russia, **Christianity did not undergo any paradigm shift**. Rather, Russia essentially **took over the Hellenistic Byzantine paradigm (P II)** and adapted it in a more or less organic development to its own social and political conditions.

But because now in the second millennium Christianity had largely assumed a traditionalistic character in Byzantium – indeed everything was already strongly canonized, from dogmas and prayers to morals and icons – in Russia, too, **from the beginning the Orthodox paradigm had a markedly traditionalistic and monastic character:**
– liturgical texts as in Byzantium;
– hagiographies as models for some biographies of saints in the Byzantine spirit;
– ascetic and spiritual literature in the Byzantine style;
– monasteries everywhere as strongholds of conservatism.

So everywhere it was simply a matter of going by the well-tried past and preserving what existed. It was a matter of observing certain rules and practising rituals which were always the same – all this very much more than in the Western Middle Ages, as we shall see. There was no call for creativity and criticism, innovative thought and knowledge, communicated through books and printing houses (the first printing house in Moscow was at first closed again, and the two printers were accused of heresy). Unexplained circumstances led to the printers leaving Moscow in 1565 and beginning work again in Poland–Lithuania.

That makes the question all the more urgent; why in Russia did no one, as in the West, raise the question how things had originally been in the church? Why did no one in Russia demand a 'root and branch reform' when this was being called for in Germany? Why did no one refer to the Bible as the critical norm for church tradition, with the aim of reforming this tradition? In a word, why was there in general no Reformation in Orthodoxy?

Why no Reformation in Orthodoxy?

To some Orthodox the very question of a Reformation might seem quite out of place, almost blasphemous. Isn't the Orthodox Church the old, original church of the apostles? Has it allowed itself innovations and aberrations like the papal church of the Middle Ages (P III)? But it may help to survey present-day problems if we first of all consider the relationship of Orthodoxy to the Protestant Reformation (P IV) in historical perspective and ask why the Protestant Reformation (and Counter-Reformation) stopped at the frontiers of Russia and the Turkish empire. Different perspectives need to be taken into account.

First, can a church reform itself which is not free but is oppressed by the state, especially when the state rulers are of another religion? We should be clear that except in Russia, the Orthodox Church had come completely **under the rule of an alien religion,** Islam.[261] The very first Patriarch of Constantinople after the conquest of the city, Gennadius Scholarius, a theologian and monk hostile to union, was elected by the bishops but appointed by the sultan – now in place of the emperor – completely in accordance with Byzantine ceremonial. Of course this situation did not only have disadvantages. For the sultan, who as a Muslim did not separate religion and politics, the patriarch as supreme head of all Christians in the Ottoman empire was at the same time a political leader. That explains why the Patriarch of Constantinople was not only the religious head of the Orthodox Church, indeed of all the Orthodox churches (in part with their own patriarchates) under Muslim supremacy, but also at the same time the civil head of the Greek nation. In this way the Greek world had its own religious and political organization, which moreover was maintained in Turkey until the year 1923. Thus the Greek nation could survive for four centuries under Turkish supremacy. However, despite everything, considerable problems arose for the church.

Certainly the Muslims were considerably more tolerant towards the Christians than the Christians of the Reformation period were towards one another. Christians, according to the Qur'an 'people of the book', who had received their own revelation through the great prophet Jesus, were not to be persecuted. So the Muslim rulers largely left the church untouched as long as it proved to be politically compliant. But at the same time, in practice there were many abuses and much discrimination: the sultans required a large sum of money from each new patriarch, gave the patriarchate to the highest bidder, and often deposed or appointed patriarchs for purely financial considerations. The newly elected patriarchs for their part attempted to exact the sums of money they had to pay from their bishops, who in turn extracted them from their clergy and people. Christians, who were not required to convert, but had to pay a poll tax and wear different clothing, were clearly second-class citizens under Islamic law, who could not marry Muslim women, make converts or have posts in the army. Only their own conversion to Islam could have relieved them of the constant social pressure and decisively improved their social status. Doesn't that make it understandable how a church in such a battle for survival should have concentrated on its own tradition and be disinclined to make any fundamental change? The churches of Orthodoxy now truly had other concerns than internal reform.

Secondly, can one church (the Protestant) communicate reformation to another church (the Orthodox) if it has itself so little understanding of the different paradigm? At any rate initially, on the Reformation side there were **illusions** about the possibility of transferring the new Protestant paradigm to the Eastern churches. For Luther and the Reformation had much sympathy for the Orthodox churches – and not just on the basis of a shared opposition to Rome. Like other humanists, Melanchthon and Calvin in particular were stamped with a love of Hellenism and felt solidarity with the church suffering under the Turkish yoke. Melanchthon had a Greek translation of the Augsburg Confession made as early as 1530. But relations between the Reformation churches and those of Orthodoxy were not at all developed.[262] Most of the Orthodox churches, persisting in a relatively low level of education, did all they could to ward off the influences of the great church revolution in Germany and Europe, so that individual contacts were limited to humanistic scholars and clergy on their travels, to students in the West and diplomats above all in Istanbul.

Is it any wonder that in these circumstances attempts at approaches to the Orthodox churches of Turkey (Anatolia) on the part of the Jesuits and the papal missionary authority Propaganda Fide in the sixteenth century also remained unsuccessful? So did the correspondence from the two professors Jacob Andreae and Martin Crusius, who in 1573 on behalf of the **Protestant Faculty of Tübingen** made contact with **Patriarch Jeremias II** through the Protestant embassy preacher Stephan Gerlach and finally presented him with the Greek version of the Augsburg Confession mentioned earlier.[263] They, too, did not succeed in convincing the patriarch of the necessity of this teaching for salvation. Rather, he persisted in the almost scholastic argumentation of the Orthodox tradition – the different evaluation of which is 'the fundamental difference between Tübingen and Constantinople',[264] and ended the correspondence after three written answers (1576/79/81) with the request that there should be no more writing about doctrines but at most out of friendship. Already in the last two decades of the existence of the Byzantine empire people in Constantinople had to grapple with the theology of Thomas and the influence of scholastic thought.

The concentration of the Protestant dialogue partners on the themes of scripture and tradition, freedom of the will and grace, sacraments and prayers to the saints, made it clear that they were arguing from a completely different paradigm (P IV), which at that time was incomprehensible to Orthodoxy (we shall have to discuss this at length later). Later the patriarch of Constantinople, **Cyril Lukaris,** was the only one to attempt to reform Orthodoxy in accordance with Calvin's teaching, in the face of a Roman threat (Union of Brest); in 1629 he sent to Geneva an 'Anatolian Confession of Christian Faith' which was regarded as Calvinistic. But he finally fell victim to wide-ranging intrigue. Falsely denounced for political high treason by the man who was later to succeed him, he was strangled on the Sultan's orders in 1638.[265] A condemnation of the Confession followed at the synod of Jerusalem in 1672, the last synod of the Anatolian church before 1923.

Thirdly, can a church critically examine its own tradition if it has no criterion for this examination? As we heard, the Russian church of the Kiev period had taken over the Orthodox paradigm from its mother church of Byzantium in a highly consolidated state, and the Russian church of the Muscovite period also had an utterly traditionalist orientation. Everything **Russian** (for example the 'dogma' of wearing beards, which was similarly taken over from Byzantium) was regarded as **Orthodox** and everything **foreign** as **heretical.** Moreover the shaving off of beards was condemned by a synod under Ivan IV the Terrible and punished with refusal of Christian burial.

Indeed even a slight change in the liturgy was regarded as sacrilege by people and clergy. In the seventeeth century the powerful **Patriarch Nikon** attempted a radical return, not to the gospel but to the Greek model, and a restoration of the old 'Greek laws', to show, in accordance with the will of the Czar, that Moscow was clearly the Third Rome, the new capital of the Orthodox world.[266] But when at the Council of Moscow in 1667 the patriarch attempted a reform of corrupt liturgical texts and an alteration to some liturgical customs, there was a passionate unrest among the Russian people. This was in contrast to, say, the Ukraine, where people, literate and accustomed to dealing with printed books, went along without any great difficulty. Although Nikon, who attempted to set his patriarchal authority over the Czar, was finally deposed, the people worried in an almost apocalyptic way about the **infallibility of the old Russian tradition.** For, it was thought, if there should be errors and disfigurements in the holy tradition of Moscow, this last bulwark of Orthodoxy, one almost had to believe the Antichrist was coming!

No, no one had any idea that in the church of Jesus Christ everything had once been completely different. The Russian view of history did not make use of a critical comparison of then and now, but transfigured and perpetuated tradition. The **Bible** did not play **any normative role** for an innovative theology or a church practice which needed to be reformed. So even the reformers did not have any ultimately normative criterion for a reform of the tradition. And the 'Old Believers' ('Staroverzy') who were hostile to reform did not shrink even from schism;[267] despite harsh state persecutions, executions and forcible conversions – the death of their champion, the proto-pope Avvakum, at the stake – they could not be exterminated. Thinking in terms of a salvation history and not a critical history, they felt that the Russian words and rites were important not just as externals but as the Orthodox faith itself, and bore witness to this in some circumstances even by setting light to themselves. It is in keeping with this, however, that the Russian pastoral clergy in this phase were generally ignorant, in other words less capable of being spiritual pastors than sacramental functionaries, even if from the seventeenth century on efforts were made to improve their education.

Nevertheless, this development was not an inevitable one. That is shown by the history of the Orthodox under the Roman Catholic domination of Poland–Lithuania in the Ukraine and in White Russia.

The special role of the Ukraine

After the move of the Metropolitan to Moscow, the Orthodox outside the Moscow empire formed an **independent hierarchy**.[268] As a result of their need constantly to fight for equal rights with the Catholic ruler and in the imperial parliament (*sejm*), the Orthodox **laity** developed considerable self-awareness here. To further their aims they combined with the clergy in brotherhoods. These maintained schools and printing houses, supervised the life-style of their members and fought for the preservation and renewal of Orthodoxy locally. They took part in synods for the election of bishops and to regulate church life.

There was no **rigid traditionalism** nor any xenophobia after the Moscow fashion. They quite naturally went to Catholic and Protestant universities in Western and Central Europe, grappled with Western ideas and took over much which seemed to them to be compatible with Orthodox faith. They often revised their liturgical books – without the traditionalistic reaction there was in Russia.

So theologically they maintained quite a high level. In constant dialogue with Roman Catholic and Reformed theology they learned from both, above all about form and style of argument, but in principle remained loyal to the Orthodox tradition. They negotiated over church union with both the Catholics and the Reformed. The **union** with Rome on the basis of the union council of Ferrara-Florence which took place in Brest-Litovsk in 1596 was primarily a matter for the bishops and senior clergy; the people, above all the brotherhoods, were for the most part opposed to it. Only later did the union become something like a 'third confession' in the spirit of the Roman Catholic paradigm. By contrast, in 1699 there was a confederation of the Orthodox with the Reformed on the basis of an eighteen-point programme which recognized the supreme authority of the Bible; the Reformed did not require further concessions or changes!

The most prominent representative of this West Russian Orthodoxy was Petru Movila, in Ukrainian **Petro Mohyla** and in Russian Petr Mogila (c.1595-1647), the son of a Rumanian priest who had a Western education. As early as 1631/32, as abbot of the Crypt Monastery of Kiev he founded a college. As Metropolitan of Kiev from 1633, he indefatigably worked for the reform of the church, and held annual synods in which clergy and laity took part. The Kiev General Synod of 1640 approved a draft catechism presented by him which achieved pan-Orthodox recognition two years later in Jassy.

However, soon after Mohyla's death the **Muscovite conquest** of the Western territories began: White Russia in 1654, East Ukraine in 1659, Kiev and Smolensk in 1667, West Ukraine apart from Galicia in 1772. Moscow suppressed the united church and Russified the Orthodox Church; indeed in 1685 it abolished the independence of the Metropolitans of Kiev. The Ukrainians and White Russians played a key role in the modernization of the Russian church between the sixteenth and the eighteenth centuries. However, they also brought with them to Moscow Western ideas of an absolutist state church.

At all events, for a long time the policy of the Russian church was opposed not to the technical but to the cultural progress of the West. This was an exclusion, not of course of Western techniques of armaments and weapons, which the Czars of the sixteenth and seventeenth centuries introduced immediately, but of **Western culture, world-view and religion**. Yet the culture of the West exercised a tremendous fascination on the Russians, who had increasingly come into contact with it since the Italian Renaissance. In the sixteenth and seventeenth centuries the influence of the advancing Lithuanians and Poles also increased substantially in the Western Russian empire. For protection against the Latins, and as armament and defence against the 'Latins' and the 'union' with Rome, people were compelled to read Western (and not least German) books and to invite countless 'Westerners' (even educated Jesuits) to Russia. Russia increasingly underwent Western influence – more than the completely simple-minded Russian theology of the time noticed – long before Peter the Great opened the door wide to the West and ordained a secular Enlightenment rather than a religious reformation for Russia.

Petersburg: the third phase of Russian history

What **Peter the Great** prescribed for Russia was a revolution – given the blatant social abuses and the enormous cultural deficits. As a representative of Western state absolutism, the young Czar (1672-1725), who had come into contact with the foreign community in Moscow at a very early stage and later had made incognito journeys especially to the Netherlands and England, was firmly resolved to bring about an **internal Europeanization** in Russia, which historically was long overdue. In other words, for the first time Russian Christianity was confronted with a new post-Reformation, **modern paradigm** (P V) which was just emerging.

Thus began the **third, Petersburg phase** of Russian history, which brought a deliberate secularization and rationalization of the Russian state. The abolition of beards, the introduction of the Western calendar[269] and the encouragement of schools as specialist educational institutions affected everyday life deeply. But the centre of Peter's reforms was the formation of a standing army, a modern fleet and a new capital (from 1712 St Petersburg). He also **reorganized** the civil administration and **the church** – a tremendous undertaking, given the traditionalism of Russian Orthodoxy.[270] Peter was advised by Archbishop Feofan Prokopovic, who was a Ukrainian, had even studied at the Gregoriana in Rome, and was a champion of the Enlightenment view of the grace of God which was modern at that time. Peter used the absolute power over state and church which had been given him and, with the assent of the Eastern patriarchs, in 1721 again abolished the Patriarchate of Moscow, so rich in tradition, which was a possible rival focus to his power. It was replaced, with reference to the Byzantine *synodos endemousa* (in the imperial palace), by a permanent collegial organ, the 'Holy Synod'. This was pledged to the Czars as 'the supreme judges of this Spiritual College', to whom it was subordinate in every way.[271] Otherwise the hierarchical and sacramental structure of the church was maintained, but *de facto* the German Protestant church order, in which churches were governed by local rulers, was taken over.

So now the Orthodox Church, which had not been able to arouse itself to any religious reformation, was quite directly confronted with a **political and secular** Enlightenment which made the church administration a 'department of the Orthodox confession' that could be controlled easily. Now the state also increasingly called for the confessional unity of Russia, as a result of which, in the Czar's empire, even non-Russians were to become Russian and convert to the Orthodox Church: the more pliable Lutherans in the Western provinces suffered rather less under this policy than the Roman Catholic Poles, who constantly tended to rebel.

Of course the Orthodox Church outside the capital, far into the gigantic country, was very much less affected by the modern development; here monasticism continued to shape the spiritual life even of the laity, much more than the hierarchy directed by the Czars.[272] It is no coincidence that 'Heaven is high and the Czar is a long way off' is an ancient Russian proverb. In the eighteenth century in particular, not only Neo-Hesychasm but also the **Startsy movement**, mentioned above, came into being.

However, then as now, church critics of Peter the Great asked whether the new Russian concept of a 'symphony' of state and church did not make the church completely dependent on the state. In reply, we must ask: hadn't that already been the case previously? Wasn't the marked dependence of the church on the state since Constantine the Great part of the Hellenistic paradigm, and hadn't it also long been characteristic of Moscow? Didn't the **state absolutism of modernity** which was now breaking through with Peter's rule represent a consistent development? There is no disputing the fact that the absolutist administration and police state in the spirit of Peter the Great (unlike the modern legal and constitutional state) sought to regulate the whole political, economic and social life of its 'subjects' on its own authority – through adminstrative ordinances and repressive measures of control. In this way not only state but also church administration was to be rationalized, centralized and disciplined. To what end? To make the church an enlightened moral instrument of education.

So the **state** was no longer the 'protector' of the church but an **absolute authority** which was responsible for everything. The church and the clergy were also entrusted with tasks which seemed necessary for the advancement of the common good – a central concept of the Enlightenment. On this basis the number of monasteries was reduced, their economic activities were put under state authorities, and their social and charitable purposes (not least for war veterans!) were brought into the foreground. Monasteries were to run schools or hospitals; only mature adults were to become monks or nuns. These were all 'reasonable' things. Didn't the critics in the church, then as now, fail to note sufficiently that the Western cultural influences called for by Czar Peter, for all their ambivalence, were having a positive effect not only on literary but also on church life? At all events, not only were foreigners allowed to practise their religion freely, but a revision of the Church Slavonic translation of the Bible was ordered. Moreover, up to 1750 no less than twenty-six priestly seminaries were founded and the education of priests was considerably improved – as mentioned above, under Latin influence. Education and training, knowledge and theology, were modernized in the Petersburg period, albeit within narrow limits.

But part of the ominous **ambivalence of this new 'symphony' of state and church** was that here two paradigms, the traditional Hellenistic Byzantine paradigm (P II) and the modern Enlightenment paradigm, were in part being unconsciously interlocked. The theocratic Byzantine church law was overlaid by modern natural and constitutional law, according to which the will of the people became the will of the rulers. A religious basis was fundamentally superfluous for the autocracy grounded in natural law. There was a highly paradoxical situation: a monarch with a modern disposition, who appealed to natural law, as always had himself theocratically celebrated as 'God's anointed' in the ceremonial Byzantine liturgy; at least for a day he wore sacral garments with the cross on his head, the icon of God venerated by the people! And the church still regarded the Czars as spiritual figures and sacral anointing as a limitation of their absolute power. But this limitation was an illusion, and the 'symphony' a fiction. For the Czar himself regarded anointing as a sacral legitimation of his unlimited power. That explains how, a century later, in the Metternich era, the militaristic Czar Nicholas I could proclaim as a domestic political maxim: 'Autocracy, Orthodoxy, Narodnost' (nationality and popular piety[273]); at the same time, the foreign policy was that all Orthodox living outside Russia should show their solidarity with the Czar's realm.

So as time went on, the **Orthodox Church** inevitably came to seem to the people not just a prisoner but, along with the nobility, the army and the police, a **guarantor and support of the Czar's regime** – despite isolated attempts at reform and the beginning of a lay theology.[274] And the more the Czars, who now no longer saw themselves just as the supreme administrators and judges of the church, as Peter did, but as its head, despite isolated reforms brought the old Russian 'party' (also backed by the church hierarchy) to the fore and disappointed all hopes of modernization and liberalization, the more not only the Raskolniki and the very different religious sects, often social protest movements in religious garb, but also (after the Polish rebellion of 1861) the idealistic youth were frustrated, and the more even the state church itself was compromised; indeed, the more the freethinkers (Voltaireans) and then the **nihilists** found a following: that terrorist revolutionary party which worked for the radical overthrow of all values and conditions. They were responsible for the murder of Czar Alexander II in 1881 and then, with other trends critical of society (the Socialists), in 1905 initiated a highly dangerous revolution during the Russo-Japanese war. When after this revolution Czar Nicholas II – who was to be the last Czar – finally promised a constitutional reform of the state and freedom of conscience for the individual, yet again disappointed expectations, he ensured that of historical necessity the revolutionary prelude of 1905 led to the great Revolution of 1917, which has proved an utter catastrophe for Christianity in Russia down to the present day.

12. The October Revolution – and the Orthodox Church?

It can hardly be disputed that in the course of Russian history religion had largely become opium for the masses of ordinary people. Certainly it was comfort in a life often full of deprivation, but often even more consolation. And particularly after 1989 we may ask: what might the Russian world, and indeed the whole world, have been spared had the Russian Orthodox Church in the nineteenth century made itself the passionate advocate of the social reforms in Russia which were so bitterly necessary! After all, there was not a little social criticism and impetus for reform, above all on the part of various lay theologians – a new phenomenon in Russian Orthodoxy.

Christian social criticism before the Revolution

I shall mention only three of the most famous nineteenth-century Russian thinkers, all **representatives of an alternative Orthodoxy**. First there is Count **Leo Tolstoy** (died 1910),[275] the most famous social utopian of Russia in a Christian spirit. He was the advocate of a universally human Christianity strongly influenced by the West, with an emphasis on love of neighbour and non-violence. And he clashed increasingly strongly with the state church, which in the eyes of its critics was doing more to stupefy the people than educate them. Indeed, in 1901 Tolstoy was 'excommunicated' for blasphemously mocking the Orthodox liturgy in his novel *Resurrection*. Then there was **Fyodor Michaelovich Dostoievsky** (died 1881), who already in his first work *Poor People* (1846) had made the social situation his theme. As a member of a revolutionary terrorist group he had been condemned to death, but his sentence was commuted immediately before his execution to a four-year banishment to Siberia. In his great novel *The Brothers Karamazov*, in a unique way Dostoievsky brings the church which has become the Grand Inquisitor face to face with a Jesus who has returned, and at the end shows the hopeful vision of an alternative Orthodoxy through the figure of Alyosha Karamazov.[276] Finally, there is **Vladimir Solovyev** (died 1900), who developed not only religious and social ideas but also a complete and well-grounded system of Christian social ethics. Because he interceded for a pardon for the murderers of the Czar in 1881, Solovyev was forbidden to teach; in his social ethical demands he is no less radical but at the same time more deeply and comprehensively Christian than Tolstoy.[277] His philosophy of religion, based on love and aimed at a universal unity, a synthesis of religion, philosophy and science leading to a holistic life, recalls Origen in the framework of our paradigm analysis.

Through these laity we hear as it were the **Orthodox Church from below**. Social reform thinking also spread through the **spirituality** of the Orthodox **parish clergy**, especially after Czar Alexander II, who in 1861 abolished serfdom. Above all in the sphere of education and welfare, vigorous activity was developed within the Orthodox Church by the local communities and particularly by their clergy, but this was much hampered by the legal situation at the time and by imperial bureaucracy.[278] The Protestant theologian Ernst Benz, who has paid special attention to the social, ethical and political problems in Russian Orthodoxy,[279] has emphasized that ideas of social reform were rife among the clergy and the laity – especially among the 'Old Believers' and the 'Slavophiles'. In particular the **seminaries for priests**, which often gave highly gifted young men from priestly families and the lower classes an opportunity for education and a rise in life, were seedbeds of ideas for social reform and indeed social revolution. However, they also produced the supporters of Russian nihilism and Russian Communism. Can we ever forget that one of the greatest criminals of the twentieth century (alongside Adolf Hitler) was the product of a priests' seminary in Tiflis, namely that Georgian Josef Vissarionovich Dzhuhgashvili, who later took the name **Stalin**?

However, a **social critic** who is unfortunately largely forgotten even in Russia also emerged from a priests' seminar – the priest **Grigori Petrov**. He similarly represents a widespread social unrest even among the clergy and long before the Revolution brought out a *Pravda* (= truth), namely the Christian Socialist *God's Pravda* – which met with a great response among Orthodox people and much mistrust in Marxist circles. Petrov, at first tutor to two grand ducal families, was to be tutor to Alexei, the successor to the throne. But he came to oppose the ruling system and was elected independent deputy in the first Russian popular assembly, the Duma.

It was Petrov who subjected the politically and socially uncommitted clergy of the state church to sharp criticism. In 1908 he had written to Metropolitan Antonij: 'There is no Christian emperor, no Christian government and no Christian order of society. The upper classes rule over the lower classes; a small group dominates all the rest of the population . . . They have excluded the lower classes from everything: from power, science, art, even religion; they have made religion their servant . . . The church did not transfigure the state but robbed it of outward splendour . . . Christianity became the state religion, but that did not mean that the state ceased to be pagan . . . The explanation for this is that the influence of Christianity was not directed at the political and social order. The Gospels were diverted from their broad mission of establishing the kingdom of God in society and state along the narrow path of personal virtue and personal redemption.' And Petrov's conclusion? It consists in a requirement that the Christian church should be detached from the Czarist system: 'The church is a universal human organization transcending the nation and the state. For the church, none of the existing political systems is complete, finally valid and unassailable. Such a state system is a thing of the future.' Thus Petrov in 1908.[280]

What was the reaction of the church authorities? For his criticism Petrov was excommunicated, like Tolstoi before him. And the popular procession of the priest **Georgii Gapon** with icons and pictures of the Czars, which on 'Bloody Sunday' 1905 sought to renew the damaged religous bond of the Russian people with the Orthodox Czars, was dispersed by salvoes from the regimental guards with numerous deaths, a response which was interpreted by many people as the definitive dissolution of this bond.

A mere decade after Petrov's exclusion from the church, the **Revolution** broke out. This **February Revolution of 1917** (without Lenin) brought the resignation of the Czar and – here historians today are agreed – represented the real, democratic Russian revolution. Now it was of little use to the Orthodox Church that some church leaders, too, referred to ideas of Soloviev, Petrov and other critics.

– Certainly there had been freedom of speech in the Russian Orthodox Church since the 1905 Revolution, and thus also great **discussion** over reforms.

– Certainly under the provisional democratic government of Kerensky an Orthodox **Council** held in Moscow in August 1917 had resolved on internal reform of the church: the re-establishment of the patriarchate abolished by Peter the Great, election of bishops by the faithful, the representation of the laity in parish, diocesan and patriarchate councils.

– But this council, too, made **no** statement about **social reforms**. Rather, it supported the continuation of the war against the Germans and spoke out against the peace of Brest-Litovsk which was concluded (unfortunately only by Lenin on 3 March 1918).[281]

Lenin's and Stalin's hatred of religion

The February Revolution of 1917, with the democracy which dawned in it, could have had incredible consequences – for state and church. But in the **'October Revolution'**, in fact an anti-democratic coup against the provisional republican government, the leader of the Bolsheviks (= maximalists), Vladimir Ilyich Ulanov, called Lenin, came to power. He had only returned to Russia in April, and on 8 December 1917 with his

Bolsheviks had only gained 23.5% of the votes (as compared with the 62% for the Socialists and the 13% for the bourgeois parties), but at the same time he had already founded the secret police, the Tcheka. On 18 January he brutally dissolved the constitutional assembly when it refused to recognize the 'Soviet power' unconditionally.

Lenin was possessed by an indescribable hatred of everything religious. He, too, had had bad experiences with the state and religion in Czarist Russia. Above all the execution of his brother Alexander in connection with the murder of Czar Alexander II on 1 March 1881 had deeply shaken him, indeed stamped his whole life. Though showing political wisdom by outwardly restraining himself, once he had come to power Lenin initiated a vigorous campaign against religion, which for him was not only 'the opium of the people', to which people devoted themselves to mitigate their misery, as it was for Karl Marx, but also opium for the people, which was deliberately given to them by their rulers in state and church: 'a kind of spiritual booze in which the slaves of capital drown their human image, their demand for a life more or less worthy of men . . . But the modern class-conscious worker . . . contemptuously casts aside religious prejudices, leaves heaven to the priests and bourgeois bigots, and tries to win a better life for himself here on earth.'[282]

We know – many of us still as eye-witnesses – that it was only a small step from the massive verbal repudiation of religion to a massive practical persecution of it. This mass persecution already began under Lenin, and then continued above all under Stalin. The worst years of the Stalinist terror for the Russian church were 1927 to 1943, until Stalin introduced a national turning point in the distress of the Second World War. Thousands of clergy had been imprisoned and deported, thousands of churches devastated or closed, millions of people, believers and unbelievers, sent to the 'Gulag archipelago' (Alexander Solzhenitsyn!).

But the Russian Orthodox Church survived even this, not without numerous martyrs on the one hand and even more opportunists on the other (collaboration with the KGB). Despite everything, numerous people kept faith. Indeed since 1988/89 this church – profiting from the perestroika of Mikhail Gorbachev, the then head of the Communist Party – has been able to open up again and fulfil its task without constant state reprisal and discriminations. However, what the future of Orthodoxy will be in Russia in particular after the end of the Cold War and the Soviet empire, and in what direction a specifically Russian theology, spirituality or even social ethics will develop, is still quite open. In a further volume on Christianity I hope to be able to develop rather clearer perspectives on this.

What are the strengths, dangers and possibilities of Orthodoxy?

A theological evaluation of this second, Hellenistic ecumenical paradigm of the early church is urgently needed at the end of this long section.[283] This Christianity shaped by the early church Hellenistic paradigm (P II) essentially deserves our respect and **admiration**. By comparison with the Christians in the Jewish Christian paradigm (P I), this Christianity has safeguarded its survival – despite often life-threatening crises, despite the conquest of most of the Christian Orthodox countries by Islam, and despite Communist oppression. Christians in Eastern Europe have been spared the fate of the Christians in North Africa. And as I have continually stressed, compared with Latin Christianity, in many respects **Orthodox** Christianity is the **form of Christianity which is nearer to the origins**. Abiding Orthodox achievements are:
– a significant theology,
– a liturgy which speaks to both spirit and emotions at the same time,
– a *koinonia, communio,* fellowship of churches with equal rights preserved through state oppression and political persecution, represented by its spiritual (not legal) supreme head, the Patriarch of Constantinople.

However, the **dangers** of this second paradigm of Christianity have similarly become clear. First of all, attention must be drawn to the danger of **liturgism**. Where it established itself, this in fact reduced the life of the church to liturgy, crippling a contemporary proclamation and hardly inspiring social and political reforms. There may be no criticism of the Orthodox liturgy, but can there be also none of Orthodox liturgism?

Down to most recent times it has been the **Orthodox liturgy** in particular[284] which has won the hearts of countless people even in the West. Here we should not overlook the fact that even the liturgy of Orthodoxy has undergone a tremendous development, in two respects: in the course of time the simple **celebration of a meal in memory of Jesus** has become what Fairy von Lilienfeld has called an **imposing 'Solomonic' temple worship,** in which it is no longer the earthly or risen Jesus who occupies the central position but – against the background of incarnation and exaltation – the Christ Pantocrator as he is depicted in the incomparable mosaics: the omnipotence of the divine Logos. And to the present day the bearded bishops and presbyters with their mitres, gold-embroidered robes, crosses and icons make a powerful impression on Western observers as well; even today they give us some idea of the dignity and splendour, the style and taste of ancient Byzantium.

At the same time the simple **psalm-singing and hymns** of the early

Christian communities became an art form, indeed in Byzantium a highly developed, if still unison, form of artistic choral singing (with extended coloraturas), though for dogmatic reasons all instrumental music was forbidden (because it was pagan?). Not dead wood and metal, but the living voice should praise God. And through contact between unison Byzantine church music with polyphonic music, above all Venetian church music (Gabrieli!) on the islands of the Mediterranean occupied by the Italians or via Poland and the Ukraine, an attractive **polyphonic choral singing** finally developed in Russia which today speaks deeply to East and West and can unite them in worship.

But even in the face of these very significant changes we in the Western church, too, should concede today that in many respects the **Eastern liturgy has preserved nearness to its origins better** than the mediaeval Latin liturgy. In the East there is

– no exclusive fixation on seven sacraments as in the West, but **concentration** on **baptism** (which also includes anointing or confirmation) and **eucharist**. Otherwise there is openness to an indeterminate multiplicity of sacred actions for pastoral purposes;

– no dogmatic fixation of the celebration of the eucharist on the words of institution nor a 'transformation' of the elements of bread and wine understood in a substantive way. Rather, there is a spiritual presence of the exalted Lord in the general course of the celebration from the beginning, and after the account of the Last Supper an invocation of the Holy Spirit (**epiclesis**) on the gifts of bread and wine;

– no eucharistic celebration by the priest alone without the community being present ('silent mass') as in the West (before Vatican II), but always **a celebration of the priest with the community**, which itself receives the Christ who comes and appears, and has a right to communion in both forms, bread and wine.

Now in the West it has often been claimed that the Eastern liturgy is '**rigid**'. The answer to that is that the Eastern liturgy, like the Western, distinguishes between 'fixed' parts (basic structure) and changeable parts which are adapted to the relevant feasts or saints and in which the different scriptural readings, prayers and hymns give room for variation and alternation. Particularly in most recent times the Orthodox liturgy has represented for many people a happy contrast to the grey ugliness of everyday Soviet life, a contrast which automatically raises questions about a 'wholly other', about God. To this degree the Orthodox liturgy automatically had and still has a missionary function. In this way it was also, amazingly, possible for the Orthodox Church to survive not only under alien Mongol rule, which was relatively well-disposed to the church, and Arabic and Turkish rule, which was relatively tolerant, but also under the totalitarian Bolshevik regime of violence (at a time when the printing of religious books was forbidden, many faithful knew the liturgy by heart) and to preserve authentic Christianity in the various state church systems.

But that does not remove the problem. It is not so much that the liturgy is rigid; it is isolated. Even so benevolent a Western observer of Eastern Orthodoxy as Ernst Benz thinks that the way in which it makes the liturgy independent must be cited as one of the main weaknesses of Orthodoxy: a 'liturgical isolationism' in which 'the liturgy becomes a shell into which the church withdraws like a tortoise, only rarely sticking its head out'.[285] So here – particularly in view of the secularized society in Russia and other Orthodox countries – important questions arise for the future:

Questions for the Future

Shouldn't a liturgy which really claims to be a Christian liturgy

– be **grounded** in the **proclamation of the Christian message** (preaching), which has to be in keeping with the gospel and the times, and has not yet been replaced by a hymn of praise to a Holy One at the end of the liturgy, which was to follow when a restriction of the church to as solemn a liturgy as possible was all too welcome to those in political power?

– have **consequences** in the **realization of a Christian ethic** which could not be restricted to private life but would also have a realistic social dimension, and, particularly in times of a new freedom, would permeate the spheres of economics, politics and culture? In the future shouldn't the social and political impulses again come from the church itself rather than primarily from opponents of the church?

A further danger to the Orthodox Church lies in the **state church system**, in which under emperors, Czars and General Secretaries the church could become a pliable instrument of the state or the party. The whole development of the 'symphony' model which I have depicted shows abundantly clearly that the dependence of the Russian Orthodox Church (even in many spiritual matters) on the political regime at any time – a dependence which has not yet been abandoned even in the present – has a tradition which has been hallowed for a particularly long time. It is not only in line with the Muscovite state church system which developed in the fifteenth and sixteenth centuries, but has deep roots in the Byzantine tradition, indeed already with Constantine. The Byzantine Slavonic state church tradition also explains why most Orthodox churches are mistrustful of the ideas of 1789, the ideas of democracy, the separation of church and state, freedom of conscience and religion.

This danger emerges in an acute form in modern **nationalism.** Certainly, for the Slavonic people under Ottoman rule, for centuries the church was the last bastion of the recollection of their own identity and independence; and so the church had the function of constituting and legitimizing the nation. But in the more recent history of Orthodoxy the nationalistic ideology which emerged from this has often enough served to inflame ethnic rivalries instead of damping them down and taming them. So not least, developments in the former Yugoslavia have become so fanatical because for centuries the churches have encouraged nationalism instead of taming it: the Catholic Church the nationalism of the Croats, the Orthodox Church that of the Serbs. Indeed there is also nationalism in Poland, Ireland and certain Protestant countries. But if there is a particular temptation and danger in the world of Orthodoxy, it is not so much authoritarianism (Catholic) or subjectivism (Protestant) as in the West, as nationalism.

However, this danger of too close a link between nation and religion exists beyond Orthodoxy in all Christian churches, indeed beyond Christianity in all religions, especially the prophetic and monotheistic ones. So here questions arise for all three religions.

Questions about the Relationship between Religion and Nation

Judaism is a religion which has an extraordinary influence on human history. At the same time there is an indissoluble link between the religion and a people and a land. But is there not a danger here that the religious foundation of the land will become a state ideology which seeks to deny others their right to live in the same land? Is there not a danger that the ideology of the state will become a substitute religion? Militarism instead of the military, nationalism instead of the nation, turning the state into an idol?

There are also state churches in Protestantism, Anglicanism and partly also in Catholicism, which for their part criticize Orthodoxy. But does criticism of the Eastern 'symphony' model (P II) justify Western papalism (P III), Protestant churches under the control of the authorities, and Protestant synodicalism (P IV)? Indeed, can any state church be shown from scripture to be of Christian origin?

☾ Islam understands itself as a universal religion transcending all nations and cultures. At the same time there has never been a separation of religion and society in Islam. Doesn't that always lead to the danger that Islam may be misused for the purposes of the political rulers and wars legitimated by religion? Is the function of prophetic protest in religion still possible for Islam in Muslim countries in the face of those who rule and hold property in them?

It is impossible to end this chapter on the analysis of the second great paradigm of Christianity, the Hellenistic early church paradigm, which goes over into the history of Eastern Byzantine and Slavonic Orthodoxy, with all its triumphs and defeats, without expressing a wish. This relates to the account of the challenges of the present and the possibilities of the future which are to be depicted in a further volume. It is a wish:

That after the collapse of the idol of the 'Communist Party' the churches of this paradigm may succeed, without anxiety about modernity and its authentic achievements, in making a decisive contribution to what in the states of the former Eastern bloc is so needed in the transition to a new world era:

– a **renewed faith** in the one true God, which excludes any cult of persons, parties and nations;

– a **renewed ethic** in the face of so much passivity, laziness and cynicism;

– a **renewed spirituality** in the face of such a lack of spirituality and the moral decline which is so bewailed;

– a **renewed liturgy** which does not abolish the old but renews it from the power of the gospel;

– a **renewed Christian humanity** in unity with the other Christian churches, in peace with the world religions and in collaboration with all people of good will.

III. The Roman Catholic Paradigm of the Middle Ages

The Middle Ages of Western and Central Europe which will be discussed in this chapter, those 'middle ages' between antiquity and our own modern times, are an era which is still extremely alien to us, in many respects more alien than the antiquity which preceded it. For a long time, moreover, the assessments of this period by historians differed completely. Only in our day is a twofold consensus emerging, which can be sketched out briefly like this:

– The Middle Ages is **not simply that 'dark time' of decay** so despised ('monks' Latin', 'Gothic') by the humanists of the 'Rinascimento' (the rebirth of antiquity as a model in language and the arts);

which the Reformers then condemned even more as the papistic period of apostasy from the true Christian faith;

and which therefore the Protestant church historians of the nineteenth and twentieth centuries still regarded as unfruitful for the church and theology – apart from some 'pre-Reformers' like Wyclif and Hus.[1]

– Nor are the Middle Ages that **ideal time of exemplary Christianity** to which an almost normative force for church, theology and society is attributed,

such as was dreamed up by an anti-Enlightenment Romanticism (Novalis and some converts to Catholicism);

such as was enthused over patriotically by the German nationalistic historians of the nineteenth century, at least in connection with the mediaeval emperors (culminating in the Hohenstaufens);

such as Neo-Romantics, Neo-Gothics, German pre-Raphaelites and also Neo-Gregorians and Neo-Scholastics hoped to renew against a papalist ultramontanism;

finally such as even today the anti-conciliar Roman reaction, which dreams of the old 'Christian Europe', envisages as a model for its 're-evangelization campaign'.[2]

1. The change in mediaeval scholarship

But down to the present day there is dispute over the question how long the Middle Ages lasted. The division into 'Antiquity – Middle Ages – Modernity' has become customary in Europe only since the seventeenth century. The key dates are still set differently by historians, and it is clear that such historical **periodizations** are governed by national, confessional and sometimes also personal perspectives.

Key dates of the mediaeval paradigm

No matter how the questions of dating are to be solved, there is no doubt today that the mediaeval Roman Catholic paradigm (P III) which is to be analysed here differs clearly from the Hellenistic early church paradigm analysed in the previous chapter (P II), though it developed only slowly. Indeed any **paradigm shift** – even a relatively sudden one like the Reformation – has its makings in the previous paradigm.

Essential **presuppositions** for the mediaeval paradigm were already emerging in late antiquity, which still remained largely governed by the early church Hellenistic paradigm. What we saw in the making from our so to speak distant perspective, from Byzantium and the East, is now to be analysed in detail from close quarters, from Rome and the West, namely: there would have been no new mediaeval paradigm in the West
– without the division of Constantine's Christian Roman empire into an Eastern empire (Byzantium) and a Western empire, a division which became definitive after the death of Theodosius the Great (395);
– without the theology of Augustine (died 430), who was to prove to be the father of Western theology;
– without the policy of the Roman Popes of the fourth and fifth centuries who, appealing to the apostle Peter, accrued to themselves more and more power in the church and finally also in the state.

Furthermore, in connection with the **advent** of the new mediaeval constellation we must take into account the fundamental developments through which the paradigm shift was **initiated**:
– the Germanic migrations of the fifth and sixth century; the downfall of the Western Roman empire in 476 and the Catholic baptism of Clovis, the Merovingian king of the Franks, in 498/9;
– the rise of the prophet Muhammad (622 marks the beginning of Islamic chronology) and the Arab conquest of the eastern and southern Mediterranean countries which once formed part of the empire;
– the renewal of the Christian empire under Charlemagne (who died in 814).

But it will prove that it was the Gregorian reform in the eleventh century which brought the definitive **breakthrough** of the Roman Catholic paradigm in the Western church and thus **completed** the paradigm shift – though at the cost of a split with the Eastern church. This mediaeval paradigm then reached its climax and finally its turning point in the twelfth and thirteenth centuries, so that already in the fourteenth and fifteenth centuries it was utterly in crisis, and by the beginning of the sixteenth century – with Martin Luther's Reformation and a split now also in the Western church – was showing how rigid it had become.

However, it will also become clear that this paradigm is still the conscious or unconscious framework for the thought and feeling not only of the Catholic Counter-Reformation and anti-modernism but for many traditional Catholics down to the present day. So we must analyse this paradigm, too, more closely, always with a view to the problems of the present – not therefore with the historian's detachment but with historical involvement. I must stress once again that my purpose here is not to relate the **history** of the Roman Catholic Middle Ages in detail, but – though not without any narrative – to analyse the mediaeval **paradigm** of Christianity, in other words to describe 'the **entire constellation** of beliefs, values, techniques, and so on' **which still holds today**. This will become evident when we first turn to a preliminary question.

A Germanic paradigm?

Is Christian Europe a product of 'Christianity, Germanhood and antiquity', as has been assumed since Leopold Ranke? Quite apart from the fact that, as we saw, the Byzantine and Slavonic elements also belong to Europe, the contrast between the Germanic and Roman antiquity which the nationalistic German historiography of the last century played up even in church history and the history of canon law may now be regarded as an outdated opposition.

In his critical survey of the state of mediaeval scholarship, the German church historian Arnold Angenendt points out how historiography since the Second World War has 'experienced a fundamental liberation from the complex of Germanism' and 'research has been internationalized'.[3] At any rate it is no longer possible to speak of an 'essence of the Germanic' which is alleged to remain the same – a historical foundation for 'Germanic man', 'German politics' and the 'German way of life' – all in contrast to the Romanic 'Welsh'. But why is such a historical Germanism outmoded? Historians draw attention to two things.

On the one hand, Germanism was no more a uniform entity than Germanic religion. 'The Germans' may certainly be said to be linked through a linguistic affinity, but already in the early Middle Ages this linguistic affinity could not form the basis for any shared social awareness. And neither the 'distinctively Germanic church' (a church which both legally, in terms of its property, and ecclesiastically was the property of the ruler[4]) nor the 'Germanic popular character' and 'Germanic religion', allegedly characterized by 'Germanic virtues' like honesty, independence, loyalty, allegiance, inwardness, soul and awareness of community, proved to be exclusively Germanic.[5]

On the other hand, at least the everyday culture of late antiquity continued, despite the collapse of the administrative and organizational superstructure of the empire in the early Middle Ages – albeit in different ways in different zones and periods. This made it possible for the Germans to have a link with the ancient world, despite all the confusion. Thus it is impossible to make a neat distinction between the Germanic and the Romanic elements of late antiquity. So many of the notions, conceptions, modes of action and institutions formed in late antiquity – like the divine grace of the ruler, the dynastic idea and the great estates with their landowners – persisted. But in the early Middle Ages these were often intermingled with the **archaic beliefs and practices** of the Germans: more rite than ethic, more *mythos* than *logos*, magical thought, witchcraft, belief in demons, a piety of relics, oaths and magic spells. Still, all this is not specifically Germanic nor indeed specifically Celtic (in large parts of Western Europe), but simply archaic – characteristic of the mentality of certain people at a particular primitive level of culture.

A Latin paradigm?

We may conclude from this that although 'the Germans' had an essential part in shaping the mediaeval paradigm, it cannot be said to be typically Germanic. Rather than being Germanic, the Western paradigm primarily had a **Latin** stamp, to the degree that **Latin** was the **official language** of the Western church and theology, law and the state, and remained so all down the centuries.

As we know, in the first centuries *koine* Greek had been the language of Western Christianity also. This was an international language of the urban population throughout the Roman empire, used not only by educated people but also in trade and commerce, and thus quite naturally also the language of the church and worship. Not only were the Bible, creeds and the first theological works written in Greek; even the liturgy of the city of Rome was celebrated in Greek. It was only after a lengthy transitional period that **Latin** was universally and finally introduced **into worship** following the model of Milan, between 360 and 382.[6] The East, which, as we saw, after Constantine's foundation of the new imperial capital Constantinople was stronger in terms of population, economy and military power, naturally preserved Greek in both state and church and increasingly neglected Latin. Precisely the opposite happened in the church: here Greek disappeared during the third and fourth centuries in favour of Latin, which was now given an even greater significance as a result of Christianization.

This Christian, ecclesiastical Latin had meanwhile developed in North Africa, as also had specifically **Latin theology**. This began almost a century after Greek theology – with **Tertullian** (*c*.150–155 – after 222). Granted, this skilful theologian and lay theologian first still published works in Greek, and because of his material and the problems he tackles he is sometimes called the last Greek apologist. But in Tertullian for the first time we have a typically Latin theology of a kind which has been precisely described by the church historian Hans von Campenhausen: 'In the powerful, non-speculative and practical orientation of his theology, Tertullian appears beyond dispute as the first Latin father of the church. The same applies to the realistic, legalistic and psychological bent of his intellect, to his inclination towards social issues, and towards the congregation and church as a firm political society, and also to his emphasis on will, standards and discipline.'[7] First of all, however, Latin theology remained completely under the wing of Greek theology: the Spirit blows as it were from East to West, and this is already reflected in the number of Latin translations from the Greek, which are hardly matched by the number of Greek translations from the Latin.

From the beginning the **theological interest of Latin Christianity** lay in a different direction. To what degree?

- **Greek theology**, which had more of a philosophical disposition, concentrated above all on theoretical questions of christology and the doctrine of the Trinity. It was mainly interested in metaphysical and speculative problems: the relationship between the Father, Son and Spirit and the possibility of the incarnation of God and the deification of human beings.
- **Roman theology**, with its practical orientation, centred on pastoral questions of penitential discipline, the Christian way of life and church order. Its main interest was in psychological and ethical problems and problems of discipline: guilt, atonement and forgiveness, church order, ministries and sacraments.

And yet, despite such a towering Bishop of Carthage as **Cyprian**, a generation after Tertullian, despite this great spiritual leader of the African church, defender of episcopal autonomy against Rome and a popular writer of edifying works, around the middle of the fourth century Western Latin Christianity still appeared to be an appendix to the Greek Christianity of the Eastern Roman empire which was spiritually in the lead. One significant indication of this is that all the ecumenical councils took place in the East with very meagre participation from the West (legates from the Bishop of Rome). Only in the fourth century do we find theologians who deliberately went to school with the Greeks: for spiritual exegesis to Philo, Origen and Gregory of Nyssa; for speculative theology to the Cappadocians. These included Hilary, Rufinus, Jerome and above all **Ambrose**, Bishop of Milan, who was best able to make an organic combination of Greek and Latin. But by the middle of the fifth century the Latin West had caught up theologically with the Greek East. Why? This was thanks to the life work of a theologian who was to become **the** theologian of the Latin church: Aurelius Augustine.

2. Augustine: the father of the new paradigm of theology

No figure in Christianity between Paul and Luther has exercised greater influence in theology and the church than Augustine.[8] I have already described the life, work and influence of this man in a previous book, *Great Christian Thinkers*. So here I can concentrate on the question how far Augustine laid the theological foundations for the paradigm of the Latin mediaeval West. What made him the father of the new paradigm of theology?

A Latin theologian

I begin from two basic theses:
– Augustine **shaped Western theology and piety** more than any other theologian; in this way he became the theological father of the mediaeval paradigm.
– Augustine is **repudiated by the East**[9] to a greater degree than perhaps any other Western church father – a further indication of the shift in Christianity from the early church Hellenistic paradigm to the Latin mediaeval paradigm which in fact begins with him.

Today, both these facts must be taken equally seriously. Augustine must not go on being ignored, as he is in Eastern theology, but he must not be spared virtually all criticism, as he is in some Western accounts; rather, a balanced judgment must be passed on him as the **initiator of a new paradigm**. For a paradigm shift never means just progress, but also gain and loss. And indeed a new paradigm came about in theology when this originally extremely worldly man, this real intellectual genius and acute dialectician, gifted psychologist, brilliant stylist and finally passionate Christian, set out to develop his very varied experiences theologically into a powerful synthesis.

Origen was – as we may recall – a **Greek** through and through (with some knowledge of Hebrew). But from the beginning and with all his heart Augustine was a **Latin**:
– Augustine, born precisely a century after Origen's death, in the year 354, was a Roman citizen and son of a city official in the Roman province

of Numidia, in present-day Algeria.

– His language, of which he had a sovereign command, was Latin; he hated learning Greek; he was the only significant Latin philosopher who knew almost no Greek.

– He felt no solidarity with Carthage, far less with Athens or Byzantium, but with Rome, which for him was still the capital of the world and now also the centre of the church.

– Augustine sought hardly any contact with the great Greek church fathers of the East, the schools of Cappadocia, Antioch and Alexandria. In short, 'Augustine's education was essentially, if not quite completely, grounded in the Latin language.'[10] He took the writings of the Greek church into account only when Latin translations were available to him.[11]

There is one more thing: whereas Origen went his way from his youth up as a convinced Christian ready for martyrdom in a world which was still pagan and hostile, Augustine at first, as a young man, rejected Christianity in a world which was already largely Christianized. Only after many wanderings did he find his way from worldliness to being a Christian: in 391 he became a priest and in 396 Bishop of Hippo Regius (in present-day Algeria). But at that point the time of crises was by no means behind him. For in the course of his church career Augustine was to be entangled in epoch-making controversies. For us that is a further indication that any new paradigm, including the new Latin paradigm, emerges from a **crisis** which leads to a new constellation.

Crisis of the church I: Which is the true church?

Augustine was to remain bishop for thirty-five long years. Unlike the other bishops, most of whom were married, until his death he lived a strictly regulated communal life with his priests, deacons and other clergy. Outwardly he was separated from his people by vows of celibacy and poverty and by the wearing of black robes; however, the monastic ideal was not seen primarily as asceticism, as in the Greek world, but as a common life in harmony and love; here was a herald of the Middle Ages with its communities of canons on the Augustinian pattern. As bishop, Augustine was now to become the leading figure in the two crises which shook the church beyond North Africa; these also compelled Augustine himself to make new changes, and were finally to have their effect on the whole Latin church of the West. It was here in Africa that the form of the church in Europe was to be decided.

First there was the **Donatist crisis**, which was to have consequences for **Augustine's** emphatically **institutional and hierarchical understanding of the church and then that of the whole West.**[12] The background was this.

In the fourth century the Catholic Church had already become a quite secularized church of the masses. But in North Africa in particular, some circles remembered very clearly the time of martyrdom and the strict church discipline, and the more spiritual understanding of the church and sacraments in Tertullian and Cyprian. According to them, baptisms and ordinations which had been performed by unworthy bishops and presbyters, above all those who had 'lapsed' in persecution, lacked the Holy Spirit and were therefore invalid; so they had to be repeated. For this reason, even before the change under Constantine, there had already been a schism with the rigorists for about a century: they accused the mainstream church of laxity. Indeed after the Constantinian change, the majority of the North African bishops were rigorists, and were now called **Donatists**, after their leader, Bishop Donatus (who died in 355).

When Augustine became bishop of the Catholics in Hippo, eighty-five years after the start of the schism, the tensions within the church had not yet died away. And the **persecuted church** was now to become a **persecuting church**. How did this come about? After the Catholic Church had been declared a state religion under Theodosius, and orthodoxy had been established, Theodosius's successor Honorius then decreed that the Donatists were to be brought back into the Catholic Church by force. He summarily banned their worship and threatened to confiscate their goods and banish them. Only the Catholic Church was to be recognized by the state. The subordination of the individual to the church as an institution which was the means of grace and salvation – this was to become a characteristic of Latin Christianity.

The crucial test came soon, for in Hippo, with its Donatist majority, from the beginning Augustine had worked intensively for the **unity of the church**. As a Christian he was tormented by the broken unity of the African church, and as a Neo-Platonist more than most he found the idea of unity a sign of the true and the good. For him, the one true church could in no way be represented by a particular church which encapsulated itself, but only by the universal church – in communion with Jerusalem, Rome and the great Eastern communities: the great **Ecclesia catholica**, expanding further and further and absorbing the world, endowed with sacraments and led by orthodox bishops, that church which Augustine calls the 'mother' of all believers. The 'catholic', which Augustine so stressed here, was to become of the utmost significance for the paradigm of the Middle Ages.

Of course Augustine, too, was well aware that this one, holy, catholic church will never be perfect on this earth. Some belong to the church only with their body (*corpore*) and not with their heart (*corde*). The real church is a pilgrim church, and will have to leave the separation of chaff and wheat to the final judge. To this degree the true church is the church of those who are holy, predestined, saved, a church contained in the visible church but hidden from human view. As for the **sacraments** of the church, a distinction must be made between validity on the one hand and legality or efficacy on the other. The decisive thing is not what is done by the bishop or priest (who is perhaps unworthy), but what is done by God in Christ. The sacraments are objectively valid (though they may not always be legitimate and effective), quite independently of the subjective worthiness of the one who dispenses them, provided that they are administered in an orderly way as provided for by the church. *Ex opere operato* was to be the term used in the Middle Ages: a sacrament is valid simply in the dispensation.

This great controversy certainly led to fundamental clarifications, and in it Augustine largely gave the whole of Western theology the **categories, solutions and neat formulae for a differentiated ecclesiology and doctrine of the sacraments**: that the church is at the same time both visible and invisible, two entities which do not simply coincide; the understanding of the unity, catholicity, holiness and apostolicity of the church which follows from this; how word and sacrament go together: the word as audible sacrament and the sacrament as visible word; how in sacramental theology a distinction must be made between the chief dispenser (Christ) and the instrumental dispenser (bishop, presbyter), on which the question of validity can be decided.

Force in matters of religion

Despite numerous compulsory measures, even the death penalty, the mainstream church and the state (which from the time of Constantine had always been interested in 'unity') did not succeed in completely eliminating the schismatic and heretical subsidiary churches which kept springing up. Finally Augustine – impressed by the success of crude police actions – felt that he also had to justify theologically the use of force against heretics and schismatics. This he did with a saying of Jesus from the parable of the great supper in its emphatic Latin translation: *Coge intrare*, 'Force (instead of 'compel') those who are outside in the alleyways and hedgerows to come in.'[13]

The consequence of this was that with his fatal argument in the Donatist crisis, the bishop and Christian Augustine, who could talk so convincingly about the love of God and human love, had to be summoned as a key witness. For what? For the **theological justification of forced conversions, the Inquisition and a holy war** against deviants of every kind. Indeed this was virtually to become a characteristic of the mediaeval paradigm, far removed from what the Greek church fathers had advocated.

Moreover Peter Brown, who has written the most informed and sensitive biography of Augustine, rightly remarks: 'Augustine, in replying to his persistent critics, wrote the only full justification in the history of the Early church, of the right of the state to suppress non-Catholics.'[14] Certainly Augustine could not exterminate the all too numerous non-Catholics in Hippo (as the Inquisition later exterminated the small sects), nor did he want to; he simply wanted to correct and convert. So – again according to Peter Brown – 'Augustine may be the first theorist of the Inquisition; but he was in no position to be a Grand Inquisitor.'[15]

Crisis of the church II: How are human beings saved?

There is no doubt about it: Augustine, an indefatigable preacher and interpreter of scripture, changed profoundly as a bishop – as so many were to do after him. More than before he now tended towards institutional thinking, towards harshness, impatience, even pessimism. And this is even more evident in the second great crisis in which he was again one of the main agents: the crisis over the highly-respected lay monk **Pelagius**, who came from England. This **Pelagian crisis sharpened and narrowed Augustine's theology of sin and grace**,[16] but found decisive spokesmen not only in the Middle Ages, but also in the Protestant Reformation and in Catholic Jansenism.[17] What was the issue?

Pelagius, personally an ascetic and an educated moralist, utterly opposed to Arianism, was active in Rome between 400 and 411, above all among lay people. He passionately attacked Manichaeism and the immoral paganism which was still widespread, but was equally critical of the lax nominal Christianity of well-to-do Roman society. And in order to be able to combat this evil, Pelagius, inspired by Origen, attached great importance to the human **will**, human **freedom**. Personal responsibility and practical action were important to him.

Certainly Pelagius also affirmed the necessity of the grace of God for every human being, but he understood grace in a more external way and not, like Augustine, as a force working within a person, almost a fuel. For Pelagius, grace was the forgiveness of sins, which for him was also an unmerited gift of God. The moral admonition and example of Christ were also grace. There is no question that for Pelagius, too, men and women were justified in baptism without works or merits. But once they had become Christians, they had to make their own way to salvation by their own actions with the sword of the free will – in accordance with the commandments of the Old Testament and the example of Christ. That was Pelagius' concern. And wasn't that an utterly reasonable theology?

However, Pelagius' teaching touched Augustine on a sore spot in his experience, indeed struck at the heart of his faith. Hadn't he experienced through all the wearisome years before his conversion (which are described in his *Confessions*) how little human beings can do of themselves? How weak their wills are? How much fleshly desire culminating in sexual pleasure (*concupiscentia carnis*) prevents them from doing the will of God? And therefore how much human beings need the grace of God right from the beginning – not just afterwards, to support their wills, but already for the willing itself, which can be intrinsically evil and perverse? From this perspective we can understand Augustine's massive counterpoint.

Original sin and double predestination

This counterpoint is all the more fundamental since Augustine was convinced that behind all the misery of the world lurks a great sin which is having an effect on all human beings. This, of course, was also the conviction of many pagans in late antiquity, but Augustine accentuates it through a theology of the first Fall, by historicizing, psychologizing and above all sexualizing this 'primal event'. For according to Augustine, human beings have been deeply corrupted right from the beginning by Adam's fall. '**In him** all have sinned' (Rom.5.12). What Augustine found in the Latin Bible translation of his time was **in quo**, and he referred this 'in him' to Adam. But the original Greek text simply has *eph'ho* = 'because' (or 'in that') all sinned! So what did Augustine read out of this sentence in Romans? Not only a primal sin of Adam but an **inherited sin,** a sin which every human being has from birth, an original sin. For Augustine, this was the reason why every human being, even the tiny infant, is poisoned in body and soul. All would incur eternal death unless they were baptized.

And worse still, because of his personal experience of the power of sex and his Manichaean past, Augustine – in contrast to Paul, who does not write a word about it – associates this transmission of '**original sin' with the sexual act** and the fleshly (= selfish) desires, concupiscence, connected with it.[18] Indeed Augustine puts sexuality generally right at the centre of human nature. And which theologian in fact understood more about this than Augustine? Who could give a better description of what goes on inside human beings?[19] No other author of antiquity had such a capacity for self-analysis as Augustine.

But this attempt at a solution raised a further question: if it is God who brings about all that is good in human beings (who are corrupt), the **problem of grace and freedom** arises. What becomes of human freedom if everything happens through the grace of God and even the good will must be given by God? Augustine was convinced that God's grace is not motivated through human freedom; on the contrary, the human will is first moved to freedom by God's grace. Grace is not acquired; grace is given. It is God's gift alone which brings about all things in human beings and is the sole basis of their redemption. Human beings constantly need this gift, freely given, until their end, but it requires their constant co-operation.

But in that case why are there so many people who will not be saved? The deeper Augustine got into the controversy with the Pelagians, the more his position hardened. This becomes clearest in his doctrine of **double predestination,** predestination to bliss or to damnation.[20] It was to have a quite uncanny effect in Western Christianity. According to Augustine, to fill the gap caused by the fall of the angels God a priori predestined only a fixed, relatively small number of people to bliss, in contrast to the great 'mass of damnation'. But is this compatible with the assumption of God's goodness? Certainly, since:

– God's **mercy** is revealed in human salvation, which bestows eternal **bliss** without any legal claim (though envisaging human merits).

– God's **righteousness** is revealed in the rejection of the majority of human beings. God does not will evil but does allow it (because of human free will), and thus lets the majority of human beings go on their way to eternal **damnation**. What a difference from Origen and his teaching of the reconciliation of all things! This is a terrifying doctrine, which Calvin was to think through to the end. It raises urgent questions.

Questions: suppression of sexuality – reification of grace?

It is indeed greatly to the credit of Augustine that he energetically directed **Western theology,** which was tending towards righteousness by works, to **the Pauline message of justification,** which with the disappearance of Jewish Christianity in Hellenistic Christianity had lost all topicality, thus **indicating the significance of grace.** Whereas Eastern theology continued to have a very marked Johannine stamp and largely neglected the Pauline problems associated with justification, with their antitheses, in favour of talk of the divinization of human beings, because of his personal experiences and his intensive study of Paul Augustine made grace virtually the central theme of Western theology. In this sphere, too, he found numerous neat Latin formulations. Against the moralism widespread in the old Latin church, which built all too much on human achievements, he demonstrated how everything is founded on God's grace: 'What do you have that you did not receive?'[21] So according to Augustine Christianity should be presented not as a religion of works and the law but as a religion of grace.

Augustine's great achievement has often been praised and need not be emphasized further here. Indeed, it is impossible here to come anywhere near assessing this epoch-making work and all the wise and profound, brilliant and moving things he wrote about the human longing for happiness in the world, under the rule of sin and the rule of grace, all his deep thoughts on time and eternity, spirituality and piety, surrender to God and the human soul. Once again, I must emphasize that in the framework of this paradigm analysis the prime concern must be to work out the difference which gradually developed between the Hellenistic way of thinking and the Latin way of thinking in Christianity, and which brought about the change from the early church Hellenistic to the Latin mediaeval paradigm. So we cannot be concerned here with the theological content of Augustine's thought in all its breadth and depth; however, we do have to examine the paradigmatic shifts in this great theologian, which can be traced into the Middle Ages and their crisis, the Reformation, and then on into modern times. And here there can be no doubt that Augustine, who so impressively advocated the primacy of the will, of love, in the face of the Greek primacy of the intellect, and who ventured so bold a statement as *Dilige, et quod vis fac*, 'Love, and do what you will';[22] who could write in so grand a style on the grace of God, is also responsible for highly problematical developments in the Latin church, at three decisive points:

1. The **suppression of sexuality** in Western theology and the Western church. More than other Latin theologians (e.g. Jerome), Augustine stressed the equality of man and woman at least on a spiritual level (in respect of their rational intelligence) because both are in the image of God. But at the same time he maintained the physical subordination of the woman which was general at the time – according to Genesis 2 the woman is created from the man and for the man.[23] In all this Augustine's theory of sex and sin remains problematical.[24]

This is because for Augustine it was clear that ideally sexual intercourse should take place only for the procreation of children. Sexual pleasure purely for its own sake is sinful and to be suppressed; it was inconceivable for him that sexual pleasure could even enrich and deepen the relationship between husband and wife. This Augustinian legacy of the vilification of sexual libido represented a tremendous burden for the men and women of the Middle Ages, the Reformation, and far beyond. And still in our own day a Pope has proclaimed in all earnestness the view that even in marriage a husband can look on his wife 'unchastely', if he does so purely for pleasure . . .

2. The **reification of grace** in Western theology and piety. Whereas the East did not develop any notion of a 'created grace' corresponding to the Latin Western doctrine of grace, and remained interested in the hoped-for total 'divinization' of human beings and their 'immortality' and 'incorruption', the Latin Tertullian already understood grace less in biblical terms as God's disposition and remission of sins than – following Stoic notions – as a *vis* in human beings, a 'power' stronger than nature (*natura*: in Tertullian we find for the first time the contrast between nature and grace).

So for Augustine, too, the 'grace of forgiveness' is merely the preparation for the 'grace of inspiration', which is poured into human beings as a healing and transforming dynamic substance of grace: *gratia infusa*, something like a supernatural fuel which drives the will (which is incapable of driving itself). Here by grace Augustine means not so much the living God who is gracious to us as a 'created grace' distinct from God himself, independent and usually attached to the sacrament. There is nothing about this in the New Testament, but the Latin theology and church of the Middle Ages – a church of grace and sacraments – was to concentrate on it, in complete contrast to Greek theology.

3. The anxiety about **predestination** in Western piety. Whereas the Greek church fathers maintained the human capacity for decision before and after the Fall, and did not recognize any unconditional divine predestination to salvation or damnation, indeed in part even believed in a reconciliation of all things, like Origen and the Origenists, Augustine as he grew old adopted a mythological Manichaean idea in an over-reaction to Pelagianism. In addition he neutralized the universal significance of Christ and in a completely un-Pauline way interpreted what the Letter to the Romans says about Israel and the church[25] in individualistic terms. But what kind of a God is it who has a priori destined countless human beings, including even countless unbaptized infants, to eternal damnation (though perhaps in a milder form) simply for the sake of his 'righteousness'?

Augustine's Byzantine contemporary John Chrysostom had explicitly emphasized that small children are innocent, since in his community some people believed that they could be killed by witchcraft and their souls be possessed by demons. But Augustine also made quite a substantial contribution to the fear of demons in the Western church. His doctrine of predestination, though already repudiated by Vincent of Lérins as an innovation (offending against the Catholic principle of 'what has been believed everywhere, always, by all') and thus by no means fully accepted by the mediaeval church, instilled in many people up to Martin Luther an anxiety about the salvation of their souls which does not match the teaching of Jesus and contradicts God's will for universal salvation. Even the French patristic scholar Henri Marrou, who interprets Augustine so benevolently, cannot avoid stating: 'If serious errors have often distorted his real thinking, as the history of his influence shows, Augustine himself bears a great deal of the responsibility.'[26] At the latest from the time of the Synod of Orange (529) and its endorsement by the Pope (530), Augustine, suspected of heresy, began to become the undisputed father of Western theology.

By contrast, Augustine provided little stimulus for the Christian life of 'lay people' in the world or for a cosmic piety, though he did stimulate speculation on God. Indeed he set completely new accents not only in matters of sexual morality or the theology of grace and the sacraments, but also in the doctrine of God, above all in rethinking the Christian tradition about the Trinity. Here he goes far beyond what we have heard so far about oneness and threeness in God from the Greeks, and especially the Cappadocians.[27]

Paradigm shift in the doctrine of the Trinity

Augustine's *Confessions* and *Commentary on Genesis* already show that he did everything possible to **bring together the Neoplatonic and biblical understanding of God,** to reconcile faith and reason, differing from most Latin theologians from Tertullian to Jerome in his high esteem for theology. For Augustine, God, understood in Neo-Platonic terms, is the supreme good, truth and beauty itself, the eternal light, the infinite being, and at the same time biblically the personal 'You', who may be addressed and spoken to: at the same time God is more inward to us than our innermost being, and higher than our highest being: *'interior intimo meo et superior summo meo'*.[28]

Was Augustine a **mystic**? Only if one uses this word in a vague sense: for any religious feeling of personal surrender, immersion in and communion with God. But not if one uses it strictly in the sense of a unitive mysticism, a real experience and doctrine of unity of the kind that appears above all in religions of Indian origin. Augustine never speaks of an ecstatic fusion which brings unity with the divine being. To this degree, like Paul and John he remains basically in line with the prophetic religions, which take seriously the qualitative difference between God and human beings, between the holy and the sinner, and know only a union with God's 'will'. Augustine, too, knows the enthusiastic feeling of surrender to God in knowledge, in will, in love, in prayer, a momentary flash of happiness, but this does not grasp the being of God directly. The *fruitio Dei*, the 'enjoyment of God', remains reserved for the other, eternal life. And for all the gloomy things he wrote about human predestination, we will grasp his understanding of the Trinity only if we take seriously the fact that for him **God himself is most profoundly love.** In the fifteen books of *De Trinitate*, written between 399 and 414, and often held up by other tasks, Augustine develops this thought for his readers.

But precisely in this great speculative work, almost the only one which he had begun without any external occasion, Augustine was clear that he was presenting an **innovation**. So it is by no means a rhetorical gesture when right at the beginning of the first book he remarks: 'Let me ask of my reader, wherever, alike with myself, he is certain, there to go on with me; wherever, alike with myself, he hesitates, there to join with me in enquiring; wherever he recognizes himself to be in error, there to return to me; wherever he recognizes me to be so, there to call me back.'[29] But hardly any readers did this; they were far too fascinated by the depth of the speculative notion of God which Augustine had set out like no one before him in Christianity.

The background to Augustine's innovation was this. As a Latin who always primarily wanted to see a clear emphasis on the **unity of God**,[30] he was unsatisfied with the Greek theory of the Cappadocians, originating with Origen, though he knew it only superficially. This theory began from the three different 'hypostases' and put far too much emphasis on the plurality of the three divine 'persons'. So what was the really new feature of Augustine's doctrine of the Trinity compared with the Greek Hellenistic doctrine? Was it perhaps that Augustine thought through and deepened the logical and ontological co-ordination of Father, Son and Spirit in a brilliant way with the use of anthropology and psychology? Certainly, but before that had come something more fundamental:

- Augustine no longer thought like the Greeks in terms of the **one God and Father** who is 'the God': the one and only principle (the *arche*) of the Godhead which the Father also gives to the Son ('God from God and light from light') and the Holy Spirit (the proceedings not understood as actions but as gifts).

- Rather, Augustine now begins with the one Godhead: with the one divine essence, glory, majesty common to all three persons. **The starting point and foundation** of his doctrine of the Trinity is thus the **one divine**

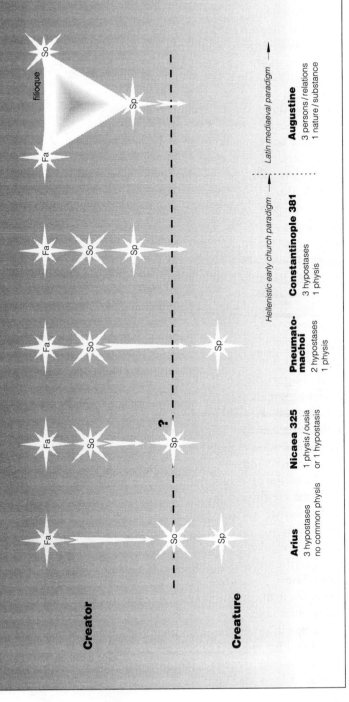

Triunity of Father, Son and Spirit

Creator

Creature

filioque

?

Hellenistic early church paradigm

Latin mediaeval paradigm →

Arius
3 hypostases
no common physis

Nicaea 325
1 physis/ousia
or 1 hypostasis

Pneumato-machoi
2 hypostases
1 physis

Constantinople 381
3 hypostases
1 physis

Augustine
3 persons/relations
1 nature/substance

nature, which for him is the principle of the unity of Father, Son and
Spirit.

● Within the unity of the one divine being, Father, Son and Spirit differ
only as **eternal relationships** (these are the foundations of life within
God), which are identical with God's being and do not appear
outwardly as such in any way.

But how does Augustine interpret God's being in anthropological and
psychological terms? Of course Augustine does not want simply to
speculate for the sake of speculation. The basis of this speculation is to
be the biblical revelation and – an important factor – the Catholic faith
(*fides catholica*). So in the first four books Augustine discusses the
scriptural evidence, in the next three dogma, and in the other eight he
offers his own thinking. That means that for Augustine, on the basis of
church teaching the Trinity is established beyond any discussion; his
sole concern is to demonstrate how a threeness is possible at all on the
philosophical and theological presupposition of oneness. That is not
very easy to understand, and continued to be difficult down to the most
recent Catholic and Protestant Western dogmatic theology (!). Here I
shall briefly sum up the essential points.

The psychology of the Trinity

According to the book of Genesis (which, however, speaks only of one
God and not of a Trinity!), human beings were created in God's image
and likeness. So God (and for Augustine, in a quiet un-Jewish way, this
is the threefold God) is the original on which human beings are based.
Augustine, who is here taking up ideas of the philosopher and convert
Marius Victorinus, therefore sees an analogy, a similarity (though in it
the dissimilarity is greater than the similarity), between the threefold
God and the three-dimensional human spirit (*mens*): memory (*memoria*
as the centre of the person), understanding (*intelligentia*) and will
(*voluntas*).

From this, Augustine constructs the **Trinity as an unfolding of God's
self** with philosophical and psychological categories:

– The **Son** is 'begotten' according to the intellect (in the divine act of
thinking) from the substance of the Father: he is the Father's personal
word and image.

– The **Spirit** 'proceeds' from the Father (the one who loves) **and** the Son
(the one who is loved – hence the famous *filioque*) – according to the
will in a single breathing (*spiratio*): so the Spirit is the personified love
between Father and Son.

– Therefore Father, Son and Spirit represent three subsisting relationships (*relationes*), really different from one another but at the same time coinciding with the one divine nature: fatherhood, sonship and spiration itself. This trinity clearly expresses not only the unity of the one divine nature but also the interrelationship of the three persons.

– One important consequence of thinking in terms of the one divine nature is that all activity of the Godhead 'outwards' (whether in creation or redemption) does not proceed from one of the persons but from the one divine nature, and is common to all three persons (*opera trinitatis ad extra sunt unum*).

These, quite briefly, are the basic notions which Augustine developed at length in his treatise. And even a superficial comparison with Origen and other Greek church fathers indicates that here in the framework of his new Latin macroparadigm Augustine has brought about a **paradigm shift in the doctrine of the Trinity,** so to speak the shift of a micro– or mesoparadigm. Moreover, the Greeks could never have gone along with this theology.

On the contrary: the Greeks reacted vigorously when the Latins, referring to Augustine's doctrine, from the sixth/seventh centuries gradually and then under Pope Benedict VIII finally, in 1014, introduced the procession of the Spirit from the Father 'and the Son' into the Niceno-Constantinopolitan Creed – moreover, against Augustine's intentions. For it would never have occurred to Augustine himself that his doctrine of the Trinity, although it was clearly a basis for the *filioque,* could ever have broken up the Niceno-Constantinopolitan Creed and thus become a main reason for the split between the Eastern and Western churches. Right down to the present day this inserted *filioque* – which the West then elevated to the status of a dogma – has seemed to the East to be a falsification of the ecumenical creed and thus clear heresy. In the East the original wording was strictly adhered to: the Spirit proceeds from the Father (through the Son). Hence the requirement, still maintained, that the *filioque* should be removed from the ecumenical creed. Is all this just a dispute over words?

We in the West will never understand the importance of the question for the East if we think that this is just a matter of a different terminology or the subtleties of a theological theory. No, what is at issue here is no less than a new **overall constellation in the understanding of God.** For the Greek fathers, the principle of unity between Father, Son (Word) and Spirit was and is not just one divine nature common to all three persons. The principle of unity is the one God and Father, who is 'the principle of Godhead' (*tes theotetos arche*), the root and the source of the Son and the Spirit, on whom he bestows the Godhead. He is the origin, who reveals himself 'through the Son (Word) in the Spirit'. The Godhead (the divine nature) is not defined independently of three persons, but only with them and in them.

A century ago now the French historian of the dogma of the Trinity, Théodore de Régnon SJ, illustrated the difference between the Latin paradigm of the Trinity usual in the West and the Greek paradigm in his four-volume work with an enlightening image.[31] In the Western constellation we see three stars illuminating one another in a triangle on the same level (even if for other reasons Augustine protested against the trinitarian interpretation of the triangle by the Manichaeans). However, in the Greek paradigm these three stars appear precisely one after another in a straight line, so that they cannot be distinguished by the human eye. The first star gives light to the second (the Nicene Creed's 'light of light, God of God!'), and finally to the third, though to the human eye – as it were from below – these three stars appear only as one star and their radiance only as one radiance. But anyone who sees the Son in the Spirit, also sees the Father.

The Trinity as the central dogma

Now the Eastern side should also have recognized that in its way the anthropological-psychological interpretation of the Trinity gives clear expression to the great old concern of Western theology. For here there is primarily a defence of the **unity of God** against all tritheism, against all the belief in three Gods which kept breaking out in the practical piety of both churches. Now we have seen in connection with paradigm II how the Cappadocians had demonstrated a clear and consistent solution to the problem '1 = 3?' (on the basis of the development in dogma which had now taken place), a solution which is now praised as the royal middle way between modalism and tritheism, oneness and threeness, indeed monotheism and polytheism. Yet earlier we already had to raise the question: is the contradiction between oneness and threeness really resolved simply by introducing a conceptual distinction: 'one' denotes God's 'nature', 'three' the 'persons'? With such a threeness, isn't the oneness of God merely asserted, since in purely philosophical terms there can only be one God, but the Bible seems to speak of three divine entities? Thus this is a purely conceptual, intellectual 'solution' which contrary to the will of the fathers of Nicaea in fact abandons monotheism, despite all assertions to the contrary, so that this 'solution' also can never convince either Jews or Muslims, as I have emphasized.

Now Augustine provided a new solution compared with the Greeks, in so far as he wanted to understand Father, Son and Spirit not as three different substances but only as three different relationships within the one Godhead. Relation is, after all, the weakest of all the Aristotelian categories, only an *esse ad*, a 'being related to' (say, the Father to the Son and vice versa). Accordingly, three relationships would not add anything substantial to the divine nature, but only represent the relationship of the three entities within the one Godhead which is common to all three, though in different ways: God the Father as the one who begets, God the Son as the one who is begotten, and the Holy Spirit who is the divine love common to both.

This is certainly an ingenious theory, which we can admire even more if we have thought through its inner logic with all its implications. But if we compare it with what we read in the New Testament about Father, Son and Spirit, here too we cannot avoid asking some critical questions. Here are just three, which are interconnected:

– In Augustine, aren't Father, Son and Spirit volatilized, so that they become three relationships, and levelled down into one nature, so that fundamentally there is only one God with different relations, aspects or countenances, whereas in the New Testament Father, Son and Spirit are three very different and quite distinctive entities?

– In Augustine's world, isn't the activity of Father, Son and Spirit combined and channelled into one action in such a way that both creation and incarnation, crucifixion and resurrection, must always be the joint work of all three persons? But doesn't scripture speak of a special activity of the Father (e.g. in creation), of the Son (in the crucifixion), and of the Spirit (at the feast of Pentecost)?

– So in the last resort isn't this doctrine a free-floating conceptual construction remote from scripture? Even a Catholic dogmatic theologian like Karl Rahner, whose theology deliberately remains within the system, speaks of 'a seemingly almost gnostic speculation about what goes on in the inner life of God'.[32] Certainly great psychological inferences are made from the designations 'Father', 'Son' and 'Spirit' with apparently compelling logic, but the different experiences of the activity of the Father or the Son or the Spirit as reported in Scripture have little real relation to them. Certainly here we have an extremely subtle theology, which has time and again fascinated subtle minds, but can it really be preached? Or doesn't such a theology also contradict especially the old liturgy, where even in the Roman mass from its Greek beginnings it was never 'the Trinity' which was worshipped, but the Father through the Son in the Holy Spirit: '*Deus pater omnipotens . . . per Dominum nostrum Jesum Christum . . . in unitate Spiritus Sancti*'?

However, unconcerned with any objections, **in the Latin West**, where Greek now faded right into the background, **Augustine's doctrine of the**

Trinity was very soon **regarded as** *the* Catholic doctrine, to some degree as the central Christian dogma. The introductory catechesis that begins **Quicumque** ('Whosoever would be saved'),[33] which originated only in the second half of the fifth century in southern Gaul or Spain, was now given out and popularized as the Athanasian Creed. And this although it does not indicate the slightest connection with Athanasius and the Greeks, far less the New Testament. Its origin remains obscure, but in the question of God, in an utterly Augustinian way the oneness of the divine nature is stressed before the threeness. From the eighth century in Gaul (at first against persistent Roman resistance) a Latin **Liturgy of the Trinity** was also propagated. Finally, in 1334, the Avignon Pope John XXII even introduced a feast of the Trinity – the first festival to be dedicated not to a 'saving event' but to a church dogma. Augustine's theology had triumphed completely.

Thus Augustine's doctrine of the Trinity established itself in the West, totally and exclusively; Thomas Aquinas and the Neo-Thomists, the Reformers and Karl Barth with his pupils in fact also accepted it as the central dogma, modifying it slightly, refining it, and translating it into another language (some into Aristotelian, others into a more recent terminology). But is it much help if instead of three 'persons' or 'subsistent relationships' (Thomas) one speaks of three 'modes of being' (Barth) or 'distinct modes of subsistence' (Rahner)? In the West the Greek doctrine of the Trinity, in so far as it was known at all, was regarded as superseded, and the New Testament was used only as a quarry for the doctrine which had already been sanctioned by the church for so long.

Question: In which God should the Christian believe?

Now as Peter Brown has demonstrated in detail,[34] Augustine wrote the masterpieces of his middle period – and these include *De Trinitate* – as a priest and bishop in 'splendid isolation', a 'cosmopolitan *manqué*'. Moreover his relations with Greek theology and the culture of the Hellenistic world were of a somewhat 'Platonic' nature. Augustine soon lost his original longing for Greek books, so that he now wrote his books only in contact with local North African authors. We may regret that, for Augustine was the only figure whose powerful mind could have mediated between the two cultures of the Latin West and the Greek East. So unfortunately because of Augustine's limited cultural horizon, the Latin theology which followed him also had hardly any inner connection with the world of Greek culture.

In this way the **originally simple triadic confessional statements** of the New Testament about Father, Son and Spirit developed into an **in-**

creasingly demanding intellectual trinitarian speculation on $3 = 1$. It was almost like a higher trinitarian mathematics, but despite all attempts at conceptual clarity, lasting solutions were hardly reached. We might ask whether this Graeco–Latin speculation, which, far removed from its biblical basis, boldly attempted to spy out the mystery of God in vertiginous heights, did not perhaps, like Icarus, the son of Daedalus, the ancestor of Athenian craft, come too near the sun with wings made of feathers and wax.

Of course all these critical questions should not give the impression that nowadays the classical Latin doctrine of the Trinity belongs on the rubbish heaps of history. Rather:

- The classical doctrines of God and Trinity, Christ and redemption, grace and sacraments must not be dismissed unthinkingly. But they must not be repeated unthinkingly either, and forced on people who cannot understand them as the 'heart' and 'central dogma' of the Christian faith. What would Jesus and his disciples have understood by them?
- Rather, the classical doctrines are to be assessed in the context of the paradigm by which they were formed and the time by which they were conditioned; they must be examined critically in the light of their origins and not just modernized with the help of current sociological, indeed gynaecological, insights.[35]
- Christians are to believe in Father, Son and Spirit, but they need not believe in either a Greek-Hellenistic or a Western Latin **trinitarian speculation**. This is **not part of the essence of Christianity**. It is not divine revelation, but church teaching, and thus a human work which came about – as we heard – under particular paradigmatic conditions.

In the light of the New Testament, no more is required than that the relationship between Father, Son and Spirit should be interpreted in a critical and differentiated way for the present. The 'heart' of Christian faith is not a theological theory but belief that God the Father works in a revealing, redeeming and liberating way in us through his Son Jesus Christ in the Spirit. Any theological theory must not complicate this basic statement; rather, it must be seen simply as an instrument for clarifying it against differing cultural horizons.

Moreover, Augustine, unlike Origen, did not work out any all-embracing system, but put forward a unitary conception. And he had not yet completed his work on the Trinity when as a bishop he was confronted with an event which now clearly signalled a crisis not only for the church but also for the empire, and thus a change in world history.

Crisis of the empire: What is the meaning of history?

On 28 August 410 Rome, which had believed itself to be 'eternal', had been stormed by the army of Alaric, king of the West Goths, and plundered for days on end. In North Africa, now refugees told of horrific atrocities: numerous fires, women raped, even senators murdered, the rich hunted, whole families exterminated, houses plundered, valuables of all kinds carried off by the barbarians by the cartload, the old government and administrative centre of the Western world destroyed. Uncertainty and defeatism were abroad: if 'eternal Rome' could fall, what was still safe?

Augustine reacted with a last gigantic work, on the *City of God* (*De civitate Dei*), in which he attempted to come to terms intellectually with the fall of ancient Rome.[36] How? By pointing to the Christian –Byzantine New Rome which was still intact? That never occurred to Augustine. Rather, by presenting a great interpretation of history which went beyond the immediate occasion. There was no argument which Augustine did not take up in the course of his work to offer a **theodicy** in the grand style, a justification of God in the face of all the insoluble riddles of this life, all with the aim of helping to strengthen unconditional trust, faith in God.

Augustine's concern is the destiny of human beings, indeed the destiny of humankind. So in the last twelve books his apologia issues in a large-scale **interpretation of history**: a battle between the *civitas terrena*, the earthly state, the world state, world citizenship, and on the other hand the *civitas Dei*, the city of God, the state of God, the citizenship of God. The great controversy between world state and God's state is the mysterious **foundation and meaning of history**, which is at the same time a history of salvation and disaster. Augustine describes its origin and beginning, then its progress through seven ages, and finally its outcome and goal.

Where is the origin of the two civil communities? It lies in primal times, when the apostasy of proud angels led to a second realm alongside **God's state** – the **devil's state**. Consequently there was a need to make good the gap torn open by the fall of the angels, from those predestined from the human race, until the full number of the citizens of God was attained again. However, through the primal sin of Adam the angelic sin of pride has repeated itself, so that now among human beings an earthly **world state** has developed over against God's state. Its first representatives were on the one hand Abel, the just, and on the other Cain, the builder of cities and fratricidal murderer; then Israel and the Gentile world; then Jerusalem the city of God and Babylon the city of the world. In the end time all this culminates in the fight between Rome, the new Babylon, and the Catholic Church.

So the city of God and the city of this world are **fundamentally different** right from the beginning:
– their Lord and Governor is different: on the one hand God, and on the other the gods and demons.
– their citizens are different: the elect worshippers of the one true God – the repudiated worshippers of God and the selfish;
– their basic attitude is different: the love of God rooted in humility, going as far as despising the self – the self-love grounded in pride, going as far as despising God.

Of course Augustine is not a historian in the modern sense, but a theological interpreter of history; he is not primarily interested in the development of humankind, but in God's plan.[37] Yet unlike Homer and Virgil, he is concerned not with a mythology of history but with real history and its deepest ground. With the help of the Bible and ancient historians, Augustine wants to achieve two things: first, to present numerous historical details with every possible parallel and analogy, allegory and typology; and secondly, precisely in this way to offer a **meaningful overall view of world history** as the great clash between belief and unbelief, humility and arrogance, love and striving for power, salvation and damnation – from the beginning of time until today. So it was Augustine who created the first monumental **theology of history** in Christianity – which had a deep influence on the whole of mediaeval Western theology and the theology of the Reformation, up to the threshold of the modern secularization of history. Before Augustine, in antiquity, there was neither a philosophy of history nor a theology of history. Augustine thus took seriously the fact that in the Jewish Christian understanding – so completely different from the circular Hellenistic, Indian understanding – history is a movement towards an end, guided and directed by God: the eternal city of God, the kingdom of peace, the kingdom of God.

No politicization and clericalization of the city of God

However, the Roman rule of the world had collapsed in North Africa as well; Augustine's theology was to make world history on another continent, Europe. No wonder that the grandiose and dramatic *City of God* became the favourite book of the Middle Ages, far more so than the intimate and poetic *Confessions*, since it vividly presents its readers with the issues in the great, perplexing battles of world history. Charlemagne is said to have read the *City of God* every day. No wonder, too, that different political powers and trends later attempted to use the *City of God* as an instrument for their own power struggles. For what was more natural in the great dispute between Pope and emperor over investiture and power in Christianity than to discredit the German emperor and empire as the 'world state' and to glorify the Pope and the Roman church as 'God's state'?

However, we must not blame Augustine for that. He was thinking of individuals and not of institutions. So such **politicization and clericalization of the city of God** was far from his mind. For Augustine, all bishops are equal in principle and all priests are servants of the church. And what is more important to him than visible church organization is the church as the hidden body of Christ, given life through the one Spirit, united in the eucharist. In the Middle Ages, those critical of the hierarchy were also constantly to refer to the 'invisible church' and the more spiritualistic elements in Augustine's theology. At any rate Augustine provides no impetus for papalism; only the Bishops of Rome were concerned about that.

Now in fact it was the **Roman** church in particular which was increasingly to take on its own profile in the Latin paradigm of the Middle Ages, so that this Catholic paradigm, when completed, would present itself as Roman Catholic. But what a long way it was from Pope Damasus, Augustine's contemporary with so much self-esteem, to Pope Gregory, who in a life-and-death battle with the German emperor established the Roman view in the Catholic Church and the German empire, even if personally he came to grief! We now have to turn to the further development of this Roman Catholic paradigm.

3. The Bishop of Rome's claim to power

Instead of Jerusalem, Rome was now the centre and leading church of Christianity: this is a clear indicator of the paradigm shift from Jewish Christianity (P I) to Gentile Christianity (P II), as we already saw.[38] The increasingly active **role of the Roman church** is impossible to overlook even in the second and third centuries, as is the constantly growing significance of the law.[39] What is the basis for the Roman position of power?

Does the biblical promise to Peter apply to a Bishop of Rome?

The church of the imperial capital, as old as it was powerful, had always been notable for its good organization, legalistic procedures and comprehensive charitable work. But it had also shown its faithfulness in different persecutions and was quite rightly seen as a **stronghold of orthodoxy**. Had it not proved itself in the battle against Gnostics, Marcionites and Montanists? The notion of the apostolic tradition and succession gained an early footing here, and as early as about 160 this was given expression with the erection of monuments to Peter and Paul. The influence of Rome had also been important in the formulation of the baptismal creed and the demarcation of the New Testament canon. In matters of doctrine the Roman church always wisely adopted a middle, mediating position. And it was equally to be expected that the genius of the Roman church, the Roman talent for organization and sense of real politics, would have a particular effect. In short, the Roman church had **high moral authority** and all the makings of a leading role.

But something else should equally be stated for the record: in the first centuries there could be **no question of a legal primacy** – or even a position of pre-eminence based on the Bible – for the Roman community or even the Roman bishop. As we heard in connection with the so-called Letter of Clement, at the beginning of the Roman community there was manifestly no monarchical episcopate. We know hardly more than the names of the Roman bishops of the first two centuries. Historians regard the year 222 (the beginning of the pontificate of Urban I) as the first certain date in papal history. The first collection of papal biographies (*Liber Pontificalis*), which brought together some earlier traditions, was probably made after 500.

One piece of evidence for the original Roman modesty is the fact that the **promise to Peter** from the Gospel of Matthew – 'You are Peter, and on this rock I will build my church' (16.18f.) – which in giant black letters on a golden background now adorns the basilica of St Peter, and which is so central for the present-day Bishops of Rome, does not once occur in full in the whole of the Christian literature of the first centuries – apart from a text in Tertullian. This quotes the passage, but for Peter, not for Rome.

Only in the middle of the third century does a Bishop of Rome named Stephen refer to the promise to Peter, in a dispute with other churches over whose is the better tradition. He does not hesitate to slander Africa's most significant metropolitan, Cyprian, as a pseudo-apostle and a pseudo-Christian. But it was to be long after the shift under Constantine, only from the second half of the fourth century on, that Matt.16.18f. was to be used (especially by Bishops Damasus and Leo) to support a Roman claim to leadership and authority. Eastern Christianity never went along with such an interpretation of the Peter passage. For up to the eighth century and beyond, the whole of Eastern exegesis sees Matt.16.18 only as **Peter's personal confession of faith** and Matt.18.18 as an authority to forgive sins ('binding and loosing') which is also given to the other apostles; at all events, this is not seen as a personal authority of Peter in the juridical sense, far less as a primacy in matters of jurisdiction, exercised specifically by a successor to Peter in Rome. So can a position of institutional power be built on the figure of Peter in Rome?

Roman power politics in the name of the apostle Peter

Conflicts become evident at a very early stage. The well-founded **moral authority** of the Roman church became problematical wherever it was understood in **legal** terms and attempts were made to establish it in **authoritarian** fashion, without respect for the character and independence of the other churches in doctrine, liturgy or church order. And the problems increased as time went on. Two striking cases of conflict involving an emergent Roman **authoritarianism**, which was unable to win through at that stage, are known from as early as the period before Constantine.

– Towards the end of the second century Bishop **Victor** of Rome already excommunicated the whole of Asia Minor for the sake of a single (Roman!) date for Easter; but bishops of the East and West, in particular the highly respected Irenaeus of Lyons,[40] protested, and Bishop Victor suffered a defeat.

– Around the middle of the third century Bishop **Stephen**, whom we have already met, wanted to exclude wide areas of the church from communion because they had a different assessment of heretical baptism, now for the first time referring to the biblical promise to Peter; however, the Bishops of Alexandria and Caesarea joined Cyprian and the churches of Africa in defending the practice.

So neither Victor nor Stephen could carry through their demands. Again still **in the time of Constantine** it was the emperor who continued to bear the title and the authority of Pontifex Maximus (supreme priest) and had the monopoly of legislation even in church matters (*ius in sacris*). Even in Rome **nothing** was known of a **legal primacy of Rome**. Certainly, as a result of Constantine's incorporation of the Catholic Church into the state order the Roman community, like all other Christian communities, became a corporation under public law and the bishops of the provincial capitals (metropolises) became metropolitans. But the aim of the emperor, who in Bishop Ossius of Cordoba had an important adviser on church policy from the West, was the unity of the church. He did not negotiate with any Roman 'Pope' (the forged 'Donation of Constantine' came later), and summoned the First Ecumenical Council of Nicaea on his own authority, without asking for any advice. There the Roman Church was represented among several hundred bishops only by Bishop Ossius of

Cordoba, mentioned above, and two presbyters, and did not play the slightest role in the proceedings. Granted, the council itself already recognized metropolitan sees set over the other churches, the later patriarchates, but not the primacy of Rome over the whole church, and this is also confirmed by Eusebius' *Church History*. In Rome itself, too, at this time there is still no reference to a biblical basis for a special position of the Roman church.

Things are different in the **period after Constantine**, above all after 350. Now we have a development which is characteristic only of the West: the **rise** of the community of Rome and **the Bishop of Rome to a position of monarchical pre-eminence in the West**, which was to become typical of the Latin mediaeval paradigm. What contributed to this special development in the West?

– **The transfer of the imperial residence** to Constantinople: the position of the Bishop of Rome, who enjoyed particular imperial gifts (the Lateran palace and the new Lateran church and the church of St Peter) was indirectly strengthened.

– The rule of the one emperor over the church as well: in time this called for a **church counterpart**.

– **Tendencies towards centralization in the church**: the metropolitans over the bishops, and the super-metropolitans (patriarchs) – who became increasingly important – over them. In the latters' contest for the primacy in the end only Rome and Constantinople (and for a time also Alexandria) were left.

– **Monarchical tendencies in the Roman church**: these were encouraged both by philosophical and religious monotheism and by the political monarchy.

– **Adoption of imperial structures of organization**: the creation of an efficient chancery and an archive, with the registering of all incoming and outgoing post.

– **Exemption of the Roman clergy** from taxes and their own ecclesiastical jurisdiction in questions of faith and civil law.

The development of the Roman idea of the Pope

The Roman bishops of the fourth and fifth centuries purposefully extended their official competence, with the intention of establishing a patriarchate over the West, and soon also of achieving a primacy over the whole church. One institutional development of the Roman primacy began at that time which was significant for the future; the Cambridge historian Walter Ullmann has played a leading role in analysing it.[41] The presuppositions for this, which had no biblical foundation, entered church law over the course of the centuries. Papal Rome, too, was not built in a day.

Stage 1: **Julius** (337–352): Rome becomes a **court of appeal**. A canon of the Western rump synod of Sardica (Sofia) of 343 allowed deposed bishops to appeal to Rome. At a very early stage Rome presented this as a universally valid decree of the Ecumenical Council of Nicaea and interpreted it extensively.

Stage 2: **Damasus** (366–384): Rome applies the New Testament **promise to Peter** to itself. It was Damasus who for the first time used Matt.16.18f. as a foundation for Roman claims to power and at the same time interpreted it in a legalistic way. This was the background. 137 people had perished in the turbulent election involving him and Ursinus. He owed his enthronement to the city prefect of Rome and moreover was accused under a new city prefect of instigation to murder; only the intervention of rich friends who went to the emperor saved him from being condemned. This power-conscious Bishop of Rome, a princely host who was called 'the matrons' ear-tickler', had every occasion to strengthen his weak moral and political authority – by a novel emphasis on his dignity as **Peter's successor**. Now he spoke constantly and exclusively of the Roman church as the '**apostolic see**' (*sedes apostolica*) and thus raised for the Roman church the claim to a higher status than that of the other churches, grounded in a monopolistic position for the church of Rome, allegedly God-given through Peter and Paul. So it is no coincidence that Damasus had the tombs and churches of Peter and Paul, along with those of the Roman bishops and martyrs, richly decorated and provided with beautiful Latin inscriptions in their honour, all to make it clear that the true Rome was now Christian Rome. It was also in line with this policy that he gave the learned north Italian Jerome the task of making an easily understandable and modern Latin translation of the Bible (instead of the Old Latin Itala or Vetus Latina). Moreover this naturally rendered many expressions, especially in the Old Testament, with terms drawn from Roman law, and later became the **Vulgate**, normative in both church and theology, the liturgy and the law. So what was the 'achievement of Damasus', who like all the other fourth-century bishops of Rome was involved with the Roman upper class nostalgically dreaming of the great pagan Rome? With Henry Chadwick, we may note matter-of-factly that he fused 'the old Roman civic and imperial pride with Christianity'.[42] Anyone who wanted to write a history of the mentality of the Roman Curia would have to begin here.

Stage 3: **Siricius** (384–99): Rome adopts an **imperial official style**. Damasus' followers continued along the same lines. It was all the easier for them to fall in with this since in the West (!) Rome was the only 'apostolic' foundation and here the metropolitan constitution was less developed than in the East. At the same time, from the start the Roman church was better organized than the other churches in the empire. Bishop Siricius – his contemporary Bishop Ambrose of Milan is more significant as a theologian, churchman and politician – was the first to call himself **'Pope'**: **'Papa'**, from the Greek *pappas*, was a loving and honorific name for father, but in the East it was used by Christians everywhere for their own bishop. From the end of the fifth century the Bishops of Rome claimed the term exclusively for themselves. The process of a Roman **monopolizing of titles** originally belonging to many churches and bishops (priests) had begun.[43] But what was of even greater significance for the future was that Siricius began to call his own **statutes** without further ado **'apostolic'** and was the first to take over the **official style of the imperial chancery**. It was as though the requests for advice and help from the different churches were enquiries from Roman provincial governors, to which the Bishop of Rome had to reply to with an imperial rescript, with *decreta* and *responsa* ('answers'). And so it still is today.

Stage 4: **Innocent** (401–417): Rome encourages **centralism**. This bishop, who had already published a whole series of decrees, wanted to have any **important matter presented to the Roman bishop for a decision** after it had been discussed at synod. In so doing he claimed – one of the historical fictions in Rome's favour which were now becoming increasingly numerous – that the gospel had reached the other Western provinces exclusively and solely from Rome (North Africa, southern France and Spain are manifest instances to the contrary), so that all the Western churches should follow the Roman liturgy – regardless of the fact that Milan, which was quite near, had its own independent liturgy. Moreover Ambrose, Augustine and later also Gregory the Great pursued another policy in liturgical matters. But liturgical uniformity remained a Roman aim.

Stage 5: **Boniface** (418–422): Rome forbids further **appeals**. The development of the hour was not just that Rome was regarded by other churches as a court of appeal and established itself as a court of appeal. Rome also regarded itself as the 'apostolic pinnacle' (*apostolicum culmen*), and its verdicts and decisions as ultimately binding. There could no longer be any appeal beyond Rome to another authority. *Prima sedes a nemine iudicatur* – 'The first see is not judged by anyone' – a principle later formulated in general terms, already began to emerge here.

But all these were primarily **simply Roman claims and postulates**. Even Augustine, the great contemporary of Bishops Damasus, Siricius, Innocent and Boniface, who was truly a friend of Rome, knows nothing of a Petrine primacy of jurisdiction. The Catholic Augustine scholar Fritz

Hofmann has more recent scholarship behind him when he writes: 'The question of a Petrine primacy of jurisdiction, the foundation of which was left to a later theological development, did not even occur to him.'[44] Indeed, for Augustine, Christ and belief in him, not Peter as a person (far less his 'successors'), is the foundation of the church. This is also confirmed by the young Joseph Ratzinger in his dissertation on Augustine's ecclesiology: 'So if the church is founded on Peter, it is not founded on his person but on his faith . . . The foundation of the church is Christ. "*Non enim dictum est illi: tu es petra, sed: tu es Petrus. Petra autem erat Christus*" (For he was not told "You are the rock", but "You are Peter", and the rock was Christ), this sentence shows that the Christ (*petra*) accepted in faith (*Petrus*) is the true foundation stone of the church.'[45] For Augustine, it is not the Bishop of Rome who is the supreme authority in the church but the ecumenical council, and he does not attribute any infallible authority even to that.[46]

Far less did anyone take the Roman claims and postulates seriously in the East. Who in the new Second Rome was interested (theologically and legally) in the old imperial capital which had gone under? The supreme authority alongside the emperor was not the Pope, but the universal, ecumenical council, which only the emperor could call and to which of course even the Bishop of Rome had to submit.

The objection of the ecumenical councils

Anyone who studies the decrees of the First Ecumenical Council of **Nicaea in 325**[47] will discover (as I have already indicated) that Rome, like the other great ancient episcopal sees of Alexandria, Antioch and Jerusalem (the patriarchates), enjoyed privileges, but did not exercise any primacy over the whole church. That also applies to the most significant bishops and theologians of the Western church, alongside Augustine above all Ambrose, who similarly did not derive any privilege for the Bishop of Rome from the saying about Peter in Matt.16.18, but followed Cyprian's episcopal line throughout. However, their contemporary, Pope Damasus, whom we have already met, was already making insolent and untruthful claims. He argued that Nicaea enjoyed unique authority only because his predecessor Silvester had approved the resolutions of the ecumenical council.

The polarization increased. Whereas the fundamental decree of the emperor Theodosius in 380 which made Christianity a state religion declared the faith of both the Bishop of Rome and the Bishop of Alexandria to be the criterion of orthodoxy (against the Arians), a resolution of the Second Ecumenical Council of **Constantinople in 381** gives the Bishop of New Rome, the seat of the emperor and the imperial government, the second place after the old Rome. At the same time the council forbade all bishops to intervene in other dioceses (a thrust against Rome!). However, this did not prevent a Roman synod summoned by Bishop Damasus in 382 from stating that the Roman church had not been founded by synodical decrees but by the apostles Peter and Paul. The Roman church derived from a special divine dispensation, from which it followed that the Roman church had a primacy!

Similarly, at the Third Ecumenical Council of **Ephesus in 431** a three-member Roman delegation argued that Peter was the head of the apostles and the current Pope (Celestinus) his successor. However, these great Roman claims found no echo at the council, especially as the Roman contributions to the christological discussion played a completely subordinate role. Still, this Roman proposal is also faithfully preserved in the papal archive for future times, though it is purely theoretical. The fact remains that all attempts by the Roman bishops in the fourth and fifth centuries to draw conclusions from the saying to Peter for a divinely willed Roman jurisdiction over the whole church and to establish such a claim came to grief. The papacy as the source (*fons*), origin (*exordium*) and head (*caput*) of Christianity? For a long time all this remained Roman wishful thinking. Even the most significant Bishop of Rome in the fifth century, Leo I, had to experience this.

The first dispute between Pope and council: Leo the Great

No one was fuller of the Roman consciousness of mission than **Leo**, whom historians call 'the Great'.[48] In his twenty-one years in office (440–461) this man proved to be a solid theologian (his letter to the Council of Chalcedon) and a brilliant lawyer, but also a pastor and a preacher. His statesmanship became legendary. For in 451 a Roman delegation (including Leo as bishop) succeeded in persuading Attila's Huns in Mantua not to sack Rome – though of course the situation was different in 455, when Leo could not prevent the conquest and plundering of Rome by the Vandals.

It was this Leo who created the **classical synthesis of the idea of Roman primacy** from elements which had been prepared in the fourth century.[49] For with theological clarity and legal acuteness he combined the biblical, historical and legal arguments to support the primacy of Peter and thus that of the Bishop of Rome:

– The **biblical** basis for a **primacy of Peter** over all the other apostles was now a massively legalistic understanding of the classic Petrine passages in the New Testament:[50] the New Testament already meant a '**fullness of power**' (*plenitudo potestatis*) to govern the whole church of Christ (later called the 'power of jurisdiction', 'pastoral power'), which was given to Peter. But had Peter ever nominated a successor, a successor even in Rome?

– The **historical** basis for the Bishop of Rome as Peter's successor was established with the help of a letter from Pope Clement to James the brother of the Lord in Jerusalem. According to this letter Peter had transferred to Clement in a last dispensation the power to bind and to loose (in Roman legal terminology *solvere* and *legare*), thus making him his sole legitimate successor – excluding the other bishops. At least nowadays we know that this letter is a forgery from the end of the second century which had only been translated from Greek into Latin at the end of the fourth or the beginning of the fifth century. But from now on it was the constant justification for the Roman claim.

– **Legally** the position of Peter's successor was defined precisely with the help of the **Roman law of inheritance**. The Bishop of Rome takes the place of the testator, Peter, as his heir, though of course he does not inherit Peter's personal characteristics and merits (subjectively, the Pope is an 'unworthy heir'). But he does inherit the official authority and function transferred by Christ to Peter (objectively the Pope, if not an 'apostle', is 'apostolic'). That means that even a completely unworthy successor to Peter – and there were to be many of them – nevertheless remains his legitimate successor, whose decrees are valid, independent of any personal moral quality. The main thing is the office, which is entered into the moment the election has been accepted, even if the person elected should still be a layman and not an ordained priest (this was often the case and the practice remains legitimate to the present day).

On the basis of these constructions Leo was convinced that Peter personally spoke and acted through his person. Moreover, as far as was possible at the time he governed the Western church in this spirit. He also got political support; for opportunistic reasons in 445, under Leo's influence, the West Roman emperor Valentinian III formally confirmed the legal pre-eminence of Rome in an edict, though this did not apply in the East. So because of his theory and practice in church history this Bishop of Rome is rightly the first to be given the title '**Pope' in the real sense**.

However, it should be noted that all these fine constructions continued to be treated throughout the church as Roman wishful thinking. Certainly, with his proposed solution to the bitterly disputed christological questions Leo had met with great approval at the Fourth Ecumenical Council of **Chalcedon in 451**, which was almost exclusively an Eastern affair ('Peter has spoken', the council said).[51] But the claim of the three papal legates – who together with two African bishops were the only Western participants – that they should preside was rejected outright by the imperial executive committee at the council. And contrary to Leo's explicit prohibition, his letter was examined by the council to see if it met the norms of orthodoxy. In other words, no one even in Chalcedon thought of according the city of Rome, now in any case in danger and ruined, and its bishop any privileges or even a position of pre-eminence over the whole church, self-conscious though this synod with its 600 members was. And it was of little use to Leo that he was the first bishop to adorn himself with the title of the pagan supreme priest, 'Pontifex maximus' – once Tertullian had applied it to the Bishop of Rome in mockery and the emperor had now discarded it! – and with a reference to the saying to Peter required obedience also from the Eastern churches and even the submission of the ecumenical council. Quite the contrary.

Leo, of all people, had to watch the Council of Chalcedon, without the slightest hesitation, in canon 17 making the ecclesiastical rank of a city dependent on its civil status. And in the famous canon 28 the seat of **New Rome (Constantinople)** is accorded **the same primacy** as the old imperial capital.[52] The Roman legates protested in vain. Leo's subsequent sharp protest against this revaluation of the Second Rome, which moreover had been accompanied with a demonstrative acclamation of the Emperor Marcian as a 'new Constantine', as 'king and priest', resounded unheard. Deeply hurt, Leo then hesitated for an unforgivably long time – until 453 – before recognizing Chalcedon. In so doing, he unintentionally helped the enemies of the two-natures formula in Palestine and Egypt, where the popular fury against the christological definition of Chalcedon was indescribable, so great that Proterius, the then patriarch of Alexandria, was later torn to pieces by a fanatical mob. However, Leo himself was the first Roman bishop to be buried in St Peter's – another symbol.

At the end of the fifth century an interim climax was reached in the Roman claim to power – under **Gelasius I** (492–96).[53] Already very influential as secretary to his predecessor Felix III, who, with a full sense of his power, in 484 had thought that he could 'depose' and excommunicate the Byzantine patriarch Acacius (of course to no effect), Gelasius was completely under the thumb of Theoderic, the Arian king of the East Goths. But in this way he became largely independent of Byzantium. With impunity he could venture not only to reject the Caesaropapistical interference of the emperor in questions of doctrine, but in addition develop the **claim to an unlimited supreme priestly power over the whole church completely independent of the imperial power.** According to Gelasius, the emperor and the Pope have different functions in one and the same community: the emperor has only secular, the Pope only priestly *auctoritas*; but the spiritual authority is far superior to the secular authority. It entails responsibility for the administration of the sacraments and before God even responsibility for the secular ruler.

No *infallibility of the Bishop of Rome*

However, we must ask: is this battle over papal authority already one about the infallibility of the Pope's decisions? No! For this was not claimed at that time even in Rome. Certainly, the ecumenical councils of the early church did not want to make any decisions on matters of faith without or contrary to the Bishop of Rome. And how could they? After all, he was the only patriarch of the great Western church and the first patriarch of the imperial church. But as we saw, the four classical councils made their decisions on their own authority. There was no talk of their having to be summoned by the Bishop of Rome and guided by him. There was no question of their resolutions having to be confirmed by Rome. And how little the Roman claim to orthodoxy was understood as 'infalliblilty' can be seen in a vivid way after the phase of the expansion of papal power in the fourth and fifth centuries from **two 'classic' cases of erring Popes in the sixth/seventh centuries**. Moreover these cases were cited at the First Vatican Council against a definition of papal infallibility, but were ignored by the majority, as were so many other facts:[54]

– Pope **Vigilius** adopted conflicting positions over Monophysitism at the Fifth Ecumenical Council in Constantinople in 553 under Justinian. He lost all credibility there by his worthless fickleness, so that later he was not even buried in St Peter's, and down the centuries continued to be despised even in the West.

– Pope **Honorius I** was condemned at the Sixth Ecumenical Council in Constantinople in 681; this condemnation was repeated by the Trullan Synod of 692 and the Seventh and Eighth Ecumenical Councils, and moreover also accepted by Honorius' successor Pope Leo II, and again confirmed by subsequent Popes.

So there were at least two clearly heretical Popes! Infallible? An enquiry is needed. Down to the twelfth century, outside Rome the significance of the Roman church for doctrine was **not** understood as a real **teaching authority in the legal sense**. The Catholic theologian Yves Congar, who has summed up all the research in his rich volume on the ecclesiology of the High Middle Ages, states: 'The teaching role which was accorded explicitly to the Pope was more a matter of a religious quality which Rome owes to the fact that it is the place of the martyrdom and the tomb of Peter and Paul. Peter stands for faith, Paul for the proclamation of the faith. People are fond of asserting that the Roman church has never erred in the faith. Here it appears as a model, since it is the church of Peter, who was the first to confess Christ and is therefore an example . . . But this is not to concede what we call, inauthentically, the infallibility of the papacy or, more exactly, the infallibility of the judgments which the Pope can make in the last instance as universal and supreme pastor. Occasionally the magisterial statements of the Popes have been disputed.'[55] Here Congar refers to the work of J.Langen, who gathered together all kinds of facts and texts to demonstrate that the decisions of the Pope were not regarded as infallible at least from the seventh to the twelfth centuries.[56] Indeed it was still to be a long road to Vatican I (1870). This road was built with an unflagging Roman concern for power, which did not hesitate even over the use of forgeries.

Papal forgeries with consequences

For nowadays there is no denying the fact that particularly after the fifth century, clear **forgeries** favouring Roman and papal prestige accumulated: false acts of martyrs and false acts of synods, the latter in particular which were to be put to good political use. Historically, the most significant of these was the **'legend' of the holy Pope Silvester**,[57] narrated in a most skilful way with a clear political intent and elaborated down to the smallest detail. Deriving from an unknown author between 480 and 490, it has no authentic historical content whatsoever. It runs like this: Constantine, the furious persecutor of Christians, was smitten with leprosy and not only healed in Rome by Pope Silvester, but also converted and baptized. Indeed the emperor, who on his own initiative was planning to move the seat of government to Constantinople, threw himself to the ground before the Pope in remorse, without his imperial robes and insignia, did penance and then, when his sin had been forgiven, made the move with the Pope's consent. The whole point was that Rome's arch-rival Constantinople, the city of the emperor and the councils, owed its rise to the favour of the Bishop of Rome! Just a touching story?

No! In the eighth century this tendentious product of the imagination, which was much read in the Middle Ages, stimulated one of the most influential forgeries in church history: the story of the **'Donation of Constantine**[58] (*Donatio* or *Constitutum Constantini*). It goes like this. Before departing to Constantinople, Constantine not only bestowed on Pope Silvester I the right to wear imperial insignia and robes (the purple), to pattern the title and rank of the papal Curia on the imperial court and nominate consuls like patricians, but also bequeathed to him Rome and all the provinces, places and cities in Italy and the Western regions. The Pope's position thus became like that of an emperor. Indeed Constantine had bestowed on the Roman see the primacy over all the other churches, especially those of Antioch, Alexandria, Constantinople and Jerusalem.

This forgery came into being in the circle of papal politicians who wanted to provide 'historical' justification both for the independence of Rome from Byzantium and for the foundation of a church state. The inauthenticity of the 'Donation of Constantine' was demonstrated only in the fifteenth century by a Renaissance member of the Curia, Lorenzo Valla,[59] along with the inauthenticity of the works of '**Dionysius the Areopagite**', alleged to have been a disciple of Paul (which also come from the fifth/sixth centuries!). 'Dionysius' had introduced the concept of earthly 'hierarchy' ('holy rule'), which is unbiblical in every respect, based it on extravagant speculations about a many-tiered heavenly hierarchy, and praised the bishop as the bearer of mystical powers.

Nor is that all: the 'Symmachian Forgeries', those highly successful forgeries from the entourage of Pope Symmachus, the second successor of Gelasius, also derive from the sixth century. These fabricated the acts of a fictitious Council of Sinuessa in 303 which included the statement '*Prima sedes a nemine iudicatur*: the first see is not judged by anyone'. In other words, as the supreme authority the Pope may not be judged by anyone, even the emperor.[60] What was the significance of all these forgeries? Here is one historian's answer: 'The forgeries which were produced at that time sought to provide historical justification for the proceedings of the council (a Roman synod) and to liberate the one who held papal dignity for ever from any worldly or spiritual court. This was the conclusion to a lengthy development: however, it was for the future to show whether the legal claim *Prima sedes a nemine iudicatur* was capable of establishing itself and gaining general recognition.'[61]

Be this as it may, despite these legal definitions and the ever-increasing claims to primacy of jurisdiction, papal history lists 'from the earliest times to the fifteenth century a whole series of "**papal trials**" to which occupants of the *prima sedes* were summoned as defendants and as a result of which they were often even deposed'.[62] The papal trials of the sixth and seventh centuries clearly tell against a general recognition of the legal statement *Prima sedes a nemine iudicatur*, although this statement may have been known. And although this sixth-century forgery already appears in ninth-century collections of papal law and was often used in arguments, the papal trials from the middle of the eighth century to the investiture dispute were quite effective proceedings. Even in Rome, the old church order was still largely in operation: those involved in the election of a Pope, namely the clergy and people of Rome and the emperor, also pronounced the sentence of deposition – especially in the case of heresy or *invasio* of the office.

The historical **conclusion** to be drawn for the **West** is that even though there is a wide gulf between Rome's claims and historical reality, with Gelasius at the end of the fifth century the development of the church community into an independent corporation with a monarchical focus which his predecessors had been promoting for 150 years was already complete. In principle, by now not only had a theological foundation been laid **for a new paradigm of the church** (by Augustine) but also a **church-political foundation**: the paradigm of a **Rome-centred Catholic Church (P III)**. In deliberate contradiction to the East Roman doctrine of the emperor as the protector and legislator of the church, with the backing of Augustine's doctrine of two kingdoms Gelasius had already formulated the doctrine of the two powers, the worldly power and the spiritual power which was superior to it. So the Leonian–Gelasian doctrine has rightly been called the Magna Carta of the mediaeval papacy. This doctrine detaches the clergy from the worldly order and jurisdiction ('exemption' as a clerical privilege), and is the theoretical foundation for the supreme authority of the Pope as leader and the claim of the papacy to absolute rule.

However, for the whole of the **East** this paradigm remained highly **offensive**: how can the Bishop of Rome, a fallible man and only a successor of Peter and no more, identify himself with Peter in an almost mystical way? What a presumption for an individual bishop in the church to want to attribute to himself the whole personal responsibility and authority of the apostle Peter! It was quite unacceptable, above all, that by a refined combination of theological, allegedly historical and especially legal arguments, every possible legal conclusion should be drawn from the apostolic authority of Peter, in a completely one-sided way, in favour of an claim to absolute power by Rome.

Down to the present day (as we saw in connection with P II), the Roman claim to primacy of rule clearly remains an unresolved question between the Eastern and the Western churches, which has so far never been discussed at an ecumenical council between East and West – and Eastern Orthodoxy shares the blame for this since it has never explicitly taken up this question. Far less has it been resolved in a way that is binding on East and West, although, as we may recall, the theory and practice of Roman primacy is the main cause of the split between the Eastern and the Western churches.

If we want to have a better future, can we avoid raising here some **questions** which have been postponed all too long? Here I start from the biblical evidence that in the New Testament not only is the word 'hierarchy' consistently and deliberately avoided, but so too are all secular words for 'office' in connection with church functions, as they express a relationship of power. Instead of this, an all-encompassing term, *diakonia*, service (really 'serving at table'), is used, which can nowhere evoke associations with any authority, control or position of dignity and power. Here Jesus himself had evidently set the irrevocable criterion. There is hardly any saying of Jesus which has been handed down in so many forms (six!) as that about **serving** (in the dispute between the disciples, at supper, the foot-washing): the highest is to be the servant (servant at table) of all! Quite certainly a Bishop of Rome will never do justice to this demand of Jesus if he merely calls himself the 'servant of the servants of God' and moreover attempts to dominate these servants with every possible means and method. No, in the light of this saying of Jesus there cannot be any office among the disciples of Jesus which is simply constituted by law and power and corresponds to the office of those who hold power in the state: 'The kings of the Gentiles exercise lordship over them; and those in authority over them are called benefactors. But not so with you; rather let the greatest among you become as the youngest, and the leader as one who serves.'[63]

This is not the place to develop a theology of the Petrine service which the church needs. That has been done elsewhere.[64] Many Protestant theologians, too, nowadays affirm that the church of Christ needs a Petrine service to mediate, inspire, lead and promote unity.[65] Here it is possible only to raise basic questions for the future with a view to a reform of the papacy (something that was also avoided by Vatican II) and for the sake of the ecumenical understanding which depends on that. These are questions for the future which should be discussed at a Third Vatican Council (or a second in Jerusalem).

Questions for the Future

The following questions arise over any reform (not abolition) of the papacy:

• The papacy has increasingly become an **institution of power**. It has remained so to the present day – despite Vatican II. But does such an institution of power have any right to go on existing in a faith community which should be governed only by service, and in a democratic society which repudiates all institutional, uncontrolled authoritarianism? Can the papacy go on being the last absolutist monarchy in Europe – allegedly by God's grace, after the example of the Roman emperors? Shouldn't it rather be a Christian institution at the service of the Catholic Church and the ecumene, as was shown in our century by John XXIII?

• The papacy developed more and more **power structures** by adopting highly developed Roman jurisprudence and imperial legal practice. In view of the completely different structures of the New Testament community and, again, of our modern democratic society, does the papacy have a future if it seeks to remain a centralistic legal and administrative institution and regards the faith-community of the church as a corporation which is to be understood and ruled primarily in legal terms: *populus docendus, non sequendus*, as they have said in Rome since the fifth century – 'the people are to be led, not followed'? So is the church still to be a community regulated by law, with a centralistic rule – or a faith community led by servants? An *Imperium Romanum* – or a Catholic 'commonwealth'?

• The papacy has preserved the **trappings of power** which it developed at that time down to the present day: an imperial style in its offices and its letters; Latin as the official and legal language; a papal archive which can cite any papal or conciliar declaration as an ideological treasury for any Roman appropriation of office; a *Codex Iuris Canonici* which in its decisive canons ultimately goes back to mediaeval forgeries. So should the Catholic Church go on being flooded incessantly with Roman *decreta* and *responsa*, instructions and declarations, *motu proprio*s and encyclicals – or should Rome, in the spirit of the New Testament and modern democracy, form a mediating and inspiring centre of unity?

However, there should be no disputing one thing: by resulting in an enormous concentration of power on Rome and a tremendous legal system in the church, the development of the papacy as a powerful institution handed down to the rough and uneducated barbarians, who now flooded into the Roman empire from all sides, the idea of ancient constitutional law. And after analysing the theology of Augustine and the Roman Popes with their powerful institution, we must now investigate a third element of the Latin Roman Catholic paradigm of the Middle Ages: the new piety and church practice of the Germans.

4. Constants, variables and the shift from East to West

Despite all the continuities between late antiquity, brilliantly represented in theology by Augustine, and the early Middle Ages, we cannot for a moment overlook the **migration of the Germanic tribes,**[66] which immediately before Augustine's death had even reached his North African Hippo. This represented a **revolution of epoch-making extent** for the Christianity of the West. Already in the fourth century they had infiltrated increasingly heavily into the Roman empire, forcibly settled there by the Romans or taken into service in the army as good soldiers. Driven on by the Huns advancing from the steppes of southern Russia, the Vandals, Alanni and Suevi had crossed the Rhine on 31 December 406 when it was frozen, and marched *en masse* into Gaul, and two years later over the Pyrenees to Spain, in search of pasturage and food.

The migrations and their consequences

What became of 'eternal Rome', unconquered since earliest times, which as we heard was first captured in 410 by those West Goths who were later to settle in Spain? Over the next few centuries the city of Rome, which had numbered almost a million inhabitants, became a city of hardly 20,000 (as it was in the Carolingian period). In the fifth century the Germans, first of all seen as a temporary scourge, founded kingdoms on Roman soil: not only the West Goths but also the Alemanns, Burgundians, Franks and Vandals who, coming from Spain, had invaded North Africa as early as the time of Augustine in 429; by 439 they had captured Carthage and formed the first state on imperial territory to be recognized by the Romans. However, this recognition did not prevent these wild hordes of warriors from launching a new Italian campaign, including a further plundering of Rome in 455. In 476 the last emperor of the West, still a child, Romulus Augustulus, was deposed by Odoacer, general of the German army. In this way the West Roman emperorship, already long dominated by barbarian army commanders, was finished; this caused hardly any stir at the time, unlike the first fall of Rome.

However, we must be quite clear that the stage of development of the Germanic peoples invading the empire was primitive – by comparison with ancient civilization. Encapsulated, without a universal perspective or even a sense of being part of Europe, these tribes, which were underdeveloped both intellectually and culturally, concentrated only on the life of their own peoples. The consequence was not just a collapse of the superficial Roman civil and military administration, only part of which the new peoples could take over, but a process of dissolution of the Roman state and Roman law generally, indeed a collapse of ancient civilization. Of course this differed depending on the region and sphere of life, but generally speaking it was beyond question a tremendous **economic, social and cultural relapse**. It was to take centuries for it to be made good again. The most recent historiography, which aims at an integration of research from the spheres of social history and the history of structures, religions and mentalities, has given an impressive description of the effects:[67]

– **The loss of many techniques of safeguarding life** and thus minimal agricultural produce, often miserable food, clothing, living conditions and hygiene;

– **A collapse of the infrastructure,** the road systems, bridges and aqueducts, and thus increasingly difficult conditions for trade and communication;

– **A drop in the population** of a quarter or a third down to the eighth century: the depopulation of the cities, which became large villages, and thus the development of a small-scale village-agricultural world;

– **A decline in the ability to write:** neither Odoacer nor the East Goth Theoderic the Great, neither Charlemagne nor Otto the Great could write. For the warrior aristocracy throughout the Middle Ages the art of writing remained a suspect business; there was a decline in literary capabilities and higher education generally;

– **The retention of a class society:** a permanent division of society into those who were free and those who were not, and slavery down to the Carolingian period;

– **A degeneration of the security provided by the law:** of the constitution, public law and the legal system; blood vengeance and the personal exacting of justice (for example in the case of adultery, murder and violations of marriage) were again the order of the day;

– **the leading role of the nobility** (instead of a trained officialdom!): state property and money came into the possession of the king and the nobility. The new rulers even took over rule of the church (apart from what was really a sacrificing priesthood) and exercised their rights as sacral persons; so the appointment of bishops and the control of synods lay with the secular rulers up to the time of the mediaeval investiture dispute;

– **a general provincialization** and thus different regional developments of Latin – now often written completely wrongly and stylistically run wild – into different '**national languages**' (Italian, Spanish, French, Rhaeto-Romanic); now Latin became a language which had to be learned specially, though it was then the educated language used throughout the West in state and church.

And the Catholic Church? In the convulsions, wars and destructions of the migration at first there was nothing for it to do but to retreat, since all the Germanic tribes were pagan. Cities like Cologne, Mainz, Worms and Strasbourg, which had become Frankish, along with other cities on the Rhine and Danube, in northern Gaul and in the Balkans, had now lacked a bishop for more than a century. It was only later that Christianity returned, first among the East Goths in present-day Bulgaria, to which Christianity found its way as early as around the middle of the fourth century, through the activity of Bishop Ulfilas, who created a Gothic form of writing, literature and a translation of the Bible – albeit in the form of the Arian faith at that time favoured by Byzantium. And from the East Goths this **Arian Christianity** also found its way to the West Goths, and through them to most of the other Germanic tribes, including the Vandals in Spain and Africa.

The Neo-Latins of the Western province, whose Latin now passed over into the national languages, kept to their inherited Catholic faith. But what was to be even more important for the future was that the last Germanic tribe to achieve unity under a monarch, which was nevertheless to create the most significant kingdom of the West, the **Frankish kingdom**, also became **traditionally Catholic.**[68] Unlike the Vandal kingdom in North Africa, the kingdom of the West Goths in Spain and the Langobard kingdom in Italy, which did not last and need not be discussed further here, the kingdom of the Franks was to inherit the Roman empire. The **baptism of the Frankish king Clovis** of the Merovingians is regarded as a basic date for the history of mediaeval Christianity: this took place in 498/9, in fulfilment of an oath which brought him victory over the Alemanns, and certainly also with a view to winning over the Neo-Latin Catholic population. At that time the Byzantine emperor Anastasius had recognized the new power, which, as we have already heard and will hear in more detail later, to the dismay of the Greeks was to bring forth a new rival Western emperor with whom the papacy opportunely allied itself.

So what was the difference between the early church (Graeco–Latin) paradigm and the mediaeval Latin paradigm of the church which was now increasingly taking shape? First of all, it has to be said that it was not a different substance of faith.

What was preserved of the substance of faith

Scholars argue over whether we do better to speak of the Christianizing of the Germans or the Germanizing of Christianity. But at least today there is no dispute that in this epoch-making revolution **the church** represented a, indeed the, **decisive factor of continuity**. It was not the princes but the clergy who could read and usually also write, and so in time they could again develop a new written culture. What ancient literature, profane and theological, was handed down to the Middle Ages usually came through the church and above all through the monasteries, which were now becoming increasingly numerous even in the West. But the episcopate, which was now taking on more and more administrative and political functions, and the high constancy of the episcopal sees, were also important for the continuity. And even more important: despite all the decline and silence in theology between Gregory the Great (who died in

604) and Isidore of Seville (who died in 636) in the sixth and seventh centuries, and Anselm of Canterbury in the eleventh, and despite all the grisly primitive paganism in popular piety, even in this period there was a fundamental **continuity of Christian faith, rites and ethics.**

Indeed, despite all the truly epoch-making differences, in the new mediaeval paradigm (P III) we still have **the same constants** of Christianity as in the Jewish Christian primitive church paradigm (P I) and the Hellenistic early church paradigm (P II). Moreover this holds not only for the 'clerical elite' but also for 'ordinary people':

- Though most of the Germanic peoples who were converted to Christianity were Arians, at least they all believed in one and the same **God**, the God of Israel, his Son Jesus Christ and the Holy Spirit: the same **gospel**!
- And although the motive of the stronger God often played the decisive role in conversion to Christianity, and a collective baptism accompanied the baptism of the ruler, this was still the same **baptism** for the forgiveness of sins and for incorporation into the Christian faith community: the same **initiation rite.**
- And although an unbiblical notion of sacrifice and clericalism came into the foreground in the liturgical celebration of the mysteries of the faith, in essence it was still the old **eucharist** in memory of Jesus that was celebrated (Sunday, as the day of resurrection, had been declared a day of rest by Constantine since 321): the same **community rite**!
- And although since Constantine's victory the cross – originally a sign of Christian unselfishness and powerlessness – had increasingly become a prophylactic against enemies and even a sign of victory in war, and 'barbaric cruelty' became even proverbial in the early Middle Ages, the basic notion of **discipleship of Christ** was not abandoned; indeed, as a result of a social activity which had not previously been customary, and the widely organized care of the poor and liberation of prisoners, it took on new dimensions: the same **ethic**!

So basically, this continuity in gospel and ethics, initiation and community rites, did not just involve some sacred customs, pious practices and unthinking piety, but the **substance of Christian faith**, which was **preserved** even in the new mediaeval entire constellation. Moreover it did a great deal to shape the world of images, the intellectual ideas, different forms of life and practical behaviour, of countless mediaeval men and women – and not just some 'pre-Reformers'. So for all their justified criticism of the Middle Ages, Protestants, too, should recognize today that despite a tremendous revolution in mentality, the Christian identity was maintained.

On the other hand, Catholics should no longer dispute that in the Middle Ages a **fundamental revolution** also took place within the church, which simply embraced everything – from the proclamation of faith through the understanding of the sacraments to the papacy. The most significant liturgical historian of our century, Josef Andreas Jungmann, did not exaggerate when he wrote: 'In the two thousand years of church history there was probably nowhere a greater revolution both in religious thought and in the corresponding institutions as there was in the five centuries between the end of the patristic period and the beginning of Scholasticism.'[69]

What changed in devotion, discipline and organization

It has already become clear that this revolution in Christianity took place not so much, as later in the Reformation, in the form of an abrupt break, as in slow and basic shifts and reinterpretations. The following **three constituent elements** of the new **mediaeval Latin entire constellation (P III)** have emerged from the paradigm analysis so far:

- the Latin **theology of Augustine**, which differs from Greek patristics,
- the development of the **Roman papacy** as the central controlling ecclesiastical institution in the Western church,
- the novel piety and church practice of the **Germanic peoples**.

This last point needs to be clarified. Already in the period after Constantine, those momentous new accents and new forms began to emerge which were to have a broad influence on the early Middle Ages through the presence of the Germans:[70]

– After tribal baptism, adult baptism disappeared completely from the church's consciousness. The passive-unconscious **baptism of infants** became the rule.

– While even in the period after Constantine the **eucharist** was increasingly celebrated not just weekly, but daily, the universal reception of communion now declined more and more. Instead of the people's liturgy of the early church, an explicitly **clerical liturgy** (except for singing) also developed in the West, a sacred play in a sacred language, in which the people were only passive spectators who no longer took part in the meal itself. For now the priest offered 'the sacrifice' 'for' the people. This encouraged a magical understanding of the sacrament.

– Even in late antiquity the **public penance** of the early church, which was possible only once in a lifetime and under the control of the bishop, was almost always postponed to the death-bed because it was compromising, and it increasingly disappeared. But from distant Ireland, which was never part of the empire, had accepted the Christian faith only in the fifth century, and had been largely shaped by a monastic rather than an episcopal order, at a later stage itinerant monks on a mission brought to the European continent a novel form of **private penance** practised in their monasteries, which we have already encountered among the monks of the East. This could also be used for everyday sins, and repeated as often as desired; it was no longer controlled by the bishops but by priests. This originally monastic penance now spread quickly, first in Western Europe, as **auricular confession for everyone**.

– From the **veneration of martyrs** at their tombs, practised in the early church, in the early Middle Ages there developed in the churches a massive **veneration of saints and relics**. In anti-Arian polemic and piety the '**one** mediator between God and men, the man Christ Jesus',[71] was increasingly caught up into God in a practical Monophysitism and simply identified with God (the God Christ won the victory over the god Wotan). So he was no longer in much demand in practical piety and was displaced by other mediators standing closer to men and women, who could obtain almost anything from God (Christ): Mary and the saints.

– Because of their archaic mentality the Germans introduced an almost boundless degree of **superstition** into Christianity: as in all primitive societies, popular piety was governed by a belief in spirits. Good and especially evil spirits were thought to be around everywhere, also behind natural phenomena, and people attempted to ward them off or win them over with works, gifts and practices of very different kinds. A **primitive piety of works** developed which was largely remote from the Bible, externalized and reified.

– Whereas the great **theologians** of Greek and Latin patristics worked hard to penetrate Christian truth with independent thinking and thus often corrected popular piety, the theologians of this transitional period limited themselves to repeating sentences, making excerpts from them and collections of them. There was hardly any educated clerical elite, since this presupposed urban conditions and appropriate schools.

– Instead of **education**, not only among the clergy of the religious orders but increasingly also among the secular clergy the **obligation to celibacy** became increasingly important for deacons, priests and bishops, although in the early Middle Ages a married priesthood was still largely the custom. At the same time the **ordination of women** as deacons, which was still customary in the fifth century, was abolished, so that women were denied any ministry at the altar. But the church hardly dared to intervene in manifestly pagan situations, for example in the Frankish kingdom, in the sphere of marriage (the ruler's concubines), the legal system (cruel ordeals instead of a clarification of guilt) and slavery (which continued down to the Carolingian period).

– Yet alongside the hierarchical structure of the bishops and their dioceses, as a result of the Irish–Frankish movement sparked off in Gaul by the Irish monk Columba the Younger (who died in 615), a gigantic **network of monasteries** developed (at the end of the seventh century there were around 550 in Gaul alone). As a sign of obedience to the abbot these had mostly combined Columba's rule with the Benedictine rule and disseminated the Irish penitential system, but they also developed a lively written culture in good Latin. At the same time they gained a special legal status: contrary to the regulations of the Council of Chalcedon (the subordination of the monasteries to the bishop), the monasteries now had freedom from the bishop: exemption in appointing abbots and correcting monastic discipline, often combined with immunity from state intervention.

Above all the **episcopate** emerged strengthened from these developments. For in the confused times without state organization the bishop was often also responsible for social welfare, justice and the collection of taxes, with the result that in the fifth and sixth centuries he often also had political control of his city. Thus the office of bishop became the monopoly of leading families and rose to be the highest office. In particular the Gallic episcopate controlled by the king and its primate, self-confident and little concerned for Rome, opposed various papal instructions. Had not primate and synodical activity disappeared with the downfall of the Merovingian monarchy, the Gallic episcopate – after the collapse first of Christian North Africa and then Christian Spain under the Islamic onslaught – would have been a real counterbalance to the Roman centralism which was then already clearly taking shape.

So **in the West the Bishop of Rome** remained **unrivalled** from an ecclesiastical perspective. And after the final downfall of the West Roman empire in 476 the development of the Christian community into an independent corporation was also advanced by the Bishops of Rome after Leo I – still under Byzantine supremacy – though these were not so significant. Their aim was leadership not only of the Roman church but of the whole church by a right which was based on faith. But what did the situation really look like?

The humiliating dependence of the Roman Popes

For a long time the discrepancy between the highly-developed papal theory of power and the weakness of papal power itself still remained considerable. For after the downfall of the last Roman shadow emperor and his Germanic mercenary leader Odoacer (the 'king of Italy'), the **East Goths of Theoderic the Great** (489/93–526) formed the dominant political power in the West. Thus began a period of a humiliating dependence of the Popes on the Arian East Gothic rulers. These rulers established themselves in Ravenna, erected splendid buildings there, and as sole rulers of Italy appointed Popes who obeyed them completely as a matter of course. So Theoderic, who himself pursued a policy of religious tolerance even towards the Jews, summarily sent Pope John I to Constantinople to mediate for the supporters of Arianism, and had him thrown into prison on his return because he had failed; there he died in the same year as Theoderic (526).

Even after the downfall of the East Gothic kingdom, there followed a period of oppressive dependence on the **Byzantine emperors,** who saw the Bishop of Rome as no more and no less than the patriarch of the old imperial capital and thus of the West.[72] With a view to a restoration of the unity of the Roman empire, the Emperor Justinian I in particular was quite interested in a revaluation of old Rome alongside new Rome which was not political, but limited to the church sphere. So he was prepared to grant the Roman church a *primatus magisterii* = 'primacy of the teaching office' in faith and questions of doctrine, a primacy of doctrine, though this at first had no practical consequences. It developed only in the high Middle Ages and was to come to a climax almost 1500 years later at Vatican I in the definition of papal infallibility.

However, the last thing in the Emperor Justinian's mind, too, was a primacy of jurisdiction for the Pope. On the contrary, during his largely absolutist rule over state and church which lasted for four long decades (from 527 to 565 – as we saw at length in connection with the Hellenistic paradigm) he developed his power in every respect – in politics, law, ritual and symbols – and gave it a sacral aura. An infallible Pope alongside him was inconceivable. Justinian, who thought himself as pre-eminent a theologian as he was a ruler, acted as his own legislator, with reference to God's will and inspiration, even in questions of faith. He ordered the Bishops of Rome whenever necessary to his court, where their orthodoxy was formally examined.

In Italy the Greek-speaking, Byzantine re-conquerors with their exarchs (first resident in Rome and then in Ravenna) and their arrogant officials, who called themselves 'Romans', were soon as unpopular as the East Goths before them. And when Justinian died in 565 and the pagan or Arian **Langobards** invaded Italy and completely overran wide areas of the imperial system, the dream of the rebirth of a Roman empire and a single imperial church within the framework of the Hellenistic Byzantine paradigm went out of the window once and for all.

But the papacy attempted to exploit its hour. Under the Langobard counts it had been able to hold on to the Roman duchy (*Ducatus Romanus*: only southern Italy remained nominally Byzantine). So now it could mediate both politically and linguistically between the Langobards and Byzantium and attain a *de facto* political independence. At the same time, because of its estates (*patrimonia*), which were administered in good Roman fashion and had increased, in due course it could develop into the largest private landowner in Western Europe, whose incomes benefitted not only the Roman Curia and the city of Rome, but also the indigenous population. But Byzantine control remained, and if need be could be imposed with violence and terror. One sign of this was the presence of a Byzantine garrison in Rome. We should be clear that since Justinian's decree in 555 the imperial *fiat* had to be obtained (later this was at least the *fiat* of the Exarch of Ravenna) for any election of a Bishop of Rome – a procedure which remained valid constitutional law until the break with the imperial regime in the eighth century. However, slowly the balance in the West began to shift in favour of Rome.

Gregory the Great: the first mediaeval Pope

A significant figure of this period, Pope **Gregory I**, called the Great (590–604), played a key role in the unstoppable political continental shift.[73] The Great? There is good reason for not including Gregory in a series of 'classics of theology',[74] although officially he is counted the fourth of the Western *Doctores ecclesiae* after Ambrose, Jerome and Augustine, since he was not a great, original theologian. But he also could not be left out of a series of significant 'Figures of Church History' edited by a Protestant church historian – and not just because this series included all the Popes.[75] For because of his tremendous influence on mediaeval cultural and church history, Gregory is even one of the 'greats of world history'.[76]

Gregory's **theology** – popular theological literature, sermons and interpretations of the Bible – was already subjected to sharp criticism by Adolf von Harnack: 'Under the shell of Augustinian words,' Gregory was said 'again to have expressed the vulgar Catholic type, but reinforced by superstitious elements, and to have brought to light the old, Western view of religion as a legal order.'[77] Here Harnack was referring above all to Gregory's *Dialogues on the Life and Miracles of the Italian Fathers* modelled on the *Apophthegmata patrum*, which had been translated from the Greek just beforehand, and his propagation of a crude belief in miracles, visions, prophecies, angels and demons, along with his theological sanctioning of a massive veneration of saints and relics, of purgatory and masses for souls, his excessive interest in sacrifices, penitential orders, categories of sins and punishments for sins, and finally his emphasis on fear of the eternal judge and the hope of reward instead of trust in God's grace in Christ and love.

But we may leave on one side the question whether Gregory in particular and above all did or not create the 'vulgar type of Roman Catholicism'.[78] Without doubt Gregory reduced the distance between the culture of the later Roman elite and barbarian popular culture and as **the last of the Latin church fathers** at the same time **ushered in the Middle Ages**. Because he was simple and popular, he was read more than his master Augustine, whose stark doctrine of predestination he rightly toned down. Even the Protestant historian of dogma, Ulrich Wickert, who is well disposed towards Catholicism, thinks that Gregory handed on the great tradition in simplified form, and that his thought world, compared with that of his spiritual forebears (above all, Augustine), is 'duller, sadder, flatter'. 'But,' he adds, Gregory 'was called, eschatologically tuned by oppression, to be the pioneer of a new age'.[79] An English expert says that he was engaged in 'an indefatigable quest for that which is not transitory'.[80]

Indeed, however much Gregory's simple and often primitive theology incurs criticism, his **pontificate** has found recognition. Even Harnack spoke in extremely warm terms of Gregory's personality. He was a 'wise, energetic monk, a skilled politician and a lovable and imposing pastor'.[81] Although he came from a rich Roman senatorial aristocracy and was already city prefect of Rome in his early thirties, three years later – just like Augustine – after a conversion he decided for a life of asceticism. His family palace became a monastery and he also founded monasteries on his estates in Sicily – six in all.

However, the monastic peace did not last long, for Gregory, who had not become a Benedictine, was appointed by the Pope regional deacon and finally plenipotentiary (apokrisiar) at the imperial court in Constantinople, an official post which all the patriarchs had there. But here the limitations of the old Roman Gregory became evident: he made little use of his opportunity for mediation. Instead of learning Greek in the course of his stay of more than six years there, in this splendid city by the Bosphorus he wrote a commentary for his people on the book of Job with every possible moral application – of course in Latin (later, under the title *Moralia*, it became the moral handbook of the Middle Ages). In any case he only half trusted the Greeks, since he was stamped by the traditional Latin view that the Greeks were too intelligent to be honest.

590 was the year in which Gregory was appointed Pope – still by the community, but in reality more by the clergy and aristocracy. But turned fifty, he was by no means the aristocratic prince of the church and

'political Pope' that might have been expected. Granted, Gregory's tombstone bears the title *consul Dei*, but at heart he remained a **monk and ascetic** whose personal piety, orientated on pastoral work and mission, was rooted in trust in God and thus at the same time had an inner side directed towards solitude and contemplation.

On the other hand Gregory was a highly energetic **bishop with a very practical disposition** who was in full control of the already considerable institutional apparatus of the papacy. He also administered the gigantic papal estates, mostly worked by colonists, not only in Italy, Sicily and Sardinia but also in Gaul, Dalmatia and North Africa, with a sure eye and a sense of reality. Indeed he had such an outstanding understanding of reorganization that he was able to use the produce to relieve the need of the population and provide abundant food, in particular for the people of Rome, which had now sunk to being a disaster area with barely 100,000 inhabitants, no more than a country town.

To avert further plundering of Rome Gregory paid an astronomical ransom of 500 pounds in gold to the still largely pagan or Arian Langobards, whose royal couple had meanwhile become Catholics. Thus he devoted himself in every way to his people and to peace with the Langobards, especially in time of war and plague. No wonder that as a result he took over the **responsibility for administration, finance and welfare** which was strictly that of the imperial exarch. However, for Italy's Romanic population Gregory, and not the Byzantine exarch, was the supreme authority. Indeed he was more: by his administrative skill in what for him were apocalyptic times, Gregory imperceptibly laid the **foundations for the secular power of the papacy**, which was still barely developed in his time.

And yet practical politics did not lead this Pope to forget a concern for the **spiritual good** of the church. This can be seen in particular from his encouragement and protection of monasticism. Just as Athanasius wrote about the desert father Antony, so Gregory now wrote in the second book of his **Dialogues** about the life and miracles of **Benedict**, the founder and abbot of Subiaco and Monte Cassino, who was only a shadowy figure. Gregory first made Benedict **the** exemplary Roman abbot and monastic father, here too weaving in fantastic and scurrilous stories about miracles and visions in a way typical of his world of faith. And with his practical and pastoral bent, right at the beginning of his period in office he presented the church officials with a **Regula pastoralis**, a monastic 'pastoral rule' focussed on the world to come, which the emperor also had translated into Greek. To the secular clergy of the Middle Ages this document on the ideal pastor of souls was to mean what the rule of Benedict of Nursia (*c*.480–547) did to the religious orders.

Furthermore, Gregory also took great pains over **cultural work**: over the library in the Lateran, adorned with a picture of Augustine, and over the cultivation of liturgical singing. He probably founded or reorganized a special institution for this purpose, later called the *Schola cantorum*, song school. However, that he himself composed a 'sacramentary' and invented 'Gregorian chant' belongs in the realm of legend. But this legend was skilfully utilized in the ninth century to establish a single form of the *Cantus Romanus* in the Frankish kingdom.[82]

Still, all these well-intentioned activities could not disguise the fact that the **spiritual and cultural situation** in Rome and Italy was **miserable**. The great culture of antiquity was now in decline and was increasingly forgotten; philosophical knowledge was minimal, and in Rome there was hardly anyone who could translate the Greek texts flawlessly into Latin. Literary culture, too, had declined. Gone was the Indian summer of classical education during which in a work *De doctrina Christiana* Augustine had to recommend that Christians should study the Bible so to speak as a 'corrective'. Now everything had been condensed into the study of the Bible along with all the relevant auxiliary sciences. Indeed a reduced **clerical culture**, focussed solely on the Bible and at the same time on clergy and monks, who were the only ones who could read and write, was in the making. Moreover it was clergy and monks whom Gregory, the monastic Pope, wanted above all to address. And yet, is all this enough for world-historical 'greatness'? No, a decisive factor must be added.

The beginning of a political shift from East to West

On the one hand we should note that Gregory, still a subject of the Byzantine emperor, had been clear since his stay in Constantinople that it was **impossible to establish a Roman primacy of jurisdiction in the East** and that a rebellion against the emperor could be punished at any time as high treason. So he had waited quite correctly for seven months until consent to his consecration as bishop came from Byzantium. For not only the emperor but also all the Greek bishops took it completely for granted that the position of the Bishop of Rome corresponded to that of an Eastern patriarch. And indeed in political and legal terms Rome was still a Byzantine city with a Byzantine garrison, and the Roman church was part of Justinian's imperial church. The political fate of insubordinate Popes was shown only a few decades later in the case of Martin I, who had not opposed a revolt against Byzantium in Rome. He was imprisoned, deposed, transported to Constantinople and after a great show trial banished to the Crimea, where he died (a similar fate to the condemnation and cruel mutilation of the most significant theologian of the seventh century, Maximus, later called 'the Confessor', who was well disposed towards the Pope).

On the other hand, Gregory was the first Pope to have recognized the potential and creative powers of the Germanic peoples, who had settled in Western Europe since the second half of the fifth century. And so his **radius of action** extended **above all northwards and westwards**. Gregory made an effort
– to revive the church in the **Frankish kingdom**, which had already become Catholic in 498/9 under Clovis (though here he had limited success);
– over the **kingdom of the West Goths** in Spain which had converted from Arianism to Catholicism in 586 under Reccared, and above all
– over **Britain**, which was to become one of the countries most supportive of the Pope after Gregory had initiated a mission here in 597.

The English historian Edward Gibbon is said to have remarked that while Caesar needed six legions to conquer Britain, Gregory, who had entrusted the leadership of the mission to his pupil Augustine (later to become Archbishop of Canterbury), needed only forty monks. In fact, in the seventh century the new Anglo-Saxon church with its Roman orientation (and metropolitans in Canterbury and York) was able to establish itself in the face of the two older Celtic churches, the old British church and the Irish monastic church, both of which had existed without any legal connections with papal Rome. And from the end of the sixth century to the middle of the eighth the Irish/Scottish and Anglo-Saxon monks were to undertake from Britain the missions, above all to Germany and central Europe, which have already been mentioned.

So Gregory once for all broke open the narrow sphere of influence of the Roman bishops. And wherever his missionaries went, of course they spread **Christian faith with a Roman stamp**: the Roman church as the source and foundation of this Christianity. Gregory could address the 'barbarian' rulers in the West in quite a 'paternal' way as 'sons' and give them instructions in a way the emperor had never dared to. For as in Gaul and Spain, the primacy of Peter and Rome was recognized from the start by the Anglo-Saxons as a divine foundation. And in the subsequent period the Roman papacy was to exploit increasingly the opportunities for political control which were offered here.

So historically it is beyond dispute that as a result of the extension of Christian faith with a Roman stamp, Pope Gregory laid the foundations for the spiritual and cultural unity of 'Europe': a Europe made up of the south, west and north. However, Greece and the Eastern countries were lacking, for here as we know the typically Roman belief in a divinely given Roman primacy of jurisdiction and teaching was firmly rejected. But conversely, this meant that the more the Pope lost in the East, the more he gained in the West and North. The separation of the two Christianities which was in the making became increasingly deep.

So was Gregory the 'father of Europe'? No, for Europe is more than the West under Roman domination. With his two-track church politics Gregory was a spiritual father, not of Europe, but of the new specifically Roman Catholic paradigm, the theological foundations of which had been laid by Augustine and the legal and programmatic foundations of which had been laid by Popes Leo and Gelasius. By his missionary efforts, Gregory had transformed a mere programme for Western Europe into an ecclesiastical reality. And now already it is becoming evident that a **paradigm shift from the Hellenistic Byzantine (P II) paradigm to the Roman Catholic paradigm (P III) was unavoidable.** So was the schism also unavoidable?

Another image of the papacy

The **need** for a paradigm shift still in no way implied a particular **version** of the paradigm, and so a split between the Western and the Eastern churches was by no means a necessity. In principle, at the beginning of the seventh century there were still two possible constitutions for the church in the mediaeval paradigm (P III) which was now developing:

- a Catholic communion embracing both West and East to the same extent, with a Roman primacy of service following the pattern of the primitive church (P I) and the early church (P II), or
- a hierarchical church with an authoritarian and monarchical constitution and a controlling Roman primacy following the pattern of the Roman emperors and dictators, which would inevitably lead to a split between the Eastern and Western churches.

To this degree the papacy now stood at a crossroads. And it is strange to reflect what course history might have taken had the papacy understood itself more along the lines of Gregory the Great – for all his limitations and weaknesses – than along the lines of Leo the Great. We need to be clear that:

– Whereas Leo was ardently interested in developing a theology of primacy, Gregory, who was no doctrinaire figure, was more interested in the **pastoral and missionary work** of the church.

– Whereas for Leo the *plenitudo potestatis* ('fullness of power') was the central concept, even officially Gregory followed the New Testament in calling himself *servus servorum Dei*, 'servant of the servants of God'. Gregory had already used this title as a monk and a deacon, and now he was to describe the **Pope as the supreme servant** in the church,

though this could also be interpreted in the sense of a universal claim.
– Whereas Leo advocated the proud primacy of a ruler and time and again emphasized the pre-eminence, distinction and authority of Peter, Gregory advocated a **humble and collegial understanding of the primacy** by often emphasizing in his reflections on penitence even the errors and failure of Peter. One characteristic saying of his is: 'The one who is in the supreme position will rule well if he is more master of his vices than of his brothers.'[83] Thus Gregory was far from having his predecessor's tendency towards a complete centralization of the church administration. And his instruction to Augustine, whom he had sent out as missionary to the Anglo-Saxons, to reject any liturgical uniformity is in keeping with this. He did not want to force the local Roman liturgy and the local Roman customs on other churches. 'For things (customs) are not to be loved for the sake of place, but places for the sake of things (customs).'[84] He censured the bishops of southern Gaul for wanting to baptize the Jews forcibly.[85] Instead of this, he insisted on respecting the protection which had been legally guaranteed to the Jews.

Now that certainly does not mean that Gregory could not also make an authoritative defence of the Roman primacy. His good relations with the Patriarch of Constantinople, John IV, which had lasted for many years, finally came to grief because Gregory felt that he had to protest against the title 'ecumenical patriarch', which had been used since the beginning of the sixth century. A title containing the attribute 'ecumenical' made a universal claim and detracted from the other patriarchs. Even the apostle Peter, so greatly revered in West and East, had not called himself a universal apostle.

So Vatican I shows signs of a highly manipulative historiography when it quotes Gregory, of all Popes, in its definition of the primacy of jurisdiction of a 'supreme and **universal** pastor', who said to the bishops: 'My honour is the honour of the universal church. My honour is the solid vigour of my brethren. Then am I truly honoured when the honour done to all and each is not denied them.'[86] For in Gregory's own work the sense of this passage is precisely the opposite: in the letter to Patriarch Eulogius of Alexandria which is quoted here, Gregory protested against the form of address '*universalis papa*', just as he did not want his letter to be regarded as a jurisdictional *iussio*. And the previous sentences, which were glibly passed over in the council text, read: 'I did not command, but was desirous of indicating what seemed to me to be profitable . . . I do not regard that as an honour whereby I know that my brethren lose their honour.' It is in this perspective that the sentences quoted by the council, 'For my honour is the honour of the whole church . . .' follow. In turn they are followed by a further sentence about new titles which again is not quoted by the council: 'Away with words which inflate vanity and violate love.'[87]

Throughout the Middle Ages Gregory was regarded as an **exemplary Pope**. And even Martin Luther stated succinctly: 'Gregory the Great was the last bishop of the Roman church; those who came after are Popes, in other words high priests of the Roman church.'[88] So is it completely beside the point to ask whether the further development of the papacy might not have been different in the ecumenical spirit of Gregory the Great, which was so in keeping with the gospel? Could not so much, not least the split between the Eastern and Western churches, have been avoided? Be this as it may, it is worth pausing here in our account at least for a moment. Much as some Orthodox, Protestants, Anglicans and even Catholics would like to abolish it, the primacy of the Bishop of Rome has a tradition behind it which, while ambivalent, is highly significant. So its abolition is not desirable, nor are we to expect that it will automatically disappear in the course of history. The problem seems to be not so much the fact as the specific constitution of the Roman primacy.

Questions for the Future

The following questions should be asked in aid of a better ecumenical future:

• Should the Roman primacy remain a **primacy of domination**, which lays claim to a God-given direct jurisdiction of the Bishop of Rome over the individual churches and individual Christians? Without any prospect of future realization, nearer or more remote, in the Christian ecumene – in Eastern Orthodoxy, in Protestantism or in Anglicanism?

• Or should the Roman primacy be a **primacy of service**, which in succession to the biblical Peter and after the model of Gregory the Great (and John XXIII) is a truly pastoral primacy with a sense of spiritual responsibility, providing internal leadership and showing active concern for the well-being of the whole church? A papacy which could serve as a centre of inspiration, an authority for mediation in the church, and a possible authority for arbitration? In other words, should it be a primacy of unselfish service, responsible to the Lord of the church and in humble brotherhood with all? Should it be a primacy, not in the spirit of Roman imperialism, but in the spirit of the gospel?

However, to begin with, everything did not seem to indicate a rule by the Popes as primates. For Gregory's successors – in the roughly 150 years between 604 and 751 there were eighteen Romans, five Greeks, five

Syrians and one Dalmatian – had little opportunity to announce their claims to primacy or extend them further. They were completely under Byzantine control. This was 'the age of the "Byzantine captivity" of the papacy',[89] which again produced the clear case of a heretical Pope – Honorius I (625–638) – who has already been mentioned . . . But this did not halt the now increasing devotion to Peter, especially among the Germans (Peter as the gatekeeper of heaven, now always depicted with the keys; his relics; and his representative in Rome), and now became significant for the piety of individual Christians in the West. In the eighth century circumstances were to change fundamentally in favour of the papacy, so that it could soon dare to challenge Byzantium. But none of that would have been possible with the great counter-force which suddenly appeared on the stage of world history and represented a political catastrophe above all for Eastern Christianity: Islam.

5. The great counter-force: Islam

It already became clear in the seventh century that the real opponents of Catholic mediaeval Christianity were not the pagan and then the Arian Germans but a new religion which had become unprecedentedly powerful: **Islam**. At first Christians hardly took any notice of it, or attempted to dismiss it quickly as a Christian heresy. But this was no use, for Islam developed into a powerful world religion which above all won military victories; it taught Christianity fear, and drove it into a great historical confrontation. The whole of the third volume of this trilogy 'The Religious Situation of our Time' is to be devoted to Islam, so here I can limit myself to a few remarks.

The unprecedented triumph of Islam

The Prophet Muhammad had died in 632, but although the *hijra*, his migration from Mecca to Medina, had taken place only a decade earlier, he had united Arabia in faith in the one God of Abraham, whose definitive prophet Muhammad himself was taken to be. The Arabs exploited the power vacuum which had arisen through the mutual weakening of the great powers of Byzantium and Persia.

First of all they thrust northwards. In a **first wave of conquest** under the four 'just' Caliphs beginning in 634 they captured the Byzantine kingdom of Syria with Damascus (634) and Palestine with Jerusalem (638). And after they had also conquered the Sassanid kingdom of Persia, they

Arab Conquests

Frontiers of the Caliphate 632

Conquests of the four Caliphs (to 661)

Conquests of the Umayyads (to 750)

Medina Residence of the Caliphs

Places and regions

Samarkand
Bukhara
Kabul

Sassanid Empire
Isfahan

Baghdad
Basra
Kufa

Tiflis
Aleppo
Damascus 635
Jerusalem 638

Medina
Mecca
Aden

Akhsumite Empire

Khasar Empire

East Slavs

West Slavs

Bulgars

Southern Slavs

Byzantine Empire

Constantinople
Athens

Rome
Naples

Fustat
Alexandria 642
Barqa
Asswan
Tripolis

Frankish Empire
Aachen
Paris
Tours
Lyons
Poitiers 732

Oviedo
Toledo
Cordoba
Jerez 711
Tangier
Fez

Tunis
Kairouan

Magreb

attacked Egypt and conquered Alexandria (642). Here the oppressed Monophysite Copts were the only Christians to support the Arabs against the hated Chalcedonian Greeks. In exchange they were recognized as the only legitimate Christian group, and have been able to safeguard their existence in Egypt down to the present day. In the West the Arabs then advanced along the coast to Libya (647) and across the sea to Cyprus (649), Rhodes (654) and – on their first plundering campaigns – Sicily (652); now the whole of the eastern Mediterranean was lost to Byzantium. In the north they finally advanced as far as Armenia (653).

A **second wave of conquest** under the Umayyad Caliphs led to a second great confrontation between Islam and Christianity, but this time in the extreme West. By 683 the first Arabs had reached the Atlantic in their conquest of North Africa; the conquest of Spain followed in 711 and meant the downfall of the Christian West Gothic kingdom there. Furthermore in the East, too, that same year the Umayyads achieved a breakthrough, into the Indus valley. A few years later they were already in Central Asia: Samarkand and Bukhara, present day Uzbekhistan. So finally – barely a century after the death of the Prophet – the Muslim kingdom literally extended from the Pyrenees in the West to the Himalayas in the East, indeed far beyond the Roman empire in the southeast. Only the northern Mediterranean countries formed an exception; they could not be conquered. First of all Byzantium resisted a second siege (672–678 and 717–718), and finally the Muslim hordes were also stopped in Gaul by the Franks in 732.

What does the Islamic conquest represent for **Christianity**? Beyond question a **catastrophe of world-historical dimensions**. Christianity no longer had a chance in North Africa – apart from the Egyptian Copts – and in a lengthy process it disappeared almost completely. The great Latin churches of Tertullian, Cyprian and Augustine went under. The Patriarchs of Alexandria, Antioch and Jerusalem sank into insignificance. In short, from that time the area in which Christianity originated (Palestine, Syria, Egypt and North Africa) was lost to Christianity – the conquests of the Crusades were to remain episodes.

The question cannot be avoided: why did this Christianity – apart from remnants which fused together – allow itself so easily to be absorbed by Islam?

Why Christianity failed

Even compared with Judaism, which was incomparably weaker, Christianity could in fact offer little inner resistance to Islam. If we leave aside the manifest military, political and organizational power of the Islam of the time, and the cultural, economic and geostrategic factors which also applied to Judaism, a main cause of the failure of Christianity seems to have lain in the **inadequate foundation of the dogmas of christology and the Trinity**. The Catholic theologian Hermann Stieglecker, who gives an admirable account of the theological controversies between Christians and Muslims in his book on *The Doctrines of Islam*,[90] rightly regards this lack as one of the most serious causes of the collapse of Christianity, particularly in its homelands, in the Near East and North Africa. It was in fact simpler to believe in the One God and Muhammad, the Prophet after Jesus. In addition, however, there were also the lamentable internal divisions within Christianity, and the anxiety and shock caused everywhere by the rapid onslaughts of the hosts of Muslim horsemen.

But these '**inner divisions** within Christianity' are equally connected with Hellenistic dogmas: here is clearly a second theological reason for the lack of any internal resistance within Christianity, in which both West and East Rome were notable for their lust for dogmatic supremacy and their impatience, especially towards the churches in the Near East and in North Africa. It is evident that Islam – just like Judaism – did not have the unfortunate **urge to give the most precise definition of everything, even in the understanding of faith**. And if we go on to consider the world religions of Indian and Chinese origin in this respect, it becomes even clearer that this desire to 'dogmatize', i.e. to decree legally, as many aspects of faith as possible is a 'Christian', or more precisely a Graeco–Roman, speciality.

The feeling for philosophy and aesthetics, for polished language and the harmonious presentation of faith is **Greek**; so too is the intellectualizing of faith in often extravagant speculation and unfruitful conceptual mysticism which is expressed in the dogmatizing. The feeling for form, law, and organization, for tradition and unity, the useful and the practical, is **Roman**; so too are an efficient power politics and authoritarian methods of leadership even in religious matters, and the traditionalism, legalism and triumphalism which keep breaking through in definitions.

Islam regards theology as a peripheral philosophy of religion which is hardly necessary. It has limited definitions and dogmas to the legal sphere. Instead of orthodoxy it has concentrated on **orthopraxy**, though here the preponderance of law in Islam is hardly less problematical than the preponderance of dogma in Christianity. At any rate Islam has preserved unity very much better – despite the great split between Sunnis and Shi'ites, for which there are other reasons. In Christianity people praise the great christological-trinitarian councils, but usually forget what I have brought out clearly: that the names Nicaea, Ephesus, Constantinople and Chalcedon were associated not only with disputes which went on afterwards, but also with great splits in the church which have persisted in Egypt and the Near East to the present day, despite the fatal threat from Islam.

A shift of focus in world history

Hardly any victorious progress has taken place in world history so rapidly and extensively, and at the same time so persistently and permanently, as that of Islam. And even today all the Muslim feelings of pride ('a religion of victors') and inferiority ('why not today?') are based on these historical experiences of the early period.

In his famous book on *Muhammad and Charlemagne*,[91] written in 1937, the Belgian economic and social historian Henri Pirenne for the first time pointed out the significance of the Islamic invasion of the ancient Mediterranean world and the shift of the focus of Christian European history northwards which followed as a result. In terms of economic history this may be problematical, but certainly not in terms of political and cultural history. Rather, the consequences of the victorious Islamic progress should be noted for the **formation of the mediaeval paradigm of Christianity**:

- The **East Roman empire** had been decisively weakened compared to the West by the loss of its southern and south-eastern lands; Justinian's dream of a Christian restoration of the united Roman empire was over once and for all.
- The **unity of the Mediterranean world** was shattered for ever; to the present day the Mediterranean Sea has ceased to be a Christian *mare nostrum.*
- The **Frankish kingdom** had the historical opportunity of forming the new Christian empire. As Pirenne pointedly put it: Muhammad made Charlemagne possible.
- Finally, the **papacy** was offered the possibility of definitively detaching itself from East Rome with the help of the Franks and attaining **state independence**; without the Franks there would have been no church state with the Pope as spiritual and secular supreme head. And without the church state Rome would not have self-confidently demonstrated its power against Byzantium.

In a word, the **shift of political focus northwards,** to northern Central Europe, was of fundamental significance for the formation of the Western mediaeval paradigm of Christianity (P III).

The religions and wars

However, we should note that the victorious progress of the Islamic Arabs was not primarily an Islamicization, at least as far as non-Arab peoples were concerned. In other words, Islam was not imposed as a religion; the conquered peoples were 'merely' subjected politically. Conversion was not usually required of those who had been conquered; what was required of them was a poll tax and unconditional political obedience. Nevertheless, we cannot overlook the fact that religious motivations played an essential role in these campaigns of conquest. So people talked and still talk of the Islamic 'holy wars'. Is that right?

'Holy war' is a Western formulation of uncertain origin which does not exist in Arabic as such. For the Arabic equivalent *jihad*[92] means neither 'war' nor 'holy'. In principle this one word simply means 'effort, dedication'. In some circumstances this can be understood not only in moral terms (the 'lesser effort') but also in terms of war (the 'great effort'). And the word has often been understood in the latter sense already in the Qu'ran, with the result that it has justified every possible kind of violence against non-Muslims (especially Jews) and against apostates and rebels. Be this as it may, the idea of *jihad* certainly underlies the victorious progress of Islam. And the division of the world in principle into the 'sphere of Islam' (*dar al-Islam*) and the non-Muslim 'sphere of war' (*dar al-harb*) doubtless furthered the view that Muslims are not content with defence and passive resistance against attackers but if there is a favourable opportunity will also go over to the attack, in order to help the law of Islam to victory. So the goal remains the victorious extension of their religion throughout the world. The present-day Islamic revivalist movement also propagates the maxim: 'Islam rules, it is not ruled over.' So isn't Islam, as is often claimed, the most aggressive of all religions, at any rate more aggressive than Christianity?

Here at the latest I must pause in this account and once again insert a critical/self-critical interim reflection. 'Triumph'? Whether Muslim or Christian, today this word has a fatal ring about it. In our present-day perspective with the efforts of present-day humankind to achieve a global peace, do we want to wish or grant any religion a new 'triumph'? An Islamic 'holy war' or a Christian 'crusade'? Should a religion, any religion, ever devote itself to wars, wage wars?

This question arises for all three prophetic religions, which are often so aggressive. Of course it arises least of all for **Judaism**, which had the possibility of motivating or inspiring wars only up to the destruction of the Second Temple (135), though it has regained this possibility in most recent times. Moreover Judaism, as a religion concentrated totally on its people and its land,[93] has never made a universal claim.

Things are different with **Islam** and **Christianity**. Christians, including Christian experts on Islam, often overlook and ignore the fact that Islam is not the only religion to have made an aggressive claim to universality and advocated an ideology of war rather than peace. The same is true of Christianity.[94] Not only Muhammad's armies but also those of Charlemagne waged 'holy wars' of the utmost cruelty for centuries. Historically there is no disputing the fact that not only in Islam but also in Christianity (above all in the mediaeval paradigm), people began from the assumptions:
– that their own religion was the best form of community for human beings, a perfect society;
– that a 'city of God' was desirable on earth and that their own order of life, sanctioned by divine authority, had universal validity and therefore was in principle binding on all societies and states;
– that therefore one had an obligation to extend one's own sphere of religious control as far as possible and use political and, if need be, even military means for this mission in order to produce a uniform religious society which embraced as many human beings as possible, with the final goal of the victory of one's religion throughout the world.

But at a time when, in contrast to antiquity and the Middle Ages, humanity can destroy itself with new technological means, must not all religions, and especially the three prophetic religions which have often been so aggressive, make new efforts to see how wars can be avoided and peace furthered? A re-reading, a differentiated re-reading of our own religious traditions, is unavoidable here. And a double hermeneutical change of direction is needed:

(a) The **warlike** words and events in our own traditions should be interpreted historically, in terms of the situation at the time:
– the cruel 'wars of Yahweh' and the inexorable psalms of vengeance in terms of the situation of the conquest and the later situation of defence against over-powerful enemies;
– the Christian missionary wars and the 'Crusades' in terms of the ideology and theology of the early and high Middle Ages;
– the summons to war in the Qur'an in terms of the particular situation of the Prophet in the Mecca period and the special character of the Mecca surahs.

(b) But the words and actions in our own traditions which **make peace** are to be taken seriously as impulses for the present. Christians should really find that easiest, since their original memories do not point to warrior heroes or kings or a general, but to a preacher of non-violence and an original community which spread through the Roman empire not by force but by a message of justice, love and peace. Yet beyond doubt all religions, and especially the three prophetic religions, face challenging questions in view of the threats and dangers to world peace.

Questions for the Future

✝ By its missions in the early Middle Ages and the Crusades in the high Middle Ages, by the wars of religion at the time of the Reformation and by colonization and mission in modern times, Christianity has left enormous trails of violence, blood and tears in history.

Is it not necessary to reflect once again, above all on the Sermon on the Mount, in which the peacemakers are praised, and violence and retaliation are rejected? 'Blessed are the peacemakers' (Matt.5.9); 'Recompense no man evil with evil' (Rom.7.12).

☾ From the beginning Islam appeared in the world as a religion of military combat and victory, and at the time of the Prophet and the four 'just Caliphs' it already produced a number of cases of cruel violence.

Is it not necessary to reflect once again on the peacemaking words which can also be found in the Qur'an? 'If they (the enemy) incline to peace, make peace with them, and put your trust in God' (Surah 8.61).

🕎 Judaism, for almost two thousand years not a religion of victors, as at the beginning, but rather a religion of sufferers, has rightly created a home for itself in the State of Israel, which must and should be defended with all political and military means to prevent new pogroms and a new holocaust.

But finally, is it not necessary here to reflect once again on bringing peace to the whole of the Near East? For the sake of safeguarding the existence of the State of Israel, instead of concentrating on a retaliatory morality of 'an eye for an eye', is it not therefore necessary to concentrate on the prophets' message of peace and those words in the Hebrew Bible which call for peace? 'Seek peace and pursue it!' (Psalm 34.15); 'And they will beat their swords into ploughshares' (Isa.2.4).

Now let's turn once again to Christianity: to the further history of Western Christianity and above all to the development of the papacy, which after a lengthy period of external dependence was finally able to establish itself as the determinative religious and political power in the West. Here the fact that the church had its own state and that there was a Western emperor, backed by Rome, who could protect the Roman papacy against Byzantium and under whose protection it was able slowly but surely to rise to control of the world, was of key importance. Now the elements of the mediaeval Roman Catholic paradigm took on concrete forms.

6. Elements of the mediaeval Western paradigm

In the eighth century the focal point of Christianity had shifted definitively westwards. The Germanic peoples developed a tremendous dynamic, while the East tore itself apart in the iconoclastic dispute, retreated increasingly into itself and became isolated from the West. An epoch-making paradigm shift in Christianity is in fact often also connected with a geographical **shift in the centre of church power**: now from the East, which was politically, ecclesiastically and culturally dominant in the early Hellenistic Mediterranean world, to the **West**, which was above all ecclesiastically and then also politically and culturally coherent.[95]

There was a new fusion of the vital West Germanic Catholic population with the old worn-out Latin population from which the vigorous Romanic nations emerged. At the same time there was to be missionary work among the Germanic tribes east of the Rhine, above all under the influence of Iro-Scottish and Anglo-Saxon monks. Christianity had already spread throughout southern and south-western Germany before Boniface, though there was little ecclesiastical orgnaization. And in the north, too, paganism was now forced further and further back.

The church is given a state

At this point we must realize that only the **Catholic Church**, the heir to the education and organization of antiquity, was left in the West as a cultural force. Under the leadership of the **papacy** and with the help of **monasticism** it was in fact the only cultural force which in the long run was able to put a stamp – cultural, moral and religious – on the Germanic and Romanic peoples, who in many respects were primitive. So for many centuries the church was quite naturally the institution which dominated the whole of cultural life, though it did not avoid taking on numerous Germanic influences: polytheistic elements in the veneration of the saints, a belief in souls and demons in the 'masses for souls' and 'purgatory'.

The order of Benedict of Nursia,[96] the **Benedictine order**, was of great assistance in the church's cultural work. It combined old monastic traditions with the Roman military spirit in a rule which in the face of the numerous itinerant ascetics committed its members to *stabilitas loci*; to obedience to the abbot; to a renunciation of possessions and marriage;

and to manual work (agricultural work, household tasks, crafts and, increasingly, teaching and the copying of ancient and Christian manuscripts). Thus there was at least a minimum of cultural tradition in an otherwise rather uncreative period.

However, despite a growing common awareness of the church and despite all the respect for the Roman Pope, initially among the Catholic Germans it was still **impossible for a universal Western church to develop**. For in the Germanic 'particular churches' of tribes, countries and rulers it was not the Pope but the king (and the nobility) who had the say. That was also true of the **Frankish kingdom**, which came to play a leading role in the eighth century and which, after the conquest of the more highly developed Spanish kingdom of the West Goths by the Arabs (in 711), with the Italian Langobard kingdom became the only kingdom on the Western European continent between the Pyrenees and the Elbe. But in the Frankish church, too, it was the king and not the Roman Pope who ruled.

The rise of the Frankish kingdom and the creation of a great European empire thus did not begin from the Mediterranean region and the culture of late antiquity there, but from the **north**, from northern central Europe. And now the Roman **papacy** for its part took the **epoch-making** decision to detach itself from the constitutional framework of the Roman Byzantine empire and turn to the kingdom of the Franks. So there was a break with the Byzantine emperor and an association with the Frankish ruling house. Why? The underlying hope was for freedom both from Byzantium and from the Langobards and speculation about a **separate papal state**.

Now the occasion proved favourable: Byzantium was completely absorbed in the iconoclastic dispute; the imperial Byzantine rule in northern Italy and Rome was in decline; the Langobards had expelled the Byzantine exarch from Ravenna; because of the papal resistance in the iconoclastic dispute the emperor put the territories in southern Italy and Sicily ruled by Byzantium under the Patriarch of Constantinople, and confiscated the papal possessions. However, already by the time of the royal major-domo **Charles 'Martel'** (a military 'hammer', 714–741), the papacy had sought and cultivated ties with the Frankish kingdom. Charles had inflicted a famous defeat on the Arabs at Tours in 732 and thus secured the existence of Christianity north of the Pyrenees and generally safeguarded the Frankish heartlands.

There had been a fearful neglect of morality under the Merovingians, who had ruled in the Frankish kingdom since Clovis' conversion. But already in the time of Charles Martel the Anglo-Saxon Willibrord (of the diocese of Utrecht) had begun work among the Frisians, and the Anglo-

Saxon monk **Boniface** (really Winfrid) among the Germans on the right bank of the Rhine. Finally consecrated archbishop by Rome and even nominated papal vicar for all of Germania, he established a whole series of German bishoprics. First of all he pressed for the observance of the Roman canons among the clergy, with celibacy for all, and after Charles Martel's death in 741 effectively embarked on the reform of the Frankish church which was so urgently needed. This 'apostle of the Germans', as he was later called, did more than others to establish papal control in the Frankish kingdom. At the Frankish synod of 744 Boniface had even obtained from the bishops a written submission to the Roman church: in 754 he was killed by pagan Frisians in a mission to Friesland.

Whereas Charles Martel had refused to intervene in Italy against the Langobards who were threatening Rome, his son **Pepin** the Younger (741–768) was very interested in a rapprochement with the Pope. Why? For the Pope to sanction his *coup d'état* against the shadowy and decadent Merovingian kings and sanction the elevation of the major-domo to be the Frankish king. This in fact happened in 751 on 'apostolic authority'. Note that in this way the **foundation was laid in the West for the Christian idea of the king**; for the first time a Pope (at that time Zacharias) acted so to speak as kingmaker. Here suitability for office ('idoneity') had been given preference over dynastic legitimacy. As a substitute for the 'royal blood' which he lacked, the Carolingian Pepin was anointed the first Frankish king with holy oil (possibly by Archbishop Boniface). The 'grace of God', *Gratia Dei Rex*, had replaced alleged descent from the pagan gods and blood affinity. One became king by the grace of God, whose 'representative' on earth in the Roman view was none other than the Pope.

Thus Pepin's elevation to the throne brought advantages to both sides: to the Carolingians, since they had their rule in a way divinely legitimated; to the Popes, since in future nothing happened without their blessing. A coalition of interests between the Franks and the papacy began to develop which was to have consequences, and a test case soon occurred. It happened after the first journey of a Pope westwards instead of eastwards: in 753/4 Pope Stephen II, threatened by the Langobards and left in the lurch by Byzantium, travelled in search of help to the Frankish court and there put Rome under the permanent protection of the king of the Franks. Conversely, Pepin pledged himself to reconquer the territories conquered by the Langobards, the exarchate of Ravenna and other lands which the Pope had never previously possessed. Here, too, it should be noted that this was the first intervention of a power outside Italy in favour of the papacy. After two campaigns, in 756 Pepin then in fact donated these territories to 'St Peter': the **Donation of Pepin**.

The Roman understanding was, however, that the 'donation' was more of a 'restoration', since according to the **Donation of Constantine** these territories in any case belonged to the Pope. But as the Donation of Constantine was a **Roman forgery** – perpetrated only fifty years earlier – in this way a forgery became the foundation for a fact: for the real donation by Pepin. What a game! The document which was the foundation for the donation was solemnly put in the tomb of St Peter in St Peter's church; with it the Pope established his rights to possession once and for all. The emperor was to bear the title 'Patricius Romanorum', which virtually amounted to 'military guardian of the Romans'. The advantage for the latter was that they could now reject the political claims of Byzantium. Moreover Pepin resolutely refused to restore the conquered territories to the Byzantine emperor, whose special emissary had arrived at the last minute. After all, according to his understanding of the Donation of Constantine too, this was not the emperor's possession, but that of the apostle Peter.

Thus were laid not only the theological and ideological but also the economic and political foundations for the **church state**, a 'state' which was to last for more than eleven centuries, until the year 1870. For a time the papal coins still bore the emperor's image and papal documents were dated by the years of the emperor's reign. But these formal signs of Byzantine supremacy were soon to disappear when under Pepin's son Charles a second great blow against Byzantium followed: the establishment of a second, now Western, emperor.

Charlemagne: a Christian emperor of the West

In 798 Pope Leo III had fled to the Franks because of the opposition of the nobility of the city of Rome to him; in distant Paderborn, in the midst of what was formerly pagan territory, he gained the support of the powerful ruler of the Franks, presumably already promising there to crown him emperor. Thereupon **Charlemagne**[97] (768–814) undertook an expedition to Rome. According to the reckoning 'after the birth of Christ', which had become customary since Dionysius Exiguus in the sixth century, this was the year 800. In Rome, Charles summoned a Roman synod very much in the style of the Byzantine emperors, which also included many Roman and Frankish laymen. He himself presided over it and directed it. The Pope had to swear an oath purging himself of all the crimes of which his opponents accused him. But he did this with an appeal, which had previously been accepted by the synod, to the sentence from the Symmachian Forgeries which had never previously been put into practice, that the Pope could not be judged by anyone.

Charles' attitude becomes comprehensible if we realize that the king of the Franks and the Frankish church accepted, as being in their own interest, the view of the Pope as the divinely chosen successor and administrator of St Peter which prevailed in Rome – in clear contrast to the Byzantine emperors and the church of the East. But Charles had certainly not thought originally of an imperial power which would be a kind of counterpart of Byzantium. For when on 23 December 800 the same synod resolved to elevate Charles to be emperor, Charles quite naturally saw himself as a new **emperor of the West**: the king of the Franks as a king over the Western kings – not superior to but with the same rank as the Byzantine emperors.

But here too the Pope was pursuing his own interests. Two days later, at the beginning of the Christmas Eve liturgy in St Peter's in the year 800, with a precious crown Leo II crowned the Frankish Charles simply and without formality '**Emperor of the Romans**', which could only mean all the Romans, in the West and in the East. For the Pope this was an increase in prestige and a consolidation of his position in the city of Rome, but at the same time it was an unimaginable affront to the emperor in Byzantium. And Charles, too, was annoyed. So later it was with his own hands that he put the crown on the head of his son and successor Louis, later called the Pious, in the Palatinate Chapel in Aachen (813).

But at that time Leo was acting quite consistently on the basis of the Donation of Constantine.[98] For according to this the Emperor Constantine had personally handed over the imperial crown to the Pope; out of sheer modesty the Pope had not wanted to wear it, and had left it for the emperor to use, whereupon the emperor had gone to Constantinople with papal consent. So here for the **first time a Pope was claiming the right to crown the emperor**: the crown of the Caesars (which really belonged to him!) was given at a time when the throne was vacant (though at that time in fact a woman, Irene, was reigning in Constantinople!) to an utterly strange barbarian ruler, and all this without a special ceremonial, since in this case the Byzantine imperial ceremonial was inappropriate. But the deficiency was soon made good. After Charlemagne's death, in 816 a Pope travelled specially to Rheims to crown Charles' son Louis, too – with his own ceremonial and a crown which he had brought with him: with prayers and above all a special anointing for the 'special son of the church'. Moreover anointing (deriving from the Old Testament) also became fundamental for the emperors of the West: as they had no historical legitimation, the grace communicated through papal unction gave them a theological legitimation. Louis' son Lothair was then invited to Rome for his coronation in

823, and from then on, St Peter's was the place of imperial coronations (with the bestowal of the sword), for which on each occasion subsequent Frankish kings had to beg humbly.

Thus from the time of Charlemagne there was a second 'emperor of the Romans', who was not a Roman at all. For Byzantium, where of course the throne had never been vacant, this was a ridiculous measure, not to be taken seriously. But more quickly than they thought there, it made history and finally led to the schism in the church which I described earlier, the empire in any case having long since been divided politically. Granted, in 812 the East Roman empire offered 'brotherhood' to the newly created Frankish emperor, who in his turn wisely dispensed with the Roman character of his emperorship, calling himself merely *imperator et augustus*, while the Byzantine *basileus* (king) deliberately called himself 'emperor of the Romans'. Nevertheless, the process of detaching Old Rome from New Rome which had begun fifty years earlier was now complete.

In the West: Christian = Catholic = Roman

So now all at once there were **two Christian emperors**. Were they of equal status? Not at all, since in the West with its Latin stamp, the new Germanic emperor was regarded as the true and legitimate emperor because he had been anointed by the Pope, while the Eastern 'Greek' emperor was increasingly regarded as illegitimate and finally as schismatic. Thus in the West that ecumenically pernicious equation **Christian = Catholic = Roman** was established, a further decisive step in the course of the development of what I am calling the **Roman Catholic paradigm of Christianity**. So in the eighth and ninth centuries the foundations were laid not for the unity of Europe, but for the **division of Europe**.

Charlemagne also proved generous to the Popes. Now also 'king of the Langobards', he confirmed and enlarged the **papal state** and gave 'back' further Italian lands to the Pope: Venice, Istria, parts of the duchies of Spoleto and Benevento and the island of Corsica. Charles rejected papal claims documented in the papal archives which went even further. He felt himself in no way to be a Roman subject, but rather half a Pope. For although Charles as lord of the empire gave priority to politics, as lord of the empire he also regarded himself in a completely theocratic way as **lord of the church**. Imperial politics were church politics and church politics imperial politics. So without any moral or religious scruples he forced his form of Christianity on the tribes he subjected (Frisians, Saxons, Slavs, Avars) and did not shrink from costly wars which, in the case of the Saxons, were to last around thirty years and brought executions and deportations to thousands of people. The 'unity of the empire' came first. This Frank regarded the Pope as the guardian of the apostolic tradition, responsible for questions of faith, dogma and liturgy, but limited to purely spiritual functions.

Moreover, in the style of Byzantine emperors Charles did not allow any autonomous interventions of Rome in his empire. Rather, he was personally involved in all ecclesiastical and even theological questions, for example opposing the veneration of images and the Seventh Ecumenical Council of Nicaea (787) under the Empress Irene, which favoured this, with his own imperial synod in Frankfurt in 794; in another synod (Aachen 809) he required the Pope to include the *filioque* in the Creed. At that time Leo III insisted on the still unaltered original ecumenical text, but he could not prohibit the Frankish version, which was becoming increasingly established in the West. In a *Corpus Christianum* Charles understood himself like the Byzantine emperors as *rex et sacerdos*, as 'king and priest', as *defensor*, defender, and *rector*, governor of the church, whereas the duty of bishops and clergy was above all that of sacrifice and prayer. So Charles has been called a 'Frankish Justinian'.

But the Frankish ruler by no means had a static view of society. Although illiterate, he encouraged schools and libraries and understood himself as a **renewer of education and culture**, of the Latin language and historiography, of architecture and illuminated books. Moreover, **fascinated by the myth of Rome** (empire, language, culture), Charles ushered in his own '**Renaissance**'. Supported by an international team of capable scholars, he thus brought about the rebirth, if not of classical antiquity, at least of Christian late antiquity. As a result, the first independent Germanic European culture had a deeply religious and at the same time a Latin and Roman stamp. This was a first, still rudimentary, mediaeval 'Renaissance' with its centre in the imperial palace at Aachen, whereas the second Renaissance in the high Middle Ages was to emanate from Paris and its university and the third late mediaeval Renaissance from the Florence of the Medicis.

In all this the king and emperor understood himself as a reformer of the church, who was trying to complete the reform of clergy and people introduced by Boniface and continued under Pepin:

– hence the correction of the Latin translation of the Bible by the Anglo-Saxon monk Alcuin, the most important figure in Charles's circle of scholars;

– hence the duty of the bishops (all no longer elected by the people but nominated by the king) to preach and visit without holding court;

– hence the establishment of parishes also in the country, and of communities of canons at cathedral and collegiate churches;

– hence a concern for regular participation in worship, frequent preaching and inculcating the Lord's Prayer and the Creed in the vernacular, and finally also the building of churches. However, there was another side: the 'tithe' (a tenth of annual income, derived from Old Testament) for the support of the bishops (who were now largely drawn from the nobility) and the clergy was widely hated, and was one of the main reasons why the Saxons rejected Christianity.

Yet despite all the shadow side, Charles appeared the ideal ruler and new founder of the Roman empire. In his universal Western empire (from Schleswig-Holstein to far beyond Rome and from the Ebro to the Elbe) there was a Frankish state church under the direction of the emperor – but still **no papal universal church** under the leadership of Rome. As in the East, so too in the West there was not a trace of a papal primacy of jurisdiction. Only in one respect did Charlemagne, along with Pepin, do decisive preliminary work towards a papal universal church: by adopting the Roman liturgy among the Franks for the sake of the unity of the empire. Here we must turn from the paradigm shift outside the church to the paradigm shift within it.

A paradigm shift also in the liturgy

We have seen how the Christian celebration of the eucharist, which was originally so simple, consisted of a prayer of commemoration and thanksgiving (including the account of the institution of the Lord's Supper), with the communion of all present, and of the liturgy of the word in the style of the synagogue, which was combined with it at a very early stage. In the new and splendid hall-churches (the basilica was originally a secular hall!) of the Constantinian period this worship of the earliest church (P I) had very soon turned into the **basilican liturgy of the early church** (P II): the bishop or presbyter still celebrated the old liturgy of commemoration and thanksgiving at the table, facing the people, in ordinary 'civilian' clothing.

But in time it had all become bigger, longer and **more ceremonial.**
Intercessions had been inserted into the old simple prayer of thanksgiving, for the living, the dead, various concerns, and these had been linked with the names of martyrs. Outside the prayer of thanksgiving, the **singing of psalms** had been introduced, particularly at three points:
– at the beginning at the entry of the clergy: entrance psalm/introit;
– at the offering of bread and wine and other gifts by the faithful: sacrificial psalm/offertory;
– at the communion of the faithful: communion psalm/communio.
But already at that time a whole series of ceremonies had been taken

over from Roman and especially Byzantine **court ceremonial**, even ceremonies which earlier Christians had rejected as pagan: genuflections, bowings, kisses; features like incense and candles; and special distinguishing marks like stoles, rings and so on. In addition there was **artistic** singing by specially trained singers, which had often suppressed the popular singing of the whole community. As we heard, from as early as around 250 the liturgy had no longer been celebrated just in Greek, but also in **Latin**, because the people in Rome no longer spoke Greek, but Latin again. However, in the sixth and seventh centuries theological learning had sunk to such a low level that the presbyters in the communities could no longer formulate the liturgical texts themselves: they required pre-formulated texts, so now liturgical.texts were increasingly collected and codified. Thus what was originally an extempore liturgy had finally become a **liturgy of the book,** in which increasing importance was to be attached to a faithful rendering of word and rite. On the whole there was no preaching. The designation 'mass' (*missa* = sending, prayer of blessing, blessing) became established for the eucharist.

It was under **Charlemagne** that there was to be a paradigm shift in the liturgy as well: from the early church ecumenical paradigm (P II) to the typical **Roman Catholic liturgy of the Middle Ages** (P III). For the introduction of a uniform liturgy was of the utmost importance for the unification of the Frankish kingdom. Thus Charles carried through what Pepin had probably already decreed in 754. And this **transplanting of the Roman liturgy into the kingdom of the Franks,** carried out above all in the imperial interest, had momentous consequences for the whole liturgy of the Western Middle Ages down to the Reformation, indeed to the eve of Vatican II. We have full and detailed information about this as a result of the historical researches summarized by Josef Andreas Jungmann:[99]

– For the first time in church history, towards the end of the first millennium the liturgy was celebrated by the Germans (unlike the Slavs!) not in the vernacular but in **Latin**, an alien language which was the only one sanctioned, since it was now alleged that there were only 'three sacred languages' – Hebrew, Greek and Latin. And as the clergy were virtually the only ones to understand Latin (at first the only written language), the liturgy became their preserve. There was no German-language liturgy.

– As the liturgy adopted among the Franks was not the relatively simple Roman parish liturgy but the solemn papal liturgy (shaped by Roman and Byzantine court ceremonial), the over-zealous Franks made the liturgy even more **solemn**, with an increasing number of genuflections, signs of the cross and censings.

– As the Germanic emotionalism also sought expression in worship through the uninterrupted prayer of the priest in a language which was no longer understood, numerous 'silent' prayers came into being (once again especially at the beginning, at the preparation of the gifts and the communion), and finally there was even the '**silent mass**' of the priest without the people, in which the eucharistic prayer in particular (which was sung in the East) was only whispered mysteriously ('hocus pocus'), and the account of the Last Supper was no longer understood as a proclamation for the community, but as 'words of consecration' for the gifts.

– Thus in time **altar and congregation** became completely **alienated**. As altars were built higher and higher, the altar table was finally pressed up against the wall of the apse ('high altar') and the priest's eucharist was no longer celebrated 'with' the people but 'for' the people ('the sacrifice of the mass'); no longer facing the people but facing the church wall.

– Thus what had originally been the simple celebration of a meal of thanksgiving increasingly became a **sacral play** which was interpreted allegorically for those who could not understand the language as the drama of the life of Jesus. In the period of the Franks, sacred scripture (Hebrew, Greek, Latin) was not translated into the unholy ('barbarian') vernacular any more than the mass texts were. Only the 'Lord's Prayer' and the Creed were translated into Old High German, in isolation, in the eighth century.

– Thus the **activity of the people** was completely **limited to seeing**: the garments retained by tradition from the late Roman period were now worn in specific alternating colours. Since the sacred forms could no longer be seen behind the priest's back, they were elevated and veneration was offered by genuflections. From the high Middle Ages the 'bread of life', formerly eaten in loyalty to the biblical legacy, was primarily looked upon and worshipped (later even a 'monstrance' was introduced). The normal bread became an unleavened, snow-white 'host' which looked little like bread, placed into the mouths of the 'laity' by the priest with his 'pure' hands instead of into their hands (which were 'impure'). In any case the communion of the faithful became the exception; indeed it became so rare that in the high Middle Ages a rule had to be made that it was to be made at least once, at Easter; finally communion from the chalice for the laity fell completely out of use.

– Whereas in the paradigm of the early church all presbyters celebrated one and the same eucharist, together with the bishop, in the Middle Ages each priest celebrated his own mass (for remuneration in the form of a 'mass stipend'). Then because of the **many masses, many side altars** were build in churches alongside the single altar, so as at the same time to make possible the private masses endowed by the faithful (especially masses for the dead, Gregorian masses and votive masses). Thus the sacrifice of the mass was offered as frequently as possible – to obtain 'grace' for the living and the dead, for help in all need, to fulfil every possible wish and petition, for every conceivable concern and need from a woman's infertility to a blessing for the harvest. Now the mass was **the** pious practice of the Middle Ages, and those who could pay could have hundreds of masses read for themselves and others, for their temporal or eternal salvation, without ever being present – an almost infallible means, superior to any prayer.

– **Baptism** was now administered exclusively to **infants**, and instead of the 'I believe' said by the person being baptized (which was now spoken by the sponsor) the priest's 'I baptize you' came into the foreground; the Christian became the passive recipient of the sacrament, the object of numerous rules. The anointing which was originally given after baptism split off at this time because it was reserved for the bishop, and became a separate rite, **confirmation**. Indeed, it finally became a separate sacrament, which now bestowed its own grace.

Gregorian chant – Roman?

Also in the Frankish period that **mediaeval tradition of singing** of the Roman rite developed which is known as **Gregorian chant**; however, this term has been in general use only since the choral restoration in the nineteenth century led by the Benedictine abbey of Solesmes, which was refounded in 1833. But as we have already heard, this chant had nothing to do with Gregory the Great. For in reality this is not, as the restorers of the time with their Roman and Romantic orientation claimed, 'old Roman' chant (P II) and thus the 'authentic' chant of the Roman church, the supreme model for all church music (Pius X, *Motu proprio*, 1903). In fact it is a **Frankish mediaeval transformation** of the chant of the early church – a paradigm shift (P III) in the micro-sphere, something that in our day traditionalist representatives of Roman *Musica sacra* long sought to deny.

Both German and French scholars have made a thorough investigation of this. Thus after the younger Solesmes monks M.Huglo and E.Cardine, the leading Gregorian scholar Professor Helmut Hucke of Frankfurt has stated: 'The concept of a *cantus Romanus* did not originate in Rome but in the Frankish kingdom, when Pepin the Younger and Charlemagne decided to introduce the Roman liturgy there "for the sake of the unity of the empire and union with the Apostolic See". What they received from Rome was the liturgy of the papal court. The earliest tradition of the mass chants of this liturgy appears in ninth-century Frankish manuscripts, but these only contain the texts and no musical notation.'[100]

So is there no original repertory of melodies in the church? No, melodies and above all modes of performance were handed down aurally. There was still no uniform liturgical chant in the Middle Ages. To quote Hucke once again: 'Down to most recent times Gregorian chant has been treated as though it had always been handed down in writing. In fact the written tradition of the melodies only begins at the beginning of the tenth century. However, the chant books of the ninth, tenth and even eleventh century without musical notation which have come down to us indicate that the dissemination of Gregorian chant in the Frankish kingdom still began with oral tradition; in Rome, its own tradition was set down only in the eleventh century, in an alien notation.'[101]

What is true of the Western liturgy as a whole is also true of liturgical chant: its Frankish redaction eventually found its way even to Rome. In other words, what was propagated in the nineteenth century as a genuinely 'old Roman' creation (or inspiration) was in reality a **Frankish re-creation**, and in the end this became the **mediaeval Roman tradition**. No wonder that all the more recent and most recent quest for an 'original version' of Gregorian chant has not led back 'to a musical opus'. Gregorian chant has proved to be 'a tradition which has constantly been understood in different ways, which becomes all the more varied and impossible to grasp, the further back one follows it. There can never be a historically correct performance practice.'[102]

In this connection we should reflect that the paradigm shift in the liturgy is to be seen in connection with important **shifts of accent in christology**. Josef Andreas Jungmann noted in the Carolingian period not only a transition from congregational worship to priestly worship, but also a shift from the theme of Easter to that of Christmas and the feasts of Mary, to Incarnation and Trinity. The shift in emphasis which had already emerged among the Greek fathers in the fight against Arianism now also came to influence the Franks through the Spanish church of the kingdom of the West Goths: a concentration on '**Christ our God**', the '**mother of God**', the '**most holy Trinity**'. So in the West, too, there was 'a retreat of the mediation of Christ, an emergence of the trinitarian element and the rise of the cult of Mary, and for this reason alone, in the West, too, we are compelled to take the fight against the Arian heresy into account as a main factor in the development'.[103]

Thus increasingly in the Carolingian period **Christ** is identified with God (*ho theos*) and **absorbed into the Trinity**, so that in certain prayers (e.g. the *Confiteor*) he is no longer mentioned at all as a mediator alongside Mary and the saints. At the same time the *Heliand* (the title of a heroic epic of a Jesus in German garb, which was composed around 830) appearing on earth becomes **the** manifestation of God. The festivals of the incarnation and the passion therefore now stood in the foreground and sought to instil a believing disposition, wonder and compassion, gratitude and penitence in the face of the incarnate God. And at a time which knew grave moral transgressions and abuses, particular importance was attached to penitence, not least in respect of sexual morality.

Private confession and rigorism in sexual morality

As we heard, the new **private confession which could be repeated without limit**, made to an individual priest under the seal of silence, did not come to the European continent from Rome but from the Celtic **monastic church** via Irish and Scottish missionaries. But then it spread amazingly quickly throughout Europe. It forced the public penance of the early church to the periphery and became a **characteristic element of the mediaeval Roman Catholic Church**. It is a further clear indication of the paradigm shift (P III). Alcuin, in the time of Charlemagne, already states that the eucharist is not to be received without the confession of sins. The Fourth Lateran Council in 1215 was to prescribe confession before Easter communion as a universal obligation, and Thomas Aquinas finally elevated confession theologically to a sacrament which was in fact necessary for the salvation of every Christian and firmly inserted it into the doctrine of the seven sacraments.[104]

When laying down the conditions of penance (which were originally very strict), the priest usually went by **penitential books** (*libri penitentiales*), which determined the degree of punishment (penitential tariffs).[105] These were mostly attributed to Irish saints (Patrick, Columba) and had their heyday between 650 and 850. Though in many respects they were contradictory and never approved officially, they soon came to belong among the office books of any priest and confessor: they were an expression not only of the widespread spirit of penitence but also 'documents of an extreme legalization and externalization of penance and an oppressive treatment of the penitent'.[106] Towards the end of the ninth century, penances were increasingly completed after confession, and finally they could even be replaced with payments of money; this inevitably led to injustices and numerous abuses.

Particular attention was paid in the penitentials to **sexual sins** at a time which did not take these seriously. The sexual morality of Charlemagne was certainly not what one would have called that of a 'model Christian' of the time. He had entered into several marriages by Frankish law, and in addition he had numerous associations which were illegitimate in the church's eyes; the number of his legitimate children is known approximately, but even he probably did not know how many illegitimate children he had. As with kings and emperors, so too with the nobility and the people, there was a great divergence between the moral demands of the church and actual circumstances. But there is no mistaking one thing: now the **paradigm shift also** became established **in church morality**.

We noted how in contrast to the Greek fathers, who were still moderate (P II), a **negative evaluation of sexuality** had become established **as early as Augustine** (the doctrine of original sin). As was pointed out by the Catholic moral theologian Josef Georg Ziegler, who went on to investigate the penitential tariffs which later came to be attached to the penitential books, 'The devastating effect of Augustine's association of original sin and sexual pleasure was that over the centuries it ruled out any open approach to marital intercourse and thus to marriage generally.' Following the African church teachers, early scholastic theology put forward the view that original sin is transmitted by the sexual pleasure of the marital act.'[107]

There is no mistaking the fact that in the face of increasingly marked moral degeneration as early as the Merovingian period, in the Carolingian period a **sexual-moral rigorism** established itself on a broad front, influenced by numerous primitive sexual tabus associated with sexual anxiety.[108] It governed less the official than the unofficial doctrine and penitential practice of the mediaeval church.

– For the **clergy**, who since Boniface's church reform had been required to observe sexual continence under threat of harsh penalties, this meant that anyone who wanted to come into contact with sacred things had to have 'pure', 'unsullied' hands (hence, even now, the anointing of hands at the ordination of priests). Sex, even if involuntary (emissions of semen) or permissible (in marriage), excluded them from encounter with the holy.

– For the **laity** this meant that they were excluded from preparation of and contact with the holy forms (hence no communion in the hands), indeed that women even had to be kept out of the sanctuary. Male semen, menstrual blood and blood lost in childbirth brought moral impurity and excluded those concerned from receiving the sacraments.

We need to reflect on the sexual repression that those countless penitentiaries with their often contradictory catalogues of sins or punishments created – all in the name of God and the church. 'Continence', in late antiquity the ideal of particular elites, was now as far as possible imposed on the whole population as an ideal. This **morality, hostile to pleasure**, stipulated with merciless casuistry that:

– during the days of their menstruation women were not to enter the church nor receive communion, and that after giving birth they should have a special blessing;

– the emission of seed, especially if it was caused deliberately, made men impure;

– married couples must refrain from sexual intercourse not only during menstruation and in the period before and after giving birth, but also on all Sundays and high feast days along with their vigils and octaves, on certain days of the week (Fridays), and in Advent and Lent. There is no doubt that the intention here was a **rigorous limitation of marital sexual intercouse**, and the giving of pleasure even in marriage was put in the background. For sexual stimulation was intrinsically bad, even if it was involuntary. Only in the course of the thirteenth century was at least the view of the sinfulness of any sense of pleasure overcome. But enough of a rigoristic pessimism about sex and marriage remained: sexual pleasure was legitimated only by other motives – principally the purpose of procreation.[109]

Here too – though one might hardly expect it – an **inter-religious problem** arises which also affects Judaism and Islam, and which should be briefly reflected on here. Not least because of the Christian sexual morality of the Middle Ages, there has been talk of a '**Judaized Christianity**', often in a historicizing way but often also polemically. Is this right?

Granted, there is no disputing the fact that in particular the Christianity of the Carolingians, at whose court Charlemagne was celebrated as the new David, Moses or Joshua, and scholars often addressed one another with biblical names, had features reminiscent of the Old Testament. And it is also beyond dispute that the commandment to tithe, the sabbath (Sunday) rest and the instruction about unleavened bread occur in the Hebrew Bible but not in the New Testament, and that the Hebrew Bible also contains explicit regulations about **sexual pollution and cultic impurity**.

Nevertheless it is **wrong** here simply to speak of a **Judaizing**. For in the Hebrew Bible, as also in the New Testament and the Qur'an, sexuality and human love are affirmed as the gift of the creator: man and woman are created for each other in their bodily nature as well, and are to become 'one flesh'.

– Not only the Hebrew Bible but also the New Testament and the Qur'an contain certain restrictions on sexual intercourse. For example, the Qur'an, too, forbids it during the wife's menstruation, during the day in times of fasting and also during the pilgrimage to Mecca. And even though no such restrictions are prescribed in the New Testament (in any case some were assumed as a matter of course against the Jewish background), here in particular (in contrast to the Hebrew Bible and the Qur'an) celibacy is praised by Paul, even if it is nowhere required.

Nowadays cultural anthropologists have been able to demonstrate the degree to which sexual customs and modes of expression have become norms and patterns of orientation required by a culture; how notions that the emission of seed and menstrual blood are intrinsically defiling are not specifically Jewish notions but widespread archaic pre-ethical notions, some of them also part of ancient natural medicine, and thus not specifically Jewish, Christian or Islamic. And nowadays, isn't the **question posed to all the religions** of Near Eastern origin this: should, can, the present-day view of sexuality in religion still proceed from notions and attitudes involving an archaic understanding of human beings and God? Or from an ancient natural medicine which, for example, has the erroneous view that blood lost in menstruation and in giving birth is a poisonous emission, and that sexual intercourse during pregnancy damages the child? A cultic sexual purity has long, all too long, been advocated for clergy and laity. In contrast to Judaism and Islam, in Christianity a depreciation of sexuality and marriage has been encouraged by the high esteem associated with a religiously motivated celibacy.

If we look back, we find all the elements of what we might call a **typically mediaeval piety** only from the Carolingian period: a piety that eventually embraced the whole of human life visibly from the cradle to the grave, from early in the morning until late at night, and which was constantly reactivated not only on Sundays but also on all the feast days, which became increasingly numerous. Scholars have even spoken of a Carolingian 'age of liturgizing' based on a combination of structures, forms and formulae from the early church with extremely archaic or more recent Germanic habits, rituals and customs.

But by now all this should have been made sufficiently clear. All these early mediaeval developments, and especially the **Carolingian innovations and changes** – a liturgy of the clergy and the sacrifice of the mass, private masses and mass stipends, the power of the bishop and priestly celibacy, auricular confession and monastic vows, the monasteries and the piety of All Saints, the invocation of saints and the veneration of relics, exorcisms and blessing, intercessory chants and pilgrimages – are **not constants, but variants – mediaeval variants of Christianity**. Certainly all this now stood in the centre of a piety of works, and increasingly overgrew the originally Christian element. However, this is not part of the original essence of Christianity, but rather an ingredient of the mediaeval paradigm. These are variables which could be encouraged, tolerated and even abolished again, depending on the pastoral situation. And it was precisely these early mediaeval developments of Christianity which, having become more and more excessive, were increasingly criticized in the late Middle Ages. Most of them were finally to be abolished again by the Protestant Reformers.

7. Romanization at the expense of Catholicity

Charlemagne's great empire did not last. Held together politically, militarily and culturally by Charles' powerful character, it fell apart only a generation later. In the conflict between his son Louis 'the Pious' and Louis' sons, three important groups of lands developed which were important for the future of Western Europe (the Treaty of Verdun, 843): **France, Italy and Germany.** However, all of them suffered an economic and cultural decline and devastating plundering raids: the Normans kept invading from the west, the Hungarians from the east and the Saracens from the south, which had become Islamic (after Sicily was also conquered).

It is not necessary for an analysis of the Roman Catholic paradigm to pursue the extremely varied political history of these groups of lands. For whereas the political and military stucture of the Carolingian empire collapsed, its spiritual and ecclesiastical foundation, **the paradigmatic Roman Catholic framework, was preserved**: beginning from written and spoken Latin, through Roman liturgy, dogmatics and morality to church order and the papacy in its mediaeval form. The view that the Pope bestowed imperial dignity became established. Indeed, as early as the period of the downfall of the Carolingians in the middle of the ninth century there was a kind of prelude to a total Romanization of the Catholic Church: to the degree that on the one hand a further major forgery once again decisively strengthened the ecclesiastical power of the Roman papacy, and on the other the Roman claims to power from the fifth century were now put forward by a Pope with extreme boldness and resolution – though even then without any abiding success.

Widespread forgery in Rome's favour

Barely a century after the foundation of the papal state it was Pope **Nicholas I** (858–67) who, with the political collapse of the Carolingians in his favour and in full awareness of his Petrine office, dared for the first time to impose the ban (exclusion from the church for disregard of a doctrinal or papal decision). For this Pope, the papacy was the divinely willed foundation of the social order. He already wanted to put the

Petrine theory into practice. He already attempted to replace the self-administration of the churches of the lands with a Roman central administration. Moreover, fully aware of the power which had been allegedly bestowed on him by Christ, he treated bishops, archbishops and patriarchs, kings and emperors, as though they were there to do his bidding. He unexpectedly threatened the king of the Franks with excommunication because of a difficult marriage situation and deposed the powerful Archbishops of Cologne and Trier who supported the king.

In keeping with this, Nicholas was the first Pope – possibly in good faith – to **appropriate** not only the Donation of Constantine but yet other monstrous **forgeries**. Granted, in the ninth century they did not yet have any great effect on the politics of church or empire, but in the eleventh century they were to come fully into their own. The documents in question were the **Pseudo-Isidorian Decretals**,[110] a collection of canons which were attributed to an otherwise unknown Isidorus Mercator. In their extended version they comprise more than 700 closely printed pages and contain papal decretals, synod resolutions and Frankish imperial laws including the Donation of Constantine. They begin with the forged letter of Clement of Rome to James the brother of the Lord, now further extended.[111]

What was **the historical reality?** It seems to be this: here 115 texts were given out to be documents of Roman bishops from the first centuries, although for the most part they had been fabricated not long beforehand, in France. In addition there were 125 authentic documents with later interpolations and alterations. Presumably these crude forgeries (it is conjectured that they were made in the diocese of Rheims, the heart of Frankish imperial territory) were the work of a whole group of highly skilful forgers who were probably clergy.

– What was their **main purpose?** To strengthen the position of the **bishops** against the powerful archbishops and the provincial synod, and also against the king and secular forces. Here for the first time we have a manifestation of that Frankish episcopalism which was to play a major role throughout the Middle Ages.

– Their **main argument?** The early church had allegedly been ruled even in detail by papal decrees.

– Their **main beneficiary?** Not the bishops, but the papacy, which at the time when the forgeries were made was weak and not yet to be feared as an opponent of episcopalism. For what to the forgers was a means to an end – the **exaltation of the power of the papacy**, designated *caput totius orbis* – for the papacy later became the end which justifies many means.

Their **strategies?** The right which the Frankish kings had exercised hitherto to hold and confirm synods was promised to the Pope alone; accused bishops could appeal to the Pope; in general all 'serious matters' (*causae maiores*) were reserved for the Pope's final decision. Indeed, state laws which were in conflict with the canons and decrees of the Pope were regarded as null and void.

Pseudo-Isidore's handy collection soon spread throughout Western Europe. For centuries these documents were regarded as largely 'authentic'. But Nicholas of Cusa and Lorenzo Valla already doubted their authenticity, and in the time of the Reformation the *Magdeburg Centuries* (edited by Matthias Flacius and others, from 1559 on in Magdeburg), and comprehensively the Reformed theologian David Blondel (who died in 1655), demonstrated the inauthenticity of the decretals. And understandably these Reformation critics were already unsparing in their accusations against the forgers and the Pope, some of which were unjustified. By contrast, modern mediaeval historians have taken no little trouble to understand the numerous forgeries 'in terms of their time', among them Professor Horst Fuhrmann,[112] a specialist in Pseudo-Isidore, until 1993 professor of the *Monumenta Germaniae Historica*, in his *Introduction to the Middle Ages*.[113] He gives a summary answer here to two fundamental questions about the forgeries.

The ethical question: '**Was there a lack of morality in the Middle Ages?**' The historian's answer is, no, since what made a law valid at that time was 'not the fundamental act of institution, as with us, but only its intrinsic justice'. The forgeries would have been made to serve justice, as the authors 'subjectively felt'[114] it. Indeed, they were to serve the order of salvation, and some forgers indeed 'really served heaven'.[115]

However, we may ask in return: in the Middle Ages might anyone who felt himself to be in the right or who wanted to serve 'heaven' make forgeries without any moral inhibitions? In the great majority of cases, weren't legitimate clerical or curial interests also at issue, which the forgers 'served', rather than 'intrinsic justice'? And where was the 'intrinsic justice' in the case of the universal ecclesiastical claims of the papacy? Shouldn't papal historians in particular ask more critical questions here?

The intellectual question: '**Did the Middle Ages lack a critical capacity?**' The historian's answer is: no, the weaknesses of mediaeval criticism do not stem from 'a lack of intellectual capacity, from a lesser mental capacity'. The forgeries were often 'embarked on in a different spirit which attached no special weight to a formal state of authenticity'.[116]

However, we may ask in return: given the material significance of the forgeries, what does 'formal' mean here? Moreover, didn't the church authorities defend the formal authenticity vehemently when it was doubted, and at the same time investigations were made of the church's power structures by the mediaeval 'heretics', above all in relation to the Donation of Constantine and other Roman claims to power?

Now beyond question, at all times and in all places there have been forgeries which have to be understood in terms of the time.[117] And the pseudo-Isidorian decretals are perhaps not forgeries in the modern sense of being written deliberately to mislead. Yet it was precisely these Middle Ages, alleged to have been so deeply religious, which more than any age before them or after them – even according to their defenders – were a **'time of forgeries'**. Marc Bloch, the founder of the French 'new history', whom we have already met, has even spoken of a 'mass episode of forgery' between the eighth and twelfth centuries. But does stating this at the same time excuse it? Even after the event, may we not ask critical questions about this practice, although it was now to have an enormous political effect? Can at least a committed Christian today be indifferent to what was done to the church of Jesus Christ in the name of these forgeries, which are certainly not just a **curiosity 'of that time', but a power factor down to the present day**?

A historicization of the forgeries?

As a Christian theologian of today, one looks on the attempts to 'historicize' those major forgeries with mixed feelings, especially when in particular historians of status pull out all the apologetic stops to excuse them and trivialize them by a hermeneutic of acquiescence. This is what happened in the concluding lecture given by Horst Fuhrmann at the 'Sixteenth International Congress of Historians' in Stuttgart in 1985. In a way which I find incomprehensible, he seethes with polemic against historical criticism, against the Enlightenment and modern 'demystification', culminating in a plea for mediaeval thought forms and a postmodern 'remystification of the world'. In this context the historian concedes:
– that even in the Middle Ages forgery was in no way a transgression which went unpunished;
– that Pope Innocent III (the workshop of a group of forgers had been discovered immediately after his elevation to the papacy) enacted rules for examining a document and proclaimed that forgeries might in no way be tolerated under a mantle of holiness;
– that the papal chancery attempted in its own interest, in the face of professional falsifiers, formal bureaus of falsification and rings of forgers, to track down, prosecute and prevent forgeries.

No, for all the justified historical rehabiliation of 'mediaeval thought-forms', committed theologians must ask historians to understand that in the case of such historical evidence a few further questions concern them which might perhaps also be interesting to the historian.[118] Certainly we may not simply measure the Middle Ages by the criteria of modern rationality and historical criticism. So these are no false moralizing accusations, but **critical questions** for the sake of the truth:

– Why did the papal chancery only attempt to track down forgeries when this was in its own interest?

– Since it was in a better position than any other institution, why did it never bother to investigate forgeries which told in its favour, above all the major forgeries of the Donation of Constantine and the Pseudo-Isidorian Decretals, which are unique in world history?

– Why didn't the Pope and Curia draw conclusions at the latest at the very beginning of the second millennium, when the Emperor Otto III for the first time in the Middle Ages declared the Donation of Constantine to be a forgery and in a solemn document pronounced all the donations built on it to be null and void (though he then went on to hand over to the Pope, by virtue of his own imperial power, the lands which constituted the papal state)?

Or to ask a more fundamental question: Were all the Roman claims really a 'God-given truth' which one might 'help to victory'[119] even through forgeries? Do fictions so simply become facts if they are recognized by the church? Does a lie become the truth if one lies in the name of or in favour of the church? And was the forger's art ever morally justified as 'an action for the common good and pleasing to God',[120] because the end justifies the means? Indeed, may the cynical saying which probably first went the rounds in the sixteenth century, '*Mundus vult decipi, ergo decipiatur*' ('The world wants to be deceived, so let it be deceived'), simply be presented as the expression 'of a basic feature of human existence', even as 'the longing for a sphere free of reason, which gives meaning'?[121] Are we at the end of the day to justify even the mediaeval forgeries with the argument that 'all believers' nurture 'an area in which they do not allow rational proof to prevail'[122]? Even the worst possible deceptions and crimes of history can be justified with such an apologetic, provided that they have been committed in the name of a reality which cannot be proved rationally.[123]

But what makes these forgeries so pernicious? The fact that they still have an effect on the way in which the church understands itself. As early as 1955 the papal historian F.X.Seppelt already remarked on the effect of the Pseudo-Isidorian decretals that 'the denial of the notion of development in church order' was 'a bad influence', as it was expressed 'in the backdating of many later definitions to an earlier time and the introduction of the ideas and demands of a church party of the ninth century into the post-apostolic period'.[124]

In fact these are the decisive **influences on the self-understanding of the church**. These ninth-century forgeries
– give the papal claims to power which had been made since the middle of the fifth century the aura of great antiquity and the halo of the divine will;
– create for these claims to power that theological and legal foundation in the first three Christian centuries which they had previously lacked;
– 'perpetuate' a quite particular form of the church which had come into being in history;
– thus serve to cement a 'constitutional life' of the church which was historically by no means unchangeable and irreformable.

No, there is no disputing the fact that the exaggerated claim of the papacy to power, which was to result in the schism with the East and the protest of the Reformers in the West, was established in the eleventh and twelfth centuries essentially with the help of these forgeries. And if we reflect that down to our day the control of Rome over the whole Catholic Church, over local, regional and national churches, over bishops, clergy and individual believers, indeed even over the ecumenical councils, was given a legal basis unscrupulously by means of these forged decretals,[125] this debate ceases to be a trivial historical matter. Its effects, though carefully concealed today, can be traced right down to the *Codex Iuris Canonici*, which was revised under curial control and promulgated once again in 1983. For as our examination so far has shown, the curial system of power cannot appeal to the New Testament and the old Catholic tradition. It is based on ever-new appropriations of power down the centuries, and on forgeries which provided legal confirmation of them after the event.

In fact later Popes adopted such forgeries, and in so doing gave them a pseudo-legitimacy. Pius IX, the infallibility Pope of Vatican I, who did not lag far behind some of his mediaeval predecessors in his sense of clerical rule and who yet lost the church state, could praise a collection about the Romanus Pontifex which reprinted the false decretals as authentic evidence for the papacy. And in support of the legal principle that the Pope alone has the right to summon an ecumenical council, which is still important today, the *Codex Iuris Canonici* which was valid up to Vatican II cites 'six passages from earlier legal sources: three come from the Pseudo-Isidorian forgeries, and three are derived from them'.[126]

So what is to be done with such a *Codex Iuris Canonici*? Is it to be historicized and thus simply accepted? No, that would be to renounce any fundamental reform of the Catholic Church. So should it be overturned?

No, it should not be concluded from all these historical insights that today the *Codex* needs to be overturned completely rather than being reformed radically. But certainly we must see that the regulations mentioned (as I have already indicated previously[127]) are not divine but human law, and can be and indeed should be altered in the church at any time, wherever this seems justified by the criterion of the gospel and the demands of a new age.

For that time, the result of the Pseudo-Isidorian decretals was now to **concentrate the image of the church and church law completely on Roman authority**. The Pope now appeared virtually as the *norma normans*, the norm which is the norm for all other norms, and indeed for the whole church. So the Catholic French ecumenical scholar Yves Congar is right in noting a lack of tradition here, against all the appearances: 'Pseudo-Isidore attributes to the *magisterium* and the disciplinary authority of the Pope an autonomous character which is not bound by the norms of the tradition. To a contemporary of Cyprian, Pope Lucius, he attributes the statement that the Roman church, "mother of all the churches of Christ", has never erred.'[128]

As for the mediaeval forgeries, there is therefore no getting round the sobering **conclusion**: the Symmachian Forgeries prepared the way for the Donation of Constantine, and both were taken up and brought to completion in the third and greatest forgery, that of Pseudo-Isidore. Together they form **the legal basis for a future total Romanization of the Western church and simultaneous excommunication of the Eastern church**. They contributed to the development of common thought structures in the West which were less theological than legal, less originally Christian than mediaevally papal, and which had not so much a Catholic as a Roman stamp.

From now on **Europe** was **identical with the Latin West**. As the historian Walter Ullmann rightly comments, 'The idea of Europe was held to apply only to that part of the Continent which manifested the basic Latin substructure. Europe was an ideological concept, and no longer a merely physical term. It was welded together by the Roman Christian faith fixed by the papacy. But because the empire governed from Constantinople did not accept this faith enunciated by the successor of the prince of the apostles, it no longer belonged to Europe and therefore was heretical.'[129] In fact Nicholas I, through his bold deposition of the Patriarch of Constantinople, which was followed by his own deposition by Byzantium, was the main cause of the 'Photian' ('Nicolaitan') Schism – the prelude to the definitive schism two centuries later.

But while Nicholas' successors maintained these lofty claims, they were weak and often morally corrupt, just as the last Carolingian emperors were also weak and decadent. The West was in a process of decline. However, the leading ideas of the Carolingian period – the one universal empire, the one imperial church, the single Latin-ecclesiastical culture – remained in force, and new things were to emerge from this.

From decadence to reform

The second Christian millennium begins with an almost terrifying church disorder. I need not dwell at length here on the notorious tenth century of church history (extending into the eleventh) which even the Roman cardinal and historian Cesare Baronio, writing in 1607, called the '**dark century**' (*saeculum obscurum*). In any serious history of the Popes one can read dozens of pages about all the intrigues and battles, murders and acts of violence, in which the aristocratic parties of the city of Rome, the Popes and anti-Popes, were entangled. What is so to speak symbolic of the whole century is the macabre exhumation of Pope Formosus by his successor immediately before the turn of the century.[130] But this century makes virtually no constructive contribution to the new paradigm. The only thing to reflect on is that all these crimes, shameful acts and abuses did not essentially shake the authority of the Romanus Pontifex. Why? Since the time of Augustine, people had been accustomed to make a distinction between the office and its holder, between personal worthiness and official authority, between personality and institution. For emperors and princes, for bishops and clergy, as for the always numerous pilgrims to Rome, what counted was the 'objective', not the 'subjective'. So however great the moral perversion of individual Popes, it could not shake the papacy as an institution. And didn't the impressive coronation ceremonies for the Germanic emperors make it clear to the whole world that there was no imperial dignity (Western and Latin) without the papacy?

Evidently it was still difficult at this time for the papacy to assert itself without an imperial patron. Only when around the middle of the tenth century the kingdom of the East Franks again emerged from the collapse as the first of the three kingdoms to succeed that of Charlemagne, under the Saxon kings (Henry I), and rise to be the leading European power under Henry's son **Otto the Great** (936–973), was the papacy at least for the moment to be snatched from the collapse. In his kingdom Otto relied on the church instead of on the rebellious tribal dukes and made the bishops and imperial abbots princes of the realm (since they were unmarried, they had no dynastic interests!). They were all nominated by him and all bound to him by an oath of allegiance, making military, economic and political contributions. Thus mediaeval Germany became a land of clerical principalities, which were to exist until their secularization under Napoleon in 1803.

Fascinated by the example of Charlemagne, Otto was also interested in **renewing the role of emperor**, without having any inkling of the burden he would thus place on the German monarchy. His hour in history struck when – as now the most powerful ruler in Europe – he was summoned for help by Pope John XII against a self-proclaimed 'king of Italy' (Berengarius), and Byzantine forces advancing from southern Italy. Thus there came about the first of the Italian campaigns of German kings which were to stretch over five centuries. Otto was little concerned here with the moral stature of John XII; the powerful Saxon prince was far too interested in imperial coronation, for which he needed the Pope. This took place in 962. But John XII, who had been elected Pope as an immoral sixteen-year-old and was the first Pope to change his name (Octavian) on entering office, exercised a cynical rule and turned the Lateran into a den of immorality. And such a Pope did not hesitate to give the emperor, after the coronation, a lavishly embellished copy of the Donation of Constantine.

However, Otto had made the Pope and the people of Rome swear an oath of loyalty to him at the coronation, and only after that did he confirm the Donations of Pepin and Charlemagne. And when John XII broke his oath of allegiance soon after the emperor's departure, Otto returned to Rome, held a synod in St Peter's, and simply deposed the Pope (who had fled), who was accused in a letter of every possible vice, including incest. As his successor he appointed Leo VIII, a layman, who received all the orders in one day. This was another of the numerous **depositions of Popes** of which we have heard, but the first by a German king. They all show that the forged Symmachian legal principle 'The first see is not judged by anyone' had not found general recognition, even in Rome.[131] On the contrary, with the frequent absence of the emperor from Rome, depositions and appointments of Popes, Popes and anti-Popes, murdering and murdered Popes, were no rarity.

The **reorganization of the papacy** – the presupposition for a final shaping of the Roman Catholic paradigm (P III) – took place in three historical thrusts from three different sides: from French monasticism, the German monarchy and the Roman papacy itself. Let us look at this more closely.

On the way to a new world order

The **first phase** was initiated by the reordering of the church and the papacy **by monasticism**. The ascetic ideals of the early church revived again in the tenth century, above all in France (Cluny), in Lothringia (Gorze and Brogne) and in Italy (Camaldoli, Vallombrosa). In particular the monastery of **Cluny**[132] in Burgundy (founded as early as 910) became the cradle of a **monastic reform** orientated on Rome (and, in contrast, say, to Gorze, strongly centralistic), following the original ideals: strict observance of the rule of Benedict, reform of the economy of the monastery and, in reaction to the Germanic particular church, liberation from the supervision of the episcopate and direct submission to the protection of the Pope (*Petri*). For a long time the papacy, unconcerned about the decree of the Council of Nicaea, had begun to grant 'exemption' from the jurisdiction of the bishops as a papal 'privilege', and as in the first half of the eleventh century a number of monasteries in Western Europe and Italy now attached themselves to the reform association of Cluny, they all received the privilege of exemption, for which, however, they had to send a *'census'* to Rome. This was a lucrative enterprise for Rome, for such papal privileges had to be paid for time and again. So in time the papacy had under its control a fine-meshed network of bases, usually very well endowed, later also in the Germanic lands, indeed throughout Europe. Monasticism and the papacy supported each other; indeed, long before the papacy had imposed its centralism this was achieved by Cluny: strict submission to the monastery under its central government and at the same time the imposition of spiritual authority.[133] At the time, and not only in Rome, this was seen as an army of men of prayer on the spiritual battlefield!

The more the notion of reform pervaded the clergy in the eleventh century, the more the movement for monastic reform became a movement towards **church reform**, which concentrated above all on two points:
– strict discipline for the clergy: a fight against the marriage of priests which was still traditional and widespread, and concubinage ('nicolaitism'[134]):
– liberation of the church from the uncanonical intervention of the laity: a fight against the purchase of offices ('simony').[135] But the papacy itself was still in a lamentable condition.

The second phase: the reform of the papacy was **carried through by the German monarchy**. The deeply religious King Henry II, influenced by Cluny, had already devoted himself to reforms. Given two rival Popes, he decided for Benedict VIII, who crowned him emperor; in 1022 he then held a great reform council with Benedict in Pavia for the renewal of clergy and people. But it was above all **Henry III** (1039–1056), towards the middle of the eleventh century, who, faced with three Popes reigning at the same time, finally achieved the reform of the papacy by having all three rival Popes deposed at the synods of Sutri and Rome in 1046.[136] Nominated by the king, Bishop Suitger of Bamberg was elected Pope by the clergy and people of Rome (Clement II). The next three Popes – German and also outstanding men – were also nominated by the emperor, so that the Popes drawn from the Roman nobility were now followed by a series of imperial Popes. Probably no German king had a greater influence on the Western church than Henry III. But by committing himself to the reform of the papacy, he unintentionally set up the greatest enemy to his imperial status.

The third phase: the reform of the **papacy was completed by the papacy itself.** Under Henry's kinsman **Leo IX** (Bishop of Toul in Lothringia, 1049–1054), the reform movement was extended to the Pope. This created the foundation for an incomparable rise of the papacy and the Western church. Granted, the papal administrative apparatus with its different offices and divisions had functioned automatically even in the time of the morally corrupt Popes, and had issued countless decreta and responsa in the same elevated Latin all over Europe. Even a newly missionized area (and at that time such areas included, as we heard, not only Bohemia and Moravia but also Scandinavia as far as Iceland and Greenland) could not be incorporated into the ecclesiastical organization of the Western church without Roman assent. But this was so to speak routine.

In the brief and extremely hectic five years of his pontificate, the Lothringian Leo IX not only reformed the Roman city clergy but also decidedly helped on the reform by introducing regular synods. Furthermore, by his travels in Italy and to France and Germany he made the living successor to Peter effectively present at gatherings of clergy and synods. Everywhere he fought against simony and the marriage of priests. He tightened and strengthened the papal central government by making the cardinals – originally the most important representatives (from *cardo* = hinge, turning point) of the Roman city churches – into a kind of papal senate, and also summoned to this body prominent advocates of reform from beyond the Alps: these included the Lothringian Humbert (now Cardinal Archbishop of Silva Candida), a learned and shrewd theoretician of papal reform; then Frederick of Lothringia, chancellor of the Roman church; finally the Camaldolese Peter Damian, and, initially in a subordinate position, Hildebrand. Only in this way could the papacy become an institution representative of Europe, which in more delicate matters soon also intervened directly throughout Europe by 'legates' (personal representatives of the Pope).

These highly intelligent and deeply committed new men in Rome were concerned with no more and no less than **a new world order.** And this was to be achieved by a revolution (which they saw as a restoration of the order of the early church) from above. For they were firmly convinced that only through the unshakable, indefatigable and consistent emphasis on the papal primacy could the clergy, the church, indeed the world, be renewed and the divinely-willed world order be restored. Every possible means was to be used: the inexhaustible resources of the Pseudo-Isidorian Decretals, the developed Roman apparatus of control and administration (from now on we can talk of a real Curia), the college of cardinals, the novel system of embassies, indeed the Roman system which was now arising.

What was fundamental in this connection was the novel and learned polemic, aimed at public opinion, which was practised by **Humbert of Silva Candida** (*c.*1006–1061),[137] who is already known to us as an impetuous papal legate in Constantinople. Humbert, the Pope's closest confidant, was a skilled and often ironic and sarcastic stylist, lawyer and theologian, who in the fragment *De sancta Romana ecclesia* and in his passionate three books against the simonists in fact set out a whole political programme for the church. In practice Humbert was the second man in Rome, author of countless papal letters and bulls, the pioneering theoretician of papal politics, whose loyal pupil the Pope himself was. Indeed, Humbert was the perceptive and imaginative theoretician of the **Roman principle**, which was the foundation for the Roman system that would soon take shape:

– The papacy, the first and apostolic see, is the source and norm of all church law, the supreme authority, which can judge all but cannot itself be judged by anyone.

– The relationship between Pope and church is like that between hinge and door, foundation and house, source and river, mother and family.

– The relationship between church and state is like that between sun and moon, soul and body, head and members.

In the name of the Petrine authority this representative of the new world order, who was both extremely wise and extremely terse, called for the **freedom of the church**. What did he mean by that? Free election of bishops, and abolition not only of the Germanic proprietary church system but also of simony and married priests (here, with extremely effective verbal strategy, he was able to extend fatally the concepts of both simony and celibacy):

– By '**simony**' (originally the transfer of a church position for a payment of money or material gain) he understood any transfer of office ('investiture') by a **lay person**, whether for payment or not; this was the signal for the 'investiture dispute'.

– He regarded **any priestly marriage** as '**concubinage**': this made any priest's wife a concubine and any priest's child an illegitimate child, in fact without rights, and met with resolute resistance from the clergy, especially in Germany.

This loyal papalist programmer and uninhibited propagandist of the Roman principle, who in 1056 provoked the break with Constantinople and in 1059 enforced a crudely realistic understanding of the eucharist against Berengarius of Tours, this passionate fighter, died in 1062 and was given honourable burial in the Lateran. But at his side there had always been a younger administrator, an expert financier and a bold, purposeful politician. He was similarly seized with the notion that the Pope was none other than the apostle Peter of the day. He was that legate, archdeacon and finally Pope who twelve years later was to put Humbert's new programme into pratice boldly and purposefully, with tremendous energy: Hildebrand.

The establishment of the Roman system

If we think of the drama of the many pontificates, how long the way had been between Leo I and Leo IX! Yet how short it was if we look at its programme! Finally, after so many setbacks and defeats, the papacy was in a position to put into practice the programme that had already been developed around the middle of the fifth century, and to establish in the church the rule of the Pope, which had allegedly been founded by the apostle Peter. Equipped with a wealth of documents and decretals, the Pope's primacy of rule (primacy of jurisdiction), now supported by history and dogma, given legal form throughout and with a developed organization, could now be brought to bear against archbishops and bishops, national and diocesan churches, and finally against each individual Christian: the humblest believer and kings and emperors alike. Only now, after 600 years, could the **Roman programme** be established in Christianity as a **legal and political system,** as a form of church determined by having institutions and persons dependent on it. Only now, in the eleventh century, did the Latin Catholic paradigm for which the foundations were laid by Augustine and the Bishops of Rome in the fifth century appear as the **developed Roman Catholic paradigm** in the strict sense.

However, an important qualification needs to be made immediately: this Roman system was unable to establish itself throughout Christianity, throughout the church; that was possible **only in the Western church.** Still, it now emerged with increasing self-confidence and consciousnes of power in the form of the papacy. It was not only that papal decreta and responsa had never been requested from Eastern Christianity; not only that no Eastern monastery had ever asked to be granted exemption by the Pope; not only that the East – except in crises like that under Nicholas I and the patriarch Photius – had continued to live in the traditional early church paradigm, largely unconcerned about Rome, which for such a long time had been decadent. No, the differences go deeper.

We already heard in connection with the Hellenistic early church paradigm (P II) that when Eastern Christianity was now directly confronted with a Roman primacy of rule which was fully developed not only historically and dogmatically but also legally and politically, in the person of Pope Leo IX who so delighted in shaping it and his passionately impetuous legate Humbert of Silva Candida (Humbert in Constantinople!), it had rejected it out of hand. And when in 1054 Humbert then pronounced in the name of the Pope an excommunication of the patriarch Cerularius and his followers which had been prepared beforehand, the Byzantine counter-excommunication followed without delay, and the other Eastern principalities (Bulgaria, Serbia and Russia) fell into line with it. The result was that the break between the Eastern and Western churches, which was now open and was never again really healed, made quite clear what had already been developing in a long and highly complex process of alienation: the **new Roman Catholic paradigm** (P III) had clearly proved **incompatible with the Hellenistic early church paradigm** (P II). The rise of the Roman primacy was at the expense of the **episcopal synodical structures** of the early church, which in the West had been largely **destroyed**.

Indeed, given its thousand-year-old traditions, how could Eastern Christianity ever have accepted that primacy of Roman rule which had already been long proclaimed in old Rome but never really taken seriously in new Rome, a primacy which in the eleventh century was now being propagated actively by the Pope personally and his legates in all the centres of Western Christianity? How could it have accepted what had been defined five years before the break at a council in Rheims (1049) under the personal presidency of Leo IX: that the Pope alone is the apostolic universal primate? Certainly the heavy military defeat which Leo incurred when he went in person at the head of an army in an attempt to impose his claim to primacy on the Normans in southern Italy who had settled there since 1016 should have been a warning to him. But a 'renversement des alliances' between the Normans and the Germans was closer than the world thought at that time. For the realization of the supremacy of the church under the slogan '*Libertas Ecclesiae*' – 'Freedom for the Church' (as a papal institution), which was now part of the programme called for, not to be confused with the 'freedom of the

Christian' or 'freedom in the church!' – now made rapid progress. The liberation of the papacy from the influence of the German monarchy, by which it had been elevated, and its **rise to become the central institutional power in Europe** took place with impressive speed. Here are some short notes on those dramatic years.

1054: Leo IX dies and his successor Victor II is to be the last Pope nominated by a German emperor;

1056: the emperor Henry III dies unexpectedly at the early age of thirty-nine, leaving a son, Henry, who is only six years old, and thus a power vacuum;

1057: Stephen IX (the Roman chancellor Frederick of Lothringia, not very well disposed to the Germans, who had accompanied Humbert to Constantinople) is elected Pope at Humbert's suggestion, only four days after Victor's death, ignoring all the historical rights of the German king – a *fait accompli* of which Hildebrand as papal legate later brings news to the royal court;

1058: Nicholas II, also a Lothringian, is elected Stephen's successor, probably the first Pope to be crowned like kings and emperors – a symbol of the now monarchical character of the papacy which could be recognized all over the world.

1059: a Lateran synod under Nicholas II and Humbert resolves:

– the **college of cardinals** is to be the exclusive organ for **electing the Pope**, independent of interventions by the Roman nobility and the German king (the clergy and people of Rome may assent subsequently); this now also functions as an advisory organ for the Pope ('consistory') and occupies the most important posts in the papal administration.

– a ban on laity from taking part in services conducted by **married priests** and the threat of excommunication on priests who do not divorce their wives.

– a prohibition against any priest receiving a **church office at the hands of a laymen** – whether or not in exchange for payment.

Over all these years one man had already been playing a key role in the background, Hildebrand the archdeacon. His greatest hour was still to come. In 1073, still during the funeral rites of his predecessor, he was elected Pope to tumultuous acclaim with a blatant failure to observe the decree relating to papal elections. He named himself Gregory VII – after Gregory I, the model Pope of the Middle Ages. The structural conflict between monarchy and papacy, which had long been simmering, now came to a climax.

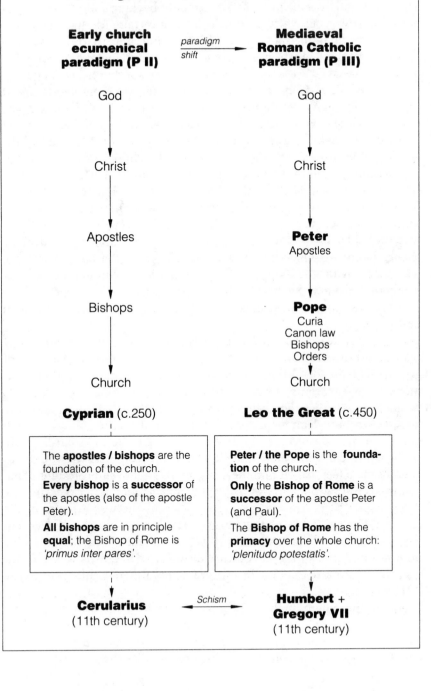

Two Systems of Church Order

Early church ecumenical paradigm (P II) → *paradigm shift* → **Mediaeval Roman Catholic paradigm (P III)**

Early church ecumenical paradigm (P II)	Mediaeval Roman Catholic paradigm (P III)
God	God
↓	↓
Christ	Christ
↓	↓
Apostles	**Peter** Apostles
↓	↓
Bishops	**Pope** Curia Canon law Bishops Orders
↓	↓
Church	Church

Cyprian (c.250)   **Leo the Great** (c.450)

The **apostles / bishops** are the foundation of the church.	**Peter / the Pope** is the **foundation** of the church.
Every bishop is a **successor** of the apostles (also of the apostle Peter).	**Only** the **Bishop of Rome** is a **successor** of the apostle Peter (and Paul).
All bishops are in principle **equal**; the Bishop of Rome is *'primus inter pares'*.	The **Bishop of Rome** has the **primacy** over the whole church: *'plenitudo potestatis'*.

Cerularius (11th century) ← *Schism* → **Humbert + Gregory VII** (11th century)

The Pope over all in the world: Gregory VII

The place and year of birth and the family background of this **Hilde-brand**,[138] now around fifty years of age, are uncertain. All that is certain is that he grew up in the sphere of the Roman church. Perhaps he had been entrusted to the Roman monastery on the Aventine where he probably made his monastic vows. At all events, it is certain that he accompanied the deposed Pope Gregory VI to Cologne, and presumably also lived for a time in Cluny before he returned to Rome in 1049 with the new Pope Leo IX. Here he increasingly became the decisive figure, as papal legate getting to know the European centres well; from 1059 he had the best possible insight into the inner life of the church as an influential archdeacon and administrator of the possessions of the Roman church (and his own!). Indeed, at the time of Nicholas II and the Lateran synod of the same year it was already being said of Hildebrand's role that he fed 'his Nicholas in the Lateran like an ass in the stable'.[139] He was probably also behind the reversal in foreign policy, the decisive change of course which was now embarked on: in the same year peace was made with the Normans, on whom in an unprecedented act southern Italy and Sicily, which had previously been imperial, were bestowed as a papal 'fief', in order to shake off the rule of the German kings.

Even today he is a disputed figure, this physically small and rather ugly man, who however had a passionate and convinced faith and a heart of granite. Did Gregory VII not so much think in institutional terms but, as more recent historians like A.Nitzschke and C.Schnieder assume, divide people into whether they belonged to God or the devil? A man of rare honesty, without fear, impatient and unscrupulous, he could be rough even to his friends and even more cruel to his enemies. His hardly more gentle fellow cardinal Peter Damian, who finally threw his see of Ostia at Hildebrand's feet, called him the 'holy Satan', but even Protestant papal historians followed Thomas Carlyle in admiring him under the category 'hero as priest'. Be this as it may: at all events he was a figure of the century. For with his name are associated not only the 'Gregorian Reform' (although, as we saw, this had already begun before his pontificate), but also the 'investiture dispute', which, as is well known, was about far more than the investiture (appointment to office) of clergy by laymen.

For our paradigm analysis Gregory VII must be rated the Pope who **radically and irrevocably put the Roman Catholic paradigm of the Middle Ages into political practice**. The French theologian Yves Congar could find general assent among historians when he remarked: 'The understanding of the church held by the reformers of the eleventh century, Gregory VII and the canonists around 1080 and later, can be described in a word: it is by nature Roman.' And he adds: 'Not only in the sense that it again adopts the standpoint which Rome itself had occupied since the time of Leo I, but also in so far as it makes the pre-eminence of the see of Peter, the Roman church, the axis of all ecclesiology: the words *caput and cardo*, of which Humbert of Moyenmoûtier was so fond, are a good summary of this understanding.'[140]

In fact, the **paradigm shift** introduced with Augustine and the Bishops of Rome in the fifth century **is now definitively complete**, in so far as the **Roman** element seems **fully expressed** in this constellation. What had previously often been only a theoretical and abstract programme put forward in Rome, now became a practical and concrete reality throughout the Western church. Walter Ullmann, who has given a more acute analysis than others of this whole development up to Gregory VII in terms of institutional history, remarks: 'What had hitherto been merely programmatic and an idea, was to be made concrete in the world at large. The papacy under his intrepid direction was propelled by its own inner strength and programme to become an institution of European dimensions. The papacy had made Hildebrand, and Gregory VII was to make it the focal establishment of Europe. The fifth-century view that the Roman church was the mother of all churches from now on began to approach reality, though at time she was a harsh mother and the pope as monarchic ruler an exacting father.'[141]

Gregory VII and the Gregorian party were concerned to establish all over Europe an explicit 'mysticism of obedience' which 'at the same time has very spiritual and very institutional and legal features'. Once again Congar describes it very precisely: 'To obey God means to obey the church and that in turn means to obey the Pope, and vice versa.'[142] Here Congar has made the decisive point. For at the latest from this time the obedience of all Christians is a central virtue for Rome, and to give orders and compel obedience (by whatever means) is the Roman style. Already in his second year of office Gregory VII made quite clear to himself what the equation **'Obedience to God = to the church = to the Pope'** meant in theological and dogmatic and above all in legal and disciplinary terms: in 1075 he wrote his *'Dictatus Papae'*,[143] **twenty-seven pregnant principles of papal primacy**. Their original purpose is disputed, and at first they were hardly known outside the Curia; scholars today believe that these **Dictates** represent chapter headings of a planned[144] or lost[145] collection of laws or privileges: at all events a strategic draft of prime importance which was to be realized successively.

More than any other document of the time, these 'Dictates' bear witness not only to Gregory's unbounded sense of mission but also to the **overthrow of the early church constitution** (P II) which had now become possible. Who are Gregory's key witnesses? They will come as no surprise to us: some remarks of Augustine in *The City of God*, then the pontificate of Gregory I, but above all the Pseudo-Isidorian forgeries and Nicholas I's understanding of office. Probably on Hildebrand's instigation Humbert had compiled a *Handbook of Church Law*, almost five-sixths of which comes from Pseudo-Isidore, in which the rights of the Pope are for the first time put at the head, and the whole of the legal standing of the church is almost exclusively based on decrees of the Bishops of Rome (with an almost complete suppression of the councils). Gregory's 'Dictates', which make statements from the tradition more pointed and formulate completely new ones, once again brings all this into sharp focus.[146] Thus the conflict with secular power was pre-programmed. And Gregory, here with Augustine's ideas in his head, in any case suspected this power of being of the devil.

The 'Dictates of the Pope' express three basic ideas, all of which are grounded in the fact that as Peter's successor the Pope now has the divinely given *plenitudo potestatis* (Leo I), that fullness of power from which all legal prerogatives logically follow. The Pope
– is **the unqualified lord of the church**: he stands not only above all believers, clergy and bishops, and over all local, regional and national churches, but also over all councils;
– is **the supreme lord of the world**: not only all rulers but even the emperor (as a 'sinful man') are subject to him;
– becomes undoubtedly **holy** by taking up office (on the basis of the merits of Peter): the Roman church, founded by God alone, has never erred and will never err.[147]

These 'Dictates of the Pope' represent the clearest legal description of the papal primacy of rule before the definition of the primacy at Vatican I (1870) and assert – not least with an eye on Byzantium, in connection with Gregory's plans for a crusade and a union – an **unlimited competence of the Pope in ordination, legislation, administration and jurisdiction**. However, as the 'Dictates' also apply the authority to bind and loose to dealings with worldly rulers (which in theory was maintained in Rome down to the nineteenth century) and in their blatant claims to power are often painful even to papalists today, they are not mentioned at all from first edition to last in Denziger, that collection of church doctrinal definitions, including random papal letters, which is otherwise so fixated on the Pope.[148] So I shall print them in full here.[149]

A Papal Programme

1. The Roman Church has been founded only by the Lord.

2. Only the Bishop of Rome is legitimately called universal bishop.

3. He alone can depose or reinstate bishops.

4. His legate presides over all bishops in council even if he is of lesser rank, and can pronounce the sentence of deposition on them.

5. The Pope can also depose those who are absent.

6. Among other things we may not even live in the same house as those who have been excommunicated by him.

7. He alone is permitted, if the age requires it, to decree new laws, establish new bishoprics, transform chapters of canons into monasteries and vice versa, divide rich sees and combine poor ones.

8. He alone may use imperial insignia.

9. All rulers have to kiss only the Pope's feet.

10. His name alone may be named ceremonially in the churches.

11. This name is unique in the world.

12. He is permitted to depose emperors.

13. He is permitted to transfer bishops from one see to another if this is urgently necessary.

14. He can ordain clerks from any church at will.

15. One ordained by him can also preside over another church, but may not perform more lowly duties; he may not receive a higher degree of consecration from any other bishop.

16. No synod may be called general without his instruction.

17. No legal statement and no book may be regarded as canonical without his authorization.

18. His decision may not be revised by anyone; he is the only one who may revise the decisions of all others.

19. He himself may not be judged by anyone.

20. No one shall dare to condemn anyone who appeals to the apostolic see.

21. The more important affairs of any church are to be brought before the apostolic see.

22. The Roman church has never erred, and according to the testimony of scripture will never ever err.

---

23. The Roman pontiff, if he has been consecrated canonically, is beyond doubt sanctified through the merits of St Peter.

24. On his instruction and with his permission, subordinate persons are permitted to make accusations.

25. He can depose and reinstate bishops without convening a synod.

26. No one who is not in accord with the Roman church may be regarded as a Catholic.

27. He can release subjects from their oath of loyalty to evildoers.

The 'Dictatus Papae' of Gregory VII

Of course it should not be disputed that during his lifetime Gregory required a radical form of Christianity of himself. He was beyond doubt upheld by the deeply felt experience that he too was poor and that his person too was dependent on God's power, love and gracious mercy.[150] But precisely because of this, he could be a shrewd politician for the church, who did not hesitate for a moment to put his programme into practice. Moreover, as was granted him after the decree of election, according to which even a lay person is Pope immediately on accepting the election, from the first day of his election on Gregory ruled the church as virtually a reincarnation of St Peter, at all events in mystical identification with him. Fully convinced that the whole world owed obedience to 'Peter', as in heaven so on earth, as the new Peter he took the offensive against the political powers outside ('external policy') as well as in the church ('internal policy').

In his '**external policy**', Gregory attempted right from the beginning after the Normans to bring yet further kingdoms under his power with reference to every conceivable hodge-podge from history. And of course for this privilege these princes had to pay annual tribute to Rome. For the recognition of papal supremacy, the homage of a vassal, the acceptance of a fief and the payment of annual interest belonged together. The papal policy was successful over Sardinia, Corsica and Spain, but not over France, England and other states. Gregory VII was a 'world politician' like no other Pope before him.

In his '**internal policy**', already at his first Lenten synod of 1074 Gregory VII concentrated on the **fight against the marriage of priests**. He wanted to enforce the prohibition of the marriage of priests (celibacy) which had been made earlier – but hardly followed, especially in

Germany – with the sharpest possible means. Contrary to all the law of the early church he declared the actions in office of married priests invalid and called on the laity to rebel against married priests. Even before his own pontificate, in order to implement papal aims, as necessary he had entered into an alliance even with the lower and the lowest classes, above all with the social revolutionary mass movement of the cities of northern Italy, the pataria (= 'flea market', riffraff), with whose help and armed rebellion he attempted to impose on Milan the candidate he wanted in the face of the bishop nominated by the German king.

The historical test came when Gregory, an incomparable fighter, wanted to shift the dividing line between Roman internal and external policy in keeping with his programme. For the so-called '**investiture dispute**'[151] was ultimately about no more and no less than a new definition of the relationship between spiritual and worldly power, between the clergy and the laity, fundamentally about the question who ruled over the clergy. The German king and (at least future) emperor was the representative of the laity. And this Pope required obedience even from king and emperor. The German king of the time was **Henry IV** (1056–1106). At the time of Gregory's accession he was only twenty-three, but for all his inexperience, rashness and lack of concern he was a ruler with a marked sense of his royal dignity. And after his victory over the rebellious Saxons, Henry, too, felt ready for battle: 'The German crown should be subject to the commands of the Pope. But that touched on a point on which even Henry . . . could never willingly yield. Therefore the battle between king and Pope was unavoidable, and from the start it was a life and death struggle.'[152]

Gregory VII began the conflict at the Lent synod of 1075 by a sharp renewal of the **prohibition of lay investiture**, the appointment to office of the clergy by the laity, combined with a clear warning to the king. And when Henry IV continued with the appointment of bishops in imperial Italy, neighbouring on the papal state (not only Milan but also Spoleto and Fermo), in December 1075 Gregory sent an ultimatum to the king. He threatened him with excommunication and the fate of Saul if he continued with the nomination of bishops. King Henry reacted at a Reichstag and imperial synod held simultaneously at Worms in 1076: badly advised, he responded by **deposing the Pope**: 'Hildebrand,' as he addressed him, was 'no longer Pope but a false monk!' This was a disastrous over-reaction, accompanied with personal taunts which proved counter-productive. In any case it was a mistake to want to depose a Pope to some degree at a distance; moreover it was a mistake to make his papal assailant a victim in the eyes of the world, the victim of an arrogant German. True, Henry's father, Henry III, had already deposed and appointed a whole series of Popes, as we heard. But Henry IV failed to recognize how much the situation had changed in the meantime in favour of the newly formed papacy. For the Pope now had ideological and above all legal instruments with which to assert himself, and not least effective publicity to sustain the battle for public opinion, of a kind which had not existed since the downfall of antiquity.

A few weeks later Gregory VII reacted at the Lent synod of 1076 in a highly dramatic way: **he excommunicated and deposed the king**, suspended all the bishops involved in the decision against his person (unless they recanted) and indeed **released Henry's subjects from their oath of loyalty**! This was a monstrous, unprecedented event for the world of the time, with the result that the bishops and rulers, with their own power in mind, after long hesitation left their king in the lurch and in October resolved to depose him if he were not absolved from the ban within a year. There was nothing for it: Henry had to submit.

In order to avoid a Reichstag and day of judgment in Augsburg, Henry IV travelled with his young wife, his two-year-old son and his court over the Alps – in the midst of the worst winter of the century: even the Rhine was frozen over. Gregory VII, already on his way from Augsburg to the Reichstag, over which, on the suggestion of the rulers, he was to preside, fearing a *coup d'état* took refuge in **Canossa**, the impregnable fortress of Countess Mathilda of Tuscany, who was well-disposed towards him, at the foot of the Apennines. Here, quite pitifully, bare-footed and in traditional penitential garb, the king appeared before the castle gate, on 25 January 1077, asking for pardon. After an unprecedented three-day penance – and only after the pleading of the mistress of the castle and Archabbot Hugo of Cluny, Henry's godfather, who asked Henry for a written promise, the Pope, having forced Henry to prostrate himself on the ground in the form of a cross, graciously raised him up and released him from the ban. In this way, while Henry's royal status was restored, it was at the same time stripped of its sacral character and its ideological basis was shaken: Canossa was the turning point! No wonder the 'journey to Canossa' has become proverbial beyond German lands for the hubris of an immovable hierocrat and the deepest humiliation of a German ruler, who had to recognize the Pope as the supreme judge (as Bismarck was to remark in the Kulturkampf in 1872: 'We are not going to Canossa!').

But Canossa also proved a turning point for Gregory's pontificate. For Gregory, lacking political moderation, had manifestly taken upon himself too much power, and his first active and successful period was soon followed by a second more reactive and largely **unsuccessful period**. The Lent synod of 1078 again decreed a universal prohibition of all investiture and extended this even to the king. But Germany had been cast into civil war by Henry's excommunication; for the first time there was now a German anti-king, Rudolf of Swabia, supported by Gregory. However, this hardly helped him. Henry's second excommunication and deposition by Gregory (1080) ran out of steam, and Gregory's bold prophecy of Henry's downfall by the feast of St Peter's Chains remained unfulfilled. Instead, the anti-king died, after his 'accursed' (treacherous) hand had been struck off in battle. Henry now had the Archbishop of Ravenna elected Pope (Clement III), and in 1081 came with an army to Rome. Gregory's active reign came to a standstill, the money ceased to flow in, and the Romans finally took Henry's side. But the gates of the city were only opened in 1084: now Clement II was solemnly enthroned in St Peter's and King Henry was crowned emperor. Gregory VII had already fled at an early stage to the impregnable Castel Sant'Angelo, where he remained until the Normans, summoned to help him in his deep distress as their liege lord, freed him. The emperor had returned to Germany. So for three days the Normans (and Saracens from Sicily) plundered and burned the city so terribly that, faced with the indignation of the Romans, Gregory had to withdraw with the Normans to southern Italy, where Salerno was assigned him as an abode. There he died the next year, abandoned by almost all the world, on his lips the words: 'I have loved righteousness and hated iniquity, so I die in exile.'

But despite this defeat Gregory VII, this unloved Pope, who found neither an appropriate biographer nor the honour of altars in the Middle Ages, had an epoch-making effect. Now he personified the ideals of those who shaped the church in the eleventh century, and to this degree it is right to speak of the 'Gregorian Reform', which indeed Hildebrand had been carrying out even before his pontificate. A local cult was first founded in Salerno in 1606, but it was banned in some countries up to 1728, when it was extended to the whole church. Yet even today there are historians who believe that 'with good reason' one can even describe the Gregorian reform as a 'second Christianization', because people 'began to take seriously church regulations which hitherto had been observed casually'.[153] But such a basic evaluation calls for historical and theological reflections.

Romanization instead of Christianization

'The Christian Middle Ages'? Right at the beginning of our reflections on the mediaeval paradigm I raised fundamental objections to the Middle Ages being seen as a 'dark' age of Christianity. And I demonstrated in detail the degree to which the substance of Christianity was preserved

The Development
of the Roman System

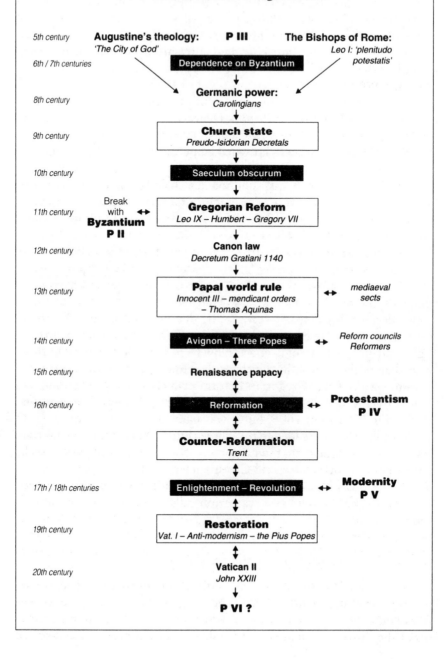

5th century	**Augustine's theology:** 'The City of God'	**P III** **The Bishops of Rome:** Leo I: 'plenitudo potestatis'

5th century — **Augustine's theology:** 'The City of God' — **P III** — **The Bishops of Rome:** Leo I: 'plenitudo potestatis'

6th / 7th centuries — Dependence on Byzantium

8th century — Germanic power: *Carolingians*

9th century — **Church state** *Preudo-Isidorian Decretals*

10th century — Saeculum obscurum

11th century — Break with **Byzantium P II** ↔ **Gregorian Reform** *Leo IX – Humbert – Gregory VII*

12th century — **Canon law** *Decretum Gratiani 1140*

13th century — **Papal world rule** *Innocent III – mendicant orders – Thomas Aquinas* ↔ *mediaeval sects*

14th century — Avignon – Three Popes ↔ *Reform councils Reformers*

15th century — Renaissance papacy

16th century — Reformation ↔ **Protestantism P IV**

Counter-Reformation *Trent*

17th / 18th centuries — Enlightenment – Revolution ↔ **Modernity P V**

19th century — **Restoration** *Vat. I – Anti-modernism – the Pius Popes*

20th century — **Vatican II** *John XXIII*

P VI ?

even in the epoch-making change from late antiquity to the early Middle Ages. I need not repeat what I said about the early Middle Ages in connection with the high Middle Ages. So it is all the more astonishing to find the concept of a 'new Christianization' used in connection with the Gregorian reform. Historians lightly write that church precepts which had long been observed loosely now begin to be taken seriously. But as a theologian one cannot suppress the critical question whether these **church precepts** which had previously been observed loosely were really **Christian precepts**. Moreover, even if historians should lack serious criteria for what is Christian, they must not presuppose that all church precepts are a priori truly Christian precepts.

Gregory VII himself would doubtless have pointed out here that the church precepts which he urged with so much passion were divine law and ancient Christian decrees, laws and notions formulated by early Popes and synods. That is the only reason why he could have put forward his demands so fearlessly and unyieldingly. He was concerned to reshape contemporary life in the Christian spirit, to Christianize it: a new Christian world order arising out of reflection on the old. As the much-quoted saying of Tertullian has it, Christ did not say that he was the custom but that he was the truth. And that is why as Pope, Gregory had to use every means to free especially the clergy from customs and traditions – *libertas Ecclesiae*, 'freedom for the church' – which had imposed a totally un-Roman, Germanic order on the church. Indeed, Gregory would doubtless have agreed had he been told that his essential concern was a consistent **Romanization** of the church and thus of Christianity. For *Christianitas* and *Romanitas* had so fused into a unity, the Christian and the Roman had become so identified, that he was convinced that the Roman church in particular had never erred in the faith and never could err.

Now historical research has brought out quite clearly that the world-historical conflict between Pope Gregory VII and King Henry IV was a **conflict over two quite different views of law:**
– **Henry IV** represented **Germanic customary law based on loyalty and allegiance,** which since the conversion of the Germans to Christianity had also found expression in the German **proprietary church system,** in Gregory's view the most offensive element in the Germanic system and still in force all over Western Europe. But how could such a form of rule be in force unless a king or another lay lord had appointed the incumbent even to clerical office by investiture? Without this investiture there would be no homage and giving of oaths by the clerical vassals, indeed the archbishops, bishops and abbots would be princes independent of the king: free of the economic, military and political obligations which were

essential for king and realm. To yield to Roman demands to abolish investiture by the king amounted to destroying the basis of existing society.

– By contrast, **Gregory VII** represented the specifically Roman Latin view of the church as a **monarchical hierarchy appointed by God**, the foundation of which had been laid by the Bishops of Rome since the fifth century and which Gregory VII had once again summarized in his *Dictatus Papae*: a new world order in justice, orientated on Rome, to which of course opposing Germanic customs and traditions had to yield. And to the degree that Gregory fearlessly and immovably made an attempt to implement radically and consistently the Roman principle and Roman ideas about church and society which had matured over a long period, he himself represents **in person the consistent and radical embodiment of the Roman system**, though as the product of a particular historical development (in the context of P III) this is by no means identical with the Catholic Church or even the essence of Christianity.

For in theological perspective, for the historian too the question arises whether this Roman system is right in constantly appealing in its claims to power in church and society to the apostle Peter and the early church, indeed to Jesus Christ himself. In other words, in some circumstances isn't the Roman use of power more inspired by Roman Caesars, Byzantine emperors and Frankish forgers than by the gospel of Jesus Christ? I shall illustrate and test this by some characteristics of the Roman system which still hold today.

8. Characteristics of the Roman system

In estimating the historical consequences it might be advisable to include the period of church history following Gregory VII, up to its climax at the end of the twelfth century with **Innocent III** (1198–1216). For it was not Gregory's pontificate but Innocent's which, according to the papal historian F.X.Seppelt, was 'probably the most brilliant in the long and varied history of the papacy'.[154] In it **the claims and reality of the papacy fully coincide.** What Augustine laid the foundation for, but certainly did not want, and what Leo I did not dare to dream of, seemed to have been achieved: the twofold identification of city of God and church on the one hand and church and papacy on the other. At the early age of thirty-seven, Lotario of Segni was the successor to the ninety-two-year-old Celestine III; he was an acute lawyer, a capable administrator and a refined diplomat. The son of a Langobard nobleman and a Roman patrician, he was moreover a theological writer, a skilled orator, indeed a born ruler, who beyond question marked the climax and at the same time the turning point of the mediaeval papacy. The question here is: what developments can be established in comparison with the early church paradigm (P II)? I want to indicate five momentous processes in the mature paradigm III which were consolidated as permanent marks of the Roman system.[155]

Centralization: the absolutist papal church as mother

Romanization meant **centralization**. Here the person of **Gregory VII** plays a key role. Together with Humbert, from the beginning he called for this Roman centralization in an almost fanatical way and promoted it, fought for it and achieved it by making already old demands specific and radical. His aim was a total orientation of the whole of the Catholic Church, i.e. in faith, law, liturgy, discipline and organization, indeed a total orientation of European Christianity, on the Roman Pope as Peter's successor and the absolute spiritual monarch. Only now can we speak of a **papal universal church in the West** – not yet in the time of the Carolingians and the Ottonians. Soon the bishops everywhere were to complain that the Pope was giving them orders as though they were his administrators; he summoned them to Rome and deposed them if they resisted him. There was papal authority instead of episcopal collegiality, Roman uniformity instead of Catholic plurality.

Gregory VII regarded the apostle **Peter** (= the Pope) as the **father** and the Roman **church** as the **mother and teacher** of all the churches. The Roman papal historian Michele Maccarone has seen Gregory's formula from the Salerno Appeal of 1084 as the 'heart' of Gregory VII and has summarized his view of the Roman primacy like this: 'The blessed Peter, prince of the apostles, is the father of all Christians and the first pastor after Christ, and the Holy Roman Church is the mother and teacher of all the churches.'[156] We must discuss this at a later stage: the more authoritarian and rigoristic the way in which a monastically orientated church isolates itself by celibacy, the stronger become the sublimations and spiritual projections on 'the church'. Papal authoritarianism and an idealization of the church go hand in hand at a very early stage.

And more than any of his predecessors, **Innocent III** shows how far the Popes had already gone in their more than earthly consciousness of mission.[157] He preferred the title '**Christ's representative**' (*vicarius Christi*), used for any bishop or priest up to the twelfth century, to 'Peter's representative', 'because it gave him the basis for a more radical and extended authority'; his successor Innocent IV was even to call himself '**God's representative**' (*vicarius Dei*), 'which made it possible for him to exert his authority beyond the circle of believers'.[158] Indeed Innocent III, a master of papal ideology, had such an consciousness of his role as a great religious ruler that on the day of his consecration he simply preached about himself. He saw himself 'as the representative of Christ set between God and human beings, below God and above human beings, less than God and more than human beings, judge of all and to be judged by no one (except the Lord)'![159] Here was a Pope above and outside the church, but Vatican II would be the first to oppose this, with its remarks about the collegiality of bishops.[160]

No wonder that Innocent, who thought in extremely patriarchal terms, loved the title '*mater*' = '**mother**' which Rome had favoured for the church since Innocent. But Innocent gave a further twist to this symbolism. For obvious reasons, he used 'mother' not so much for the universal church as specifically **for the Roman church**. Why? In order to 'express the primacy of the Roman church'.[161] The title of mother had the advantage of being applicable quite generally 'to the *ecclesia Romana* and also to the *sedes apostolica*: Innocent seems to have distinguished between two different ways in which the Roman church is mother. First, the Roman church is mother of all other churches and therefore also their head. But as *mater omnium Christi fidelium* she is in a direct relationship with every individual believer and therefore is ultimately identical with the *ecclesia universalis*'.[162]

Moreover Innocent, who was certainly a man of honest piety and moral earnestness, was able to display the fullness of Rome's power more than any Pope before him. The **Fourth Ecumenical Lateran Council** of 1215 gave him the occasion. In fact this was a purely papal synod, which demonstrated both the complete power and central authority of the Pope and the practical insignificance of the episcopate. Around 200 bishops, abbots and plenipotentiaries or secular rulers were summoned by the Pope and assembled under his presidency to pass decrees which the Pope wanted – seventy of such decrees bear witness to the extent to which legalism had taken root in the church. They were intended above all as a reform of the church,[163] but (apart from a papal tax on all the clergy and a requirement that all believers should go to confession and make communion at Easter) they largely remained paper.

However, the resolutions directed **against the Jews**, which despite the papal guarantees for their worship in many respects anticipate later antisemitic measures, did not remain paper: distinctive clothing, a ban on holding public office and going out on Good Friday, a compulsory tax to be paid to local Christian clergy.[164] I have commented on this in my *Judaism*.[165] As already under Gregory VII, who had enacted the first decrees against Jews in state offices, under Innocent III authoritarian papalism and anti-Judaism went hand in hand. Here too, however, unfortunately the mendicant orders which had then been approved, above all the Dominicans, emerged as the executors of the new anti-Jewish Roman policy, which fundamentally changed the situation of the Jews both legally and theologically (Jews as unbelievers = 'slaves of sin' = now slaves of Christian rulers).

Be this as it may, the Fourth Lateran Council was a synod domin-ated by the Pope in a way which would have been inconceivable in the early church Byzantine paradigm. As far as centralization was con-cerned, in fact an essential difference emerged between the early church Byzantine paradigm (P II) and the mediaeval Roman Catholic para-digm (P III):

- In the early church Byzantine paradigm to the present day the church forms a fellowship (*koinonia, communio*) of churches without a centralized authority for all churches.
- Since the Middle Ages the Catholic Church of the West has represented a church completely focussed on the Pope in faith, law, discipline and organization: there has been a centralization of the church and a fixation on an absolute monarch who alone has supremacy in the church. However, this is not in keeping with the New Testament origins as we have come to know them.

Legalism: the legalistic church and its science of canon law

Romanization meant **legalism**. It was first in the Gregorian reform that the legal postulates of former Popes and the Pseudo-Isidorian forgeries were translated into ecclesiastical reality. **Gregory VII**, who had Humbert's papalistic-canonistic handbook distributed everywhere, claimed an unprecedented right to legislate. Some of his decisions in fact took on the power of law, even if strikingly his decrees and letters are hardly ever cited in the *Corpus Iuris Canonici* (and in Denziger). At any rate, at the time of the Gregorian Reform, especially in Rome, **collections of laws** (unlike earlier ones thorough and completely professional) were made in the Roman spirit – they were necessary in this new era of papal legalism. For it has been calculated that the Popes of the twelfth century promulgated more legal decisions for the whole church than all their predecessors put together.

In view of the existence of various older collections of law and the obscurity and uncertainty that they caused, the publication around 1140 by the learned Camaldolese monk **Gratian** from the University of Bologna, the stronghold of legal studies in the Middle Ages, of his textbook *Concordantia discordantium canonum*, still misleadingly called the *Decretum Gratiani*,[166] was generally welcomed. This is without doubt an outstanding summary of existing law, which removes the numerous contradictions by means of the dialectical method. Moreover it was immediately used for teaching in the two most famous law schools, in Bologna and Paris. However, what went unnoticed – a fact which has burdened the science of canon law to the present day – was that up to a fifth of this lawbook of Gratian's, which was fundamental in the subsequent period, consists of forgeries: 324 passages from Popes from the first four centuries are quoted from the Pseudo-Isidorians, 313 of which are demonstrable forgeries.

For a long time the laity, untrained in the law, and indeed many clergy and even bishops, had ceased to be capable of using church law. And just as in the state sphere professional 'legists' were needed, who predominantly followed Roman law, imperial law, so in the church sphere, from the eleventh century there were the professional **canonists**, who went completely by the papal canons and now became an inestimable ideological support for the Roman system in Rome as in numerous chanceries and courts.[167] In Bologna, by his lectures Gratian had founded the school of canonists (decretists) who glossed canon law; alongside the school of Roman law, which mostly had an imperial orientation, were the church lawyers, who in fact were 'papal lawyers'. Canon law study or the science of church law was born as a separate branch within scholasticism.[168]

For there was indeed more than enough to comment on. The church lawyers saw all the many individual papal decisions as supplements or alterations to the *Decretum Gratiani*. Thus in time three official (and one unofficial) collections of decretals were made, which together with the *Decretum Gratiani* formed the **Corpus Iuris Canonici**. The **Codex Iuris Canonici**, which is still in force today, worked out under curial direction, published in 1917/18 and then only lightly revised after the Second Vatican Council and republished in 1983, is based on it. From the twelfth century, for most Popes (and those seeking a career in the Curia) the main qualification for office was less a theological than a legal training, and this gave the Popes an inestimable advantage over contemporary rulers. It was only through legal learning that the papal monarchy had the legal equipment and personnel to make the Roman claims a reality. Moreover from all over the world Rome was flooded with requests for decisions on even third-order disputes. This already led Bernard of Clairvaux, with many others, in his famous admonition *De consideratione* (around 1150) to chide Pope Eugene III, his pupil: 'Here you have not followed Peter, but Constantine.'[169] On the other hand, it was the same Bernard who in the same work was the first to put forward the pernicious theory of the two swords given to the church by God: the spiritual sword for its own use and the secular sword for the emperor to use in accordance with the Pope's will.[170]

Under **Innocent III**, who had studied theology in Paris and church law in Bologna, and also proved a master of papal law and a reformer of the curial apparatus, what Gregory VII could only call for in the *Dictatus Papae* was in fact already achieved. The Pope was now in fact the unrestricted lord of the church: any influence of worldly powers on church affairs was excluded. Rome has never known a separation of authorities, and rejected it even when it was realized in modern states in modern times. The Pope is and remains **supreme governor, absolute lawgiver** and **supreme judge** of the church. And Innocent III in particular did everything he could to bring Rome into play in every possible case as the supreme court of appeal, even in secular affairs; Innocent, who was the first Pope to have an official collection of church law published. But already at that time appeals to Rome were the cause of the worst abuses. Even then the tendency towards a legalistic trade in privileges, the arbitrariness and partisanship which can be seen in Rome even now, became evident, in a way which is characteristic of all absolutist regimes and also of current Vatican practice.[171]

As we saw, there was also marked legalism in Byzantium, which was above all advanced by the emperors (Justinian!). Nevertheless, there is a further important distinction between the early church Byzantine paradigm (P II) and the mediaeval Roman Catholic paradigm (P III) in respect of the church:

- In the early church Byzantine paradigm, from the beginning the church was and legally remained incorporated into imperial state law.
- But from the Middle Ages on, the Catholic Church of the West developed its own church law (along with its own science of church law), equivalent to state law in complexity and differentiation but now totally orientated on the Pope as the absolute ruler, lawgiver and judge of Christianity, to whom even the emperor was subordinate.

Politicization: the powerful church and its rule over the world

Romanization meant **politicization**. And in this respect, too, it was **Gregory VII** who engaged in a direct power struggle with the most significant ruler of Europe, the German king and emperor. This monastic Pope had increasingly come to think that if Peter's successor may already loose and judge heavenly and spiritual matters, even more may he loose and judge earthly and worldly matters. Peter has the right to rule the world! And with reference to the well-known dubious 'legal titles', this Pope attempted to persuade all the world, even William, England's conqueror, to swear fealty, pay tribute and offer homage – though William in particular (because he was completely new) coolly refused. In the papal view, as 'sinful men' even emperors and kings were subordinate to the Pope: *sub ratione peccati* (from the perspective of sin = morality); in the coming centuries, too, the Popes were to intervene indirectly or directly in secular matters. And because this power struggle at first remained unresolved, after Gregory's death the passionate political and public dispute in Christianity continued for another whole generation, with fluctuating success.

A compromise was first reached over the investiture question in 1122 (the Concordat of Worms): the king renounced investiture with ring and staff, and retained only investiture with the sceptre. In future the **election of bishops** was made by the clergy and nobility of the diocese, and from the thirteenth century by the **cathedral chapter**, though of course this hardly ever chose a bishop who was not acceptable to Rome. Moreover the power of the papacy was hardly ever disputed in the decades after the Concordat of Worms. In any case the pre-eminence of the German church had been replaced by that of France. The most powerful spiritual personality in the first half of the twelfth century was now **Bernard of Clairvaux** (1090–1153), counsellor and admonisher of Popes and princes, called the secret emperor of Europe, a great mystical interpreter of the Song of Songs, who unfortunately also acted as the self-appointed guardian of orthodoxy, as an evil agitator against other theologians (especially Abelard, the brilliant early scholastic) and as a fanatical preacher of the 'holy war'.[172] In Germany the brilliant rule of the self-confident Hohenstaufen emperor **Frederick I Barbarossa** (1152–1190) formed a climax in the second half of the twelfth century.[173]

But only when Barbarossa's son Henry VI unexpectedly died at the age of thirty-two, leaving behind an heir, Frederick (II), who was only three, was there a great dispute over the throne in Germany itself between the Hohenstaufens and the Welfs, and thus a power vacuum. This was a political opportunity of the first order for **Innocent III**, who is already well known to us – an unattainable model for most Popes down to our own century, so much so that Leo XIII, whose guide Innocent was, wanted to be buried opposite his tomb in the Lateran. Unlike Gregory VII, Innocent combined boldness and resolution with cool consideration, statesmanlike wisdom and tactical flexibility. Through his skilful anti-German policy of 'recuperations' ('repossessions') he became the **second founder of the papal state** (now almost double in size).

In Innocent's time Rome was beyond dispute the dominant and busiest centre of European politics. Indeed Innocent really was **ruler of the world**, if we understand that not in the sense of absolute domination but as the supreme arbitrator and the greatest liege lord: 'In his letters and addresses he often put forward the claim that he stood over the peoples and nations.'[174] The 'dualism' of Pope and emperor, church and state, which of course still existed, was wholly subordinate to the 'papal hierocracy': 'The papacy and canon law find the unity in a subordination of the state to the church, in the incorporation of secular rule into the hierocracy of the papal church.'[175]

But despite all the successes, this triumphal pontificate proved not only a climax but also a **turning point**: more than Innocent could guess, with his power politics carried on by spiritual sanctions, by ban and interdict, and also by deceit, deception and oppression, he was undermining for the future the love of the nations for the see of St Peter. Innocent, who was so concerned for ordered legislation and collections of legal decretals, attempted to destroy by his ban the epoch-making state law, the *Magna charta libertatum*, which the English nobility and clergy had exacted from King John – but in vain. And by his regime of regulations and charges, Innocent, who reorganized the Roman Curia almost on business principles, strengthened the impression that Rome was less concerned with the *Evangelium secundum Marcum* than with the *Evangelium secundum Marcam*, the gospel of the mark, the silver mark. Even at the end of the Fourth Lateran Council every prelate who took part had to deposit a respectable 'donation' for the Pope, who was always thinking of new means of raising money. Indeed, under Innocent those terrifying **phenomena of decay** began which were then to be among the main complaints of reformers and the Reformation, but which in part have remained characteristics of the curial system right down to our day:

– Nepotism and the favouring of relatives and officials of the Pope and the cardinals,

– Avarice, corruption, the excusing and concealing of crime,

– financial exploitation of the churches and peoples by an ingenious system of offerings and dues.[176]

There is also a significant difference between the early church Byzantine paradigm (P II) and the mediaeval Roman Catholic paradigm (P III) in the politicizing of the church.

• In the early church Byzantine paradigm the power of the church was incorporated into a system of symphony and harmony in which in fact the secular power dominated the spiritual power.

• But from the Middle Ages on, as a result of the papacy the church of the West presented itself as a completely independent ruling institution of the very first order, which at times succeeded in getting almost complete control even over secular power.

Militarization: a militant church and its 'holy war'

Romanization meant **militarization**. And here, too, it was beyond doubt **Gregory VII** who was the first to occupy himself intensively with the plan for a great campaign to the East – to enforce the obedience of Byzantium and to conquer Jerusalem – twenty years before the First Crusade. Under his personal leadership as Pope and general, the Roman primacy was also to be established in Byzantium, and the schism ended. Indeed, Gregory was a defender of the 'holy war', who not only sent 'Peter's standard' (= Peter's blessing) to the warring parties which he favoured and thus blessed war, but also was the first Pope to grant an 'indulgence' remitting punishment for sins to those engaging in war – for example in the reconquest of Spain: as always, quite naturally with the 'full authority' of Peter. Thus Gregory VII has not unjustly been called the most warlike Pope ever to have occupied the throne of Peter. He constantly recruited troops, engaged in warlike enterprises and even rode into battle in person, splendidly arrayed. He seems to have forgotten the early principle that the church does not shed blood. He was fond of quoting a saying from Jeremiah: 'Cursed is he who keeps back his sword from bloodshed!'[177]

So it was no coincidence that the First **Crusade**[178] took place only ten years after Gregory's death – into and for the 'Holy Land', to liberate the holy places from the 'unbelievers'. Obviously a Crusade is essentially different from a pilgrimage, an adventurous expedition or an emigration, although the element of pilgrimage played an essential role and the desire for adventure (fairy-tale ideas about the East) and escapism (from debts and other wretched circumstances at home) was not negligible. By nature a Crusade is a **holy war** under the sign of the victorious cross – we may recall Constantine. Bernard of Clairvaux was the first Christian theoretician of the holy war, and provided theological justification for the killing of unbelievers.[179] But this could not come about without the initiative and the blessing of the papacy, which helped with privileges for Crusaders (indulgences, immunity from taxes and tolls, a moratorium on private debts). From the beginning the Crusades were papal undertakings, even if the papacy then often avoided carrying them out in practice.

So Crusades are no historical accidents or chance by-products of church history. They are a **typical phenomenon of the Roman Catholic paradigm.**[180] In the West people were generally convinced that a Crusade was a deeply Christian undertaking:
– The Crusade was regarded as a matter for the **whole** of (Western) **Christianity**, even if the First Crusade took place under French leadership, the Second under French and German leadership, and the Third under German leadership.

– The Crusades were thought to have been **approved by Christ himself,** since the Pope as Christ's spokesman had personally issued a summons to them. Here the papacy could only gain increased significance, since the Crusades emphasized its primacy at the head of the West.[181] And the stronger an external enemy of Christianity was, the closer the solidarity of the Christian under the one supreme pastor.

– The Crusades, which usually led men through hostile territory without any basis for provisions, over thousands of miles and with indescribable hardships, would not have been possible without authentic **religious enthusiasm,** passion, often almost a mass psychosis. The Crusades were presented to the Crusaders as a kind of pilgrimage, and some even took part on them on the basis of a specific oath to go on pilgrimage. And particularly for this time 'Jerusalem', the holy city of the beginning and end of the history of Christianity, had a magical ring about it. Indeed the unspeakable suffering, anxiety, losses and, despite everything, the amazing success of the First Crusade in particular seemed to confirm to them that this was God's will.[182]

The role which **Innocent III** played in the politics of the Crusades in particular is difficult to understand: he may have been concerned to integrate particular heretical groups. He became the **Pope of Crusades even against fellow-Christians.** Here he took seriously Gregory VII's principle that 'anyone who is not in accord with the Roman church should not be regarded as a Catholic', and thus in legal terms is so to speak an outlaw. As we heard within the framework of P II, Innocent, who praised the Crusade as a 'means of salvation', initiated the Fourth Crusade (1202–1204), which led to the disastrous conquest and three-day plundering of Constantinople, to the establishment of a Latin emperorship with Latin church organization, and to the servitude of the Byzantine church. Granted, this was not originally Innocent's intention, but after the event he praised the development as the work of divine providence: the papal goal which had been striven for since the fifth century – the establishment of the primacy also in Constantinople – seemed to have been achieved. But the opposite was the case: this in fact sealed the schism.

Only a decade later, at the Fourth Lateran Council of 1215, the same Pope promulgated a decree for a further Crusade to Palestine; he would have led it personally had he not died the very next year (1216). But what did transpire after the murder of a papal legate was the first great Crusade against other Christians, Christians now even in the West: against the Albigensians (neo-Manichaean Cathars) in southern France. This cruel twenty-year Albigensian war, accompanied by bestial cruelties on both sides, led to the extermination of whole parts of the population, put the cross to shame, and was a perversion of Christianity. Nevertheless it gained a following.[183] No wonder that already in the time of Innocent evangelically minded protest groups established the notion that the Pope was the Antichrist.

Of course we must understand the Crusades, too, 'in terms of their time', without thus excusing them. Behind them lay Augustine's theology that the use of force by the lawful authority was legitimate if it was for a just reason. The 'cause of Christ' was to be defended or established, and this Christ, although he was now seen with his human features, was now understood as a 'political Christ'. So contemporary criticism was at most directed against the Crusaders, whose sins were regarded as a cause of the failure, but hardly at all at the Crusades, at any rate not as long as people believed in their success.[184] Certainly the Crusades indirectly contributed to an expansion of the spiritual horizons of the West, to the economic boom in Mediterranean trade and in the Italian cities, to the formation of a nobility based on common ideals (chivalry) and a raising of living standards in urban life (a middle class). But at the same time we should reflect that in the face of this manifest political and military reinterpretation of the Christian message, while there was increasing doubt about the utility of the Crusades and the high taxes connected with them, and doubt whether the Christian faith was the only right faith, from the beginning, hardly a voice could be heard raising the obvious **critical questions**:

– whether the Jesus of the Sermon on the Mount, who proclaimed non-violence and love of enemies, would ever have approved such a warlike enterprise;

– whether the cross of the Nazarene had not been turned into its opposite, if instead of inspiring Christians really to bear the cross every day, it legitimated the bloody wars of the Crusaders who bore that cross on their garments;

– whether the Pope really was the spokesman of Christ if he presented such a warlike expedition as an act of Christian 'love' and 'penitence' and as a 'meritorious work', particularly for laity and especially for knights, since monks and priests were not allowed to shed blood;

– whether the bloody persecution of Jewish communities in France, in the Rhineland, in Bavaria and Bohemia, which was already connected with the first wave of Crusaders, should not have been a warning sign that there was more hatred, vengeance and avarice here than penitence and love;

– whether the strategy of massacring or expelling the non-Christians in important places that were conquered (in the expectation of Western settlers) and the fearful bloodbath of Jews and Muslims after the entry into Jerusalem did not stand in blatant contradiction to the Jesus who entered Jerusalem without violence, riding on an ass;

– whether the newly founded Crusader states and the orders of knights who gave armed service (the Knights of St John and the Templars) were not from the start disowned by the preacher from Nazareth, according to whom only the non-violent will possess 'the land';

– whether contrary to the ancient tradition, fallen warriors should have been regarded as martyrs who went directly to paradise.

No, in connection with the militarization of the church, too, the early Christian message (P I) had been completely transformed by the now prevailing paradigm (P III). But a difference from the early church Byzantine paradigm (P II) also stands out:

• The Orthodox churches of the East were also entangled in most of the political and military conflicts of the secular power and often gave theological legitimation to wars, indeed inspired them.

• But only in Western Christianity was there that (Augustinian) theory of the legitimate use of force to achieve spiritual ends which finally allowed the use of force even in the dissemination of Christianity, against all the tradition of the early church: in wars of conversion, wars against pagans, wars against heretics, indeed, as a complete perversion of the cross, in Crusades against fellow-Christians.

Clericalization: a church of celibate men and the prohibition of marriage

Romanization meant **clericalization**: under the influence of the monks Humbert and Hildebrand, in a kind of 'pan-monasticism' Rome required unconditional obedience, the renunciation of marriage and communal life for all the clergy. The resolutions of the Lateran Synod of 1059 on the **prohibition of priestly marriage** were followed more in France, the cradle of monastic reform, than in **Italy**. At any rate the prohibition against priestly marriage was not proclaimed by the bishops of Lombardy – except by the Bishop of Brescia, who was almost beaten to death by his priests for doing so. But this perseverance of the clergy in legitimate priestly marriage led to another revolt of the powerful movement of the Patarini (from *pattari*, 'old clothes dealers', 'scrap dealers') against them, again encouraged by the Pope. There were repulsive drives against wives of priests in the clergy houses.

The indignation over the prohibition of marriage was even greater in **Germany** than in Italy. There only three bishops (those of Salzburg, Würzburg and Passau) dared to proclaim the Roman decrees, one of them (the last) at Christmas: he was driven out, almost lynched by the clergy.

The lesser clergy were particularly affected by the condemnation, and they protested in their thousands (3,600 clergy at a synod in the diocese of Constance alone) against the new laws and the stirring up of the church people against their spiritual leaders. In a petition the German clergy argued:

1. Does the Pope not know the word of the Lord, 'He who is able to receive it, let him receive it' (Matt.19.12)?

2. The Pope was compelling men by force to live as angels; he wanted to forbid the course of nature. This would only lead to unchastity.

3. Faced with the choice whether to give up the priestly office or marriage, they would decide for marriage. Let the Pope recruit angels for the ministry of the church.[185]

Here again it was **Gregory VII** who introduced the definitive decision by accepting the petitions of the Patarini and endorsing the resolutions of 1059 at his first Lenten synod in 1074. Indeed, he suspended all the married priests (who were censured as 'concubinarians') and at the same time mobilized the laity not to accept any priestly functions from them. This was new: a **boycott of the clergy** by the laity staged by the Pope himself. However, the Second Lateran Council of 1139 was the first to draw the conclusion for church law by declaring the receiving of higher degrees of consecration (from the sub-diaconate on) to be a hindrance to marriage. This meant that priestly marriage which, while forbidden, had been legally valid was now a priori invalid; all wives of priests were regarded as concubines, indeed the children of priests were made the property of the church, slaves. So from now on there was a **universal and compulsory law of celibacy**, though in practice it was only observed to a limited degree up to the Reformation, even in Rome.

More than anything else, the mediaeval, typically Roman Catholic law of celibacy – over which there is again much dispute today – contributed to the 'clergy', the 'hierarchy', the 'priestly state' being removed from the 'people' (who became the 'laity') and set completely above it; now the state of celibacy was beyond dispute regarded as morally more 'perfect' than that of marriage. Indeed **clericalization** was now so extensive that the 'church' and the 'clergy' were virtually identified – terminology which has lasted to the present day. For the exercise of power, this meant:

– The laity were excluded from the church, which hitherto had consisted of clergy and laity.

– As those who administered the means of grace, the clergy alone formed 'the church'.

– The church of the clergy had a hierarchical and monarchical organization with the Pope at its head, so that *Ecclesia Catholica* and *Ecclesia Romana* became synonymous.

– The clergy ('church') and laity formed 'Christendom' (*Christianitas*), but in it, according to the Roman view, Pope and clergy had to dominate.

Now in the high Middle Ages the clergy consisted more than ever of two powerful branches: the secular clergy and the clergy in religious orders. And it was in the time of **Innocent III** in particular that the significance of the clergy in religious orders was decisively to increase. Not only were the monks in the West now increasingly priests (*patres*), with lay brothers (*fratres*) only for more menial services. It was Innocent III in particular who wisely domesticated the poverty movement in the church and approved those novel orders in which discipleship of the poor Jesus was the leading idea: the **mendicant orders** of the Franciscans and Dominicans, as we shall see in more detail.

Over **clericalization**, too, a striking difference between the early church Byzantine (P II) and the mediaeval Roman Catholic paradigm (P III) is evident:

● In the Eastern churches the clergy, apart from the bishops, remained married and therefore seemed very much closer to the people and more assimilated to the structure of society.

● But the celibate clergy of the West seemed totally removed from the Christian people, above all because they were unmarried. They had their own, dominant social status, totally superior to the lay state and totally subordinate to the Roman Pope, who was now for the first time supported by an omnipresent, centrally organized, available and mobile celibate troop of auxiliaries: the mendicant orders.

Gains and losses

In subsequent years the militancy of the papacy was to become evident time and again, from the last phase of the fatal battle with the Hohenstaufen emperors through the Italian Renaissance and the Counter-Reformation to the downfall of the papal state with its 'Papa-Ré' (Pope- king) at the head. Indeed up to the Second Vatican Council people in Rome were fond of speaking of the church as an *acies ordinata*, a 'battle line' against all possible enemies, real or imagined, all of course under the supreme command of the Summus Pontifex, who called for unconditional obedience.

If we survey the development in the high Middle Ages in order to **take stock**, we may ask: could this clerical and centralist system, safeguarded in every respect by law, politics and the army, still be seriously threatened? But if we look closely, this whole development not only had gains but also considerable losses. A dialectic of history becomes visible, which can be demonstrated vividly, in particular in the papalist system.

For what **positive conclusions** could the papacy draw from the clashes between the Popes – latterly also Gregory IX (the nephew of Innocent III) and Innocent IV – and the highly gifted Hohenstaufen emperor Frederick II, which were both warlike and highly publicized?

– The **papacy** clearly won a victory over the **Hohenstaufen emperors**: Conradin, barely sixteen years old, grandson of Frederick II and the last Hohenstaufen, was defeated by the Pope's ally Charles of Anjou (the brother of Louis IX of France, who was rewarded by the Pope with Naples and Sicily), and despite his petition for intervention from the Pope, was beheaded in Naples along with his companions as a traitor. Now lay investiture was finally abolished, and the papacy with its legal system became the central institution of Europe.

– The **German emperor was ruled out as a force capable of shaping history**: in fact the empire in Italy and Germany dissolved into a whole series of independent territories.

– Within the Latin church the **papacy** with its centralistic system of control established itself totally as the **absolute institutional power** (legislative, executive and judicative at the same time), in a way utterly at odds with the episcopate and the synodical structures of the early church.

– In the framework of the Roman Catholic paradigm the **independence of the church from the state** and an autonomy of the spiritual sphere from other spheres of life became possible – something that was inconceivable in the East Roman Orthodox symphony paradigm from Byzantium to Moscow. This was a presupposition for the later process of the secularization of politics, law, the economy and culture, which with good reason originated in north-western Europe.

However, these gains contrast with considerable **losses**, caused by both external and internal pressures:

– The more time went on, the more the **Crusades** proved to be a **fiasco**: King Louis IX of France was defeated and taken prisoner in Egypt on the Sixth Crusade; indeed on the Seventh and last Crusade in 1270 he died of the plague with the bulk of another army before Tunis. **Islam** remained the great hostile power for Christianity.

– The papacy, acting in a legalistic, monarchical and absolutist way, **permanently lost the churches of the East** with their sacramental, collegial and conciliar constitution through its excommunication of the Patriarch, the Fourth Crusade and the establishment of a Latin emperorship.

– By destroying the German universal emperorship, the papacy at the same time undermined its own position as a Roman universal papacy: in this way it gave a boost to the **formation of modern nation states**. Utterly fixated on Germany, it left the monarchies in England and France largely undisturbed to develop their power. But in this way it now became increasingly and openly dependent on **France**, the country of the theocratic 'most Christian' kings (because according to the legend of Clovis, which had been exploited for propaganda purposes, they had been anointed wth oil directly for heaven). France, which was often host to Popes in political difficulties, also became a threat to the papacy, at first imperceptibly.

However, the threat from within was to be no less dangerous to the papacy than the threat from outside by the nation states: it took the form of organized opposition within the church, of a kind that had not emerged for five hundred years in the West, since the overcoming of Germanic Arianism.

Opposition and Inquisition

Previously there were at best a few deviants (like for example the poor monk Gottschalk of Orbais in the ninth century, who was condemned for his Augustinian doctrine of predestination and held captive until his death), and these were quickly disciplined and isolated. But from around 1170–80 two great **non-conformist penitential and poverty movements** developed which threatened the Roman system.[186] In the face of a Christianity which had been made rigid by canon law, rich monasteries and a senior clergy living in luxury, and which neglected the duties of preaching, they adopted the slogans 'itinerant preaching and apostolic poverty' as their programme.

First there were the **Cathars** (from the Greek *katharoi* = the pure). They spread from the Balkans (the Bogomils, whom we have met) around the middle of the twelfth century through itinerant apostolic preaching and strict asceticism: they rejected the eating of meat, marriage, war service, taking oaths, altars, saints, images and relics. They found a large following especially in the south of France and upper Italy, even among the nobility, clergy and monks. After the Council of St Félix de Caraman near Toulouse in 1167, at which a high Cathar dignitary from the East, Papa Niquinta (Nicetas), ordained new bishops, questions of doctrine and organization came into the foreground. The Cathars, who were also called Albigensians after one of their centres, the city of Albi in southern France, now increasingly advocated a doctrine with a Manichaean structure, the doctrine of a good and an evil principle, of God the creator of the invisible, good world, and Satan the creator of the visible, evil world. Here they now made a sharp distinction between two degrees of membership: 'believers', for whom the ascetic demands were moderated, and the 'perfect', who alone might pray the 'Our Father'. In time, here too a real anti-church developed with its own hierarchy and dogma, which was to gain many adherents from all classes, especially in developed areas with abundant cities.

Then there were the **Waldensians**. They are a product of the West and emerged from an ascetical lay brotherhood gathered around Peter Waldo, a rich merchant from Lyons. He had been converted by a Provençal translation of the Bible and had distributed his wealth among the poor. The early Waldensians preached and wrote especially against the Cathar orthodox. But the dispute with the hierarchy came over lay preaching. Despite episcopal and papal prohibitions the Waldensians (often women as well) went around the country in pairs as preachers, like the apostles. They proclaimed the 'law of Christ', Holy Scripture, large parts of which they knew by heart, in the vernacular. Many of the nobility of southern France supported this movement in the spirit of the gospel. Many became radical only because they were excluded from the church: already in the time of Innocent III a branch of them fell in with the church and from then on called themselves 'Catholic poor'. But after the death of their founder another branch took a radical course, and now resembled the Cathars. A real lay church emerged, with its own services, administration of the sacrament, lay eucharist and lay preaching (also by women); like the Cathars, these Waldensians rejected taking the oath, war service and also altars, church buildings and the veneration of the cross, purgatory and the death penalty.

And what was the **answer of the official church**, which had the support first of the bishops and then of the Pope, and throughout of the emperor? As a rule it responded by **banning lay preaching**, indeed by **condemnation of the 'heretics'**. But excommunication and the use of legislation against heretics simply drove these religious movements underground and now made them even more widely known. Moreover they spread as far as Bohemia, where they were to influence the pre-Reformation movements of the Hussites, Taborites and Bohemian Brethren. The first general law on combating heresy (enacted by Pope and emperor at the Synod of Verona in 1184) defined failure to accord with the decrees of the papacy as a mark of heresy. At the same time it called on the secular power to eradicate heresy by force at the church's bidding.

In other words, although a man like Innocent III took the trouble to differentiate between some 'heretical' groups (groups of 'Humiliates' and Waldensians who had already been condemned were reintegrated into the church[187]), on the whole Popes and bishops persecuted opposition within the church without mercy. Force increasingly ruled in the church, safeguarded by the theory of the two swords, according to which the 'secular arm' had to lend its sword to the spiritual authority against heresy and schism. Bishops and Popes, kings and emperors, had prepared the way for what was then to fill many of the darkest pages of church history under the deterrent name of the **Inquisition:**[188] the systematic legal persecution of the heretics by a church court (*inquisitio haereticae pravitatis*) which had the support not only of the secular power, but also wide circles of the people, who often greatly enjoyed the executions of heretics.

Basically, Inquisition now became a **specific characteristic of the mediaeval Roman Catholic paradigm**. For what was an isolated instance in the early church (P II) became a regular institution in the church of the high Middle Ages (P III): the universal and more effective papal Inquisition as relief for, supplement to and intensification of the episcopal inquisition (which had already been practised in the early Middle Ages). What the church of the fourth century had abhorred thus became a command in the church of the twelfth and thirteenth centuries. But how did the papal Inquisition come about?

With the growth of a powerful church, understandably the opposition groups 'from below' had also grown, and both church and state believed that they could defend themselves against these groups only by reprisals. One cruel example is the Crusade proclaimed by Innocent against the Albigensian Cathars, which led to a war of persecution lasting twenty years (1209–29). The consequence was, on the one hand the extermination of large groups and the annihilation of the leading families of southern France, but on the other hand the strengthening of the central authority in Paris over this region. In the middle of the war, in November 1215, the Fourth Lateran Council (as we heard) promulgated harsh general decrees not only against Jews but also against heretics: in condemnation of them a lengthy confession of faith was proclaimed right at the beginning of the constitutions of the council, and in a long section on the heretics even unauthorized preaching was forbidden as heresy in order to tame them.[189]

Without question the emperor Frederick II had a decisive influence on the formation of the Inquisition in the Middle Ages. In his coronation edicts (1220) he decreed death **at the stake** as punishment for heresy. So did Pope Gregory IX, who through the constitution *Excommunicamus* (1231) took upon himself the whole fight against the heretics which had previously been organized above all by local bishops. He nominated **papal inquisitors** principally from the mendicant orders to track down the heretics. Heretics condemned by the church were to be handed over to the secular court – for punishment through death by fire or at least for their tongues to be cut out: the laity were not to discuss the faith either in private or in public, but to denounce all those suspected of heresy (which was treated as an infectious disease). The church authorities alone were competent in decisions on matters of faith, and they allowed no freedom of thought or speech. Innnocent IV, a great lawyer Pope, then went yet one stage further. He empowered the Inquisition even to allow the use of torture by the secular authorities to extract confessions. The real torment this meant for the victims beggars all description.

Is all this 'past times'? Today, it will be said, even in the Roman Catholic paradigm there is no longer any torture or death by fire; after all, these barbarisms were done away with after the Reformation and the Enlightenment. But the Roman Inquisition, founded in the Middle Ages, continues. Its name has often been changed (Holy Office, now Sacred Congregation for the Doctrine of Faith), but essentially it still acts in accordance with the same mediaeval principles, which have little to do with generally recognized legal principles (and at that time were even advocated by the papacy as an alternative to others). Indeed they have little to do with the most primitive requirements of justice.[190] This is because:

– proceedings against the suspect or the accused are secret;
– no one knows who the informants are;
– there is no cross-examination of witnesses or those laying charges;
– no inspection of documents is allowed, so that a knowledge of the preliminary proceedings is hindered;
– prosecutor and judge are identical;
– appeal to an independent court is either ruled out or useless;
– the aim of the enquiry is not to discover the truth but to achieve submission to Roman doctrine, which is always identical with the truth ('obedience' to the 'church').

The question is: what does such an Inquisition, which very often leads to the spiritual torture and psychological burning of those entangled in such procedures, have to do with the message and behaviour of Jesus of Nazareth? Clearly nothing at all. Such an Inquisition mocks not only the gospel but also the sense of justice, widespread today, which has found expression, say, in the declarations of human rights.[191] But mustn't we understand even the Inquisition (I mean the mediaeval Inquisition!) in terms of its time? Wasn't any heresy at that time a threat to the common foundation of the faith of mediaeval society, a treasonous rebellion against the 'full authority' of the Pope? Didn't the individual who cast doubt on an article of faith forfeit all rights? Didn't he or she have to be sacrificed for the well-being of the whole community, for the sake of which individuals existed?

Yet measured by Jesus Christ himself, even then people could see that the Inquisition was a profoundly un-Christian enterprise. For even in the Middle Ages the approach could have been quite different. In an extremely important case we are indebted to a shift in Innocent III's policy against heretics that the person and the cause were not excluded as heretical but remained incorporated into the church: the evangelical and apostolic poverty movement of the so-called mendicant orders. Whereas Innocent had stubborn, unteachable heretics like the Cathars exterminated with fire and sword, he gave the newly-founded movements of Dominic[192] and Francis of Assisi (as before them the Waldensians and Humiliates) a chance to survive within the church, although the Fourth Lateran Council prohibited the formation of new religious orders.

The alternative? Francis of Assisi

Amazingly enough, it was the great Innocent who found himself directly confronted with so insignificant a man as Francis of Assisi. The result was that in 1209 there was a truly **historic encounter**: Francis of Assisi face-to-face with Innocent III, the world ruler face to face with the 'poverello', the little poor man. Wasn't the great alternative to the Roman system embodied here, in the person of Giovanni di Bernardone, once the worldly son of a rich textile merchant from Assisi with a great delight in life?

Perhaps Innocent's concession was not so amazing. For Francis, who had renounced 'the world', in other words family, wealth and career, and had even given all his clothes back to his father, had fled in his nakedness into the bosom of the church. H.Grundmann has the right insight here: Francis always had a 'believing trust in the church and its sacraments'; always an 'unerring veneration for the priestly office, to which as a layman he himself never aspired'.[193] Moreover Innocent III was also well aware of the urgent need for reforms in the church, and indeed was to summon the Fourth Lateran Council for this purpose. For he was sensitive enough to note that the church which was outwardly powerful was inwardly weak, that the 'heretical' trends within it had increased considerably and that they could hardly be countered with force alone. Would it not be better to tie them to the church and meet their wish for apostolic preaching in poverty? So a priori Francis of Assisi could by no means have been unwelcome to him, nor in the event was he.

But precisely what was the **concern of the 'poverello'**? What did the twenty-four-year-old, who saw the 'rebuilding of the fallen church' as a call to himself in a vision of the crucified Jesus (1206), mean by the phrase? In a sentence: an end to self-satisfied bourgeois existence and the beginning of true discipleship of Christ in poverty and itinerant preaching in accord with the gospel, indeed authentic conformity to the life and suffering of Christ and identification with Christ (*alter Christus*, 'another Christ').

This controversial approach of the young drop-out, hardly in conformity to the church, has not always been brought out with the necessary self-critical sharpness by scholars from the Franciscan orders like Hilarin Felder[194] and Kajetan Esser,[195] as though there had been no fundamental difference between Francis and the Curia, and from Francis to the Franciscans there was at best an 'organic development' with hardly any contradictions. The Tübingen historian of theology Helmut Feld,[196] taking up the researches of the Strasbourg historian Paul Sabatier[197] and the Marburg religion expert Ernst Benz,[198] paints a different picture. On the basis of a critical re-reading of the sources he has not only worked out **three indisputable core points of the Franciscan ideal** but also examined the subsequent development critically:[199]

– *Paupertas*, poverty: Francis of Assisi aimed at a life in uncompromising poverty. He was prompted to this by a saying of Jesus which he heard in a service in 1208: 'You received without pay, give without pay. Take no gold, nor silver, nor copper in your belts, no bag for your journey, nor two tunics, nor sandals, nor a staff; for the labourer deserves his food.'[200] The conclusion which he drew from that, as can be read in his Testament, is that not only the individual member of the brotherhood (as with the earlier orders) but the community as a whole was to have absolutely no possessions; it was forbidden to have money or to build great churches and buildings, even forbidden to seek any privileges from the Roman Curia. But the brothers were to work hard in the fields: so they were not a mendicant order (they were to beg only in an emergency)!

– *Humilitas*, humility: Francis of Assisi aimed at a life which renounced power and influence, extending to extreme forms of self-denial and self-mortification. He preached the virtue of patience in all situations and a basic mood of joy which can endure even taunts, humiliations and blows. Here the suffering and poverty of Jesus were a model for him; indeed Francis identified with the suffering Jesus.[201]

– *Simplicitas*, simplicity: Francis of Assisi aimed at a discipleship of great simplicity in every action. Science and scholarship seemed to him more like obstacles. Instead, he sought a new relationship to creation, as is indicated in some accounts and legends and above all in the 'Hymn to the Sun': a new relationship to animals, plants and inanimate natural phenomena, even to 'our sister, the death of the body'.[202] He called all creatures brothers and sisters because he saw them, like human beings, as beings ensouled and filled with divine life.[203]

Thus Francis, who regarded his way of life 'after the form of the holy gospel'[204] as a revelation of God and composed a brief rule exclusively made up of quotations from the Bible, went to Rome in 1209 with eleven 'lesser brothers' (*fratres minores*) to seek from Innocent III the **church's**

approval of the life of poverty and lay preaching. In conformity with Jesus, but not in confrontation with the hierarchy, not by drifting into heresy but in obedience to Pope and Curia, he and his followers sought to put their aim into practice and, like the disciples of Jesus, proclaim the ideal of the gospel life through itinerant preaching. Though outwardly barely distinguishable from 'heretics', they wanted to live out their ideal of poverty, not in opposition to orthodox teaching – nor in remote monasteries, either – but by proclaiming the gospel in the cities of Italy (which were becoming increasingly prosperous and powerful at this time of the Crusades).

And what about the hierarchy? The Benedictine cardinal John of St Paul, a Colonna who was a friend of the Bishop of Assisi, played a key role for Francis in Rome. Convinced of the need for church reforms, he welcomed the brothers into his house and had lengthy conversations with Francis. While John, too, could not convince Francis to lead a monastic or eremitic way of life, he influenced the Pope positively: God could reform the faith of the church through this man who conveyed the gospel to all the world. So the link was made between Francis and Innocent III. After a lengthy admonition, Innocent seems to have given Francis permission for penitential preaching. His only hesitations were whether the ideal of a life in absolute poverty required in the rule could be fulfilled. Francis was to seek out the will of God over this in prayer, which Francis indeed did. According to tradition, on the basis of a vision in a dream – for Innocent as for Francis, visions played a great role – in which a small insignificant member of a religious order was able to prevent the papal Lateran basilica from collapse, the Pope finally approved Francis' rule and made it known in the consistory. But nothing was fixed in writing.

All this means that Francis, dangerous though he appeared, committed himself fully to the church. He promised the Pope obedience and reverence and bound the brothers by the same promise. At the wish of Cardinal John he had himself and his eleven companions elevated to the status of clergy by the tonsure; this made preaching easier, but encouraged the clericalization of the young community. Moreover priests now joined the community. The process of the 'ecclesiasticization' of the Franciscan movement had begun, and Francis, who would have liked to detach himself from everything in poverty, was now all the more dependent on 'holy mother church'. Nor was he spared another paradox: the more he abased himself, the more he was revered by the people.

Now at least we have once again to address the substantive problem which the appearance of Francis of Assisi raises. Was he the **alternative to the Roman system**? What would have happened had Innocent III for his part taken the gospel seriously, and applied to himself the key points made by Francis of Assisi? What would have happened had the Fourth Lateran Council (1215) put the reform of the church on this basis?

Here there could have been quiet reflection on the fact that what Jesus said on sending out the disciples was addressed to itinerant preachers, and cannot simply be generalized. And in our reflections on the earliest community we have seen how those who wanted to follow Jesus and share his free itinerant life necessarily had to leave everything behind. Certainly Jesus did not require the surrender of possessions to the community (as did the Essene monastery of Qumran by the Dead Sea). He let Zacchaeus distribute only half his possessions; he did not lay down any laws and paragraphs; various of his followers, including Peter, had houses of their own. But Jesus required everyone to be content and undemanding, to have trust and a carefree spirit, inner freedom from possessions. In the earliest community, the conditions in which were later idealized, an ideal social utopia may not have been achieved, but a 'community in social solidarity' certainly was.

So we must ask once again: what would have happened had the message of Jesus been taken seriously once again at that time – not *in imitatione Christi* but *in correlatione cum Christo*? The answer can only be: had Francis's demands, which were so in keeping with the gospel, been understood, not literally but spiritually, they could have powerfully put in question the centralized, legalized, politicized, militarized and clericalized **Roman system**, which had taken over the cause of Christ. And in the subsequent period such demands were to become louder and louder. Francis of Assisi represents a reflection on what the cause of Jesus Christ originally meant, and this reflection inevitably seemed all the more radical, the further the Roman system had removed itself from the original message.

However, in barely two decades the **Franciscan movement,** which was spreading strongly all over Italy, had **almost completely domesticated itself in the church,** so that it was soon at the service of papal policies as a normal order. This was quite essentially the work of the nephew of Innocent III, Cardinal Hugolino of Ostia,[205] whom we have already met; even in Francis' lifetime he had made himself Francis' intimate friend and protector and he ascended the papal throne as Pope Gregory IX a year after Francis' death. How did he achieve this? As early as 1228 he canonized Francis, who had already long been beatified 'from below', and thus turned him into a man who had been pronounced a saint 'from above'. He also allowed Brother Elias of Cortona,[206] the Vicar whom Francis himself had appointed, to build a splendid basilica resting on a powerful substructure above Francis' tomb. Here were a lower and an upper church and a monastery building, before the walls of Assisi – all contrary to the express prohibition of the saint against building large churches and buildings. And in 1230 Gregory IX issued a bull in which, at the wish of the Franciscan community, now already organized as an order that had become increasingly sedentary, he 'interpreted' the rule: the brothers were allowed, not the possession (*proprietas, dominium*) of property, but its use (*usus*) – a fictitious distinction which Francis himself would have rejected as resolutely as he rejected the indirect use of money in the form of bills of payment, which was now also allowed.

So for more than a century there was to be a dispute in the Franciscan order – I cannot go into the details here – between the rigorists and those who were laxer in their understanding of poverty. But the more priests, scholars and students in need of training joined the Franciscans, the more the 'lesser brothers', too, turned to the sciences, so that even Francis himself said in his Testament that theologians were to be respected highly. Soon in Bologna the Portuguese Antony of Padua, and in Paris the famous professor from Britain, Alexander of Hales, and his no less famous pupil the Italian Bonaventure, later Minister General and Cardinal, joined the Franciscan community.

Innocent III was probably the only Pope who by virtue of his unusual qualities could have shown the church a fundamentally different way, one which could have spared the papacy division and exile and the church the Protestant Reformation. However, this would then have resulted in a further paradigm shift for the Catholic Church as early as the thirteenth century, and not first in the sixteenth century, though this shift would not have split the church but really renewed it, and would also have brought the Western and Eastern churches together again. So the three key concerns which Francis of Assisi derived from earliest Christianity – *paupertas, humilitas, simplicitas* – still remain questions for the future of the church, particularly if we do not idealize his person, which has its one-sidednesses and weaknesses.

Questions for the Future

What should be the face of the church? Should the church of the future be a **church in the spirit of Innocent III or in the spirit of Francis of Assisi**? Even if we are aware of the complicated questions of economy, exercise of office and law which a church cannot ignore in enthusiastic idealism; even if we accept a legitimate form of bestowal of office, exercise of law, and financial transactions in the church, this basic question always remains a live one, which stems from the gospel as the foundation of the church. What should be the face of the church?

• A church of riches, pomp and splendour, avarice and financial scandal? Or a church of transparent financial policies, a modest church, an example of inner freedom from possessions and a Christian generosity, which does not suppress but encourages life in accord with the gospel and apostolic liberty?

• A church of power and domination, bureaucracy and discrimination, repression and inquisition? Or a philanthropic church, a church of dialogue, of brotherliness and sisterliness and hospitality even to nonconformists, of unpretentious service to its leaders: a community of social solidarity, which does not exclude new religious forces and ideas from the church but makes fruitful use of them?

• A church of immovable dogma, moralistic censorship and legalistic protection, totally ruled by canon law, omniscient scholasticism and anxiety? Or a church of the good news and of joy, a theology orientated on the simple gospel, which listens to people instead of merely indoctrinating them from above, a church which does not only teach, but keeps on learning?

Francis of Assisi, betrayed by his ideals but without having spared his body, which had been weakened by excessive asceticism, died on 3 October 1226 as poor as he had lived, at the age of only forty-four. Innocent III, who had succeeded in increasing the power, possessions and wealth of the Holy See like no one before him, had already died ten years earlier, quite unexpectedly, seven months after the triumphant conclusion of the Lateran Coucil, at the age of fifty-six. He too died in human poverty and wretchedness. On the evening of 16 June 1216 he was found in the cathedral of Perugia, forsaken by all and completely naked, plundered by his own servants: the corpse of the one who at the beginning of his meteoric career had already as a young theologian written *On Despising the World, or The Wretchedness of Human Existence.*

Innocent III was a moderate theologian. And his writing contributed hardly anything to that *Credo ut intelligam,* 'I believe in order that I may understand', which had already been sketched out a century earlier by that Benedictine abbot born in Aosta (Piedmont), who via Burgundy and Normandy finally attained the chief archepiscopal see of England, **Anselm of Canterbury** (1033–1109).[207] To begin with totally indebted to the Augustinian tradition, Anselm sought to explain the Christian faith without recourse to Bible and authorities – a demand which was now typical of the time. **Faith in search of understanding** was now the programme, and to it Anselm – along with a quite problematical legalistic theory of redemption as the satisfaction of God – contributed a proof of

God, the famous 'ontological' argument: 'God' is that greater than which cannot be conceived. Such a God cannot exist only in thought but must also exist in reality, otherwise what really exists would be greater than that greater than which cannot be conceived. The probative force of this argument did not go undisputed from the beginning, but it has fascinated theological thinkers down to the twentieth century.[208]

On the basis of this programme Anselm has been called the 'father of scholasticism'. However, a century after Anselm another figure became the 'prince of scholasticism'. He rejected any argument from the concept of God to the existence of God, criticized the compulsion to make the doctrine of satisfaction a system, and rose to be one of the greatest Christian thinkers: Thomas Aquinas. We must now turn to him.

9. The great theological synthesis: Thomas Aquinas

Thomas Aquinas (1225–1274) represented that **third** force alongside emperor and Pope which replaced the monasteries in the thirteenth century as centres of education: the **universities** and thus the **science** which was to serve the universities in research and teaching. And from this context ultimately a really new paradigm was to emerge which would be dominated by neither emperor nor Pope. Would perhaps the brilliant man from Aquino work out this new overall constellation in a scientific way, at least for theology? This is the question on which we shall concentrate on this instance. For all biographical details see my *Great Christian Thinkers*.[209]

Thomas Aquinas – he is the *Doctor communis*, the 'universal teacher of Christianity', and down to the present day continues to bear this name at least in the Catholic Church. But that was by no means the case from the beginning. For only since the period after the First Vatican Council around the end of the last century has Thomas occupied this almost impregnable position. Popes now promote not so much Thomas as Neo-Thomism with all the power at their disposal: encyclicals about Thomas, the naming of Thomas as the authentic teacher of the church and patron of all Catholic schools, a new critical edition of Thomas, the obligation of Catholic theology to accept twenty-four normative and basic philosophical theses. Indeed even the *Codex Iuris Canonici* of 1917/18 imposed the binding condition that in Catholic institutions of education, philosophy and theology should be 'treated after the method, teaching and principles of the Angelic Teacher' (= Thomas Aquinas).[210] Moreover up to 1924 one can count 218 commentaries on the first part of the *Summa theologiae* and 90 on the whole *Summa*. Granted, Thomas Aquinas played virtually no role at the Second Vatican Council, which was about *aggiornamento* and the newly emergent problems and hopes of Christianity; since then there has no longer been a Thomistic school. But Thomas is still 'especially' commended in the new 1983 *Codex Iuris Canonici*,[211] and in the Roman *World Catechism* published in 1993 he is in the end again quoted by far the most frequently of all church writers (63 times), with the exception of Augustine (88 times) and John Paul II (137 times!).[212]

However, this forced Roman concentration of the whole of Catholic theology on Thomas Aquinas, who is still thought to be directly relevant, a concentration born of a defence against modernity (and connected with this, as has been customary since the high Middle Ages, cruel sanctions against deviants), demonstrates two things:

– that despite the Reformation (P IV) and Enlightenment (P V) the mediaeval paradigm of theology (P III) could persist in the Catholic Church in practice up to the Second Vatican Coucil, though it is now manifestly on the defensive;

– that condemned heretics can become normative church teachers. For despite all the neo-scholastic absolutizing of 'St Thomas as teacher', there can be no forgetting the fact that the original historical content of his theology was not orthodox, nor was the basic approach of his theology. Why not? That has to do with the acceptance of a 'pagan' philosophy which was thought to be too dangerous – that of Aristotle.

The new challenge: Aristotle

When Thomas, aged twenty, arrived at the study centre of his order in Paris, he had the inestimable good fortune to meet a uniquely learned teacher, around twenty-five years older, who rightly bore the title *Doctor universalis*: the Swabian **Albert the Great** (1200–1280). At this point in life very much more famous than Thomas, Albert was a pioneer in two respects. By researching into nature, through his writings on the natural sciences and the philosophy of nature he produced new results especially in biology and in the physiology and classification of plants; indeed he was even suspected of magic because of his chemical (and alchemical?) experiments. But as a philosopher Albert was a pioneer because of an encyclopaedia of Aristotelian thought on which he had worked for twenty years. He also bravely disseminated and evaluated the Aristotelian, Arabic and Jewish writings which had been rediscovered in the twelfth century; since some of them were still banned at the time, Albert did not develop them further but paraphrased them. His view was that while in theology Augustine was the master, in astronomy the master was Ptolemy, in medicine Galen and in natural philosophy Aristotle. However, Albert left the task of a synthesis of Aristotle and Christian faith to his pupil Thomas, who was philosophically far more gifted.

What we take for granted today was not at all the case at that time. For many people thought that a pagan philosopher like **Aristotle** was extraordinarily **dangerous** and disturbing. And with good reason. Didn't Aristotle advocate the eternity of the world instead of a creation and thus the temporality of the world? The blind compulsion of history instead of a divine providence? The mortality of the soul, tied to its body, instead of its immortality? Generally speaking, didn't this philosopher embody such a concentration on empirical and visible reality that heaven, God and his revelation seemed to be being neglected? As late as 1263 Pope Urban IV had once again banned the study of the writings of Aristotle – but in vain. For already in 1255 the Paris Faculty of Arts had decreed the whole of Aristotle teaching material. This was the hour of the birth of the philosophical faculty, which wanted no longer to be just the portal to theology but to be independent; it was also the hour of the birth of the scholar, the professor, the intellectual.[213]

This complex of problems was further accentuated by the fact that Aristotle had by no means been handed down 'purely', but often was mediated, commented on and supplemented by Arabic and Jewish philosophy above all from Spain, which had progressed very much further. The Muslim philosopher, theologian, lawyer and doctor from Cordoba, Ibn Rush, in the West called **Averroes** (1126–1198), played a key role here; he was the commentator on Aristotle *par excellence*, one of the most powerful defenders of the independence of reason and philosophy over against religion. And this Averroes was later to have a skilful ally in the Paris Faculty of Arts, Siger of Brabant, who like Averroes accepted only a single intellect in all human beings and emphasized the independence of philosophy from theology.

So I need not spend long explaining how both Aristotelianism and Arabism posed a tremendous intellectual **challenge to the young Thomas**. Furthermore, even if Thomas did not say so, traditional **Augustinianism**, which hitherto had governed everything, was in a **crisis**. In this new time one could no longer solely refer in questions of faith to the previous authorities – Bible, church fathers, councils and Popes – which were often contradictory. Rather, one had to make much more use than before of reason and conceptual analysis to achieve clarity. At all events, Thomas did this both resolutely and boldly, with not a little objectivity and logical acuteness, but also often uncritically, and reinterpreting the statements of the authorities unhistorically – in the *expositio reverentialis*, respectful exposition, customary at the time.

Rational university theology

However, we should be clear that Thomas' theology – unlike the more contemplative monastic theology of the church fathers and still that of Augustine – is quite essentially a **rational university theology**, composed by the professor in the *schola*, the school, and intended primarily not for the people and pastoral care, but for students and colleagues in theology. All the works of Thomas Aquinas – whether the *Summas* or the questions for disputation, the commentaries on Aristotle, Pseudo-Dionysius, Peter Lombard and Boethius, or those on a variety of Old and New Testament books, or finally the various *opuscula* – are utterly stamped with the 'scholastic' approach to learning. They are all exclusively composed **in Latin** (Thomas did not learn either German in Cologne or French in Paris); all are very clear, terse and compact. But there was a price to pay. They are impersonal and monotone compared with Augustine, because their procedure is constantly analytic, with numerous divisions and subdivisions, with sharp definitions of concepts and formal distinctions, with objections and answers, with all the means of grammar, dialectic and disputation.

But there is no doubt that for all his tremendous use of highly developed and often over-developed scholastic technique, Thomas Aquinas never lost sight of the great task of his life. Right at the beginning of the *Summa contra Gentiles* he put it like this: 'I am aware that I owe it to God as the first task of my life to let him speak in all my discourses and senses.'[214]

So for Thomas, the university professor, as for Augustine, the bishop, 'theo-logy' was responsible talk of God. It was what the Flemish Dominican Edward Schillebeeckx[215] has described as a '**theological life project**': the whole life of Thomas understood 'as **priestly service of the Word** in a reflected, thought out, responsible contemporary form'. God's Word was to be neither curtailed nor evacuated, mutilated nor brought down to the level of one's own understanding. No, God's Word was not to be interchangeable with some human, time-conditioned garb or invention which exposed the 'articles of faith' to the *derisus infidelium*, 'the scorn of unbelievers'. So Thomas was concerned to serve the truth in a way which 'always fights **on two fronts at the same time**': 'against different species of a conservative integralism' (represented by the Augustinian traditionalist Bonaventure) and 'against different forms of exaggerated progressiveness' (represented by the Aristotelian Averroistic progressive Siger).

The power of reason and the shift in theology

The influence of Aristotle was particularly evident in the fact that Thomas gave, had to give, knowledge gained by **human reason quite a different value** from that which it had in the theological tradition. For there was no disputing the fact that reason has its independence, its own right, its own sphere, over against faith. The new desire for knowledge, for science, had to be taken seriously. Earlier theologians had had things easier here: they proved as it were the justification for reason alongside faith. But as he shows in the introductions to his two *Summas*, Thomas felt compelled to prove the justification for faith alongside reason (*rationem fidei*). This was a completely new challenge, which forced him to think through the relationship between faith and reason in a new, fundamental way. How?

Thomas' starting point was that philosophy exists in its own right alongside theology. Not by permission of the church, but because of the nature of the order of creation. The creator God himself has endowed human beings with understanding and reason. Science is a 'daughter of God' because God is the 'Lord of the sciences' (*Deus scientiarum dominus*). If one takes this seriously, the result is a liberating **shift for all theology**:
– a shift towards the creaturely and empirical,
– a shift towards rational analysis,
– a shift towards scientific research.

So we can understand Thomas only if we have understood his basic hermeneutical and methodological decision. Whereas Bonaventure, his famous colleague of the same age at the University of Paris and founder of the earlier Franciscan school, ultimately derives all science from theology,[216] Thomas in principle makes a **distinction** between modes of knowledge, levels of knowledge and thus sciences:
– There are two different human **modes of knowledge** (directions of knowledge); it is important to analyse precisely what natural reason is capable of and what comes from faith through grace.
– There are two different human **levels of knowledge** (perspectives of knowledge): it is important to distinguish precisely what human beings know as it were 'from below', within the limits of their horizon of experience, from what they know 'from above', from God's own perspective through inspired Holy Scripture. In other words, it is important to distinguish what belongs on the lower level of natural truths from what belongs on the upper level, that of revealed, supernatural truth.
– So there are two different **sciences**: a precise distinction must be made between what philosophy can know in principle and what theology can

know. What are we to learn from Aristotle 'the philosopher' (hence the commentaries on Aristotle), and what are we to know from the Bible (hence the Bible commentaries)?

Thus according to Thomas, human **reason** is given a wide sphere in which it can be independently active in knowledge. For even the existence and properties of God, God's work as creator and God's providence, the existence of an immortal soul and many ethical insights, are natural truths which human beings can know, indeed demonstrate by reason alone, without revelation. And **faith**? Faith in the strict sense is necessary for the acceptance of certain higher truths of revelation. These include the mysteries of the Trinity or the incarnation of God in Jesus of Nazareth, and also the primal state and the last state, the fall and redemption of human beings and the world. These truths transcend human reason; they cannot be proved rationally but are beyond reason, though they should not be confused with irrational 'truths', which could be refuted rationally.

Two Summas – an organizing principle

Because of this twofold possibility of knowing God, and the twofold mode of knowing the truth about God, while **philosophy** (including the philosophical doctrine of God) and **theology** are not to be separated, since they speak of the same God, they are to be distinguished, since they speak differently of God. Here philosophy proceeds rationally 'from below', from the creation and creatures, while theology proceeds in faith 'from

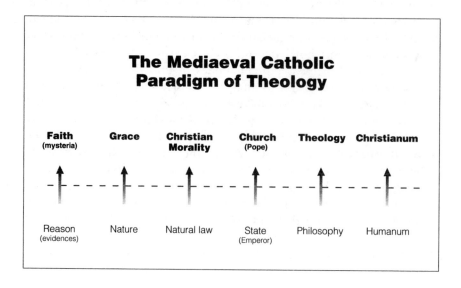

The Mediaeval Catholic Paradigm of Theology

Faith (mysteria)	**Grace**	**Christian Morality**	**Church** (Pope)	**Theology**	**Christianum**
Reason (evidences)	Nature	Natural law	State (Emperor)	Philosophy	Humanum

above', from God. Nevertheless, reason and faith, philosophy and theology, should support each other. In this theology, *intelligo ut credam*, 'I know in order to believe', rather than Augustine's *credo ut intelligam* ('I believe in order to know'), stands in the foreground.

The very first part of the *Summa theologiae* – beginning with twelve long chapters on the one God[217] and then sixteen chapters on the threefold God[218] – makes it clear that the starting point is to be two spheres, two levels of knowledge, metaphorically **two storeys**, which are clearly distinguished but not simply separated: one of higher certainty, the other fundamental and rationally clearly superior, yet both of which are in the last resort not contradictory but in fundamental accord. The First Vatican Council in 1870, 600 years later, was to define the relationship between faith and reason in a similar Neo-Scholastic, Neo-Thomistic way.

Thus beyond question Thomas Aquinas **created for theology the mature, classical form of the mediaeval Roman Catholic paradigm.** His re-structuring of all theology includes a **revaluation** of
- reason as compared with faith,
- the literal sense of scripture as compared with the allegorical, spiritual sense
- nature as compared with grace,
- the natural law as compared with a specifically Christian morality,
- philosophy as compared with theology; in short,
- the *humanum* as compared with the distinctively Christian.

So it was quite consistent that Thomas should work out **two different** *Summas*, two overall accounts of theology for two different purposes, though this did not prevent him from expressing in both also the **same cyclical formative principle, understood primarily in spatial terms,** which come from Neo-Platonism. For in their first halves, both of Thomas's overall outlines deal with the *exitus*, the issuing of all things, from God (God as origin), and in the second with the *reditus*, the return of all things to God (God as goal) – however, they do so without the cosmic determinism of the Neo-Platonists. All things are to be understood from God, their supreme ground of being and their ultimate goal. So why two *Summas*, despite the same basic pattern? Because the two *Summas* serve different purposes and could operate at different levels:

1. The *Summa* against the Gentiles. It was written for Christians who found themselves arguing with Muslim (and also Jewish and heretical) opponents, whether with Muslims in Spain, Sicily and North Africa, or Jews and heretics in Christian Europe. In the thirteenth century, Islam, which was advanced culturally, was not only a political and military but

also an intellectual and spiritual challenge. Therefore an alternative
had to be provided to the Graeco–Arab world view. This was the aim
of the *Summa contra Gentiles*: an overall view of Christian convictions
with an apologetic, missionary and scientific purpose. But precisely
because it is aimed at convincing non-Christians, except in the fourth
apologetic part[219] it largely operates at the level of **natural reason**. In
the introduction Thomas says that one cannot discuss God, creation
and the moral life (the three themes of the first three parts) with
Muslims and pagans on the basis of the Old or New Testament, 'so it
is necessary to resort to the natural reason, to which all are compelled
to assent'.[220]

2. The *Summa theologiae*. This is intended for theologians, indeed
for 'beginners' in theology (a typical professorial overestimation of the
capacities of students). The theological *Summa* is a handbook with a
clear pedagogical and scientific aim within the church, which is meant
to provide a systematic survey of the whole of 'sacred doctrine'. Here,
despite all the rational arguments, in principle the biblical message and
thus **Christian faith** is constantly presupposed. But Thomas succeeds
impressively in interpreting personal language about God, the Father
who speaks and can be spoken of, in contemporary terms with concepts from Greek philosophy: God as the supreme being (*summum
esse*), being itself (*ipsum esse*), the greatest truth (*maximum verum*),
the truth itself (*ipsa veritas*), the supreme good (*summum bonum*). In
his two *Summas* Thomas certainly does not think unhistorically, as has
often been claimed. However, it would be wrong now to swing to the
opposite extreme and stylize him as a theologian of history.

A theology of history?

Augustine, as we saw, was a theologian of history. So too was the
abbot **Joachim of Fiore** (1202),[221] the founder of an order in the
century before Thomas, the forerunner of modern political messianism
– in a prophetic apocalyptic and trinitarian way. He had developed a
great vision of God's progressive revelation in world history: the age of
the Father (the old law: Israel) is followed by that of the Son (the new
law: the church of Peter), and will be replaced by a third age to be
expected soon, that of the Holy Spirit ('the third empire'). A church of
John will come – it was forecast for 1260 – a monastic church, in
which the papacy will die away and the gospel will really be lived. No
wonder that the Franciscan movement applied this prophecy to itself,
although the Fourth Lateran Council in 1215 had naturally rejected it
because of its threat to the hierarchy.

The sober Thomas Aquinas, who was on his way from Paris to the Roman Curia in 1260, the year of the change forecasted, also rejected this view with unusual sharpness as 'utter nonsense' and a 'vain hope', referring to Christ as the fullness of time: 'this state of the new law is not followed by any other state' (of the Holy Spirit).[222] For Thomas' system of order is not orientated on the eras of history but on the stages of philosophical being and causation.

So from the start Thomas refrains from making a synthetic theology of history out of elements of salvation history.[223] That this does not mean any neglect of the Bible is shown by his many commentaries on scripture; at all events his *Summa theologiae* contains long sections on the six-day work of creation,[224] the old law[225] and the mysteries of the life of Jesus,[226] all topics which Neo-Thomists tend to neglect almost completely in their textbooks; the sections orientated on the Beatitudes, the fruits of the Spirit, the Decalogue and the charisms, which are also less philosophical than biblical, should also be noted.

Beyond question, with his two *Summas* Thomas set a high standard for theology. And today even his opponents will no longer dispute that he created a grandiose new theological synthesis for his time. A synthesis, yes – but also a new paradigm? The answer is, no. Why not?

Tied to existing Augustinian theology

Why couldn't Thomas – like Augustine – create a new paradigm, make possible a truly new entire constellation of theology and the church? Why didn't he become – as Luther did later – the initiator of a paradigm shift (P IV), although he did not lack either a new milieu (the university), or knowledge, perceptiveness and courage? The answer is that while with his philosophical theological system Thomas Aquinas quite substantially **modified Augustine's Latin paradigm**, he did not replace it.[227] Indeed, despite its encyclopaedic (but ultimately fragmentary) greatness, his theology has its indisputable **limitations** and **defects**. They are connected above all with his imprisonment throughout in the world-view of Greek antiquity, and especially with his problematical dependence on Augustine.

For however much Thomas may have corrected Augustine in some details, modified him and sometimes even ignored him, at the level of the truths of faith he remained essentially bound to the prevalent Augustinian theology. Certainly Thomas was no Neo-Augustinian (and Neo-Platonist) like Bonaventure. He was never able to accept that the human intellect is in some way in contact with the eternal divine truths. For him, in good Aristotelian fashion – knowledge comes from the senses. No, in

his epistemology and metaphysics, despite the fact that he retained certain
Neo-Platonic notions, Thomas was a convinced Aristotelian. Moreover
he never wrote as Bonaventure did about the mystical 'ascent of the soul
to God',[228] nor did he at the same time succeed in becoming a cardinal.
Thomas, constantly averse to ecclesiastical honours, remained a man of
the academy. He could have become Abbot of Monte Cassino or
Archbishop of Naples. He rejected both posts. He remained a scholar, a
researcher, to his last breath – almost.

Nevertheless, little though Thomas was an Augustinist as a
philosopher, he was one as a theologian, loyal to the distinction in his
system. He largely retained the second 'storey', the theological superstructure, the sphere of the 'supernatural' and the mysteries of salvation,
in the Neo-Platonic Augustinian tradition. Certainly he constantly
pointed out that the theology of Augustine and the church fathers use
Platonic conceptuality. But neither in the doctrine of the Trinity nor in
christology, neither in soteriology nor in the doctrine of the church and
the sacraments, did he fundamentally investigate behind the patristic
positions. Certainly he reflected on them with his Aristotelian conceptuality, in order to bring them up to date, refine them and confirm them. But
only rarely, and more tacitly, as in his doctrine of predestination,[229] did
he fundamentally correct them.

The French Dominican Marie-Dominique Chenu, who has written one
of the best historical introductions to the work of Thomas Aquinas, rightly
says: 'Thomas is very careful not to reject Augustine's texts even where he
has to say that Augustine is following the view of the Platonists; rather, he
respectfully uses the procedure of *expositio reverentialis* (respectful
interpretation) . . . In the mediaeval Renaissance Thomas can decide
against certain of Augustine's Neo-Platonic sources – in his theological
statements and his spiritual nature he is Augustine's loyal disciple.'[230]
Moreover Chenu can note a 'basic Augustinian stratum' in many details,
'without which Thomas cannot be understood, and which moreover is the
abiding world of all of mediaeval scholasticism as a common and
unchallenged possession of all the masters of the thirteenth century'.[231]

But Chenu, this great Thomist (wrongly condemned by Pius XII) who
performed such a great service in the renewal of French theology and the
French church,[232] does not go on to a critical evaluation of this evidence.
On the contrary, for him Augustine represents 'the embodiment of the
highest and purest Christian character and at the same time the religious
spirit in the original sense of the word'.[233] He is certainly not completely
to be contradicted here, since our account has also shown that Augustine
was the initiator of the Latin Roman Catholic paradigm and the father of
Western theology.

However, with such a 'canonization' of Augustine Chenu misses the fundamental **weaknesses** of the theology of Thomas Aquinas, which he unconsciously shares with Augustine:

– Thomas, although he had read some works by Greek theologians which had just been translated, did not see through either the one-sidednesses and defects of Augustine's 'psychological' **doctrine of the Trinity** (starting from the one divine nature[234]) or the further narrowing of the **doctrine of redemption** by Anselm of Canterbury's legalistic doctrine of satisfaction.[235]

– He did not criticize Augustine's notion of an **original sin** handed down since Adam to all human beings through the sexual act, and defends against the Greeks the doctrine of a **purgatory** which was similarly developed by Augustine for Latin theology.

– He took the reification of the understanding of grace (a concentration on 'created grace') considerably further, though at the same time, within the framework of his doctrine of grace,[236] he happily developed a *Quaestio* of his own on the 'justification of the sinner'.[237] But he neglects 'grace' as God's disposition, benevolence, graciousness[238] – as his teacher Albert the Great had already done. Instead, with the help of Aristotelian physiology and psychology, he analysed the different kinds of that *gratia creata* (which cannot be found in the New Testament), that created grace or 'gift of grace' (to be understood as sommething like a 'supernatural fluid or fuel'), and its effects on the substance of the soul, the intellect, the will, before, during and after the act of knowing and willing. These were all very impersonal, over-complex distinctions, which would already be obsolete in Luther's time.[239]

The problematical separation of reason and faith

A further question relates to the **split** which Thomas made **between reason and faith, philosophy and theology,** and focusses on the **subsequent influence** of Thomas. Already at that time not only was a distinction justified, but there was also the danger of a fundamental separation of research and piety, inwardness and externality, spirituality and corporeality, pastoral care and care for the world. Modernity was to draw conclusions from this: a belief in God apart from the world and a worldliness without faith, an unreal God and a godless reality. That was of course the last thing that Thomas himself had intended. But was his grandiose and balanced synthesis between reason and faith, nature and grace, philosophy and theology, secular and spiritual power sufficiently protected against this split? More precisely:[240]

– Is the lower level of the 'natural' truths of reason (the meaning of life, first principles of being, the existence of God, a natural law ethic) in fact demonstrated by such indisputable 'evidence' as Thomas Aquinas assumes?

– Is the upper level of 'supernatural' truths of faith (Trinity, Incarnation) in fact to be secured at a particular point as 'mysteries' against questions from reason or in the light of the New Testament, as Thomas secures it? And is the Bible on which Thomas commented so zealously not all too integrated into the strict system of apparently timeless doctrinal principles and in this way domesticated?

Certainly, Thomas Aquinas was a mediaeval man, not only in his view of the world but also in his faith, and he took it as a matter of course that reason is subordinate to faith, nature to grace, philosophy to theology and the state to the church. No truth of the upper sphere might or could ever be contradicted in the lower sphere, in philosophy or other disciplines. Thomas did not want any philosophy or ethics completely independent of theology. Yet in connection with the history of his influence the fact cannot be overlooked that the Christian mediaeval synthesis presented by Thomas is one of extreme tension, and in the dynamic of historical development had effects which were to prove self-destructive: there was to be an unprecedented and all-embracing **movement of secularization and emancipation** 'at the lower level'. We shall have to report on this later (P V).

A court theology nevertheless: support for papalism

There is yet another intrinsic weakness in Thomas' theology, which one can easily overlook if one first (rightly) emphasizes the innovative power of this theology and even refers to the history of his conflict with the *magisterium* of the church. But this weakness cannot be concealed, sobering though that may be for Thomas' admirers. For in his understanding of the church and above all the papacy, Thomas Aquinas differs both from Origen, who as a theologian remained critical of the hierarchy, and Augustine, who even as a bishop was anything but fixated on the Pope (as a papalist), but was more an episcopalist like Cyprian. In the end – and this must be said quite clearly – Thomas became the great **apologist of the centralist papacy** in the spirit of Gregory VII and Innocent III, and remains so today. His may not have been a court theology in the sense of subservient praise and glorification of those in power, but it was one in the sense of being a theological science which made an extremely effective contribution to the Roman system of power.

Certainly the man from Aquino claimed a **magistral** teaching office for theologians, which in contrast to the **pastoral** teaching office of the bishop was not to proceed authoritatively but by argumentation, and to rest on the academic competence of the magister. But at the same time he was able to incorporate the new political and legalistic development towards an absolutist papacy in the second half of the thirteenth century into the dogmatic system of theology. To what degree? One can compare him with Augustine:

– Whereas Augustine still does not even begin to think in terms of a primacy of jurisdiction of Peter, this primacy is at the centre of Thomas' view of the church.

– If for Augustine Christ himself and belief in him is the foundation of the church, for Thomas this supreme authority is the person and office of Peter.

– Whereas for Augustine the ecumenical council is the supreme authority, for Thomas it is the Pope, who alone may convene such a council.

– In short, contrary to the early church paradigm (P II) and even still to Augustine, this is a Gregorian **picture of the church derived completely from the papacy.**

What is the evidence? It is to be found in the little work *Contra errores Graecorum*, which Thomas wrote in 1263 in Orvieto at the behest of Pope Urban IV for his union negotiations with the emperor Michael VIII Palaeologus. Here Thomas, who knew virtually no Greek but now studied new Latin translations of the Greek fathers more punctiliously (especially those of W.von Moerbeke OP), presents to the Greeks, who were then politically weak, their 'errors' in the matters of the *filioque* and the **primacy of jurisdiction** of the Roman Pope. For towards the end of his work, in a number of chapters which teem with quotations from the Pseudo-Isidorian and other forgeries, Thomas 'demonstrates' with compelling logic 'that the Roman Pope is the first and greatest of all the bishops', 'that the same Pope has the pre-eminence over the whole church of Christ', 'that the same has the fullness of authority in the church', 'that in the same authority bestowed by Christ to Peter the Roman Pope is Peter's successor'.[241]

Thomas also demonstrates with reference to the papal **teaching authority** 'that it is for the Pope to define what faith is'; and all his chapters culminate in the fatal sentence, evidently formulated dogmatically for the first time by him and then included by Boniface VIII in the bull *Unam sanctam* ,'that it is necessary for salvation to submit to the Roman Pope'.[242] Thomas then also took his theses over in the *Summa theologiae*, which he began in 1265, where they were even more to make church history.[243] Cannot it be understood that this Thomas was not a faithful representative of the early church tradition for the Greeks, cannot be a teacher of the church, and is only to a limited degree a model for our present theological situation?

Nevertheless, it is an irony of history that few theologians made such an indirect contribution towards the destabilization of the papacy as Thomas of Aquino. He did so, of course, involuntarily, through his political philosophy.[244] How is that to be understood? Thomas, who also wrote a commentary on Aristotle's *Politics*, not only **revalued** nature over against grace, natural ethics over against Christian morality, and political philosophy over against theology, but also the **state over against the church**. This was a particularly important element for the process of secularization and emancipation, the foundations of which were laid at that time. Granted, in his work *De regno* Thomas regards the monarchy (moderated by aristocratic and democratic elements) rather than democracy as the best form of the state. But he does not advocate any theocracy ('one God – one Christ – one Pope – one emperor') either. Here we find independent talk of 'human law',[245] of the natural being of man, of human nature. And by thus attributing innate qualities, rights and duties to the individual, at least indirectly, Thomas laid the foundation for a humanism which was to develop subsequently.

The human individual is not simply a being subject to authority – the state or the church – nor simply an obedient subject who receives his rights in the church ultimately from the Pope, but rather a free citizen with natural rights and duties. Such a view became established above all in the cities with their ambitious classes: the city or the state is to be understood as a natural corporation of autonomous citizens, who alongside the supernatural church could make their own human laws. There is no doubt that in the long term this view of the state and society contributed to the downfall of the mediaeval papacy, as did the development of the idea of a national consciousness which was connected with it. Here of course the vernacular (completely neglected by Thomas in favour of Latin), which was becoming established everywhere (along with popular songs, popular literature and finally hymns), and the natural sciences which were soon to awaken, played their part.

So who would dispute that Thomas Aquinas, with no little courage and great openness, also accepted the challenge of non-Christian thinkers, posed by the 'pagan' philosophers of antiquity and above all by Aristotle. But what about contemporary Muslim and Jewish philosophers, like Averroes and Moses Maimonides?

Dialogue with Judaism and Islam

Thomas Aquinas was involved in **living discussion of the challenge of Judaism and Islam**. Nor did he content himself with the ignorance that was customary in the early Middle Ages, and ugly polemic against Islam and the Qur'an.[246] In particular his *Summa contra Gentiles* cannot be understood unless we sense the pressure that must have burdened some Christian intellectuals of the time: Isn't Islam both spiritually and culturally far in advance of Christianity? Doesn't it have the better philosophy? How can the option for Christianity rather than Islam and Judaism be justified?

'Thomas did not travel to Morocco nor to the land of the Mongols, and he did not utter a single remark about the Crusades' – thus Chenu, who continues: 'But he always had the works of the great Muslim philosophers on his desk, and he measured the dimensions of a Christianity which, having hitherto been included within the geographical and cultural frontiers of the Roman empire, now suddenly became aware that it embraced only a part of humankind and discovered the immeasurably secular condition of the cosmos.'[247] That is admirably put, but it is correct only if precisely at this point we once again take note of Thomas' limitations.

These limitations do not lie so much in the fact that Thomas 'did not travel to Morocco nor to the land of the Mongols' (Spain and Sicily would have been far enough). The limitations are substantial ones, and lie in the fact that Thomas did not know any Muslims personally, and did not engage in personal dialogue with any of them. But it is even more suspicious that Thomas did not write a single word about the Crusades, though Dominicans were also active in Palestine and though it had already proved that the Crusades were not having the hoped-for effect on the Muslims. Yet what is most dubious is that Thomas knew Islam at best from the works of the great Muslim philosophers, who were in any case more philosophers than Muslims, and not from the Qur'an itself, although on the initiative of Peter the Venerable (= 1156), the last significant Abbot of Cluny, the Qur'an was now available in Latin translations (more than one). So unfortunately Thomas had only a **rudimentary knowledge of Islam**; he had no access to the self-understanding of Muslims, who regard the Qur'an as the definitive revelation of God. His main informants may have been Christian missionaries who had evidently had difficulties in arguing against Islam. Whereas the Franciscans only attempted to influence the Muslims by simple preaching and practical example, at a very early stage the Dominicans also engaged in intellectual argument with Islam.

Moreover that explains the enquiry of a cantor from Antioch to Thomas about the Muslim doctrine of the unity and oneness of God, the Muslim denial that Jesus was the Son of God and of the crucifixion, and the problem of freedom of action. This is an enquiry to which Thomas responded with his usual acuteness, terseness and clarity, shortly after finishing the *Summa contra Gentiles*, in his short work **On the Grounds of Faith** (*De rationibus fidei*). However, significantly in his arguments he does not go back to the Bible itself. Rather, he presupposes the dogmas of the Trinity and Incarnation, formulated in the Hellenistic paradigm (P II) and understood in Augustinian terms (P III), as revealed by God himself. Then while he does not attempt to give a positive demonstration of the rationality of these dogmas, he does defend them in a critical and negative way against all Islamic objections. Christian faith is not irrational (contrary to reason), but it is not rational either (it cannot be proved); it is only reasonable (in keeping with reason).

This of itself tells against still using this short work or the *Summa contra Gentiles* as a model for Christian apologetic towards Islam, though Thomas doubtless seeks to adapt to the horizon of understanding of his conversation partner. Certainly in contrast to most earlier apologists of Latin or Byzantine origin Thomas argued in a way which was pleasantly neither polemical nor argumentative. But all this was not an *apologia ad extra* but at best an *apologia ad intra*, i.e arguing to the converted.[248] At that time only isolated individuals thought of an authentic inter-religious dialogue;[249] indeed in twelfth-century Paris the dialogue with the Jews which had still been going on had now been interrupted as a result of the Crusades, the expulsion of the Jews, pogroms and all their atrocities.[250]

So questions of a fundamental kind which arise from our analysis of the religious situation of the time are unavoidable about dialogue between Jews, Christians and Muslims:

Questions for the Future

✝ Is it sufficient, after the manner of Thomas Aquinas, to demonstrate that the dogmas of the Trinity and the Incarnation (P II) are not contradictory, rather than going back to the Qur'an, the Hebrew Bible and the New Testament? Shouldn't they in particular be understood in the Semitic context common to Jews, Christians and Muslims (P I), which displays a consistent monotheism? Shouldn't there be a critical re-reading of the dogmatic statements of the church in the light of its origins, taking into account the many things which Bible and Qur'an have in common and the relations between them, without disqualifying the dogmatic and magisterial rules of language a priori as apostasy from the gospel?

> **C** But conversely, is it convincing when Islamic theology starts in a purely dogmatic fashion from the absolute authority of the Qur'an (that the revealed book is uncreated, perfect and therefore immutable) and accuses the Hebrew Bible and the New Testament of falsification and corruption of the texts? Couldn't a comparison easily establish that the Hebrew Bible and the New Testament give historically more original accounts, with more authentic content, both of the history of Israel and the person and cause of Jesus, than the Qur'an? So isn't there also a need for a critical re-reading of statements in the Qur'an in the light of the Hebrew Bible and the New Testament, which need not contradict the basic Qur'anic mesage of the one and only God?

We have to reflect on one last point, which was to have a fatal influence: the position of women.

A problematical assessment of sexuality

By way of excuse, it has been said that for all his universality, Thomas did not understand three things: art, children and women. Because of his monastic and celibate way of life that is at least understandable in the case of women. But didn't he say quite basic and historically influential things about women and their nature? Defenders of Thomas point out that he only dealt with women here and there throughout his work, as it were incidentally. But at two crucial points even in the *Summa theologiae* there are quite basic statements about women: within the doctrine of creation a whole *quaestio* with four articles on the 'bringing forth' (*productio*) of the woman (from Adam),[251] and within the framework of the doctrine of grace an important article on the right of women to speak in church.[252]

Now it must be said straight away that for Thomas Aquinas there was no doubt:
– that **woman**, like man, is **created in the image of God**;
– that woman therefore in principle has the same dignity and the same eternal destiny for her soul as man;
– that woman was created by God not only for procreation but also for a shared life.

So Thomas Aquinas may not simply be depicted as a dark mediaeval misogynist. But is that a reason for playing down his other statements? In matters relating to the 'theology of the feminine', didn't Thomas **accentuate** and refine many of **Augustine's remarks** and as a result not tone down but intensify the contempt for women? Didn't he assert with reference to the biblical account of creation that man is the 'starting point and goal of woman', and that there is **something deficient and unsuccess-**

ful (*aliquid deficiens et occasionatum*) about woman?[253] Woman – a man who by chance is defective and unsuccessful, a *mas occasionatus*?[254] This remark of Thomas' has been much quoted.

This finding from the doctrine of creation explains why **women** had absolutely no say at all in the **mediaeval church**. Granted, in the light of the Old Testament they could not in principle be denied the gift of prophecy. But the **ordination of women** as priests? While Thomas was not able to discuss this in more detail in the *Summa*, since he broke off working on it, in his younger days he had come to a negative conclusion on this question in the commentary on the *Sentences*.[255] Not only the illegitimacy but even the invalidity of such an ordination is asserted here, and moreover this view was promptly taken up in the posthumous supplements to the ***Summa*** (***Supplementum***) as Thomas' valid position.[256] The same applies to women's preaching.[257]

But anyone who on the basis of all these negative statements immediately wants to pass a definitive, negative, judgment on Thomas should remember three things. First, Thomas is anything but original in many of his remarks; rather, in many cases he is simply expressing what people (men) thought at that time. Secondly, in some of his statements Thomas is simply basing himself on the Bible, on the Old Testament (for example women inherit only when there are no male descendants; no men in women's clothes) or even the New Testament (for example, woman created for the sake of man, women to keep silent in church). Thirdly, as a 'progressive theologian', for his knowledge of women Thomas followed the greatest scientific and philosophical authority of his time, to whom there was hardly any alternative: **Aristotle**. And it was Aristotle who in his treatise *On the Procreation of Living Beings* provided the biological basis for a fatal 'sexual metaphysics' and 'theology of the sexes'.

For already according to Aristotle a woman is a 'failed man'. Why? Applying his theory of act/form and potency/matter to physiology, Aristotle asserts that in the procreation of a new human being the **male** is the **sole active, 'procreative' part** by virtue of his sperm (the *virtus activa*). By contrast the woman is the **exclusively receptive, passive part**, the receptive matter which merely makes available the disposition (*virtus passiva*) for the new person. Thomas, too, asserts just this, and also follows Aristotle in replying to the difficulty why it is that in one case the male begets a boy and in another case a girl. This can be due to a weakness in the male procreative power or the female disposition or to an external influence: the north wind for a boy and the (moist) south wind for a girl, so that in one case a full man and in the other only a 'failed' man is born. We can imagine the devastating effect that such view had for centuries. For it was only in 1827 that the existence of a female ovum was demonstrated, and even later the precise way in which ovum and spermatozoa come together in procreation. All this is no excuse (Galen, the most famous doctor of Roman antiquity, had assumed an active biological role of the woman in the production of the foetus), but it does explain some things.

Nevertheless, for the sake of historical justice it must be added that in the face of the prevailing Augustinianism Thomas Aquinas contributed more than others of his time to a universal philosophical and theological **revaluation of the material reality of creation** (corporeality) and was more positive about sexuality than his teacher Augustine. However, that does not fundamentally alter the anthropology of Augustine and Thomas, which the Norwegian Catholic historian of theology Kari Børresen has investigated thoroughly in various fundamental works.[258] Her conclusion is that both Augustine and Thomas without any doubt advocate an **androcentric anthropology centred on the man**. Both regard the theory of the relationship between the man and the woman not from the perspective of a reciprocal relationship but from the perspective of the male. The male is seen as the exemplary sex and the nature and role of the woman are understood in terms of him. So there is hierarchical superiority and subordination instead of reciprocal complementarity. Thomas corrected Augustine in different ways without explicitly adopting a standpoint opposing him.[259]

If we now look back on Thomas' theology as a whole, above all his ecclesiology and anthropology, we cannot avoid noting that, leaving aside the philosophical substructure, his system is only qualifiedly a new theology. It is a systematic and speculative reshaping of the Roman Catholic paradigm with Aristotelian categories and arguments, but unfortunately also a **consolidation, accentuation and completion of the Roman Catholic paradigm** (P III) already initiated by Augustine and Leo.

However, Thomas would have been the last person to strive for any form of 'canonization' or even 'absolutization' of his theology. Within certain limits he was well aware of the contextuality of statements of faith and thus of their relativity.[260] The crisis in systematic speculative scholasticism had to come first – in late mediaeval nominalism (Ockhamism) it had become increasingly remote from the Bible and alien to the world, and had neglected the basic truths of faith and its existential character in favour of purely rational criticisms – for a new paradigm shift to be created: the paradigm shift to the Reformation (P IV).

The problem of the status of women, which we have just addressed critically in connection with Thomas, must concern us again because of its fundamental significance: the role of women generally in the Middle Ages, which are commonly called 'Christian'.

10. Christian Middle Ages?

Pope and emperor, power struggles and the fight against heretics, Crusades and mendicant orders, excommunication and Inquisition, university and theology: is that the whole of the Christian Middle Ages? Of course not. What else should be reported at the same time? One could report how in these selfsame high Middle Ages, in the time of the Hohenstaufens, the heyday of chivalry, the Minnesingers and the popular epic, the high Romanesque cathedrals of Worms, Mainz and Speyer were built and the breakthrough to Gothic had already been achieved with Notre Dame of Paris, with Chartres, Laon, Canterbury and Marburg. With their unique combination of reason and faith, with their refined vaulting technique and their mysticism of light, with their enormous variety of sculptures and stained glass and the strict unity of the architecture pointing upwards, these cathedrals have been called a 'scholasticism of stone'.[261] And the Middle Ages is in no way only the light age of cathedrals, universities and castles, but also the dark age of the great famines and epidemics, the hordes of the poor and the helpless sick. And above all it is not only a time of men but also of women, of princesses, nuns and madonnas.

Everyday Christian life

Christian life in the Middle Ages? Are the Middle Ages at the same time Christendom? Beyond question the Middle Ages were stamped by a unitary Christian world-view, as the Russian historian Aaron Gurjevich in particular has brought out.[262] Nevertheless they were not a uniform block, to be blackened as 'dark' or gilded as 'Christian'. They were **the living of a varied and colourful life.** That is already true of the history of **private life,** of the central tendencies, structures and milieux of the kind that Georges Duby and his team analysed and illustrated with pictures,[263] not chronologically, but typologically by means of different kindred relationships, customs, forms of abode, rites of piety and experiences of intimacy among the nobility, peasantry and citizens from the feudal age to the Renaissance (eleventh to fifteenth centuries). It is true of the various **types of mediaeval people** from monk and knight through peasant and city-dweller to artist and outsider, as ten distinguished contemporary mediaevalists under Jacques Le Goff have depicted them.[264] It is also true of the **culture** of the German **nobility,** under French influence, the literature of which has been analysed by the Cologne mediaevalist Joachim Bumke: from eating habits to court love or 'Minne'.[265] And finally it is also true of the **intellectuals,** among whom those thinkers and trends not connected with the university must be taken seriously, as Ruedi Imbach[266] and Alain de Libera[267] have brought out. Indeed, how complex these Middle Ages were (they were by no means a unitary Christian culture!), how inquisitive (about Arab, Jewish and Greek thought), how innovative (what bold new approaches not only from Thomas but also from Ramón Lull, Dante and Eckhart)! This was a century of faith, certainly, but as can already be seen right at the beginning, from Wolfram of Eschenbach's *Parsifal* epic, the most famous German poem of the Middle Ages, it was also an age of doubt. This was made clear by the great Abelard, author of the doubting, questioning *Yes and No*, who was violently castrated because of his love for his student Eloise, niece of a canon of Paris.

Indeed, how much could be told of 'barbarians, heretics and artists', of the 'worlds of the Middle Ages', and is told by the mediaevalist Arno Borst, a specialist in the Cathars[268] and in forms of life in the Middle Ages! In his book[269] he skilfully and colourfully illustrates not only the mediaeval interpretations of language, power and history, not only the religious, social and spiritual movements, but also the mediaeval experiences of art, science and play, of nature and finally also of mortality. All this of course is part of what we now call the 'Christian Middle Ages'. Indeed we must say even more basically and self-critically that what has necessarily concerned us for the most part in the analysis of the mediaeval paradigm so far is by no means the main axis of everyday mediaeval life. What did the normal Christians of the time, who could hardly read and write and had no access to any authentic news, know of the great battles between emperor and Pope, all the decretals and controversial writings? And how far in their everyday life were they interested in whether the emperor or the Pope ruled the world? The power or supremacy of the local bishop was much closer to them, and the citizens of the mediaeval cities, who had become self-confident, often rebelled above all against their bishops.

What was not part of **Christian life**, which quite practically and concretely was **dominated by the church**? The church was already present **acoustically**, with every stroke on the bell, which constantly announced the time and important events. And it was no less present **optically**: the churches and their towers (and in cities like Paris or Cologne there were whole landscapes of towers) stood out above citizens' houses, which were still modest, and even the above town hall: there were as yet no buildings for entertainment. Indeed for a long time the church also dominated mediaeval life **intellectually**, through its schools and its certainly impressive contributions to culture. The richly adorned church porches and the stained-glass windows and frescoes, as 'Bibles of the Poor' (*Biblia* pauperum), constantly displayed the most important saving events from the history of Israel and Jesus Christ – above all the proclamation, birth, miracles, passion and resurrection of Jesus. And there was the then still unrivalled liturgy with its splendid colour, its golden vessels and its unsurpassable solemnity, the processions, singing and soon also the playing of the organ: a true feast for the senses and the hearts of old and young, rich and poor.

There is no question that the great festivals of the church in particular were **community events** which interrupted the social and economic wretchedness of the populace in mediaeval cities in a welcome way. But there is also no question that the regular Sunday and feast-day liturgy at the same time represented a form of **social control** which gently forced everyone into a collective from which they could hardly escape at a time of limited mobility. Society and church were too interwoven, social life was too much also church life and vice versa. It is only modern times which have a disentangling of religion and society, a differentiation of the social sectors, of which the church is finally becoming just one. By contrast, in the Middle Ages society and the church were still undivided – as today is sometimes still the case with Islam in some places.

In any case, the great masses had no need to escape the church. Why? After all it was not only **collective joy** which kept people together but also **collective anxiety**. Wasn't it understandable that at a time of poverty, dirt, a lack of hygiene and medical provisions, of invasions wars, famines, plagues, early mortality and a high death rate generally, people welcomed any way of coping with their distress, their guilt and their anxiety? We have already heard about all the pious superstition, in part taken over from the Germanic period, and the pious works of the sacrifice of the mass, the veneration of saints and relics, the exorcisms and auricular confession, the blessings, litanies and pilgrimages. In particular, at that time ideas – often abstruse ones – developed about heaven, hell and **purgatory**. Jacques LeGoff describes in great detail – against the background of earlier notions of the next world – the 'birth of purgatory' in the twelfth century, where with the heyday of feudalism and the rise of a new middle class the noun *purgatorium* emerged for a place midway between heaven and hell and was clearly localized as an intermediate state in which men and women would have to withstand trials. Here is an originally Augustinian doctrine which was then made a dogma by the church, contrary to Greek theology, at the councils of Lyons (1274) and Florence (1439), and given unsurpassed poetic form by Dante Alighieri (died 1321) in the 'Purgatory' of his *Divine Comedy*.[270]

But mention should also be made – positively – of the mediaeval *ars moriendi*, an art and culture of dying. It did not let people die alone; they died in the midst of the community, surrounded by members of their family and strengthened by prayer and the church's rites for the dying.[271] To mediaeval people death was near and familiar, a constant companion, especially as in the twelfth century there was a new experience of personal, individual death, and in the fourteenth and fifteenth centuries death had become an unprecedented mass phenomenon as a result of the waves of pestilence. At that time people were aware of the meaning of life, because they were aware of the meaning of death. Is this the reason why in the Middle Ages not only atheism but also suicide was extremely rare? Certainly mediaeval religion was very strongly orientated on the next world, but people by no means forgot this world and all its needs because of the constant presence of the next world on the horizon.

Christian charitable work and the peace of God

Of course in the face of this sometimes cheerful, sometimes oppressive mediaeval piety of works we can ask: what is really Christian about it and what not? What is simply habit and what is inner conviction, what pure tradition and what Christian faith? What is a contemporary façade and what the truly Christian substance? But in our reflections on the change from late antiquity to the Germanic Middle Ages we could already see how[272] the typically mediaeval forms of piety which emerged newly in the Carolingian period were **variables** which cannot be absolutized and perpetuated as such. At the same time there is no disputing the fact that the **Christian substance** was preserved: the same gospel, the same entrance rite (baptism), the same community rite (the eucharist) and the same ethic (discipleship of Christ), however much these were overlaid, shifted and obscured. To claim anything else would be to suggest that the Roman Catholic paradigm is simply apostasy from Christianity.

Was there also the same ethic, discipleship of Christ? Perhaps not only Protestants will doubt this, of all things, and not be content with a reference to the men and women of the religious orders. Certainly there is no denying the fact that in the Middle Ages, too, indeed precisely then, discipleship of Christ was misunderstood. The discipleship of the cross was often confused with a cult of the crucifix, with mystical immersion in a private, obsequious sharing in the suffering of Jesus or even with copying the way of the crucified Jesus in his passion (the flagellant movements). And yet there were similarly countless mediaeval people who wanted to live out an **authentic discipleship of Jesus** unpretentiously in everyday life: not in an imitation of Christ but in a correlation, a correspondence to Christ. Christ had not in fact sought suffering nor just endured it, but had fought actively against it: committed to the weak and marginalized, of whom our history constantly knows so much less than of the upper classes. He actively attacked the powers of evil, sickness and death in a world which was not at all whole. And his message? Didn't it find its climax in the command to love one's neighbour, imperishably inculcated in the parable about the care of the man who fell among thieves? Wasn't there the story of the last judgment (Matt.25) in which the returning Christ judges people by the criterion of their commitment to the hungry, the thirsty, the naked, the strangers, the sick and imprisoned? Countless people lived out this form of Christianity in the Middle Ages as a matter of course, and all this belongs in a history of Christianity which is more than a history of the church. Truly the **history of authentic Christian life** and the history of the establishment of the church as an institution in a political power play are two different things!

So there is no disputing the fact that mediaeval Christianity in particular recognized active **charitable** work as its special task, the care of the suffering and the poor.[273] And the question arises whether the systematic care of the sick for the sake of Jesus has not become a specifically Christian concern which marks Christianity out from the other world religions. In fact at a very early stage bishops and deacons organized the **care of the sick** in the communities. Hospitals (*nosokomiai*) were created as early as the fourth century. And in the Middle Ages the care of the sick developed everywhere through the monasteries, especially after the Cluniac reform, but also as a result of the knightly and civil orders of Hospitallers. It was from this that the modern care of the sick by Catholic and Protestant orders and congregations developed. And there is no question that from the beginning to the present day women in Christianity have shown a special commitment to the care of the sick.[274]

Nor should the concern for **peace** in an unpeaceful time be forgotten: the high Middle Ages first of all saw a fight by a Christian peace movement in southern France against archaic customs widespread in the early Middle Ages like blood vengeance and feuds (often lasting for many years), the consequence of a Germanic law of self-help. Then these feuds were finally curtailed to a considerable degree all over Europe by bishops who proclaimed the *treuga Dei*, the 'peace of God', for all 'holy times': for Advent and Christmas, Lent and Easter, and for weekdays from Friday to Sunday. This was a 'peace of God' from the bishop which the king then made the '**peace of the land**'. Brutality disappeared, customs became more refined, and between 1100 and 1300 the robber knights of old often became the gallant knights of the Minnesingers and the tournaments. Now the attitude of contempt for the world increasingly disappeared, and art took a turn towards realism.

But we cannot discuss all this in more detail within the sober framework of our paradigm analysis. I must repeat that, first, we have to concentrate on Christianity (and not on culture generally). Secondly, it is impossible to depict all the colourful and varied life of Christians, important though it is for the way in which individuals have lived out their Christianity. The aim of our enterprise is to work out the dominant, paradigmatic basic structures which still persist even today. Some basic comments on everyday Christian life which identify the paradigm shift must suffice. And it becomes particularly specific in a decisive issue which has already occupied us in the context of P I and P II and which now also becomes a test case in respect of P III: the problems experienced by women, which became acute in the Middle Ages. Wasn't it in the Middle Ages in particular − quite apart from theology − that women clearly suffered a setback?

Women in the Middle Ages

Women in the Middle Ages: even more than in other eras, here research is in flux − driven on by feminist scholars who are convinced that above all in the churches the self-understanding and behaviour patterns of women today are still under the influence of the Middle Ages, which in a basically patriarchal way was still accustomed even when praising women to measure them by male criteria ('the weaker sex'!). However, it is proving easier for feminist research to reconstruct mediaeval theories, discourses and models than to rediscover how women really lived.[275]

Now we have indeed discovered the reasons[276] why despite all the beginnings made in antiquity and early Christianity women were prevented from having truly equal status even in the early church. They include the establishment of hierarchical structures and male domination specifically in the sacramental sphere; a hostility to sexuality which was typical of the time even outside the monasteries, in church and society; and finally the disparagement of education, which for women in particular was sometimes openly scorned. And we have similarly heard[277] how then in the Carolingian period a rigoristic sexual morality, both for the clergy (the prohibition of marriage) and for the laity (the prohibition of touching the sacred forms and the exclusion of women even from the sanctuary), broke through on a broad front. Nor should we forget the pernicious influence of the penitentials disseminated on the continent of Europe by Iro-Scottish and Anglo-Saxon monks, which attempted to repress sexual intercourse. 'A mediaeval world'? In the ideal view of the church that meant **a world governed by priests, monks, nuns and their ideal of continence.** These were not just the only vehicles of a written education but also occupied the highest rank on the Christian scale, because they already embodied the kingdom of heaven even now, without marriage and (private) property.

However, for the **married** this meant that precisely because the body was now regarded as a sacrosanct temple, it might only be united with a body of the other sex, if at all, if this union took place for the purpose of procreation. Contraception was therefore put on the same level as abortion and the exposure of children. So we can understand how Jacques LeGoff can speak of a great 'cultural revolution' (I would call it a paradigm shift) involving the body: after antiquity, which with its theatres, baths, stadia and arenas was so positive about the body, there was now a Middle Ages which despised the body (and especially the female body) as a prison of the soul, because it was the seat of sexuality and the 'infection of the flesh' by original sin. Here a '*déroute doctrinale du corporel*', 'a doctrinal derailment of the bodily',[278] became evident. All in all, this was a defeat for the body and the woman's body in particular, since this was seen as being particularly prone to the temptations of Satan; the beginnings of the witch-craze.

At the end of antiquity, when at least upper-class women had great opportunities, Roman law and culture still gave them some freedom. However, we might ask, didn't the free German woman originally also have a greater degree of personal self-determination, sexual freedom, economic independence and right to consent in marriage than has long been assumed? There is a discussion about this in contemporary feminist scholarship in connection with the **early Middle Ages.** This research is rewarding in providing a picture of how women really lived.[279]

For feminist scholars today are no longer content with the well-known fact that women could play a by no means insignificant role as **rulers:** women like Adelheid, Theophanu, Agnes or Constance, and also abbesses (e.g. Mathilde of Quedlinburg, the sister of Otto II) and other women of the aristocratic upper class already among the Merovingians, the Carolingians and the Ottonians. This was especially true of the 'first lady' of the empire (*consors imperii*), whose position was a considerable one, from the coronation liturgy to *de facto* regency or (if there were no descendants) even sole regency. Statues from the early Middle Ages portray king and queen side by side on equal terms. Even in the second half of the twelfth century the women in aristocratic lay society were usually more educated than their husbands, who were usually illiterate (as was even the Emperor Frederick Barbarossa). In France and Italy, too, these aristocratic women could always exercise considerable *de facto* political influence (but not constitutionally), in particular in **widowhood**: we may recall the widowed Margrave Mathilda of Tuscany, the mistress of Canossa, who was an indispensable ally to Gregory VII in his historical struggle. Women could administer dowries and possessions inherited from their husbands and freely decide to remarry.

But what does all this say about the social status and self-understanding of the mass of women at this time? Not very much. That noblewomen could in some cases become as significant as noblemen is merely the exception which proves the rule. For there is no overlooking the fact that even in the **high Middle Ages** the **social structure** continued to have an utterly **patriarchal** stamp. Granted, the fact that slavery had been abolished at least since the time of the Carolingians and had been transformed into 'serfdom' had a positive effect. But in the Christian Mediterranean, and especially in ports like Genoa, there were still countless slaves (male and female, not least from Muslim countries). So to the degree that women in the Middle Ages were free at all and not slaves or serfs, they were usually neither capable of holding a fief, nor could they swear an oath before a court, so they were not regarded as eligible for military service.

In the family and the home the will of the master of the house prevailed. Certainly women had their share of civic freedoms. But these were not personal freedoms in the modern sense; they were the corporate freedom of the middle class, the civic community, guilds and other corporations. Certainly the fully developed city offered women more possibilities than before, in crafts, retail and on occasion even wholesale trade. But we need to note that it did not offer them the same rights and the same rewards, nor did it offer them **any political say** – unless they belonged to a small class of regents and noblewomen. If we follow the study by the Bonn mediaevalist Edith Ennen of women in the Middle Ages for the area between the Seine and the Rhine, that second focal point in the development of mediaeval cities alongside the cities of upper Italy, we find 'that the woman had only a passive share in the great development of urban life in the twelfth and thirteenth centuries, as the consort and helper of the man'.[280] Specifically, that means: 'She was not one of the jurors in the cities of northern France, nor did she sit on the city councils which formed as urban organs in thirteenth-century German cities. She shared the risk of the serf, the small man who went to the city and started a new life there with the money that he had raised by selling his property or simply with his own labour. She contributed to her social rise, as far as the profits of a city merchant allowed her, by wearing valuable clothes, having maids, and living in and running a large and well-equipped house.

She already worked professionally in city trade. But we know little of that before 1250.'[281]

Of course circumstances varied greatly, depending on time and place. And anyone who does not pass a monocausal judgment will concede that there were several causes of the **gender-specific division of work** which resulted in a stereotyping of the roles of the sexes to the detriment of women:

– the **increase in the population** since the seventh century, possibly favoured by a warming of the climate between the tenth and twelfth century (a surplus of women is disputed);

– the development of **new techniques**, the heavy plough which went deeper and the use of horses which were shod and harnessed;

– the redevelopment of the Roman **cities** in the West which had contracted since the fifth and sixth centuries, and the marked influx from the country;

– the rise of a **middle class** with legal (not social) equality and free from the control of the lord of the city (who was usually a bishop).

– the development of an urban, mercantile, business **market economy** which deprived agriculture of its previous significance as the means of securing survival; but on the whole the crafts and trades were men's work, and the household was a household of women;

– the **university** and thus all the academic professions continued to be closed to women for centuries; the (male) scholars educated at the universities pervaded the authorities of land and city and were now indispensable as doctors, notaries and procurators. This forced women into merely auxiliary posts because they lacked academic training. For example, women could not become professional doctors, but could become assistants, nurses, midwives.

As the historian Annette Kuhn reports, much research into women in the Middle Ages revolves around the 'central question of the conditions and the reasons for the exclusion of women from the development of the capitalist economy'.[282] Following the American historian Martha Howell,[283] Kuhn distinguishes two interconnected but different systems which cross in women's work: the first system describes a 'sphere of work in which the woman works in her own capacities as mother, sexual partner, creditor, guarantor of subsistence (food and clothing) and for the market'. But a second system crosses with this: 'the economy in the sense of an economic movement starting from the capitalist market which among other things also leads to a hierarchy of work and an unequal evaluation of work, e.g. as productive and less productive work'.[284] Certain contradictions in women's lives can be explained from this duality of traditional household economy and the new mercantile capitalism. But so much for economics. What about the church?

Repression of women in the church

The church, too, presents a deeply ambivalent picture. Certainly it must be recognized that through its theology and practice of **marriage** the church contributed to the **revaluation** of woman in society. Thus in the twelfth century the church established that the mutual declaration of intent, in other words the **consent** of the partners, was an essential part of a marriage, and this presupposed their fundamental equality.[285] The church also saw to it that – contrary to a persistent abuse in the form of clandestine (secret) marriages – marriage was formally concluded in public. Indeed at this time, when the doctrine of the seven sacraments was developed, above all by Peter Lombard and Thomas Aquinas, marriage was given the status of one of the seven sacraments: this was the foundation for the indissolubility of marriage and strengthened the self-awareness of women.

On the other hand, the same church, in which the Pope appeared as the 'father' and the 'church' (hierarchy) as the 'mother' of Christianity, in which celibacy was forced on the secular clergy, and the codification of church law took on dramatic proportions, encouraged an intensified **patriarchalization** of the power structures and norms. Now there was a **repression of women** (in part also legal) which has remained a characteristic of the Roman Catholic paradigm to the present day. A symptom of that at the time was that the **ruler's wife** now had to be at a due distance behind her consort, accompanied by her ladies in waiting. The **abbesses**, who also had spiritual authority, were restricted to their jurisdictional authority. With an argument from the Old Testament, the **law of inheritance** was limited to the male (patrilinear) succession (unless male descendants were lacking). But even more important:

- **Canon law** (already the *Decretum Gratiani*) prescribed that women were subject to men with an argument from natural law.
- The **church's ideal** for women's existence was primarily **the nun**, who leads a continent life, well pleasing to God, free of earthly ties. Yet the lay culture and court poetry which arose in the twelfth century already shows a new secular ideal for women which was expressed by the Minnesingers, who were not only men but women (the existence of the latter is often overlooked), and was to be developed further in the Italian Renaissance.
- Women remained excluded from all **church offices**, and were even

repeatedly forbidden to preach because of the attractiveness of the Cathars and Waldensians, with their positive attitude towards women.

Unfortunately things were no better in the religious orders. Some monastic orders even opposed parallel foundations for women. The new religious **communities of women** which came into being in the spirit of Dominic and Francis (sometimes at the request of the women themselves and mostly by papal decree) were finally put under the corresponding male orders in order to integrate them into the established forms of church religious life. Other communities 'of virgins and widows dedicated to God', living in the world, which first formed in the Netherlands for religious and economic reasons and worked for a living with crafts and charitable activity, were even declared heretical. Their name, '**Beguines**', may be a truncated form of 'Albigensians', i.e. heretics (they were suppressed by the Council of Vienne in 1311). Here again we have a history of church persecutions which also affected the parallel male communities, the Beghards.[286]

Here, too, we certainly must not overlook the fact that within the sphere of the church at that time women had **space and possibilities of influence** which society did not offer them. There was space for unmarried women and widows who in their attachment to religious orders and the church found a safe, fulfilled existence with rich possibilities of education and influence and a new feminine self-awareness. Here, too, Edith Ennen may be right: 'In the dawn period of the twelfth and thirteenth centuries women thronged into the convents of their own free will purely to become disciples of Christ.'[287] That the nobility often used the convents as welfare institutions for daughters and widows is less important here than that the womenfolk of well-to-do parents received a basic education in reading, writing and doctrine in the cities, even outside the convents; however, only in exceptional cases could they get a specialist education.

But this **thronging into the convents** must not be confused with a political freedom movement for women. It derived from a pious movement which increasingly also took hold of the grass roots, from the mediaeval male world of the Benedictines, Cistercians and Premonstratensians, and finally the Franciscans and Dominicans, also taking over the world of women. But we should note that in the early Middle Ages the convents were virtually only for women from the aristocracy. And how deeply this class thinking was rooted is shown by the most significant woman religious of the time, **Hildegard of Bingen** (1098–1179).[288] Even in the twelfth century she wanted to maintain the privilege of the nobility, although leading monasteries like Cluny, Hirsau and later Citeaux had long since given up the privileges of birth. However, such class-specific separation could not be maintained any longer. For now an increasing number of urban patricians, daughters or wives of estate officials and citizens entered convents – to attain perfection in keeping with the gospel and certainly also to attain economic and social security and independence outside marriage. Still, for women from the middle and lower classes at this time it was sometimes difficult to get a place in a convent – either because the convents were full or because the women had no dowry.

Women religious were only rarely active in church politics: outstanding examples like Hildegard of Bingen, Birgitta of Sweden, Catherine of Siena and later Teresa of Avila are only the exceptions which again prove the rule. But there was one area in the high and late Middle Ages – apart from poetry (Hroswith of Gandersheim) and the crafts (weaving, embroidery) – in which women were not only men's equals but often showed more imagination and creativity: mysticism. Hildegard of Bingen was already a versatile writer and visionary mystic. And she not only published mystical books interpreting the world – that famous book *Scivias*, or 'Know the Ways' – but also composed works on nature and medicine which today are the most important sources for the knowledge of nature in Central Europe in the early Middle Ages. She composed seventy spiritual songs and undertook three great preaching journeys; she was a unique woman, in whom spirituality and empirical sensitivity, wide-ranging interests and mystical depths were combined. Mysticism – let us look at that more closely.

Mysticism under suspicion

Beyond question, **women** played a quite special role **in German mysticism**,[289] the significance of which has often been suppressed by men like Meister Eckhart, Johann Tauler, Heinrich Suso and Jan van Ruysbroeck. But like the Benedictine convent at Bingen by the Rhine under Abbess Hildegard in the twelfth century, in the thirteenth century the Cistercian convent of Helfta (close to Eisleben, later the place of Luther's birth and death), which was regarded as the 'crown of German convents', was an important centre of mysticism. Here Gertrude of Hackeborn, who was elected abbess at the early age of nineteen and was to lead the convent for forty-one years, was active, and here too lived a young sister who also had mystical gifts, Mechthild of Hackeborn. Gertrude of Helfta (later called 'the Great') was also accepted into the convent at a very early age. The convent was also the scene of the activity of Mechthild of Magdeburg, who had already become famous as a mystic with her six books of the

Flowing Light of the Godhead. Living as a Beguine in accordance with the rule of Dominic, Mechthilde had made enemies in the Dominican order in particular as a result of her reports of mystical experiences (for the first time in German!) and her criticism of the religious and secular clergy. She had every reason to complain bitterly about injustices and calumnies and finally to enter the convent of Helfta.

So what was the position over **mysticism in the church**? There is no question that it often represents a reaction to the way in which in the late Middle Ages the church was becoming increasingly worldly, theology increasingly academic and piety increasingly externalized. But didn't mysticism, which developed so richly especially in the late Middle Ages, in addition perhaps offer a new paradigm of theology and the church? What was its fascination? Certainly many people were attracted by:

– the tendency towards internalization, spiritualization and a concentration on essentials,

– the inner freedom from institutions, pious works and the compulsions of dogmatics,

– the overcoming of dualism, formalism and authoritarianism.

It should already have become clear that the '**mystical**' can no longer be identified – as it still is in popular terminology – with the enigmatic, strange, mysterious or simply religious ('mysticism' and 'politics'). It does not just involve phenomena like levitation, visions, ecstasy and stigmata, which since the second half of the nineteenth century have prompted physicians, psychologists, neurologists and philosophers, from the Paris psychiatrist J.-M. Charcot through William James to Sigmund Freud, to point to mystics as extremely interesting abnormal figures who need psychiatric clinical care; philosophers like Henri Bergson and theologians like Joseph Maréchal have effectively guarded them against this.

There is agreement at least among scholars that 'mysticism' – understood in the original meaning of the word – derives from the Greek word *myein*, which means to close one's mouth. Therefore the 'mysteries' are 'secrets', 'secret teachings', 'secret cults' about which one keeps as quiet as possible to those who have not been initiated. So not every form of spirituality is 'mystical', but precisely that form which closes its mouth about its hidden mysteries to profane ears, in order to seek **salvation within itself**. That presupposes a readiness to turn away from the world, though this does not necessarily mean a flight from the world, but an inward detachment and freedom in the spirit. It thus means inwardness, and finally, in ecstastic moments, the surging feeling of direct unity with the universe, with the Absolute – these are the characteristics of mysticism. And all this does not happen in a wild and arbitrary way, but in an ordered and methodical progress:

– first of all an often tense and deliberate **concentration** induced with various physical and psychological means;

– then relaxed, passive, self-forgetful, rapt **contemplation**;

– finally, elevated or profound **ecstasy** in which the person loses himself or herself in the immeasurable fullness of the Absolute.

Thus – leaving aside abnormal, simulated, projected, pathological phenomena and all forms of pseudo-mysticism in which the Absolute is replaced by a surrogate – mystical experience can be defined quite generally as a **direct and intuitive experience of unity**: as the intuition of a great unity with nature or the absolute ground of Being, which transcends and abolishes the split between subject and object. But none of the mediaeval mystics, women or men, is concerned with just any kind of romantic nature-mysticism, with unity with nature, the cosmos, 'life', or with a pantheistic experience of identity. The experience is not one of immanence but of transcendence, which brings happiness, yet is transitory and incomplete. The moments of ecstasy are about the unity of the whole person with the primal ground of reality, with that embracing, comprehensive, all-determining, first and last reality before which our understanding begins to stutter, our concepts fail and our ideas vanish away. So this is **the** 'mystery', the 'mystery' of reality, the flowing 'light' of the Godhead.

Thus the Christian mystics in no way want to turn the things of nature into God (the divinization of the universe) or necessarily to see God 'from within' (his trinitarian 'processions'). But they do often experience the Absolute directly, by contemplating either scenes from the Bible or even nature. However, they do not understand this experience to be self-generated; it is 'granted', 'given': the **presence** of God, **fellowship, unity with God** as overpowering grace and love.

Moreover, already for Thomas Aquinas, the Absolute, Being itself, is present in every grain of sand and every flower, though Thomas would never have allowed world and God, soul and God, to flow into each other. This happens first under the influence of Christianized Neoplatonism after Thomas' time: in addition to the women mystics, with Dietrich of Freiberg and his great pupil **Meister Eckhart** and his school. Whether Dietrich of Freiberg, Albertus Magnus or Thomas Aquinas was the starting-point for Eckhart is as disputed today as the assessment of the Inquisition process, which forced this highly respected preacher, professor of the University of Paris, provincial and Vicar General of the order, at the age of sixty-seven to make a journey to Avignon, where he was interrogated, but died before his condemnation could be pronounced.[290]

But the 'German mysticism' which gained international influence through Latin works (or in translations) is by no means a singular phenomenon. In the Middle Ages – if we leave aside the early more intellectual Areopagitic mysticism in the monastic school of St Victor of Paris under its Flemish (or Saxon) leader Hugo and his pupil Richard, a Scot, in the twelfth century – there were numerous **waves of mysticism** througout Europe which, as Otto Karrer,[291] an sympathetic expert in mysticism, noted, take place with remarkable time-lags:

– **Italian** mysticism in the thirteenth century (Francis, Clare, Angela of Foligno, Margaret of Cortona);

– **German** mysticism in the thirteenth/fourteenth centuries (its three stars, Meister Eckhart, Tauler and Suso) and the **Flemish-Dutch** mysticism of Jan van Ruysbroeck and his pupil G.Groote, who with Thomas à Kempis was author of the much-read *Imitation of Christ*;

– **English** mysticism in the fourteenth/fifteenth centuries (Richard Rolle, the anonymous author of the *Cloud of Unknowing*, Julian of Norwich);

– **Spanish** mysticism in the sixteenth century (Ignatius of Loyola, Francis Xavier, Teresa of Avila, John of the Cross, Luis de León);

– **French** mysticism in the seventeenth century (not only the Oratorians Bérulle and Condren but men and women from the Carmelite, Ignatian and Dominican schools).

And yet we must realize that mysticism is **not a specifically Christian phenomenon**. Not only is mysticism older than Christianity; it also comes from far away. Mystical religion already came into being at a very early stage – in the late Vedan period – in **India**. Thus a doctrine of unity is formulated in the Upanishads, and meditative practices aimed at a direct experience of union are handed down, promising redemption from ignorance through knowledge: through the knowledge of Atman, the essential core of the individual, and its identity with Brahman, the world principle that pervades all things. Possibly (this can only be guessed at) the broad stream of mysticism in Asia Minor, Greece and the Hellenistic world which finally leads to Christianity also issues from India: beginning with the pre-Socratic Ionian metaphysicians, Orphism and the Pythagoreans, through Plato and the late-Hellenistic mystery cults to the other Neoplatonists. We have already met that mystical philosopher who under the mask of Paul's disciple **Dionysius the Areopagite** in the fifth and sixth centuries wrote his book *Mystike theologia*, from which our word 'mysticism' derives. He, at any rate, learned more from Plotinus and Proclus than from Paul and John, and the Latin translation of his book made by John Scotus Eriugena (in the ninth century) largely governed mystical piety in the Christian West. Down to the nineteenth century Dionysius was regarded as an authentic disciple and his writings were thought to date from the first century and thus from earliest Christianity. But the decisive question for our paradigm analysis is:

Was earliest Christianity mystical?

Were Jesus and his apostles and disciples mystics? Certainly there were mystical elements even in early Christianity, in Paul and John, to the degree, for example, that we find talk of possessing the Spirit. And we have seen that Alexandrians like Clement and Origen, contemporaries of Plotinus, and then also the North African Augustine, combined the originally biblical and prophetic religion with Hellenistic mystical elements and tendencies. However, here one can hardly yet talk of mysticism in the strict sense. There is **mysticism in the authentic sense of a unitive mysticism** only where the experience of unity between God and the human soul is striven for. And who could overlook the fact that this unity is not to be found either in **Paul** or in **John**? What is normative for them is trusting faith in God and active love of the neighbour, not the mystical vision or the possession of God. Indeed what matters for them is a hope orientated on the future rather than bliss in the present. Despite his use of mystical thinking, Augustine, too, explicitly opposed the Neo-Platonic pantheistic flowing together of soul and God, however much he in particular knew the desire of the human heart which is restless until it rests in God. In him we find no being taken up into God but rest in God through being free, seeing, praising and loving without end.

But the most important thing is that **Jesus** himself was **no mystic**. Only two visionary states are related in connection with him (which are not historically certain), but this does not alter the decisive fact: for Jesus the world was not a vanity from which one had to withdraw, the nothingness of which was to be seen in the act of immersion; far less was it simply to be identified with the Absolute. Rather, the world was the good creation, even if it is constantly corrupted by human beings. What did Jesus require of people? Extraordinary ecstatic experiences, ruminating speculations about God's nature, psychological self-dissection and unhistorical techniques of immersion? No, love of God and love of neighbour. Beyond doubt Jesus stands in the line of the Old Testament prophets[292] and not that of the Indian mystics, and the saying 'I and the Father are one' which is constantly quoted does not come from Jesus himself but from the Fourth Evangelist. Nor does it denote any mystical unity between God and his Christ but a unity of will, action and revelation between the man Jesus and God, between the Son and the Father: 'Whoever sees me sees the Father.'[293]

Thus Jesus is understood adequately only when he is understood as an **emissary and pioneer in the prophetic spirit** who is seized with a passion, as God's anointed ('Messiah', 'Christ'). He does not teach any spiritual technique for redemption from guilt and all evil, but calls on people to repent. Instead of requiring the surrender of the will he appeals specifically to the will, which he calls on men and women to bring into line with the will of God, intent solely on the comprehensive well-being, the salvation, of humankind. So he proclaimed a love which makes personal demands, which includes all who suffer, are oppressed, sick and guilty, and even opponents and enemies: a universal **love** and an active **beneficence**.

Here may be the most profound substantive theological reason why mysticism has never become paradigmatic in Christianity, in complete contrast to India. Indeed it is quite striking how **in India mysticism** has a recognized place, at the centre of many of the great classical traditions. There mysticism is not regarded at best as an enrichment, as it is in Christianity, but constitutes the innermost essence of religion. There extraordinary experiences beyond normal consciousness form the climax of the life of mystical piety: new dimensions of perception and know-ledge, ecstasies and ecstatic visions and auditions, in which the stimulation of the senses is combined with purely spiritual experience. Such mystical experience in Hinduism is never merely naive, but is usually associated with a high degree of reflection, regardless of whether this is philosophical speculative thought, as in the Upanishads, or precise psychological self-analysis as in Yoga.

If we follow the ideal-typical profile constructed by Friedrich Heiler here,[294] the basic experience of **prophetic piety**, which is characteristic also of Jesus, is quite different. We find it at every step in the Bible. It is characterized by a strong will for life: an urge towards assertion, a being grasped by values and tasks, a passionate effort to realize particular ideals and goals. So prophetic piety is primarily directed outwards; it is in confrontation with the world and seeks to become established in it. To this degree the person with a prophetic orientation is a figure who struggles to move from doubt to the certainty of faith, from uncertainty to trust, from the consciousness of sin to the attainment of salvation by grace. Even the most devotional psalms know of no ecstatic unity, but only of trusting security in the God of grace and mercy.

So is it entirely surprising that wherever mysticism in Christianity threatened to be the main thing instead of an enrichment, it came up against resistance? Moreover, **conflicts with the official Roman Catholic Church**, which feared the loss of its monopoly of the communication of word and sacrament, accompany the rise of mysticism like a shadow. But why here (P III), in contrast to the East (P II), was there always repression and excommunication? As we heard, the translator of the works of Pseudo-Dionysius, John Scotus Eriugena, was condemned by a council in Valence in 855 for his views of predestination. The writings of the mystics, men and women, were constantly suspect; indeed, many great mystics like Meister Eckhart, Teresa of Avila, John of the Cross and Madame Guyon (and her protector Fénélon) were pursued by the Inquisition. And that Beguine, the mystic Marguerite Porete, who around 1300 had written the *Miroir des simples âmes* ('mirror of simple souls'), was not just condemned as a heretic by the Bishop of Cambrai in 1306. Marguerite, whose work lived on after her condemnation in four languages and six versions, but anonymously, and apparently had an important influence on Meister Eckhart,[295] was again accused in 1308, transported to Paris, interrogated by the Inquisition (here she refused to say anything about her teaching) and was finally burnt at the stake in 1310.[296]

Nor is it surprising that – for all the influence of Tauler and the *Theologia Teutsch* (by a secular Frankfurt priest around 1400) on Martin Luther – mysticism did not feature in the paradigm shift of the Reformation (P IV) either, and that subsequently almost all **Protestant mystics stood outside established Protestantism**, either because they were compelled to or because they themselves wanted to. Moreover, to the present day mysticism has met with anything from mistrust to rejection in the Protestant sphere. The early 'dialectical theology' of Karl Barth, Emil Brunner and Friedrich Gogarten rejected it radically at the beginning of our century. Here, too, the reasons were its hybrid identification with God (self-divinization, pantheism, 'righteousness by works'), unchurchly inwardness (subjectivism), and a contempt for creation ('Manichaeism', 'Quietism').

Although these charges often lack a substantive basis, they do explain why mysticism still leads a marginal existence in the sphere of theology and the church. In this way it could never form a paradigm, an entire constellation, for theology and the church. Mistrusted and suspected, vilified, sometimes even suppressed, at best it could survive in the sphere of monasteries and convents and small circles of 'initiates', without really renewing the church fundamentally. At any rate the **Roman Catholic paradigm,** as it had already become established in the Middle Ages, was **at best disturbed, but never shaken** by mysticism.

Moreover in the late Middle Ages, as in the Reformation, what was normative for Christian spirituality was not mystical immersion but **prayer** – the expression of believing trust in God. Indeed prayer in the Bible is amazingly natural and uncomplicated – in the midst of life and from life: often a naive 'outpouring of the heart' in simplicity and unbroken realism. And it is all utterly addressed to God: a petition for hearing, help, mercy, grace, salvation for oneself, for others, for the people. It is a petition which develops freely, and also a wish and a protest, but above all thanksgiving and praise.

And however much in the course of history biblical prayer, too, can become fixed in formulae, liturgically stylized, refined and sometimes even combined with ascetic efforts, remarkably the Bible knows
– no talk of methods, systems, a psychological technique of prayer;
– no stages of prayer to be gone through, no uniformity of religious experience;
– no psychological reflection on prayer, for all the prophetic criticism of prayer and sacrifice, no self-examinations and ascetic efforts to achieve particular states of the soul.

Instead of this there is a naively unreflecting 'conversation with God': expressions of faith, hope, love, thanksgiving, praise and intercession – in great individual variety.

All this means that a mystical attitude of prayer can be important for Christians, but **it cannot claim normativity**, as if mystical immersion were the highest form of prayer. So for all the admiration for the great **Teresa of Avila**, that brilliant woman who is one of the most significant mystics in the history of religion, in neither the Old nor the New Testament is there any ideal of an inner prayer or a prayer of the heart; there is no invitation to observe, describe and analyse mystical experiences and states. No stepladder of mystical prayer leading to ecstasy can be recognized, and there is no emphasis on any prayer which presupposes a special religious gift. Mystical prayer is a charism, just one charism among others, and not the highest. It can serve the discipleship of Christ which culminates in love, but it can also – if it becomes an end in itself – lead away from it.

So not all great religions derive from mysticism as the 'real' religion, the 'essence' of religion, as philosophers and psychologists of religion have constantly attempted to demonstrate. Artificial harmonizations between the religions are no more help than the exclusiveness bred by dogma. In our time a **mutual interpenetration of these two basic types of religion**, the mystical and the prophetic, is possible, desirable, even necessary, not just at the periphery but at the centre of the understanding of God. For example, Thomas Aquinas' understanding of God beyond doubt needs to be supplemented by that of the Christian mystic, his brother religious **Meister Eckhart**. According to the latter's intellectual view God creates the world and human beings **in himself**, and God's own being extends into things, so that the deep unity of all entities in God can be experienced in the 'ground of the soul': this is not a substantial but an 'energetic' unity. And according to **Nicholas of Cusa**, God's abundant fullness contains all opposites in itself, so that God is at the same time the greatest and the smallest, centre and periphery, past and future, light and darkness, indeed even being and non-being. These are opposites which are one in God but separate in the world: in that world which is to be understood as *explicatio Dei*, as the unfolding of that God who himself is the many without multiplicity and the opposite in identity.[297]

As we saw, mediaeval piety is unthinkable without mysticism, especially women's mysticism, although this mysticism could never become paradigmatic for theology and the church. But mediaeval piety is also unthinkable without the growth of Marian piety, in which the paradigm shift can once again be demonstrated vividly – to some degree in the micro-sphere.

Veneration of Mary on the increase

Here we must note in advance that much as veneration of Mary increased in the Latin high Middle Ages, not only in church customs, in church festivals and ceremonies, but also in poetry and art, it must nevertheless be recognized that **veneration of Mary first** developed **in the Hellenistic Byzantine paradigm** (P II).[298]

For in the **East** there was an age-old tradition of the cult of mother deities, particularly in Asia Minor, which could be fruitfully used for veneration of Mary: in the form of a cult of the 'perpetual virgin', the 'mother of God' and exalted 'queen of heaven'. It was in the East that Mary was first invoked in prayer ('Under Your Protection', third/fourth centuries), and the commemoration of Mary was introduced into the liturgy. It was in the East that legends about Mary were first told and hymns to Mary composed, churches were first named after Mary, Marian feasts introduced and images of Mary created.

The dogmatic statements about Mary can only be explained against this background. For only a council in the East could arrive at the idea of committing the church to belief in Mary as 'Mother of God', namely the **Council of Ephesus** in 431. We know now that this momentous christological statement particularly corresponded to the political interests of a man who knew the grandstand ploys with which to manipulate this council: Cyril of Alexandria. Even before the arrival of the other party in the council from Antioch, which had spoken of Mary as '**Mother of Christ** (*christotokos*), he had succeeded in carrying through his definition, 'Mother of God' (*theotokos*).[299] This was a new title, remote from the Bible, which was to provoke formulae even more open to misunderstanding.

So only in the East, in Ephesus, had it been possible to establish such a mariology, in a city whose inhabitants in any case worshipped the 'Great Mother' (originally the virgin goddess Artemis, Diana) and accordingly welcomed the substitute 'goddess' Mary with enthusiasm. The theological price paid for this did little to disturb such enthusiasm: the fact that the formula 'Mother of God' was suspect of Monophysitism (which was then corrected by Chalcedon) and led to a reification of the understanding of the divine Sonship and the incarnation. As if 'God' could be born, rather than a human being who as God's 'Son' is God's revelation for believers! This talk of a 'Mother of God' is partly responsible for the Jewish mistrust of Christianity even now and the present misunderstanding of many Muslims that the Christian Trinity is a triad consisting of God (father), Mary (mother) and Jesus (child).

By contrast, in the **West** Eastern forms of piety connected with Mary did not become established without resistance. For example, in Augustine, at any rate, the theological father of the Latin mediaeval paradigm (P III), we find neither hymns nor prayers to Mary; not even feasts of Mary are mentioned. That is striking. Only in the fifth century do we find the first example of Mary being addressed in a Latin hymn ('*Salve sancta parens*', Caelius Sedulius). From this an increasingly rich Latin and later also German body of poetry to Mary developed in the late sixth century.[300] Rome, too, now followed: in the sixth century Mary's name (and the title '*Mater Dei*') was incorporated into the text of the mass; in the seventh century the Eastern feasts of Mary (Annunciation, Visitation, Birth, Purification) were introduced; towards the end of the tenth century legends were in circulation about the miraculous power of prayer to Mary.

Beyond doubt the climax of the mediaeval cult of Mary came in the eleventh/twelfth century; it is inconceivable without the influence of the Cistercian monk Bernard of Clairvaux. In the meantime the theological accents had increasingly shifted. It was no longer the role and activity of Mary as the earthly mother of Jesus as depicted in the New Testament that now stood in the foreground. What was now decisive was **Mary's cosmic role** as the virgin mother of God and queen of heaven. Coupled with this was a process of idealization and exaltation. Whereas earlier church fathers still had spoken without hesitation about moral faults in Mary, now a perfect sinlessness of Mary was increasingly asserted, indeed a holiness even before her birth.

Here it was only logical that from the twelfth century on there were even individual voices which explicitly asserted that **Mary** had been **preserved from original sin** – which since Augustine had now become something like a basic dogma of the Catholic Church. Granted, at first such an exception to the fate of all humankind could not be established because of the opposition of the theologians, and especially of Thomas Aquinas. But this did not prevent the significant Franciscan theologian Duns Scotus (1308) later from seeking a 'speculative solution' and arguing: how can one maintain the dogma of the universality of original sin and at the same time declare Mary the exception? So Scotus invented the term 'anticipatory redemption' (*redemptio praeservativa*) of Mary – a purely theological construction. But now it was even harder to stop the process of the exaltation of Mary. Formally, distinctions were still maintained and were made between the general veneration of saints (*doulia*), heightened veneration of Mary (*hyperdoulia*) and worship of God (*latria*). But in practice Mary's creatureliness and humanity often played a slight role.

However, the Mary of doctrine was one thing; the Mary of piety was another. In **popular piety** Mary, like Jesus himself – not least under the influence of Bernard and especially Francis of Assisi – took on more markedly human features. Mary appears in many prayers, hymns, songs and in many pictures and statues as the embodiment of mercy, as the intercessor who can obtain virtually anything from her heavenly son, as a lovable figure who stands nearer to human cares than the ascended and exalted divine Christ. Gothic style created an impressive 'cloaked Madonna' for this piety. She expresses in a unique way what millions of people often felt about Mary: she is the helper particularly of ordinary people, the oppressed, the anxious and the marginalized. A piece of mariology 'from below' becomes visible here, which contrasts with the dogmatic super-theories of 'Mary' among theologians, monks and hierarchs. This also explains the popularity of the biblical *'Ave Maria'* from the twelfth century on; together with the 'Our Father' it became the most widespread form of prayer, though only since 1500 has it been prayed in its present form with a petition for support in the hour of death. It also explains the popularity of the 'Angelus', rung three times a day since the thirteenth century, and the prayer of the rosary, which has been practised since around the end of the thirteenth century.

An ecumenical image of Mary?

The church in the Middle Ages guarded only against one thing: proclaiming any new **Marian dogmas**. This was reserved for the Popes of the nineteenth and twentieth centuries, Pius IX and Pius XII. Pius IX in particular immediately burdened the church with two dogmas by his policy. Having already formally elevated to dogma, without any biblical foundation, Mary's Immaculate Conception (preservation from original sin) in his counter-revolutionary conservatism opposed to the Enlightenment, science, democracy and freedom of religion, sixteen years later with the help of Vatican I (1870) he also forced on the whole church the primacy and infallibility of the Pope. Pius XII continued this line after the

Second World War. Unconcerned in his Roman triumphalism about Protestant and Orthodox reservations and reservations within Catholicism, he had the ambition also to promulgate Mary's bodily assumption to heavenly glory as a dogma; and did so in 1950 as the climax of a 'Marian Age' which he himself then proclaimed.[301] Numerous appearances of Mary which 'took place', hardly by chance, in the nineteenth and early twentieth century (Lourdes, 1858 and Fatima, 1917) also fit in this 'Marian climate'.

Thus what was not yet so clear in the Middle Ages was plainly demonstrated by the Pius Popes: here and only here **papalism and Marianism** go hand in hand as typical of the Roman Catholic paradigm. The background is doubtless the **celibacy** which – as we heard – is deeply rooted in the mediaeval world. In the face of this development, the leading Catholic professor of feminist theology in Europe, the Dutchwoman Catharina Halkes, asks doubtfully: 'Is Mary a possible model which was exploited against women, which was not critical of men and which was to legitimate the gulf that the church had left open between (female) sexuality and the mediation of the saints?'[302] Beyond question a mediaeval Roman Catholic hierarchy which has remained mediaeval down to the twentieth century (with a Pope like John Paul II, who has replaced the cross in the middle of his coat of arms with an M), which propagates celibacy for the clergy even in the face of thousands of parishes without pastors, and wants to tie sexual pleasure in the sphere of marriage to the procreation of children, created in the form of Mary a compensatory figure for unmarried clergy with whom in a 'spiritual way' one could experience intimacy, kindness, femininity and motherliness. Eugen Drewermann has described and analysed, with many examples, the fatal psychological consequences that this policy can and does have.[303]

It is also important to reflect on the effect of this Roman Catholic Marianism on the Christian **ecumene**. Thus the Protestant theologian Jürgen Moltmann rightly points out: 'We have to note honestly and soberly that so far mariology has been more against ecumenism than for it. Mariology, as it has been developed further and further, has alienated Christians from Jews, the church from the New Testament, Protestant Christians from Catholic Christians and Christians generally from modern men and women. But is the madonna of the church's mariology identical with Miriam, the Jewish mother of Jesus? Can we find the one in the other? Given the splits and separations which have been perpetrated in the name of the Madonna of the churches, should we not ask about the Jewish mother Miriam herself?'[304]

Indeed, given this development in the framework of the mediaeval paradigm, it is appropriate to pause to reflect on what might be the **future for the church**. The figure of Mary needs to be liberated from certain images – from both the fantasies of a male celibate priestly hierarchy and the fantasies of women engaged in a compensatory search for identification. There can be no question here of spiriting away, indeed of destroying, the significance of Mary for theology, the church and the history of piety. Rather, the figure of Mary must be interpreted for our time in terms of her origins and liberated from so many misogynistic clichés and paralysing stereotypes. The aim must be to make the way free for a truly **ecumenical image of Mary**, so that the saying in Luke, 'Behold, from henceforth all generations shall call me blessed', can again hold in all the Christian churches.[305] There is still dispute among feminists as to whether Mary can be an inspiring figure with whom they can identify. But at all events the following guidelines for an ecumenical picture of Mary seem to me to be important.

- According to the New Testament Mary is an utterly **human being** and not a heavenly being. The picture of Mary in the New Testament is extremely matter-of-fact and in part also contradictory. The earliest evangelist tells us only of a conflict between mother and son; Jesus' mother, like his family, thinks him crazy.[306] The earliest Gospel also knows no legendary story of Jesus' birth, says nothing about a virgin birth, of Mary standing by the cross, or Mary at the resurrection. It is only the later Gospels, depicting a believing, obedient Mary, which recount all that has become so deeply impressed on Christianity through the history of Christian art.[307] So already in the New Testament a distinction must be made between Mary as a historical figure and Mary as a symbolic figure[308] – as virgin, mother, bride, queen, intercessor.[309]

- According to the testimony of the New Testament Mary is above all the **mother of Jesus**. As a human being and a mother she is a witness to his true humanity. And this testimony to Jesus' humanity is not in contradiction with the faith also expressed in the New Testament, that Jesus' existence can ultimately be explained only in the light of God, has its deepest origin in God; that for believers he is the Son sent by God and chosen by God.[310]

- Mary is the example and **model of Christian faith**. Already according to the evangelist Luke, her faith, which is not spared the sword of offence, division and contradiction, and which experiences its greatest tribulation in the face of the cross, is in fact an example for Christian faith.[311] So Mary does not display any special faith, any special insight into the mysteries of God. Rather, her faith, too, undergoes a history and thus marks out the way of Christian faith.

- Mary points to the cause of her Son, to the **cause of Jesus of Nazareth.**
Mary's cause is none other than Jesus' cause, which is God's cause.
Here too Luke has set the right emphases. Mary's key words *Fiat* and
Magnificat still make sense today. Mary praises a God who 'casts down
the mighty from their thrones and exalts the lowly'.[312] And Mary's son,
Jesus, does not have 'typically male' or 'patriarchal' features. Mary's
son is more the friend of women, whom he calls to follow him as
disciples and helpers, among them Mary Magdalene, who was
venerated in the early communities as an intimate friend of Jesus.[313]

So those who attack the discrimination against women in the church
which has lasted since the Middle Ages cannot appeal to Miriam/Mary
and her son. No commands for women to be silent or submissive issue
from the lips of Mary and Jesus. Neither knows any 'Eve myth' which
makes women responsible for all the evil in the world. Neither knows any
vilification of sexuality, any degradation of the woman as an object of
pleasure or defamation as a universal seductress. Nor does either know
any law of celibacy, though strikingly Jesus was unmarried; nor do they
know any fixation on marriage. To this degree the apostle Paul
interpreted the cause of Mary and Jesus sympathetically when he wrote
about Christ, the exalted Lord, 'For freedom he has set us free.'[314] And
'Where the Spirit of this Lord blows, there is freedom.'[315] In the sphere of
this freedom there is no place for sexual discrimination, devaluation of
women, making sex tabu, emotionality, feminine corporeality, submission to a male hierarchy. In the sphere of this freedom which Christ
embodies, 'There is neither male nor female, for you are all "one" in
Christ Jesus.'[316]

But the crisis of papalism, marianism and celibacy, which is manifest
today even to traditional Catholics, was already developing in the late
Middle Ages. We must now turn to it.

11. The crisis of the Roman Catholic paradigm

No one suspected that the change from papal world power to papal
powerlessness could take place so abruptly. At the beginning of the
thirteenth century Innocent III was still reigning in glory, while now at the
end of the century **Boniface VIII** was wretchedly languishing in prison.
This Pope, who was fond of displaying himself with great pomp (i.e.
with crown or tiara) as master of the world, did not even notice how the
papacy was making claims which he himself had undermined, and was
fighting with weapons which had become blunt. The title of his first

important bull, *Clericis laicos infestos*, was to prove an ominous prophecy: 'Antiquity already tells the city that the laity are hostile to the clergy.'[317] But who was to blame for this?

The change from papal world power to papal powerlessness

There are no monocausal explanations: there is only a whole complex of factors. As Walter Ullmann has convincingly demonstrated,[318] the **hierocratic papacy** appears as **the 'declining system'** and the independent, autonomous powers, soon to be **nation states**, appear as **the 'rising system'** of rule and law. To be specific:

– The papacy waged a war to the death against the German emperors and their claim to universal power, and the mediaeval empire met its end as a European institution intended to be universal. The French monarchy long favoured by the papacy, which produced the French nation state, backed by a new French national consciousness, had grown to be the supreme European power. It would now put the papacy radically in question as the universal ruling authority of Europe. The evacuation of the idea of universal imperium resulted in the evacuation of the idea of the universal papacy.

– The papacy attempted to defend its supremacy with traditional theological and legal arguments, but had fewer and fewer creative intellectuals on its side. By contrast, with the help of effective counsellors, university professors and publicists, the French (and English) kings developed and disseminated constitutional criteria which were later to lead to Gallicanism and Anglicanism.

– The papacy attempted to transform the Western universal church into a theocratic universal state. But its moral credibility had been deeply shaken, even among the laity, and its roots in the religious convictions of the peoples permanently damaged.

– The papacy attempted to maintain its universal primacy (of jurisdiction and doctrine) with diplomacy and excommunications, interdict, inquisition and holy war. But critical spirits increasingly distanced themselves from the papal church; the clergy, who in the thirteenth century dominated learning, were displaced from their leading literary position by the knights and retreated into Latin; a secular lay culture and also an increasingly strong opposition to the clergy and the Curia began to form.

– In the high Middle Ages the reconciliation of faith and reason was the prime theological problem. However, in the late Middle Ages the problem was increasingly the new view of human beings as natural beings, of natural law and the state as the natural corporation of citizens introduced by Thomas, along with the development of the natural sciences, natural language and popular song (instead of Latin), and finally the development of the idea of the 'individual'. The result of this was necessarily a new subjectivism in the face of an objective church order which had been laid down once and for all.

And how did the papacy develop against this background? Dramatically in every respect. Events now followed blow by blow.

1294: In July, after a vacancy in the see of more than two years, an eighty-year-old pious, well-meaning but completely unworldly Benedictine monk from the Abruzzi is elected Pope: **Celestine V**. In a completely secularized church, though welcomed messianically by some as the 'angelic Pope', he was to become the first Pope in papal history to resign of his own accord (after only five months)!

1294: In December Cardinal Benedetto Gaetani is elected his successor: **Boniface VIII**. Acute lawyer and reckless man of power as he was, he seems to have played a major part in the resignation of his predecessor. Moreover after his election he had Celestine imprisoned for safety in the fortress of Fumone, where he died in a small triangular cell a few metres in dimension. Historians also describe Boniface as a proud guardian of his own interests, an experienced but fortunate politician who shamelessly increased his family fortunes, and who had clear pathological traits.[319]

1296: In the **bull** '*Clericis laicos*', which has already been mentioned, Boniface declares the taxation of the clergy the sole right of the Pope, challenges the royal jurisdiction over the clergy and threatens with excommunication and interdict. However, this does not intimidate either France or England.

1300: Boniface inaugurates with pomp and jubilee indulgences (rich takings for the Curia from countless pilgrims) the first '**Holy Year**', which since then has been celebrated every century, indeed every fifty and sometimes every twenty-five years.

1301: His confidence strengthened by the 'Holy Year', Boniface risks a conflict with the French king Philip IV the Fair (who was also an unscrupulous man of power, but brilliantly advised). He launches the bull *Ausculta fili* ('Hear, my dearest son, the commands of your father') against him, and indeed summons the French prelates and scholars for counsel in Rome.

1302: Philip goes on the offensive in his publicity. In any case the arguments, derived from the Pope-emperor ideology (the sun and moon simile), cannot apply to a 'mere' king (Gregory VII: *regulus* = little king): the 'most Christian king', *rex christianissimus*, of France sees himself as directly anointed by God. Boniface reacts with the **bull** '*Unam sanctam*'. Basically, it simply repeats the Roman doctrine of supreme spiritual power, abruptly referring to every possible theological authority, and follows Thomas Aquinas in defining obedience to the Pope as 'completely and utterly necessary for salvation for every human creature'.[320] In a skilful propagandist ploy the king now appeals to the French estates, nobility, clergy and representatives of the 'third estate' (from the urban middle class), who, with extremely well orchestrated publicity, take the side of the king in national unanimity. For the first time the papacy is confronted not just with a king but with a whole people. Philip appeals to a general council.

1303: Boniface prepares for 8 September the excommunication of the king and the release of subjects from their oath of loyalty. But an unprecedented event takes place the night before: the Pope – lord of the world – is taken prisoner in his castle at Anagni by a host of armed men under the king's counsellor Guillaume de Nogaret and Sciarra Colonna, who knows the place: **the Anagni attempt**. Called on to resign, instead he offers his life. Though freed by the people of Anagni, Boniface dies in Rome only a month later, on 12 October, a broken man after this humiliation.

1309: Boniface's next successor but one, Clement V, previously Archbishop of Bordeaux, is enthroned in Lyons, remains in France, primarily for health reasons, and after long vacillation takes up his residence in **Avignon**. The 'waning of the Middle Ages'[321] had begun; the end of papal world rule had come, but not that of papal claims.

Papal exile – public criticism of the Pope

What is now thought of in Rome as the **'Babylonian captivity' of the Popes in Avignon** lasted around seventy years.[322] At any rate it is a fact that the Popes were now all Frenchmen and politically to a great degree dependent on the French crown, though this did not disturb the smooth functioning of the central administration. On the contrary, the apparatus of papal officials, financial administration and ceremonial were powerfully developed (as also was nepotism). And despite their political dependence on France, the Avignon Popes, too, maintained the Roman claims. Indeed in Avignon – because of the decline of the papal state, the erection of a new papal palace and the 'chapel' for palace worship, and finally the acquisition of the county of Avignon – papal centralization and legalization culminated in a curial fiscalism, almost unimaginable today, which knew no bounds: an unparalleled **exploitation of the whole church** and thus also a dangerous **alienation of the papacy from many countries**. The Roman papacy – previously the leading religious and moral power – became the **first great financial power in Europe**, which mercilessly enforced its spiritually-based secular demands by every means: papal executors, excommunication and the interdict.

And yet in the fourteenth century the Popes had to reckon increasingly with an opposition which had its base in the many universities, colleges and schools (now also newly founded), and in the middle class of the flourishing German and Italian cities, among the Italian Ghibellines and among the influential **public critics of the Pope**:[323]

– In his political confession *De monarchia* (*c*.1310),[324] **Dante Alighieri**, who in his *Divine Comedy* condemned Pope Boniface VIII to hell,[325] denied world rule to the papacy as an institution: it was not to the Pope, but to God alone that the monarch was accountable. As a result this book by the creator of the Italian national language remained on the papal index of forbidden books until 1908.

– Even more important, above all for state and church lawyers, was the polemical work *Defensor pacis* (1324), written by the famous Paris doctor and former university rector **Marsilius of Padua**.[326] For the first time, with philosophical and biblical-patristic arguments it presented an unclerical theory of the state which, with its separation of secular and divine right, law and conscience, prepared the way for modern theories of the state: the sovereignty of the people; the independence of state power from church power; the independence of the bishops from the Pope and also of the community from the hierarchy. This 'defender of the peace' with his acute arguments saw the main cause of unrest and disturbance in political life in a fullness of papal authority (*plenitudo potestatis*) which lacked any biblical or theological basis; disputed questions should be dealt with in general councils, convened by worldly rulers.

As Germany had had the interdict imposed on it for almost two decades, and religion and morality were suffering serious damage in Europe, the most influential advocate of imperial rights against the papacy, who joined Marsilius at this time, was the head of the *Via moderna* (nominalism), the English philosopher and theologian **William of Ockham**. Denying that faith had any foundation in reason, William was also to have a great influence on Luther through Gabriel Biel: he castigated the personalities of contemporary Popes and criticized the papal 'full authority' over worldly things.[327]

Remarkably, however, Ockham, who in 1328 had escaped papal arrest along with the General of the Franciscan order, Marsilius and others by fleeing to the royal court of Ludwig of Bavaria in Pisa, and who was to die in Munich in 1347, was one of the defenders of a papal infallibility. How did such a doctrine, which had never been taught anywhere in 1200 years, arise particularly at this time?

The infallibility of the Pope – originally a heresy

This was the situation: even Gregory VII, who by no means excluded error among Popes, had only claimed that the **Roman church as such** could never err in faith. And even the canon lawyers well disposed to the Curia strictly maintained the traditional Catholic teaching incorporated in the **Decretum Gratiani** that even a **Pope could err in the faith.** Even Thomas Aquinas had not explicitly asserted an infallibility of the Pope any more than the other great scholastics. But now such a doctrine emerged. From where? What were its origins?

This riddle has been answered in our day by a book by the American historian Brian Tierney.[328] He notes two things about the origin of **papal infallibility:**

– The **origin** of this doctrine is **not orthodox**: the canon lawyers and canonist Popes of the twelfth century, often extreme papalists, do not offer, as was previously assumed, a foundation for such a doctrine; rather, in accordance with strict legal logic they had to reject it. Why? Because the absolute authority or sovereignty of the Pope (ruling at a particular time) was limited specifically by infallible and thus irreformable degrees (of previous Popes).[329] So in his own interest, properly understood, no Pope could be interested in such a claim to infallibility.

– The **origin** of this doctrine is even **heterodox**: it was an eccentric Franciscan accused of heresy by the name of Peter Olivi (1298) who around 1280 propagated papal infallibility against the background of the apocalyptic of Joachim of Fiore. Why? In order to bind all the subsequent Popes once and for all to a decree of Nicholas III in favour of the Franciscan order from 1279. Thus the Pope had to be obeyed by all Catholics in all matters of faith and morality *tamquam regulae inerrabili*, as an 'infallible rule'. And a Pope who acted against himself? This would be the false Pope expected by Peter Olivi and some others for apocalyptic times.

– But this early doctrine of the infallibility and irreformability of papal decisions – from the beginning both belong together – was not taken particularly seriously by the church, nor even by – indeed particularly by – the Pope. Indeed when the Franciscans used it against another Pope, around forty years later, a corresponding counter-reaction followed: in 1324, in the bull *Quia quorundam*, the Avignon Pope John XXII consistently condemned the docrine of papal infallibility as a work of the devil, the 'father of all lies'.[330]

– What does that mean? It means that there was no slow 'development' and 'unfolding' of the doctrine of papal infallibility, but rather its sudden (but politically explicable) creation at the end of the thirteenth century –

by a Franciscan accused of heresy. And in the subsequent period it was defended only among Franciscan dissidents, in order to prove that John XXII was a heretic. For in the period of the Western papal schism which now followed, with two and then three Popes, there was not the slightest prospect of establishing such a doctrine in the church. Even the council of the Counter-Reformation (Trent) did not dare to take up the theme for fear of conciliar demands for reform. As we heard, it was to be left to the restoration papacy in the late nineteenth century to give this originally heretical doctrine the aura of Catholic super-orthodoxy. We shall be returning to this.

– But now first of all we must look back again to Avignon, the residence of the Popes since the fall of Boniface VIII. What had happened there in the meantime? There had been a split in the papacy itself!

What is to be done about two, indeed three, Popes at the same time?

In Italy the situation had become more and more difficult. In the meantime the demagogic tribune of the people, Cola di Rienzo, with utopian dreams of ancient Rome in his head, had come to hold sway in Rome. And as in Rome, so all over Italy there were the wildest partisan struggles. There was even a threat to the existence of the papal state. So in 1367 Urban V returned to Rome for three years, and then went back to reside in Avignon again. It was only in 1377 that Gregory XI – at the urging of Catharine of Siena and Birgitta of Sweden, but probably above all for political considerations – transferred the papal residence back to Rome. However, he died the very next year, in 1378.

Gregory's legally elected successor Urban VI soon showed such incompetence, megalomania and indeed mental disturbance[331] that even according to the traditional canonistic view there was reason for him automatically to lose office.[332] At any rate, some cardinals saw occasion enough to elect another Pope that same year, 1378. This was Clement VII of Geneva, who after the defeat of his troops before Rome again took up residence in Avignon. Thus all at once there were two Popes, since Urban VI would not consider giving up his office. And worse still, the two Popes now excommunicated each other.

The **great schism of the West** was now a fact. This was the second schism in Christianity after the break with the East, and was to last for almost four decades – until 1415. Specifically, the split in the Western church meant that now not only France but also Aragon, Sardinia, Sicily, Naples and Scotland, and also some western and southern German territories, were **obedient to Avignon**; the German empire, central and northern Italy, Flanders and England, the eastern and northern countries, were **obedient to Rome**. The conflicts of conscience this produced for individual Christians, too, were almost unthinkable. Even 'saints' differed in their views: for example Catharine of Siena was for Urban VI, while the ecstatic ascetic Vincent Ferrer, instigator of the famous flagellant processions, was for Clement VII. Now two colleges of cardinals, Curias and financial systems duplicated the financial abuses of the papacy.

No wonder that all the world called for a '**reform of the church, head and members**'. And it was the University of Paris, which during the Middle Ages acted as a kind of *magisterium ordinarium* in the church, that produced the most significant spokesmen of reform: the professors Pierre d'Ailly, Chancellor of the University, and Jean Gerson. The *via concilii* finally became established. Only a **universal council** could help, a council which was no longer to be an emanation of the papal *plenitudo potestatis*, like the Fourth Lateran Council 'under' Innocent III, but one which was thought of as a **representation of all Christianity**.

In recent times, as a result of dogmatic narrowness, an attempt has been made cheaply to brand all conciliar ideas and the conciliar theory which now developed in the Western Schism as a 'conciliarism' tending towards heresy. But after preliminary work by F.Bliemetzrieder,[333] A.Hauck[334] and M.Seidlmayer,[335] Brian Tierney has again demonstrated that the view that the conciliar theory originated only with dissidents like Marsilius and Ockham is untenable. There can be no question of a break with tradition. Rather, the conciliar ideas are already grounded in the completely orthodox official canon law of the twelfth and thirteenth centuries.[336] I myself demonstrated on the eve of the Second Vatican Council that already in the patristic tradition the ecumenical council is a real representation of the church. The very first report of church councils which we have in Christian literature bears witness to this understanding of the council with amazing clarity. Tertullian reports: '. . . in Greek countries those councils of all the churches are held in particular places by which the more important matters are discussed in common and the **representation of all Christianity** is made in a reverent way'.[337]

But neither of the Popes would think of retreating. And when the cardinals of both sides held a general council in **Pisa** in 1409, which deposed the two previous Popes and elected a new one (Alexander V), the church suddenly had **three Popes**. The 'accursed papal binity' had unexpectedly become an 'accursed papal trinity', especially as a John XXIII[338] was to follow Alexander V in the Pisan line. Now the question was even more dramatic and urgent: how could this rule of the three Popes be overcome and the unity of the church be restored again? The answer was given by the **Council of Constance**,[339] the only ecumenical council which has been held in Germany so far, but perhaps the most impressive of the mediaeval councils.

Often people only notice a century later what historical opportunities have been missed, what capital has been squandered and what a disastrous direction has been taken. I am not speaking here about the period after the Second Vatican Council, whose reform decrees Rome has increasingly attempted to neutralize, whose ecumenical openness Rome has increasingly attempted to block and whose new proclamation of faith Rome has again sought to channel into a traditionalistic *World Catechism*. I am speaking – in the sense of a 'lesson of history' – of the period after the great **ecumenical reform council** which met from 1414 to 1418, for around four years, like Vatican II. The council had already set itself a threefold task:

- The *causa unionis*: the question of church unity.
- The *causa reformationis*: the question of church reform, head and members.
- The *causa fidei*: the question of church proclamation and the administration of the sacraments.

No reform without a council! That was the general conviction outside Rome. And at the same time, the council, not the Pope, was in principle the supreme organ in the church. That was the early church tradition. In fact, despite serious compromises and disastrous historical false decisions which Luther later criticized (the prohibition of the chalice for the laity and the shameful burning of the Bohemian patriot and reformer Jan Hus, contrary to all promises of safe conduct), generally speaking the Council of Constance was a **success**. For in the famous decree *Haec sancta* of the fifth session (6 April 1415), the council solemnly declared: **the council is above the Pope**. The gathering understood itself to be a general council legitimately assembled in the Holy Spirit, representing the whole church. Its authority was directly bestowed by Christ, and everyone, even the Pope, had to obey it: in matters of faith, the abolition of the schism and church reform. Anyone – even if this should be the Pope – who refused to obey the commands and resolutions of this council and any legitimate ecumenical council on the points mentioned was to be duly punished.

This was a clear defeat for the Roman curial system, which had taken the Catholic Church of the West to the edge of the abyss. Authority in the church does not lie in a monarch but in the church itself, of which the Pope is the servant, not the master. As silence has been maintained over this fundamental solemn definition of this ecumenical council (though it is inconvenient for the Roman Curia) down to the most recent edition of Denzinger's officious *Enchiridion*,[340] I am reproducing the key passages here.[341]

The Council is above the Pope

'This holy Synod of Constance, which forms an ecumenical council, legitimately assembled for the eradication of the present schism and for the unity and reform of the church of God, head and members, to the praise of almighty God in the Holy Spirit: in order to achieve the unity and reform of the church of God more easily, safely, richly and freely, ordains, defines, decrees, decides and declares the following:

First, this synod, legitimately assembled in the Holy Spirit, which forms an ecumenical council and represents the Catholic Church in dispute, has its authority directly from Christ; everyone, of whatever estate or dignity, even if this be papal, is bound to obey it in matters relating to the faith, the eradication of the said schism and the universal reformation of this church of God, head and members.

Similarly, anyone, of whatever condition, estate and dignity, even if this be papal, who stubbornly refuses obedience to the commands, resolutions, ordinances or precepts of this holy synod and any other general council legitimately assembled in respect of what is said above and all that has happened and is to happen in respect of this, shall, if he does not come to his right mind, be subject to the appropriate punishment and be duly punished, by other legal means should this be necessary.'

Decree 'Haec sancta' of the ecumenical council
of Constance, 6 April 1415.

Thus equipped, the council both coped with the past (the removal or resignation of the previous three Popes) and looked forward, in order to institutionalize the reform process for all time. This was done by the decree *Frequens* of 9 October 1417. It designates the *frequens generalium conciliorum celebratio*, i.e. **the frequent celebration of general councils**, as the best means for a reform of the church. For this reason it was ordained that the next council was to be held only five years after the conclusion of the Council of Constance, the one after that seven years later, and subsequent councils at intervals of ten years.[342] The voting here was not by nations – as in some universities – which would doubtless have suggested the notion of national churches. Finally Martin V was elected the new Pope – on the basis of these decrees!

The Council of Constance: still normative

The Council of Constance is the only ecumenical council in conciliar history to have succeeded, after unspeakable trouble, in **permanently abolishing a great schism**. And we should note that the legitimacy of Martin V and all subsequent Popes to the present day depends on the legitimacy of the Council of Constance and its procedure over the question of the Pope. And yet, strangely enough, apart from its condemnation of the Oxford scholar John Wyclif and the Prague professor Jan Hus, this council enjoys no great popularity in the dogmatic treatises of Roman scholastic theology. Doubtless the fault for that lies less with Constance itself than with the one-sided orientation of more recent Roman ecclesiology. This cannot cope positively with the decrees of Constance and often cites them only as 'difficulties' against particular ecclesiological theses. Anyone who knows the Roman system from within knows that **Constance** was **always inconvenient to a papalist theology centred on Rome**, and remains so today.

No wonder that advocates of a curial ecclesiology did not hesitate to claim that the decrees of Constance were not binding, with often very strange, pseudo-historical arguments. Constance, it was said, had not been 'approved' by the Pope, so its decrees are not formally in force. But I already demonstrated in *Structures of the Church* (written in 1962, before the Second Vatican Council) how threadbare such an argument is. For in the real ecumenical councils of the first millennium, in any case the question of a formal papal approval was never raised; the approval of the emperor was decisive and people were content with the general consent of the Bishop of Rome as patriarch of the West. Papal consent only arose at the mediaeval general synods, which were wholly dominated by the Popes. But at the Council of Constance, which again understood itself to represent the whole church, explicit papal approval was no longer thought necessary. Precisely because the council derived its authority directly from Christ, precisely because it stood above the Pope (or rather above the three Popes), **the question of papal approval never arose from the start**: 'On 22 April 1418 Martin V closed the synod. There was no question of a special papal confirmation, and historically speaking it is wrong to regard only the last sessions under the new Pope as ecumenical.'[343]

And how did the new Pope himself relate to the council? Had **Martin V** not at least to some degree been an advocate of the conciliar theory in these circumstances he would never have been elected Pope. He too was a 'conciliarist', the **advocate of the superiority of councils**. However, he was not a professional theologian or writer but a Curia cardinal, and more on the conservative wing. And while this conservative wing, too, affirmed a 'superiority' of the council, it interpreted it in a restrictive way. Whereas the **radical** advocates of the conciliar idea wanted to transfer the ordinary government of the church fundamentally to the council, the **moderate** representatives wanted to transfer it again to the Pope and the cardinals; in the view of these moderates the council was only to intervene in a crisis. They, too, were in favour of a limitation and control of the power of the Pope; however, this was to be not primarily by the bishops, but by the cardinals.

But the opposition between a moderate and a radical 'conciliarism' (if we are to use at all a term which is often employed to discriminate against an utterly orthodox conciliar theory) had become sharper after the removal of the three Popes. The radicals wanted to introduce a universal conciliar church government and reform the church before any papal election. The moderates were concerned above all to preserve papal authority and legitimacy. A **compromise** was reached as early as 1417. The radicals achieved the publication of the **reform decrees** (including the decree *Frequens*), and the moderates the **election of a new Pope** for the whole church, whom they expected to channel radical conciliarism. Nor were they disappointed. For the very skilful new Pope very soon did all he could to strengthen his position again and force back the influence of radical conciliarism.

Indeed, there was a **restoration of papal absolutism** amazingly soon **after the council**, and the reform of the church constitution which was so urgently needed was thus prevented. Granted, the binding character of the decrees of Constance was not put in question at the subsequent councils of Pavia and Siena. Granted, the ecumenical council of Basel renewed the general decrees of the fourth and fifth sessions of Constance immediately on convening, in 1431. Granted, in a letter of 5 June 1432 to the newly elected Pope Eugene IV, Cardinal Julian Cesarini, to whom Martin V had entrusted the presidency in Basel, made it very clear that the legitimacy of Martin V and any subsequent Pope depended on the validity of the decrees of Constance. But the Curia as a regular authority and constant force proved stronger than the extraordinary institution of the council. It acted in accordance with the slogan: councils come and go, but the Roman Curia remains!

Rome was able to re-establish the mediaeval theory and practice of the church constitution to an amazing degree. But the re-establishment of papal absolutism was not just a consequence of Roman policy. Other **factors in favour of central authority** played a part (and again recall what happened after Vatican II):

– Some of the most loyal and vociferous advocates of the conciliar idea (like Enea Silvio Piccolomini, later Pius II) went over to the papacy for opportunistic reasons.

– Especially the cardinals (created by the Pope and addressed by him not as 'brothers', like the bishops, but as 'sons') often preferred the Curia to the council.

– But even bishops and abbots, who at the council claimed to represent 'the church' (= *congregatio fidelium*, 'community of the faithful'), never dreamed of allowing the 'lesser clergy' and the laity (especially the learned laity) to take part in the church's decision-making processes.

– Finally, some theocratic rulers with their advisers and publicists also thought that the conciliar ('democratic') ideas and the movement 'from below' which followed from them could be dangerous and disturbing for all those 'above'. The monarchs, too, were all for the *status quo* and thus had only a limited interest in the reform of the papacy, which made considerable concessions to them. 'Both the papacy and the secular monarchies were confronted with a common adversary, the rising educated and urban classes of the city. Hence the readiness on the part of of the papacy and the monarchies to conclude the concordats.'[344]

With the renewed reinforcement of curial power the **Popes** also pressed on **with renewing their earlier claims**. Indeed it was a convinced representative of the conciliar idea, Enea Silvia Piccolomini, on becoming Pope (Pius II), who in his bull *Execrabilis* of 1460 **officially forbade the appeal from the Pope to a council** and threatened excommunication for this, in order to strand the conciliar theory. Successfully? No, the papal prohibitions failed to **gain acceptance** in the church.[345] People took them for what they were, threatening curial gestures, and continued to go by the decrees of Constance. These were emphatically defended outside Rome: by bishops and theologians throughout Europe. Thus outside Rome the church of the fifteenth and indeed of the sixteenth century was still largely dominated by conciliar ideas, even if the conciliar movement had lost its force since the middle of the fifteenth century.

But the **Decrees of Constance** continued to be **ignored and suppressed**: although decisively weakened and politically one force among others, the papacy worked indefatigably to restore its old absolutist claims. At the Fifth Lateran Council of 1516, on the eve of the Reformation, Leo X bluntly declared: 'The Roman pontifex now existing, who has authority over all the councils . . .'[346] But already at that time the ecumenicity of this papal council was disputed, since it had been made up almost exclusively of Italians and members of the Curia, and like the mediaeval general synods was completely under the control of the Pope so that it brought no church reform.[347]

In later centuries, too, there was to be constant chafing over Constance.

Roman court theologians of the seventeenth century, above all Cardinal Robert Bellarmine SJ, left no stone unturned to disqualify the ecumenicity of this council.[348] It was now thought scandalous that Constance had foisted on the Roman Curia inconvenient reform decrees and above all the supremacy of the council over the Pope and the periodic holding of councils. The First Vatican Council of 1870 was the final climax of a policy away from Constance, indeed against Constance. For in opposition to Constance this council attempted to make the supremacy of the Pope over the council a dogma for all eternity – until the Second Vatican Council (1962–65) again powerfully reinstated the conciliar idea and in its constitution on the church magisterially laid down the collegiality of bishops and Popes. Moreover today the fundamental **binding character of the decrees of Constance** may not be evaded. No Pope has ever dared to repeal the decree *Haec sancta* or to declare that it is not generally binding.

So what remains if we see the decisive result of the Council of Constance as also relevant to our time? Questions arise for the future of a church which has often had bad experiences with the Popes, questions about a curial authoritarianism and a concilar radicalism.

Questions for the Future

• The Council of Constance **defined a superiority of the council** along the lines of at least a moderate conciliar theory. In the future, doesn't the ecumenical council therefore have the function of a kind of 'controlling authority' over the Pope, beyond the emergency of the time?

• What was **not defined** was a **conciliar parliamentarianism** (along the lines of radical conciliarism). Would it really be good for the Catholic Church if the usual ordinary government of the church were simply transferred by the Pope to the council and the Pope was demoted to being a subordinate executive organ of the conciliar parliament?

However, at any rate since the Council of Constance it has been impossible to extinguish one insight: the **mediaeval form of church government is not the only one,** nor even the only right one. Since then the old principle *Quod omnes tangit, ab omnibus approbari debet* ('What affects all must be approved by all') has become topical again. And the church could have avoided much unhappiness after the Council of Constance had the basic position of the council – papal primacy **and** a definite 'conciliar control'! – been maintained. But just as Martin V and his successors tried their hardest to recapture a primatial authority without heed to any control, so on the other side the extreme conciliarists in Basel (1431–37) increasingly strove for the *de facto* evacuation of the primacy in favour of everyday leadership of the church by the council. But extreme conciliarism without authentic primatial church government led (along with many other factors) to the abuse of office by the Renaissance papacy and (indirectly) to the Lutheran Reformation. Historical developments are illuminating.

The Renaissance – a new paradigm?

Rinascimento, Renaissance, rebirth: **Italy** now took over the leadership of art and culture in Europe. And who would not admire the Italian Quattrocento, the Florentine early Renaissance (*c*.1420–1500), with the cathedral of Brunelleschi, the David of Donatello, the frescoes of Fra Angelico, the paintings of Botticelli? Who would not regard the Italian Cinquecento, the Roman High Renaissance from 1500 to the Sacco di Roma in 1527, as one of those rare highpoints of human culture? The names and works of Bramante, Raphael, Michelangelo and Leonardo da Vinci, the artist, natural scientist and poet, are only some of those which come to mind. And who would not be reminded by the mention of the Renaissance of the revival in the study of Latin and Greek which preceded the rise of the graphic arts, and the historical-critical interest in and discussion of the ancient writings of the Romans and then the Greeks, encouraged in Florence by the Union Council with the Greeks there (1439), the flight of Greek scholars after the fall of Constantinople (1453) and the Platonic Academy (1459)? So did a link develop with Graeco –Roman traditions of painting and art, with its ideas and depictions, in a move away from mediaeval scholasticism and Gothic? A completely new combination of art and philosophy with humanism?

Beyond question, the Rinascimento, beginning with Giotto and ending with Michelangelo, represents a new era for Italian art history, a paradigm shift from mediaeval painting, still strongly influenced by Byzantium, to a new style which was finally also to radiate to Germany, the Low Countries, France and England, though there mostly only to penetrate, clarify and bring late Gothic to maturity with new formal elements. It is also understandable that the Italian art historian Vasari (1674) was the first to use the term '*rinascità*' = 'rebirth' in his biographies of artists to distinguish the new art of Italy, orientated on antiquity and interested in natural forms, from barbaric, Gothic, mediaeval art. Finally, it is also understandable that the Enlightenment was to take the term Renaissance from art history and generalize it into a historical term for the whole of the fifteenth and sixteenth centuries, regarding the Renaissance as a prelude to its own, 'modern' age. Here already individuals recognized in the mirror of antiquity their distinctive value as earthly and historical personalities; here already a free, responsible, progressive humanity appears; here already there was the discovery of the natural person and the free citizen. Now Renaissance and **humanism** became largely parallel, analogous terms.

This was a picture of history which was made more profound and specific in the nineteenth century by the seventh volume of Jules Michelet's *Histoire de France* (1837)[349] and above all by Jakob Burckhardt's *Die Kultur der Renaissance in Italien* (1860).[350] Renaissance was now no longer understood solely as a stylistic concept from the history of art but also as a **concept describing an era in the history of culture**. It was characterized by a new interest in human beings, nature and the world. The Renaissance – a new age, marked off against the 'dark' Middle Ages and its narrow world of belief on the one hand and 'enlightened' modernity and its new picture of humanity and the world on the other. So first of all it seemed natural to assume that this was a new period, a new entire constellation of convictions, values and procedures, in short a new paradigm, not only for Italian but also for European art and culture – the European Renaissance.

And yet what seems quite clear at first sight gets much more complicated when examined closely. The term Renaissance in fact proves to be one of the **most controversial** in history. Why?

– The **basic definition** of the term is disputed: for some it denotes an era of world history and can be applied to all spheres of life at the time; for others it is only the name for a movement above all in literature and art (just as there was a 'Carolingian' or an 'Ottonian' Renaissance, now there is the Italian Renaissance).

– The regional **extent** of the Renaissance is unclear: for some it is a specifically Italian phenomenon (especially the Quattrocento), which proved fertile for other cultures but did not lead to the development of a pure Renaissance style in them. For others it is a phenomenon affecting the whole of Europe; a priori the great Flemish painters of the fourteenth century (the van Eyck brothers) and the old school of Cologne (Lochner) must already be incorporated into it, and in parallel to the great Italians of the high Renaissance (and yet so different from them) the German masters Dürer and Grünewald.

– Its temporal **limits** are indefinite: for some the Renaissance begins with Cimabue and above all with Giotto; for others already with Joachim of Fiore's 'third age', with Francis of Assisi and his nature piety, with Dante's heightened interest in antiquity and a move away from the monastic ascetic negation of the world and towards an individual piety which is already becoming evident in the court culture of the thirteenth century. And those who conversely want to see the Renaissance simply as the 'cradle of modernity' overlook something that Nietzsche, an admirer of Cesare Borgia, already noted (and regretted): the Renaissance was very soon countered, indeed broken off, by the Reformation and the Counter-Reformation. It does not seem to fit into any overall European synchronism.

Three important insights emerge from the discussion for our paradigm analysis:

1. The Renaissance cannot be detached from its mediaeval context: there is **no break** between the Middle Ages and the Renaissance, as there is **between the Middle Ages and the Reformation**. For all the discontinuity, the continuity with mediaeval thought is greater. So we can speak of the Renaissance as a late mediaeval period of transition and change leading to a still undefined new time, which embraces a series of aesthetic, social, economic and political changes.

2. Here the enthusiastic return to **antiquity**, to Graeco–Roman literature and philosophy (Plato!), art and science, plays a decisive if not exclusive role. Now these were not only studied but imitated and in the end also developed very much further. A classical education became the common property of the Italian elites and displaced mediaeval scholasticism. However, antiquity was less an end than a means; above all it provided a **criterion**. Men and women came to be detached from many mediaeval norms of life, and for many people, especially the artist but also the pious individual (the mystic), this brought a new self-awareness.

3. For all the widespread church indifference and inner alienation, with few exceptions the Renaissance cannot simply be set over against Christianity as a 'new paganism'. Open opposition to the church was rare. The Renaissance, supported by many Popes and many clergy (including Francesco Petrarch, the model poet of the Renaissance), developed externally within the **social framework of Christianity**, even if the new artistic and scientific experience of nature resulted internally in a release from the bonds with the hierarchical Christian thought of the Middle Ages. Not only the great penitential preachers Bernardino (in Siena) and Savonarola (in Florence), who found a great response among the people, but also the greatest humanists, beginning with Nicholas of Cusa, through Marsilio Ficino and his Platonic Academy in Florence, to Erasmus of Rotterdam and the statesman Thomas More in London, were interested in a '*renovatio Christianismi*' and a lay piety in the spirit of the humanism of the Reformers and the Bible. For some the Bible – now since the fourteenth century increasingly available in the vernacular – was the real source of inspiration; we shall be returning to this in the context of the Reformation.

So how is the Renaissance to be fitted into our paradigmatic consideration of Christianity? It is better not to see it as an era which can be defined both backwards and forwards, embracing all spheres of life, but as an important **intellectual and cultural stream within the late Middle Ages**. Its rise shows how much the Middle Ages was in deep crisis, pressing towards something new. To this degree one can subscribe to Jacques LeGoff's plea '*pour un long Moyen-Âge*': 'I suggest that this period should be reduced to the right proportions; a brilliant but superficial event. Far from marking the end of the Middle Ages the Renaissance is – the Renaissances are – a characteristic phenomenon of a long mediaeval period, a Middle Ages always in search of an authority in the past, backwards towards a golden age. Not only has the "great" Renaissance no relatively precise chronological origin – in Europe it fluctuates between three, if not four centuries – but it is overtaken by numerous significant historical phenomena.'[351]

The Renaissance papacy and its inability to reform the church

For the church and Christianity, at any rate, the Renaissance did not have any general epoch-making influence (apart from art), unless one wants to put into this category the increasing Italianization of **the Pope and the Curia** that was to develop later. The Popes from Nicholas V, the last Pope to crown an emperor, in 1452, under whom the resignation of the last anti-Pope and the terrifying conquest of Constantinople (1453) took place, to Leo X, under whom the Fifth Lateran Council was held with so little results for reform, followed immediately afterwards by the Reformation – these Italian Popes in particular were zealous supporters of the spirit of the Renaissance. The St Peter's of Bramante and Michelangelo, along with Raphael's stanzas and Michelangelo's Sistine Chapel in the Vatican, shows this clearly enough.

However, all that was now left of the ambitions of former Popes to rule the world was a middling Italian territorial state, again with a completely Italianized government. After the peace of Lodi in 1454 the papal state was only one of five major Italian powers ('Cinque Principati'), along with the duchy of Milan, the republics of Florence and Venice and the kingdom of Naples. In these circumstances the Popes wanted by their gigantic **building activity and patronage of art** to give visible expression to the fact that the capital of Christianity was at least also the centre of art and culture.

But all this was purchased at the cost of a **refusal to reform the church** which would have presupposed a fundamental alteration to the disposition of the Popes and the members of their Curia. However, no one thought of that at a time when even the Popes were quite ordinary **Italian Renaissance princes** – Machiavelli had plenty of contemporary illustrative material. They pursued their self-interested policies unscrupulously, did not shrink from any intrigue or meanness, and ruled the papal state as if it were an Italian principality belonging to them: their own kinsfolk or legitimized children (bastards) were preferred; an attempt was made to create dynasties in the form of hereditary petty princedoms for the papal families of the Riarios, della Roveres and Borgias.

Of course there was an awareness of the need for a reform programme even among the Borgias. But the more time went on, the more insolently these 'Renaissance Popes' (the name became proverbial) led a life of tremendous luxury, boundless sensuality and uninhibited vice. No historian will ever discover how many children these Popes had, though of course for 'their' church they still maintained celibacy with an iron hand. All that is certain is that, say, the corrupt Sixtus IV (a Franciscan and promoter of the 'Immaculate Conception' of Mary) looked after whole hosts of nephews ('*nipoti*') and favourites at the church's expense and elevated six relatives to the cardinalate, including his cousin Pietro Riario, one of the most scandalous wastrels of the Roman Curia, who succumbed to his vices at the early age of twenty-eight.

We need not go into all this here. Nor into the shamelessness of Innocent VIII, who with his bull *Summis desiderantes affectibus* of 1474 gave powerful encouragement to the witch-craze and had witches tried, but on the other hand did not hesitate to recognize his illegitimate children publicly and have their marriages celebrated in the Vatican with pomp and splendour. Nor the policy of the shrewd Alexander VI Borgia (1492–1503), who maintained his office by simony in the grand style and had four children by his mistress (and others with other women when he was a cardinal), but did not shrink finally from excommunicating the great penitential preacher Girolamo Savonarola and seeing to it that he was burned at the stake. We would not need to waste words on all this had not attempts been made down to our day to 'historicize', indeed 'rehabilitate', this wretched, immoral and criminal figure, trivializing him by highly superficial political criteria.[352]

Venus ruled under Alexander VI – so ran a proverb in Rome at the time. And Mars under his successor Julius II della Rovere, who was constantly waging war. And under Leo X Medici? Minerva. In 1513 this completely unclerical son of Lorenzo the Magnificent ascended the papal throne, having been made cardinal at the early age of thirteen (along with four other Medici nephews) by his dissolute uncle Innocent VIII. He loved art above all, enjoyed life, and politically concentrated completely on acquiring the duchy of Spoleto for his nephew Lorenzo. So he failed to realize that in 1517 an epoch-making event took place, involving a monk who was unknown at the time, named **Martin Luther**. A **paradigm shift** *par excellence* had been introduced, putting an end even in the West to the universal claim of the Pope, which in the East had never been recognized anyway. But how did Rome react? Rome did not react to the Lutheran Reformation with its own reformation, but with the Counter-Reformation. However, present-day Catholics are careful about using this term, because of the notion of the use of authority in religious matters which is associated with it.

12. Counter-Reformation? Back to the mediaeval paradigm

I shall be devoting a separate long chapter (C IV) to the Reformation Protestant paradigm (P IV). In the framework of our paradigm analysis (and following the present state of international historical discussion), in fact the origin and development of a paradigm are more interesting than its late phases and possible reinforcement and hardening: as I already said in the Introduction, equal treatment throughout this book would make it impossibly long. So here in the context of the Roman Catholic paradigm (P III) we must concentrate on the way in which **Rome** reacted to Luther's thrust and the process of religious and ecclesiastical change in the early sixteenth century, which was to change not only church and theology but also the whole of social life and the political power structure. Should we speak of a 'Counter-Reformation', as has been usual since Ranke? As early as 1946 Hubert Jedin, who in his four-volume history of the Council of Trent was to raise the Catholic interpretation of this period to a new academic level, proposed that this period should be described by the unabbreviated term 'Catholic Reformation and Counter-Reformation'.[353] This distinction is helpful, as long as we do not overlook the fact that after the Reformation, in fact any Catholic reform also had a Counter-Reformation stamp.

Reformation instead of reforms

For a long time Rome had blocked real reforms, so now instead it got the Reformation. All at once in the West, alongside the papal church there were new Christian **churches**, which in their first phase were to develop a **powerful religious, political and social dynamic**. In the eyes of Rome this was a catastrophe. For generally speaking the Protestant Reformation cost the Roman Catholic Church roughly the northern half of its *Imperium Romanum* – from Protestant Zurich, Bern, Basel and Geneva and large parts of Germany to Holland, England, Scotland and Scandinavia – not to mention North America, which came later. At the end of the Reformation period four large and very different types of Protestant Christianity had developed within this Reformation paradigm: Lutheran, Anglican, Reformed and Free Church. We shall be turning to them later.

Certainly at this time Christianity still remained the decisive religious, cultural, political and social framework of Europe. But historically speaking the papacy was forced on to the **defensive** and condemned to **reaction**. The Roman Catholic paradigm, which at first was so innovative, became rigid in its mediaeval strait-jacket. How it was 'kept pure' first against the powerful forces of the Protestant Reformation and then against enlightened modernity can be reported here only in the broadest outline. For despite all the later reforms within the church, most of the really epoch-making, paradigmatic innovations and 'modernization effects' in church, theology and society are not to be found within the Roman sphere of rule (P III) but within the Reformation (P IV) and then the modern paradigm (P V). They will be discussed there.

Certainly, since the 1530s it had also become increasingly clear to Protestants that the mediaeval Roman Catholic paradigm was offering more resistance than Luther and his like-minded allies had originally assumed. Granted there was no longer the one Catholic Church of the West, but the **collapse of the Roman system** expected by the Reformers in their apocalyptic and eschatological mood **failed to materialize**. Rather, as time went on, a **Mediterranean Catholicism with an Italian and Spanish stamp** developed in characteristic opposition to the Protestant Christianity of northern and western Europe (and later also of North America). At a very early stage this not only influenced the German Catholic lands but was also transferred to Latin America – with all the consequences which we shall be considering in a separate investigation. In the face of an initially powerful Reformation movement which now, however, often lost its élan, there was a Roman system and instrument of rule which, though halved, had again become a force in history. For in contrast to the increasingly pluralistic Protestantism it was now held together by a hierarchy organized even more tightly, in the framework of an absolute monarchy, which, as we shall see, remained equipped with authoritarian power, censorship and Inquisition in matters of faith and morals.

But how did the shift in the Roman Catholic Church from the late Middle Ages and Renaissance to the 'Catholic Reformation and Counter-Reformation' come about?[354] Like the Reformation, the Counter-Reformation also had its political dimension, though it would be wrong to regard this as primary. For the **basis** not only of the Reformation but

also of the Counter-Reformation was primarily **religious**: the renewal of the Catholic Church from its own substance.

How the Catholic reform came about

It was not primarily Reformation but **pre-Reformation impulses towards reform**, mostly along the moderate, humanist line of Erasmus of Rotterdam, the 'prince of the humanists', and his programme of 'back to the sources' (scripture and the fathers), which first influenced the Roman Catholic Church. There was an 'evangelism' which could primarily be noted in the sphere outside the Reformation, in Spain and Italy.[355]

The Catholic reform originated, not in Rome, but in **Spain**. Spain, united by the marriage of Isabella I of Castille-León with Ferdinand II of Aragon, had completed the Christian *reconquista* in 1492 with the conquest of Muslim Granada. At the same time it had mercilessly driven out both the Jews and Muslims who would not be converted and in the same year laid the foundation for a colonial empire rich in precious metals with the discovery of America (later the conquest of Mexico in 1521). This Spain now competed for Italy and even for the German imperial crown with the leading continental power, France. Immediately after the outbreak of the Lutheran Reformation this had been won by the grandson of Ferdinand and Isabella, the young Spanish king Charles I, known in the world as the **Emperor Charles V**. A convinced Catholic Habsburg with a high sense of European mission, he had an empire – from the Balkans through Vienna to Madrid, Mexico and Peru – on which the sun literally never set. In this decisive period between 1519 and 1556 Charles now attempted, against all religious and national particularism, to re-establish the mediaeval universal monarchy, and in so doing involved himself in a permanent struggle with France, which was similarly striving for European hegemony.

But what about Spain and reform? Mustn't we associate the strict Spanish Catholicism stamped by the *reconquista* primarily with the disastrous renewal of the **Inquisition** under the Grand Inquisitor Thomas de Torquemada, under whom around 9000 auto-da fés (= *actus fidei*, 'acts of faith', punishment usually inflicted by burning at the stake) were carried out? Mustn't we associate it with the secret state police and courts which had often raged against Jews converted (often only superficially) to Christianity and the Muslim Moors, and which were later to turn even against Erasmian humanists? That is one side.

But we also must not forget the church **reform** which was given powerful impetus particularly by Erasmus, and which under the leadership of the humanist Francisco Ximénez de Cisneros, an ascetic Fran-

ciscan who was made Archbishop of Toledo and Primate of Spain by
Isabella, led to a renewal of the monasteries and the clergy with the
support of the secular power, to the foundation of universities in Alcalá
and elsewhere, and to a much-admired polyglot edition of the Bible. The
sixteenth century was generally to become Spain's proud '*siglo de oro*', its
'golden century'! In the second half of the century Spain (relatively
independent of Rome on the basis of concordats) under Charles' son
Philip II (1555–98) became the most significant power in Europe,
although Charles' brother Ferdinand and the German Habsburgs
retained the title of emperor.

In **Italy**, too, the foundation for Catholic reform was laid, partly under
the influence of Spain and even more under that of Erasmus: first of all in
small, insignificant circles reflecting on the gospel, where a deep
humanistic and evangelical piety was fostered. From them emerged – to
reform the clergy – Gaetano of Thiene's Theatine order, and also the later
'reform' Pope Gian Pietro Caraffa, a Neapolitan nobleman. In Venice
there was the reform circle around Gasparo Contarini, who as Venetian
ambassador had witnessed Luther's appearance at Worms in 1521 and
who unlike Caraffa was stamped by the ideals of the earliest church.

But while the catastrophe of the plunder of Rome for many days by
unpaid imperial troops, the **Sacco di Roma** (1527), put an end to Roman
Renaissance culture, it did not bring the reform of the Roman church.
Charles V missed the unique opportunity of the imprisonment of the Pope
to summon a reform council, as his brother Ferdinand urgently recommended him to do. The papacy remained unreformed. Only under the
following transitional Pope, **Paul III** Farnese (1534–49),[356] did the
reform finally also affect the papacy. Only now did partial reforms
become an effort at reform by the whole church. Paul III, with his four
children and three grandsons between fourteen and sixteen as cardinals,
was still a Renaissance man through and through, but he introduced
reform in Rome with three actions:

– He appointed the leaders of the reform party, a series of very capable
and profoundly religious men, members of the **college of cardinals** (the
layman Contarini, then Pole, Fisher of Rochester, Morone and Caraffa),
and they worked out the famous reform document *De emendanda
Ecclesia* of 1537 for the Pope.[357] In this way moral and religious
earnestness slowly set in again in Rome and the Vatican.

– In 1540 Paul II confirmed the novel 'Companía de Jesús' formed by the
Basque knight and officer Inigo/Ignatius de Loyola, who had had an
experience of awakening after a war wound: here was the **Society of
Jesus**, bound to the Pope in special obedience.[358] The Jesuits, with a
strong religious motivation as a result of the Ignatian 'exercises', at the

same time carefully chosen, thoroughly and scientically trained and strictly organized under a general, became the powerful elite order of the Counter-Reformation. Its members, like the Protestant pastors, mostly came from an urban milieu, from the middle and upper classes. With no religous dress, no fixed abode, and no choral prayer, under strict religious discipline and owing unconditional obedience to God, the Pope and their superiors, they were to concentrate on the conversion of heretics and pagans and establishing the rule of the Catholic Church (in pastoral and educational activities, in higher schools and universities, in the confessional at princely courts and in missions). Popular preaching and pastoral care were to be even more the tasks of the **Capuchins** and **Oratorians**, who with other new religious communities bore witness to the new spirit in the old church.

– Finally, in 1545 – almost three decades after the outbreak of the Reformation and two years before Luther's death – the Pope opened the **Council of Trent**, which was not an autonomous action on the part of the church but a central element in the political calculation of the European powers. But which direction would the reform take?

Renewal or restoration?

Even Catholics do not recognize sufficiently that at the beginning of the Catholic reform under Paul III the question whether there was to be a real renewal or only a restoration was still undecided. And there was a strong trend even in the highest circles of church government which argued for a positive renewal. It had a positive attitude towards some concerns of the Reformers, was open to dialogue, and thus in the end tended towards some arrangement with Protestantism.

There is no doubt that the young **reform movements within Catholicism** were decisively influenced by the controversy over Protestantism. But for the most part, in Italy in particular, as we heard, they drew their ideas from grappling with the Bible (especially Paul). The gospel stood at the centre. And originally Erasmus was more important than Luther. Problems like justification, *theologia crucis*, the invisible church and so on were as much in the air as the Reformation. But this reform within Catholicism emphatically wanted to retain the sacramental and hierarchical church. This group included not only the Viterbo circle (with Michelangelo and Vittoria Colonna) and the two Camaldolese Quirini and Giustiniani (who had already addressed a bold proposal for reform to Leo X!), but bishops like Giberti of Verona and Lippomano of Bergamo, and above all Cardinals Contarini, Sadoleto, Cervini, Pole, Morone and the Augustinian general Seripano, who were already allied with humanists beyond the Alps, especially with Erasmus and German Catholic theologians (Pighius, Gropper and Pflug) and politicians (above all those around the emperor). The reform proposal *De emendanda Ecclesia* had emerged from this group. Its leader was the Contarini who as papal legate had come to an understanding with Melanchthon over the doctrine of 'double righteousness' at the religious dialogue in Regensburg in 1541 – though this was problematical for both sides.

But the development took a fatal course and the reform group did not win through. Erasmus had died in 1536: his potential as a reformer, which is often not valued sufficiently, will need to be considered more thoroughly in the framework of the Reformation paradigm (P IV). And the year 1542 was to be ominous for Catholic renewal. For in that year (apparently at the instigation of Ignatius of Loyola), the Inquisition was reorganized and a centre for the Inquisition for all countries was established in Rome by Paul III: the famous and notorious **Sacrum Officium Sanctissimae Inquisitionis**.[359] Now Contarini was suspected of heresy and died. The key figure in this cruel game was the conservative zealot Cardinal Gian Pietro Caraffa from Naples, which was then Spanish; he also published the first *Index of Forbidden Books*. That same year the famous Capuchin preacher and Vicar General of his order, Bernardino Occhino, fled in desperation to Calvin. With him some of the most ardent advocates of Catholic reform fell away, some of them succumbing to radical heresies (anti-trinitarianism, etc). Others, in danger, had to keep silent. And when Caraffa was elected Pope in 1555 as Paul IV and attempted once again to set up a mediaeval theocracy in the style of Boniface VIII, the Restoration had definitively become established.[360] Just one symptom of this is that the Caraffa Pope even had an Inquisition process launched against Cardinal Pole; Cardinal Morone, similarly suspected of heresy, was kept prisoner in Castel Sant'Angelo for almost two years until the death of the Pope in 1559.

The Council of Trent, in which Pole had initially taken part as one of the three presidents and legates, had meanwhile come to follow the conservative line completely. We must now look at its role more closely in connection with the great dispute over the paradigm of church and theology: was it a council of Catholic reform or of the Counter-Reformation?

The two faces of the Council of Trent

The place where the council assembled was the imperial city of Trent in Upper Italy. Opened in 1545, with interruptions and transfers it was to be in session over three periods up to 1563.[361] So long desired by

Christianity, continually called for by the emperor, it had kept being postponed by the Curia for fear of reforms and political entanglements. And unfortunately the Italian friends of reform had hardly anything to say here from the beginning. In contrast to the previous reform councils, abbots, theologians and all laity, even rulers, were excluded. Only the papal legates had the right to make proposals, and in this way they could block in advance all resolutions which were unacceptable to Rome. Although this council is counted as the Nineteenth Ecumenical Council in the Catholic Church, it was in no way an ecumenical council after the model of the old ecumenical councils or the Council of Constance. Rather, it was again a **papal council** following the example of the mediaeval Roman general synods, in which at first almost exclusively Italian and Spanish prelates took part; the Protestants therefore a priori rejected it.

What were the debates about? With establishing true doctrine (desired by Rome) and practical reforms (called for by the emperor). The two issues were discussed in parallel. The **doctrinal decrees** ('*de fide*') dealt with the sources of faith, original sin, justification, the sacraments, the sacrifice of the mass, purgatory, indulgences . . . The **disciplinary decrees** ('*de reformatione*') related to marriage, the training of the clergy and the establishment of episcopal seminaries for priests; the duties of bishops in residence and on visitations; the prohibition of the union of several bishoprics, benefices or livings in one hand; the nomination of bishops and cardinals and their duties in office; the holding of annual diocesan synods and triennial provincial synods; reform of the cathedral chapters and religious orders; mission tasks in territories overseas.[362] And the reform of the papacy? Not a word about it!

These **efforts at reform** in the narrow sense made by the council are beyond question not just the expression of a Counter-Reformation but of a Catholic reform. One thinks of the creation of new forms of training for priests, of the religious life, and of preaching. One also thinks of the organization of pastoral care, the missions, catechesis, the care of the poor and sick, and later the renewal of religious customs, church culture, art and mysticism. But all this is so to speak only the inside of the Tridentine Reform. For the demarcation from, indeed the fight against, Protestantism forms the external framework and thus also the substantive limit to this positive internal renewal. The breakthrough of Catholic reform had only come about at all under pressure from the Reformation. But the Reformation was not just the occasion for the Council of Trent, as some Catholic historians think; it challenged the council, accelerated it and was its permanent opponent. In other words, the Counter-Reformation does not first begin, as the Catholic historian of the council, Hubert

Jedin, suggests, **after** the Council of Trent (with Gregory XV, 1621–23, i.e. seventy years after the council was convened[363]); it begins **with** the council. How else are we to understand the fact that every doctrinal statement of Trent has an anathema against the Reformers? What the Reformers did not dispute (the doctrine of the Trinity, christology), was not discussed at all.

All this means that this council was **not** the long-expected universal **union council** of all Christianity. Nor, with its dozens of threats of excommunication, was it a peaceful Catholic reform council either, **but on the whole it was the particular confessional council of the Counter-Reformation**. It was to serve to re-Catholicize Europe (an aim which was never lost sight of) against the background of the violent clashes over 'Catholic' or 'Protestant' territory which had already begun.

So Jedin's historical double concept easily becomes an apologetic double ploy in two phases. There was by no means first a Catholic self-reform and then a militant Counter-Reformation. At Trent both already went hand in hand from beginning to end, and are like two sides of one and the same coin. Moreover, recently, instead of the often unsatisfactory double concept,[364] 'Catholic confessionalization' has been proposed as a blanket term for this period.[365]

In fact it seems to me beyond dispute that this is the Counter-Reformation of a confessional church, with a conciliar foundation and definition, which would almost unavoidably also encourage political and military clashes, really 'confessional wars'. Certainly the Marxist interpretation of the Counter-Reformation as a feudalistic bourgeois reaction or counter-revolution falls far short of reality. But there is no overlooking the fact that for all its novel baroque triumphalism, within the sphere of the church the Catholic reform bears the stamp of **Restoration**. It is the mediaeval spirit in Counter-Reformation garb! In any case this council did not take up reform *in capite*, i.e. of the Pope and the Curia – the central point for all Catholic reformers. The most prominent Catholic papal historians Ludwig von Pastor and Joseph Schmidlin therefore rightly prefer the term 'Catholic Restoration'. And even Jedin in fact emphasizes the continuity of the Tridentine reform with the mediaeval papal church (and its distance from the Reformation). He therefore should really have agreed with the evaluation that the Council of Trent and the whole of the Counter-Reformation **remain within the framework of the mediaeval Roman Catholic paradigm (P III)**!

There is no disputing the fact that whereas the emperor and many people in Germany still wanted an arrangement with the Protestants and had not yet given up the reconciling *via media*, the Council of Trent, like the Roman Curia, adopted an unambiguously anti-Protestant attitude and took up the positive stimuli from the Reformers only by way of exception. Certainly there was finally a recognition of the danger in which a church which is completely incapable of reform finds itself; there was a recognition that it was possible to oppose Protestantism only if the church reformed itself, i.e. did away with the worst abuses. But there was now no longer any thought of an understanding with the Protestants. Rather, there was a concern to prevent the further expansion of Protestantism by every means, to win back the 'lost' territory, indeed to win new mission lands in the continent that had been discovered. In short, there was an attempt to stop the power of Protestantism by a **double strategy** of reform and containment. For precisely this reason Trent was the council of the Counter-Reformation: here **reform within the church is not a means of reconciliation and reunion but the programme for a battle against the Reformation.**

So we can understand why the Catholic Church at that time – for all of its purging of itself in some spheres – primarily concentrated on preserving what already existed and on repristinating the past, and thus ran the danger of failing to do justice to the Catholic breadth and fullness which had truly existed previously, or of making it too rigid. An example? One need think only of the **celebration of the eucharist**, which was not reformed creatively out of an inner understanding of the concerns of the Reformers, but was simply 'restored in its purity'. However, the primary model for that was not, say, the celebration of the eucharist described in Holy Scripture and practised in the apostolic church, but the mediaeval liturgy.

Given the demands of Luther – highly justified in the light of scripture and ancient tradition – for the vernacular and a liturgy for the people (with the chalice also for the laity!), this continuity was quite fatal. For in this way, up to the Second Vatican Council the **mediaeval Latin mass** was to remain the basic form of the Catholic liturgy, which moreover was fully **restored** in 1570 by the Roman mass book (missal), on the basis of the resolutions of Trent. Certainly the Council of Trent cut back the most monstrous accretions to the mass, which had crept in particularly in the Middle Ages. On the other hand, the same council had stipulated the order of the mass to the last detail, which had never been done previously. So this mass was now called the 'mass of rubrics', those countless little instructions printed in red which were inserted everywhere between the text of the mass proper. Everything was now officially regulated, to the last word and the way in which the priest held his fingers. No room was left for spontaneity, emotiveness and creativity; there could be no question of the people playing an active part in the celebration. They remained spectators of the sacral, clerical sacred play, now increasingly decked out musically with baroque splendour: a **clerical liturgy** which was increasingly **regulated and ceremonialized**.

So as a result, private personal piety with all its feeling and living power engaged in the various and finally ever more numerous **devotions** for every possible saint and occasion. All too often in the following centuries the mass was regarded as one devotion among others (perhaps still the most important); more candles burned at the devotions than at the mass. But finally in Europe, what has been called the exodus from the Sunday mass was quietly to begin. It would be noted with horror in very different countries of Europe what a small proportion of the faithful still regularly went to the tedious Sunday mass, and how conversely the celebrations of the small churches and sects with their quite different emotional atmosphere were proving increasingly attractive. But even more basic questions arise, not only about the celebration of the eucharist but about the sacraments generally, to which the majority of the doctrinal decrees were devoted.

The system of seven sacraments – critical questions

The Council of Trent defined the number of sacraments as seven – under threat of excommunication. This question may seem peripheral to some people today. But as the whole of Roman **canon law** is built on it and is thus basically **sacramental law,** it is of central significance for the Roman Catholic system. From baptism onwards it is the express duty of Catholics, repudiating the freedom of a Christian, to observe all the commandments of the church (even those which are not contained in scripture).[366] Doctrinally it was the clear aim of the Council of Trent to define Catholic doctrine over against Reformation doctrine and separate off the Reformers. But despite all that was anti-Protestant (and especially anti-Lutheran), we must not overlook the positive side of the internal reform. The really fundamental dogmatic definitions were created at the first session of the council (1545–46). We must grant that to a decisive degree they are formally stamped by a rejection of the scholastic disputes and the not wholly unsuccessful concern for a formulation of Catholic doctrine in a language which is more biblical than scholastic. Even Protestant historians of dogma like Harnack regard the decree on **justification**, which takes up the Reformers' concerns to a surprising degree, as a credit to the council.[367]

However, considerably less trouble was taken in the decrees on the seven sacraments: the proceedings of the council bear witness to that. Already in the preceding decree on **scripture and tradition** the opportunity had been missed to emphasize that while the church tradition was a norm, it was a norm normated (*norma normata*) by scripture (as the *norma normans*), and instead scripture and tradition were set on the same level (to be treated 'with the same feeling of piety and the same reverence').[368] So the traditional **number of seven** sacraments allegedly instituted by Christ himself was simply asserted in an almost unthinking way in canon 1 of the decree on the sacraments, and those who denied it were threatened with the anathema, exclusion from the church.[369] Could not, should not, the work here have been more careful? For Luther had posed the problem that the number of seven sacraments does not come personally from Jesus Christ, but is a **product of history**. Unknown throughout the first millennium and put forward for the first time in the twelfth century, at first without any claim to exclusiveness, it became established *de facto* and was first adopted in an official church document around three hundred years before the Reformation, but subsequently was treated even by councils (especially the union council of Florence) as a matter of faith. To this degree the concept of sacrament proved not only an analogous but also a very variable concept, defined in different ways at different times. This should have been discussed.

Moreover, biblically and theologically there is no disputing the fact that the traditional seven sacraments are not all on the same level. They do **not** have **the same dignity**. In the New Testament, baptism and eucharist are always derived directly from Jesus Christ and play a significant role in all the communities right from the beginning. **Ordination**, as we saw, is quite a different matter.[370] In particular, the undisputed letters of Paul say nothing about it, and these are the most important witnesses to early church order. Only the Acts of the Apostles thirty years later and the Pastoral Epistles fifty years later mention the ordination of leaders of the community. And centuries were to pass before ordination was to be counted a sacrament similar to baptism and the eucharist. However, even Trent – and here that canon 1 can easily give a wrong impression – did not want to put all the sacraments on the same level. On the contrary, the priority of the **eucharist** over all other sacraments is emphasized in the decree on the eucharist. At the same time the fundamental significance of **baptism** for justification as the sacrament of faith is emphasized. The distinction between main and subsidiary sacraments may be said to be traditional.

The number of sacraments in fact depends on the **definition** of what is to be designated a sacrament:[371]

– If (like the Council of Trent) one recognized institution by Christ as an essential element of the sacrament, the great majority of the thity sacraments which were accepted, for example, by Hugo of St Victor

had to be ruled out a priori as sacraments; these were then no longer called sacraments but sacramentals. At best seven sacraments remained.
– If (like Luther and the Reformers) one accepted institution by Christ in the strictest historical sense (as explicitly attested in the New Testament), then a further distinction had to be made in the seven sacraments of the high Middle Ages; some were then no longer called sacraments but church customs or the like. All that were left were baptism and the eucharist (in some respects also penance).

However, **Trent** had no understanding of the new problem posed by the Reformers. The mediaeval definition was taken over regardless, and with it the **mediaeval numbering**. The holy number seven was normative. But Trent could not demonstrate in the strict historical sense that Christ instituted either confirmation or last unction, or the sacrament of marriage or finally ordination. Nevertheless people continued regardless, with the help of some distinctions and doubtful exegesis, to claim that the sacraments had been instituted by Christ and to draw important conclusions from this. But that can no longer be accepted uncritically today, any more than can the **Reformation solution**, which at the time was illuminating in many ways. For meanwhile **historical-critical exegesis** of the Gospels in particular has demonstrated that despite all the fundamental significance of baptism and eucharist for the life of a Christian, that they were 'formally' instituted as sacraments by Jesus is highly questionable. The New Testament does not think in such institutional categories. Only a general 'empowerment' by Jesus' words and actions can provide a basis for baptism and eucharist in the light of the New Testament.

All this means that the question of an 'institution' by Jesus and thus the conceptual definition of a sacrament and with it finally also the number of the sacraments is raised again today and must be given a new answer – taking into account all the results of more recent exegesis and the history of dogma. A speculative derivation of all seven sacraments from the church as a 'primal sacrament', which has been attempted by individual Catholic theologians, and which is arbitrary in its fixation on the precise number seven, obscures this question rather than solving it. Only a constructive criticism of the dogmatic statements in the light of the Christian message illuminated by exegesis, which will involve more than particular conceptualities, can help here. But this goes beyond the framework of our investigation.[372] Here I shall keep to some basic **critical questions** to the Council of Trent.

In retrospect we need to ask, **first**: can the Council of Trent, because of its minimal *de facto* representative character (mostly only a small number of Roman Catholic Italian and Spanish prelates and theologians), claim the same **theological quality and authority** (we are not concerned here with legal 'validity' in terms of Roman church law) as a council fully representing all churches, nations and theological trends? One need only compare Vatican II. There can be no question of Trent having had a similar representation of theology from the countries concerned, Germany above all, or even of Reformation theology. Moreover, in the Roman perspective it was a priori concerned not with integration but with the condemnation of the new Reformation approaches.

That raises, **secondly**, the question: did Trent also really **understand correctly the Reformers** whom it condemned? Did it not only quote the Reformers, but also understand the basic approach of their criticism and their positive basic intentions? This is not to be expected, given the defensive and polemical methods (anathemas) used in the Tridentine decrees on the sacraments, which mostly lay down negative dividing lines. And to judge from the whole debate and its results, this can in no way be said to be the case. The council did not submit the new Reformation paradigm as such to any examination. Indeed, given its composition, that would have been beyond it.

And **thirdly**, we must ask: did Trent take note of the **historical development in the doctrine of the church and the sacraments** which was emphasized so strongly by Luther and the Reformers? Did the council really investigate scripture? It had honestly tried to do so in the decree on justification. But in the decree on the sacraments – a central theme of Luther's polemical work *On the Babylonian Captivity of the Church* (1520) – without any self-critical questioning of scripture and history it a priori stated that all seven sacraments had been instituted by Jesus Christ, something that can be affirmed only with many qualifications even for baptism and the eucharist (not to mention confirmation, the sacraments of penance and of marriage and the ordination of priests). There was no serious discussion of the arguments against, because already in the previous century the number seven had been defined by the Council of Florence in the decree (!) for the Armenians (!).[373] So with dozens of condemnations, which were often extremely problematical in the light of the Bible and the great Catholic tradition, the individual sacraments were defended against the attacks of the Reformers, and these demarcations were then used to consolidate the endangered sacramental system as a theological foundation for canon law for some partisan supporters. That raises a fundamental question about the historical and theological status of Trent: was Trent a catalyst for the new paradigm?

The Roman Catholic bulwark

It can certainly be demonstrated in very great detail that, compelled by the Protestant attacks, the Council of Trent abolished many crass abuses (e.g. the office of preacher of indulgences, and papal provisions) and countless superstitious practices (e.g. votive masses for sick cattle). But did the council in so doing display a serious grasp of the new Protestant Reformation paradigm? No – and this is not just the verdict of Protestant theology. What then? Generally speaking, the council brought about a **restoration of the mediaeval status quo ante**. Individual Reformation concerns were incorporated into the mediaeval paradigm, as in the understanding of justification ('justified freely, by faith alone'), but no conclusions were drawn from them, say, for the conscience of the individual and the freedom of the Christian or for the understanding of the church, the universal priesthood of believers, church office and its authority. The mediaeval **system of indulgences**, the occasion for Luther's protest, was solemnly confirmed, along with the excommunication which went with it.[374] There was no understanding of three purely disciplinary, but extremely urgent requests also of countless Catholics, including the emperor: the **vernacular** in the liturgy, **the marriage of priests** and the **chalice for the laity**, let alone any deeper theological concerns. There was an absolute intent to maintain the particular features of the mediaeval paradigm, indeed to accentuate it further: legally, **marriage** was now solely a matter for the church, and if it was to be valid it now had to take place before the pastor and two or three witnesses. And this confirms that the Council of Trent was also a theological pastoral council, indeed the council of the Counter-Reformation.

But one thing did **not** happen: the council did not recognize the **papal primacy**! Even many Catholics still regarded this as only 'human (and not divine) law'. Nor was there any interest in the recognition of a papal **infallibility**. The members of the council still had too vivid a memory of the rule of the three Popes and the decrees of the Council of Constance on the supremacy of the council; the more anti-curial 'conciliarist' bishops and theologians who had opposed the curialist party were too numerous even at this Counter-Reformation council. And indeed, when leading German bishops and delegates from Protestant territories appeared at the reopening of the council in 1551, they all called for the renewal of the resolutions of Constance on the supremacy of the council over the Pope and for bishops present to be released from their oath of loyalty to the Pope – though in vain. Because the Pope dominated the council through his legates, the Roman Curia astutely prevented any discussion of the question of the papacy. At best this would have led to further demands for reform. But as already at the Fifth Lateran Council on the eve of the Reformation, and later at Vatican I and Vatican II, the Roman Curia was able to block this. Doctrinal decrees against the 'enemies of the church' were preferable. And it was a final triumph for Rome that at its conclusion the council asked the Pope to confirm its resolutions.

But even so, the **effects** of the small assembly of the church at Trent were enormous, although in some countries its results took some time to be received. Now faith and theology, liturgy and canon law, were unified as never before: a **confessionalizing** in every respect! Just consider all that was decreed with reference to this council, what was established step by step by the Roman Curia in a church which now consistently manifested itself as a **Roman Catholic confessional church** (contrary to all its theoretical claims, one confession alongside others) or as **Roman Catholicism:**

– the Tridentine **confession of faith** (*professio fidei Tridentinae*[375]) with the oath of allegiance to the Pope and the **Roman Catechism** (*catechismus Romanus*, a handbook for pastors);

– the **priestly seminaries** for the training of a strictly orthodox celibate priesthood and the Catholic **religious orders**, both the reformed ones and the newly founded ones (Capuchins, Jesuits); the systematic establishment of church study centres in Rome after the model of the Collegium Germanicum for the training of foreign priests and future bishops;

– the uniform **Latin mass book** (*Missale Romanum*), the **Book of Hours** or breviary (*Breviarium Romanum*), strictly prescribed for all secular clergy, and finally a revised official Latin **translation of the Bible** (the 'Vulgate'), described as 'authentic' (but twice a failure);

– the revaluation of the **confessional**, the confessor and penitential morality, on which a now increasingly voluminous moral theology was erected;

– renewed **popular piety** with new saints, new miracles and also new superstition.

But the implementation of the Tridentine reform took almost another century in Germany – in view of the resistance even of many bishops: 'All in all it can be said that Catholic confessionalization, if we sum up Catholic reform and the Counter-Reformation under this term, is clearly visible only towards the end of the sixteenth century, and first led to success in the seventeenth.'[376] Here it was most of all the state which pressed forward reform in the secular or clerical princely states. In practice, here there was almost a reversal of the phases claimed by Jedin: no reform without Counter-Reformation. According to the most recent investigations, in German cities and territories 'the Catholic counter-offensive took place in the following stages: 1. the purging of officialdom, the city councils and guilds of anything Protestant; 2. an oath on the Council of Trent by officials, teachers and graduates; 3. the expulsion of Protestant preachers and teachers; 4. the admission of only 'tested' Catholic priests; 5. the sequestration of Protestant books and a ban on taking part in Protestant services abroad; 6. visitations to re-Catholicize the population; 7. the banishment of notorious Protestants.'[377]

Here we must note that the Tridentine restoration was able to establish itself more quickly in the Romanic countries than elsewhere. However, it is difficult to make reliable statements because here the life-style of clergy and the way in which they behaved in office, sermons and catecheses, priestly celibacy and popular piety, have still not been investigated very much by historians or sociologists. But one thing is clear: bishops from these countries were represented at the council itself, and thus got something of the will for reform. Moreover, the religious renewal in Italy, Spain and France in the sixteenth and seventeenth centuries – helped on by reformed old and new religious orders – produced many significant figures. To mention only three who were of the greatest influence in reform: **Ignatius of Loyola**, whose *Spiritual Exercises* with their active spirituality, directed towards the world, had a formative effect far beyond the Jesuit order and still do today; **Teresa of Avila**, the reformer of the Carmelite order, who like Ignatius could combine mysticism with a capacity for organization; and finally **Philip Neri**, the founder of the Oratory and of new methods of pastoral care. Moreover, all three were highly suspect to the Inquisition as 'Alumbrados' (enthusiasts), though the content of their preaching, pastoral work and teaching was hardly new (Ignatius, who had a theological fixation on Thomas and a quite practical bent, had hardly read anything by Luther). What were new were the forms of influence and methods.[378]

However, where the council resolutions did not suit the Roman Curia, the implementation of them was selective: thus the council decrees on regional synods were simply not carried out. At first the **central Inquisition authority** already established in Rome before the Council by Paul III acted with restraint, but under Paul IV Caraffa it was active even against cardinals and Philip Neri. The Tridentine **Index** of books forbidden to all Catholics was published in 1564, and in 1571 even a Congregation of the Index was appointed. In 1600 the Inquisition was to burn Giordano Bruno in Rome on the Campo de' Fiori, in 1633 to compel Galileo to bend the knee, and so to intimidate Descartes that initially he did not dare to go on publishing. This laid the basis for the disastrous rejection of the empirical natural sciences by the Catholic Church; the works of Copernicus and Galileo were to remain on the Index until 1835. However, at the time this seemed less important than the Catholic plans of reconquest which were being forged above all in Madrid and Rome, but also in Cologne, Munich and Vienna.

Wars of religion and baroque culture

The Curia was tightened up and reorganized into fifteen ministries ('Congregations'), and thus the powerful consistory of cardinals was largely disempowered. Collegial structures in the church were dismantled further, in part contrary to what had been laid down by Trent, and **mediaeval centralization** was advanced to an unprecedented degree with new means. Wherever possible, permanent **nunciatures** were established – to influence the state and supervise the church, its bishops and theologians (in addition, at the time of Ignatius' death there were 100 Jesuit settlements with around 1000 members in all the important Catholic centres). What had not been provided for by Trent were the 'apostolic **visitors**' sent out by the Pope, the obligation on bishops to pay regular **visits to Rome** (*ad limina apostolorum!*) and the requirement of persisting questions to be put to the Roman Congregations – all of which still apply today. For the missions, in 1622 the Congregatio de Propaganda Fidei was founded by Gregory XV, and all the territories which had become Protestant were also put under it.

Wherever possible, the Restoration within Catholicism was implemented politically, and wherever necessary also by military means. Diplomatic pressure and military intervention: in the second half of the sixteenth century in Europe this confessional strategy had led to a real flood of acts of violence, 'battles of faith', '**wars of religion**' (what an abuse of 'religion'!) with different outcomes:[379]
– in **Italy** and **Spain** the small Protestant groups were relatively quickly throttled by the Inquisition (except for the Waldensians in Piedmont);
– in **France**: eight civil wars, the mass murder of 3,000 Protestants in the 'St Bartholomew's Eve' massacre in Paris (approximately 10,000 throughout the province), which Gregory XIII, the Pope of the improved 'Gregorian Calendar' had celebrated with a *Te deum* and commemorative coins – cruel preludes to the great Revolution;
– in the **Netherlands**: the freedom fight of the Calvinist Dutch against the Spanish rule of terror under Count Alba (around 18,000 executions) and a war between Spain and the Netherlands which lasted for more than eighty years, only being ended by the Peace of Westphalia in 1648;
– in **Germany**: the re-Catholicization of large Protestant areas with the help above all of Jesuits (the Collegium Germanicum in Rome for the training of elite priests; the establishment of an educational system in Germany; Peter Canisius, the spiritual leader of the Jesuits and his widely

disseminated catechism); semi-Protestant Austria was again completely Catholicized;

– in **Poland**: a Counter-Reformation which was finally successful, though it failed in neighbouring Sweden;

– in **Scotland and England**: the beheading of the Catholic Queen of the Scots, Mary Stuart, ordered by her kinswoman Elizabeth I, led to the great military campaign by Philip II, the leader of the Catholic world, against England, the supporter of the rebel Dutch, and to the downfall of his 'invincible' Armada in the English Channel in 1588.

I must not and cannot say any more about all this here. The important thing to note is that with the outbreak of the Bohemian rebellion, the political and religious antagonisms finally led to the fearful **Thirty Years' War** (1618–48). This made Germany a battlefield not only of Catholics and Protestants but also of Danes, Swedes and French, and left it in ruins. The result was a tremendous impoverishment, a disquieting decline in the population, a destruction of cultural values, a degeneration in morals, an increase in superstition and a witch-craze. The **Peace of Westphalia** which was finally negotiated in 1648 regulated affairs in Germany on the principle of the parity of the two confessions (against which the papal nuncio and Pope Innocent X vainly protested) and with the recognition of the Reformed as well (against which the Lutherans vainly protested). Switzerland and the Netherlands were recognized as states independent of the empire. The territories of the confessions in Germany were now demarcated and constitutionally remained essentially as they were down to the twentieth century – resulting in a rigidly confessionalistic state church system to the present day.

Not only politics but also **art** was put at the service of the Counter-Reformation. And without doubt the Counter-Reformation was at its most original and creative here – because it was at its most free. In their monumentality, wealth of movement and exuberance the triumphal architecture, statues and paintings of the **baroque**[380] in Italy (Bernini, Borromoni, Pietro da Cortona) – a great framework for the *theatrum ceremoniale* of the baroque liturgy – very well reflect the regained self-confidence and the claim to rule of a 'church militant and triumphant'. And just as Pope Urban VIII Barberini or King Louis XIV could produce a self-portrait of their absolutist rule elevated to theatrical ceremonial and at the same time ruin the state finances (with Bernini's Cathedral, Confessio and St Peter's Square, and the chateau and court of Versailles respectively), so too did many princes, bishops and abbots.

But this **art style** of the 'barroco' (Portuguese 'barucca', used for misshapen, irregular pearls) even less represents a new distinctive paradigm of Christianity than the Italian Renaissance and the mannerism from which it emerged. Although 'barroco' was originally a designation for anything bizarre and unusual, this art style – already abhorred by the representatives of classicism – must not be seen simply as the decay of the Renaissance and an aberration of taste (as initially Jacob Burckhardt still thought, and as his great pupil Heinrich Wölfflin worked out decisively in his book *Renaissance and Baroque*, 1888).[381] So only from the second half of the nineteenth century does 'baroque' develop into a term for a style or period.

This artistic tendency which emerged from the Counter-Reformation (Il Gesù, the mother church of the Jesuits in Rome, was consecrated in 1584) did not of course remain limited to Catholic Italy, Spain, Portugal and the South American colonies. It also overtook southern Germany, Austria and the Netherlands, indeed France and Italy, where it was further combined with elements of classical style and became the art of princely absolutism in both Catholic and Protestant areas, extending as far as northern and eastern Europe. To this extent, only a qualified distinction can be made between a Roman (Catholic) culture of form and a German (Protestant) culture of writing.

There is no mistaking the fact that baroque, incorporating literature and music, for all its adaptations to the different regions, is the **last unitary style** to spread through **all of old Europe**, still dominated by court and church, until in 1720 there was a transition to refined, dainty and asymmetrical rococo and it vanished a couple of decades later in classicism. To this degree we can speak of a 'baroque age' or a 'baroque culture'. It is still hard to say what constitutes this, since because of chronological overlaps of stylistic elements and marked geographical differences, baroque, like Renaissance, is a difficult term to define; moreover French art history prefers the reigns of individual rulers (Louis XIV, XV, XVI).

However, at least it can be said that here, on Renaissance lines, Christianity and antiquity were linked: the unity of a divine world order was depicted artistically with a balance of reason and faith, a juxtaposition of the sacred and profane worlds, Christian legend and pagan myth. In many respects this was **a synthesis of artistic illusion**: just fifty years after the condemnation of Galileo (one might think of Andrea Pozzo's giant frescoes in S.Ignatio in Rome), indeed a century afterwards, people were still being presented with a baroque vision of how things were in heaven, with Father, Son and Spirit, Madonna, angels and saints, as though the Copernican shift had not taken place, as though the telescope had not been invented, as though the way had not been laid for a further highly momentous and epoch-making paradigm shift in astronomy, physics and philosophy,[382] which we shall have to investigate separately (P V).

No wonder that this last overall European style could not unite in politics and religion a Europe split up into confessions and nations and respond to the stimuli of the beginnings of modernity. For the Roman Catholic Church, too, baroque represented more a splendid renewal of the religious façade and a ceremonial self-portrait with many illusory elements than a renewal of religious substance which, as we saw, continued to have a thoroughly mediaeval stamp. Everywhere there was much artifice, glorification, apotheosis, display and a pathos heightened in an illusory way with – even in such significant painters as the Spaniard Murillo, the Italian Guido Reni and the Dutchman Peter Paul Rubens – relatively little authentic religious inwardness. Like the Renaissance, 'baroque' certainly represents a new artistic style in architecture, sculpture and painting, and also in literature and music, indeed a new sacred or profane 'total art work' in an indissoluble combination and interweaving of architectural, sculptural and artistic effect. But a comprehensive **new entire constellation of theology, church and religion?** No, it did not offer a new paradigm of Christianity.

Apologetics, battles between schools, popular Catholicism

Despite the grandiose development of the arts, at least today, even in the Catholic Church and theology, there is no mistaking the fact that the 'new' Counter-Reformation paradigm of Christianity remained basically the 'old' one! The paradigm of the Counter-Reformation is the **mediaeval Roman Catholic paradigm** (P III) enriched with various new elements and sometimes brilliantly **restored**; now – since the north largely fell outside it – it had very much more of a Romanic touch. The still undivided mediaeval Catholic Church had never been as authoritarian, monolithic and triumphalist as Counter-Reformation Catholicism was. Compared with Protestantism (P IV), this Roman Catholicism:

- was the conservative confession;
- no longer had an international stamp, but was largely Romanized;
- was increasingly fixated on obedience to the Pope, by comparison with whom scripture and tradition, church fathers and ecumenical councils faded into the background and were used above all to defend the threatened church system.

If the Counter-Reformation had been most original in art (because there it was most free), it was least original in **theology** (because there it was most tied). There was essentially a **'revival of scholasticism'**:[383] above all in Salamanca with the Dominican Francisco de Vitoria (died 1546: he introduced Thomas' *Summa theologiae* in place of the basic *Sentences* of

Peter Lombard as a text book), then in the Collegium Romanum (the later Pontifical Gregorian University) of the Jesuits with Suárez, Maldonado, Vázquez (Rome for the first time was a centre of theological studies; a majority of the clerical elite was trained in Rome), and finally also in Germany (Ingolstadt, Dillingen). True, the Jesuit and Cardinal Robert Bellarmine – whose constitutional theory of a merely 'indirect authority' of the Pope in secular matters had been condemned by the Pope – gave classical form to the new theological genre of **controversial theology** with his multi-volume *Disputationes de controversiis christianae fidei* based on Trent. But with its one-sided polemic and largely uncritical self-affirmation this in particular made an essential contribution towards the consolidation of confessional fronts.

Controversial theology was also behind the '**boom in positive theology**'[384] which began later, though of course it remained within limits – the narrow limits of Tridentine orthodoxy. Now on the Catholic side, too, there was certainly a tremendous expenditure of historical learning. But if we look closer, we see that all these academic enterprises served to defend the prevailing church system against a Protestant scholarship which was more advanced in both exegesis and history. Thus everything ultimately culminated in **historical apologetic**:

– in the new editions of councils and church fathers and

– in the twelve-volume *Annales ecclesiastici* of the Oratorian Caesar Baronius (who died in 1607), which were praised in the Catholic camp as the beginning of a church history based on the sources: in confrontation with the church history of the Protestant *Magdeburg Centuries*;

– in the history of the Council of Trent by the Jesuit Pietro Pallavicino Sforza (died 1667): in confrontation with the conciliar history of the Venetian Paolo Sarpi,[385] which disclosed the background;

– in the patristic studies of the French Jesuit Dionysius Petavius (died 1652): in confrontation with the theological position of the Protestants. At any rate from the middle of the seventeenth century the Bollandists (Jesuits) and the Maurians (Benedictines), beginning from a critical examination of the legends of the saints, developed the first auxiliary scientific instruments and methods with which the first critical collections of sources were to be edited.

The teaching of Thomas Aquinas, so long underestimated, became the norm for the Jesuits and at this time established itself on a broad front. Indeed in 1567 Pius V declared Thomas the teacher of the church. Spanish baroque dogmatic theologians, now leading in the Catholic sphere, produced a giant library, but today it can no longer be appealed to even by more traditional Catholic theology. The greatest of them – the last complete edition of his works numbers twenty-eight large volumes[386] –

was the acute Jesuit Francisco Suárez (died 1617), professor in Rome, Alcalá and Coimbra, who also incorporated Augustinian and Scotist elements. Vitoria and Suárez exercised most influence in colonial ethics, in **constitutional philosophy and international law**: Vitoria provided the first definition of international law not only as the 'law of the peoples' (*ius gentium*) but as 'law between the peoples' (*ius inter gentes*) and thus became the founder of international law. In the footsteps of Thomas, Vitoria and Suárez affirmed the right of the nations to self-determination (we shall return to this in connection with Latin America). With his doctrine of **natural law** and national sovereignty (including resistance aginst unjust rulers), Suárez later influenced the European view of law and even Protestant orthodoxy.

And what about Spanish **mysticism**? Here, too, for all our admiration, we must note that despite all its acute psychological observations and eloquent descriptions of the sevenfold mystical way, the mysticism of Teresa of Avila (died 1582), the great reformer of her order, and John of the Cross (who died in 1591, having been thrown into prison by the Inquisition) remained marginal to the church and theology. By contrast, for decades **battles** raged between two theological schools over the problem of **free will and grace**. On one side were the **Jesuits** who put more emphasis on human freedom of will (in a 'modern' way which seemed Pelagian to their opponents) and on the other the **Dominicans**, who in traditional Augustinian fashion emphasized the efficacy of grace. But all the battles ended with a pact: the Pope did not want to decide between the two orders and their theologians, and finally forbade the two parties to engage in further polemic (1611).

The only ones not to be pardoned were the members of the strict religious and moral reform movement of the **Jansenists**, whom their not over-particular Jesuit opponents could easily associate with Calvinism as a result of their forced Augustinian doctrine of grace (we shall be returning to the extraodinary figure of the mathematician, scientist and philosopher Blaise Pascal in connection with modernity). After long controversies and several papal condemnations, the dragoons of Louis XIV finally razed the Jansenist centre of Port Royal to the ground in 1705. But all these disputes – which were carefully repeated in theological lectures down to the time of the Second Vatican Council – remained completely within the framework of mediaeval scholasticism. And woe to any student of Roman theology (even in my time) who dared to seek any other foundation for his theology than the mediaeval Counter-Reformation theses brought to him with strict methods, and the casuistic penitential moral theology that went with them.

However, dry theology was one thing at that time and living **popular piety** was another. For of course to describe and evaluate this restoration Catholicism from a present-day perspective is not to claim that a Catholic of the Counter-Reformation period did not feel utterly at home in his or her 'unreformed' church. On the contrary, the average Catholic in any case had little to do with the disputes between theological schools. In many areas mediaeval colour, movement and sensuality largely prevailed. Here not only was there prayer, sermons and hymns (at best church music), as in the Protestant liturgy; there was also the drama of pontifical masses, the splendour of great processions, pilgrimages which were a rich experience, the great spectacles of the Jesuit and Capuchin preaching aimed at mission and conversion, and perhaps the Jesuit baroque theatre. All this now had a Catholic confessional character and an anti-Protestant focus. There was no more splendid festival in the year than the Feast of Corpus Christi, on which church and state combined to show all that they could offer, in order to give a public acknowledgment of their Catholic faith.

But there were also quieter occasions for practising piety. In time the rood screen which divided clergy and people in the church was again removed (except in Spain). Granted, the average Catholic did not play an active part in the **liturgy of the mass.** Only once in the year at Easter, faithful to the commands of Pope Innocent and the Fourth Lateran Council in 1215, did Catholics go to 'communion'. Before doing that, they would purify themselves with confession (now tabu in Protestantism); what was formerly a public and mobile confessional now became a fixed part of the church furniture, artistically decorated. And day by day Catholics had an opportunity to venerate in a special way the eucharistic host (a practice similarly tabu to Protestants). Instead of the small sacramental aumbry, set at the side, there was now the tabernacle, raised up in the middle of the choir and usually dominated by a giant baroque painting. Before it there was always an 'eternal light' which admonished the faithful to offer silent worship to the 'holy of holies'; but at any occasion, even during the mass, it was solemnly 'exposed'. The 'forty-hour prayer' before the holy of holies was becoming established,

In addition there was the heightened **veneration of Mary,** promoted by the Marian congregations of the Jesuits and by places of pilgrimage like Loreto, from which the Lauretian litany spread. The rosary was vigorously promoted by brotherhoods of the rosary, as was a feast of the rosary, newly introduced after the naval victory at Lepanto over the Turks. Nor was there a lack of new saints, above all Romanic saints (the Jesuits Ignatius and Francis Xavier, the Franciscan Antony of Padua). Soon there were small devotional pictures everywhere, with prayer books and postils. Truly, Catholics could be proud of all the things that the church offered for piety and everyday life. The Middle Ages had reached a baroque heyday. Didn't this church offer a spiritual home, a firm direction in life, security, despite much personal failure? Indeed there was still largely a unity of church and culture, religion and society.

And what was the price? In and after Trent, Catholics had set themselves apart from Protestants, in both dogma and morality, liturgy and canon law, even if the resolutions had been carried out only partially in the different countries. And time and again after Trent they had imprisoned themselves spiritually in the Roman Catholic 'bulwark' (*Il baluardo* – thus the title of a book by Cardinal Alfredo Ottaviano, still chief of the Inquisition authorities during Vatican II). From there, as always firing in all directions – though now **with old-fashioned weapons** (condemnations, prohibitions of books, excommunications and suspensions) – they defended the Roman Catholic paradigm against all the attacks of the 'enemies of the church', who were now to become increasingly numerous in subsequent centuries.

But these weapons increasingly failed: for example, when Pope Paul V Borghese (his name now proudly adorns the splendid new façade of St Peter's, which was completed under him), in dispute with the Republic of Venice, pronounced a papal ban on the Doges and the authorities and put the whole city under the interdict, the clergy there simply continued to administer the sacraments. Since then, no Pope has dared to pronounce an interdict on a whole country. After some significant Popes of the Catholic restoration from Pius V (566–72) through Gregory XIII (1572–85) to Urban VIII (1623–55) in the Thirty Years War, the **papacy** was now increasingly **overshadowed by history**. And the attack of the sixteenth-century Reformation soon appeared harmless compared with that of modernity, which began around the middle of the seventeenth century and was to reach its climax with the Enlightenment, the great revolution of the eighteenth century and the modern achievements of the nineteenth century.

13. From anti-Protestantism to anti-Modernism

After the age of the wars of faith, confessions or religion, the religious forces which had been at full stretch in the Reformation and Counter-Reformation were largely exhausted. Now a new secular culture was developing along the lines marked out by the Renaissance. It was able to free itself from supervision by the church, indeed it even influenced church life and teaching in many ways. We shall have to analyse later how from the middle of the seventeenth century a new epoch-making paradigm shift took place above all in France, Holland and England: from the Reformation (P IV) and Counter-Reformation (P III) to the **modern Enlightenment paradigm** (P V). This was a process which changed politics and state theory as radically as it changed philosophy, the natural sciences, history, art, literature and culture generally – with powerful effects on religion and morality, church and theology. In the framework of our analysis of the mediaeval Counter-Reformation paradigm (P III) which now has so much of a Mediterranean stamp we are primarily interested in only one question: **how did the official Catholic Church**, how did Rome in particular, **react to** what is now called **modernity** (P V)?

The Roman reaction

The mediaeval paradigm had once been in many respects progressive – by comparison with the early church Byzantine paradigm: it was a new response to a new challenge in world history. But the climax with Innocent III was also the turning-point. And already in the late Middle Ages and decisively at the time of the Reformation this Roman Catholic paradigm had fallen behind the times. In European modernity it was increasingly seen as a relic of the 'dark' Middle Ages.

The innovative spirit of the Middle Ages had now become a **demon of apologetics and reaction:**[387]
– Reaction against the **conciliar theories** which, following Constance, had argued for the supremacy of the council over the Pope. By contrast, there was a reinforced emphasis on papal primacy even over councils and the episcopate.
– Reaction against the **spiritualism** of the Wycliffites in England and the Hussites in Bohemia who in the face of the ruthless exercise of power emphasized the invisibility of the church. Over against this there was an emphasis on the ecclesiastical and externally visible character of the Christian community.
– Reaction then above all, time and again, against the **Reformers** and their successful new paradigm. Over against this there was an emphasis on the objective significance of the sacraments, the importance of hierarchical authorities, of the priestly office, of Latin, celibacy and the episcopate.
– Reaction against **Gallicanism**, which again emphasized the traditional independence of the French church under Louis XIV through Bishop Bossuet (the last representative of an Augustinian theology of history), stressed the supremacy of the council, and challenged papal infalli-

bility (unless it was confirmed by the church). Against this was set a theology of hierarchical and especially papal authority and the understanding of the church as an empire organized from and dominated by Rome, alongside (and in moral matters even over) the state.

– Reaction against **Jansenism**, which was allied with Gallicanism, and its rigorous interpretation of the Augustinian doctrine of grace. Over against this there was special emphasis on the papal 'teaching office' ('magisterium').

– Reaction, finally, against the **state absolutism** of the eighteenth and then the '**laicism**' of the nineteenth century which first indirectly and then quite directly advanced secularization. Over against this was a propagation of the church as a 'perfect society' equipped with all rights and means.

Of course the **Enlightenment** – which we have still to discuss in detail (P V) – did not simply stop at the gates of the Catholic Church, well preserved and well guarded though it was. Granted, in Germany the Enlightenment could not have such an intensive effect as in the freer Protestant territories – where in any case there were clear time-lags. It had its effect above all on the clergy, members of the orders, officials and the educated, and in addition to the standard themes of superstition and Jesuits affected especially questions of pastoral care, the liturgy and the relationship between the bishops and Rome. The traditional Counter-Reformation Roman Catholic paradigm – now not only under sharp criticism from outside but also undermined from within – showed considerable tensions and rifts. There were invasions by the hated 'spirit of the time'. If we look more closely, it is evident that in the seventeenth and eighteenth centuries the Roman Catholic paradigm was in deep **crisis**.

The shaking of the Roman Catholic paradigm

Several factors contributed to the shaking:

– In the age of enlightened princely absolutism the **Popes** had sunk into political insignificance (there was a praiseworthy exception between 1740 and 1750 in the human and socially concerned, learned and enlightened Benedict XIV Lambertini, a vigorous promoter of archaeology, history and liturgical study, and also of chemistry, physics and anatomy, who was highly respected even among Protestants).

– **Conversions** of Protestant rulers (Augustus the Strong of Saxony to gain the Polish throne) to Catholicism remained isolated instances which had no effect on the territories concerned.

– **Persecutions of Protestants** (in France, the Palatinate, Salzburg, Hungary and Poland) often damaged the lands concerned the most: first of all the exclusion of all non-Catholics from state offices in Poland, and later the division of the Poles, who for a long time had been extending so far East, under a Russian Orthodox and a Protestant Prussian rule.

– The **Inquisition**, especially the fight of the Jesuits against Jansenist 'Protestantism' and against mysticism, severely weakened the church of France and also of other countries.

Another exacerbating factor was that ideological pillars of the Counter-Reformation system had themselves been made shaky by the pressure of the Enlightenment:

– Even in Catholic Germany the **papalism** of the Roman Curia came under fire with criticism from revived **episcopalism** in the spirit of the early church paradigm (P II: Febronius was the main representative). Its demands were that the council should again be set over the Pope as in the ancient tradition and that the church primacy need not unconditionally be associated with the Roman see. It saw curialism as the great obstacle to church unity (the resistance of the German archbishops to interventions from the nuncio in Munich).

– **Jesuitism**, which, remote from the ideals of its founder, had entangled itself in the politics and trading of this world, now itself came under the pressure of the Enlightenment as an ideological chanpion of the mediaeval Counter-Reformation paradigm. Hated particularly in the Romanic countries as an agent of the papacy and an exponent of anti-modernity, the Jesuit order was banned by the absolutist regimes of Portugal (the Jesuits were expelled from the admirable Indian reductions in Paraguay), France, Spain and Naples (which were of course pursuing their own advantages) and finally banned personally by Pope Clement XIV 'for ever' (only the Prussia of Frederick II and the Russia of Catharine II offered asylum).

– **Scholasticism** was tacitly demolished by German theologians through more 'reasonable' interpretations of dogmas, openness to historical criticism, disregard of confessional conflicts and the dissemination of German translations of the Bible.

– **Canon law** in its mediaeval Counter-Reformation form equally came under criticism, above all over compulsory celibacy, monastic life and its general intolerance. Especially in Austria, the Emperor Joseph II intervened massively in church affairs – not very skilfully, and in the spirit of absolutist state supremacy ('Josephinism'): an edict for the Jews, toleration of the Protestant and Orthodox churches, the abolition of numerous monasteries, the reform of the training of priests, the purging of the cult, in other words an effort to create a national church largely independent of Rome.

The **Catholic rulers** – highly interested in maintaining the political and religious **status quo**, were sometimes almost the only supporters of the papacy, but precisely in this role they forced through a right of exclusion in papal elections (thus Spain, the German Empire, Austria, France until 1904). They supported the prevailing Roman system where necessary by the violent suppression of Catholic opposition within the church (for example the Jansenists and Port Royals) and through the persecution and expulsion of Protestants (in the Rhineland Palatinate, in the Archbishopric of Salzburg, in Habsburg Hungary and Silesia, in Poland and finally also in France). It was this in particular that provoked the witty and sharp-tongued Voltaire, pleading for toleration of confessions and religions, and the herald of an unprecedented revolutionary onslaught.

And what about **Rome**? Most Catholic church historians today will agree with the judgment of the Dutch church historian L.J.Rogier: 'Generally speaking, the actual influence of Rome on world history was extremely slight; and its relation to the development of thought was exhausted in stereotyped and sterile protests. Anyone who surveys the cultural history of the eighteenth century will constantly miss the participation of the church and its supreme government in discussions of burning issues of the time. If Rome intervened at all, it was in a completely negative way, with a *monitum*, an anathema, or by imposing the obligation to keep silent. Regrettably Rome neglected to enter into dialogue with, indeed systematically avoided, a generation so strongly caught up in the stream of time as that of the eighteenth century. Would it not have made sense to hold a council in the middle of the period of "crisis of conscience" and later, in the middle of the eighteenth century?'[388]

But we shall have to clarify in our analysis of the modern paradigm (P V) what the Enlightenment, the French Revolution, the imprisonment of Pope Pius VI, Napoleon's concordat with Pius VII and finally his abdication meant for Christianity. How did events develop?

Restoration again after the Revolution

In the Catholic Church of the nineteenth century there was beyond doubt a new awakening of religious forces among the clergy as among the laity, among the religious orders and in the missionary movement, in charitable work and education, and in popular piety, to which we shall be returning. But in the framework of an analysis of the mediaeval Counter-Reformation paradigm (P III) we must be primarily interested in the attitude of the papacy, which was still dominant in the Catholic sphere. From the beginning, Counter-Reformation Rome was against modern philosophy, against modern science, against the modern theory of the state and of course also against the slogan 'Freedom, Equality, Brotherhood'. What the Louvain historian Roger Aubert says of Pius VI, the Pope of the age of the Revolution, can also be applied to the Popes of the age of the Restoration: 'When the storm of revolution broke loose in France, the greater part of Catholic Europe eventually became involved. At that moment there sat on Peter's throne a Pope who was conscientious but who lacked precisely those characteristics which which were needed under such trying circumstances.'[389]

In Rome and in the **papal state** – in the nineteenth century politically and socially the most backward state in Europe – there was fundamental opposition to all the modern developments. Rome was

- against the sovereignty of the people and constitutional democracy,
- against tolerance and human rights, freedom of religion, of conscience, of assembly and the press,
- against new scientific discoveries, historical criticism, and later also against the biological theory of evolution,
- even against the railways which were now being built, gas lighting, suspension bridges.

In this state of monsignors only one lesson had been learned from history: that one had to defend one's own legal positions and positions of power – some of which had been gained in highly dubious circumstances (the Donation of Constantine, the Pseudo-Isidorian forgeries) – or even simply appropriated. Roman Catholicism, which had suffered particularly under the French Revolution, regained its strength. The hierarchical structures, parts of which had been destroyed, were restored. As early as 1799 Mauro Cappellari had proclaimed 'the triumph of the Holy See', more than three decades before his election to the papacy as Gregory XVI. After the unprecedented revolutionary upheavals '**Restoration**', now in an eminently political sense, had become the great European slogan, proclaimed by the 'Holy Alliance' of the powers which had gained the victory over Napoleon. And what institution could have had a greater interest in the return to pre-revolutionary and authoritarian conditions than the papacy, which had behind it the abolition of God in Notre Dame in Paris and the replacement of the papal state by the Roman republic?

Nevertheless, would not a self-critical and constructive rather than a purely restorative answer to the revolutionary upheavals a priori have been conceivable? Here one might recall three significant dates in the first half of the nineetenth century: 1806, 1830 and 1848.[390]

In **1806** the 'Holy Roman Empire of the German Nation' ceased to exist – after the end of the clerical princedoms in Germany as a result of the secularization of the dioceses, foundations and monasteries three years earlier. Since Charlemagne, the political substratum of the mediaeval Roman Catholic paradigm had shaped it. The last representative of the *Imperium Romanum nationis Germanicae*, the Habsburg Francis II, laid down the German imperial crown and now called himself simply 'Emperor of Austria'.

And Rome? At the Congress of Vienna the Cardinal Secretary of State Ercole Consalvi did all he could to restore the Holy Roman Empire and church conditions as they existed in Germany before 1806, but without success. All he succeeded in doing was to re-establish the papal state within its old frontiers. Was this a real success? The notorious backwardness and blindness of Pope and Curia were again demonstrated for all the world to see: the modern Napoleonic Code was immediately abolished and the former papal legislation reinstated; 700 cases of 'heresy' were investigated by the Holy Office, all significant state offices were put in the hands of churchmen. The **economic abuses of the monsignori** were **restored** – one of the main reasons why the Pope could not make any stand on social questions until the end of the century. More than anyone else he should have criticized and admonished himself. But in the age of the Austrian State Chancellor Metternich, the stirrings of freedom in Europe were suppressed anyway. And a Romanticism orientated on the Middle Ages, a revival of traditional religious feelings and the restoration of the Jesuit order seemed to suppress Enlightenment and democratic ideas again for ever. But:

In **1830** the Paris July Revolution brought the victory of the liberal middle classes over the reactionary Bourbons, who had returned to power after the fall of Napoleon – with revolutionary consequences from Belgium and Italy to Russian Poland.

And Rome? The Roman church (Gregory XVI) obstinately rejected all changes made in the spirit of political liberalism, and thus liberalism became radically anti-clerical. Now one anti-modern Roman measure followed another: a renewal of the Congregation of the Index, the condemnation of all Bible societies (including Catholic ones), a new emphasis on confessional differences, an attempt to transfer the training of clergy from the enlightened universities to Tridentine priestly seminaries. No wonder that instead of the unity in faith between Catholics and Protestants aimed at in the Enlightenment there was a **split between clericals and anti-clericals** (conservatives and liberals/radicals) which was disastrous above all for the Romanic lands and which was also transferred to the new world of Latin America, where it has persisted in part to the present day (under a variety of different party labels). But:

In **1848** the revolutionary wave flowing from the Paris February revolution also reached the papal state. Pope Pius IX, elected two years before, first of all fell into line with liberal reforms and was hailed enthusiastically by the people. But then, because he shrank from more radical reforms, he was compelled to flee to Gaeta.

And Rome? Pius IX returned to Rome after the defeat of the Italian revolution with the help of French and Austrian troops and now became the implacable opponent of all free ('liberal') political, intellectual and theological streams. It was under him that **'Ultramontanism'** spread in northern and western Europe, an emotional and sentimental veneration for the Pope 'beyond the mountains' of a kind that had never existed either in the Middle Ages or in the Counter-Reformation, but which had gained prominence at the beginning of the nineteenth century in reaction to Gallican and Josephinist enlightened ideas. Countless new congregations of men and women loyal to Rome, the Catholic associations ('Pius Association'), and organizations of all kinds which in the second half of the century were increasingly active in the spirit of the Roman restoration and unconditional obedience to the Pope, rather than overcoming the political polarization in society, reinforced it to the point of causing a 'Kulturkampf'.

What a short-sighted strategy: internal consolidation and external isolation! Under the emotional inspiration of Pius IX, who was untroubled by any intellectual doubt but probably had psychopathic features, the mediaeval Counter-Reformation Catholic fortress was now **strengthened against modernity** with every possible force. How? By a reinforcement of a papalism, dogmatism and Marianism which supported one another in the face of increasing religious indifference, hostility to the church and loss of faith. Within the fortress, there was emotional security and unburdening through popular piety of every kind, from pilgrimage, through devotional objects for the masses to May devotions.

At this time **Catholicism became a specific social form** which Catholic sociologists, above all Franz-Xaver Kaufmann[391] and Karl Gabriel,[392] have analysed in the last two decades. Karl Gabriel has summarized this social form of the Catholic in a very recent publication: 'There are three characteristic complexes of features:

1. The involvement of various Catholic social milieus in a closed, confessional group milieu with its own "world-view", its own institutions and a specific ritualization of the everyday;

2. The centralization and bureaucratization of the structures of church office with a sacralization of modernized forms of organization and a disciplining of the clergy, who were separated from the "world";

3. The development of an ideologically closed system which legitimated both the distance from the modern world and the claim to a monopoly of ultimately valid interpretations of the world.'[393] For

Catholics in the modern democracies this meant a march into the ghetto.[394]

The old dogmas, and also new ones, were of special importance for this closed ideological system. At that time the great event was in 1854, in the midst of the tremendous industrial revolution, when Rome manifested a new 'creative' understanding of its magisterium by the solemn papal definition of the '**immaculate conception of Mary**' (Mary herself conceived by her mother without original sin), a 'luxury dogma', as John Henry Newman, later a cardinal, was ironically to comment. In fact for the first time a dogma had not been resolved on in a council in a situation of conflict to ward off a heresy. Rather, it was solemnly proclaimed by the Pope alone from the perfection of his power, to further traditional piety and support the Roman system. For whom, why? In the closed Roman Catholic group milieu, even dogmas long rejected outside retained their plausibility, as they were constantly repeated and taken for granted as the only valid dogmas. And what about Catholic theology?

The repression of modern Catholic theology

The situation got worse and worse for Catholic theology in the second third of the nineteenth century. At the beginning of the century, at least in German Catholic theology and among the clergy generally, under the impact of the Enlightenment there had been relative openness towards a critical discussion with modernity. In southern Germany clergy associations for the abolition of celibacy had formed. The Catholic theological faculty at the **University of Tübingen**, the first Catholic faculty alongside a Protestant faculty in the same place, founded after the Napoleonic wars, aroused great hopes.[395] Here, under the leadership of Johann Sebastian von Drey and Johann Baptist Hirscher, there was an intensive and constructive discussion with both the Enlightenment's idealistic philosophy and its practical concerns for reform. What was called for above all – as it had already been by Martin Luther – was a reform of the ordained ministry (abolition of compulsory celibacy) and the liturgy (introduction of the vernacular). A beginning was also made in applying the historical method in exegesis and the history of dogma.

But at the same time – first in Italy and then also in Germany – a neo-Scholastic counter-movement had begun which in the face of modernity attempted once again to revive the mediaeval and Counter-Reformation paradigm in philosophy and theology. Parallel to **neo-Romanticism and neo-Gothic** in architecture and **neo-Gregorianism** in church music there was a **neo-Scholasticism** which – apart from its historical investigations – proved considerably more superficial than Spanish baroque scholasticism. But after some delay the Roman Curia recognized its opportunity and gave powerful support to the rise of neo-Scholasticism. Here was a new success for curial centralism: Neo-Thomism finally became the **normal Roman Catholic theology** prescribed by law even for all Catholic schools. There had never been such a fixation on a single school even in the Middle Ages. Its main representative in Rome was the Jesuit theologian Giovanni Perrone, who made the theological preparations for the definition of the dogma of the 'Immaculate Conception of Mary' in 1854 by Pius IX. This Roman Catholic theologian had removed himself beyond the horizon of general interests and questions and now quickly got left further and further behind.

Since the July revolution of 1830 Rome had been acting with increasing resolution and purpose against the movements for theological renewal, especially those in Germany, but less against conservative 'fideism' in France. There is no mistaking the fact that in the face of the threat of a paradigm shift in Catholic theology and the church, it was resolved on to introduce a **phase of repression**, and woe to those affected by the purging!
– The Catholic theological faculty of **Marburg**, barely founded, was liquidated by the church itself, as later was that of **Giessen**.
– The faculty in **Tübingen** clearly shifted to the Roman line when the wind changed (there are parallels to very recent events here), under the pernicious influence of **Johann Adam Möhler** and the 'Möhlerians' in the faculty (Möhler's confessional *Symbolics* appeared as early as 1832); this led to a split in the faculty and finally to resignations which went deep.[396]

In the 1830s the Roman ban also hit the faculty in **Bonn**, where the thoroughly Catholic professor **Georg Hermes** and his pupils had been discussing constructively with Kant and other philosophers: Hermes' works were put on the Index and the 'Hermesianism' of the Bonn faculty was brutally suppressed by a new Archbishop of Cologne, who was also essentially responsible for the Cologne dispute over mixed marriages with the Prussian government: half a dozen professors were removed from office.[397]
– In **Vienna** in the 1850s, the 'Güntherians', the utterly Catholic Viennese secular cleric **Anton Günther** and his pupils, then suffered the same fate as 'Hermesianism' in the 1830s and 1840s, and were forced to submit.
– Germany's outstanding church historian **Ignaz von Döllinger**, who opposed the Roman repression at a very early stage, was dogged by suspicions and the now usual denunciations long before the break came over the definition of infallibility.

Now German Catholic theology was on the defensive all down the line. In 1863, in **Munich**, under the leadership of Döllinger, for many the most significant theologian of his time, there was a **congress of Catholic** scholars that showed a completely different tendency from the neo-Scholastic theology which was the norm. However, this German congress of Catholic scholars only took place this once, and not again. Why?

The general condemnation of modernity

Already in the following year, 1864, Pius XII published a *Syllabus errorum modernorum*, a 'collection of modern errors' (eighty in number).[398] It represented the absolutely uncompromising defence of the mediaeval Counter-Reformation structure of doctrine and power, and moreover was regarded everywhere as a general **declaration of war against the paradigm of modernity** (P V). Granted, today some Catholic apologists want to play down all that was condemned there in a pose of *de facto* papal infallibility, but the facts speak for themselves. There was a condemnation of liberal clerical associations – with an eye to Munich (Döllinger) – along with Bible societies and secret societies (Freemasons: Opus Dei did not yet exist at that time). Human rights generally were condemned: freedom of conscience, religion and the press, and civil marriage. So too – always given a blanket label – were 'pantheism', 'naturalism' and 'rationalism', 'indifferentism' and 'latitudinarianism', 'socialism' and 'communism'. The whole list of errors, which also included any rejection of the papal state, culminated in the general condemnation of the statement that the Roman Pontifex can and must 'be reconciled to and accept progress, liberalism and the new civilization'.[399]

In the German Catholic milieu there was satisfaction with this general reckoning, but that was not the case in a considerable part of French Catholicism. After the emigration of the reformers and then the modern natural scientists and philosophers, an **emigration of intellectuals** from the Catholic Church had now become largely unavoidable. After all, Rome had opposed modernity – ultimately without success – with all the means of ideology, politics and the Inquisition. This Catholicism no longer had anything to offer at the level of science and education, which were fundamental for modern men and women. One important symptom of this disastrous development was that the **Index of Books forbidden to Catholics** now contained a majority of the representative spirits of European modernity: alongside numerous theologians and church critics and the founders of modern science, Copernicus and Galileo, were the fathers of modern philosophy: Descartes and Pascal, Bayle, Malebranche and Spinoza, and the British empiricists Hobbes, Locke and Hume, and also Kant's *Critique of Pure Reason*; of course Rousseau and Voltaire were there, and later Cousin, John Stuart Mill, Comte, and also the great historians Gibbon, Condorcet, Ranke, Taine and Gregorovius. In addition there were Diderot and d'Alembert with their *Encyclopaedia* and the Larousse *Dictionary*, Grotius the constitutional and international lawyer, Pufendorf and Montesquieu, and finally an elite of modern literature: Heine and Lenau, Hugo, Lamartine, the Dumas, father and son, Balzac, Flaubert, Zola, Leopardi and D'Annunzio – and in our day Sartre and Simone de Beauvoir, Malaparte, Gide and Kazantzakis.

All this confirms impressively how far Rome had gone **on the defensive** with the mediaeval Roman Catholic paradigm. For the **modern world** had largely come into being **without and against Rome** and moreover went its way, not at all impressed by the backward-looking utopia of a papal state bureaucracy dreaming of the Middle Ages and hostile to the Reformation and to reform generally. Hardly any attempt was made to engage in a critical constructive discussion with modern atheism, which was reaching a climax in the figures of Feuerbach, Schopenhauer, Marx and Nietzsche. With their backward gaze, church and theology in the Roman ghetto hardly perceived how much the world had changed around them. What was true of the intellectual sphere was also generally true of the spheres of the natural sciences, technology, industry and society. Since 1848 the rebellious intellectuals had been joined by the rebellious proletariat, and in the last third of the nineteenth century the pastor's son Friedrich Nietzsche was to proclaim the 'death of God' and the monistic scientist Ernst Heckel the materialistic solution to the 'riddle of the universe', a logical climax to a modernity which had begun to make human freedom, autonomy, reason and progress absolute.

Rome, helpless, did not recognize the signs of the times but blockaded itself. Now a closed mind, submission, humility and obedience to an increasingly narrow-minded and arrogant hierarchy were regarded as central Catholic virtues. The church was an *acies ordinata*, a battle line with closed ranks, admired and praised by some Catholics, who of course would never dream of joining it. But the more that erroneous judgments were given by the Roman 'teaching office' on matters of science and biblical exegesis, democracy and public morality, the more the opposition grew and the more fixated Rome was on trusting in its own infallibility. I have already discussed this elsewhere,[400] but must return to some decisive points.

The Counter-Enlightenment council

Oppressed as he was by all the 'errors' of modernity and all the attacks of the 'enemies of the church', Pius IX could not resist the temptation, three hundred years after the Council of Trent, to summon a new 'ecumenical council', though this was to be even more markedly Roman than Trent. If

Trent was dominated by the Counter-Reformation, in accordance with the will of this Pope this council was to be completely dominated by the **Counter-Enlightenment**.

That was the position in 1869, and it is more than symbolic of the reinforced Roman centralism that the council now took place not just in Rome, but in the Vatican. Could the council ever be free in this curial 'frame'? Moreover, this was doubted, and not without reason, before, during and after the council.[401]

Neither in Trent nor at Vatican II, which was held a good four hundred years later, would a **definition of papal infallibility** have been conceivable. That makes all the more interesting the question why such a definition could have been arrived at by the First Vatican Council, a century before Vatican II. According to historical research,[402] several factors played a role:

Factor 1: The majority of council fathers had grown up in the age of **political restoration** and anti-Enlightenment and anti-nationalistic Romanticism during the **first half of the century**. That meant that after the confusions and excesses of the French Revolution and the Napoleonic period a majority of Europeans had an irresistible longing for peace and order, for the good old days, indeed for the 'Christian Middle Ages'. And who could better guarantee the religious foundation for maintaining the political and religious status quo or the restoration of the status quo ante than the Pope? Moreover, the majority of leading Catholic churchmen in the various countries were regarded as loyal supporters of political and social reaction; some were close to the fashionable philosophical trend of 'traditionalism' (at that time a title of honour).

Factor 2: In the **second half of the century** the foundations of this work of restoration had again been threatened by **Liberalism**, which established itself rapidly with the onrush of industrialization, and its no less modern counterpart, **Socialism**, which in many respects was similar. With their belief in reason and progress in economics, politics, science and culture, these philosophies seemed to do away with all religious authorities and traditions. Clericalism and anti-clericalism egged each other on. Enlightenment rationalism had returned in the form of anti-Idealistic and anti-Romantic positivism, along with the aspiring empirical sciences, the natural sciences and history. The persistence of the church authorities not only in the established political system but also in the traditional 'biblical' view of the world often drove both politicians and scientists into a vigorous aggressiveness against anything religious.

Factor 3: In the Rome of the **1860s** the '**Roman question**' overshadowed everything: whether the **papal state** restored in 1849, but already reduced to Rome and its environs as a result of intervention by the

Piedmont government, was to be abandoned. Could it hold out permanently with French support alone against the movement for Italian unity? As finally a united state, didn't Italy need Rome as its capital? All this was looked on in the Vatican with the utmost concern. And the opposite calculation was: would anyone dare to take Rome from a Pope whose universal primacy and papal infallibility an ecumenical council had proclaimed *urbi et orbi* in a solemn and definitive form? This was almost the only ray of hope for all those who at the culmination of modernity were fighting for the preservation of the mediaeval papal state – with reference to Matt.16.18.

Factor 4: The more time went on, the more openly Pope **Pius IX** pressed for a definition of papal infallibility as his **dearest concern**. The one who had been greeted at his election in 1846 as a liberal and a reformer but who after his political failures and his exile in 1848 had turned into a political and theological reactionary now hastened to say his intransigent 'no' to the Italian movement for national unity as well: Rome must for ever remain the city of the Pope. At the same time the ultramontane press and numerous bishops and faithful, especially in France, promoted a vigorous campaign against Italy and for the Pope threatened in his papal state.

The consequence was that while Pius IX involved the Italian Catholics in unnecessary and severe conflicts of loyalty between state and church, he played the role of the 'persecuted victim of un-Christian powers' brilliantly and thus gained the applause for his person and his office that he had aimed at. The dogmatic bond between Catholics and the Pope which in any case already existed now also took on sentimental overtones. A completely new phenomenon developed: a **'veneration of the Pope'**, arousing deep feelings, which was considerably reinforced by the papal audiences and mass pilgrimages to Rome that were now becoming usual. Pius IX himself saw the crisis over the papal state as a further act in the world-historical battle between God and Satan, which with a completely irrational trust in the victory of divine providence he hoped to win. In any case, this friendly and very eloquent man was dangerously emotional, had a superficial theological education, was unfamiliar with modern scientific methods, and was surrounded by narrow-minded advisers.

This setting alone explains the Pope's urge to dogmatize his own primatial authority and infallibility. And only the papal veneration offered to Pius IX explains at the same time why a **definition of infallibility met with a favourable mood** in wide circles of the Catholic clergy and people, and not with rejection. The process of ultramontane indoctrination and administrative centralization of the church which had been rapidly and systematically advanced since the middle of the century was accepted largely without resistance. The Syllabus, the condemnation of German theologians, the placing of all writings with a Gallican and Febronianist tendency on the Index, were accepted without protest. So too were the now increasing influence of Rome on the election of bishops and the constant interventions of the nunciatures in the internal affairs of dioceses, the invitation to bishops to strengthen their contacts with Rome, the deliberate advancement of priests propagating Roman ideas even against their own bishops, and the constantly new instruction of the faithful in the doctrine of the primacy of the Pope, the foundation of the church. So everything had been well prepared, and the First Vatican Council could take place.

Two dogmas for the Pope

The council summoned by Pius IX first of all did not delay to supplement yet further with the magisterium the anti-Protestant and anti-modern paradigm of church and theology which had been defended for so long and with so many sacrifices. That explains the 'Dogmatic Constitution on the Catholic Faith', which concentrated on the relationship between faith (revelation) and reason defined in a thoroughly Thomistic way: this combated both rationalism and fideism.[403] None of this was particularly controversial. But there was a vigorous controversy for weeks when on the personal urging of Pius IX the council was to decree the **definition of papal privileges**. For many of the council fathers were quite clear what that meant: instead of the ecumenical council (as in the early church, at Constance, and in the conciliar tradition), the Bishop of Rome (as in the Middle Ages) would be promised supreme, indeed now even **infallible**, authority in the church. Moreover the most prominent representatives of the opposition departed before the decisive vote: in addition to the Archbishops of Milan and St Louis, Missouri, the representatives of the most important metropolitan sees in France, Germany and Austria-Hungary, whose successors a century later were to make up the nucleus of the now progressive majority at the Second Vatican Council.

Pius IX was not impressed by this. Despite all opposition, on 18 July 1870 **two papal dogmas** were formally proclaimed by the vast majority of the council (above all from Italy and Spain), dogmas which are still the object of controversy between churches and within the church:

- The Pope has a legally binding **primacy** of jurisdiction over every individual national church and every individual Christian.
- The Pope has the gift of **infallibility** in his own solemn magisterial decisions. These solemn (*ex cathedra*) decisions are infallible on the basis of a special support from the Holy Spirit and are unchangeable ('irreformable') of themselves, not by virtue of the assent of the church.

The Authority of the Pope

Accordingly we teach and declare that by the ordinance by the Lord the Roman Church has the pre-eminence of ordinary authority over all others, and that this **authority of jurisdiction** of the Bishop of Rome, which is truly episcopal, is direct: to it the pastors and faithful of every rite and rank – both individually and all together – are obligated in hierarchical submission and true obedience, not only in matters of faith and morals but also in such matters as concern the discipline and leadership of the church spread throughout the earth, so that through the preservation of unity both of communion and of the same confession of faith the church of Christ with the Bishop of Rome may be one flock under one supreme Shepherd (cf. John 10.16). This is the teaching of the Catholic truth, from which no one can deviate without harm to faith and salvation...

If the Bishop of Rome speaks *ex cathedra*, in other words if he decides in exercising his office as pastor and teacher of all Christians by virtue of his supreme apostolic authority that a doctrine of faith or morals is to be maintained by the whole church, then by means of the divine support promised him in blessed Peter he possesses that **infallibility** with which the divine Redeemer willed to see his church equipped in the definition of doctrines of faith or morality; therefore such definitions by the Bishop of Rome are of themselves unalterable, and are not based on the assent of the church.

If anyone – which God forbid – should undertake to contradict this our definition: let him be excluded.

Constitution Pastor aeternus of the
First Vatican Council, 18 July 1870

So Pius IX succeeded; and the price was high. But despite everything there was one matter in which he did not succeed: he could not save his **papal state**. Just two months after the end of the council this collapsed when on 20 September 1870 Italian troops marched into Rome. And the Pope? His secular power had been lost. An overwhelming Roman popular vote opposed him, and he postponed the council *sine die*, for an indefinite period. Thus a further important element in the mediaeval Roman Catholic paradigm had dropped away, which the Pope had defended to the end with tooth and claw.

Politically the power of the Pope was thus reduced to that over a dwarf state of around 1000 inhabitants, in surface area barely a fifth of the principality of Monaco. But instead of understanding the new situation, Pius IX took on a new role, that of the much pitied 'prisoner in the Vatican'. This could only give powerful impetus to the emotional veneration of the Pope and the pilgrimages which had already developed – now no longer as fifteen hundred years earlier to the tombs of the apostles, but above all to the 'Holy Father'. Only now did the great popular audiences in Rome begin. '*Non possumus*', 'We cannot', ran the rigid formula with which the Pope had ensconced himself behind the walls of the Vatican in the face of the new state of Italy, backed by the definition of primacy and infallibility. Moreover, for decades the Popes refused to accept the new situation between state and church.

Did this dogmatic '*non possumus*' rule out any reconciliation for ever? No. At the very point when the Fascist leader Mussolini came to power the Vatican resolved on a *possumus* ('We can'). At an earlier stage Pius IX's wiser and more liberal successor **Leo XIII** had first settled the 'Kulturkampf' sparked off by the German imperial chancellor Otto von Bismarck, which had done even more to set political Catholicism on its feet. Leo XIII had also – while maintaining the papal dogmas and the necessity of a church state – corrected Rome's negative attitude to modernity to a considerable degree; towards democracy, the liberal freedoms, indeed in part even towards modern exegesis and church history, but above all on the social question. The loss of the papal state finally freed the way for a long overdue social encyclical (*Rerum novarum*, 1891). And many people in the Catholic Church had already been given some hope that a fundamental change could come about. They were called 'reform Catholics'. But such a change was still a long way off.

The twentieth century saw two more **anti-modern purges** in the Catholic clergy, at the beginning and around the middle of the century, both started by Rome, before the Second Vatican Council was to take up essential concerns of both the Reformation and modernity:

– At the beginning of the century **Pius X** condemned all reform theologians (especially historians and exegetes) in France, Germany, England, North America and Italy under the label '**modernism**',[404] which had been created by the Curia to defame them. They were punished with sanctions of various kinds (the Index, excommunication, dismissal). A new Syllabus, an anti-modern encyclical (1907) and an 'anti-modernist oath' forced on all the clergy (1910) were meant to eradicate the 'modernists' definitively in the Catholic Church.

– After the Second World War **Pius XII**, who had kept silent over the

Holocaust,[405] dismissed and in part even excommunicated the reform theologians, above all in France (the Jesuits P.Teilhard de Chardin, H.de Lubac, H.Bouillard and the Dominicans M.D.Chenu, Y.Congar and H.Féret), this time under the label '**Nouvelle Théologie**'. Others, like Karl Rahner in Germany, were put under special censorship. A further encyclical (*Humani generis*, of 1950) condemned all the 'errors of the time'. The culmination of this policy was a new Marian dogma, now declared 'infallible' (the bodily assumption of Mary into heaven, 1950). It manifested to all the world the authoritarian approach of this Pope, the last unchallenged representative of the pre-conciliar mediaeval Counter-Reformation anti-modern paradigm, who attempted to suppress all opposing or even alternative voices in the church – beginning with the worker priests in France.

It was to be a good ten years later that an epoch-making change took place with John XXIII (1958–1963) and the **Second Vatican Council**. The significance of this council in the light of the paradigm theory will only become clear when we have also analysed the other two paradigm shifts, those of the Reformation and modernity. For it is this which now once again puts the history of the Catholic Church in quite a different light. With Vatican II – despite all the difficulties and constraints of the Roman system – it has attempted to catch up with two paradigm shifts, and incorporated basic features of both the Reformation (P IV) and the Enlightenment-modern paradigms (P V). So in discussing these two further paradigms we shall also indirectly be discussing the Catholic Church. But here we must pause, first, for a brief interim stocktaking.

The Roman Catholic Church: strengths and dangers

A theological evaluation of this third Roman Catholic paradigm is not very simple, since in time the Roman system increasingly overlaid the Latin paradigm of the Catholic Church and bracketted itself with it, so that the Roman element concealed the Catholic element. However, despite all the interweaving a fundamental distinction needs to be made:

- between the **Catholic Church**, which preserved the substance of Christianity in the mediaeval Counter-Reformation anti-modern paradigm and which again came clearly to light with Vatican II;
- and the **Roman system** which, having broken through in the eleventh century, attributed to the Pope and his Curia an absolutist supremacy in the church which was strictly rejected by the Orthodox churches of the East and the churches of the Reformation, was criticized all down the centuries by reform currents within Catholicism, weakened by the loss of the church state, and was shaken for all the future by Vatican II.

Here there is no question that the **papacy,** which is an essential element of this paradigm, did tremendous **service to the unity and freedom** especially of the Western church of late antiquity, the early Middle Ages and the high Middle Ages. In the time of the migrations, the general collapse of state order and the fall of the old imperial capital, the Roman church not only did a cultural service to the young Germanic peoples in preserving an inestimable legacy of antiquity but also a real pastoral service in building up and preserving these churches. And down to modernity the Catholic Church owes a debt to the papacy for not simply falling victim to the state but being able to preserve its freedom: not only in the face of the Byzantine emperors and the German rulers who were heads of their own churches, but also in the face of the absolutist ambitions of the modern nation states. On the basis of old Roman tradition, which always had a great sense of practical issues, law and order, time and again Rome exercised true pastoral authority at a universal level. Nor should there be any dispute that a pastoral preaching authority of the Pope along with the bishops often performed a meaningful function in the church: wherever it was exercised in accordance with the norm of the gospel and took account of its own functional limits over against scientific theology and science generally.

So in all sobriety we can share something of the admiration for the Catholic Church which is to be found among many non-Catholics, admiration of so much historical continuity, trans-national ubiquity and identity of faith. We can share the admiration for the efficient organization, the well-ordered structure of offices, the liturgy with its rich tradition and the contribution to secular culture without which Europe would be the poorer. We can share the admiration above all for the countless people who in (and often despite) this church live out their life as Christians all over the world in a concrete and active way, in dedication as priests or laity, men and women, for the needy, the marginalized and the underprivileged, who indeed experience God and Christ in this church despite everything: in the sacraments, in the life of prayer, in service to neighbours.

On the other hand, the development of the **Roman system** in particular has now shown what **dangers** there also are in this third paradigm of Christianity. Instead of authentic Christian authority we all too often find an **ecclesiastical authoritarianism** which – as we saw – results in a dogmatism. But isn't this also the problem with other confessions and religions? We shall be talking about biblicistic fundamentalism in connection with the Reformation paradigm (P IV). But the two other prophetic religions do not have the problem of dogmatism in this form. For dogma does not play a central role either in Judaism or in Islam.

Neither religion has to the remotest degree the developed dogmatics which found its cornerstone in Catholicism with the First Vatican Council. Jews can content themselves with the simple confession of faith, the 'Shema Israel', which they say morning and evening and as they are dying: 'Hear (*shema*), O Israel, Yahweh is our God, Yahweh alone.'[406] And the simple Muslim confession of faith ('Shahada'), 'There is no God but **God**, and Muhammad is his prophet,' is also known beyond Islam. Compare these lapidary confessions of faith with the Tridentine confession of faith (and all its Vatican additions) – not to mention 'Denzinger' (with 4858 sections) and the Roman *World Catechism* (with 2865 sections).

Unfortunately there is a form of authoritarianism which has also developed in Judaism and Islam: legalism. For there is no question that all three prophetic and monotheistic religions have increasingly orientated the realization of the relationship between God and human beings on the law (*ius*). And all three incur similar problems with their faithful. What in Catholicism is canon law, is to an even greater degree the system of religious law in Judaism (the halakhah) and in Islam (the Shari'a). So God's truth and direction finally appear in all three religions in a form safeguarded by law – legalism as a distortion of God's revelation. This raises questions for all three religions.

Questions about the Relationship between Legalism and Religion

No believing Jew will fundamentally put in question the significance of the Torah as God's instruction. For human beings as the unique covenant partners of God, created in God's image, are not allowed any anarchical autonomy or individualistic libertinism. God's ethical commandments are still binding on men and women today. But today in particular, are men and women as God's covenant partners to be asked to show a pious servility and blind obedience to the law? Are God's ethical commandments simply identical with the halakhic system which has developed in the course of a long history and then survived in many respects? In Judaism, too, isn't the watchword, 'Ethics and law, yes; legalism, no'?

No believing Christian will seriously put in question the Jewish ethical commandments (the 'Decalogue'), which are confirmed in the New Testament, and the instructions which follow from Jesus' message; as disciples of Christ, Christians know specifically what their ethical behaviour should be. But in Catholicism in particular, hasn't church authority been idolized over and beyond scripture and tradition? Hasn't any criticism of authority been rejected and suppressed as un-Catholic for the sake of an unavoidably Catholic orthodoxy? And here in particular, instead of concrete talk of Pope and bishops, isn't there abstract and anonymous talk of 'teaching office' ('magisterium'), a term which is grounded neither in scripture nor in the old tradition, which presupposes the completely unbiblical distinction between the teaching church (*Ecclesia docens*) and the 'learning church' (*Ecclesia discens*), and which was reintroduced only in connection with Vatican I's doctrine of infallibility in the last century? And are God's ethical commandments identical with a system of church law? For Christians, too, isn't the watchword, 'Ethics and law, yes; legalism, no'?

C No believing Muslim will fundamentally put in question the basic ethical instructions of the Prophet, laid down in the Qur'an, which correspond with Jewish and Christian tradition. God's will has also been made concrete through the Qur'an in commandments and prohibitions. But in the course of Islamic history hasn't the ethical and prophetic message of the Qur'an all too often become an oppressive system of religious law, a legalistic authoritarianism, which does not liberate men and women but enslaves them in the everyday world? Hasn't the Shari'a largely concealed the original prophetic instructions? So for every Muslim, too, isn't the watchword, 'Ethics and law, yes; legalism, no'?

The future of the Roman primacy

But if this is the case; if the great Catholic tradition was often enough absorbed by the Roman system; if the mediaeval paradigm was progressive and varied in the first phase but in time became reactionary; if the Roman system thus made the mediaeval paradigm of the West more uniform and poorer through legalism, centralization, politicization, militarization and clericalization, and bears responsibility for the division of Christianity into East and West, North and South, here too the famous question arises. How long still? How long will this system go on like this? For ever? No one can overlook the fact that with time the **absolutist papacy** has become the **ecumenical problem number one.** Paul VI was the first to concede this himself with ecumenical openness: instead of being a rock of unity the papacy is a block on the way to ecumenical understanding.

In view of this situation of Roman Catholicism, doesn't Catholic theology in particular have the right and the duty to **criticize the church** openly? Doesn't it have the duty, in view of the fundamentally distressing historical development, to make objections wherever in official preaching, liturgy, discipline and pastoral care the biblical accents are consciously or unconsciously shifted, the original proportions distorted, and thus the incidentals are made the main issue and the main issue is made incidental. Mustn't Catholic theologians also protest if the Christian truth is concealed or forgotten by the church authority itself, and its own errors and half-truths are ignored, denied or even disseminated further? Time and again they in particular will point in a radical way to the main point, the 'centre of scripture', the 'hierarchy of truths', '**the essence of Christianity**'. That is their task. The authority of the church is not undermined in this way but is again expressed credibly against all authoritarianism. That is true particularly in the question of the future of the Roman primacy. What can be said here with theological responsibility?

On the basis of our paradigm analysis we must reflect that from the standpoint of contemporary, even Catholic, exegesis and history, any argument about the existence of a Petrine **primacy of jurisdiction**, even more of a **continuation** of such a primacy, and most of all its continuation in the **Bishop of Rome**, faces almost insuperable **difficulties**. After all the evidence I have presented, the possibility of a convincing demonstration of a direct **historical** succession of the Bishops of Rome in a Petrine primacy seems extremely questionable.

However, the questionable character of any exegetical historical demonstration of a succession does not exclude the possibility that even in the view of many Orthodox and Protestant theologians the **primacy of an individual in the church as a whole** is not only not contrary to scripture but can even be scriptural and **meaningful**. This can be so if this is a **succession in the Spirit**, in the Petrine mission and the task, in the Petrine testimony and spirit (which is in principle also possible in a charismatic way), in other words succession in a **primacy of service for the sake of the unity and edification of the church**, one which is really lived out. 'The modern papacy represents only **one** possible model of Petrine authority in the church. There are also others.' So says the American papal historian Brian Tierney in a special issue of the international theological journal *Concilium*, in which under the editorship of the Italian church historian Giuseppe Alberigo possible programmes are developed for *Church Renewal and the Petrine Office at the End of the Twentieth Century*.[407] And the Catholic dogmatic theologian, now Bishop of Rottenburg-Stuttgart, Walter Kasper, writes: 'Even in a careful interpretation of church teaching, the difference between the biblical beginnings and the historical development remains manifest. We may not overlook the epoch-making breaks and changes: there are not only developments but also constraints, not only heretical challenges and underestimations but no less damaging exaggerations, to the point of almost blasphemous forms of papolatry.'[408]

But wouldn't such a primacy of service in the service of unity merely be a primacy of honour? No. It would be a pastoral primacy in the spirit of the Gospel (along the lines of the classical passages about Peter in Matt.16.18; Luke 22.23; John 21.15–17), modelled not on Leo I, Gregory VII, Innocent III, the Pius Popes or John Paul II, but on Gregory the Great and John XXIII.[409] Such a Petrine service would have primarily to be concerned for the unity of the individual churches and at the same time would involve action not only as the spokesman of the Roman Catholic Church but also as a representative voice of the whole ecumene, of all Christianity in the one world today. Even many Orthodox and Protestant theologians would have no objection to such a pastoral primacy of service.[410] Anyone who is serious about the ecumene, anyone who is concerned with true catholicity, will reflect on the dogmatic and legalistic assertions in the Roman system both critically and responsibly in the light of the gospel. The Catholic Church needs a Petrine service and, in my view, so does the ecumene. But the Roman system came, and one day (like the papal state) it will go again. It is not part of the essence of what is Christian, indeed Catholic.

So it is superfluous to repeat here all the historical-critical questions which I justified in great detail in my book *Infallible? An Inquiry*, published in 1970 on the centenary of the Roman papal definitions. I surveyed the results of the wide international and interconfessional discussion with other theologians in *Fallible? A Stocktaking*, in 1973. In Rome it was thought that there was no need to respond to the substantive questions which had been raised; they could once again be suppressed with repressive measures (which had no theological basis and were legally questionable).[411] However, this proved counter-productive.[412] For it succeeded only in achieving the rejection of papal infallibilty today, at least in the developed industrial countries, not only by Protestants, Orthodox and non-Christians, but also by the great majority of Catholics.[413] So here – after a historical and systematic clarification of the problems, I need only repeat in the form of 'questions for the future' those requests which I made in all modesty in 1979 at the end of my book *The Church – Maintained in Truth?*, to which that same year Rome gave an authoritarian rather than an argued reply. Numerous Catholics all over the world – laity, pastors, theologians and bishops – are convinced that a constructive solution can and must be arrived at on this point, which is eminently important for the whole ecumene.

Questions for the Future

• Under a new pontificate might not and should not the **question of infallibility be investigated again**, with objectivity, scientific honesty, fairness and justice?

• Could not an **ecumenical commission** be appointed for this question consisting of internationally recognized experts in the different disciplines (exegesis, the history of dogma, systematic theology, practical theology and the relevant non-theological disciplines)?

• In the investigation, should not the emphasis be placed less, as previously, on the negative points than on the positive and constructive points? Surely the **abiding of the church in truth despite all errors** has a better foundation in the Christian message and the great Catholic tradition, and it would be better to live by this in the church today?

Combined with that is my wish that the Catholic Church may succeed in again showing more **evangelical catholicity**[414] in the Roman Catholic paradigm:

– Catholicity in **time**: my wish is that contrary to any destructive radicalism, from the perspective of the gospel it may shed new light on the **continuity** of faith and faith community which persists through all the breaks. There is a need for more authentic evangelical radicalism, trusting in the indefectibility, the indestructibility of the truth.

– Catholicity in **space**: my wish is that contrary to all the dissolution caused by particularism it may realize from the true centre, from the gospel, the **universality** of faith and faith community which embraces all nations and regions, races and classes. There is a need for more legitimate multiplicity, collegiality, plurality, brotherliness and sisterliness.

The urgency of these questions is manifest. But they will become very much clearer if after the analysis of the mediaeval Counter-Reformation anti-modern paradigm (P III) we turn to an analysis of the Reformation paradigm (P IV).

IV. The Protestant Evangelical Paradigm of the Reformation

No break since the Gregorian reform of the eleventh century and the breakthrough of the Roman Catholic paradigm in Western Christianity was deeper and more momentous than the Lutheran Reformation. In the sixteenth century **Martin Luther** initiated a new era: a further paradigm shift for the church, theology and Christianity generally, away from the Roman Catholic paradigm of the Middle Ages (P III) to the Protestant Evangelical paradigm of the Reformation (P IV). Here too historical research is in flux, so I also want to begin this chapter with a few hermeneutical reflections.

1. A changed image of Luther

In present historiography there is much discussion of the question whether persons make history or vice versa. Who is right?

A dialectic of structures and persons

The current trend is towards long neglected **social history**, which concentrates on structural conditions and historical change. This now tends to put what Hegel called the 'individuals of world history', who so long occupied centre stage, into the historical shade. And indeed a history of the church and theology without social history lacks any view of the grass roots of the church, the history of simple believers. In particular, social histories of individual cities or territories – an investigation of church ordinances, visitation reports, the records of moral courts and of schools have made it clear that the 'Reformation' is an extremely complex social phenomenon and that it took very much longer for this Reformation to break through than for a long time was assumed.[1]

Now in the framework of a social history, in a period which has been called the time of a 'concentrated Christianity', **religion** takes on central significance: here it is not yet one 'sector' alongside others (science, business, politics, culture), as it was later to become in modernity, but an all-pervading 'dimension' of social life which social historiography, too, neglects at its peril. In the framework of the Reformation paradigm in particular, it can be shown what a mobilizing, motivating and inspiring factor religion can be – with positive or negative consequences.

So the description of social forces functioning over the long term is of basic significance. But it seems to me that this approach must not neglect specific individuals acting within its framework. The activity of Martin Luther in particular in fact shows impressively how the **factual history** of contingent individual events and the actions of individuals by no means simply lies on the surface, but is rooted in the process of social history. Certainly the Reformation is not simply **Luther**; he must be seen together with a whole series of Reformers: Erasmus, Carlstadt, Melanchthon, Zwingli, Bucer. But Luther is and remains the figure who **embodies the Reformation programme** more than any other. He is a model example – of the kind I have demonstrated for Judaism in the case of King David[2] – of the dialectic of structures and persons which is at work throughout history.

Only since Leopold Ranke's *German History at the Time of the Reformation* (1839/47[3]) has the term **Reformation**, which down to the eighteenth century was by no means attached to the church sphere and even the Lutheran movement, become a term clearly defining an era, associated with the name of Martin Luther. Here we must reflect self-critically that the **image** of persons who were influential in history is also exposed to historical change and often to fashionable adaptations, and to an amazing degree this has been the case in particular with the man from Wittenberg. Historical facts and historiography, the historical person and his or her image are not the same. The image of persons can change. And both the Protestant and the Catholic images of Luther have changed markedly in the course of the past five centuries.[4]

The Protestant image of Luther

The Protestant image of Luther changed with the ideals of the times – how could it be otherwise? Luther, the prophet of the original gospel sent by God: that is how his Protestant contemporaries saw him, in a quite existential and at the same time idealistic way. Luther, the restorer of 'pure doctrine': that is how Lutheran orthodoxy saw him, in a more intellectualist way. Luther, the opponent of an orthodoxy growing rigid, the man of prayer and hero of faith, the model of a piety of the heart and trust in the God's gift of mercy, who issued a call to conversion: in this way he became important for Pietism.

The Enlightenment saw him in quite different terms again: Luther as the one who brought liberation from the pressure of the conscience, the champion of reason and the opponent of superstition. And he was different again for the Sturm und Drang: Luther as a genius of language. Then he was different for German classicism, idealism and romanticism: Luther as the pioneer of modernity; and later in the move back towards restoration he was the conservative. In the nineteenth century there were thus the most varied species of conservative Lutheran and liberal Neo-Protestant interpretations. And Luther increasingly came to appear as the great instigator of German culture, so that in the time of nationalism and National Socialism he could be praised as the 'eternal German'.

However, at the beginning of this century the advances made by Karl Holl and especially Karl Barth led beyond the liberal-conservative contrast and created an image of Luther remote from the national myth. Since then Luther has been understood again theologically as the man of God: as witness to the Word, to the grace and freedom of God, as the advocate of a *theologia crucis*, indeed theologically as a 'speech event' (thus Gerhard Ebeling). And it was the historical research of our century which made Protestant theology capable of basing its understanding of Luther on a precise investigation of the sources instead of on an idealizing transfiguration. Extensive material has been discovered in our century: from the period of the mature Luther (copies of lectures, sermons) and especially the young Luther (manuscripts of his early lectures).

All this has made possible a **differentiated judgment on the development of the complex personality and theology of the Reformer** in their different phases and polarities. Moreover historical research also forms the ecumenical crossroads at which the Protestant and Catholic images of Luther can be increasingly reflected upon today.

The Catholic image of Luther

The Catholic image of Luther was for a long time stamped by hatred or at least ugliness. For a long time Luther was not forgiven for splitting the church, as if that were above all his fault. So for a long time the account by the decided anti-Lutheran theologian John Cochlaeus was followed. All the Catholic accounts right down to the twentieth century were directly, and even more indirectly, dependent on him. Fortunately these times are past. But it was a long way from Cochlaeus, Eck and Bellarmine in the sixteenth century, through Möhler, Döllinger, Janssen, Denifle and Grisar in the nineteenth century, to Merkle and Kiefl and finally Herte, Jedin, Lortz and Iserloh in the twentieth century.

Specifically, that means that whereas for Cochlaeus and his numerous following in four centuries Luther was above all the perverted monk and demagogic libertinist, the revolutionary and arch-heresiarch, the man who split the church and the empire, for Döllinger he was still a criminal and in our century for Denifle a man with nothing godly in him, for Grisar a psychopath, and finally for Joseph Lortz, the pioneer of a new Catholic image of Luther, a brilliant, tragic, *homo religiosus* caught up in almost inextricable inward and outward difficulties, a man living from a deep faith and a man of prayer, a personally pure Christian and Reformer.

Whereas Janssen (in response to Ranke) attempted to depict the Reformation as a political and religious revolution in the framework of a collapse in all spheres of life, with destructive consquences for the church, culture and freedom, by an unrelenting disclosure of the abuses of the late mediaeval church Lortz exonerated Luther from a great part of the blame for splitting the church. Here he advanced to a **positive understanding of the Reformer as a religious figure** and the Reformation as a religious event. Furthermore, Johannes Hessen saw Luther not only as a religious person but as a representative of that 'prophetic type' which is always needed, who fought a legitimate battle against intellectualism, moralism, institutionalism and sacramentalism in the church. So it is important for a new Catholic understanding of Luther not to accuse Luther over-hastily of a subjectivism which broke up unity or of theological one-sidedness, as even Lortz still does.

The interesting attempt by the American psychoanalyst Erik H.Erikson to derive the theological development of 'young man Luther' through depth theology from a father complex does not lead much further, for all the increase in our knowledge of decisive matters. For the study of theology and his monastic life are more important for Luther's shift than his childhood and youth. And more important for him than the problem of his father was the question of God against an apocalpytic horizon, as has well been demonstrated by the Dutch Reformation historian Heiko Oberman in his book on Luther. That means that Luther may in no way be interpreted merely in biographical and psychological terms; rather, he must be understood in historical and theological terms, from the centre of his work. And what is this centre? There is agreement that the centre of Luther's theology is the theology of the justification of the sinner.

However, we can only understand this centre of Luther's work if we remember all the causes of the Reformation. We have already seen these in the account of the late mediaeval crisis of the Roman Catholic paradigm, so here I can sum them up briefly (for biographical details about Luther again see my *Great Christian Thinkers*).

2. The basic question: how is one justified before God?

For a long time, then, there had been much pressure towards a far-reaching transformation of the existing entire constellation. Thus hardly one of Luther's reform concerns was completely new. But the time had not been ripe for them. Now the time had come, and it took only the religious genius to bring together these concerns, put them into words and embody them in his person. Luther was this man of the time.[5]

Why the Lutheran Reformation came about

What had been the **preparation** for the new **paradigm shift in world history** before the Reformation, which had introduced the structural conditions that had to be fulfilled for an epoch-making change to come about? It was a whole syndrome of manifestations of crisis:[6]

– the collapse of papal rule of the world, the split in the church between East and West, then the twofold, later threefold, papacy in Avignon, Rome and Pisa along with the rise of the nation states of France, England and Spain;

– the lack of success by the reform councils (Constance, Basel, Florence, Lateran) in 'reforming the church head and members';

– the replacement of the natural economy by a money economy, the invention of printing and the widespread desire for education and Bibles;

– the absolutist centralism of the Curia, its immorality, its uncontrollable financial policy and its stubborn resistance to reform, and finally the trade in indulgences for rebuilding St Peter's, which was regarded in Germany as the pinnacle of curial exploitation.

However, even north of the Alps, as a result of the Roman system, some of the abuses were quite blatant:

– the domination of the nobility among the higher clergy and their distance from the lower clergy, and the consequent secularization of the rich prince bishops and monasteries;

– the hair-raising abuses caused by compulsory celibacy; the clerical proletariat, which was far too numerous, uneducated and poor;

– the retrograde state of church institutions; the ban on levying interest, church exemption from tax and jurisdiction, the clerical monopoly of schools, the encouragment of beggary, too many church festivals;

– the way in which church, theology and society were overgrown by canon law;

– the radical critics of the church – Wycliffe, Hus, Marsilius, Ockham and the humanists – and the theological uncertainty and lack of orientation;

– finally, a terrifying superstition and cult of relics among the people, a religious nervousness which often took enthusiastic-apocalyptic forms, an externalized liturgy and a legalistic popular piety, a hatred of work-shy monks and clerics, a malaise among the educated people in the cities and despair among the exploited peasants in Germany. This whole complex of symptoms shows an abysmal **crisis for the whole of society** and at the same time the inability of traditional theology, church and society to cope with it.

Everything was ready for a paradigm shift, but there was need for someone to present the new paradigm credibly. History was ripe for the man who then also made history. He was a lowly monk and yet became an epoch-making prophetic figure: **Martin Luther** (1483–1546). Although this young doctor of theology first of all understood himself not as a prophet but as a teacher of the church, intuitively and inspirationally he was able to meet the tremendous religious longing of the late Middle Ages. He could begin to purge the strong positive forces in mysticism, and also in nominalism and popular piety, confidently centre all the frustrated reform movements on his brilliant personality, which was stamped with a deep faith, and express his concerns with unprecedented eloquence. In Arnold Toynbee's terminology, Luther gave the 'response', the appropriate historical answer, to the great historical challenge. Without Luther there would have been no Reformation.[7]

But first of all we must ask: in his understanding of the event of justification was Luther a priori un-Catholic? No. We must see Luther's continuity with and discontinuity from the theology of the previous period.[8]

The Catholic Luther

An **uninterrupted train of tradition** binds Luther to the church and the theology of the preceding period precisely in his understanding of justification. We must look briefly at four lines of historical continuity, all of which are important for Luther's understanding of reformation and which in part overlap: the Catholic piety which Luther encountered in the monastery; in connection with that mediaeval mysticism; then Augustine's theology; and finally late mediaeval nominalism in the form of Ockhamism.

Catholic piety? Granted, the traditional Catholic piety caused a crisis for Luther in the monastery. And so all his life, for him the monastic way of perfection remained the way of legalistic works, of wanting to be something before God, which did not bring him peace of mind and inner security, but anxiety and desperation. Nevertheless, Luther salvaged the best of Catholic piety through his crisis. For the doctrine of justification, it is particularly significant that it was Luther's superior in the monastery, Johannes von Staupitz, a man with a concern for reform, who diverted him from his heart-searchings over his own predestination and pointed him to the Bible, to God's will for salvation and the picture of the crucified Jesus, before whom all anxiety about whether or not one is elect disappears.

Mediaeval mysticism? Granted, the pantheizing features of mysticism and its tendency to blur the line between the divine and the human were quite remote from Luther. Nevertheless, it is known that Luther had knowledge of the mysticism of Dionysius the Areopagite and Bernard of Clairvaux. Moreover, he discovered the mystical work *Theologia Deutsch*, studied it with enthusiasm and brought out an edition in 1515/16 (completed in 1518). Furthermore he called the mystic Tauler one of the greatest theologians and continued to commend him. There is no doubt that Luther's sense of being humble, small, nothing before God, to whom alone honour belongs; his insight that piety by works leads to vanity and self-satisfaction and thus away from God; and finally his faith in the suffering Christ, particularly as he took this from the words of the Psalter – that all these ideas which were decisive for his understanding of justification are the traditional material of mediaeval mysticism.

Augustine's theology? Granted, it was not least the doctrine of predestination and the understanding of the perfect love of God as developed by the old anti-Pelagian Augustine which were responsible for Luther's crisis. And all his life Luther understood grace differently from Augustine, in a more personal way. Nevertheless, insight into the deep corruption of sin as human selfishness and a distortion of the self remained decisive for Luther's understanding of justification, as did insight into the omnipotence of the grace of God, which he learned above all from Augustine. So Luther remained tied to one of the basic components of mediaeval theology, the theology of Augustine, whose *Confessions* and great treatises *On the Trinity* and *The City of God* he had studied at a very early stage; Augustine, who was not only dominant in pre-Aristotelian early Scholasticism and in the high Scholasticism of Alexander of Hales and Bonaventure, but who also could not be overlooked in Thomas Aquinas and his school (though there he had clearly been forced into the background) and finally also in the late Middle Ages. The continuity was much stronger than Luther himself realized, not only in the doctrine of the Trinity and in christology, but also in the theology of grace. It dawned on Luther that Romans 1.17, the passage about the 'righteousness of God', which was decisive for his breakthrough to the Reformation, does not speak of the inexorable judgment of God's righteousness, before which no sinner can stand, but of God's righteousness as a gift. The passage was understood in this way not just by Augustine, as Luther thought, but, as Catholic scholars have demonstrated,[9] by the majority of mediaeval theologians.

Ockhamism? Granted, in his doctrine of justification Luther reacted most vigorously against the Pelagianism of the late-Franciscan Ockhamist school which is found both in Ockham himself and in his great pupil Gabriel Biel, as also in Bartholomew Arnoldi of Usingen, Biel's pupil and Luther's teacher. Nevertheless, there is also a way from Ockham and Biel to Luther's doctrine of justification. The Thomistic school was certainly not right in slating late mediaeval theology in general and Ockhamism (nominalism) in particular as a disintegration of mediaeval theology. But on the other hand Protestant Reformation scholarship has been equally wrong in treating late mediaeval theology only as the dark background against which Luther's doctrine of justification could shine out particularly brightly. Attention must not be limited, as it usually is in the Protestant sphere, to Luther's dependence on Paul and Augustine; his positive connection with Ockham and Biel must also be considered: for example with respect to particular aspects of his concept of God (the absolute sovereignty of God), his view of grace as favour, of sin, of the acceptance of human beings by free divine choice which has no ground in humankind.

In view of this rooting of Luther in the Catholic tradition, is a **sweeping condemnation of Luther** still possible for Catholics? No, it is **impossible!** The mediaeval Catholic understanding of justification and Luther's new understanding of justification simply have too much in common for that. The mediaeval understanding of justification is not a priori contrary to the gospel, and conversely the Lutheran understanding is not simply non-Catholic. In other words, only a differentiated and nuanced judgment does justice to both sides. And this differentiated and nuanced judgment will not harmonize everything. Rather, it will at the same time see the discontinuity in all the continuity: Luther's decisive new beginning.

Luther the Reformer

The decisive **theological** discussion, which primarily has to be carried on not by church historians but by systematic theologians, may not be carried on only with the 'Catholic' Luther – with a Luther who is still Catholic or who remained Catholic. As the Catholic expert on Thomas and Luther, Otto Hermann Pesch, has pointed out,[10] in particular it must be carried on theologically with the **Luther of the Reformation**, who with Paul and Augustine was against Scholasticism generally and Aristotelianism in particular. Especially Luther's authentically Reformation teaching deserves not only to be explained psychologically and historically in terms of church history, the history of theology and his own person, but also to be taken seriously theologically.

However, the decisive question is: by what **criterion**? That is a question on which unfortunately even Catholic church historians have seldom reflected in passing judgments on Luther's theology which in fact are less historical verdicts than dogmatic evaluations. They have often simply taken as the criterion for their judgment the Council of Trent, the fundamental theological weaknesses of which have been overlooked: thus Hubert Jedin. Or the theology of the high Scholastic period (Bernard of Clairvaux, Thomas Aquinas), the Catholicity of which has not been examined critically: thus Joseph Lortz. Or Greek and Latin patristics, whose distance from scripture has manifestly not been seen: thus French theologians. Or finally the school theology which historians have often brought along uncritically with them since their student years and which in fact represents a conglomerate of neo-Scholastic, Tridentine, high Scholastic and patristic elements, enriched and polished up with the results of a more recent theology and exegesis only at particular points.

Here we must ask: if church historians do not want to suspend their **theological** judgments – which we would have to respect, since every discipline has its limits – may they evade a purely **exegetical** examination of Luther's theology and especially his understanding of justification? Aren't Luther's doctrine of justification, his understanding of the sacraments, his whole theology and his explosive effects on world history grounded in one thing: the return of the church and its theology to the gospel of Jesus Christ as it is originally attested in Holy Scripture? So can we engage with Luther at all in the most authentic way if we avoid this particular battleground, whether out of superficiality, convenience or a lack of capacity? This is where a decision is finally made over splitting the church and uniting the church.

After Vatican II, Catholic theology will also concede that Neo-Scholastic school theology or Trent, high Scholasticism or patristics, are now secondary criteria compared with this **primary, fundamental and abiding, binding criterion: scripture**, the gospel, the original Christian message. Indeed, the Greek and Latin fathers refer to this just as much as the mediaeval theologians, the fathers of Trent and the Neo-Scholastic school theologians do. And of course Luther, too, is responsible before it. That means that what is decisive is not whether this or that statement of Luther's also already appears in this or that form in Thomas Aquinas, in Bernard of Clairvaux, in Augustine or some Pope, but whether it has the gospel, the original Christian message, behind it or not. So:

Where Luther was right

Does Luther have the New Testament behind him in his basic approach? Of course I cannot give a comprehensive answer to this question here. But I can indicate an answer which is based on my previous work in the sphere of the doctrine of justification.[11] And here it seems to me beyond dispute that with his basic statements about the event of justification, with the *sola gratia, sola fide, simul iustus et peccator*, **Luther has the New Testament behind him**, and especially Paul, for whom the doctrine of justification is crucially important. I shall indicate this simply by key words:

- What is '**justification**'? According to the New Testament it is not in fact a process of supernatural origin which is understood physiologically and takes place in the human subject, but is the verdict of God in which God does not impute their sin to the godless but declares them righteous in Christ and precisely in so doing makes them truly righteous.
- What is '**grace**'? According to the New Testament it is not a supernatural endowment of power, a quality or disposition of the soul, nor a series of different quasi-physical supernatural entities which are successively poured into the substance and faculties of the soul, but is God's living favour and graciousness, his personal conduct as made manifest in Jesus Christ, which precisely in this way determines and changes people.
- What is '**faith**'? According to the New Testament faith is not an intellectualist holding truths to be true but the trusting surrender of the whole person to God, who does not justify anyone through his or her grace on the basis of moral achievements but on the basis of faith alone, so that this faith can be shown in works of love. Human beings are justified and yet always at the same time (*simul*) sinners who constantly need forgiveness afresh, who are only on the way to perfection.

Catholic theology today will be able to **take note** of the **evidence of scripture** and thus also Luther's doctrine more openly than a few decades previously. Why? 1. Catholic exegesis has made considerable progress and displays virtually no confessional differences in its interpretation of passages from, say, Romans or Galatians, which were disputed in the Reformation period. 2. The time-conditioned nature of the Council of Trent and its formulations have been demonstrated to all by the Second Vatican Council. 3. The Roman Scholastic theology, the almost exclusive domination of which in the Catholic sphere between the two Vatican Councils made ecumenical understanding largely impossible, has clearly manifested its inability to solve the new problems of today and is manifesting it again in the 1993 *World Catechism*, which has been criticized everywhere. 4. The changed atmosphere since the council has opened up incalculable possibilities which were hardly dreamed of before Vatican II. 5. While the discussion over justification carried on in recent years has shown great differences in the interpretation of the doctrine of justification, it has not brought out any irreducible differences between the Catholic and Protestant doctrines of justification which would **split the church**. A number of officially agreed documents from both sides have confirmed that **the doctrine of justification no longer divides the churches**.[12]

One last thing must be said quite clearly about Luther's doctrine of justification, which hithertho has hardly been said from the official Catholic side. Luther found a direct existential approach to the apostle Paul's doctrine of justification in a way which no one, even Augustine, had achieved in the previous 1500 years. This **rediscovery of the original Pauline message of justification** under the shifts and over-paintings of 1500 years is an amazing, a tremendous theological achievement. For that reason alone there should be a formal **rehabilitation of Luther** and a lifting of the excommunication by Rome. But his achievement would not have been possible without a basic spiritual experience brought on by the mediaeval piety of the law, which Luther himself attributed not to his ingenuity but to a certainty given graciously against all doubt and against all despair. Why was it given to him in particular and not to someone else? We must not speculate on that – but perhaps it happened to humiliate a theology which had become all too certain of its orthodoxy.

All this does not mean that there were not already differences between Paul's and Luther's doctrines of justification, simply on the basis of their different starting points: Protestant scholars themselves often note them; in particular too individualistic an orientation on Luther's part. Nor does it mean that in some statements of his doctrine of justification Luther did not lapse into **one-sidedness and exaggeration**: some formulations with *solum* and works like *De servo arbitrio* or *On Good Works* were and remain open to misunderstanding and need supplementation and correction. But the basic approach was not wrong. This approach was right, as was its implementation, despite some defects and one-sidedness. The difficulties and problems (which are not insoluble) lie in the further conclusions drawn, above all in questions of understanding the church, ministry and the sacraments. Let's look more closely. What does 'a return to the gospel' mean? I shall demonstrate this from the great programmatic writings of the year 1520.

3. The return to the gospel

1520 was the year of theological breakthrough for Martin Luther; in this year his great programmatic writings for the Reformation were composed. And while Luther was hardly a man with a deliberately planned theological system, he was a man who would confidently make theological proposals to suit the situation and carry them through effectively, indeed produce a coherent and consistent programme.

The Reformation programme

The **first writing** of this year was the long sermon 'On Good Works' (beginning of 1520), addressed to the churches, written in German, in more of an edifying than a programmatic way.[13] It is fundamental, in that here Luther dealt with the basic question of Christian existence: the **relationship between faith and works**, the innermost motive of faith and the practical consequences which follow from it. Using the Ten Commandments, he demonstrated that trusting **faith** which gives God alone the glory is the foundation of Christian existence; only from faith can and should good works follow.

The **second writing**, addressed to the emperor, princes and other nobility, took up the *gravamina* (objections) of the German nation which had already been expressed so often, and is a passionate call for the **reform of the church**; it, too, is in the vernacular: *To the Christian Nobility of the German Nation Concerning the Reform of the Christian Estate* (June 1520).[14] It was the sharpest attack on the Roman system so far, which was preventing a reform of the church with its three pretensions ('walls of the Romanists'): 1. spiritual authority stands above worldly authority; 2. the Pope alone is the true interpreter of scripture; 3. the Pope alone can summon a council. At the same time a programme for reform, as comprehensive as it is detailed, is developed in twenty-eight points. The first twelve demands relate to the reform of the papacy: a renunciation of claims to rule over world and church; the independence of the emperor and the German church; the abolition of the many forms of curial exploitation. Then it deals with the reform of church life and secular life generally: the monasteries, priestly celibacy, indulgences, masses for souls, feasts of the saints, pilgrimages, mendicant orders, universities, schools, care of the poor, abolition of luxury. Here already we have the programmatic statements on the priesthood of all believers and ministry in the church, which, according to Luther, rests on a commissioning for public exercise of the priestly authority common to all Christians.

The **third writing** in the late summer of 1520 is addressed to scholars and theologians and is therefore written in Latin in a formal academic way: *The Babylonian Captivity of the Church*.[15] This work, probably the only work of strict systematic theology that Luther the exegete wrote, as it is about the foundation of Roman canon law, is devoted to a new basis for the **sacraments**. According to Luther, these are constituted by a promise and a sign of Jesus Christ himself. So if here we take the traditional criterion 'institution by Jesus Christ himself' really seriously, then only two sacraments, baptism and the Lord's Supper, remain – three at most, if one adds penance. The other four (confirmation, ordination to the priesthood, marriage, final unction) are pious church customs, but not sacraments instituted by Christ. Here again Luther makes many practical proposals for reform – from communion with the chalice for the laity to the remarriage of innocent parties in divorces.

The **fourth writing**, *On the Freedom of a Christian*,[16] published in the autumn, develops the thoughts of the first work and offers a summary of Luther's understanding of justification on the basis of I Cor.9.19 in two paradoxical statements: 'A Christian is a perfectly free lord of all, subject to no one' (in faith, according to the inner man), and 'a Christian is a perfectly dutiful servant of all, subject to all'[17] (thus in works, according to the outer man). The resolution of the paradox lies in the faith which makes someone a free person who may serve others in their works.

In these four writings we have the foundation stone of the Reformation. And now we can also answer the question of Martin Luther's ultimate concern, what moved him in all his writing, what motivated most deeply his protest, his theology and indeed his politics.

The basic impulse of the Reformation

Despite his enormous political explosive force, Luther remained a man of deep faith, a theologian who out of existential need struggled over the grace of God in the face of human fallenness. It would be quite superficial to think that he was concerned only with the fight against the indescribable abuses in the church, especially the indulgences, and in this connection with liberation from the papacy. No, Luther's personal impetus towards reformation and his tremendous historical explosive effect derived from the same source: **a return of the church to the gospel of Jesus Christ** as it was experienced in a living way in **Holy Scripture** and especially in **Paul**. In concrete, this means (and here already the decisive difference between the new paradigm P IV and the mediaeval paradigm P III emerges):

- Against all the traditions, laws and authorities which have grown up in the course of the centuries Luther sets the **primacy of scripture,** 'scripture alone' (*sola scriptura*).
- Against all the thousands of saints and tens of thousands of official mediators between God and human beings, Luther sets the **primacy of Christ,** 'Christ alone' (*solus Christus*). Christ is the centre of scripture and therefore the point of orientation for all scriptural exegesis.
- Against all pious religious human achievements and efforts ('works') to achieve the salvation of the soul, Luther sets the **primacy of grace and faith,** 'grace alone' (*sola gratia*), the grace of the gracious God as he has shown himself in the cross and resurrection of Jesus Christ and unconditional human faith, unconditional trust in this God (*sola fide*).

Compared with the 'multi-level thinking' of Scholasticism, Luther's theology represents a **sharpened confrontational thinking,** in which the accents are clear:

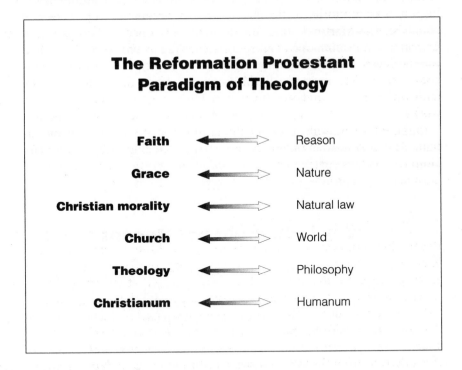

The Reformation Protestant Paradigm of Theology

Faith ⟷	Reason
Grace ⟷	Nature
Christian morality ⟷	Natural law
Church ⟷	World
Theology ⟷	Philosophy
Christianum ⟷	Humanum

Much as Luther originally came to know the private pangs of conscience of a tormented monk and aimed at the conversion of the individual, his theology of justification went far beyond the creation of privatistic peace for the soul. His theology of justification forms the basis for a **public appeal to the church for reform** in the spirit of the gospel, a reform which is aimed not so much at the reformulation of a doctrine as at the renewal of church life in all areas. In these circumstances a **radical criticism of the papacy** was unavoidable. However, Luther was not concerned with the Pope as a person, but with the institutional practices required and encouraged by Rome, which manifestly contradicted the gospel.

Now everything depended on how Rome reacted to the requirement for a radical reform. But from Rome there was no sign of a change; on the contrary. Leo X's Curia thought that they could speedily lead the heretical young monk in the far north to recant or (as in the case of Hus, Savonarola and hundreds of 'heretics' and 'witches') bring him to the stake with state help. And from a historical perspective there can be no doubt that it is not Luther but **Rome** which **bears the chief responsibility** for the way in which the dispute over the right way to salvation and practical reflection on the gospel very rapidly turned into a fundamental dispute over authority in the church and the infallibility of Popes and councils. But Martin Luther stands before us once and for all as a Christian who, summoned before the Reichstag in Worms in 1521, had the courage to keep to his faith with reference to scripture, reason and his conscience.[18] He resisted all the pressures from the state side (the emperor) and the church side (the Pope). However, for Luther it was now clear that such a Pope had to be the Antichrist announced in the New Testament. This insight was not just a product of Luther's polemic or hate, but was forced in on him because papal teaching and practice were contrary to the gospel.[19]

Why Luther did not Recant

'Unless I am convinced by the testimony of the Scriptures or by clear reason – for I do not trust either in the Pope or in councils alone, since it is well known that they have often erred and contradicted themselves – I am bound by the Scriptures I have quoted, and as my conscience is captive to the Word of God, I cannot and I will not retract anything, since it is neither safe nor right to go against the conscience. God help me. Amen.'

Conclusion of Luther's speech before the Emperor
and the imperial authorities at Worms, 18 April 1521

The Reformation paradigm

After his condemnation at the Reichstag, Luther, hidden away on the Wartburg, completed in ten months, among other things, his **translation of the New Testament** on the basis of Erasmus' Greek and Latin edition – the masterpiece of High German. The Bible was to be the foundation of gospel piety and the new community life. And Luther's Reformation paradigm, totally constructed on the Bible, was now to be the real, great alternative to the mediaeval Roman Catholic paradigm which had come under radical criticism. Here was the gospel as a motive for innovation!

The return to the gospel in protest against the false development and wrong attitudes in the traditional church and traditional theology was the starting point for the new **Reformation** paradigm, the **Protestant-evangelical paradigm of church and theology**. Luther's new understanding of the gospel and the completely new status of the doctrine of justification in fact gave the whole of theology a new orientation and the church a new structure; this was a **paradigm shift** *par excellence*, as Stephan Pfürtner has demonstrated in a comparison with Thomas Aquinas.[20] So in theology and the church, too, from time to time such **processes of paradigm shift** take place not just in the limited micro– or meso-sphere of individual questions and treatises but also in the macro-sphere: the shift from mediaeval to Reformation theology is like the shift from the geocentric to the heliocentric view:
– Fixed and familiar terms change – justification, grace, faith, law and gospel – or are abandoned as useless: Aristotelian terms like substance and accidents, matter and form, act and potency;
– Norms and criteria which determine the admissibility of certain problems and solutions shift: the Bible, councils, papal decrees, reason, conscience;
– Whole theories like the hylomorphic doctrine of the sacraments and methods like the speculative deductive method of Scholasticism are upset.

In his book on Luther,[21] Gerhard Ebeling, with his excellent knowledge of Luther and Thomas Aquinas, has given an impressive demonstration – though all too one-sidedly at the expense of the earlier paradigm – of how in Luther's theology basic theological concepts change fundamentally, and do so in the light of the new recognition of the gospel. Mediaeval theology in the tradition of the Greeks used physical and physiological categories: act and potency, form and matter, substance and accident, effective, material, formal and purposive causes; actualization, growth and so on. Luther used **personal categories**: the gracious God, sinful man, pronouncing righteous, trust, confidence. If on the one side the focus was on the static order, on the other it was more on the historical dynamics. If on the one side there was Aristotelian logic and the principle of contradiction ('then sinners, now righteous'), here there was a dialectical way of thinking and a paradoxical formulation ('at the same time sinful and righteous'). What was fundamental here was that Luther, although like Origen and Augustine an indefatigable, creative linguist and always an extremely topical commentator on the Bible, rejects, far more decisively even than Thomas, Origen's and Augustine's allegorical scriptural exegesis of the Bible. He laid the basis – and this is fundamental to his paradigm shift – for a strict **linguistic and grammatical exegesis of scripture.**[22]

It was not least the attractiveness of the theology, aesthetics and language of the new paradigm which proved decisive for clergy and laity at the time. From the beginning many were quite fascinated by the inner **coherence**, elemental **transparency** and pastoral **effectiveness** of Luther's answers, with the new simplicity and creative linguistic power of Lutheran theology. Moreover, the art of printing books and a flood of printed sermons and pamphlets, along with the German hymn, proved to be essential factors in the rapid popularization and dissemination of the alternative paradigm.

Thus the model of interpretation changed, along with the whole complex of different concepts, methods, problem areas and attempted solutions as hitherto recognized by theology and the church. Like the astronomers after Copernicus and Galileo, so the theologians after Luther got used to **another way of seeing**, of seeing in the context of another macro-model. That means that some things were now perceived which had not been perceived earlier, and possibly some things were overlooked which had been seen earlier. Martin Luther's new understanding of word and faith, God's righteousness and human justification, the one mediator Jesus Christ and the universal priesthood of all believers, led to his revolutionary **new biblical-christocentric conception** of all theology. From his rediscovery of the Pauline message of justification there followed for Luther:

- A new understanding of **God**: not a God abstractly 'in himself', on whose inner being one is to speculate, but a God who is quite concretely gracious 'for us', on whose grace one may build.
- A new understanding of **human beings**: not in the schema of nature and grace, but from the opposition of law and gospel, letter and spirit, works and faith, the lack of freedom and freedom.
- A new understanding of the **church**: not as a bureaucratic apparatus of power and finance but renewed as a community and the universal priesthood of believers.
- A new understanding of its **sacraments**: not as rituals which bestow

a quasi-mechanical 'grace', but as promises of Christ and signs of trusting faith in the gracious God.

In the light of these new theological beginnings wasn't a thoroughgoing radical **criticism of the mediaeval form of Christianity** simply unavoidable? Criticism of a church which in teaching and practice had deviated from the gospel and become worldly and legalistic? At the bottom of his heart Luther was conservative; he was terrified at the excesses of the Reformation while he was away from Wittenberg, and initially very cautious in the practical realization of his reform proposals. Nevertheless his criticism soon had revolutionary consequences:

– Criticism of the Latin **sacrifice of the mass** and **private masses**: therefore preaching was now central in worship along with a shared eucharistic celebration purged of the notion of sacrifice (with ordinary bread) in the vernacular with communion from the chalice for the laity as well; in some places daily preaching replaced the daily mass.

– Criticism of church **office**, which had in fact suppressed the one Lord and Mediator Jesus: therefore abolition of the concept of priesthood, a hierarchy appointed by God, and divine elements in church law, and instead a strengthening of the consciousness of the community and the awareness that church office is one of service (the pastor at the eucharistic table in black robes, facing the congregation).

– Criticism of **monasticism** and begging with a religious sanction: therefore an emphasis on worldly professions as divine callings and the dignity of even the lowliest work as being of equal value, indeed as worship.

– Criticism of those church **traditions** which were not justified by scripture and the pious works of everyday Catholic life, and therefore a rejection of the veneration of saints, the prescription of fasts, pilgrimages, processions, masses for the soul, the cult of relics, holy water, amulets; many festivals were abolished, above all Corpus Christi.

– Finally, criticism also of the **law of celibacy** as not in keeping with the gospel, since it devalued sexuality, women, marriage and family and violated the freedom of Christians; and therefore a fundamental affirmation of marriage for priests and a revaluation of marriage generally (not as a sacrament but as a 'secular-holy thing', solemnly performed in the church[23]).

There is no question that for traditional Roman Catholicism the Reformation amounted to an apostasy from the true form of Christianity. However, for those with a sense of the gospel it meant the restoration of its original form. They were delighted to give up the mediaeval paradigm of Christianity (P II). Rome might still be able to excommunicate the

Reformer Luther, but it could no longer put a stop to the radical new form of church life in accordance with the gospel presented by the Reformation movement, which was advancing and exciting the whole of Europe. The **new, Reformation paradigm of theology and church** (P IV) was soon solidly established. From 1525 the Reformation was implemented in numerous German territories, and after the failure to achieve reconciliation at the Reichstag at Augsburg in 1530 (the *Confessio Augustana*), it became clear to the Schmalkald alliance of Protestant German rulers that the combination of Lutheran Reformation and political power was perfect.

However, in the West, to the great schism between East and West had been added the no lesser split between North and South – a historical event of prime importance with incalculable effects on state and society, economics, science and art, which is difficult to describe here (because it is so ambivalent). Still, the theological question remains acute: was Luther's Reformation really about another, new paradigm? Wasn't it perhaps about another, new faith?

Another faith?

We really need to stop in the headlong development of history and reflect a little on this prime example of a paradigm shift embodied in the figure of Martin Luther, which represents something like a **Copernican shift in theology**: away from the all too human ecclesiocentricity of a powerful church to the christocentricity of the gospel, all under the sign of the freedom of the Christian, though this was realized to a limited degree even in the Protestant sphere. For in theology and the church, too, we can note very much more clearly than with Origen, Augustine or Thomas – because they are more rapid, radical and revolutionary (despite all the preparation for them in previous society, church and theology) – those historical regularities which Thomas S.Kuhn[24] read off the 'scientific revolutions' in the history of the natural sciences (Copernicus, Newton, Lavoisier, Darwin, Einstein) which were similarly in the making of that time. I have formulated the way in which this approach is applicable to theology in five experiential statements.[25] In the case of Luther, too, we should note:

– **The resistance of normal science to the new**: like all 'innovators', Luther was up against the authority and power of a **normative** theology (both ecclesiastical and backed by the state), its authorities, classics and doctrinal books, which did not like the new. People thought they knew what the truth was.

– **Crisis as the starting point for a change**: theology is no more involved than science in just a constant 'organic' development; rather, as in society, so in the church and theology there are always radical **crises**, which are starting points for the development of a new paradigm. Luther's theology was first of all a theology of crisis.

— **Without new candidates for a paradigm there is no paradigm shift.** The paradigm to be replaced needs a credible successor before it can be replaced, a new 'paradigm candidate',[26] a new 'form of expressing and understanding belief in the gospel . . . of a **special** novelty which marks a division between epochs',[27] 'a new **entire understanding of Christianity**'.[28] This is not just a slight correction of course, but a change of course. More than a 'scientific revolution', it represents an 'epoch-making shift'. In theology this involves a fundamental transformation of its concepts, methods and criteria, its vocabulary, the extent of its problems, indeed its overall perspective.

— **Non-scientific factors in the conversion**: as in the natural sciences, so too in theology not only scientific but also **non-scientific factors** play a part in the acceptance or rejection of a new paradigm. So the transition to a new model cannot be proved rationally; it is to be described as conversion. Rational and irrational, 'objective' and 'subjective', social and individual factors play a part here. Wouldn't the history of the Reformation have been different had Luther not been a Saxon, a German, a monk, an Augustinian, and conversely had the Pope not been an Italian, a man of the world, a Medici (afraid of a new Savonarola and a conspiracy of the cardinals)?

— **The dispute over a paradigm can turn out in three ways**: as in science, so in theology, in major controversies it is difficult to predict whether a new paradigm will replace the old, be absorbed into the old, or be put on the shelf for a long time.

The only thing that is certain is that if the new paradigm is **accepted**, in time the innovation will be consolidated and become tradition. At any rate, that is what happened in the case of Luther – and not just in Lutheranism. It happened throughout the Protestant world. And soon there was to be a Protestant 'orthodoxy' here, a new Protestant normative theology, which swore by the letter of the Bible and of Luther and which was often to be as intolerant of deviants and heretics as the Roman system.

However, outside this Protestant sphere – and above all in the southern countries of Europe – the new paradigm was **rejected**. A new split in the church which now ran, and still runs, through the world church, right through Germany and through Europe (and finally also through the 'new world' of the two Americas) was the unavoidable consequence. So just as inevitably, that raises the question: how is this paradigm shift to be assessed in today's perspective?

4. Continuity despite all the discontinuity

In the long run Luther's paradigm shift represented a 'scientific revolution' with tremendous political consequences for church and society. But Luther was **no political revolutionary**, nor was the Reformation an early bourgeois revolution, as a certain kind of Marxist historiography would have it. However we look at him, Luther is not to be compared with those great revolutionaries of world history from Spartacus through the English Puritans and French Jacobins to Marx, Lenin and Mao, who a priori aimed at a violent political overthrow of the social order, its values and representatives. As is well known, Luther was a vigorous opponent of the Peasants' Revolution and of its theological instigator, Thomas Müntzer. No, Luther wanted to be nothing but **a 'Re-former'** of the church, who went 'back' to the original 'form' of Christianity. But by doing this he in fact sparked off a 'revolution', because the 'Christian' society of the time was so remote from the gospel. So it was only against his will that he had become a political rebel, who had rebelled out of conscientious obedience to God's word – against the Roman system and the law which guaranteed this system.

The gospel as the basis for the continuity of the substance of faith

This indicates a decisive point: even in this same uniquely rapid paradigm shift of theology and the church in the first phase of the Reformation there is a discontinuity which presupposes a **deeper continuity**. Even the 'scientific revolutions' of the natural sciences by no means represent a total break; rather, even here, despite all the discontinuity there is a fundamental continuity.[29] And precisely in the case of Luther it becomes clear that the problem of continuity for theology is raised at a much deeper level. For the decisive question here is about something which the academic historians, who prefer to speak of 'conservation', usually dodge: the 'truth',[30] indeed 'the truth about life' or – as Wittgenstein put it – the 'problem of life'.[31] Existential questions are at issue here about where the world and human beings come from and where they are going, in other words about last and first meanings and criteria, values, norms, and thus a last and first reality. These are not in fact scientific questions but religious questions, the questions of a believing trust or trusting faith – which is certainly not irrational, but completely reasonable.[32] And as a discipline **theology** is responsible for them: theology as thoughtful talk or reckoning about God. However, theology is responsible in accordance with its own methods and presuppositions.

There is no such thing as a 'presuppositionless' science. And Christian theology has never been in any doubt that it cannot exist without presuppositions any more than other sciences can. Its **presupposition and subject-matter** is the **Christian message** as this is originally attested in the writings of the Old and New Testaments, has been handed down over the centuries, and is proclaimed in the church. This is the foundation, in particular, for the **continuity** of Christianity. So despite its scientific character, Christian theology is essentially not governed by a relationship with history, by historicity, but by a relationship with its origins, its originality. No, Christian theology is not about an **un**historical-mythological or a **supra**historical-philosophical truth, but about a deeply **historical** truth, about the **original** Christian truth.

Continuity: does that also apply to **Martin Luther's** theology? Truly no less than the theology of Paul, Origen, Augustine or Thomas, Luther's theology sought to be a thoughtful account of the truth of **Christian** faith: of the cause of Jesus Christ which is the cause of God in the world and thus at the same time a human cause. However, for Luther, after 1500 years of a highly divided history of the church and theology, the original testimony of faith to this Christ Jesus, the **gospel**, was once again, anew and clearly, to **become the basis and norm of Christian theology and the church**: the norm of all norms, authority of all authorities!

In retrospect, in principle could not even Luther's opponents, could not even the papal legate Cardinal Cajetan, his adversary in the disputation, Johannes Eck, and the Roman prelates, have agreed with this? In principle, yes. But in any conflict in fact they put the word of the Pope and his interests above anyone else's understanding of scripture – as we saw, this situation had slowly developed in the Roman Catholic paradigm. Only the Roman Pope and the magisterium which ruled on his behalf had a sovereign understanding of how scripture was really to be understood for the doctrine and life of the individual and the church. In fact this magisterium controlled scripture. And as we also saw, it was precisely this **Roman authoritarianism** which had long been rejected by the Eastern churches. That was what the whole dispute was now also about in Western Christianity.

Thus particularly as a result of Luther it has become clear that Christian theology is:
– not only (like the natural sciences) **related to the present**;
– nor only (like any historical science) **related to tradition**;
– but in addition (and this is its specific character) **related to its origin**.
And for Luther more than for others the **original event** in the history of Israel and of Jesus Christ and therefore the original testimony, the original documents of the Old and New Testaments, remain not only

the random historical beginning of Christian belief but its constant **normative point of reference.**

What does this mean, if not that in a fundamental revolution the Reformation **preserved the substance of Christian faith?** Despite all the radical changes there was a fundamental continuity of faith, of rite and of ethic! Indeed, despite all the truly epoch-making differences in the Protestant Reformation paradigm (P IV) there were still **the same constants** of Christianity as in the Jewish Christian earliest church paradigm (P I), the Hellenistic early church paradigm (P II) and the mediaeval Roman Catholic paradigm (P III):

- the same gospel of Jesus Christ, his God and Father, and the Holy Spirit;
- the same initiation rite of baptism;
- the same community rite of the eucharist;
- the same ethic of discipleship of Christ.

And yet the question poses itself even more sharply: wasn't Luther's Reformation nevertheless a revolution?

The gospel as the basis for the discontinuity of paradigm

Christians may and should at any time refer to the original biblical testimony. And because theologians in fact kept doing this even before Luther – in a mediated immediacy to scripture – along with the great paradigmatic schools, time and again there were also **creative individuals and groups** which went their own way in scriptural interpretation and theology and to which one can in no way deny the title of theologians. Aside from the mainstream of theology they developed their own theology with reference to the original testimony – and so German mysticism, Johannes Tauler and the little book *Theologia Deutsch* by the unknown Frankfurt 'God's Friend of the Perfect Life' (edited by Luther immediately before the dispute over indulgences) were particularly important for Luther. **In the one paradigm, different theologies** are possible, and also have always been influential alongside those which are preponderant or dominant.

In other words, the original Christian testimony, never fully caught up with by Christian theology, has time and time again developed an inspirational force which disturbs and surprises theology. The gospel as a motive for innovation! That is even more true of Luther than it is of Origen, Augustine and Thomas. For Luther the original Christian testimony – in view of the unprecedented ecclesiastical and theological consolidation and 'petrification' – developed a quite revolutionary explosive force. In such circumstances even earlier forgotten paradigms could be an inspiration, and retrospects became new insights. Just as Augustine referred particularly to Paul's Letter to the Romans, so Luther again referred to Augustine and Paul; and later with his 'theology' of crisis Karl Barth was to refer to Paul, Augustine and the Reformers all at the same time.

Thus the **gospel** itself – of course always in connection with the great contemporary social developments – can directly spark off a theological crisis: it can be the basis of **discontinuity** in theology as the impetus to a new paradigm. But as this **original** Christian witness is indeed also an abiding **fundamental** witness, while in a theological revolution it can be the occasion for a new paradigm, it **cannot** lead simply to the **total replacement**, the total suppression, of the old paradigm. And isn't even Luther's theology an instance of this? In principle, elements of the old paradigm can be taken over into the new, if and to the degree that they do not conflict with the primal and fundamental testimony. Moreover, it is seen to from the start that, as in Origen and Augustine, so also in Luther, a revolution does not lead to a total break, but preserves some common theological features with what has gone before. Moreover – and attention has been drawn to this again only recently – the affirmation of 'justification by faith alone' is to be found not only in Luther's commentary on Romans, but already in the commentaries of Thomas, Augustine and Origen.

Down to the present day that means that a theological revolution can take place in Christian theology – if it means to be and remain Christian – only **on the basis of** the gospel and ultimately **because of** the gospel, but never **against** the gospel or **apart from** the gospel! Although these texts are to be interpreted by means of historical criticsm, the truth of the gospel is never at the disposal of theologians – any more than the constitution is at the disposal of constitutional lawyers! So the **gospel** itself appears as the **foundation** not only of possible discontinuity but also of **necessary continuity** in theology. There is thus a 'theological revolution' by paradigm shift precisely on the basis of the Christian message! Isn't that exactly what Luther's Reformation was?

Paradigm shift is not a change of faith

However, Luther's opponents elevated the decision for a new paradigm (which was then further intensified as Luther reacted to them) into a decision of faith in the strictly religious sense: for or against indulgences = for or against the Pope = for or against the church = for or against Christ = for or against God. Indeed, at that time Luther's opponents could certainly have come to an agreement over the justification of the sinner by faith alone – as has been demonstrated in our century. But it was not recognized that the issue here was primarily (to put it in today's scientific language) a **paradigm shift** in theology and church (though with decisive practical consequences for the whole of theology) and **not** a **change of faith**.

But the Reformer required of Rome a 'return to the gospel of Jesus Christ'. Rome, unwilling to reform, called on the Reformer to 'return to the doctrine of the church'. From the beginning – Rome's strategy time and again – this was an invitation to capitulate: in this way **theological opponents** necessarily became **false believers** or even unbelievers. In other words, for Rome, subsequently Luther was merely the heretic, indeed, looking at Protestantism as a whole over the centuries, the 'arch-heretic'. But conversely, for Luther Rome was simply the 'whore of Babylon' and the Pope the 'Antichrist', who had set himself in the sanctuary in place of Christ. The fatal consequences of this mutual vilification are well known:
– The churches of the **Reformation** saw **Rome** as having lapsed from the true 'Catholic faith', as schismatic and heretical. Down to Vatican II the very title 'churches' was withheld from them by Rome.
– For **Luther** and for Reformation Christianity the church of the **Catholic** faith had become the unreformed Roman 'papistical church'. It was felt clearly to have lapsed from the gospel, to be heretical, even anti-Christian.

The confrontation between Luther and Roman Catholic theology also sheds bright light on the three possible outcomes of a paradigm shift:
- If a particular paradigm is **rejected** in theology and the church, the rejection easily becomes a **condemnation** and the disputation becomes an **excommunication**. This is what happened in Roman Catholicism. Here the church falsely identified its own theology with the gospel, the ecclesiastical system with the essence of Christianity, the form of faith with the content of faith.
- If a paradigm is **accepted** and innovation becomes tradition, then a theological interpretation in turn easily becomes a **truth of faith**: the theologoumenon becomes **dogma**, the tradition **traditionalism**. This was to happen in Lutheranism: a traditionalism was to develop which now no longer emerged in Hellenistic-Byzantine or mediaeval Roman garb, but in that of biblicistic Protestantism.
- If the controversy does not lead to any new decision and a new paradigm is provisionally 'shelved', then in the natural sciences such 'shelving' usually represents a predominantly scientific process in which questions remain open. However, this is not the way in which all reform theologians taking up reform concerns have been treated in the Catholic sphere over the centuries: here the shelving has often been

implemented forcibly. It has then become the imposing of a **tabu.** This is maintained by inquisition, the persecution of dissidents, psychological and earlier even physical burning, the suppression of freedom of conscience and teaching, indeed the suppression of all discussion.

Is that perhaps a malicious exaggeration? We have in fact seen in the framework of P II how for centuries in Catholic theology and the Catholic Church it ceased to be permissible to speak of certain doctrines (like lay priesthood, the freedom of Christians, *Ecclesia semper reformanda*) and certain demands for reform (the liturgy in the vernacular, the chalice for the laity, the marriage of priests). All that was regarded as Lutheran. And anyone who did this nevertheless was humbled and chastized. Centuries were to pass before **the same Christian message** and Christian church were recognized **in the different paradigms** (P IV and P III) of church and theology. Only now did people begin to see how the history of the Reformation is to be evaluated fairly;
– neither as a rediscovery of the gospel (almost completely lost since Paul and at any rate since Augustine) generally (as in the pessimistic Protestant view of history),
– nor (as in the organic optimistic Catholic interpretation of history) as the great heretical apostasy from the Catholic Church and its teaching which in principle develops organically,
– but (as in the analysis presented here) as an epoch-making paradigm shift which changes the entire theological, ecclesiastical and social constellation yet maintains the substance of Christian faith.

But now we have basically investigated only the first phase of the Reformation paradigm shift. It was to be fifty, indeed a hundred, years before the present-day confessions had formed. For a long time different options were open for particular lands and regions. People asked at that time, as we can ask today: wasn't there a third possibility, a 'third force' alongside the first force (Rome) and the second force (Wittenberg): the Catholic humanism and 'evangelism' which is above all associated with the name of Erasmus of Rotterdam? I have already discussed this 'Catholic reform' briefly in the previous long chapter (P III). Now we must look at it again, more closely, with a view to a balanced assessment of the Reformation (P IV).

5. The problematical results of the Lutheran Reformation

An alternative to Rome and to Luther? The question which we are to consider historically also has theological relevance for the present:

couldn't perhaps the humanistic reform programme of **Erasmus of Rotterdam** have prevented the split in the church had it been taken up at the right time by Popes and bishops? Church historians in both confessional camps have their doubts about this. But can we always be so confident of their historical objectivity, in view of the confessional resentment which often breaks through?[33] So quite undeterred, we must ask once again: could the humanistic reform programme of Erasmus of Rotterdam have prevented the split in the church, had it been taken up at the right time? Wasn't Erasmus' central theme, which emerged at a very early stage: 'How can one, with a good conscience, be both a man of culture and a Christian?'[34] Wasn't he concerned to be an authentic human being by being a Christian and to be a Christian by being an authentic human being – in connection with education and piety, culture and religion, antiquity and Christianity?

What the reformer Erasmus had in common with the Reformer Luther

Indeed, weren't there works like the famous **Enchiridion** (1503),[35] in which under the influence of his English friends (above all the English Lord Chancellor Sir Thomas More), the humanist took a clearer turn in the direction of biblical piety and which, according to the American biographer of Erasmus, Roland H.Bainton, contributed most of all his works towards making him the spokesman of the liberal Catholic reform movement, the counsellor of Popes and the mentor of Europe?[36]

In fact, in the controversies of his time Erasmus saw himself as 'defender of the true freedom that Christ brought and protected against the Pharisees, the freedom Paul championed against the Judaizers who wanted to take the church of the first century back to Judaism'.[37] Here 'Judaism' – not without danger – is certainly not understood as a people or a religious community, but as an attitude of externalized, legalized religion. Erasmus was deeply convinced that here he had hit on the heart of the biblical message, since so many of his notions could also be found in authors from antiquity. The more time went on, the more the **aim** of his work was **the renewal of church, theology and popular piety**, based on the Bible.

With this programme Erasmus wanted to remain a Catholic Christian; he wanted to reform the Catholic Church from within. Here was a reform programme already before the Reformation, a call to repentance even after the outbreak of the great crisis, of which of course Erasmus had had no more inkling than any of his contemporaries. What Erasmus, who had perfect command of many literary genres, gave effective and specific critical and satirical expression to in the *Enchiridion* and *In Praise of*

Folly[38] (1511), he made clear in the new edition of the *Adagia* (1515),[39] that popular, classical collection of proverbs on which he wrote a brilliant commentary. In it he argued sharply against the tyranny of rulers and the evil of wars, and pleaded for changes in church and society. A little later in his moving anti-war writing *Querela pacis*,[40] 'A Lament over Peace Persecuted in All Lands', he proposed (in vain) a European peace treaty between the German Empire, Spain, France and England, and in his *Institutio principis Christiani* (1516)[41] he composed an anti-Machiavellian **book of advice for rulers**, dedicated to the later emperor Charles V. That same year, 1516, he published the *Instrumentum Novi Testamenti*, the bold **first Greek printed edition of the New Testament with his own Latin translation** (with introductions, and not without reason dedicated to Leo X). Protesting at the traditionalists who referred to the infallibility of the church, it improved the Latin Vulgate which had been used for centuries and five years later was adopted by Luther as the basis for his German translation of the Bible.

No wonder that these outstanding works of the neat, outwardly weak and sensitive scholar, always anxious about his health and about hygiene, made him the most celebrated academic of the decade before the Reformation (the 'light of the world') and the focal point of the network of Christian humanists which spanned all of Europe (the 'prince of the humanists'). The substance of his proposed **reform of the church** can be described, in a slightly systematized form, in five points.

Like Luther, Erasmus was already concerned that there should be a **different kind of biblical scholarship.** He had nothing against an allegorical, spiritual interpretation of the New Testament, at least as long as this did not degenerate into whimsy and abstruseness – as happened particularly with preachers. But in a new age, was the mediaeval exegesis constantly to be repeated? Were people to go on swearing by the Vulgate? No, the Bible is a literary work and the foundation of its interpretation must be philology, a concern not primarily for the deepest possible metaphorical spiritual sense but for the **literal meaning of scripture.** Hence now Erasmus' more accurate translation of the Bible, first into Latin, then also into the vernaculars: 'If only the farmer with his hand on the plough sang some of it to himself, the weaver said something of it to the beat of his loom, and the traveller shortened his way with stories of this kind!'[42]

Like Luther, Erasmus was concerned, secondly, that there should be a **different kind of systematic theology.** The learned theologians, that educated and irritable breed of men, thought that they could fathom God's unfathomable mysteries, and in so doing arrived at the most impossible questions (could God also have entered the form of a woman, devil, ass or pumpkin?). Useless speculations, which had nothing to do with the apostolic orign of the church. After all, the apostles knew nothing of a transubstantiation in the eucharist, of the immaculate conception of Mary and other *quaestiones disputatae*. **Back to the sources**: that had to be the slogan of the time. Christianity and antiquity were not mutually exclusive. This new time needed a theology which recognized Holy Scripture as the only criterion, which in its understanding of the scriptures went by the church fathers instead of Scholasticism and which thus translated the original Christian message into the present in understandable terms. In such a theology **exegesis** becomes **the basic theological discipline**: in the light of the text of the Bible, church dogma, church law and church practice is subjected to criticism; everything is not concentrated on metaphysical speculations but on the saving work of Christ and the human way to salvation.

Like Luther, Erasmus was, thirdly, concerned that there should be **a different kind of popular piety**. Whether the gabbling of prayers or appeals to the fourteen helpers in time of need (Apollonia for toothache, Anthony if one was lost), whether more and more masses and pilgrimages or lucrative miracle stories, whether abuses of the confessional or costly indulgences: was superstition, were abuses to be spared irony, satire and criticism based on the Bible because some clergy and monks felt such criticism above all to be subversive, indeed destructive? Popular piety, too, was again to have a positive orientation on the biblical message, or more precisely on the Jesus of the gospel, as he went his way – a model for us – in the face of false scribes and hypocritical priests. The way **to the understanding of the true Jesus** above all for the **educated among the laity** was to be **prepared** in popular 'paraphrases' of the New Testament books.[43] If Luther started above all from Paul, Erasmus started from the Gospels. This reform movement was called 'evangelism', especially in Italy and Spain.

Like Luther, Erasmus was concerned, fourthly, that there should be **another kind of clergy**: 'as if there were no Christianity outside the cowl!', he remarked at the end of the *Enchiridion*. Erasmus criticized nothing so inexorably as monasticism – his own personal experiences keep coming through here. The impudent monks – no one stands out more for a lack of education, superstition and ridiculous pathos in preaching! For them the belly, money or honour are more important than discipleship of Jesus; the rules of the order are more significant than the gospel; the name of the order is more important than baptism; the garb of the order is worth more than anything else. Already in Erasmus such criticism culminates in a **radical questioning of previous ideals of piety**. For with reference to one and the same baptism the essential differences between clergy and laity are done away with, all traditional external features and spiritless ceremonies are relativized, and there is an argument for a contemporary, sober, everyday piety which is for everyone, concentrated on the things of Christ Jesus. And what about celibacy? It is not totally repudiated, but described as undesirable in existing circumstances: by comparison – in the *Encomium matrimonii* of 1518 – Erasmus praises marriage highly (offending greatly the clerical professors of Louvain and some preachers).

Like Luther, Erasmus, too, is concerned with a **different kind of hierarchy**. The discrepancy between the lofty claim of the 'successors of the apostles' and the reality of their life which is so little apostolic is easily demonstrated. For the hierarchy, doesn't everything focus primarily on honour, power and glory, on church law, and the splendour and pomp of the church? What a bureaucracy with countless functionaries! There is excommunication instead of communion; there are anathemas and interdicts in place of the preaching of the gospel. And in all this – as with the lower clergy, even more with the more senior ones – money lies at the centre: incomes and outgoings. Indeed, 'but if only the Popes, Christ's representatives, would attempt to live in accordance with him, namely his poverty, his work, his teaching, his cross, his readiness for death . . . whose heart would be more oppressed than theirs?'[44] Because of the confrontation between Pope and gospel, the anonymous dialogue *Julius exclusus e coelis*, immediately attributed to Erasmus – the warlike Pope Julius II who is forgotten by God and, having taken the wrong keys (the ones to his treasury), is now turned away from the gates of the kingdom of heaven by Peter, the first Pope – was understood by all of educated Europe not only as a satire on the time but as a sharp theological criticism.

In those decisive first two decades of the sixteenth century it had dawned on Erasmus with increasing clarity how tremendous the gulf had become between the 'successors of the apostles' and the apostles themselves, between the triumphalistic church of the present and the simple church of earliest times, in short between Christianity in his day and Christ Jesus then. The church and the Pope were a hindrance rather than a help on the way towards God. And it had become increasingly clear to Erasmus what true Christianity meant in his day: it meant relying on Holy Scripture and its living Christ instead of on church law, church dogma and the church system. It meant relying once again on the human, humiliated Jesus of the Gospels, who consorted with the lowly and the despised in humility and gentleness, who did not overcome the world with syllogisms (logical arguments), money and war, but with his courage to serve and his love, instead of relying on a high christology, to which the lofty hierarchy with its lofty claims could all too easily appeal. It was this practical Christianity in humility, gentleness, tolerance, readiness for peace and love which Erasmus – probably following not so much Plutarch and Cicero[45] as the Greek church fathers[46] – called the 'philosophy of Christ' or 'Christian philosophy'.

What the reformer Erasmus had against the Reformer Luther

Erasmus' reform programme – certainly presented here in a more compact form than he himself ever formulated it – was not accepted at the right time by the key political figures in church and state. For suddenly he was overtaken by events. As it were overnight, **Martin Luther** had turned learned humanistic conversation and inconsequential theological discussion into an emergency. Luther was everyone's concern, whether they wanted him to be or not. They were not content with Erasmus' admonitions to be patient and his warnings not to provoke the Pope and the rulers. A **decision** had to be made – for or against.

But **Erasmus in no way** wanted to decide. If need be, anxious and over-cautious, afraid of conflict and needing harmony as he did, he could understand his slogan *nulli concedo*, 'I yield to no one', as 'I decide for no one'. This was certainly not just weakness, even cowardice, as people often thought then and later, but in the last resort the result of his convictions and of the desire to preserve his intellectual independence. This was the foundation of his existence. Hadn't he suffered, written and fought enough for it all his life? Didn't he have to defend it – for the sake of scholarship and ultimately also for the sake of the church? Wasn't he, the church critic and scriptural theologian, regarded in public as Luther's kindred spirit, indeed spiritual foster-father? He had laid the egg which Luther had hatched.

Like some people even now, Erasmus wanted to remain above the parties. Free spirit as he was, he wanted to be free – even in the dispute. A man of the centre and averse to all extremes, he wanted to listen to both sides and mediate between them. He wanted '*et – et*', 'both – and'. So he neither condemned Luther nor identified with him. To put his dilemma more precisely:

On the one hand he wanted **no condemnation of Luther** without a thorough investigation. The man from Rotterdam could largely agree with the man from Wittenberg on substantive issues. His view was that if one wanted to suppress all Luther's teaching one would have to suppress a large part of the gospel! No, Erasmus was not ready to call Luther a heretic, and he stubbornly refused all the requests from Rome and elsewhere in the church for him to write against Luther. He also persistently ignored all urgent invitations to come to Rome to take up a post there, even when one came from Hadrian VI, the tutor of Charles V and the first Dutch (and until modern times the last non-Italian) Pope, though from the beginning Hadrian had regarded Luther's works as highly damaging. Erasmus, the great independent, did not feel that he was born to be a curial court theologian and cardinal.

But on the other hand **he would not be identified with Luther**. Luther seemed to him to be something of a crude man of power, striking out around himself in theology and the church after the manner of a German country serf. Luther had overturned so much that could well have been left standing. This German consistency was terrible! The fact that he, Erasmus, had initially approved of Luther's criticsm did not mean that he had to approve of all that Luther had written since. For example, was he to adopt Luther's quite sweeping remarks about the unfree will of sinful human beings and the impossibility of good works? No, Erasmus less and less could or would identify with such an unbridled fanatic in the faith. This highly educated, reserved, sensitive man had too much of a peaceful scholarly nature. Erasmus agreed with Luther where he was right, but where he was wrong no one could expect Erasmus to agree; here he preferred in the last resort to remain with Pope and emperor.

With his highly ambivalent policy and diplomatic skill Erasmus found himself **between the front lines**. And for many people, although he had initiated the reform movement, he soon fell far behind Luther, who had carried it out. The man of the Reformation began to displace the reformer. The one who sowed the wind became afraid of the storm; no wonder that from now on Erasmus could not get rid of the reputation of being half-hearted, double-tongued, indeed an opportunist. At first loved and admired, then wooed and sought by all sides, finally he was viewed with suspicion, slandered and scorned in both camps.

But Erasmus continued to work and publish indefatigably for **consensus, concord** between the Christian camps, which from 1520 onwards kept drifting further apart in hostility. In 1533 his last eirenic work appeared under the title *On the Unity of the Church that is to be Restored*. Now seventy, he had just over a year to live. And time and again, self-critical and introspective as he was, he kept asking himself: had he taken the right course? Should he not have written so much? Should he have written differently? But think of all that he did do, patiently, excessively patiently, day by day, to temper conflicts by understanding, to maintain endangered contacts through correspondence, to send understanding (and often apparently contradictory) answers to various questions and situations everywhere, and thus to overcome the irreconcilable and to convince people of the irreconcilable through the Bible and reason.

Erasmus died in the night of 11/12 July 1536 in Basel, in full consciousness, with words from the Psalms and finally 'Lieve God' ('dear God') in the words of his native childhood Dutch on his lips. A Catholic theologian to the end, he was solemnly buried in the Protestant cathedral in Basel by the Protestant pastor of the city in the presence of the Protestant mayor and council and the professors and students of the university. Among the less delicate heroes of his time – Luther, Zwingli, later Calvin and Ignatius of Loyola – was he, the one who was so highly-strung, perhaps the one sovereign ecumenist of them all?

The defeat of the third force

From today's perspective it is quite legitimate to ask: wasn't the cautious scholar Erasmus, to whom any display of inwardness was alien, right in his constant pleas for objectivity, the broadest tolerance possible, if need be also the recognition of differences in unity, at all events understanding and peace, as opposed to emotionalizing, hatred, fanaticism and riots? Wasn't he right when we think what the unpredictable action man Luther, who all too often seemed to replace arguments with ardour and wrath, asked too much of his church? Wasn't he right in the face of the monstrous number of victims of the Reformation in state and society, right in his slogan **Reform, yes; Reform à la Luther, no?**

So it is not an idle question to ask: what would Europe have been spared had people listened more to him, Erasmus, than to Luther, had the **third force** in Europe which he embodied, the force of reform, understanding and tolerance, come into play, first in Rome, but ultimately also in the Reformation camp, where he had so many friends? However, history, following Luther and Rome (and Machiavelli), seemed to move beyond Erasmus, the loser.

The Austrian historian Friedrich Heer, who has made 'the third force' the subject of a far-ranging and committed book,[47] is therefore right in his sorry stocktaking. The failure of the third force had bitter consequences for individual countries of Europe. This what Heer says: '**The defeat of the third force meant**: for Germany, the century-long civil war which culminated in the Thirty Years' War; for France, the hundred-and-fifty-year-long civil war, now cold, now hot, between the "royal Catholic religion" and the Huguenots, which ended with the annihilation or expulsion of the cream of the French aristocracy, the French middle classes and the French intelligentsia; for Spain, an internal separation from Europe through the annihilation or expulsion of its Erasmian humanists, its Jews, Marranos and Protestants; for Italy, the expulsion of the religious nonconformists, the chopping up into the ghetto states of the sixteenth to nineteenth centuries, which with their state police and inquisitions throttled or at least desperately oppressed intellectual life; for England, the final distancing, as an *alter orbis*, from Europe as another "continent". For Europe as a whole, the fixation which lasted until the twentieth century, on being the "West", Western Europe, in sharp contrast to the East, Russia, the Eastern church, its own masses, the lowly folk, the underground of the person.'[48]

So given this monstrous history of guilt, isn't Desiderius Erasmus of Rotterdam justified before history? However, a question may be asked in return: couldn't he, shouldn't he have chosen and practised committed **public opposition and steadfastness** in the face of Rome – given the alternatives of aggression the one hand and neutrality on the other? However, that was not the way of Erasmus and many Erasmians.

In the year of Erasmus' death, 1536, the Erasmian **Reginald Pole**, cousin of Henry VIII, whom we have already met, was nominated cardinal along with the dark zealot **Gian Pietro Caraffa**, founder of the strict order of Theatines, who is also known to us. Both then joined the famous nine-man commission which made the bold 'Proposal on Church Reform' (*Consilium de emendanda Ecclesia*) which we heard of in connection with the Counter-Reformation (P III) and which was seen generally as a shift in the Vatican towards the renewal of the church. But what a historical opportunity for the Reformers was missed years later by the failure to nominate this Erasmian Pole in a **papal election**!

How could this happen? In the papal election in December 1549, Cardinal **Pole** had received 21 and the next day even 24 votes. But because 28 votes were necessary and it seemed impossible to assemble these in the face of cardinals inclining towards the French, Pole's friends from the imperial party did all they could the next night to elect Pole *per modum adorationis*, by that means of 'homage' which would have made it possible for his opponents to assent to the election without a formal Yes. But to their great surprise, Pole, when asked whether he would accept the election – in the middle of the night *per adorationem* – fell silent and went to his cell 'dumb as an ox' (as he himself said later). The next day he did not get the decisive vote that had been promised. So, we may ask, was Pole perhaps also an Erasmian who in a decisive hour proved to be an undecided *cunctator*, a delayer, who lost the moment to act? Perhaps! At least he was an Erasmian in that instead of accepting the election and taking the reform in hand personally and practically, during the conclave which now went on for two full months, he stayed in his solitary cell writing – a book. On what? On the power and role of the Pope!

And as things went, the missed opportunity never returned, although on the seventy-first day of the conclave Pole still got the same high vote as at the beginning. But the one who probably did most to prevent his election and who had accused Pole, the foreigner, and only forty-nine, publicly of heresy, especially in matters of justification, was himself a candidate (of the French): none other than Caraffa. An exponent of the conservative restoration group and founder of the central Roman Inquisition (*Sanctum Officium Sanctissimae Inquisitionis*, 1542) as he now was, as is well known, six years later Caraffa himself was elected Pope at the age of eighty: Paul IV, the first Grand Inquisitor on the papal throne who, as we heard, even had his fellow cardinals Pole and Morone pursued by the Inquisition. The third force was played out.

The two faces of the Reformation

Finally, in December 1545, that modest small church gathering had taken place which the German 'Protestants' (so called since the Speyer 'protestation' of 1529) refused to attend and which, as we heard in connection with the Roman Catholic paradigm (P III) was to prove the historic council of the Counter-Reformation: the Council of Trent.

In the meantime the Lutheran movement had been able to spread powerfully especially in north, east and south Germany, but also beyond in Lithuania, Sweden, Finland, Denmark and Norway. In Switzerland there was a parallel to the events in Germany: from the middle of the fifteenth century Switzerland had already begun to detach itself from the empire, and there an independent more radical form of the Reformation was founded by Huldrych Zwingli, which we shall have to look at separately. Still in the 1520s, though, Martin Luther had succeeded in **consolidating the Reformation movement internally**:
– its worship through a German 'Little Book of Baptism', a 'German Mass' and a 'Little Book of Marriage'.
– its religious education through the 'Greater Catechism' for pastors and a short version, the 'Lesser Catechism', for use in homes.
– its church constitution through a new church order promulgated by the local rulers. Later Luther also devised a liturgical formulary for the ordination of pastors, and himself ordained pastors, finally also two bishops. Now within the Lutheran sphere of influence, there was largely an abolition of private masses and the host of mass priests, the countless feasts of saints and auricular confession, the monasteries and compulsory celibacy for secular clergy. Luther, too, had married: the former nun Catherine von Bora, with whom he had six sons and daughters.

Yet Germany had **split into two confessional camps**. And in view of the threat to the empire from the Turks, who in 1526 had defeated the Hungarians at Mohács and in 1529 had advanced to the gates of Vienna, Luther too had asked himself whether papal or Turkish power – both for him religions of works and the law – was the more dangerous. At the end of his life Luther did not see even the future of the Reformation churches in anything like the rosy light in which he saw them in the year of the great breakthrough. In the last years of his life he was increasingly subject to melancholy, manic depressions and spiritual tribulations, along with apocalyptic anxieties about the end time. And there were objective as well as psychological reasons for his pessimism, which grew year by year.[49] For Luther was oppressed not only by serious illnesses but by great disappointments:

1. The original **enthusiasm over the Reformation** had **run out of steam**: community life was often in ruins, not least because of a lack of pastors. In thirty years, the verve of the evangelical movement among the people had finally become paralysed. Many who were not ready for the 'freedom of a Christian' lost all ecclesiastical and thus moral support with the collapse of the Roman system. And even Luther, complaining about the ungrateful Germans, sometimes asked himself whether people had really become so much more pious and moral as a result of the Reformation. Nor could the terrifying impoverishment in art – music excepted – be overlooked.

So much that should have changed had not changed.[50] Some mediaeval abuses continued to lead a tenacious life of their own.[51] Granted, schools had been founded everywhere to educate pious Christians to read the Bible and catechisms. But visitation reports showed that ignorance and superstition, magic, curses and oaths and strange rites and customs were still very widespread, often in the form of a mixed Catholic-Protestant religion.[52] Granted, the permission for priests to marry had removed many abuses, but of course it did not prevent all sexual and other transgressions. Granted, the Lutheran pastors had lost many legal and financial privileges – a former occasion for anti-clericalism – and pastors' families became the social and cultural centre of the community. But the 'universal priesthood' of believers had by no means been realized, and the gulf betwen clergy and laity remained in many places. Indeed because of the university training for pastors which soon became universal (and because of the marriages of priests' sons and daughters), soon a new, more intellectual, clergy came into being – on the model of officialdom, heralds of an intellectualized religion far removed from popular culture.[53]

2. But the Reformation also came up against **growing political resistance**.

After the inconsequential Augsburg Reichstag of 1530 (the emperor had rejected the conciliatory 'Augsburg Confession' which Melanchthon had had the main part in drafting), in the 1530s the Reformation was initially able not only to consolidate itself in existing territories but also to extend more widely, from Württemberg to Brandenburg. However, in the 1540s the emperor Charles V, who hitherto had constantly worked at mediation, had the wearisome wars with Turkey and France behind him. Now he believed that he was again strong enough to tackle Germany. And when the Lutherans refused to take part in the Council of Trent when it was finally called (because it was under papal leadership: Luther's crude work *Against the Roman Papacy, An Institution of the Devil*, dates from 1545[54]), the emperor took this as an occasion to compel the now powerful Schmalkaldic alliance of Protestants to bend the knee by using military force. Moreover the Protestant forces were defeated in these first wars of religion in 1546/57 (the 'Schmalkaldic Wars'), and now nothing was in the way of the restoration of Roman Catholic conditions (though with concessions over the marriage of priests and the chalice for the laity) in Protestant territories.

Only a change of side by the defeated Moritz of Saxony, who made a secret alliance with France, forced the emperor to flee through a surprise attack in Innsbruck in 1552 and also provoked the adjournment of the Council of Trent, saved Protestantism from a complete military defeat. Three years later, in 1555, the confessional division of Germany into the territories of the old faith and those of the 'Augsburg Confession' was finally prescribed ('the religious peace of Augsburg'). Now on German soil, too, the end had come of the third force (*via media*), which had hitherto played a role both in princely courts and at the grass roots. Now not only religious freedom prevailed, but also the principle *cuius regio, eius religio*. Anyone who did not belong to one of the two 'religions' was excluded – and there were many of these people. For,

3. The Protestant camp had **not been able to maintain unity**. From the beginning there were countless groups, communities, assemblies, movements and individual publicists who pursued different aims and strategies in implementing the Reformation. If we look at the great camps which were at odds with one another, we can first see the division of Protestantism in Germany into a 'left-wing' and a 'right-wing' Reformation, then the division between German Lutheranism, Swiss Zwinglianism and Calvinism, and indeed finally also the divisions within both Lutheranism and Calvinism themselves – all extremely momentous developments.

The 'left-wing' Reformation: radical nonconformists

Luther had summoned up spirits, but some he could only get rid of again by force. These were the spirits of **nonconformity** ('enthusiasm'),[55] which while certainly nourished by mediaeval roots, were encouraged to an extraordinary degree by Luther's appearance. What R.H.Bainton has called 'the left wing of the Reformation' is made up of radical religious and social movements which should not be interpreted in terms of either the Middle Ages or enlightened modernity but as independent movements within the framework of the Reformation paradigm (P IV). Building up 'from below', these were lay movemnts with an anti-clerical orientation which even turned against state power when persecuted. But in other respects they show such an extraordinary difference in leaders, groups and movements that they are virtually impossible to typify.

A great variety of individual interests and individual revolts began to spread under Luther's name, and soon the Reformer in fact saw himself facing a second, 'left-wing' front. Indeed these radical groups (spurred on by Carlstadt's[56] agitation against the mass, priests and monks – there were riots and iconoclasm as early as 1522 in Luther's own city Wittenberg) soon seemed to him at least as dangerous to his enterprise of reform as the traditionalists orientated on Rome. If the 'papists' appealed to the Roman system, these 'enthusiasts' – this derogatory name is often still applied to them today, despite the corrections made by historical research – seemed to him to practise a fanatical religious subjectivism and enthusiasm. They appealed to the personal experience of direct revelation and the Spirit ('inner voice', 'inner light'), and associated this with apocalyptic, social revolutionary ideas. Now the call was for a radical implementation of the Reformation here and now, if need be by force, regardless of existing law. The establishment of Christ's thousand-year-kingdom on earth – this was already the cry of the revolutionary agitator, Luther's radical rival, the pastor Thomas Müntzer, whose roots lay in mediaeval mysticism and apocalyptic.

As is well known, two years after a rebellion by the imperial knights in 1523 the **Peasants' War** broke out; Müntzer wanted to see in it the approaching judgment on the godless and the dawn of the new order. In view of the disastrous economic conditions of the peasants this was a more than understandable political and revolutionary conflagration. It cannot be demonstrated that this was an 'early bourgeois revolution', as Marxist historiography long claimed, because in this 'Peasants' War' the great majority of the population of the cities was on the side of the feudal authorities. But it is certain that for the legitimation of their political, economic and social demands and their religious and ecclesiastical demands (e.g. free election of pastors) the peasants could now appeal again to the 'gospel' and did so, so that the direct connection between the Peasants' War and the Reformation is indisputable.[57]

However, **Luther** was afraid that his Reformation would be compromised in the eyes of the rulers by such a revolution. First calling for peace in a mediating way,[58] he was increasingly horrified by reports of abominable atrocities committed by the peasants. He reacted with his extremely passionate and striking work *Against the Robbing and Murdering Hordes of Peasants*.[59] He called on the **authorities** to **intervene regardless** ('the sword') against this rebellion which he saw as reprehensible, to hew and stab. This cost Luther much of his initial popularity.

For a long time this tragic development was repressed in Lutheranism, until after the 1848 revolution Friedrich Engels wrote the first history of the Peasants' War[60] and after the First World War Ernst Bloch[61] praised Thomas Müntzer[62] as the founder of a revolutionary tradition in Germany. But this repression was doubtless connected with Luther himself. Evidently trapped in a view 'from above', both politically and theologically, the Reformer was not ready **to draw such radical political and social conclusions** from his radical demand for Christian freedom. He did not want to support the just demands of the peasants against the princes and the nobility with corresponding clarity. For all the reprehensible excesses of the peasants, their demands were extremely reasonable and justified: their independence was threatened and they were being increasingly exploited. Nor could Luther deny their economic and legal distress. So would a plan for reform have been an illusion from the start? No. For the federal order of the Swiss confederacy, the ideal of a new order for the peasants of southern Germany, would have been a quite attainable model. But this was alien to Luther, trapped in the perspective of Thuringia. And the Habsburgs already feared an overflow of the principles of confederate political organization into southern Germany.[63]

So at Frankenhausen the **peasants** finally suffered not only a devastating military **defeat** but also a fearful legal punishment: Thomas Müntzer himself was beheaded after being tortured. The peasants, the largest social group in the empire, were now out of the running as a political factor in any wider context in the empire. The victors were again the rulers, with whom Luther too had now allied himself; with his consent they functioned in Germany as 'emergency bishops', and so very soon were also to become lords of the church.

But the currents of the radical Reformation were by no means yet exhausted. On the contrary. Against the background of the Peasants' War, in Zwingli's Zurich on 21 January 1525 in a town house the layman Konrad Grebel performed the first **adult baptism**, on the runaway monk

Georg Blauroc, without any special ceremonial, using a ladle of water.[64] This was a signal for 'revolt' to the **Baptist movement,** which then took many different forms; in it laity began to preach, to celebrate the eucharist and to baptize (even women dared to do this). Now they sharply criticized even the newly established Reformation churches with compulsory orders, because they already incorporated infants as members. On the basis of scripture the Baptists called for the conscious decision of the individual for faith and therefore for adult baptism; they regarded and practised this as the only true Christian baptism – and were therefore denounced by their opponents as 'baptizers again' (Anabaptists).

Since these Baptists, originally hovering between pacifism and militancy, turned away from Zwingli's Reformation and repudiated the integration into the ecclesiastical, political and legal community given by baptism, they were persecuted, but precisely because of this, as itinerant preachers they spread their message amazingly quickly throughout Germany as far as Moravia in the east and Friesland in the north. They regarded themselves as the only ones to be truly born again, the only ones to have been justified and sanctified. They trusted in scripture and even more in the 'inner light' that had been given them. They attached supreme importance to morality along the lines of the Sermon on the Mount, laid down by law. These groups, often apocalyptic and showing signs of early communism, continued to be extremely mistrustful of the state and the state church, and were also ready to endure patiently and heroically as martyrs all the violence and persecution inflicted on them by both the Protestant and the Catholic political authorities.

Research into the Baptist movement has grown to an amazing extent recently.[65] It has shown that we do not do justice to them if we
– vilify them as misguided, enthusiastic and unteachable disciples of Luther (thus the historians from confessional Lutheranism), or
– idealize them as a single and coherent movement for the restoration of the earliest church (thus American scholars from the free church tradition), or
– reduce them to purely social movements and neglect their religious basis (thus the Marxist Reformation historians, above all from the former German Democratic Republic).

Rather, the Baptist movement must be seen as an independent devolution of the Reformation, though in Europe it stands on the periphery of the Reformation spectrum, which has an extremely heterogeneous composition. Its 'setting in life' was a pronounced anticlericalism of lay people, who wanted an improvement in their lives and therefore markedly ethicized faith and personalized it in terms of pious individuals.[66]

It is clear that the Baptists were not going to be exterminated even by brutal persecution and the death penalty. In a report to the Wittenberg Faculty in 1531, even Melanchthon had argued for executing those of their inclination, and Luther had agreed with him. He was against these 'sneakers and preachers in corners'.[67] They came into the communities without a public calling, preached, and in so doing led numerous members away from the parish and civil community. Luther saw this simply as 'revolt'. Even Wittenberg was evidently still far from a freedom of religion in the modern sense; so far that even in Protestant Kursaxony **Anabaptists** could be **executed**, even if they were not rebels, but merely erroneous in their beliefs. However, in individual instances religious enthusiasm, too, could turn into a regime of fanaticism and terror if, as in Holland and from there in Münster in 1535 (Jan Beuckelssen, Bernt Knipperdolling) it attempted to bring in a 'kingdom of Christ' by force: with references to the Apocalypse and the Old Testament understood literally, this could involve not only legalistic rebaptism and the brutal oppression of opponents but also communism of possessions and even polygamy.

However, generally speaking the Baptists were now quiet, peaceful people, ready to suffer – like the **'Mennonites'**, moderate Baptists brought together by the former Catholic priest Menno Simons (died 1561) into communities which soon branched out. However, precisely because of the Baptist revolution in Münster they were regarded as 'rebels' and had to suffer martyrdom by the hundreds and the thousands. Only later were they were to find tolerance in Holland, in Switzerland, in some north German cities and in Moravia. However, they could only develop properly like other nonconformists in a new country, far from the old Europe. Nor is there any need to stress that elsewhere in the sphere of the Reformation too, counter-figures and counter-movements existed in opposition to the dominant structures and institutions, which became radical as a result of their opposition to the clergy, both old and new. There was the spiritualism of Caspar von Schwenckfeld or Sebastian Franck which neglected all externals, or there were the anti-trinitarians who concentrated on opposing the traditional doctrine of the Trinity. At any rate the first **free churches** developed from the Baptist and Mennonite communities; these were churches based on voluntary membership, assembling in their own churches with their own church order – but without any say with the secular authorities. More than just having a say – on the other side this was a characteristic of the right wing of the Reformation, and this brings us back again to Martin Luther.

The 'right-wing' Reformation: an official church instead of the papal church

The **ideal of the free Christian church** which Luther had enthusiastically painted for his contemporaries in his programmatic writings was **not realized** in the sphere of Lutheranism. Certainly Luther freed countless churches from the rule of worldly bishops who were hostile to reform, and above all from the 'captivity' of the Roman Curia. But what was the result?

In principle Luther had advocated the doctrine of state and church as the 'two realms'. But at the same time, in the face of all the difficulties with Rome on the one hand and 'enthusiasts' and 'rebels' on the other, he gave the local rulers (who unfortunately were not all like Frederick 'the Wise'!) the duty of protecting the church and maintaining order in it. This introduced a conservative political stamp into Lutheranism. As there were no Catholic bishops in the Lutheran sphere and their jurisdiction was no longer recognized, the princely '**emergency bishops**' soon became '**summepiscopi**', who attributed quasi-episcopal authority to themselves, took over church legislation, jurisdiction and discipline and came to control all church possessions, including the monasteries which had been abolished – and not just to use them as churches and schools. This therefore strengthened their political power considerably.

In short, the people's Reformation now became a **rulers' and magistrates' Reformation**. The result of this was that the Lutheran churches freed from the 'Babylonian captivity' could not develop any autonomous church organization, but were given a 'church government' which was that of the local ruler or city. They soon became almost completely and often oppressively dependent on their own rulers along with the latters' lawyers and organs of church administration (consistories). And as far as the imperial cities were concerned, although here it was most of all civic opposition which had forced the gospel preaching and the institutionalization of an evangelical church, it was finally the city council, the magistrate, who had the say even in the church – with very little participation from the congregation.[68]

In fact, the rulers, who even before the Reformation had worked against peasants and citizens towards a unification of their territories, which had often been thrown together in motley fashion, in order to have a coherent group of subjects, had become excessively powerful because of the retreat of the church into the religious sphere. The **local ruler** finally became something like a **Pope in his own territory**. Here it was not so much that the ruler was sacralized as that religion was politically domesticated, indeed underwent the beginnings of secularization. Here freedom of conscience and worship were still a long way off; the authorities had the say. Granted, there was some resistance in the communities, say against re-Catholicization or even Calvinism. But Lutheranism did not develop a doctrine of the right to resist the local ruler, and at best only the beginnings of a right of the pastors or superintendents to contradict. Even many Protestant scholars are now saying that the Reformation in Germany prepared the way not so much (as Protestant church historiography so often claims) for modernity, freedom of religion and the French Revolution (a further epoch-making paradigm shift would be necessary for this) as first for an authoritarian state and absolutist rule, and thus created one of the presuppositions for the modernization that was to come.

So generally speaking, what was realized in Lutheran Germany was not the free Christian church but the **rule of magistrates and princes over the church**, which was often not very Christian. It came to an end – a well-deserved end – in Germany only with the Revolution after the First World War. But even in the time of National Socialism the resistance of the Lutheran churches to a regime of terror in the state like that of Hitler was decisively weakened by the doctrine of two realms which had been applied for centuries: namely, that subordination of the churches to state authority and emphasis on civil obedience in secular affairs which had been usual since Luther. In passing, something should be mentioned here which already occupied me at length in the first volume on Judaism:[69] even Martin Luther, shortly before his death, expressed himself in such an un-Christian, hate-filled way about the **Jews** that the National Socialists did not find it difficult to cite him as a key witness in justification of their antisemitism.

On 18 February 1546, ten years after Erasmus, Martin Luther also died – preaching on a 'official visit' to Eisleben, where he had been born – after a few hours of physical weakness, in the company of his travelling companions, and making use of the mediaeval *ars moriendi*. And his cause, the 'cause' of the Reformation, went on. But even after Luther, in the long run Lutheranism could eventually establish itself only in Germany and the Scandinavian states. Yet Protestantism became a world power. That is thanks to the other Reformation, which did not proceed from Wittenberg but, having been prepared for in Zurich, emanated from Geneva. We are now entering a further phase of the Reformation paradigm shift.

6. The consistent Reformation: 'Reformed' Protestantism

Since the controversy with the 'enthusiasts', some of Luther's critics had been of the opinon that Luther was not radical enough. It was necessary to do away with the Roman Catholic paradigm more thoroughly, to follow the course of the Reformation consistently to the end in the face of Lutheran 'half measures': from the abolition of crucifixes, images and liturgical vestments to the elimination of the mass. Only what could be justified by scripture should be retained in the church. Here it was Luther's self-confident contemporary, rival and opponent Huldrych Zwingli who was to lay the foundations. I have already mentioned his negative attitude to the first Baptists briefly. Now we must look at his own approach in more detail. For Zwingli stands for that consistent type of Reformation which for Jean Calvin was then to be really **reformed Christianity**: not only a more or less thorough renovation but a systematic rebuilding of the church, a reform not only of the doctrine but of the whole life of the church.

Reformation in Switzerland: Huldrych Zwingli

In complete contrast to Martin Luther, the Reformer of German Switzerland, **Huldrych Zwingli** (1484–1531)[70] had not been an ascetic monk but was a cheerful pastor with a scholastic training, first of all at Einsiedeln, the Marian pilgrimage place, and from 1 January 1519 priest at the Grossmünster in Zurich. As an army chaplain he was present not only at the victory of the confederates at Novara and the conquest of Milan in 1513, but also at their devastating defeat at Marignano in 1515. This battle marked the end of the expansionist great-power politics of the Swiss in the direction of Lombardy and Burgundy, who since their victories over the Burgundian count Charles the Bold had the reputation of being the best soldiers in Europe.

To emphasize his independence from Luther, Zwingli subsequently put his **move to the Reformation** at a very early date, between 1516 and 1519. The earliest biographers (Myconius, Bullinger, Kessler) and some more recent ones like O.Farner have followed him here. But the most recent historical investigations by W.H.Neuser[71] and G.W.Locher[72] have made it clear that Zwingli was initially more a man of the centre, an advocate of Christian humanism and moderate church reform within Catholicism, in the spirit of **Erasmus**. Zwingli had met Erasmus for the first time in Basel in 1515 and praised him as the one who had liberated theology from barbarism (the contempt for antiquity) and sophistry (Scholasticism). At any rate, after that Zwingli no longer preached on papal authority, indulgences, purgatory, miracles, vows and the punishments of hell but on the *philosophia Christi*, the gospel of Christ, understood in markedly ethical terms. And he remained so Catholic that even in 1518 he still thought papal honorific titles important.

But in contrast to Erasmus, Zwingli was a decisive pastor and politician. So Luther's bold appearance at the Leipzig disputation and first programmatic writings influenced him deeply. First of all Zwingli – marked by his gruesome war experiences – inveighed against the abuse of Swiss peasants and citizens engaging in mercenary service abroad. Furthermore, he criticized the fixed yearly 'pensions' paid by foreign powers to Swiss aristocrats to make it possible for them to hire Swiss mercenaries at all. But along with the reading of the letters of Paul, the Gospel of John and Augustine, it was Luther's work *On the Babylonian Captivity of the Church* (1520) which stood at the beginning of Zwingli's more radical theology. And this real **transformation of the Reformer with humanistic inclinations into the supporter of a consistent Reformation in keeping with the gospel** may only have taken place in 1521–22.[73]

At any rate, now Zwingli felt encouraged – after initial hesitation because of the Roman bull against Luther threatening excommunication – to launch a **systematic attack on the Roman system**. And the years 1522–23 were to see the breakthrough of the Reformation in Zurich:

– A **ban on mercenary service** by the Zurich council.

– An open **breach of the Lenten commandments** (Zwingli's first Reformation writing was *On the Choosing and Freedom of Foods*,[74] which led to clashes with the Bishop of Constance).

– **Free preaching** of the gospel and permission for **priests to marry** (Zwingli's *Supplicatio* and apology *Archeteles*).

– The first **Zurich disputation** with Zwingli's *Sixty-Seven Theses* (his most important Reformation work[75]).

– An order from the council that all preachers must **preach the gospel**.

– **Iconoclasm** (against Zwingli's will) and the Second Zurich Disputation (on masses and images).

– A systematic **introduction of radical reforms** by a commission made up of pastors and members of the council: abolition of the mass, of organs, hymns and altars, and also of processions and relics, confirmation and final unction; limitation of the eucharist to four Sundays in the year (when the whole community was to take part).

– Finally, the adoption of **church government by the council**, which was now responsible for marriage legislation, moral discipline, care of the poor and a reorganization of schools.

However, in Zurich, too, the questions were by no means only about theology and the church; at the same time they were political and social. There were tensions between the city, where the council wanted to have the say even in the church, and the country communities, where people wanted a reform by the community itself. They wanted to abolish the hated church tithe and at the same time the domination of the country by the city. Whereas Konrad Grebel, later to become a Baptist, whom we have already met, and his friends took the side of the country communities, we find Zwingli on the side of the council. After the first baptism of adults, the Baptists' break with the Zurich Reformation and a further disputation, in 1526 the council pronounced 'anabaptism' a rebellious act punishable by death, and this penalty was inflicted on a Baptist the very next year by drowning him in the Limmat. Here Zwingli resembled Luther.

Yet Zwingli was theologically and politically more consistent than Luther. For as a man of clear rationality, practical efficiency and bold fearlessness, in his church reform he was concerned not only – like Luther – to eliminate elements which were manifestly un-Christian, but in addition to eliminate all elements which did not have a biblical foundation. In fact that meant a **completely new church order**, and did not end up finally, as in Lutheranism, with a church regulated by the local ruler, but in a synodical church under the self-government of the cities. Calvin would later develop these foundations further.

This reformation of Zwingli's, who also had many theological friends outside Zurich and increasingly developed into a statesman, rapidly also became established in Basel (where the main figure was Johannes Oecolampadius) and further in Bern, St Gallen and other Swiss cities. It also exercised a strong influence in south Germany, though there was no active political and social collaboration. Only the traditionally Catholic population of the original rural Switzerland (Uri, Schwyz and Unterwalden) and the cities of Lucerne, Zug and Fribourg offered resistance and refused to implement the Reformation. The result was that in the Swiss confederacy, too, there was now a **split** right down the middle of country and people. As in Germany, this led to political and military alliances and finally even to the civil war.

There was nothing for Zwingli but once again to go into battle as an army chaplain. The First Kappel War broke out, which was a war of religion. Zwingli fell in the second of these wars, in 1531. His corpse was quartered and burned by Catholics. However, his work lasted. Only ten years later the Frenchman Jean Calvin could develop his church in Geneva under the protection of the Reformed city of Bern. In 1549, in the *Consensus Tigurinus*, with Zwingli's successor Heinrich Bullinger, Calvin was to lay the roots of an alliance of all the Reformed in Europe. Reformed Switzerland – after Zwinglians and Calvinists combined into an ecclesiastical and theological union in the *Confessio Helvetica posterior* of 1566 – came to form the backbone of world Calvinism and thus world Protestantism. Who is this Calvin?

The completion of the Reformation paradigm shift: Jean Calvin

He was only eight years old when the dispute over indulgences broke out in Germany. A generation already separates Luther and Zwingli from **Jean Calvin**,[76] originally Cauvin, Latin Calvinus (1509–64). Yet the basic Reformation intentions remained the same: Calvin, too, essentially wanted a return to the gospel, uncompromising obedience to the word of God. For the sake of Christ, Calvin, too, had turned his back on the church of God, which for him was no longer the church of Christ: 'We have to turn away from them in order to turn to Christ.'[77]

Like Luther and Zwingli, Calvin was a man of deep piety, which was rooted in trusting faith in justification by God's grace alone. But unlike Luther, Calvin had never been a monk, and unlike Zwingli, he had never been a pastor: he was a lawyer, the son of an episcopal lawyer. Originally destined for the priesthood, at the early age of fourteen Calvin had come from Picardy in north-west France to the Collège Montaigu in **Paris** where the Spaniard Ignatius of Loyola, the future founder of the Jesuits, was studying at almost the same time. Here he was trained in philosophy and disputation. Deprived of his mother at an early stage and brought up in an aristocratic family, at the desire of his father, who had been excommunicated in a conflict with the cathedral chapter, Calvin first took a course in civil and canon law. At that time this included a by no means small knowledge of theology. At an early stage Calvin also learned Greek, for some the language of heresy. He gained his licentiate (and thus became an *extraordinarius* lecturer) in law at the university of **Orleans**.

Did he have a spiritual crisis like Luther? This earnest, self-confident man with aristocratic manners never seems to have had one. At any rate, unlike Luther, he tells us hardly anything about himself. It must therefore remain an open question whether Calvin simply turned increasingly away from the Roman church or really underwent a 'conversion experience' (which is the meaning of *subita conversio*, first mentioned in the preface to the Psalms commentary of 1557). However, it is certain that, like Zwingli, he came through humanistic reform Catholicism in the spirit of Erasmus (and in France of Faber Stapulensis) to study Greek, the Bible and the church fathers (Calvin's favourite book was Seneca's *Clementia*). He moved from Orleans to the University of **Paris**, where he came into contact with people of a Protestant disposition who quite automatically involved him in a discussion of Martin Luther. For in Paris, too, Luther had long been an issue which polarized opinions. Among the theologians of the Sorbonne there were fanatical opponents of Luther, but among the Paris humanists he had numerous sympathizers, who had already spoken of justification by grace and faith.

Beyond question, 10 November 1533 marks the decisive shift. This was the date of the inaugural lecture by Calvin's friend, the humanist and doctor of medicine Nicolas Cop (from Basel), who had just been elected Rector of the University of Paris. In this address (which Calvin perhaps helped to compose), Cop not only interpreted the Beatitudes of the Sermon on the Mount but also dared to quote Erasmus and even Luther – polemically, against scholasticism. This was bold but unwise, since on the urging of the theological faculty the police were now brought in to arrest Cop and other sympathizers, including Calvin. Calvin succeeded in fleeing Paris and avoiding prison – often moving and living under an alias. Although still by no means a 'Lutheran', Calvin was now beginning even more to study Martin Luther alongside the Bible and the church fathers.

The repression continued. Twenty Protestant sympathizers, including a friend and fellow student of Calvin's, were burnt at the stake as 'Lutherans' because of the 'affaire des placards' (ugly posters against the mass). And though by upbringing and profession he was all for order and authority, Calvin now felt driven to take the way of the Reformation. At the beginning of January 1534 he moved to **Basel**, and in a very short time this self-taught theologian was able to publish his theological *magnum opus* in a first edition (of course still very incomplete). He dedicated it to the French king Francis I, with a plea for tolerance for Protestants. This book gives a brief summary of gospel teaching and is completely based on scripture. Calvin called it *Institutio christianae religionis*. It appeared in Latin in 1536, the year of Eramsus' death, and the year in which Pole and Caraffa were nominated cardinals. Luther, who admired Calvin and with whom he exchanged friendly letters, now only had ten years to live; Zwingli had already been dead for five years. And soon Calvin was to surpass as a leader of the Reformation those who were now at the peak of their influence: Melanchthon in Wittenberg and Bucer in Strasbourg.

Was this historical providence? That same year – and in the winter of 1536 Ignatius of Loyola set off with his first companions from Paris to Rome – on his travels Calvin came to **Geneva** and here met the Reformer Wilhelm Farel, under the protection of Bern, who in the previous year had helped the Protestant movement to victory – against the Catholic Savoyards and the diocese of Geneva which was allied with them. Farel persuaded Calvin to stay, and the twenty-eight-year-old first became 'lecteur publique' for New Testament in Geneva and then also a preacher, without any official ordination. Biographers have often overlooked the fact that Calvin, although beyond question a great systematic theologian, never taught dogmatics later, but constantly produced new expositions of scripture. The Bible was translated verse by verse directly from Hebrew or Greek into Latin, to be followed by a grammatical analysis of the text and a historical and theological interpretation along with finer points of philology and philosophy.

However, Calvin's first stay in Geneva lasted barely two years. During this period Calvin wrote a catechism which was compulsory for all inhabitants, made the population swear an oath on the Creed, and with the help of a church order passed by the council introduced such strict moral discipline that Farel and he were finally banished by a new majority on the council – in 1538. Calvin again went to Basel and then to **Strasbourg**, where the Reformer Martin Bucer put him in charge of the French refugee community and where he could now gather valuable pastoral and liturgical experience. He kept up contact with German Reformers, especially Melanchthon, whom he valued highly. He even took part in the Protestant-Catholic religious conversations at Hagenau, Worms and Regensburg, though there he learned that theological compromise formulae with a church which dogmatized its mediaeval theology and church order made little sense. In Strasbourg Calvin married and had a son, but the child was to die soon afterwards. Nor did his marriage last long. After only nine years an illness took away his wife.

Meanwhile vigorous partisan struggles had broken out in **Geneva**. After three years they led to Calvin's recall, in 1541. He only returned after being given clear guarantees. But it was equally characteristic of Calvin that in Geneva he did not have a reckoning with his opponents. 'The Reformer took up the section of the Bible at which he had had to stop a few years previously and simply went on expounding this passage as though nothing had happened. He had great style.'[78] But then Calvin went on with the implementation of the Reformation in Geneva in all earnestness: all the public and private life of the city, indeed the everyday life of schools, businesses, politics and learning was to become 'worship'. Here was a total Christianization of the common life! Indefatigably, as a preacher in the cathedral, as a biblical exegete, theological teacher and writer, Calvin in fact succeeded in introducing and establishing strict church discipline in Geneva (house controls, a court on morals, a ban on dancing and playing cards) and realizing the Reformation programme laid out in his *Institutio* with unparalleled commitment and unbending consistency – inexorably strict even to his friends.

Here Calvin was always obedient to the secular authority and obeyed the laws. The more time went on, the better he coped even with the bitterest opposition group in the city council: the 'patriots', who in their xenophobia were hostile to the refugees for the faith from France, Italy and Holland. They were called the 'libertarians' because they were in favour of the exercise of moral discipline by the council and not by Calvin's consistory. For years Calvin scuffled with them at the periphery of his everyday activities: the cool, distant and humourless man (in all this very different from Luther) showed his opponents his determination, sensitivity and intelligence. But only in 1555, fourteen years after Calvin's return, did they definitively lose in the elections; after a demonstration (anti-French?) which was put down, they were exiled and some were mercilessly executed.

'Our story is of a man of order and peace who was born into a world of conflict,' writes the English historian T.H.L.Parker, who in his biography of Calvin brings out Calvin's indefatigable activity as a preacher and exegete in the light of Karl Barth and Vatican II: 'A conservative by nature, by upbringing, by conviction, his ideas became among the most revolutionary in Europe. The order, aristocratic in tendency, which he prized and which he devoted his life to establishing, became one of the platforms for democracy in succeeding centuries. His theology was fundamentally so old-fashioned that it seemed a novelty.'[79] There is no doubt that though Calvin may have had his deep shadow side as a human being and church politician, he brought the Reformation which Luther had initiated for Germany to completion for Europe, as far as it was willing to accept it.

The classic Reformed synthesis

Calvin's *Institutio* was his personal and at the same time highly objective apologia for his religious decision, as a systematic work on the same level as Zwingli's *De vera et falsa religione* of 1525 or Melanchthon's *Loci communes* in its second edition of 1535. Furthermore Calvin had provided a **basic introduction to Reformation Christianity** which was soon to make him the most significant Reformation dogmatic theologian, who more consistently than anyone else was able to ground Christian faith in the Bible and the church fathers – free of all the stereotypes of the mediaeval Roman system.[80] Its central theme was 'the knowledge of God and of ourselves'.[81] The six chapters of the first edition discussed, in accordance with the scheme of the catechism:
– the Law (the Decalogue)
– faith (the Apostles' Creed)
– prayer (the Our Father)
– the sacraments (baptism and eucharist)
– the other five sacraments (which are not true sacraments)
– Christian freedom, church authority and political administration.

But why is there nothing about the 'justification of the sinner' in this table of contents? That is no coincidence. For the very structure of the very first *Institutio* shows that Calvin, unlike Luther, is not concerned

with the quite personal struggle of sinful human beings for a 'gracious God' and an individual **certainty of salvation**. He begins from the sinfulness of decadent Christianity, which needs a better **order of salvation**. Moreover Calvin's Reformation concern is for practice, or, better, for the ordering of Christian life. In view of this it is not surprising,
– that the doctrine of justification, which for Luther is the basis of everything, only comes as final reflections in the chapter on the **Law**, after the exposition of the Ten Commandments;[82]
– that Calvin explicitly calls the Old Testament Law summed up in the Ten Commandments **good**, though human beings can only fulfil it on the basis of God's grace. This is because it above all calls for inner obedience of the heart, subjects the whole person to the rule of God and is aimed utterly at the love of God and human beings;
– that the Law not only bears witness to sin and grace and points to punishment, but is also an incentive to **progress**;
– that therefore **good works** done on the basis of faith in everyday ordinary life are to be praised and encouraged;
– that therefore emphasis must be placed on **sanctification** by works as well as justification by faith alone for the Christian life.

Luther showed the way for the Reformation with his basic intentions. And if we compare Calvin's programmatic Reformation work which he had already completely transformed and expanded in Strasbourg (1539) with Luther's programmatic works twenty years earlier (1520), we will doubtless miss the hot breath of Reformation passion and the religious existential depth of the German theologian. But Calvin's book, the most coherent systematic work of the Reformation (one can still sense the lawyer in every line), is attractive in its way: because of the Latin clarity of the account, the strict logic of the argument and the piety inspired by the Bible. Calvin was able to convince countless people by this unique synthesis, so that the *Institutes* were soon translated into all the European cultural languages and became one of the most-read books of the sixteenth century: with the 1541 translation into French Calvin became one of the classics of the French language. To meet the need of giving as balanced an answer as possible to the theoretical and practical questions which constantly arose, the book had to grow over the course of the decades. Whereas the first edition had only six chapters, the second edition of 1539 already had seventeen and the definitive edition of 1559 eventually had eighty; and whereas the first edition occupies only 248 columns in the Corpus Reformatorum, the last occupies 1,118. Calvin indefatigably supplemented and revised his book down to the last edition of 1559. Now fifty years old and threatened by a serious illness, he felt he had to complete it before his death.

Even opponents of Calvin will concede that in the last edition the *Institutes* attained such a degree of stringency and pregnancy in all questions of life and faith that it is **the most significant Christian dogmatics between Thomas Aquinas and Schleiermacher**. It has been said that what had begun as an 'oratory' ended up as a cathedral of theology, now supported and buttressed very much more strongly than before with scripture and the church fathers, but also secured at critical points on the basis of the theological controversies which had developed in the meantime. Everything still centred on two basic problems: knowledge of God and knowledge of oneself. But in the end Calvin gave his *magnum opus* another new order, now following the Apostles' Creed: the doctrines, first of God the Creator, then of God the Redeemer in Christ, then of grace imparted in the Holy Spirit, and finally the church, the sacraments and the civil regime. Each of the four books is clearly divided into chapters and each chapter in turn into numbered sections.[83]

Thus to the present day this work has remained the classic synthesis of consistently Reformation, 'Reformed' doctrine. We can probably say that it is the theological completion of the Reformation paradigm (P IV) which Luther initiated. We might perhaps compare what Calvin was after Luther with what Thomas was after Augustine. And yet, not only Lutherans would hesitate to follow Calvin in all things. For despite all the recognition of Calvin's theological achievement, the critical questions cannot be suppressed. For example, what about Calvin's distinctive famous-notorious doctrine of double predestination?

Everyone predestined

All the Reformers emphasize God's sovereignty, the uniqueness of Christ as the mediator between God and humankind, and the word of God as the norm which is the norm (*norma normans*) for all other norms (*normae normatae*). However, from the second completely revised Strasbourg edition of 1539 on, in a decisive point Calvin's theology was to diverge from the doctrine of the other Reformers: in the question of the eternal **predestination of every human being to salvation or damnation**.[84] Whereas Luther had incorporated the extremely threatening question of predestination (from the old Augustine) into a trusting faith in justification and blunted it, and whereas his master-pupil Melanchthon had deliberately not incorporated it into the fundamental Lutheran confessional document, the Augsburg Confession (1530), in Calvin the problem of predestination came into the foreground with the utmost sharpness because of his clash with his opponents.

But is the doctrine of predestination Calvin's 'central doctrine', which as a single material principle pervades all other doctrines? It is wrong to say this. It is true that predestination is a **characteristic doctrine** of Calvin's. Even during Calvin's lifetime it was formally declared a dogma in the *Consensus Genevensis de aeterna Dei praedestinatio*,[85] regardless of the criticism expressed by the physician Hieronymus Bolsec, who as a result was condemned by the magistrates and banished.[86] Later Calvinistic synods like those of Dordrecht and Westminster declared the doctrine of predestination formally binding. What does this doctrine say?

Already for Calvin himself it was a simple fact of experience that a division manifestly goes right down the middle of humankind between believers and non-believers. Some believe, others do not. Why is this so? Calvin finds the answer in scripture – where else? And there we read – for example in Ephesians: 'In him (Christ) God has elected us (the believers) before the creation of the world' (1.4). The believers. Not others. So the fact that humankind is so divided in its history stems from a decision of the eternal God himself – before all creation, right from the beginning. Unlimitedly free as God is, from eternity, in a mysterious 'decree' (which we human beings cannot see through), God has predestined some human beings to eternal life and others to eternal damnation. Was this for Calvin a quasi-Gnostic speculation on a hidden foundation to the world and its relation to creatures? No, this seemed to him to be a view of God's rule and sovereignty over the world which was well founded in the Bible and therefore indispensable. So Calvin felt that he had to accept a **double predestination** of human beings: 'For all are not created in equal condition; rather, eternal life is foreordained for some, eternal damnation for others. Therefore, as any man has been created to one or the other of these ends, we speak of him as predestined to life or to death.'[87]

That means that Calvin's theology is governed by a **radical theocentricity**. Everything has been created to the glory of God. All creatures, human beings but also Satan, are implements in God's hand, are there for the *Gloria Dei*, for the self-glorification of God.[88] And Calvin means this quite practically. Every member of the community is to help to shape the world to be a 'showplace of God's praise'. There is a striking **parallel to Ignatius of Loyola** and his principle *Ad maiorem Dei gloriam*, 'to the greater glory of God'. But whereas for the founder of the Jesuit order from the beginning human beings are wholly incorporated into the institutional church and its means of salvation, the sacraments, and remain so, in Calvin individuals first of all appear in solitude under God's unfathomable eternal counsel. They have to offer God pious fear and blind trust. The means of grace as human works are useless: they dilute the first commandment, which Calvin radicalizes. Therefore priesthood and private penance are to be rejected. 'To God alone the glory' is Calvin's slogan, and this explains why he also suppresses all sensual elements in religion and culture (except for the singing of hymns by the congregation).

Instead, the active, practical side comes into the foreground with Calvin. Although he himself ate only once a day, he in no way rejected the enjoyment of earthly life; only slavery to earthly goods. Calvin is also akin to Ignatius in active, **practical commitment in the world**, but with the necessary inner critical distance. However, it is striking that whereas the Calvinistic 'to God alone the glory' can at any time be directed against kings and rulers, the Ignatian 'to the greater glory of God' is remarkably never directed critically against popes and bishops. Rather, the *Exercises* call for a *sentire in Ecclesia*, in all things a 'feeling' with 'our holy mother, the hierarchical church'.[89]

That explains why Calvin – here following Luther – now attaches a wholly new importance to **everyday work** to the greater glory of God, especially to the fulfilment of professional gifts (one's profession is a vocation), in which they can be certain of their election. For while **good works** are not the basis of salvation, they are external, visible **signs of election** – here Calvin puts the emphasis in a completely different place from Luther. The conscience of believers 'is established also in the consideration of works, so far, that is, as these are testimonies of God dwelling and ruling in us'.[90]

In the ordering of everyday life above all a rational self-control is required of everyone (and not, as, say, in Catholicism, above all of a monastic elite), directed in **this-worldly asceticism** purely towards the proving of faith and personal calling in an unresting professional and business life in this world. Seldom did the new Reformation paradigm so clearly take a social form as here: instead of the early church or mediaeval spiritual aristocracy of the monks **alongside** the world we now have the spiritual aristocracy of the elect **in** the world. These are to dedicate themselves in their lives and callings in every respect, in a highly active, often heroic (and unfortunately sometimes even irreconcilable) way, to the fight for the glory of God. Meditation and prayer are not to be removed into a monastery, but are to take place in the midst of the everyday world.

Calvinistic ethics and capitalism

Is it surprising that so wise a person as the sociologist of religion Max Weber[91] saw this **Calvinistic ethic** as one of the most important psychological presuppositions of the typically modern '**capitalist spirit**'? Contrary to Karl Marx, Weber demonstrated that not only do economic conditions govern religious views, but conversely religious views govern economic developments. Of course Weber, too, did not deny that there were forms of early capitalism in Italy and even in Geneva long before the Reformation. Since his time the Zurich historian J.F.Bergier[92] has been able to demonstrate that the economic boom in Geneva was also connected with the political independence of the city state achieved by the 1535 revolution and the support of Reformed Swiss cities. Moreover the development of Geneva is connected with the influx of economically dynamic refugees for the faith from France and Italy: 'The opportunity for Geneva lay in the fact that the city attracted the following three factors from outside: capital, a qualified labour force, and possibilities for sales – all thanks to the Protestant refugees, i.e. a circumstance which initially had nothing to do with economics.'[93]

So Weber's thesis must certainly be refined, supplemented and corrected in many ways.[94] Religious and non-religious components overlap and influence one another reciprocally. However, Weber was less interested in the presence of capitalistic possibilities than in the new spirit, the new attitude, the new life-style, to utilize these capitalistic forms of the economy. And beyond question the Calvinistic tendency towards moral and economic activism played an important role in the formation of the consciousness necessary for this, the new collective mentality and normativity.

The Reformation doctrine could certainly also have been interpreted in a different way, and certainly there were also individual parallel developments in the Catholic Tridentine sphere. But on the whole the difference from countries with a Catholic stamp can hardly be disputed. Whereas Catholic morality concentrated (in a mediaeval way) on individual actions and (in guilty actions) on unburdening through the sacrament of penance, the Calvinistic doctrine of election required of the elect the systematic, ethical 'holiness' of their whole way of life. And whereas Luther's economic views were shaped by the barely developed small-state conditions of Germany and the fight between peasants and nobility, Calvin's were shaped by a progressive urban society and economy. In the Middle Ages rich businessmen very often returned money that they had earned with a bad conscience to the church for charitable purposes. But the Calvinist businessman could carry on his profitable business with a good conscience, trusting in his election, albeit in a disciplined way, 'puritanical' without waste. Here Calvin was entirely the practical man. In particular in his spiritual and homiletical writings one can get to know him as a man who clearly affirms the world, realistic and practical. Thus Calvin endorses private property, the productivity of capital and human labour and therefore also a variable interest rate, without following Luther in denouncing this (in mediaeval fashion) as usury.

However, this in no way prevented Calvin, anti-feudalistic and anti-clerical as he was, from sharply criticizing the pomp of the princes of the church and also the 'dead capital' of an aristocratic caste which did not want to work. Calvin deliberately brought about a spiritual **re-valuing of work**. Physical work is praised; it is not dishonourable, but honourable – to the greater glory of God. No wonder that Calvin found many supporters above all among the craftsmen and merchants who were to advance modern capitalism. Whereas the Catholic hierarchy was mostly on the side of the nobility and the established order, Calvinism was more on the side of the economic, political and indeed scientific forces to which the future was to belong. Whereas even Luther rejected Copernicus' new model of the world as contradictory to the Bible, Calvin freed himself from such a literalistic view of the Bible: the real subject of the Bible was salvation and not the world order, and now its message was proclaimed in a language adapted to human beings.

The ethic advocated by Calvin and, after him, by Puritanism, Pietism and Methodism is in some respects almost modern; however, it contains a **twofold danger**: that of either stamping all those who were not so successful in professional and everyday life as 'not the elect' and counting oneself the **class of the elect,** or (as later in the seventeenth century) of abandoning the religious motivation and becoming completely secularized in a purely worldly commitment. In a completely untheological way, faith in the gospel, the awareness of election and the notion of vocation are then turned into **purely secular thought in terms of profit**. So it often happened that Calvin's strict double doctrine of election was later thrown overboard by some Calvinists (thus in Holland by Jakob Arminius and his numerous following). But what does that count against the historical fact that it was in particular the lands under Calvinistic influence like Holland, England and France (and not, for example, the land of Luther, where Calvinism could establish itself only in the Palatinate and on the lower Rhine) which during the next century were to turn into the most highly developed civilized countries? In North America, riches and prosperity were later to be seen as a sign of divine election. At all events, the economic and social differences between northern and southern Europe, Northern Ireland and the Republic, North and South America, are also connected with religious differences. In these contexts, while Calvinism certainly did not mean a specific business ethic, it did mean a basic ethical view with a theological foundation which also succeeded in governing economic life persistently, and which between the sixteenth and eighteenth centuries was to spread in 'ascetical Protestantism'. All this is very important not only for theology but also for the history of ideas.

Church Orders
P II / P III

Fellowship (communio, koinonia) of the churches
(1st millennium)

Roman Catholic papal church (from the 11th century)

Church Orders
P IV

Local ruler
(Magistrate)

Superintendents

Pastors

People

Lutheran state churches (from the 16th century)

General synod

Provincial synod

Pastors, teachers, elders, deacons
(Consistory)

People

Reformed congregational churches (from the 16th century)

Presbyterian-synodical church order and democracy

Even before Max Weber, the Heidelberg legal scholar Georg Jellinek in a similarly pioneering article had derived civil and human rights from religious roots and referred to the 'Bills of Rights' of individual North American states; here, too, special importance must be attached to Calvinism.[95] But it is not easy to distinguish between motives and conditions outside the churches and those within them. Certainly from the beginning Calvin concentrated on a largely independent community order. Whereas Luther had left the organization of the community to the rulers, Calvin, very soon the leader of the non-Lutheran Protestant churches, took the utmost trouble to imitate the biblical community order.[96] For the city community and the surrounding villages (which for him was the 'visible church') he took over from the Strasbourg Reformer Martin Bucer a **four-office order** with a presbyterian stamp:

– pastors (for preaching and the administration of the sacraments);
– doctors (for instructing the youth and theological training);
– elders (for community discipline);
– deacons (for the care of the poor).

Pastors (preachers) and doctors (teachers) form the '*vénérable compagnie*'. Strict church discipline is to prevail, supervised by the 'consistory', made up of pastors and elders (laity). These are to control both the moral life of the citizens and the doctrine of the preachers, are to have unhindered access to all houses, and can also impose harsh penalties with the help of the council – for example for adultery and prostitution or for cursing and mockery: admonition of sinners, exclusion from the eucharist, if need be delivering over to secular justice (with imprisonment, exile and execution). Calvin maintains the distinction between clergy and laity, 'ministers' and 'people'. However, the fact that elders (presbyters, *anciens*) shared oversight of the community with the pastors and with them formed the consistory gave **lay people** in the communities a completely new significance. With an appeal to the early church (the Acts of the Apostles!), this order formed the starting point for a completely new church structure: the '**presbyterian system**'. This did not exclude a president, moderator, 'bishop' at the head of the synodical body at a local or regional level, as long as he did not claim a 'primacy' or a '*dominium*', but rather remained a member of the college.[97]

Thousands of refugees, especially from France and England, where the Protestants were being persecuted, now streamed to Geneva. But there was **no question of religious freedom** even in Geneva. That would have required precisely what Calvin wanted to prevent in all circumstances, a separation of state, society and religion. By contrast, in Calvin's city a marked compulsion in dogma and thus of conscience prevailed. In 1553 the anti-trinitarian **Michael Servetus** appeared in Geneva (in his writings he had called the Trinity a monster with three heads and emphasized the unity of God), beyond question a controversial figure everywhere. In Catholic Vienne the physician and theologian had already been condemned to death at the stake (not without incriminating material sent by Calvin to the Inquisition), but at the last minute he managed to flee to Protestant Geneva. To no avail. In Geneva, too, Servetus was put on trial: he ended at the stake as a 'blasphemer'. And Calvin? He had pleaded 'only' for beheading. Other Reformed Swiss churches, and even Melanchthon in Wittenberg, were in agreement with the death sentence. Were Reformers whose sole concern was the gospel in agreement over burning a heretic, heretics generally?

Even if it was then seen as the task of the state to establish and maintain the true religion, we cannot help noting that **even in Reformed Geneva** there was still **inquisition, torture and death by fire**, as previously under the rule of Rome; there were terrible burnings of witches – despite the abhorrence of many contemporaries who were against the killing of heretics. All this has been a heavy burden on the memory of the Geneva Reformer – who cannot be excused any more than the Roman Catholic Inquisition 'in terms of his time' – even if his influence was certainly often more practical than legal. For the lawyer Calvin with his special interest in church order and church law all too easily succumbed to the danger of identifying his view of community order with God's order.

Toleration? What Protestants had wrung out of the Pope they did not even extend to their own 'protestants', dissidents, deviants. So was the age of toleration still to come? Indeed: modernity in the real sense (P V) would come only after the Geneva Reformation (P IV).

And yet, we may not overlook the fact that just as the Calvinist doctrine of predestination was indirectly important for the development of modern capitalism, so the Calvinistic **church order** which combined with the presbyterian community order to form a synodical church order was **indirectly** of great significance for the development of modern **democracy** – especially later in North America. Calvin himself was far from being a born democrat, nor would he have wanted such a development. He felt himself far too much to be an authoritative messenger of God, and he was far too much a moral and intellectual authority superior to all his contemporaries. He sharply rejected the 'rule of the mob' and preferred a mixed (aristocratic, possibly even monarchical) constitution with the controlled and qualified participation of the people.

However, whereas Lutheranism involuntarily furthered the early absolutism of the state, the presbyterian and synodical church order created by Calvin furthered something else: the formation of an independent and self-governing **community** and then society, which **withdrew from the absolutist ruler and state**. And this was to prove significant for the future. It applied particularly where Calvinism was in the minority and survived with amazing power despite oppression. Certainly it powerfully revived the **right to resist** (which was already mediaeval), and in some circumstances even claimed the right to violent revolution: in France and Holland, England and Scotland.

Individual attributions are always difficult. But on the whole hierarchical centralistic Catholicism (and also the Lutheran churches of the rulers) may be said to show a closer affinity to political and social systems of a hierarchical and patriarchal character, whereas presbyterian-synodical Calvinism was closer to more corporate-federal systems. The presbyterian-synodical church order could be promoted as an institution required by God – as it was later in North America, against the English state church – and thus in the long term form a political order in these countries which could survive even the secularization of the states and continue to have an influence in the form of representative political democracy. Here the early Calvinistic settlers in America (like the Calvinistic Boers in South Africa later) saw their history in parallel to the ancient people of Israel: America as the promised land and the Americans as the people of the covenant newly elected by God, confirmed by successes and victories. 'God's own country', praised in national hymns like 'America' or 'America the beautiful'.

Protestantism as a world force

On 27 May 1564 Jean Calvin – after immense efforts as a preacher, professor, writer and statesman, and physically exhausted through severe illness – died in Geneva. Such a large number of people paid their last respects to his body as it lay in state that in order to avoid the veneration of a new saint it was buried the very next day, a Sunday, in the general cemetery without a tombstone – just as Calvin himself would have wanted. In any case, by his achievements he had written himself into the memory not only of Geneva but of Christianity generally.

Truly nothing should detract from Martin Luther's fundamental significance for the Reformation – its basic impulse, its programme, its new paradigm generally. But it was beyond question Calvin, this French-Swiss Reformer now famed throughout Europe, who through his deeply rooted piety, his inexorable logic, his iron will, his transparently clear and comprehensive theological synthesis, his sense of church order, organization and the international breadth of the church made **Protestantism a world power** – in complete contrast to the Wittenberg Reformer, who remained a provincial German. What Protestantism could preserve or gain outside Germany and Scandinavia it owes to Calvin. But can this recognition be an excuse for the petty-mindedness of Geneva in our century, which led it to put the figure of Calvin in the middle of the great memorial to the Geneva Reformer but simply to leave out the figure of Luther, for whose epoch-making historical achievement Calvin in particular found great words of praise? There would have been no Calvin without Luther!

Indeed – an external sign of the paradigm shift which had taken place – how the **map of Europe**, which had formerly been so uniformly **Roman Catholic (P III), was changed by Luther and Calvin (P IV)**! Now there were broad areas, from the British Isles to Siebenbürgen, from Switzerland to Scandinavia, where the Pope no longer had a say. And if any of the Reformers never **thought** in a nationalistic but in a **European** way (and at least in that respect 'papally'), it was Calvin. The city of Geneva, with its favourable geopolitical position between Switzerland, France and the Savoy, and at that time already with an international horizon because of the often economically powerful Huguenot and English refugees, was for him Europe's secret capital. From here Calvin could exercise influence as an adviser, theologian and church leader from France to Poland and Hungary. And indeed Calvin was a man who had been able to create an **international church network**. How? – through **friends and pupils** loyal to him in every possible country but especially in France, where the name 'Lutheran' was now displaced by 'Huguenot' (presumably a distortion of 'Iguenot' = 'Eidgenosse' = 'Confederate') and where Protestant communities had formed on the model of Geneva, and also in England (Archbishop Cranmer, Somerset, King Edward VI) and in Scotland (John Knox):

– by an amazingly wide international **correspondence** with theologians and churches, magistrates and individual church members throughout Europe (eleven volumes in the Corpus Reformatorum);

– by the theological **academy** founded in 1559 for training preachers for Western and Eastern Europe (not only Calvin but also his successor Theodore Beza taught there), later to become the University of Geneva;

– by **sending books** (the foundation of publishing houses in Geneva) and providing **pastors**, above all in his beloved France;

– by unresting **academic activity** (commentaries on almost all the books of the Old and New Testaments, theological treatises and polemical writing);

– by drafting basic documents like the *Catéchisme* of the church of

Geneva (1542), the *Confession de foi* (1559) and the *Discipline ecclés-iastique* for the first French national synod of the Calvinist communities in France in 1559.[98]

Only with the German Lutherans was there no union, but rather a renewed great **dispute over the eucharist**.[99] Indeed, tragically enough, the understanding of this meal of fellowship had already divided Luther and Zwingli (and the Lutherans refused a shared eucharist as late as 1929 at the quatercentenary of this religious dialogue in Marburg). But now while the new dispute united Zurich and Geneva, at the same time it split Geneva and Wittenberg. Whereas Luther had interpreted the presence of Christ in the eucharist as 'real' (even bodily), and Zwingli had interpreted it as 'metaphorical' (only spiritual), Calvin wanted to take the interests of both sides seriously and understand the presence as 'spiritual' (through the Holy Spirit): it was thus a 'real presence', but only for believers during the eating and drinking (*manducatio spiritualis*)! This made possible a consensus between the Reformed churches of Switzerland and the followers of Calvin (*Confessio Helvetica posterior*[100]), but led to a definitive separation between the Calvinist and Lutheran churches. Like Zwingli, Calvin himself had separated the eucharistic liturgy (also celebrated only four times a year) from the liturgy of the word and had left only prayer and psalm-singing alongside the sermon. Organ, altar, candles, crosses, images were removed: in Lutheranism this was felt to be dark, legalistic consistency.

But even Lutherans cannot dispute the fact that, just as Lutheranism had come up against its limits, Calvinism proved to be the great dynamic force of the Reformation movement; it also proved to be the fundamental **catalyst** in the two most serious political conflicts of this period: on the one hand in the **French wars of religion**, where even after the 'bloody wedding of Paris' (St Bartholomew's Eve) the crown policy fluctuated between extermination and toleration of the Huguenots (in 1598 the Edict of Nantes brought tolerance, creating 150 safe cities for the 1.2 million Huguenots), and on the other hand in the **Dutch revolts against Spain** and the decades-long war between Holland and Spain up to the Peace of Westphalia. Calvinism proved everywhere not only to be a Reformed Christianity of often greater vitality than Lutheranism but also a subversive movement, a political force with innovative political ideas.[101] With its spiritual conquest of the world was effortlessly combined an untroubled political involvement.

Moreover, it is no coincidence that in the subsequent period it was in the sphere of Calvinism that outside Europe, too, trends developed which were to give new features to the face of Christianity on this earth. These were different **movements** of what Max Weber called 'ascetic Protestantism', which for all their doctrinal differences (including differences over predestination) are characterized by a strict moral life. In addition to the different Calvinist, Reformed and Presbyterian churches they include:

– **Methodism,** which came into being around the middle of the eighteenth century in the context of the established Church of England and spread widely, above all in North America;

– **Pietism,** which came into being in the context of English and above all Dutch Calvinism (however, Pietism also had its own roots in Lutheranism);

– the **Baptist** movement, which although originally repudiated by Calvin, from the late seventeenth century was active in England and France and later in America, in close connection with Calvinism;

– **Puritanism,** from the seventeenth century a collective name for various 'pure' movements, i.e. movements of an ascetic character, in Holland, England and then in America (Congregationalists, Mennonites, Quakers and others).

The quest for the lost unity

More importance is attached today than formerly to the fact that at least where Protestantism was concerned, Calvin was an **ecumenical spirit,**[102] a teacher of Christianity who for all his tremendous strictness was passionately concerned about the unity of the church: he was the architect of the unity of the Reformed churches in the question of the eucharist in particular. Unity of faith only in some inalienable principles, and pluralism in secondary matters: that was his basic idea. So he worked indefatigably for an agreement over the question of the eucharist, having already assented to the Lutheran Augsburg Confession in 1530. He saw the essentials of the faith preserved in it and could accept several scholastic views. So already in Calvin's time Geneva had become something like an ecumenical centre.

However, even Calvin could not preserve the unity of Protestantism. On the contrary, there was an **increasing splintering** into different trends, churches and communities. And in the face of this splintering which was the result not only of disputes between different persons, local churches and ethnic groups, but also of theological and ecclesiastical fragmentation, now – remembering Calvin's concern for unity – questions arise.

Questions for the Future

• It became increasingly clear in the analysis of the Roman Catholic paradigm (P III) how far Roman centralism and absolutism led the church away from its origin (P I) and from the unity in multiplicity of the early church (P II), and thus prepared for splits in Christianity – between West and East, and now between North and South. However, we must ask: on the other hand, haven't the strong emphasis on the individual believer and his or her conscience and the lack of church ties and authorities extending beyond a region, which soon emerged, for.their part led to a progressive **fragmentation** and ultimately **atomizing** of Protestant Christianity, which for many people also robbed the Reformation paradigm (P IV) of its credibility?

• Reformation criticism was rightly directed against the **sacrifice of the mass**, with which a particularly large number of abuses were associated. But now isn't it the eucharist in particular – the sacrament of remembrance and promise, which the Reformers were particularly concerned to renew in accordance with scripture – that has become the main bone of contention, an issue which cannot be settled? Didn't it become the main factor in the split between the churches of the Reformation, which to the delight of Rome now even started excommunicating one another? Indeed, down to the present day hasn't the eucharistic meal – as we saw, a constant of Christianity – which is celebrated only rarely in the churches of the Reformation, often sunk to being a peripheral phenomemon, an appendix to the liturgy of the word, abandoned altogether in spiritualistic circles? Shouldn't ecumenical concerns concentrate in particular on overcoming differences and renewing the celebration of the eucharist? Instead of all the excommunications, shouldn't there be a living communion between the churches?

So here already, in anticipation, before we turn to yet another basic type of Reformation, it must be pointed out that the leading active figures of the ecumenical movement at the beginning of this century, whose thought was international, came above all from the churches with a Calvinistic orientation. Moreover it is no coincidence that the World Council of Churches was based neither in Rome nor in Wittenberg nor in Canterbury but in Geneva. And its long-serving General Secretary, Honorary President and later freeman of Geneva was the Dutch Reformed churchman Dr Willem Visser't Hooft, one of the very few really epoch- making figures of church history in the twentieth century. He was firmly supported in his efforts for the unity of the churches above all from Canterbury, by that church communion which in the Reformation period had once again gone its own way between Roman Catholicism and the Lutheran-Calvinist Reformation: the churches of the Anglican Communion.

7. The third way: Anglicanism between the extremes

From the time of Gregory the Great, the *Ecclesia Anglicana* – in the Middle Ages a geographical designation for the Catholic Church in Anglia/England – with its two archbishoprics of Canterbury and York had felt bound to Rome. With its monastic culture and learning, in the early Middle Ages it had carried on the important mission among the Germanic tribes on the European continent. With Anselm of Canterbury it had defended the freedom of the church in the English investiture dispute and introduced Scholasticism! But in this church in particular, didn't the protest against the Roman system begin earlier and become louder than on the European continent: than in Bohemia (with Jan Hus) or in Germany (with Martin Luther)?

A break with Rome, but not with the Catholic faith

Already in the fourteenth century an Oxford professor, translator of the Bible and finally itinerant preacher called **John Wyclif** (1328–84) had appeared, to give voice to a protest, first nationalistically motivated but then both religious and founded on the Bible, against the papacy as an institution of the Antichrist, against the hierarchy as contrary to scripture, against the mendicant orders privileged by the Pope, and against unbiblical customs from veneration of the saints and of images to auricular confession and indulgences. Wyclif, with his understanding of the church as the 'community of the predestined', was a 'pre-Reformer' and in many respects a Calvinist before Calvin! To this degree the church legislation introduced in 1532–34 by Henry VIII brought only a breakthrough of the late mediaeval tendency towards the national church, but at the same time it led to the **break between England and Rome.**[103]

It is idle to speculate whether this break could have been avoided. What would have happened had Pope Clement VII dissolved **Henry VIII's** (1509–47) **marriage** with the Spanish Catherine of Aragon (which was uncanonical, only concluded on the basis of a papal dispensation and odious to the king) and assented to his marriage with the court lady Anne Boleyn? Be this as it may, Henry, at one time even destined to be a cleric, had hitherto shown no kind of anti-Roman tendencies. On the contrary, lay theologian as he was, he had made a name for himself as a Catholic apologist with a work on the seven sacraments, against Luther's *The*

Babylonian Captivity of the Church, as a result of which Pope Leo X had bestowed on him the title 'Defender of the Faith' (*Defensor fidei*).

Moreover Pope Clement VII was in a precarious position when Henry's intentions got around. He did not want to damage relations either with the English king or with the powerful Catholic emperor whose aunt Catherine of Aragon was. He manoeuvred so long that the king, whose rule was *de facto* absolutist, fully a 'Renaissance man', lost patience and in an act of violence compelled the English hierarchy to recognize him as **supreme head of the Church of England**. This was in 1531. Two years later, Henry succeeded in dissolving his marriage and marrying Anne Boleyn; in 1534 he was finally recognized as 'Supreme Head on Earth of the Church of England'.

That only three years later Henry sent his second wife, who bore him Princess Elizabeth, to the scaffold for high treason, entered into four further marriages, dissolved all the monasteries and appropriated all monastic property for the crown is important here only in so far as it shows that Henry VIII was interested above all in extending his rule and not in reforming the church. Certainly his 'Reformation' was not just a matter of a divorce, as the Catholic side often presents it. But it was not, as in Protestant Germany, a popular movement either, but initially above all a decision of Parliament, forced through by the king. The need for reform was very much less widespread among the English people than on the European continent: 'The later mediaeval church was not a corrupt and repressive institution whose abuses called for radical reform.'[104]

Moreover Henry VIII's **Anglican state church** was not Protestant in doctrine and constitution after the German model, but remained largely Catholic. Despite some Protestant changes, Henry had no intention of encouraging the efforts of the Reformation. On the contrary, in the 'Bloody Statute' of 1539 he threatened cruel punishment on anyone who spoke out against the validity of the oath of chastity, against private masses, transubstantiation and auricular confession, or against the marriage of priests and the chalice for the laity. So Henry broke with Rome, but not with the Roman Catholic tradition of faith. The main difference between his church and that of the Pope was that the former Roman jurisdiction and authority now lay fully with the king or the Archbishop of Canterbury.[105]

A Reformed Catholicism

This was to change only under Henry's successor Edward VI (1547–53), a weak boy. For now the Archbishop of Canterbury who had been appointed under Henry, **Thomas Cranmer**[106] (already known to us as a correspondent of Calvin's), could implement what no bishop in Germany succeeded in doing: a **Reformation which preserved the episcopal constitution!** This was a reform of doctrine, liturgy and discipline, but without giving up the traditional structures of office.

Here Thomas Cranmer (1489–1556) doubtless played a key theological role. At a very early stage he had been convinced that the papal primacy was contrary to scripture, and he wanted to replace it with the primacy of the king with reference to Romans 13. But unlike the radical Calvin, Cranmer, this spiritual architect of the English Reformation, was not only a bishop but also a mild and cautious scholar. On the basis of his thorough theological training at the University of Cambridge, he was able to transform various ancient liturgies of Christianity into a simple English-language form of worship in such a way that for the first time in centuries the laity could take an active part in the liturgy. This came about through the introduction of the **Book of Common Prayer** (1549) as the official liturgical book, only two years after Henry's death. It brought a considerable simplification and concentration of the liturgy, and until the 1920s remained identical throughout the Anglican communion. Furthermore, Cranmer was also the main author of the 'Forty-Two Articles' (1552), which are a confession of faith with a Protestant doctrine of justification and a Calvinist doctrine of the eucharist. With few changes, both have remained the foundation of Anglican faith to the present day.

However, this Reformation within the church (albeit accompanied by royal financial misappropriations) was soon to be followed by a **Catholic reaction** under Mary Tudor (1553–58), daughter of the marriage of Henry VIII to Catherine of Aragon – known as 'Bloody Mary'. Her marriage to Philip II of Spain gave her sufficient political support to restore papal jurisdiction in England, carry out a fierce policy of re-Catholicization, indeed persecute all opponents, of whom around 300 steadfast Protestants were even executed. Even Archbishop Cranmer ended at the stake, and therefore is still venerated in the Anglican church as a martyr. It is hardly a consolation here to know that Mary's adviser, the important Dominican theologian Bartolomé de Carranza, made Archbishop of Toledo after his return from England, was now accused by the Spanish Inquisition: of Lutheranism, above all because he had defended the reading of the Bible by laity and theology in the vernacular – with the result that he was imprisoned for seventeen years (almost until his death).[107]

The Reformation had in fact split England. At that time many English Protestants had to flee to Holland or to Geneva. So too did the coming Reformer of Scotland, **John Knox**, who from Geneva published his vehement pamphlet *First Blast of the Trumpet against the Monstrous*

Regiment of Women, in which in view of the three reigning queens (in England, Scotland and France) he 'proved' the rule of women to be absolutely contrary to scripture and to nature. Knox, for whom the celebration of a Catholic mass was worse than a cup of poison, could not have suspected that the appearance of his work would coincide with a change of monarch and confession in England. And that it would be a woman who would turn the rudder around once again – in favour of the Reformation.

For in 1558 **Elizabeth I** came to the throne (she reigned until 1603), Mary's half sister, daughter of Henry VIII by his marriage with Anne Boleyn. A year later she restored the independence of the Church of England from Rome, by two acts of Parliament which were later called the 'Elizabethan Settlement'. Whereas after the return of John Knox (1560) Scotland turned radically to Calvinism and introduced a Presbyterian church order, Elizabeth succeeded in winning over all those who wanted a **Reformed Catholicism**. Specifically, this meant a church which was Reformed in liturgy and customs, but remained Catholic in doctrine and practice. The two laws were:

– The Act of Supremacy: the monarch, while not being 'head of the church', became supreme governor *in ecclesiasticis et politicis*; an oath of supremacy was required; the resistance of almost the entire episcopate was broken by the appointment of bishops loyal to the government;

– The Act of Uniformity: the reformed liturgy of Edward VI was restored and the Prayer Book reintroduced, but images, crosses, vestments and church music were retained.

The Forty-Two Articles were also subsequently revised, and above all the Calvinistic eucharistic doctrine was toned down. The **Thirty-Nine Articles** were finally approved by Parliament as the confession of the Church of England and still remain the valid foundation of doctrine. So towards the church Elizabeth pursued a wise, cautious policy, distanced from Rome and also from Lutheranism and Calvinism (only later was there sharper persecution of the suppressed Catholics and the priests who had returned secretly: in the forty-four years of her reign there were 'only' 200 executions). That Pius V finally excommunicated the queen in 1570 on the basis of false information about the successes of rebels and declared that she had forfeited her right to the throne proved both a political and an ecclesiastical mistake which caused the Catholics of England a conflict of loyalties and considerably worsened their external situation. The Elizabethan period is remembered as a heyday of literature, theatre, music and the graphic arts.

So from the beginning, the Church of England understood itself as a Catholic but Reformed church, as a **third, middle way between the**

extremes. This had been demonstrated above all by two important English theologians: Bishop John Jewel, the first to provide a methodical foundation for the Church of England over against the Roman church;[108] and **Richard Hooker**, who, following Cranmer in opposing a narrow Calvinist and biblicistic Puritanism, for the first time gave a systematic account of the *via media* of the Church of England.[109] But there were two groups in the church which were by no means reconciled to the 'Elizabethan settlement'. The one wanted a return to Rome, the other even more radical reform after the model of Geneva. So the die was not yet cast in England.

England's three options: Rome – Geneva – Canterbury

Both opposition groups had their historical opportunities and each used it in its own way. Could they win through? I cannot describe the complex path of English history and politics here; in any case our only concern is to work out what place the Anglican Church occupies in the framework of our paradigm analysis. So a more systematic approach is necessary. I shall analyse briefly the three options which initially were still quite open.

Option 1: Return to Rome. Under James I (1603–25), the son of Mary Stuart, who inclined towards absolutism, and in whose reign William Shakespeare wrote all his plays (not inspired by Reformation ideals), who ruled England and Scotland in a personal union and who again attempted to introduce episcopalianism into the Scottish church with its presbyterian constitution, the Catholics once again sensed a new dawn. But they were disappointed. Out of the bitterness in 1605 came the 'Gunpowder Plot', in which Catholic extremists planned to blow up Parliament and the king, but were thwarted. Thus the Catholics at first missed their historical opportunity. Under the Puritans, however, the suspicion persisted that England would finally be re-Catholicized again. And indeed one more attempt was made at this – but only after the Presbyterian-Puritan revolution, which must now be mentioned.

Option 2: Presbyterian-republican rule along Genevan lines. As a result of a revolution against the absolutism of the Stuarts and the English state church there was a radical reformation of the Church of England on the model of the Presbyterian Church of Scotland (John Knox!).[110] The main instigators were those radicals who for the most part had a Calvinist Presbyterian theology and called themselves **Puritans, Independents or Congregationalists.**[111] They rejected any state church and advocated freedom of religion. The only thing that counted for them was the autonomous congregation (independent of the state). Such congregations have equal rights in principle; there is no difference between clergy and laity in them; leadership is by elders (presbyters) and pastors chosen by the community. Indeed according to the New Testament, all Christians are 'the saints', and in their assembly all may speak as the Spirit inspires them, without prescribed prayers or confessions of faith.

However, this 'Congregationalism', which had already long existed in those circles which fostered an enthusiastic Puritan spirituality, only became a decisive political force when the Civil War General **Oliver Cromwell** (1599–1658)[112] began a revolution against the state and the state church. In 1642 he succeeded in gathering an army made up of Independents, with enthusiastic piety and Puritan discipline. Military successes confirmed his good Calvinist belief in divine election: the Parliamentary army joined him. Cromwell even succeeded in occupying London, seizing the king and 'purging' Parliament by force of those members who were loyal to the crown. This was in 1648, on the 'continent' the year of the Peace of Westphalia! A year later Charles I, son of James I, was executed on the scaffold (150 years before the French Revolution); shortly after that both monarchy and upper house were abolished. England was a republic!

But the 1653 **'Parliament of the Saints'** called by Cromwell and nominated by congregations of Independents, consisted of Independents who spoke and acted out of sheer enthusiasam. It was completely ineffective, so much so that it was finally dissolved personally by Cromwell. For a last time in the history of Europe an attempt had been made to build the whole social system on a purely religious basis and to square the circle: a kind of theocracy on a parliamentary basis, a parliamentary pendant to the church state. It could not work in the long run. And moreover the end of the Protestant republic came very quickly.

Oliver Cromwell had always rejected the royal crown; nevertheless, during his life he ruled monarchically and finally despotically (with constant reference to 'God's will') as 'Lord Protector' of England, Scotland and also Ireland, which was conquered with a fearful massacre that has still not been forgotten there even now. True, Cromwell's foreign policy had a deliberately Protestant orientation: it supported oppressed Protestant minorities (like the Waldensians in the Savoy) and worked in Germany, Holland and Switzerland for an alliance of all Protestant powers. But in the end he died a solitary, dark dictator, surrounded by conspirators, and his son could not preserve his heritage. The confusions following his death led in 1660 to the restoration of the Stuarts, who in 1662 gave the Church of England back its old place. Cromwell's presbyterian republican experiment had not lasted fifteen years. Since then in England the fear of revolution and antipathy to political utopias has been widespread.

The experiences under Cromwell also marked a turning point for the subsidiary enthusiastic and mystical trends of the Reformation: from militant, indeed military, engagement to a return to the self, to inwardness and non-violence. An impressive example of this is the 'Society of Friends', mockingly called 'Quakers' (enthusiastic 'tremblers'), who were brought into being by a simple cobbler named George Fox (1624–80). After a brief enthusiastic and sometimes violent phase, and now themselves persecuted, as those who had been illuminated by an 'inner light' ('Christ in us') they moved entirely towards a philanthropic practical Christianity. They were indifferent to sacraments, liturgy and confessions of faith, did not want professional pastors, and rejected oaths, military service and even laughter. They called for unconditional truthfulness and simplicity of dress and life-style, and in America were even the first to call for the abolition of slavery.

The Puritans were successful above all in England's **American colonies**. As early as 1620 oppressed English Puritans on the 'Mayflower' founded a community of the elect in the bay of Cape Cod, Massachusetts, and there were other commonwealths in Virginia, Connecticut and Pennsylvania. No wonder that of the original thirteen English colonies, finally around 85% were Puritan in spirit.

Option 3. The episcopalian state church. Restored to power in 1660, the Stuarts (Charles II and James II) not only restored the Anglican episcopal church but at the same time began a merciless persecution of the Protestant dissenters in their own land. These were thrown into prison by the thousand. By contrast they treated the Catholics with concealed and then manifest sympathy. The 'Glorious Revolution' took place in 1688 against the renewed danger of a re-Catholicization. Now James' Dutch Protestant son-in-law **William III** of Orange came to the throne. Only now was the Reformation definitively established in England.

The very next year, with the accord of Parliament, William promulgated the **Toleration Act** (1689) which made **freedom of conscience** a law for the first time in European history. However, this did not apply to Catholics and anti-Trinitarians, though it did to all Protestant dissenters. These might still not become Members of Parliament, state or civic officials, nor could they have universities and schools, but at least now they had the right to public worship. Thus from the suppressed opposition parties within the established Church of England there gradually developed **independent denominations alongside the state church, free churches**, which rejected the state church and with freedom of religion called for the autonomy of the 'congregation'. To these

'Congregationalists' – together with the Baptists and later above all the Methodists – the future was to belong in the United States.

How Anglicanism combines two paradigms

More than one hundred and fifty years after Henry VIII, the **Church of England** had finally consolidated itself and found a **basic structure** which also survived over subsequent centuries: not only in England but also in the Episcopalian Church of the United States (a separate organization since 1789!) and finally in the worldwide Anglican Communion, which formed in the non-Christian world in the nineteenth century as a result of the emigration of English men and women to the newly gained colonies and the success of Anglican missionary work (with the help of large missionary societies).

From the beginning, in an original way the Church of England had **integrated elements of the mediaeval Catholic** (P III) and **Reformation Protestant paradigm** (P IV) which now finally showed that Anglicanism was a **third way** between Roman Catholicism and Protestantism. Perhaps the whole of the Catholic Church could have looked like this had not Rome a priori ruled out Luther's concerns. In good English fashion, Anglicanism is a model of the church which is antipathetic to the extremes. These are its main structures:[113]

– **Scripture and at the same time tradition**: Anglicans believe that the Bible contains all that is necessary for salvation.[114] But at the same time they are convinced of the significance of a continuous tradition which despite all the breaks and vicissitudes in church history goes back to the old undivided church of the church fathers, indeed to the church of the New Testament itself. Richard Hooker already laid a thorough foundation for specifically Anglican hermeneutics: the truth of scripture holds wherever it is unambivalent and clear; where it is not, it must be interpreted by church tradition, or a third element, reason, must be brought into play. As for the central point of dispute, the doctrine of justification, the Thirty-Nine Articles are for justification by faith alone, but at the same time stress the importance of works.

– **A traditional liturgical order and at the same time flexible reform**: concentration and simplification in the spirit of the Bible and the early church are the guidelines of the Book of Common Prayer, and this at the same time allows revisions and adaptations. In fidelity to scripture, baptism, the eucharist and prayer stand in the foreground. 'Sacraments' with no basis in the Bible are abandoned or at best preserved as church customs. But in few churches is so much importance attached to the reading of Holy Scripture, both public and private, as it is in the Anglican

Church, and yet at the same time festivity, joyfulness and music are encouraged in the liturgy. In the Protestant spirit there are revised services for Morning and, particularly popular, Evening Prayer ('Evensong') without exaggerated liturgical uniformity.

– **An official episcopal structure of ministry and at the same time generous toleration**: the ordination of priests and the apostolic succession of bishops are maintained. What is important for the Anglican feeling of togetherness throughout the world is loyalty to the Archbishop of Canterbury; he has no real legislative or executive power outside his diocese, but he visibly represents the unity of the whole church in space and time, and to the present day maintains communion with all the Anglican bishops as *primus inter pares*, so that they all are in communion with one another.

At the same time the boundaries of doctrine are drawn wide: clergy have only to assent to the Thirty-Nine Articles, and even then in a general sense. Freedom of religion for dissidents is as much a consequence of this attitude as space for the different trends within the one Anglican Church: High Church (with a Catholic character), Low Church (Protestant biblicistic) and Broad Church (enlightened liberal). These trends continue even today: in the form of Anglo-Catholics (who emphasize the continuity with the mediaeval and early church and the unity in worship and doctrine); Evangelicals (for whom the need for constant renewal is the most important thing, today in a 'Methodistic' individualistic way through the experience of God's grace in Christ and the Spirit); and Liberals (who against all narrowness and dogmatic consolidation argue for openness to modern demands, for biblical criticism and social work). And to the present day the Anglican Church is distinguished by solid theology (significant scholars especially in exegesis, patristics, church history, dogmatics and ethics), but also by a good organization with strong lay representation and extensive educational and social work.

The Anglican Church spread into all parts of the world along with the British empire, particularly in North America, Australia, New Zealand and South Africa. In so doing it normally showed very much more tolerance to the different church communities and groups than the continental European churches. But certainly there are frictions and tensions in the complex Anglican church structure, too, above all between forces which emphasize unity and centrifugal forces, since the Anglican Church has no unchallenged organizational centre from which all important questions are decided. Nor is the Anglican model of the church free from intrinsic problems, which must be addressed in ecumenical openness.

Questions to Anglicanism: a state church – an episcopal church?

Indeed, the history of the Anglican Church itself shows that the middle position between Catholicism and Protestantism has its own problems, which have lasted down to the present. They relate above all to two problem areas: the state church and the episcopal church.

(a) **A state church for ever?** Constitutional perspectives

The problems of the state church, 'the church established by law', already emerged with the great architect of the Anglican Reformation, Archbishop **Thomas Cranmer**: his moderation in Reformation is rightly praised on all sides. But here didn't he show himself all too much to be the pliant instrument of his king? Hardly had he been consecrated archbishop than he dissolved Henry VIII's first marriage and crowned his second wife – three years later dissolving Henry's second marriage and another four years later his third. He was so involved in the personal history of his king that he was the only one thought capable of speaking out to the increasingly unbalanced king about the adultery of his happy-go-lucky twenty-year old fifth wife, who thereupon also lost her life. Cranmer was loyal to his king until the king's death. But precisely when Cranmer justifies his political pliancy with religious motives – obedience to the authorities appointed by God (Rom.13), doesn't his adaptability appear in an even more fatal light, as it can in no way be derived from the theology of Paul and the New Testament generally?

Here we need to remember at the opposite pole a man who is all too often passed over or neglected in the Anglican Church and in literature, but who is now recognized worldwide as one of the greatest Englishmen: Sir **Thomas More**.[115] In the time of Henry VIII he was Speaker of the House of Commons and then Lord Chancellor. Initially he was also a friend of the king's. At the same time, as a learned humanist he was a friend of Erasmus of Rotterdam, who moreover called him an *omnium horarum homo*, a 'Man for All Seasons' (the title of Robert Bolt's play and 1960 film). In other words, he was a man who stood by his convictions not only in fair weather but also in bad, gloomier times. This Thomas More did not adapt, like Cranmer, but was finally sent to the scaffold by Henry for his convictions. And we can see how the case of Thomas More was and is a sore burden on Anglicanism.

Now of course we have to differentiate. Granted, one can accuse Thomas More of an all too uncritical identification with the claim to papal primacy, the questionableness of which Cranmer saw at an early stage. One can attribute his resistance to the king – extremely well-considered, passive and in no way provocative – to the lack of a critical theology of the kind that the theologian Cranmer doubtless worked out for himself in the spirit of the Reformation scripture principle. And yet, can it be denied that Thomas More, unlike Cranmer,

– showed a **freedom of conscience** in the face of the supreme political authority which can only be compared with Luther's fight for freedom of conscience before emperor and Pope?

– strove for the **unity of the church**, a course of action which led him to resign as Lord Chancellor on 16 May 1532, when the Convocation of the Province of Canterbury assured the throne in a document that in future it would never pass laws or even meet without the king's consent?

– was able to mobilize against a despotic head of state a **power of resistance** rooted in the faith which enabled him to maintain a relaxed humour even up to the scaffold?

All this is in sharp contrast to those churchmen who, while they could certainly provide good theological reasons for a different relationship between church and state from the Roman one, without a word of contradiction allowed their supreme political leader (by many people increasingly regarded as a fool or a monster or both) not only to have some of his own wives and old friends but also fifty further 'traitors' and finally members of the Pole family (from which the cardinal Reginald Pole came) and the Courtenay family executed, since because of their royal blood they could have been a danger to the weakened Tudor dynasty. Indeed, in his last defence speech before the court, (his judges included Anne Boleyn's father, brother and uncles!), More gave the unity of the church ('to relieve his conscience') as the chief reason for his dissent. And he died – still humorously master of the situation on the scaffold, addressing the onlookers – 'in faith and for the faith of the Catholic Church, as the loyal servant of the king, but first God's servant'. His death was a shock for all Europe. It is a credit to the English nation that it has recently shown its respect for Sir Thomas More by monuments in the English Parliament and in the Tower.

Shouldn't Thomas More's **resistance to the whims of rulers and the state** be taken seriously, if not as a constitutive element, at least as a corrective within the framework of the Anglican Church, if that church is to represent a real third way? Resistance to the Pope certainly, wherever he scorns the cause of the gospel or human rights. But resistance no less to the state, wherever this ignores freedom of conscience and tramples down human rights. Such resistance, it is said, is necessary only by way of exception. But is it offered in the general information that one respects the state authority but does not obey it?

Richard Hooker, the great systematician of the Church of England, attached supreme importance to the unity of church and state. Moreover the church is closely bound up with the life of the English nation. To the present day the ruling monarch formally nominates all bishops and deans; to the present day there can be no alteration to church law or the liturgy without the assent of Parliament and monarch; and today some bishops have a seat in the House of Lords. On the other hand, one could ask, is not a greater distance between church and state necessary if the church is still to be able to fulfil its prophetic mission at all? At any rate the English state contributes nothing to the financing of its church, which since the Middle Ages has had rich foundations and properties. The Church of England is still the church of the English people, though some citizens do not feel it to be. So a total separation of church and state is hardly desired by the majority and would have serious effects for the state church, for state and society: not only for state rituals like the Coronation, but also for the resources of church and state. Nevertheless, even in the view of many Anglicans, instead of such a unity of state and church a greater (not hostile) distancing and thus some disentangling would be the better long-term solution.

(b) Only episcopal churches? Ecumenical perspectives

The acceptance of the **Old and New Testaments** as the rule of faith, the Nicene and Apostolic **Creeds**, the sacraments of **baptism** and **eucharist** and the historical **episcopate**: these are the four elements which are indispensable for the life of the Anglican Church and which also have to be the basis for all efforts at unity between the Anglican Communion and other churches. So this, very much in line with the Anglican tradition, was accepted first in Chicago in 1886 and then with slight changes by the Lambeth Conference of the Anglican Communion of 1888 as the so-called 'Lambeth Quadrilateral'. But whereas the first three elements are widely accepted, the demand that the episcopate should serve as the basis of the church's constitution has proved the main difficulty for reconciliation with those Protestant churches which have no episcopate. Rightly so?

That the 'Lord Bishops' represented in the House of Lords clearly belonged to the upper classes followed automatically from the very constitution of the Church of England, but also formed the social background to the rise of the most important opposition movement in England in the eighteenth century, **Methodism**.[116] This, too, was at first a nickname (because of its very methodical life and doctrine). A 'strange warming' when studying Luther's Preface to the Letter to the Romans led the Anglican minister **John Wesley**[117] to address his preaching, first in church and then in the open air, to the outcasts and the downtrodden.

Together first with George Whitefield and then above all with his brother Charles, the famous composer of hymns, he formed a 'Society' within the framework of the Church of England. This consisted of just a few priests, but many lay people and lay preachers, who in a time of economic depression helped the poor to survive spiritually and socially by preaching about the Holy Spirit who strengthens faith and gives certitude, and by a changed, well-ordered 'methodical' life stemming from that.

John Wesley saw his movement as a group within the Church of England under Anglican bishops; only in America, for want of Anglican bishops, as an emergency did he ordain two bishops for the Methodists, appealing to early Christian practice. After Wesley's death, the tensions with the Church of England became so strong that there was a **separation**. The well-placed bishops in England no more joined the new Reformation movement than those in Germany joined Luther's Reformation movement earlier. Moreover while the Methodist revival movement was strictly organized by a central authority with an effective local organization, in England, unlike America, it did not have an episcopal constitution: where bishops were appointed, of course they were not in the 'apostolic succession'.[118] Nevertheless Methodism spread rapidly, above all in North America, where the Methodists also preached on the new frontier, in the Wild West, in the open air. What had never occurred to a leading episcopalian priest or bishop thus became a hallmark of the Methodist Church. And this proximity to the people was at the same time a brilliant 'investment' in the future. For already in the middle of the nineteenth century Methodism in America was the largest individual church of all the Christian churches.

Today Methodists share with Anglicans high esteem not only for the Bible but also for the Christian tradition, yet without insisting on doctrinal conformity or being interested in theological speculation. So what today is in the way of the **reunion** of the Anglican and Methodist churches, which both have so intensively **striven for**? The partial lack of the episcopate or the lack of apostolic succession should not be a hindrance for them if, in keeping with the self-understanding of both churches, New Testament church order is taken as a criterion. As we saw, this recognizes ordination by the community or the free emergence of a charisma alongside ordination of ministers by the laying on of hands. If we accept these two basic models, the Anglican episcopal church would not be expected, say, to abandon the episcopate and apostolic succession for itself, which beyond question is an important theological sign of the continuity of the church down the ages, and for the preservation of which there is also much to be said in practice. The Anglican Church would only be expected – in good biblical fashion – to recognize forms of church ministry as theologically legitimate and canonically valid. In this way the Anglican Communion could strengthen its now already very important mediating position and its contribution towards unity in the World Council of Churches. But this is only one side of the problem.

The opportunities for Anglicanism: questions to Catholics

There is no mistaking the fact that the Anglican Church with its teaching and practice has always represented a **challenge for the Catholic Church,** as it persists in the mediaeval paradigm and attempts to ignore the justified concerns of the Reformation. This fact, too, must be addressed in ecumenical openness. For even now the Roman system is preventing the resolution of questions here and thus is increasingly causing constant irritations, tensions leading to polarization, and indeed a concealed schism between a 'church from above' ('Rome') and a 'church from below' ('the base churches'). The Anglican tradition poses the following questions to the Roman system.

– Why shouldn't it be possible for Roman Catholic dioceses, too, to make an independent **election of their own bishops** through representative organs of the clergy and laity (as happens above all in the American episcopalian churches)?

– Why shouldn't the **confirmation** of the election of a bishop by the national conference of bishops be sufficient?

– Why shouldn't it be possible for the national or regional church to be responsible for up-to-date **teaching** and religious **education** ('catechism')?

– Why shouldn't it be permissible for the **liturgy** to be developed and transformed to meet the manifest needs of a particular country?

– Why shouldn't any national church be able to define its own **discipline** in tune with local circumstances and social conditions, so that – if for the moment a world-wide consensus cannot be achieved – for example the 'women's question' (above all, ordination) could be resolved in one country earlier than elsewhere: after thorough work on theological clarification and proper consultation, and in orderly decision-making processes?

– Why shouldn't a church be able to have eucharistic communion in its country if it regards the differences as settled?

In all these points the Anglican Communion could be a model for the Roman Catholic Church. Of course unity can be endangered by greater freedoms, and it will be necessary to be careful (as is also the Anglican tradition) to see that precious elements of the tradition are not given away lightly in times of accelerated social change. Here Anglicanism is also a

warning to an individualistic Protestantism, which is more exposed to the danger of enthusiasm than other Christian traditions and which has experienced the chaos, indeed the pious terror, of 'Puritan' groups (as with Cromwell and what came after him). The **history of the Anglican Communion in particular can show Catholics,**
– that despite its loose structures the 'Anglican Communion' displays much greater cohesion than other Protestant confessional families which have founded confessional 'world federations' or 'alliances' (Lutheran, Reformed) only in modern times;
– that flexible structures and more consultative, advisory organs have many advantages over a centralistic curial system;
– that even new confessions of faith (going beyond the Thirty-Nine Articles or replacing them) need not break up church communion, but rather are the expression of a living plurality of faith which is legitimated by the Bible;
– that while liturgical revisions lead to a multiplicity of liturgical forms, this does not make common worship and a feeling of solidarity with other members of the church communion impossible;
– that separate regional or national initiatives in disputed areas like the ordination of women are often the only possible way of getting things moving and in time arriving at a new consensus;
– that entering into communion with other churches in a country need not disturb or indeed destroy relations with one's own church in other countries.[119]

Granted, in some details we can note many deviations from the Anglican ideal. But there is no mistaking the fact that over the centuries this complex and relatively well-balanced church structure has largely proved itself, even in one of the most controversial of questions, the ordination of women. For despite great difficulties, in 1994 the Church of England finally came to a positive decision on this question and even took in its stride the departure of a tiny conservative part of its clergy into the Roman Catholic Church, including the former Bishop of London, Dr Graham Leonard. That on 23 April 1994 Dr Leonard could be ordained a Catholic priest *'sub conditione'* ('on condition that he had not previously received valid ordination') makes it clear that even according to the Roman Catholic view the invalidity of Anglican orders which has been asserted for so long can no longer be presupposed automatically. Conversely, the Apostolic Letter of John Paul II *Ordinatio sacerdotalis* of 22 May 1994, prompted by the courageous Anglican step, which in quasi-infallible manner seeks 'definitively' to exclude women from the priesthood for all time, provoked an even greater avalanche of protest and renewed discussion within Catholicism.

But we cannot concern ourselves further here with the basic questions which have been raised. Within the framework of our paradigm analysis we have to ask what the Reformation paradigm shift achieved for women in church and society, in order to understand what a long process was involved in arriving at a constructive solution, even in the Anglo-Saxon sphere.

8. The hybrid position of women in the course of the Reformation

With the religious peace of Augsburg between Lutheran and Catholic territorial rulers in 1555 (the Council of Trent also ended in 1563), the real period of the Reformation was over and for Protestants the age of orthodoxy had dawned. The powerful impulses of the Reformation (P IV) and the defensive reaction of Catholicism (P III) had begun to neutralize each other, and at the same time this led to an internal stabilization. The local rulers could now determine the religion of their subjects. There was no new epoch-making paradigm change; just a further development of the paradigm that had come down. Now the orthodox Protestant paradigm – whether of Lutheran or Calvinist Reformed origin – had the same relationship to that of the Reformation as the Counter-Reformation Roman Catholic paradigm had to that of the Middle Ages. Generally speaking, it now remained a **paradigm of conservation**. Symptoms of this can be seen in the question of the status of women in the church and society.

The changed situation of women

Martin Luther wanted a return to the gospel. Did this also have consequences for the status and role of women in the church and society? Did the equality of man and woman in God's sight asserted in the apostle Paul's Letter to the Galatians (3.28) really exist? In other words, was the true equality of women with men in the spirit of the New Testament, which was already hindered in the early church (P II), as we saw, finally achieved under the auspices of the Reformation? Given all the differences of country, status, education, orientation of faith and personal circumstances of individual women, an answer to this question in the framework of our paradigm analysis will inevitably be very basic.

First of all it has to be recognized that the position of women, not only in the church but also in society, was changed by the paradigm shift which began with the Reformation. For what characterized the **new constella-**

tion (P IV) in which women now had to live in the territories of the
Reformation? If we bear in mind the earlier account of women in the
Roman Catholic mediaeval paradigm (P III) we can immediately under-
stand how epoch-making the changes were:

- The mediaeval priority of celibacy was now replaced by the **revaluation of marriage**, the primacy of priestly ordination by that of everyday family life, the ideal of the nun by that of the housewife and
mother, the vilification of sexuality by its affirmation as a natural
human drive (to be satisfied in marriage, even if it did not serve to
produce children).
- The monastic life was abolished along with the prohibition of marriage for priests: **being married to a pastor** opened up a completely
new field of activity for a woman in a particular community (Luther's
wife Catherine is an example).
- The cult of Mary, which idealized the virgin mother Mary at the
expense of other dimensions of the feminine, retreated in favour of a
secular ideal of women – which had already been taking shape since
the lay culture (Minnesingers) of the twelfth century and the Renaissance.

In other words, **the world governed by priests, monks, nuns and their
ideal of continence collapsed** – and did so definitively; exceptions today
prove the rule. This is only one example which tells against the foolish
view that history is stationary, that everything will return and that any
development can easily be reversed. Nor is there any overlooking the
social psychological change in the community structure: now that
pastors were married, the customary conscious or unconscious interest
of the female part of the community in the one unmarried 'clergyman'
(pastor or monk) disappeared, as did the often conscious or unconscious
distancing of the male part of the community.

It was one of the numerous merits of **Martin Luther** that in his
theology he saw **humanity in its physical nature and sexuality** more
clearly than his predecessors; for Luther the fellowship of husband and
wife and the relationship of wife to husband and children are a basic fact
of human existence. The Protestant theologian Gerta Scharffenorth
describes Luther's position like this:

– 'Man and woman as God's creatures are together created in the image
of God; bodiliness and sexuality are not at their disposal; they are God's
gift and are to be respected as such.'[120]

– A 'shared responsibility of man and woman' follows from the task
given by God at creation: 'for creation, for the coherence of all spheres
of life and for humane living conditions for the coming generation'.[121]

They perform this task predominantly in the state of fatherhood and motherhood, which is prior to and superior to all other spiritual and worldly states.

– By baptism, women and men are destined 'to become friends in Christ'.[122] As Luther put it: 'Since all baptized women are spiritual sisters of all baptized men, as they have the same sacrament, spirit, faith, spiritual gifts and possessions, they will be much closer friends in the spirit than through outward kinship.'[123]

So there is no doubt that Martin Luther also made a practical contribution to **the revaluation of women**, above all through his plea for the education and schooling of girls as well as boys – though this had been put previously and much more clearly by Thomas More and Erasmus: as in the latter's memorandum on schools of 1524.[124] At the same time there is evidence that women also collaborated independently in the development, dissemination and defence of Protestant doctrine and the building up of Protestant communities (Margarete Blaurer in community work, Argula von Grunbach in publicity, Elisabeth Kreuziger in writing hymns, and so on).[125] As we saw,[126] individual women had already played a leading role in the high and late Middle Ages above all as rulers (especially as widows) and abbesses. To this degree the role of Elizabeth I of England and some other women regents and nobility was not new. And yet – unfortunately all this is only half the truth.

The social structure – still patriarchal

The indisputable progress must not mislead us: in the Reformation paradigm too, **the social structure remained utterly patriarchal**.[127] Of Luther's important thoughts about the brotherliness and sisterliness, the friendship, of men and women in Christ, all that was in fact left was the duty to marry. Despite all the new possibilities of activity for women, nothing changed in their role of being subordinate to men. The hierarchical structure of obedience (man-woman, parents-children, master-servants) was preserved. Marriages were still arranged by parents. The wife remained economically, legally and politically dependent on her husband, and the choice of her spouse was usually made for practical reasons. In any case, the constant surplus of women did not make things easier for them. And though since the late Middle Ages they had had a share in civic freedoms and greater possibilities of vocational fulfilment in crafts, trade and business (and also as women doctors), they by no means yet had the same rights or the same rewards.

Moreover it was not just in society that the gender-specific division of work and the stereotyping of the role of the sexes was maintained, to the disadvantage of the woman. Within the Reformation churches, too (Zinzendorf in Pietism was the great exception), women by no means had the same share in 'sacrament, spiritual gifts and possessions'. Women still had no **say in state, education and the church**. On the contrary, under the sway of seventeenth-century Protestant orthodoxy, because of the wars, the economic recession and the increased competition for work outside the home, they were once again limited to the narrow household sphere. To what extent?

– Women continued to be excluded from all important church offices; they were accepted only as catechists and church servants.

– Not only the administration of the sacraments by women, but also preaching by women, which was practised in sects in the Middle Ages and called for by some humanist scholars, was normally forbidden.

– Space for unmarried women who had formally lived a safe, meaningful existence in convents had now disappeared, along with possibilities for educational activity, and thus unmarried women lost this basis for an independent life.

– At the same time, however, women's self-esteem was strengthened by religious instruction and the familiarity with scripture which had become possible.

As the American historian Jane Dempsey Douglass of Princeton has emphasized in an instructive study, in principle all this also applies to the sphere of **Calvinism**.[128] Calvin, too, continued the patristic mediaeval tradition. For him, too, the spiritual equality of women with men (on the basis of the same spiritual soul, the same grace in this life and the same consummation through the resurrection) went with the social inequality of women and their subjection to men. To this degree, even with Calvin Christianity by no means brought emancipation in the modern sense of the world.

And yet we should also see that unlike Augustine and Thomas Aquinas, Calvin (following the most famous physician of antiquity, Galen) rejected the Aristotelian view that the **woman plays no active biological role** in the formation of a foetus. Although even in the sixteenth century there was still widespread doubt about the physical robustness and intellectual power of women, slowly a consensus formed against Aristotle, that a woman was more than a 'defective man'. At any rate, Calvin no longer arugued in terms of physical nature when he spoke out against the ordination of women. Differently again from Thomas Aquinas, who denied women a natural capacity for the priesthood and in the light of biology and the divine law argued against women holding public office in the church, Calvin appealed 'only' to the human, church or state legal order. While this still had the same result as far as women were concerned (and to this degree Calvin is no champion of the ordination of women), it did have the decisive advantage that the possibility of changing this human ordinance could no longer be disputed with biological arguments, at least in principle. Moreover it was then adapted later to changed times.

Emancipation in the 'sects'

How different the role of the woman could be, depending on her country, confession and historical situation, becomes evident as soon as one looks at more specific research. This is attested by individual studies of 'Women in Protestant History' (Anabaptists, Quakers and Methodists!).[129] The Australian historian Patricia Crawford has also demonstrated it for **England** between 1500 and 1720 in connection with women and religion.[130] Her investigation is illuminating not least because she discusses in context individual women already investigated in earlier research, who played an important role in connection with the English Reformation – like Henry VII's second wife **Anne Boleyn**, who as guardian of bishops with a Protestant inclination, clergy welcoming reform and Protestant writers, along with other ladies was a key figure among the Reformers around the king and possibly advised him to dissolve the monasteries. And on the other side there was **Margaret Roper**, the married daughter of Thomas More, a highly educated woman who translated religious works from Greek and Latin[131] and thus also came to publish Erasmus' Latin Commentary on the Our Father. And finally there was the controversial young **Elizabeth Barton**, a nun with prophetic gifts, who is to be seen against the background of the long tradition of women to whom visions were granted.[132] She headed the opposition to Henry VIII's second marriage, was executed without a trial in 1534, and thus was the first woman martyr for the traditional faith. Nuns generally fared much worse than monks when their convents were dissolved; because monks were ordained, they could earn a living as diocesan clergy. Women like the Protestant Countesses of Suffolk and Richmond also played a major role under Edward VI, not to mention the two queens who followed later, **the Catholic Mary** who called for the dismissal of all bishops' and priests' wives, and **Elizabeth I**, who restored the independence of the Church of England from Rome.

But here, too, the other side of the coin must be considered. The classical exponent of Anglican theology, Richard Hooker, still held the customary view that women had a weaker capacity for judgment by virtue of their sex. Indeed in Anglicanism the age-old theme of the special proneness of women to heresy still persisted. Women who attempted to challenge male power could at any time be accused of violating the divine order and endangering morals. Granted, women played a special role in particular **in the religious radicalism** of the Presbyterian republican phase between 1640 and 1660, not of course because their capacity for judgment was weakened but on the contrary because with clear judgment they wanted a reformed church, and because more possibilities for activity would be granted them after the collapse of church control. A similar development had taken place a century earlier on the European continent in the Peasants' War and in the Baptist movement.[133] Now one could see and hear women teaching, preaching, celebrating the liturgy and engaging in mission. Many had joined the newer communities, like the Quakers (the most significant of them was Margaret Fell, the 'mother of Quakerism'[134]). And their role differed from that of the sixteenth-century Protestant and Catholic martyrs: 'The conflicts of seventeenth-century women were conflicts with local authorities, pastors, justices of the peace and official judges. They adopted a public role but they were not martyrs, although many of them endured prison, physical punishment and violence for the sake of their faith.'[135]

But this, too, should not lead us to exaggerate the role of women in radical Protestantism. 'It would be anachronistic to suggest that women had found "emancipation" in the sects. It should not surprise us that the customary views of the nature and place of women in the world remained essentially the same during the revolutionary period of the 1640s and 1650s.'[136] Not only did the economic possibilities remain limited, but so did views about the role of women, sexuality and childbearing. 'So the sects did not offer a fundamentally different view of women from that of the Anglican Church or society generally.'[137] Only slowly did 'the churches develop towards accepting women as partners with equal rights', and there was a 'growing readiness to allow them to speak in the churches, which finally in the most recent decades has led to a gradual acceptance of the ordination of women'.[138]

However, on one point England came off better: here too up to the end of the seventeenth century there was a belief in witches; but compared with the European continent (and Scotland) far fewer people were persecuted in England. The question is not unimportant for our paradigm analysis. How is this terrible witch-craze to be explained?

Who was responsible for the witch-craze?

Even now it is not completely clear how this witch-craze is to be explained. In time and space it emerged in bursts, interestingly enough hardly at all in southern Italy and Spain; very little in England, Ireland, Scandinavia, on the north German plain, in Bavaria and also Eastern Europe; but very widely above all in France, Northern Italy, the Alpine countries, the rest of Germany, the Benelux states and Scotland.[139] How indeed are we to explain this mass phenomena, in which 80% to 90% of those affected were women? Certainly Christianity had always had it in for witches; and the statement in the Hebrew Bible, 'You shall not allow a sorceress to live' (Ex.22.18), had been the death of many witches. But 'witch' means substantially more than sorceress, and the trial of a witch substantially more than the trial of someone performing malicious magic (*maleficium*). In the high Middle Ages the notion of people who flew through the air by night was still being combatted as a pagan error.

So the question is, how can we explain the fact that by far the vast majority of Christians from the fifteenth century, and above all in the period of the Reformation and Counter-Reformation, no longer believed in the existence of individual sorceresses but – in a combination of diffent motives – believed in a diabolical conspiracy, a new sect and highly dangerous heretical movement of witches, of malicious, lustful, devilish women who had powers over nature? According to the well-known pattern of interpretation of those who believed in witches, a whole horde of women was said to have

– **made a pact with the Devil**, almost a covenant of marriage with the Devil, abjuring God;
– **consorted with the Devil**, having slept with the Devil (usually often) to seal the pact;
– **conjured up the Devil**, an evil magic damaging the harvest and other aspects of life and killing animals or human beings;
– **danced with the Devil**, engaging in nocturnal orgies (witches' sabbath) with other witches.

The Tübingen exegete Herbert Haag, who has done a great service in combatting the belief in the Devil still rampant today, remarks that 'the church with its doctrine of the Devil' provided the 'theological justification' for the elimination of supposed witches: 'Had the Devil not been built up into an overpowering figure, such an apparatus of extermination could not have been set up, and the wave of purges would not have found this echo in a people tormented by fear of the Devil. But as it was, the stake was the simplest and at the same time the most effective means of coping with the crisis.'[140]

In church history (not to mention dogma), where it is not largely suppressed the witch-craze is often mentioned only in passing and not treated comprehensively. It was rightly brought into the centre of research by the women's movement of the 1970s, as the persecution of

witches generally had fatal consequences for women: a destruction of the
culture and the solidarity which women took for granted, a breakdown in
the handing down of specifically feminine knowledge of women's own
bodies and total submission to patriarchal domination. Once again, is
there a conclusive explanation of all this?

It is not enough to **explain** the witch-craze with reference to the use of
drugs (states of intoxication), the mass consumption of which cannot be
proved; or to mental illness, which similarly does not explain the mass
phenomenon; or even to a suppressed cult of Diana (fertility cult), which
at best can be verified only in particular places or regions. On the other
hand it is beyond dispute that there would have been no trials of witches
without a popular superstition which had a pagan stamp, without
misogyny, the Inquisition and torture. However, there was superstition,
misogyny, Inquisition and torture even before the witch trials, so the
question must be asked: what else? Who was to blame for this
development? A survey of research into witches shows that no
monocausal explanation of the mass trials of witches is possible, and that
the responsibility, as far as we can still see, lies with theologians and the
mendicant orders, with the Pope and the Curia, the emperor and state
power, and finally also with church people. To discuss these briefly:

1. In the face of the great heretical movements of the thirteenth
century, **Scholastic theologians**, especially Thomas Aquinas, developed
an extensive demonology in which, following Augustine, the doctrine of a
pact with the Devil was used as a basis for a theory of superstition.[141]
What had formerly been combatted as pagan superstition was now
incorporated into the theological system. And it was again two
Dominican theologians, the Inquisitors for upper Germany and the
Rhineland, Heinrich Institoris and (at least he put his name to it) Jacob
Sprenger, who first of all overcame the inhibitions against belief in
witches and witch trials that were widespread among the people and
the clergy. They did this with their pernicious handbook on witches, the
Malleus maleficarum (**Hammer of the Witches**).[142] With a forged
endorsement from the theological faculty of Cologne, between 1487 to
1669, in around thirty editions, it had a tremendous circulation and
became the standard work for theologians, lawyers and physicians and
for spiritual and secular courts. In the first part the concept of the witch
was focussed on women with a series of quotations (some of them forged)
from the Bible and classical authors; the second part specified all the
abominations of witches; while the third part provided guidelines for
punishment.

2. **Papacy and Curia**. It was the Popes who, as we saw, from the
thirteenth century institutionalized and intensified the persecution of

heretics and also assumed a connection between heresy and magic, both the work of the Devil. But it was then the Renaissance Pope Innocent VIII who as early as 1484, at the request of the two Dominicans mentioned above, promulgated his notorious **bull against witches**, *Summis desiderantes* (about which Denziger keeps quiet[143]), and thus gave the papal blessing to the novel doctrine of witches. On threat of excommunication the 'beloved sons' were commanded not to hinder the interrogation of them by the Inquisition. And this unfortunate bull was then promptly made a preface to the 1487 **Hammer of the Witches**. So the Pope and Curia played a key part in the origination, legitimation and continuation of the mass trials of witches in Europe. The **papal Inquisition**, no less concerned with the persecution of heretics, provided the **instrument** which was now used against the women: some denunciations, then instead of a public accusation by a private person a secret investigation (*inquisitio*) by the authorities, torture to force a confession, and finally death by fire.

3. **The emperor and the secular authorities.** The legal basis for the mass implementation of witch trials was created by the emperor Charles V's new (Roman) procedural law of 1532 ('*Carolina*'). Now the **Inquisition process was carried out completely by the state.** Here the guidelines for the trials of witches were so vague and varied that in practice almost anyone could be caught up in the inescapable mill of the machinery of the Inquisition. A mere rumour was often enough. But as this was an 'exceptional crime' (*crimen exceptum*), **torture** could also be used, without the restrictions provided for elsewhere by the lawyers. The consequence was that the names of alleged accomplices (known from the witches' dance) were extracted with indescribable torture, and a new spiral of trials was set in motion. The cruellest ordeals for witches (by water and the needle) were also customary. A complete confession usually led to the death penalty, and recantation to renewed torture (sometimes tenfold), of unspeakable human cruelty. For a long time the death penalty was primarily carried out by **burning**; after 1600 usually by **beheading**. This terror lasted decade after decade, and was to reach its climax only after the first wars of religion between 1560 and 1630.

4. **Church people themselves.** As the majority of victims came from the lower classes in the country (the nobility were exceptions), it is assumed that some **denunciations** came from the communities themselves. Simple village gossip, a person who looked abnormal or behaved abnormally, hatred, envy, enmity or avarice could be the beginning of 'petitions' to the authorities for protection from witches which then set the whole machinery in motion. However, the background to

this is the **archaic anxiety** about magical knowledge and practices which was so widespread among the people. This leads us to ask:

Why the witch-craze?

Today, little can be said in detail with any precision about the ultimate **psychological and political motives** for the persecution of witches. Scholars mention a whole series of motives:
– reactions to the bitterness and cursing of individual women from the peasantry;
– patriarchal anxieties about solitary women and their often quite real knowledge of medicine and contraception;
– the hostile attitude of the trained doctors (who first appeared with the universities), as opposed to popular medicine and the midwives and healers with no professional training who had been available to the people all down the centuries, with their often well-tried and traditional 'secret knowledge' (especially about giving birth, birth control and healings of all kinds);
– women as scapegoats for impotence and barrenness, for the failure of harvests, disease among cattle and catastrophe, sickness and death;
– a general xenophobia replacing hostility to the Jews (which after all the expulsions largely lacked any focus);
– the sexual obsessions and fantasies of celibate church inquisitors who showed interest in the alleged perversions, obscenities and orgies (even with demons) of women with an insatiable lust, vilifying the witches as followers of Satan, so that they became a dark feminine principle (this was compensated for on the other side by the idealization of women in Mary – above the senses, pure and conceived without a stain);
– the reaction of the church hierarchy and the absolutist authorities to an underground, uncontrollable popular culture;
– the confessionalizing which was interested in a far-reaching disciplining of the thought and behaviour of subjects.

For a long time the trials of witches were the subject of confessional apologetics and polemics: each side attempted to accuse the other of having the more black marks on its record. This was a vain enterprise, given the fact that **belief in demons and witches was largely common to both Catholics and Protestants.** Even if the *Hammer of the Witches* was increasingly attacked in detail, the regrettable fact has to be noted that not only within the mediaeval paradigm (P II) but also within the new Reformation paradigm (P IV) no one thought of examining belief in demons and witches critically, as one might have expected with the new orientations on the gospel. If the Catholic side was burdened by the long tradition of the persecution of heretics and witches, the Protestant side was burdened by the lack of any outrage against this inhuman and un-Christian craze.

If present-day scholarship, while no longer thinking in terms of millions of victims, at any rate reckons that there were at least 100,000 executions (and further punishments like banishment and open contempt); if, at any rate, it is clear 'that with the exception of the persecutions of the Jews these trials led to the **greatest mass killing of human beings by other human beings in Europe which were not the result of war**',[144] and if it is clear that despite all the denunciation of women by women this was a 'mass killing of women **by men**',[145] since men served as specialists, theologians and lawyers, as judges and executioners, we have to ask why at least from the Protestant side there was no vigorous protest against the witch-craze and the trials and burnings of witches – in the name of the freedom of Christians and the urgings of conscience.

It was above all the brave Jesuit and confessor to the witches, **Friedrich von Spee**, who in 1631 with his anonymously published work *Cautio criminalis* or *Legal Objections to the Witch Trials*[146] attacked all these goings on, though with little success. At the beginning of the seventeenth century, in the course of the Enlightenment, it was the Protestant lawyer **Christian Thomasius** who attacked the idea of pacts with the Devil and the whole business of judgments on witches. Now he already found much support from the public. Whereas the mass trials in the United Netherlands had ended soon after 1600 and in France in 1650, in the German empire they ended only around 1680. It is commonly thought that the last burning of a witch was that of Anna Schwägelin in 1775, in Catholic Kempten, but there were still mass burnings in Brandenburg in 1786. In other words, it was not the Reformation but the Enlightenment which put an end to the witch-craze, and the trials and burnings of witches.

9. The Reformation goes on

After the death of Martin Luther, no one could take his place in Lutheranism; no equally authoritative person emerged as his successor. So who or what was now to settle and resolve disputes? There was all too great a need for such an authority, to prevent the primal evil of Protestantism which threatened from the beginning of the Reformation: the ever-growing split.

The dispute over Protestant orthodoxy

The disputes which after Luther's death were to occupy and burden Lutheranism had in part already broken out during his lifetime. Above all there was the **dispute between the 'Philippists' and the 'Gnesio-Lutherans':** between the supporters of Philipp Melanchthon, who on the question of human co-operation with divine grace (synergism), the need for good works and the spiritual character of the eucharist advocated views which deviated from Luther and were closer to Calvin, and the 'authentic Lutherans', who under Matthias Flacius ('Illyricus') fanatically advocated allegedly 'original Lutheran positions'.

However, just as it would have been of little interest within our framework to go into the **scholastic disputes of Counter-Reformation theology** (P III) over grace and the freedom of the will, so now it would be uninteresting to go into all the scholastic disputes of **Reformation theology** (P IV): the antinomian, adiaphoristic, Osianderan, majoristic, synergistic disputes. There were countless polemical works and statements on themes like original sin and the freedom of the will, justification and good works, law and gospel, the eucharist and the person of Christ, providence and eternal predestination, topics in which questions of theological doctrine were often elevated into questions of church life.[147] Even in Protestantism the dispute did not go on without the intervention of the state authorities: punishments, dismissals, indeed imprisonments. Was this the freedom of a Christian?

Here the '**confession**' was meant to help and offer an authoritative decision on disputed matters, the **Confessio** under whose aegis the different camps of Christianity (after the Council of Trent including the Catholic camp) mustered, usually supported by the state power. The result was **confessionalizing**, which, according to the Tübingen historian Ernst W.Zeeden, who investigated the process of the formation of confessions earlier and more thoroughly than others, in the Reformation and Counter-Reformation largely took **parallel** courses, despite the differences in pace (a confirmation of what was said on P III). Confessionalizing is to be understood as 'the spiritual and organizational consolidation of the Christian confessions, which had moved apart since the split in belief, towards a semi-stable form of the church in terms of dogma, constitution, and religious and moral life'.[148] Consolidation? What was the function of the confession here? It was twofold: **internally** it was 'the sign of **unity**, which even left its stamp on the cult, the constitution and discipline'; **externally**, it was a 'sign of **distinction** from the other partial constructions, against which it dug itself in firmly'.[149] The result was that: 'In the process of the formation of confessions, the rifts in Western Christianity became deeper and harder. By the middle of the seventeenth century the major confessions had finally attained such stability that the way back to the old unity of the church no longer seemed possible.'[150]

So these new forms of being the church were about the state, the church and the people, all at the same time. Certainly the shaping of the population by the confessions was initially often very superficial in all the confessional camps, and not much progress was made with the theological education of the local clergy. However, not only in the Catholic (P III) but also in the Protestant sphere (P IV), **state power** usually gave powerful support to confessionalizing.[151] In the early absolutism, confessionalizing – whether Catholic or Protestant – meant a **social discipline** imposed by church and state (as G.Oestreich has pointed out) reaching into the villages and extending to hitherto quite private spheres, resulting in a uniform 'Christian' behaviour which had not been known by mediaeval Christianity.[152] This meant the training of those subject to it in stricter discipline: alongside the 'standing army' there was the 'sitting army' (the 'officials') and finally, through schools, church and state supervision there was control over the whole people – in fact a preparation for modern purposive rationality. Here, in Protestantism, social discipline in some respects – e.g. over dancing, gambling, the drinking of alcohol, the dedication of churches and carnival – was markedly stricter than in Catholicism. Whereas strategically the Counter-Reformation adapted itself more towards popular piety, Protestantism, led by intellectual pastors who at the same time were state officials, emphasized its distance from popular culture, so that the Reformation increasingly seemed the more rational religion, though it was far more shaped by the state. The result was not only different 'institutionalizations' of the organizations of the confessions, but also different 'forms of life' which shaped everyday existence.

At the same time, on the Protestant side, too, **controversial theology** was concerned to work out sharply the differences between the confessions, supported by a **controversial preaching** which did not hesitate to caricature opposing positions and even make use of lies and fables. Moreover, soon the various confessions had only stereotyped notions of one another. In other words, there was no trace of tolerance and freedom of conscience on either side; rather, here too church and state authority worked together in order to establish their own confession and limit minorities as far as possible.

So on the Protestant side, too, there was now by no means an unprejudiced quest for the living message of the Bible. Rather, as on the Catholic side, the concern was with proof texts (*dicta probantia*) for the 'pure doctrine' of one's own confession – against the doctrine of others, even if these were other Protestant confessions! This was called dogmatics and polemics. Very soon the **confessional writings** on the Lutheran side in particular had swollen to become an enormous volume, no smaller than the Roman Catholic 'Denzinger' (which appeared only in the nineteenth century). The *Book of Concord* contains the three creeds of the early church, the Augsburg Confession and Melanchthon's Apologia, the Schmalkald Articles, Melanchthon's treatise on the authority and primacy of the Pope, Luther's Greater and Lesser Catechisms and finally the 1577 Formula of Concord which, worked out laboriously, over dozens of pages discusses all the above-mentioned themes which are under dispute and is thus intended to end all doctrinal disputes among Lutherans.[153] This was a doctrinal consensus on a line midway between extreme Philippists and radical Gnesio-Lutherans, which 'tenaciously reinforced the **development towards a doctrinal church**'[154] in Lutheranism, made the break with Catholicism and Calvinism final and at the same time concluded the formation of the confession of the Lutheran Reformation.

In 1580 – exactly fifty years after the Augsburg Confession – the whole of the Book of Concord was subscribed to by 86 estates of the empire and around 8000 theologians. However, it was not subscribed to by all. Confessionally, despite every effort the **heartland of the Reformation** itself remained permanently **split**: into areas governed by the Formula of Concord, Lutheran areas outside the Formula of Concord, and directly Calvinistic areas which now, while keeping to Luther, called themselves 'Reformed' (along the lines of Calvin's more consistent Reformation).

Be this as it may, on the European continent in the Protestant sphere, after Luther's death for about a century **orthodoxy** prevailed. In this Protestant theology of the 'right faith' the topics of faith (*loci*) were soon treated in great dogmatic textbooks, in which reference was also made to Bernard, Tauler, some Scholastics, and above all to Augustine, and the radical doctrines of Luther were combined with the mediating doctrines of Melanchthon. The classic work of Lutheran orthodoxy is **Johann Gerhard's** (1582–1637) *Loci theologici* (published in 1610–1622), which distinguishes Lutheranism from Catholicism and Calvinism on every possible exegetical basis and with historical and philosophical arguments – in nine volumes.[155] That was how complex Lutheran faith had now become.

There is no doubt that one can have a critical and constructive discussion with all the orthodox theologians of the Lutheran or Calvinist confessions in treating dogmatic subjects even in our century, as Karl Barth has shown time and again in his monumental *Church*

Dogmatics.[156] But generally speaking, in the translation of the Christian message into a new paradigm all these orthodox dogmatic theologians can at best offer help in orientation and differentiation; moreover in contemporary Protestant theology they usually receive only grudging treatment. At any rate at that time strictly Calvinist orthodoxy (which long prevailed in Holland in particular) attached more importance to a strict life ('precision') and thus avoided the clash with the 'pietistic' piety which was in the making. By contrast, the orthodox Lutherans in their anxiety were less concerned about the 'pious life' than with the **'pure doctrine' set down literally in the Bible**, to the point of the construct of verbal inspiration (e.g. in David Hollaz). Its appointed guardians and exegetes were the preachers and theologians, so that now the Evangelical Church presented itself even more as a **church of pastors and professors** and the local church – dominated by the authorities – as a **church of the land**.

So generally speaking the theological basis of both Lutheran and Reformed orthodoxy was less the message of the Bible, the gospel, Jesus Christ himself, by which according to Luther even everything in the Bible was to be measured, than biblical statements taken literally, relating to quite definite doctrinal points and incorporated into a closed philsophical and theological system in part even with the help of Aristotle and countlesss borrowings from Scholasticism. This was a **biblicism** which in **Germany** replaced the infallibility of the living Roman Pope, claimed at least in Rome, with the *de facto* infallibility of the 'paper Pope', swearing on the inerrancy of a book inspired by God. This biblicism was to see the historical-biblical criticism developing in modernity as the work of the Antichrist.

Confessionalism and traditionalism

As in the earlier paradigms, so with the Reformation paradigm (P IV), I cannot describe the later phases in such detail as the phases of foundation and early formation. Be this as it may, research in this century has shown that even within the framework of Lutheran orthodoxy there was readiness for reform and there were ideas for reform, something like a 'reform orthodoxy', though this is difficult to distinguish from the rest of orthodoxy. But in view of all the many doctrinal documents in Protestantism, too, we may now ask: what in fact had become of the Reformation slogan *sola scriptura*? Was Protestantism really still concerned with scripture alone? Alongside scripture wasn't it, too, rigidly holding firm to its own **Protestant tradition**, young though that was?

In fact the writings of Luther and Calvin soon attained quasi-canonical status and were now expounded at great length in the theological teaching of the universities. Just as the Lutherans had their confessional writings (and the Catholics the catechism of Trent and the Tridentine decrees[157]), so the Reformed had the Geneva and the Heidelberg Catechism and the different Reformed confessions (Confessio Gallicana, Scotica, Belgica, Helvetica posterior, Westminster Confession).[158]

All this means that once its administration, church law, confession and liturgy had been formed, even Protestantism, which originally was so hostile to tradition, was not spared being stuck to its own tradition. The phase of rise, reformation and initiation which I have analysed in detail was followed by a **phase of formation, establishment and consolidation** which I can describe only briefly, **concerned with reassurance, preservation and consolidation.**[159] The nonconformity of the Reformers was followed by the conformity of their descendants. In Protestantism, too – in administration and church law, but above all also in theology – bulwarks were fashioned and built. The theological dispute (*rabies theologorum*) kept on, often degenerating into squabbles over secondary questions: in any case between Catholics and Protestants, but now sometimes even more vigorously between Lutherans and Reformed, Lutherans and Lutherans, Reformed and Reformed.

It was called the age of **confessionalism** – issuing in a thirty-year confessional war or 'war of religion' (1618–1648)! And it was also **an age of hardened confessional paradigms.** The reform movements which were still quite fluid in the first half of the sixteenth century had consolidated into rigid reform camps, which did not want any mixed marriages or student exchanges, although these could never be completely excluded. There was a 'novel political and sociological form of church life': 'particular churches clearly demarcated by doctrine, liturgy and organization, which challenged one another in their claims to be the sole representative of Christian truth'.[160] But little new in terms of theology and the church was produced for a new time; above all, the old was renovated. Moreover, in the Peace of Westphalia in 1648 – around a century after the religious peace of Augsburg – the confessional status was finally prescribed politically, as it had now been established (in the normative year of 1624). At least in Lutheranism, the combination of confession and state was followed by the subordination of confession to state.

This development forces upon us an important insight into the historical laws of the paradigm shift: what is impossible in the scientific sphere, where in the long run the dissolution of an old paradigm is enforced with the help of mathematics and experimentation, is manifestly possible in the sphere of ideas and culture, of art, philosophy, and especially theology and the church: a **paradigm already long obsolete is conserved** – albeit at the cost of liveliness and a proximity to reality!

Thus in the Reformation churches, too, a once living **tradition hardened into traditionalism** which petrified an originally living paradigm: just as in paradigm II there is an Eastern Orthodox traditionalism (to be distinguished from the true Orthodox tradition) and in paradigm III a Roman traditionalism (to be distinguished from the great Catholic tradition), so now in paradigm IV there is also a Protestant traditionalism – again to be distinguished from the good Protestant, evangelical tradition.

But here we should reflect that while the course of history cannot compel the definitive dissolution of a paradigm of theology and church, conversely, the church and theology hardened in such a paradigm **cannot hold up the progress of time.** What then threatens is a reciprocal alienation of church, theology and religion from society – with sometimes schizophrenic consequences for the individuals concerned. This also happened in the age of the Reformation and Counter-Reformation: a new paradigm shift was already becoming evident in the seventeenth century as a result of the crisis of Protestant orthodoxy. Indeed, in accordance with the experiential rules of the paradigm shift, Protestant orthodoxy itself undermined the Reformation paradigm with its ever more meticulous formations and distinctions, and increasingly got into a crisis.

Prepared for a new time?

That became evident at a very early stage in a country known for its tolerance. It had provided a home not only for Descartes and Spinoza, but alongside the Calvinist state church also for some nonconformists and 'sects': **the Netherlands.** Here, in a religious and political controversy lasting almost fifteen years (1604–1619), first of all orthodox popular Calvinism with the fierce doctrine of predestination taught by its strict preachers triumphed over its opponents, the Leiden professor Jacob Arminius and the 'Arminians'. For after the States-General Moritz of Orange had joined orthodox Calvinism out of political opportunism, at the Synod of Dort in 1618/19 all opponents were condemned – they were to be found above all in the tolerant middle classes with their humanistic education. The consequence was that many representatives of humanistic theology in the spirit of Erasmus of Rotterdam initially had to flee Holland. Indeed their leader, the seventy-two-year-old and highly respected Oldenbarneveldt, was even executed.

However, their best brain was the brilliant statesman, philosopher of law and theologian **Hugo Grotius** (1583–1643). Condemned to life imprisonment, after just three years he escaped to Paris with the help of his wife and for a while was Swedish ambassador there. As an advocate of natural law he did not allow the church any independent authority: he saw it as being subject to state sovereignty, and thus prepared for the territorial system according to which the ruler has supreme authority over all confessions in his sphere of rule, regardless of his confession. To the end of his life Grotius was the object of the sharpest Calvinistic attacks. And yet the future was not to belong to the theology of the orthodox Calvinists but to Hugo Grotius,

– who rejected a dogmatic compulsion and argued for toleration of other convictions;

– who laid the foundations for an undogmatic, grammatical-historical exegesis of the Bible;

– who attempted to interpret orthodox dogmatics rationally, especially in the doctrine of the Trinity and in christology;

– who, emphasizing the freedom of the will, argued for an undogmatic practical piety;

– who played an active part in the reunification of the Christian churches.

So still completely in the age of orthodoxy, with this great European we can already see in advance outlines of a modern paradigm of theology.

However, there is one thing that we have to concede here: despite all its traditionalism, **Protestantism (P IV) was better prepared for the new time** than triumphalistic baroque Catholicism (P II), which from the middle of the seventeenth century to the middle of the twentieth century usually lagged behind the cultural movements of the age (apart from some waves like Romanticism). Why?

● Whereas Counter-Reformation Catholicism, for all its baroque splendour, clearly represented a conservative religion of restoration, by virtue of its origins Protestantism had an **innate** tendency to press for **reform**.

● Whereas on the whole Catholicism remained the religion of the Romanic peoples, who were now often economically, politically and culturally backward (with the exception of France), Protestantism was the religion of the **Germanic and Anglo-Saxon peoples**, who were now **pressing forwards**.

● Whereas in Catholicism the Pope decided the interpretation of the Bible and did not allow any deviation from his interpretation, in Protestantism with its Reformation origins one could always appeal to a Bible read independently (and not necessarily in a Lutheran or Calvinist way) and to the **decision** of one's own **conscience** over against doctrinal statements of the church, and develop an **ethic of responsibility**.

All this will become even clearer if in our brief overall view we look beyond the bounds of orthodoxy to the broader spectrum of the religious and theological positions of the time. The age of confessionalism and orthodoxy cannot be reduced to confessionalism and orthodoxy. And it was paradoxically not least the Pietists who by their claim to individual religion with a religious motivation helped modern toleration to break through.

Internalized devotion – Protestant church music

It is amazing that in this period a **rich inwardness** of Christian faith was combined with outward dogmatic intolerance. It is expressed above all in the countless **hymns** of the period, which still form the main substance of Protestant hymnbooks. One need think only of the spiritual poems of Paul Gerhardt (1606–1676). Granted, this Lutheran regarded Catholics and even Calvinists as being excluded from eternal salvation, but in his hymns he could express the central content of Christian faith for his time in such a convincing way that the hymns were finally sung even in the confessions he had damned.

Lutheranism certainly did not succeed in creating a counterpart to the comprehensive Catholic baroque culture. But at least in music, Lutheranism (not Calvinism!) created some unique works. As is well known, the decisive musical impulses and the musical genres which were to dominate the future all came from Catholic Italy: what would the concerto have been without Gabrieli, keyboard music without Frescobaldi, oratorio without Carissimi and opera without Monteverdi? And yet – here I am following the well-founded remarks by the Tübingen music scholar Arnold Feil[161] – the **language** of instrumental music (both the instrumental imitation of vocal models and the application of instrumental techniques to vocal types) reached its climax in Germany not least because of the replacement of Gregorian melodies by hymns in the vernacular. So we can rightly speak of an **age of German Protestant church music** – a musical expression of the Reformation paradigm: 'Heinrich Schütz at the beginning and Johann Sebastian Bach at the end of this era and the many masters of a high rank alongside and between them create a new music which is no longer vocal or instrumental, no longer spiritual or secular; they produce a new view of music which is to spread

all over Europe and be fruitful everywhere, though it too will be different
in different places. Where this new music sings, at the same time it makes
instrumental gestures, and where it is instrumental it seems to
declaim.'[162] Although already situated historically in a new shift in
church history from old Lutheran orthodoxy and Pietism to the beginning
of the Enlightenment, **Johann Sebastian Bach** – together with George
Frederick Handel – brought its musical genres to their ultimate musical
height and in so doing expressed the Christian faith with a musical power,
differentiation and liveliness which was not attained before him.

Now my account so far should not give the impression that in the
transitional period between the Reformation and the Enlightenment
there were in any case only the doctrinaire orthodox who were above all
responsible for the tension between theology and piety. Rather, there
were the most varied religious and theological positions, which have been
admirably described for this 'age of absolutism' by the Protestant church
historian Hartmut Lehmann.[163] There are:

– the **apocalyptic enthusiasts**. They compensated for the tremendous
pressure of anxiety as a result of constant wars by an intensive
expectation of an imminent end to the world, for which they thought that
they could see the 'signs of the times' everywhere: the resurgence of the
papal Antichrist, the successes of the Counter-Reformation, the advances
of the Turks, but also rebellion, pestilences, natural catastrophes and
especially the appearance of comets 'bringing misfortune' (in 1664/65,
130 pamphlets about comets were published, most of them completely
untroubled by scientific knowledge);

– the **repressive fanatics**. These (often similarly against an apocalyptic
background) projected their anxieties on 'scapegoats' and thus responded
with persecution. It is no coincidence that in this century of internal and
external insecurity the persecutions of witches and Jews reached their
grisly climax: after pogroms in France, Worms and Vienna, immediately
after the middle of the century in Poland more than 250,000 Jews who
had been left in the lurch by their Polish lords were massacred by rebel
Cossacks;

– **mystics of very different stamp**. They attempted to become conscious
of an already existing unity of human beings with the abyss and primal
ground, a unity of the 'spark of the soul' with the 'flowing light' of the
Godhead. Mention should be made of theosophical ideas à la Jakob
Böhme, pansophic Rosicrucian visions à la Johann Valentin Andreae or
cosmological speculations à la Giordano Bruno.

But all these did not make up the mainstream. At this time a new kind of
religious **edifying literature** was much more important. While it was close
to a particular kind of 'reform orthodoxy', it aimed at **profundity,**

inwardness and practice rather than theological learning and the objective correctness of doctrine. As we heard, on the Catholic side (P III) there were parallels in François de Sales, Cardinal Bérulle and the Spaniard Miguel de Molinos (condemned to spend his life imprisoned in a monastery for 'quietism', as was Madame Guyon, defended in vain by Archbishop Fénélon, who was finally himself condemned). However, this edifying literature, with its often mystical orientation, had its heyday in the sphere of Protestantism (P IV), where it led to an unprecedented number of hymns, to a flood of consolatory writings, funeral sermons, poems of sorrow and collections of prayers. Indeed, for large numbers of Christians the time was a cheerless one of emergencies and crises, in which a literature of consolation and edification had a special function.

After Philipp Nicolai and his *Recipe for the Joys of Eternal Life* (1599),[164] mention should be made here above all of **Johann Arndt** with his four, later six, books *On True Christianity* (1606–10).[165] Despite his dogmatic correctness, Arndt was first expelled by the strict orthodox and even later was vigorously fought against for decades. But his notions became established, and Arndt was finally appointed General Superintendent (= Bishop) of the Protestant church in Lüneberg. Many people felt as he did, and were in search of an inward form of piety. An epoch-making paradigm shift? Perhaps not, but:

A new Reformation – Pietism

Given the hardening of church conditions in the Protestant churches and theology and the ever more externalized state churches, given this doctrinaire and institutional rigidifying of the Reformation paradigm, at the end of the sixteenth and beginning of the seventeenth centuries new movements of piety appeared simultaneously in various European countries. They aimed at a living experience of faith and the community of faith, with the disciplining and internalizing of life and the gathering of the pious into voluntary communities of the like-minded: a **pietism** *avant la lettre*, a pietism before this term existed![166]

Mention should first be made here of Puritanism in **England** with a wealth of edifying writings.[167] Translations of the writings of Richard Baxter, John Bunyan and others reached the European continent at a very early stage; no less than 1661 English treatises in German translation have been identified.[168] But the **Netherlands** also played a role with religious exiles like William Ames, who there created a particular species of Dutch 'Pietism' in reaction to a middle class which was emancipating itself; the leader who set the tone was the Utrecht professor Gisbert Voetius, founder of Dutch 'precisism'.[169]

In **Germany** all this soon led to a reform movement, directed above all against a confessionalism which was becoming rigid, and which in German Lutheranism was already taking shape in circles of 'reform Lutheranism'. Here it was most clearly expressed in the writings of Johann Arndt, so that some contemporary historians of Pietism even make it begin with Arndt: Pietism in the broader sense (J.Wallmann) or as the first phase of German Pietism (M.Brecht). But the Pietism which explicitly bears the name and formed as a special movement was only to begin a good half century after Arndt's death (521). How did that come about?

In 1675, a Frankfurt senior pastor who had migrated from Alsace wrote a lengthy preface to a new edition of Johann Arndt's sermon book *Postilla*, entitled *Pia desideria*. Soon published separately, it was to make history in German Protestantism. In it were crystallized those different impulses of the renewal movement which were alive in English Puritanism, French and Italian Jansenism and Spanish and Dutch mysticism. Indeed everywhere, for ethical reasons, open or hidden resistance was offered – long before the enlightened middle class! – to the absolutist baroque court culture, its unprecedented extravagance, its excesses and the social abuses. People distanced themselves from 'this world' (often avoiding worldly lectures, the theatre, dancing and playing cards). A 'hearty desire for an improvement of the true Evangelical Churches well pleasing to God' (thus the German title of *Pia desideria* which went with the Latin) was propagated. All this was articulated by a quiet, modest man, **Philipp Jakob Spener** (1635–1705),[170] who thus presented the programmatic work for what was first mockingly called **Pietism**.

Stimulated by Arndt, by English Puritans and Reformed Christians from Geneva and the Netherlands, Spener was intent on a quite personal, living, inward piety, the cornerstone of which was the experience of rebirth. To the great offence of the Lutheran Orthodox, at the centre of his thought was neither the promise of justification nor even word and sacrament, but the transformation of human beings, personal **rebirth to a 'new man'** willed by God and brought about by the illumination of the Holy Spirit. Spener does not see being a Christian realized simply in the judge's pronunciation of righteousness but in a rebirth to new life experienced spiritually and in a sanctification realized through action. So he understands the church not as an institution for salvation but as a community of reborn brothers and sisters. Hence 'born again' is still the decisive Christian keyword for many Christians in both Europe and America. Spener did not want to propagate a new dogma (and to this degree the incessant attacks of the orthodox dogmatic theologians missed the point), but a new life, a radical change of existence, a 'piety of the heart' lived out in practice and a commitment in the social sphere.

For anyone who seeks to accuse Pietism of both individualism and spiritualism succumbs to cliché: Spener presented not only instructions for pious individuals but also a very respectable **comprehensive reform programme** for his Protestant church. Appealing to earliest Christianity and the young Luther, he attacked established state Christianity (Caesaropapism) and aimed at no less than to complete and surpass Luther's Reformation. In the first part of the book, the sorry state of the Protestant church is illuminated in a realistic way, and in the second part the foundations are laid for the 'hope of better times' for the church (which had already long been abandoned by separatist groups critical of the church); indeed, in the third part there are even six clear and concrete demands for reform addressed to church and individual, which paint the picture of a 'hoping church'. These are:

1. An intensification of **Bible study** and the establishment of *collegia pietatis*, meetings for brotherly converse over the word of scripture.

2. The renewal of the **priesthood of all believers** because the official church of the authorities is hampered by institutionalism;

3. A concentration on the *praxis pietatis*: instead of pure doctrine, the faith is proved in the **practice of Christian life** and action;

4. An overcoming of the damaging religious disputes in the **ecumenical spirit** of brotherly love;

5. Reform of the **study of theology** by orientating it on the requirements of preaching and pastoral care;

6. Reform of **preaching**, which is not to be taught rhetorically but is to be truly edifying (the pioneers here were Arndt, Tauler, the *Theologia Deutsch* and Thomas à Kempis).

Spener, isolated in Dresden as court preacher, was brought to Berlin as Provost in 1691. Now he had enormous influence: by his widely distributed theological and edifying writings and sermons, by his promotion of youth work, social work and mission work, and also by his political position. For the early Hohenzollern rulers, intent on expansion and therefore confessionally tolerant, were already offering a home in Brandenburg-Prussia to anti-trinitarian Socinians, Jews and above all the highly-qualified Huguenots (20,000 after the Edict of Nantes in 1685). Now they took the opportunity to make the Pietists, who were persecuted in the empire, their allies against orthodox Lutheranism and the representative bodies allied with them. Now Spener no longer spoke of 'Caesaropapism', although the efforts towards a state church were manifest, at the Berlin court in particular.[171] Spener's concern was to change society by changing the individual.

At the same time, Spener's pupil **August Hermann Francke** (1663–1727) was active in Halle.[172] He was an energetic organizer who with his powerful institutions laid the basis for a major pietistic undertaking. Orphanages, schools for the poor and civic schools (the education of girls was especially encouraged!), a theological faculty with a Pietistic orientation at the University of Halle, founded in 1694, a Bible Institute with its own printing works: all this goes back to Francke. He, too, received powerful support from the Berlin court, which made him spokesman for the princely 'territorial system'. Under Francke's leadership, Pietism was now no longer on the defensive but on the offensive. This was a remarkable change: numerous Pietists attained high office in church and state, and many became army chaplains. Under the influence of Halle, soon the vast majority of north German Protestant theological teaching was on Pietistic lines; and the organizer of Lutheranism in North America, Heinrich Melchior Mühlenberg, also came from Halle.

However, the theological faculty led by Francke became involved in a dispute not only with the clergy of Halle but also with its former patron, the lawyer and opponent of witch trials, Christian Thomasius. Finally, as we shall see later, it also clashed with the famous philosopher Christian Wolff, who was expelled from Halle on the urging of the Pietists. As a result of the alliance between Prussia and Pietism, Pietism lost not a little ethical power and moral credibility. And soon under Frederick II and the Enlightenment it was to lose even its position of political power.

However, the Pietistic movement soon moved over into north-western and southern Germany, indeed also to Switzerland, Scandinavia, Eastern Europe and finally North America.[173] It also underwent a special development in eastern Germany under **Nicolas Ludwig Count von Zinzendorf** (1700–60), also from Halle, a man as emotional as he was strong in faith. He welcomed refugee Bohemian Moravian brethren on his estates in Oberlausitz, where they founded the colony Herrnhut. Here in 1727 Zinzendorf, realizing Spener's ideas of the *ecclesiola in ecclesia*, established the 'Renewed Unity of Brethren', a trans-confessional community with its own constitution, its own worship and a strong lay participation. Contrary to the intentions of Zinzendorf, who remained wholly stamped by the theology of the young Luther, a separate free church eventually developed from this. But in contrast to Halle, here in deeply emotional piety the emphasis was placed not on gnashing the teeth and penitence but – because of a strictly christocentric theology, albeit with some special features – on faith in Christ's reconciliation, joy in the new life and novel brotherly forms of worship.

Zinzendorf's opposition to every kind of defamation of human corporeality is almost unique in Protestantism.[174] So is his championing of a doctrine and practice of marriage in keeping with the gospel, along with the full involvement of **women** in the life of the community as members with equal status.[175] Here beyond question Zinzendorf's wife, Erdmuth Dorothea, née Countess Reuss, played a decisive role; she was a congenial partner and collaborator.

None of the other Pietistic groups exercised such influence far beyond Germany, to Scandinavia, Greenland and America; banished for a while, Zinzendorf himself already worked indefatigably in England, the West Indies and North America. And it was no less than the founders of Methodism, the two young Anglican clergy John and Charles Wesley, who first came into contact with the Community of Brethren there, in Georgia, before John had his experience on 24 May 1737 in one of their evening meetings, on hearing Luther's Preface to the Epistle to the Romans. But as early as 1741 the Methodists were alienated from the Community of Brethren, whereas the separation from the Church of England only took place in 1795.

From the 'inner light' to the 'light of reason'

Thus in the period between 1690 and 1730 Pietism became a determinative force in German Protestantism and was able to penetrate all social strata. Nor is there any disputing the fact that Pietism brought about an intensification of Christian life which had an effect in particular on political and social life. As the result of a living and inward religion, a renewed practical Christianity and impressive commitment in education and charitable work, it achieved a real **renewal of the already rigidified Reformation paradigm.**

The development within the churches and in the theology of German Protestantism, its biblical scholarship, its understanding of the church and its pastoral practice cannot be understood at this time without Pietism any more than can the intellectual, political, educational and social development generally. It often transcended the limits of confessionalism, emphatically in an ecumenical spirit of shared Christianity. Its stimuli were important for preaching, hymns, the practice of prayer and spirituality. In charitable work and mission it was often more active than the established churches. The deep self-examination and ascetic self-control customary in Pietism even had an effect on the psychological descriptive techniques of the new biographies, autobiographies and novels.

Here Spener himself had no separation of his pious communities from the mainstream church in mind. However, in the long run this was almost unavoidable. In fact their sectarian nature undermined the established church of the people and the state. And both the pious circles and the pious individual were now more important to the Pietists than the church as an institution. Moreover, radical Pietists left the churches and gathered again in communities of separatists or communities based on inspiration. Boundaries were often fluid.

Fame was attained by the church historian **Gottfried Arnold**, who in his learned four-volume *Unpartisan History of the Churches and Heretics, From the Beginning of the New Testament to the Year of Jesus Christ 1688* (which appeared in 1699/1700),[176] to the abiding offence of the orthodox did not depict church doctrine or the institutional church as the main factors in history but persons, whose religious truthfulness and moral integrity he subjected to an examination. In an unpartisan way, i.e. one which transcended the confessions, he launched an attack on self-righteous orthodoxy and its obsession with power, and defended the heretics and sectarians who were treated so badly in church history and often came to grief in life, and also women, so often discriminated against, arguing for permission for them to teach (privately, and where necessary also publicly). So this radical Pietist, who finally became a pastor, was a forerunner of 'unpartisan' modern church history writing.

However, in particular it was the pietistic emphasis on the subjective, individual side of religion, the practical and moral orientation of Christianity and the basically anti-confessionalist attitude which contributed to the dissolution of the ecclesiastical and theological system. Indeed it helped to bring in that movement to which the future was to belong: the **Enlightenment**. Anyone who at first does not see a connection here should note that at that time, for many people, the way from the pietistic piety of illumination, through the experiences of transcendence in English natural theology (physico-theology) fashioned by light, to Enlightenment talk of the light of reason, was not a long one.

In the face of this new constellation Pietism seemed largely defenceless and helpless. Spiritually unprepared, it refused to engage in any self-critical discussion of the modern **scientific and philosophical view of the world** and thus the modern paradigm (P V) generally. The Pietists so wanted to bring to life the traditional biblical notions and Christian content of the Bible that they opposed any modern new interpretation. In a new time they thought that they possessed the heritage, without constantly gaining it anew in the spirit.

The consequence was that soon a confrontation with the new interpretation of the world, a truly fateful challenge to European Christianity, was unavoidable. Lessing, Kant and Schiller, in part also Goethe, Fichte, Hölderlin and – especially important for future Christian theology – Schleiermacher: they were all still influenced by a Pietistic upbringing – both positively and negatively. But at the same time they belonged to a generation which had already undergone a transformation to modernity. So it was no wonder that – in contrast to the more stable Dutch Pietism and the Pietism of the lower Rhineland – even Halle Pietism largely went over to the Enlightenment in the third generation. Here the 'inner light' of mysticism had now completely become the 'light of reason'.

Revival movements – characteristic of America

I shall have to discuss the modern Enlightenment paradigm (P V) in a separate long chapter (C V). In the framework of the Reformation paradigm (P IV) we are primarily interested in the question: did Pietism die out as a result of the Enlightenment? The answer is, No. Granted, it now no longer largely dominated the cultural life of Lutheran Germany, where increasingly the spirit of reason prevailed over the spirit of piety. But in the time of the Enlightenment, Pietism survived by hibernating, in the form of a pious subculture which, however, for many Protestants meant more of a home than the enlightened churches, where even theologians and pastors no longer seemed unambiguously to hold firm to the Bible as the revelation of God. And after a time, following phases of sleep and exhaustion, a virtually new springlike awakening developed from this Pietistic soil: the **revivalist movements**.[177] These attempted once again to fill the old Reformation paradigm with new life and to give Pietism a contemporary expression.

Certainly we can discuss (as German historical scholarship in particular has done) whether the German revivalist movement of the nineteenth century was a new phase of Pietism or an independent entity. At least in the case of the revival movements in England and North America, which already begin in the early eighteenth century, something that can also be inferred from the European and especially German revival movement becomes clear; despite all their peculiarities, they are bound strongly and in many ways to earlier Pietism.[178] But how was it in **America**?

Only from the seventeenth century can one talk of Christianity in those ultimately thirteen English settlements which in 1776 were to form themselves into the 'Union', the core of the 'United States of America'. We cannot go into that within the framework of this book, and a separate investigation will be made of North American Christianity.[179] But at least one thing is important for our present context, the analysis of the Reformation paradigm: it was in North America in particular that **Protestantism** succeeded in **making up** for the lack of **influence in the 'new world'** which it had suffered from since the age of the discoveries. These English agricultural colonies were to prove by far the most important of all the European colonies. And in them – apart from 'Mary-land', the colony of the Catholic Lord Baltimore (the first commonwealth whose citizens enjoyed complete freedom of religion) – Protestantism had the say.

And what a Protestantism! It could hardly have been more varied. It was primarily a reflection of every possible European trend and group – and yet more. Since the foundation of the colony of Virginia in 1607, the first English settlement on the east coast, the immigrants had been above all **dissenters**: members of oppressed religious minorities, above all English Puritans (first the 'Pilgrim Fathers' of 1620 in Massachusetts, who have already been mentioned), who proved highly intolerant (Rhode Island was a welcome exception) and later even harshly oppressed the Catholics in tolerant Maryland. In the end the shining example of toleration was not Massachusetts, but the state of Pennsylvania, founded by the gifted and highly educated rich Quaker William Penn, who in 1682 with Philadelphia (city of brotherly love) founded a truly democratic commonwealth based on complete toleration.

However, it is already clear from this that one could talk of 'churches' only in a very limited sense in North America in the seventeenth century: by contrast there was a good deal of un-churchlike, un-Christian behaviour and soon even immorality. After the religious enthusiasm of the first decades a religious weariness had set in among many colonists. After all, down to the first decades of the eighteenth century conditions within the churches were very confusing: not only was there an indescribable lack of pastors, but also a lack of education among many of the clergy, and ordinations were disorderly. In practice there was hardly any firm church organization, and there were hardly any larger church associations.

So it was the **revival movements** which were to give North America an unmistakable stamp of its own. For even those European experts on Pietism who would like to derive every possible revivalist movement from Pietism cannot overlook the great **differences from European Pietism**:
– Pietism could presuppose a great church organization, but the revivalist movement had to create the conditions for such an organization.
– Pietism reacted to an orthodoxy which, though hardened, still had a belief in revelation. But the more time went on, the more the revivalist movements were confronted with the modernity which was breaking through in England, Scotland and America, with the self-confident rationality of the Enlightenment, and the new social distress caused by industrialization.
– Pietism was mostly active on the frontiers of its state church or local church. But the revivalist movements, often advanced by lay preachers, extended beyond the frontiers of lands, confessions and denominations.

'The Great Awakening': typically Protestant

'The world is my parish,' John Wesley could say, John Wesley who – as we heard – had founded a first great revivalist movement in England, **Methodism**, which then spread powerfully also to America. The religious and moral decline in England in the first half of the century between the Acts of Tolerance, which granted freedom of conscience to Protestants (1689), and the French Revolution (1789), which granted freedom of conscience to all, was unmistakable. There was decline not only in the Church of England and the classes which supported it (the aristocracy and the middle class) but also among the dissenters. However, here, in contrast to Catholic France with its authoritarian rule, a religious movement critical of the state church could develop freely.

At the same time there had also been a first great revivalist movement in America, **'The Great Awakening'** (1743–44). This was sparked off by the learned Puritan and powerful preacher **Jonathan Edwards** in Massachusetts; it found a great response above all among the country population of a great variety of denominations. However, the most significant preacher of the movement was to be the Methodist **George Whitefield**, who had accompanied the Wesley brothers to America. The communities and the denominations, among them especially the Baptists, grew and organized in larger associations: we have already heard of the organization of Lutheranism by Heinrich Melchior Mühlenberg, sent by the leadership of the Francke foundations, who in 1748 had established the synod of Pennsylvania (Michael Schlatter took the same action for the German Reformed).

Half a century later the situation was different yet again. Why? A **second great American revivalist movement** (1797–1805) swept over the land. It opposed the consequences of the increasing rationalism and liberalism and was led by **Timothy Dwight** at Yale College and **Charles G.Finney**. Thus there came into being a movement which this time was particularly concerned for the population of the great cities and the many people on the 'frontier', then pressing further and further West. Thousands were gathered and converted by preaching, prayer and song in large 'camp meetings' in the open air, often lasting for days. With the help of voluntary workers Finney also saw to the pastoral care of the 'new born', and finally as professor at Oberlin College, Ohio, wrote a much-noted theory of evangelization.[180]

If we survey all these revivalist movements, we can see very clearly the **characteristics** which in part are those of American Christianity generally:

– numerous **sudden conversions** of bad or indifferent Christians, often

in large groups, in sometimes spectacular circumstances (weeping, trembling, joy, ecstasy);
– an **intensive life** of faith following conversion, with numerous practical initiatives (pressure on the state in the fight against the slave trade, alcohol and capitalism);
– The rise of new **faith communities** with great power to bind and mould, of a variety exceeding that already to be found in Europe: a **pluralism** of denominations which was later to be followed by a pluralism of religions;
– very simplified preaching and **spontaneous** (not 'liturgical') emotional services **with mass congregations;**
– **deep** roots in popular Christianity, which because of the separation of church and state (which we must discuss in the context of the modern paradigm) took responsibility for financing its own churches and pastors;
– because of the legal, financial and cultural situation a strong **influence of the laity**, on whom the pastors often depended, since they were appointed by their congregations;
– an unusually large **splintering** into numerous denominations which often split again or reunited, and at the same time zealous peaceful **competition** in mutual esteem, so that the members of other Protestant denominations were normally admitted to worship and even to the eucharist – in complete contrast to the European confessions. Only the Episcopalians (Anglicans) and strict Lutherans were more restrained over intercommunion.

In themselves, such revivalist movements could break through in the framework of all the paradigms of Christianity. And indeed in the long history of the church there were always renewal movements of the most varied kinds. But 'revival'? Strictly speaking, 'revival' is not a biblical word, and it is not even found in the Reformation or orthodox Protestantism; it gains its special significance first in the framework of the movements mentioned above. So it is no coincidence that these specific revival movements are in fact **characteristic of the Reformation Protestant paradigm** (P IV). After all, they have as little to do with a mediaeval monastic reform movement or a Crusading movement than with the Jesuit order of the sixteenth century or the papal personality cult with its vast audiences, which developed in the nineteenth century.

At the same time, there is no mistaking the fact that like the Reformation paradigm generally, this Protestant revivalist movement, which was followed by parallel phenomena in a charismatic Catholicism only after Vatican II, was concerned with **renewed reflection on the gospel**. And here in fact the classical concerns of the Reformation stand at the centre: justification by faith and the rebirth of the new person in the spirit of Christ. Here a fundamental role is played on the one hand by being overwhelmed with God's grace and on the other by the believing trust of sinful men and women. 'Revival' is understood as a basic experience of the Spirit, which is to determine the whole of life. However, the other side of the coin is that the preaching of the revivalist movement often quite deliberately and sometimes one-sidedly thrust into the foreground themes meant to provoke 'fear and trembling': apocalyptic anxiety about the salvation of one's soul and therefore a dramatic confession of sin before the judge of the world who was soon to come. Be this as it may, the honest concern for a spiritual renewal in the light of the gospel is unmistakable.

From the 'revival' to ecumenism

Subsequently there were also similar revivalist movements outside North America, in Scotland and England (from the Oxford Movement to the Salvation Army[181]) and in French Switzerland, in France, the Netherlands, Germany and Scandinavia. There would be no point here in just listing all the many names, activities and organizations.[182] Soon there were centres of renewal everywhere (London, Basel, Geneva, Paris, Wuppertal). Bible societies, missionary societies, tract societies and also welfare organizations and hospitals were founded – some in opposition to the rationalistic and liberal spirit of the time and some also as part of a missionary attack.

In America in the last third of the nineteenth century 'New Revivalism' emerged again; its most successful preacher was the Chicago businessman **Dwight L. Moody**, head of the Young Men's Christian Association (YMCA, founded in London in 1844). But although the revivals contributed to a marked increase in church membership, this form of evangelization with all its concomitant phenomena increasingly faded into the twilight. Why? Many people now criticized the sometimes ecstatic features, the overestimation of personal experience and the danger of emotional self-redemption. The church, preaching and sacraments were neglected all too much. A hostility to theology was said to have developed, ending up in a basic hostility to thought and a laziness in thinking.

At all events, although these revivals had effects as far away as Australia and New Zealand, by the beginning of the twentieth century they had lost their overpowering significance in Anglo-Saxon Protestantism. And even the evangelization campaigns of people like Billy Graham, working in our century with new technologies, could no longer spark off a real popular movement, despite the great masses that they attracted. I shall be discussing the immediate present (for example the revival happenings, songs and liturgies of the 1970s) in a later investigation.

And yet it is once again characteristic of the Christian spirit of 'revival' that it was a Methodist layman whose commitment in the revivalist movement was to prove extremely fruitful for the **ecumenical movement** which was developing in the first third of the twentieth century: **John R.Mott**. Indefatigably active in the YMCA and in student work after meeting D. L. Moody, in 1896 Mott founded the World Student Christian Federation. Between 1915 and 1928 he was General Secretary of the YMCA and in 1921 he became President of the International Missionary Council; in 1900 he had written the famous programmatic work *The Evangelization of the World in This Generation*. This same John R. Mott, winner of the Nobel peace prize, was now, together with the Dutchman Willem Visser't Hooft, the driving force behind the ecumenical movement, which in 1948 had its crowning moment with the foundation of the World Council of Churches (WCC), based in Geneva. The Honorary President was John R. Mott.

But we shall be talking about ecumenism in connection with the modern or postmodern paradigm. For unfortunately, in the twentieth century a large part of the pietistic Protestantism of which we have been speaking did not turn to an ecumenism which brought the churches together, but to exclusivist fundamentalism. So after a long journey in this paradigm, too (P IV), we have come down to the present. And this is dominated by the programmatic word 'fundamentalism'. We shall have to analyse that in all its dimensions.

10. The two faces of fundamentalism

Towards the end of the twentieth century few terms have become so popular and therefore also so vague as 'fundamentalism'.[183] The term is used for certain conservative trends not only in Christianity (Protestantism) but also in Islam and Judaism, indeed in all religions. And it has meanwhile come to be used even for particular trends in politics and society. But if we want to use it meaningfully, we must first of all sharpen it up.

Why one can be fundamentalist

First of all we must note that the very origin and history of the term and the movement indicate that **fundamentalism, too, is primarily a phenomenon in the framework of the Reformation Protestant paradigm** (P IV). Between 1910 and 1915 a whole series of writings (twelve volumes) were produced by leading figures in the evangelical movement and conservative theologians from Princeton under the series title 'The Fundamentals' (meaning, of course, the fundamentals of Christian faith). So the representatives of this movement, which of course had already existed beforehand, were called 'fundamentalists' (the Baptist C. C. Law coined the term in 1920).

But a **second** point must be added immediately. Not every Protestant nor even every conservative Protestant is a fundamentalist; indeed not even every Pietist or Evangelical need be a fundamentalist. There are many conservative Protestants, Pietists and Evangelicals who, though they have a basically conservative religious attitude, seek to combine it with an openness to the social, intellectual and religious concerns of modernity. They are not modernists, but modern Protestants. So who is a fundamentalist? Answer: a fundamentalist is someone – whether from the Lutheran, Calvinist, Pietistic or Free Church tradition – who **confesses the literal inspiration and therefore the unconditional inerrancy of the Bible.**

I say 'confesses': it should be noted that this is not a scientific theory but a real **confession of faith.** Indeed it was already formulated in the first article of the so-called 'Niagara Creed' of the Niagara Bible Conference of 1878 in anticipation of the whole fundamentalist movement: 'We believe "that all Scripture is given by inspiration of God", by which we understand the whole of the book called the Bible; nor do we take the statement in the sense in which it is sometimes foolishly said that works of human genius are inspired, but in the sense that the Holy Ghost gave the very words of the sacred writings to holy men of old; and that His Divine inspiration is not in different degrees, but extends equally and fully to all parts of these writings, historical, poetic, doctrinal and prophetical, and to the smallest word, and inflection of a word, provided such word is found in the original manuscripts.'[184]

But we need to reflect on a **third** point: is this really a new confession of faith? The fundamentalist will rightly point out that none of this is new; there was already belief in a verbal inspiration and unconditional inerrancy of the Bible in the early church. And indeed, in the Hellenistic and moreover Christian view, can't the spirit of God come upon people in ecstasy? So didn't some of the **church fathers** simply see the biblical authors (quite differently from the authors themselves) as instruments of the spirit under whose guidance, indeed 'dictation', they wrote? Like a flute or a harp which is only made to sound by a breath of air? God himself through his spirit plays the melody here, determines the content and form of scripture, so that by the will of God the whole Bible is free from contradictions, mistakes and errors, or must be kept so by interpreters (through harmonizing, allegory or mystification). So everything is inspired down to the last word, *verbum*: verbal inspiration. Everything is to be subscribed to unconditionally, word for word.

That in fact is how people thought in antiquity and the Middle Ages in a quite natural, naive, so to speak innocent way, just as at that time it was taken for granted that almighty God created the world in six days and human beings from clay, that he could perform any miracle in nature and indeed did so, at least in ancient times. But this historical reminiscence leads to a third insight for defining present-day fundamentalism: for the Bible to be understood in an uncritical and naive way, literally, in a **pre- critical age**, is **not** yet **fundamentalism**. Present-day fundamentalists cannot appeal to the church fathers. But can they perhaps appeal to Martin Luther?

Martin Luther – a fundamentalist?

Luther's hermenetic once again already shows the paradigm shift of the Reformation to be a revolution of epoch-making church-historical significance. For **Martin Luther,**
– as we saw, in a revolutionary way used the scriptural principle (*sola scriptura*) critically against church tradition, scholastic theology and the philosophical alienation of theological language,
– therefore argued resolutely that the Bible interprets itself, and that in decisive matters (in its *res*) its meaning is automatically quite clear and certain,
– and therefore rejected the allegorical sense of scripture and argued firmly for taking its literal sense seriously: so Luther wanted to understand the individual biblical statements in the light of the aim of the whole: in the light of Christ, who here has to be regarded as the mathematical point of Holy Scripture.[185]

That means that according to Luther it is not the individual isolated word of scripture that is the word of God. Only in the distinction between law and gospel, in orientation on Jesus Christ himself ('what urges Christ'), can the Old Testament in particular, but also the New Testament, rightly be understood as the Word of God. In some circumstances Christ must even be set against scripture (taken literally). That means that according to **Luther the individual words of Scripture** are not intrinsically God's Word, but **in so far as they bear witness to the incarnate Word of God, who is Jesus Christ,** and are thus accepted in faith. So a present-day fundamentalism cannot appeal to Luther.

But Lutheran and Calvinist orthodoxy did not act on these liberating stimuli from their church father. They were initially too much on the offensive against mediaeval theology, and then on the defensive against Tridentine theology. In the face of a Reformation theology which was already split, Counter-Reformation theology stressed the need for the church (councils, Pope) as the decisive authority in all scriptural exegesis in order to avoid doctrinal chaos. Didn't orthodox Protestant theology then have to work out how scripture was clear and self-evident, in order to relieve itself of its apologetic burden? However, from a present-day perspective this must be doubted.

At all events, only now, and not originally at the Reformation, was there a rigorously systematized doctrine of verbal inspiration and therefore also of the inerrancy or infallibilty of scripture. And this doctrine of infallible scripture in fact became the foundation of theology and the church, a shift of the foundation which had considerable consequences. From it follows the insight that in so far as it is no longer Jesus Christ himself who is in fact 'the foundation which is laid (once and for all)' (I Cor.3.10), but rather the (orthodox) doctrine of the infallible Bible, as a result of offensive and defensive theological pressures, **Protestant theology** unwittingly **laid the foundation for fundamentalism**. The real fundamentalists could appeal to the orthodox at any time, as indeed they have.

The threat from modernity

However, for these real fundamentalists, who were no longer men and women of the Reformation period but of the modern age, the case *par excellence* in church history was now no longer that of Luther but that of Galileo (the Copernican shift in astronomy and philosophy) and then increasingly – when biology occupied the foreground in place of astronomy and physics – that of Darwin. Now no one who wanted to maintain the inherited 'faith of the fathers' could miss the new threat: in parts the **picture of the world in modern science and philosophy was in opposition to the picture of the world in the Bible**.

There was a threat that belief in the Bible, in particular the belief of 'simple believers', would be deeply shaken. Just think: the world not made in six days (possibly in six 'million-days')? No, that could not, must not, be true if one accepted in faith the divine inspiration and thus the infallibility of the Bible. Were men and women, rather than being created in the image of God (and then fallen and infected with original sin), now primitive beings allegedly descended from the apes, who didn't know the one true God at all and were incapable of a primal and original sin? No, a believing Christian couldn't accept that without putting the whole of belief in the biblical revelation in question. That kind of thing would be apostasy. For if only one stone were taken out, wouldn't that shake the whole doctrinal edifice? No, in this time blinkered by an optimism about progress, in view of the coming Last Judgment it was now important to 'save souls', even if there were only a relatively small number of them.

But the bad thing for fundamentalists was that it was not just science and philosophy which opposed the world-view of the Bible. Since the Enlightenment there was also 'unbelieving' **biblical scholarship** itself, **working with historical-critical methods.** This claimed with a tremendous expenditure of scholarship that it could discover and unveil the story of the origin, say, of the book of Genesis, the Five Books of Moses generally, and the history of the books of Isaiah and Daniel, indeed even that of the Synoptic Gospels and the Gospel of John (allegedly by no means written by the historical John). The shock caused by historical criticism was considerably greater in America than in Europe, which was better prepared for it. But in this way didn't 'Christian' exegesis itself destroy the foundation of Christianity?

Fundamentalist Christians had to take a stand and clearly identify themselves in the face of such a threat. This makes it clear to us that in the strict sense **fundamentalism is a product of defence and attack against modern science, philosophy and nature,** in order to rescue the verbal inspiration and inerrancy of the Bible from the threat posed by modernity. As the editor of the most ambitious research project on fundamentalism, Martin E. Marty, a Lutheran who is professor at the University of Chicago, says, 'the main theological hallmark of modern religious fundamentalists consists in their oppositionalism'.[186]

Thus forced on to the defensive, fundamentalism proved more Protestant than the Protestants: it protested not only against Rome and papalism but also against the modern Babylon and evolutionism, liberalism, secularism. The situation became more acute, especially in the USA. In the 1920s fundamentalists (e.g. Billy Sunday) accused liberals of heresy, and liberals (e.g. H. E. Fosdick) accused fundamentalists of falsifying Christianity. That has now led to a quite remarkable '*renversement des alliances*' which once again confirms that '*les extrêmes se touchent*': the extremes meet.

The alliance between fundamentalists and curialists

Not only Protestantism (P IV), but also, as we saw, **Roman Catholicism** (P II) had immense difficulties with modernity (P V), and as this Catholicism had already rejected the Reformation and had therefore already remained one paradigm shift behind (in the Middle Ages), its difficulties multiplied.

No wonder, then, that with the usual time lag, in the nineteenth century Roman theology similarly **largely adopted the doctrine of the verbal inspiration and inerrancy of scripture** which had already been systematized by Protestant orthodoxy.[187] And just as Rome had long maintained that the traditional Latin translation, the Vulgate (and the *Comma Ioanneum*[188]), was the only authentic version and opposed a new translation into Latin, so American fundamentalists retained the traditional 1611 Authorized, King James Version of the Bible and rejected any new Bible translation, even the Revised (American Standard) Version of 1901 and the Revised Standard Version of 1946/52. And like the American fundamentalists, so too the Roman theologians also concentrated on the questions of the biblical account of creation (six days' work, the doctrine of evolution and original sin), on the source theory of the Pentateuch, on the Virgin Birth, which was to be understood biologically, on the true divinity of Jesus, and on reconciliation through his blood, the bodily resurrection and the prophecies of the end of the world, and the return of Christ, which were all to be taken literally.

There is no doubt about it: fundamentalists and curialists also use modern means of transport, communication, healing and payment, and often the most advanced techniques of organization (Vatican Radio, the Electronic Church). Here the modernism which they otherwise identify with rationalism, progress, pluralism, materialism and secularism suits them well. But both nevertheless accuse their opponents of 'modernism'. Why? Because they see their opponents as wanting to relativize the authority of the Bible on the basis of historical research, to put in question the origin of human beings through God, and to reduce the person of Jesus Christ to a purely human level. And just as Rome attempted to establish a position by state law, so too – against the theory of evolution – has fundamentalism. Indeed it succeeded here in some southern American states. Moreover, just as the Roman Curia has kept holding heresy trials in the course of history, so too has American fundamentalism: in 1925 in Dayton, Tennessee, it provoked the famous 'monkey trial' over the doctrine of evolution, in which the biology teacher J. T. Scopes was convicted of teaching, loyal to Darwin, that human beings evolved from the animal kingdom.

But just as the Roman Inquisition discredited itself with processes against Galileo and others, so too did American fundamentalism, which failed wherever for a while it could make the teaching of its theory of 'creationism' (the direct creation of human beings by God) compulsory in state schools. This gave Protestant 'fundamentalism' the same negative connotations as Catholic 'dogmatism' or 'integralism'. That is understandable, for those who **identify** themselves **with the truth** and therefore make an **authoritarian and exclusive claim on the 'whole' truth** (*Splendor veritatis*), and thus can no longer be open to the truth of others, reveal themselves to be fundamentalists (even if contrary to scripture they like calling themselves 'Holy Father').[189]

Fundamentalism – a world problem

What the leading Jewish scholar Jacob Neusner says about the segregationalist Jewish communities applies by analogy not only to fundamentalist Christians but also to Islamicist Muslims: 'All take an exclusive view of truth, seeing Judaism (Christianity, Islam) as the only valid statement by God to humanity and, among Judaisms (Christianities, Islams), of course, only their own.'[190]

This is also the reason why most recently the term 'fundamentalism' has also been **extended to other religions** and above all to Islam and Judaism. Muslims themselves today call an exclusivist Islam which believes in the letter of the book 'Islamism', and Jews themselves call an exclusivist Judaism which believes in the letter of the book 'ultra-orthodoxy'. But anyone today who wants to describe a rigid belief in the letter and a legalistic observance of the law (often combined with political aggressiveness) in negative terms speaks of **Muslim and Jewish fundamentalism**, in the same way as Christian fundamentalism. However, theopolitical strategies are developed only by Christianity ('Crusade for Christ', 'Re-evangelization of Europe') and Islam ('Re-Islamicization of the Arab World').

Nor should we forget the religions of Indian and Chinese origin: Hinduism (against Muslims or Sikhs) or Confucianism (against non-Han Chinese) can also behave in an exclusive, authoritarian, repressive, indeed fundamentalist way. In other words, fundamentalism is a **universal problem**, a world problem.[191]

It is often asked where the enormous effectiveness and thrust of the various fundamentalisms derive from. Acording to the psychiatrist Günter Hole, a specialist in the psychopathology of religion, three factors combine:[192]

– **Consistency**: a basic religious value or basic idea is built up consistently and guarded in a perfectionist way out of a fear of forming a deviant compromise.

– **Simplicity**: thought, attitude and system are simple and transparent; variant perspectives are largely excluded.

– **Clarity**: interpretation and doctrinal structure are established unambiguously; any nuanced interpretation is regarded as a deviation from pure doctrine, indeed as heresy.

So if there can be fundamentalism in all religions, then **monotheism is not** the reason for fundamentalism, as sometimes even unenlightened Christian authors claim, saying that the traditional belief in the one and only God is an expression of structures of consciousness which are deeply incompatible with a pluralistic view of the world. As though religions could not also oppress other religions or peoples, disseminate hatred and inspire wars in the name of several gods – not to mention atheistic pseudo-religions! Isn't it rather the case that, in particular, belief in one God who embraces and governs all things could be the basis for a universalism which takes the plurality of religions seriously without giving up its own uniqueness. No, strictly speaking, it is not belief in the one God which separates the three religions of Semitic Near Eastern origin from one another, but belief in God's one people and land (Judaism), in God's one Messiah and Son (Christianity) and God's one revelation and book (Islam).

Having specified all this, however, we can concede that the **prophetic monotheistic religions** are **more prone to fundamentalism** than the others.[193] For the mystical religions of India orientated on a universal unity attempt, rather, to absorb other religions, to relativize them as preliminary stages, to include them as aspects of the one and only truth (inclusivism). By comparison, Judaism, Christianity and Islam as prophetic religions almost naturally tend to exclude other religions a priori (exclusivism), to convert them, and in some circumstances to destroy them. There is separation and conquest instead of communication and community. The specific concentration on the one God then often manifests itself not just as confrontation with the other religions but at the same time also as excommunication, indeed ultimately – through 'holy wars' – as the destruction of those of other faiths. Monotheism becomes **fanaticism**, especially when it is still bound up with visions of the end of the world.[194]

It is possible to break through this fatal interconnection only if one does not suppress the **universal horizon of the great documents of revelation**, the Hebrew Bible, the New Testament and the Qur'an, which is always the history of humankind as a whole, the history of all peoples. And if we understand these great documents of faith at the same time spiritually in terms of their spiritual centre and not in a naively literal way, we will arrive at another basic attitude to the other religions as well.[195]

Against the static understanding of revelation characteristic of an ultra-orthodoxy which regards the whole Torah (the Pentateuch, the other biblical writings and the oral Torah of the rabbinic sages) as God's literal eternally valid revelation (which is therefore also to be followed literally), with all more recent biblical research, including that of some Jewish scholars, we have to recognize that the revelation of God is a historical event. So a distinction must be made between significant commandments and those which are insignificant, even damaging, for today.[196] The same also holds for Christianity and Islam: the doctrine of the literal inerrancy or **infallibility of holy scripture**, be this the Hebrew Bible (halakhah), the Qur'an or the New Testament (or in some circumstances even the infallibility of the Pope, the Reformers or the council) must **not** be presented as a dogma of dogmas, a formal **central dogma** on which all the other truths of faith hang.

From this finding, in retrospect, questions arise for the future, for all confessions and religions,[197] not just in Christianity but also in Judaism[198] and Islam.[199] For Judaism, Christianity and Islam all want to give men and women a **basic orientation** for their lives in a period which is poor in orientation. But how?

Questions for the Future

With all its festivals, celebrations, rites and commandments, Judaism seeks to offer men and women today a meaningful framework of orientation related to practice. But what about a **fundamentalist** Judaism, which, appealing to the written and oral Torah revealed by God (Bible and Talmud), rejects any form of dealings with the world outside its own sphere of life and any collaboration in common tasks of public interest, indeed contests even any freer form of Judaism (conservative or liberal)? How can such a form of Judaism in the long run offer people such a framework of orientation in a modern democracy (as, for example, in America or Israel)? After all, democracy now presupposes a common interest of all citizens and their duty towards the common good.

With all its doctrines and dogmas, sacraments and instructions for life, Christianity seeks to offer men and women today a comprehensive interpretation of existence and the world. But in an age which is so wholly shaped by modern science, technology and culture, how is a **fundamentalist** Christianity to offer such an interpretation if it is bound to a literal understanding of the accounts of creation and the end, of fall and redemption? To the neglect of all the rules of hermeneutics, only one interpretation is allowed and claimed as absolute.

Islam seeks to offer men and women today a comprehensive view of life in which faith and action are inseparably connected. But in modern times, how is a **fundamentalist** Islam to be a meaningful influence, pointing the way, if the Qur'an may not be reinterpreted for particular challenges of the time; if the occasion, point in time and situation of individual surahs and verses of the Qur'an may not be investigated in order to establish where and for what period they are or have been valid? After all, there are also classical mediaeval interpreters of the Qur'an who distinguish between verses of the Qur'an which only apply to the time in which they were revealed and those which are valid for all times.

The Protestant theologian Jürgen Moltmann is right: 'What is nowadays termed "fundamentalism" is a secondary phenomenon: the primary religious, interreligious and areligious challege is not "fundamentalism" but the "modern world".'[200] Basically, both exclusivist Judaism, Islamist Islam and fundamentalist Christianity represent a rebellion against the modernity which threatens traditional faith. There is a concern to stop this, turn the clock back on it, in order to restore earlier religious, political and economic conditions.

But can a religion (and thus an individual believer) preserve the foundation, identity and certainty of truth at all without taking every sentence and every word of its holy scripture literally? The answer to this is: the concerns of the fundamentalists are legitimate, but their solution is fatal. In this paradigm, too, this brings us to a brief ecumenical stocktaking.

The Protestant churches: strengths and dangers

There is no doubt about it: in the face of all the detritus and silt of the mediaeval tradition, the **Reformation paradigm** pointed people of the sixteenth century back to the living source of Christianity. Thus in contrast to all the divisions in the late Middle Ages Martin Luther's Reformation programme offered a new identity and cushioned anxiety about salvation in a new certainty of faith. And Luther, the man of faith, was no more a fundamentalist than Jesus himself or the apostle Paul. The great **strength** of Protestantism lies in this ever-new confrontation with the **gospel**, with the original Christian message. Wherever Christianity is concealed, diluted, distorted or even abolished, **protest** is in place: not an empty protest only **against** abuses but a purposeful protest **for** the gospel, for Jesus Christ, the 'essence' of Christianity. **Concentration on the gospel** is the true core of 'Protestantism'. And this is quite indispensable for Christianity.

However, our time in particular has had the surprising experience of the Second Vatican Council. Here the **Catholic Church**, which was apparently totally petrified in the Counter-Reformation and anti-modernism, as I already remarked briefly at the end of my discussion of the Roman Catholic paradigm (P III), took a turn towards the other Christian churches which for all its limitations and compromises must be said to be far more epoch-making than 'Trent'. For what is it about? Prepared for by many theologians intent on the gospel and often persecuted, Vatican II in the end fundamentally followed Protestant Christianity in achieving the paradigm shift from the Middle Ages to the Reformation and, without abandoning Catholicity, became concentrated on the gospel and thus sought to **integrate the Reformation Evangelical Protestant paradigm** (P IV).

No one can overlook the tremendous difficulties that the Catholic Church had with its renewal because of the Roman system – before, during and after Vatican II. But despite all the questions that have remained unresolved (birth control, divorce, the question of ministry, mixed marriages, celibacy, the primacy and infallibility), the concrete positive results of the conciliar reform, which have fundamentally changed the Catholic Church, must not be underestimated. At the same time – one should at least indicate here – they provoke questions to the churches of the Reformation. So how far has an integration of the Reformation evangelical paradigm into the Catholic Church become reality?

First of all we should note the **fundamentally new attitude to the Reformation** which is given programmatic expression in the decrees of the council (and at the same time, at this point I should briefly recall the Catholic counter-questions, the importance of which I have increasingly come to see in long years of ecumenical activity, and which have also been described earlier):

– The Catholic **complicity** in the split in the churches is now recognized. At the same time the need for constant **reform** is explicitly affirmed: *ecclesia semper reformanda* – constant renewal of one's own church in life and teaching according to the gospel – is now also a Catholic view.

A counter-question arises: may the other churches go on understanding themselves as churches not to be reformed at all ('Orthodox', P II), or as already definitively reformed ('Lutheran', 'Calvinist', 'Free Churches')? Don't they all remain churches which still need further reform?

– The other Christian communities are now **recognized as churches**: there is a common Christian basis in all churches which is given with belief in Jesus Christ and baptism and is more important than anything that separates.

Here too a counter-question arises: mustn't the concern for the common Christian basis and 'substance' also be intensified in other churches?

– An **ecumenical attitude** is required of the whole Catholic Church, specifically: the inner conversion of Catholics themselves, a mutual process of making the acquaintance of other churches and a dialogue which is open to learning; the recognition of the faith, the baptism, the values of other Christians; and finally theology and church history practised in an ecumenical spirit.

The counter-question here would be: will the other churches also for their part recognize and realize the numerous legitimate Catholic concerns, in theology, liturgy and church structure?

It should be noted that over and above this fundamental attitude to the Reformation, in the council decrees a whole **series of central gospel concerns** has been taken up by the Catholic Church at least in principle, but often quite practically:

1. **A new appreciation of the Bible**: in worship (a more comprehensive cycle of scripture readings extending over several years); in theology (the study of scripture is said to be the 'soul' of theology); and in church life generally, instead of being forbidden to read the Bible, the laity are now invited to read it frequently.

2. **An authentic liturgy for the people**: rather than the former clerical liturgy, now the whole community worships in shared prayer, singing and communion. It is possible to hear the word of God proclaimed in the vernacular rather than as formerly in an alien Latin.

Rather than the former accretions and obfuscation there is a simplification and concentration on the essentials of the eucharist. Rather than the standardized uniform Roman liturgy there is more adaptation to individual nations. Instead of being prohibited to the laity the chalice is now allowed, at least in principle.

3. **A revaluation of the laity**: the laity have direct access not only to the Bible but also to theology. They can play many parts in the celebration of the eucharist and have far more influence through parish and diocesan councils.

4. **An adaptation of the church to the nations**: rather than a centralized system, there is increasing emphasis on the significance of the local church and the particular churches (dioceses, nations); the national and continental conferences of bishops are meant to help towards practical decentralization.

5. **Reform of popular piety**: many of the special forms of piety from the Reformation and baroque period (devotions, litanies, etc.) have disappeared again. Many regulations for fasting have been abolished and Marianism has declined considerably.

Finally, Luther's central concern: as we have heard, the **justification** of the sinner on the basis of faith alone is now as much affirmed by Catholic theologians as, conversely, the need for works or deeds of love is affirmed by Protestant theology. Once again, this Catholic realization of Reformation concerns is still far from having achieved the consistency that is to be desired – who could fail to see that? Here the Catholic Church could learn from the Anglican Church in many respects. But compared with the weak initial successes of the Counter-Reformation council, those of Vatican II may be said to be quite sensational. What church has been able to change so thoroughly, world-wide, in so few years as the Catholic Church? Despite all the imperfections, inconsistencies and compromises, the realization of Reformation concerns which it has achieved so far allows it once again to put **questions** to the Protestant churches. For shouldn't the Protestant churches be meeting Catholics with more self-critical understanding of themselves?

Questions for the Future

• There is certainly more appreciation of the Bible in Catholicism. But in Protestantism isn't there often a frequent neglect of the common **tradition** of the early church and the Middle Ages?

• The Catholic liturgy of the word and the people of God is certainly more lively. But in some Protestant churches, isn't the celebration of the **eucharist** still marginalized or neglected?

• Beyond doubt the Catholic laity, above all women, have been rehabilitated. But do Protestant churches take sufficiently seriously the significance of ordination and church **office** in the local, regional and universal sphere?

• Heightened decentralization and inculturation in the various nations is urgently necessary. But what about the international character and **universality** of the church, which is often put in question by Protestant provincialism or nationalism?

• There has been yet further reform of popular piety, particularly in certain countries. But aren't church and liturgy often kept **remote from the people** by Protestant intellectualism?

What a great new entire constellation of Christianity, newly shaped by the gospel, this paradigm of the Reformers is! But this constellation, too, has its specific **dangers**. The progressive **separatism** – splitting into smaller and smaller 'sects', groups, cells – was from the beginning the main danger to Protestantism, analogous to the danger of centralism in the Roman Catholic Church. And as far as the mainstream of Protestantism is concerned, we had to note how in time **this paradigm, too, consolidated itself and became hardened,** though in a different way from the mediaeval Roman Catholic paradigm. The result was a rigid orthodoxy which Pietism could bring to life only conditionally and partially, since, like orthodoxy, it closed itself to the new modern constellation that was coming into being. It was thought that one needed only to take the Bible literally, abandon oneself and one's reason, to be rid of all doubt. 'Only believe . . .'

And so in modern times, out of sheer opposition to modern science, society, exegesis and theology, there arose that Protestant **fundamentalism** which is only a ghostly **shadow of the great Reformation paradigm** (P IV). It is comparable to Orthodox traditionalism, which is only a weak copy of the early church Hellenistic paradigm (P II); comparable to Roman authoritarianism and infallibilism, which is a caricature and distortion of the great mediaeval paradigm (P III). It is the danger of a Protestantism which has hardened into **false protest**. For if we take a more sophisticated approach, we can see that:

1. The quest of many people for a **foundation** in times of disorientation is quite understandable. So many people no longer know what their own life and their own religion are really about. And a religion without a clear foundation falls victim to the spirit of the time, devalues itself.

But at the same time there is no disputing the fact that to hold fast to a foundation is not identical with fundamentalism. Countless people in all religions have kept or regained a foundation without accepting everything in their own holy scripture word for word. It follows from this that a foundation can be preserved even **without fundamentalism**.

2. To hold on to a religious **identity** that is threatened or to regain one that has been lost is a completely justified concern. So many people are afraid of alienation and diffusion and long for criteria and support, And a religion which does not bestow any identity but divides people and leaves them alone with their contradictions does not bind them to the Absolute but keeps them from it.

But at the same time there is no disputing the fact that maintaining one's religious identity is not identical with 'fundamentalism', which embodies a 'threatened, anxious, and uncertain identity that therefore reacts aggressively'.[201] Many Jews, Christians and Muslims attest today that identity can live with the recognition of other religions. It follows from this that identity is possible without **exclusivism**, possible in the recognition of the plurality of ways to God.

3. The need for a **religious certainty of faith** is legitimate. So many people feel deeply uncertain over the questions of where they ultimately come from and where they are going, the whole context of their life and its

long-term perspectives. And a religion which cannot offer certainty through its interpretations, symbols and criteria, but which if anything heightens the uncertainty, is not serving the truth.

But at the same time there is no disputing the fact that holding firm to the certainty of religious truth is not identical with fundamentalism. Religious certainty does not mean assurance without risk or doubt; it does not mean a fortress mentality and a strategy, but a life in ultimate relaxation, in confidence that the truth of God will establish itself even without massive human help. It follows from this that religious certainty **without fanaticism** is possible; doubt and adventure are also part of faith, as too is insight into the limits of and the need for tolerance.

Ecumenism is more than pure reform activism. Ecumenism can be found and realized only when all the churches again concentrate on the one Christian tradition: on the gospel of Jesus Christ himself. Only from that perspective will it be possible to break down again all the confessionalistic anxieties and uncertainties, to overcome the ideological fanaticism and the resentful restrictiveness, to see the economic, political and cultural links with a particular society, class, race, civilization, state which are hidden behind the theological differences and advance beyond them to a new freedom. But that means that there can be no ecumenical understanding without church renewal, and no church renewal without ecumenical understanding.

In such a basic ecumenical attitude it will also be possible to approach the new questions which arose only after the Reformation and Counter-Reformation, and which modernity put to Catholics, Protestants and Orthodox equally. We are now well prepared to look more closely at the paradigm of Enlightened modernity, P V, which has already kept appearing on the horizon in the analysis of earlier paradigms.

V. The Paradigm of Modernity, Orientated on Reason and Progress

After the Reformation and Counter-Reformation, after the age of confessionalism and the indescribable devastations of the Wars of Religion, after the Thirty Years' War on the European continent (1618-1648), followed later by the 'Glorious Revolution' and William III's 'Toleration Act' in England, **around the middle of the seventeenth century** a further great **watershed of modern history** can be noted: most of the general histories and church histories agree on that. For our paradigm analysis, this means that the crisis for both the Reformation paradigm (P IV) and the mediaeval paradigm in the form of the Counter-Reformation paradigm (P IV) which has already been described was that neither proved capable of coping with fundamentally new impulses. This is the presupposition for the transition to a new entire constellation, to the **new paradigm of modernity,** though its history cannot be written here. I shall bring out sharply just its basic features and revolutionary thrusts in terms of the way in which they influenced Christianity, the church and theology.[1] But first in connection with this new paradigm (P V), too, here are some hermeneutical reflections on history which will help us to approach the analysis of the modern paradigm, not in a naive-historical way but in line with the present historical and philosophical awareness of the problem.

1. The beginning of modernity

Historical **periodizations**, the definition of the thresholds of eras, are primarily **of our own making** and thus relative. Time can never be divided up from a standpoint beyond time; it is always divided up from a standpoint within time.[2] Historiography is a discipline of our **knowledge** of history, so it is completely determined by our standpoint and perspective and governed by our interests. It in no way merely reports, as Ranke thought, 'how it really was', but at the same time also already interprets it. So there can be no description without interpretation, nor any periodization without a decision. However, the decisions and demarcations must not be simply arbitrary if they are not to collide with reality itself. In other words, periodizations, too, must not be random. They have to do as much justice as possible to the 'facts' and not distort the view of reality.

The age of discoveries – the beginning of modernity?

One can make **modernity** begin in this or that century, depending on one's standpoint, criteria and interests. There are scholars who make it already begin in the **high Middle Ages** or the **late Middle Ages**, so that there is hardly any Middle Ages left for them. But not every possible pre-form, sign or forerunner of a new age as yet means a paradigm shift.[3] What is decisive for that is not some first instances, but the point at which the new becomes normative. That happens only:
– when the intimations of a movement shift from the private sphere to the public sphere;
– when the oppositional becomes representative,
– when ideas and examples form norms and the new has not only dawned but broken through. Only then can one speak of a change of ages, an epoch-making macro-paradigm shift.

Other historians make modernity begin with the **Renaissance**, although, as we have seen,[4] for all its forward drive the Renaissance took antiquity as its guide and not the autonomous reason or progress. Others yet again make it begin with the **Reformation**, although the Reformers, who were mostly anti-Copernican and not at all democratic, were in many ways still bound by mediaeval notions and techniques. It was not Luther, Melanchthon, Calvin, Knox and Cranmer, nor even Erasmus, the Popes of the Counter-Reformation and the baroque artists, but Descartes and Leibniz, Galileo and Newton, Hobbes, Rousseau and Kant who each in his own way were typically 'modern' figures.

But what about the historical date 1492? Beyond doubt one can make modern Europe (in the wider sense) begin with the **discovery of America**; however, for the Christianity of the time that still did not represent a pardigm shift. Why not?

Spanish and Portuguese historians are not the only ones who regard the age of the discoveries as the beginning of modern Europe. And rightly so. For the European forays on the oceans of the world and the discoveries and conquests in the fifteenth and sixteenth centuries connected with them were uniquely bold. Or is it mere chance that the other parts of the world were 'discovered' from Europe and not vice versa? Nowadays we are beyond doubt far from engaging in that arrogant, ignorant way of thinking which used to be widespread in Europe, supposing that before their 'discovery' other parts of the world had persisted in an unhistorical age or a priori were culturally inferior. How could anyone who knows Islamic culture in Persia or Baghdad or the Chinese Sung and Tang dynasties claim this? But beyond doubt in the sixteenth century, the Chinese, Indian or Islamic cultural circles seemed more inward-looking,

more static than Europe. At any rate, Europe's possible rivals did not have the motive force to develop a colonial empire overseas, whatever one may think of such a project. It is beyond dispute that:
– For all its advances towards Korea, Japan, Vietnam and Central Asia and its isolated expeditions over the sea to India, because of its universalistic view of the world and the state, the **Chinese empire** hardly showed any persistent interest in overseas trade and colonization. It did not even bring the archipelago of South East Asia under its control, so that the Pacific did not become for the Chinese what the Atlantic was for the Europeans. In the face of European expansion, China and Japan decided for encapsulation.
– Up to the fifteenth century, it is true, the **Islamic empires** did not just have a strong position on the European continent (through the Ottomans); in addition they controlled the sea trade in the Mediterranean and in the Indian Ocean as far as Java. But in the sixteenth century they were overtaken by the technically more developed voyaging of the Portuguese and Spaniards (not just coastal sailing but ocean sailng). The Muslim empires (the Ottomans and the Safawids in Persia) began to show signs of stagnation and paralysis even when there was still military expansion in the Balkans; the Indian Mogul empire broke up in the battles with the Hindu Marathas.

Certainly there were already intercontinental links in antiquity and the Middle Ages: trade, voyages of conquest and travels on land routes, migrations of larger groups of people in the Mediterranean area and in the Pacific and Polynesia. But the links between Europe and other continents which began in the sixteenth century, closer than any before, were now no longer just limited to the areas of Asia and Africa which were already known in antiquity. Rather, they opened up hitherto unknown seas and parts of the world, and made the oceans of the world no longer divisive factors but links. Geopolitically, without doubt a new time began; but does this already mark a paradigm shift for Christianity? That is quite a different question.

Still no paradigm shift for Christianity

Europe's outreach overseas had global effects: in the course of modernity the different parts of the world came to grow together into a single world by a gradual, though unequal, Europeanization – through military expeditions, trade and mission, which went hand in hand. One world, with Europe at the centre! To this degree the modern paradigm was later to manifest itself as a thoroughly **Eurocentric paradigm**. Only with the end of modernity and European colonialism and imperialism after the

Second World War were Europeans generally to become aware that this process of Europeanization was extremely ambivalent, that willy-nilly it cost tremendous sacrifice, that it meant the expulsion, deportation and annihilation of whole tribes and peoples as a result of war and epidemics and the destruction of age-old cultures and societies. The process of colonialization, like that of the de-colonialization of the parts of the world outside Europe, will therefore be described in a separate investigation.[5]

Here we shall concentrate on the fact that **for Christianity** the discovery of the new continents still **by no means amounted to an epoch-making paradigm shift**. For at that time it was primarily the Reformation which stood at the centre of political events, which with its forces and the counter-forces that it sparked off was to dominate this period of transition between the Middle Ages and modernity. So for the great masses of the European population, for a long time the discoveries outside Europe remained a marginal event. Initially the colonies overseas were important and interesting only because they put vast masses of gold and silver at the disposal of the rising Roman Catholic power of **Spain,** which it could use for its wars (against the Protestants) – not to mention the increase in the money supply, the inflation and the new types of luxuries and foods (from cocoa, coffee and tea through tobacco and sugar-cane to potatoes and vegetables of every kind). For the ordinary man and woman in the Europe of the time local conditions were infinitely more important than the discovery of distant new lands and the importation of all kinds of priceless valuables.

At all events, it was only later that the mediaeval and the Reformation faith of Christianity was to be shaken by the 'discovery' of whole continents of non-believers or peoples of other faiths. As we heard, despite reforms, in religious terms Spain in particular remained imprisoned in the mediaeval paradigm and in that same year, 1492, took extremely cruel measures against the Jews. Even at the great disputation in 1550, Juan Ginés de Sepúlveda successfully argued that the races were unequal, against the arguments drawn from natural law presented by Bartolomé de La Casas. The latter was committed to equal rights for all human beings, though these were to be established only very much later.

But wasn't **Christopher Columbus**, the bold discoverer, an utterly modern man? Hardly in his view of the world. For even this Cristóbal Colón from Genoa, a brilliant and purposeful master of seafaring and cartography, set out on his transatlantic voyage, planned for years and organized rationally, still completely motivated by partly fantastic mediaeval notions and fabulous expectations. In reality the passage westwards to India was almost twice as long as he had assumed on the erroneous information of Ptolemy (12,500 miles instead of 6,500), and as we know, the coasts which Columbus discovered were not the eastern frontiers of 'India' (China and Japan), as he firmly believed to his death, but the periphery of a hitherto completely unknown continent, America.

Moreover, in piety and ethics, too, Columbus was an utterly mediaeval man who promoted his prospecting voyage (above all for gold and other riches) as being at the same time a missionary voyage (for the traditional Catholic faith). He had looked for every possible 'prophecy' in the Bible for his enterprise, and took it for granted that those outside the Catholic Church were damned. In the old Crusader mentality he could see war against unbelievers a priori as a 'just war' and engage in colonization and Christianization in the spirit of the Augustinian *coge intrare* ('Force them to come in'). He thought that part of the gold he discovered could be used to finance a new crusade to Palestine, which he would lead personally.

In short, none of the Conquistadores were 'modern men' in the strict sense. Nor did they bring any 'modernity' to the people of the new continent, but an utterly traditional, mediaeval Roman Catholic paradigm (P III). So under the Spanish Portuguese rule (in contrast, say, to the Christian mission in the early church) it was impossible for any autochthonous, **Indian paradigm** of Christianity to develop (like the Hellenistic paradigm in the early period): mission was part of colonization and at least superficially eliminated the allegedly primitive religions of the natives and uprooted the mentalities which governed their lives.

Even the political and intellectual elites of Europe needed time just to begin to grasp the far-reaching effects of the European expansion and the global geographical, transportational, economic and political problems that it posed. Only in the seventeenth century were the discoveries of what were in fact well-inhabited giant new continents retrospectively and intrinsically to affect, unsettle and change the picture of the world and the faith held by European Christians: the **ecumene** (the whole inhabited earth) **and Christianity** were manifestly **not identical**. But this was now already the time of the Enlightenment, the time of real modernity, when after all the confessional disputes and wars, toleration was being propagated not only for the various confessions but also for the various religions.

That means that it was not the discoveries in themselves but the new philosophy and experimental science, the new natural and international law, and the new secularized understanding of politics and the state which would characterize the modern paradigm (P V) of Christianity in the real sense. We shall go on to investigate this. The course of analysing the modern paradigm will be shorter, but it will have infinite branches and be extremely difficult to survey.[6] We shall note **several major thrusts towards modernization.**

2. The new political constellation in Europe

Two well known and unique monuments, basically different, can serve as illustrations of the epoch-making change:
– the solitary, cool and grey monastic palace of the **Escorial** in the hills of Castile, which the most powerful man in the second half of the sixteenth century, the Habsburg Philip II of Spain, an orthodox Catholic through and through, had built as a residence, a seat of authority and at the same time a monastic centre of prayer and learning (with a church at the centre) and a dynastic funerary monument. To commemorate his victory over the French on St Lawrence's Day it was built on the plan of a grid (the instrument of St Lawrence's martyrdom in the third century): a monument to the battle and victory of the Counter-Reformation;
– the splendid chateau of **Versailles**, erected on marshland but now surrounded by a gigantic artificial landscape garden, which the most powerful man in the second half of the seventeenth century, Louis XIV of France (who came to power in 1661), a worldly 'Catholic' autocrat through and though, had built for himself by thirty thousand temporary labourers. It was the residence of the French kings until the Revolution, a highly representative classical state building (with the 'Chambre du Roi' at the centre and the church at the side), on which the whole of Europe was then orientated; above the gates the glory of the Sun King was proclaimed in golden letters: *nec pluribus impar*. The chateau was as it were the cult place for the absolutist monarchy and its paraliturgy.

The seventeenth century – a turning point

At the beginning of the seventeenth century Catholic **Spain** (in 1598 Philip II had died in his Escorial at the age of seventy-one) was still the greatest, richest, strongest and most feared power in Europe – despite the defeat in 1588 of the great invasion fleet against England (the 'invincible Armada') and three state bankruptcies (1557, 1575, 1596). Spanish soldiers, colonists and ships could now be encountered all over the New World. The Spanish *'siglo de oro'*, the 'golden age', extended almost to the middle of the century, particularly in culture – with Lope de Vega, Cervantes and Calderón, with Velázquez, Zurbarán and Murillo. In Europe people still read Spanish literature enthusiastically, admired Spanish wealth and Spanish culture, and imitated the Spanish court style.

Only **around the middle of the century,** with the defeat of Spain by France (1643) and the Peace of the Pyrenees (1659), with the loss of the Netherlands (1648) and Portugal (1689), did the **collapse of Spanish power** become evident. And by the end of the century Spain was no longer part of the group of major European powers. But who took its place?

Germany and Italy were out of the running; at the beginning of the seventeenth century they were irrelevant to world politics. **Germany,** in theory ruled by the emperor, was in fact a chequered realm of hundreds of electorates, principalities, duchies and cities, and moreover after the 1555 religious peace of Augsburg was confessionally divided, with the Counter-Reformation on the advance. The German empire? It was an area in which foreign powers operated, threatened by a new Islamic offensive lanched by Sultan Mehmed III, a man who had proclaimed himself as ruler of the whole world from the rising to the setting of the sun. And **Italy**? Having fallen prey to the great powers as a result of the dissension between the city states (the papal state, Milan, Florence, Naples, Venice and Genoa), at the time it was largely occupied by Spain. And Pope Clement VIII (1592–1605) was more concerned with his papal state than with Christianity and warding off the Turks, who moreover were twice in the future to advance as far as Vienna.

The **Thirty Years' War** (1648–1648) in many places turned Germany into a battlefield and a ruin, with a population reduction of fifty per cent in the country and thirty per cent in the towns. Originally a civil war and war of religion, in its later phases, especially after Sweden under Gustaf Adolf and France under Richelieu had entered the war, it had become an international, European war, purely a matter of power politics. In the end Germany was so exhausted and reduced in power that for many decades it could not recover either politically or culturally from the terrible turmoil of the war. The Netherlands and Switzerland left the imperial alliance.

Here we already have clear signs of the paradigm shift to a new entire constellation:

- The great crisis of the seventeenth century was the Thirty Years' War, which as a confessional war took confessionalism *ad absurdum.*
- The era was ended by the Peace of Westphalia (1648), which cemented confessional relationships in the German empire, domesticated the confessions and thus laid the foundations for confessional peace.
- The offensive power of Protestantism (P IV) seemed to have been broken, and the confession was subordinated to the state. However, the attempts to rebuild the imperial Catholic universal monarchy (P III) had finally failed. The papacy, which protested in vain against the clauses in the Peace of Westphalia which related to the churches, disappeared

from international law as a regulating authority and was not replaced by any institution which transcended the state.

• The confessional principle of organization was worn out, and left a vacuum in the inter-state sphere. The age of confessions was replaced by the age of absolutism (1648–1789).[7]

Given this upheaval, it seems more of a secondary question whether after the middle of the seventeenth century not only Germany but almost all of Europe did not find itself in a deep and persistent social and cultural **structural crisis**. Various investigations, first by English (E. J. Hobsbawm, T. K. Rabb, H. R. Trevor-Roper) and French (R. Mousnir), and finally also by German historians (H.Lehmann[8]), have been able to point to critical developments: a stagnation in population, a decline in agriculture, trade and commerce, a rise in prices, an increase in illiteracy, combined with a far-reaching uncertainty about moral values and norms; concern and anxiety rather than confidence and hope were predominant. However, some historians will dispute whether the different economic and political phenomena of crisis amounted to a coherent and 'universal' crisis.[9]

At all events, it is a fact that a whole series of revolts and civil wars shook the time, especially in Catalonia, Portugal and the kingdom of Naples, but also in England, France and other parts of Europe. At that time in fact the European states largely lacked police, standing armies, bureaucracy, the means of mass communication and a national sense generally. Moreover, to many political thinkers (like Spinoza and Hobbes), who argued rationally, **royal absolutism** seemed the only means of averting chaos and guaranteeing internal peace. So a strong central government was needed for the preservation of law and order. Alongside all the political disputes, there were still the late effects of the Reformation, with which even the churches could not cope, above all the disputes between the advocates of divine predestination and the advocates of the freedom of the will: between Remonstrants and Counter-Remonstrants in Holland, between Puritans and Arminians in England, and between Jansenists and Jesuits in France and the Netherlands, the Spanish Netherlands. So once again the question arises: who replaced Spain as the chief European power?

A shift of the centre of power to the Atlantic

A further indicator of the far-reaching paradigm shift was this: around the middle of the seventeenth century there was a new **shift in historical balance** in European history. This was a shift no longer just, as in the time of the Reformation and Counter-Reformation, from the Mediterranean

(P iii) to Central Europe (P IV), but now from the centre of Europe to the western peripheral zone of the **Atlantic nations** (P V). Instead of the Spaniards and Portuguese, now the Dutch, French and English controlled the 'free ocean' for their fleets, and in countless voyages of discovery and conquest advanced systematically into new parts of the earth, not only to 'discover them', but to occupy them, settle them and step by step exploit them for their own markets (colonialism). The disadvantage of being on the maritime periphery had thus proved a new advantage. A colonial five-power rule developed (alongside Portugal and Spain, increasingly France, England and the Netherlands), which for a long time felt responsible for the modern political, legal and economic world order.

In this form, this was a new phenomenon in human history: a worldwide European colonialism with highly ambivalent consequences. In the framework of earlier paradigms the Mediterranean was the geographical centre of the nations; in the seventeenth century this centre moved to the Atlantic, on the European coast of which new metropolises developed (after Seville and Lisbon came Antwerp, Amsterdam and London). Now overseas trade exceeded Mediterranean trade, and European international law also came to apply on the continents overseas. The European paradigm of modernity was a **colonialist paradigm** – and this had consequences for Christianity.

The new age belonged to the **Protestant maritime powers**. Leaving aside the Swedes and Danes in the North, now the leading maritime and colonial power was the **United Netherlands** (States General), which succeeded in gaining independence from Spain in an eighty-year war of liberation (1567–1648) ending in the Peace of Westphalia in 1648. Particularly in the period of the twelve-year cease-fire (concluded in 1609), the Netherlands, with a rich middle class which supported the state and the Dutch East India Company, succeeded in building the largest merchant fleet in the world at that time, establishing a colonial empire in East Asia and developing Amsterdam into the largest harbour and the hub of world trade. Indeed, with the founding of an utterly new discount house (1609), Amsterdam also became the centre of European currency exchange. Here the Netherlands benefitted from the flight of so many Jews from the Iberian peninsula, who were very successful in this free country.[10] At first **England**, at that time preoccupied with national problems under the Stuarts (1603–1689), still largely went its own way.

The main power to benefit from the decline of Spain and the German empire on the European continent was undoubtedly **France**. At the beginning of the seventeenth century still torn apart by the eight Wars of Religion (1562–1598) and ravaged by hunger, plague and emigration, it recovered strongly in the course of the century and became the **most**

modern state in Europe. France owed this astonishing change in fortunes to the genius of three great power politicians – Henry IV, Richelieu and Mazarin – who led France to European hegemony along the way of a centralist **absolutism** which later became the model for almost all Europe:
– **King Henry IV** (1594), as a Bourbon first the leader of the Reformed 'Huguenots', had become a Catholic in 1593 when the crown of France was to be won ('Paris is worth a mass'). By a policy of reconstruction Henry also attempted to overcome the catastrophic effects of the Huguenot wars on the basis of a new state authority and a purge of state finances, and to pacify the land both internally and externally. France remained a Catholic monarchy, but with no Counter-Reformation zeal; in the Edict of Nantes (1598) the 1.2 million Reformed were granted freedom of conscience, limited freedom of worship, equal civic rights, and indeed were ensured political and military power in 200 cities, safe places in which Huguenots were in the majority. Now in fact the Protestants formed a state within the state.
– **Cardinal Richelieu,** under Louis XIII, Henry's son, the omnipotent *'premier ministre'* (between 1624–42 in charge of domestic, foreign and defence policy, the army and the secret service which he created), developed the policy of national self-assertion further and despite an economic recession subordinated his policy to two aims. At home, he sought to establish the absolutist power of the king against anarchy, the autonomy of the feudal lords and parliament, but also against the rebellious people, above all the peasants. Abroad, he sought to establish French domination in Europe against the Spanish army, the English fleet and the German mercenary forces. He resolutely withdrew the Huguenots' special political and military (but not religious) rights and destroyed their political organization by campaigns in the west and south which he conducted personally, thus removing the existence of the 'state within a state' (1628–29). Here, cardinal of the Holy Roman Church though he was, he entered into coldly calculating alliances even with Protestant powers simply to break the grip on France by the (Catholic!) Habsburgs (in Spain, the German empire and Italy). A modern man through and through, Richelieu put 'reasons of state' above all ecclesiastical and confessional interests. As part of a systematic cultural policy he founded the Académie Française to cultivate the French language.
– **Cardinal Mazarin** (Giulio Mazarini), originally a papal negotiator, then an admirer and collaborator of Richelieu's, and finally his successor as First Minister (1643–1661), completed Richelieu's policy of absolutist centralization by abolishing the political rights of the estates and defeating the aristocratic Fronde, by developing the army and the fleet, by an alliance with Cromwell's England and by establishing French hege-

mony over Austria in the Peace of Westphalia (1648) and Spain in the Peace of the Pyrenees (1659).

So the foundations had been laid for the definitive replacement of the 'Spanish age' with the **French age**, which was to be represented by no one in a more splendid way than by the grandson of Henry IV, Louis XIV, on whose upbringing Mazarin had a decisive influence. However, we must first consider what this new European constellation of power means in the context of our paradigm analysis. The policy of the European powers, which everywhere shows features of centralization, social discipline and militarization, raises many basic questions which have only partly been resolved in modernity. I shall now comment briefly on them.

The principles of modern European politics

From a political perspective the rise of modernity displays the following characteristics which distinguish it from the mediaeval and increasingly also from the Reformation paradigm.

After the failure of the efforts of Charles V and Philip II at hegemony, the one universal empire in succession to Rome was replaced with a juxtaposition of **modern territorial states with equal rights**. These had already begun to develop in the thirteenth and fourteenth centuries, when the two greatest forces of the Middle Ages, *imperium* and *sacerdotium*, failed. But this development raised a theoretical and practical **question**: how were the state and its representative to be legitimated? And who should have the **supreme authority** in a Europe in which neither emperor nor Pope could play a dominant role?

The answer was that in place of emperor and Pope now only the **individual king** made a claim to supreme power, to a 'sovereignty' free from ties on all sides. The theoretical foundation for this was first laid by **Jean Bodin** in his novel state doctrine, *Les six livres de la République* (1576),[11] developed programmatically to overcome the anarchical consequences of the Huguenot wars. The monarch is depicted as the embodiment of state sovereignty – to avert the claims to power put forward by the French estates (internal constitutional sovereignty) and to avoid possible demands by Pope and emperor (external international sovereignty). So genuine supreme power was attributed to the national ruler – albeit under the law of God and natural law (decisions on war and peace, unlimited power of legislation), which could be replaced by no other power on earth and was therefore utterly independent.

In the next century, the English polymath and theoretician of state absolutism, **Thomas Hobbes**, a contemporary and acquaintance of Descartes and Galileo, argued in the same direction. Faced with the chaotic conditions in England, he similarly spoke out for a strong state, which he called *Leviathan* (1655), a mortal god.[12] Here was the first vision of the monster of a modern central power: freed from all restrictions by a superior idea of law and at the same time based on a quite natural social treaty (a treaty of submission) between the people and the monarch. For in order to avoid the war of all against all, according to Hobbes human beings, totally governed by the drive for self-preservation and equal by nature, had to renounce their natural rights and transfer them to a sovereign. Granted, Hobbes derived the monarchy 'by the grace of God' from natural foundations and thus forcibly robbed it of its mystique, but the power transferred to the ruler was equally inalienable and indivisible. Resistance to it was not allowed. In Hobbes (who uses arguments from scripture), religion and church appear completely subordinated to the purpose of stabilizing rule. Politics must be above religion (with its disputes). A de-theologizing and de-confessionalizing of public life seemed necessary; the result was a sharper politicization and bureaucratization.

This secularized state theory of natural law had been prepared for by the Dominican Vitoria, the Jesuit Suárez and the Spanish natural law theorists of the sixteenth century. Its foundations were then laid by Grotius, the 'secularizer' of natural law, Hobbes, Locke and Pufendorf. It is a theory which sees the state as the natural product of a treaty between people and government – in principle without any 'grace of God' and with no supernatural aims. Such a constitutional theory notionally based on a treaty would make it possible, a century later, for the sovereignty first attributed to the ruler of the state to be attributed by a man like Rousseau on the eve of the French Revolution to the people itself. However, a **question** arises: didn't the sovereignty founded on natural law in fact amount internally to an **absolutist monopolizing** of state power and externally to a dangerous **national encapsulization** from other states?

Indeed, on the scale of political values the **nation** now increasingly took over **first place** from religion. Alongside God, it became the supreme value even for the king; very much later in the revolution it would even replace God and king. The modern Europe is a **Europe of nations**. However, the awareness of an otherness and special character by virtue of descent, language, history, religion, 'mission' all too easily leads to a failure to appreciate other nationalities and to animosity towards them. Hence the **question**: isn't a fanaticism which justifies any means and which hitherto had mostly been bound up with religion, here transferred to the nation, which in modern **nationalism** justifies all means and permits what was previously impermissible?

The answer is that now in fact reason (or more precisely **reasons of state**) replaces confessional interests and ethical considerations, along with an appeal to the inherent laws of politics. The basis for this had already been laid by the Florentine Renaissance thinker **Nicolò Machiavelli** (1469–1527), though he did not seek to be the apologist for any power politics.[13] '*Ragione di stato*' (a phrase of Guicciardini's), reasons of state, mean that the good of the state, more precisely the preservation and extension of power, has to be the criterion and maxim for state action. Therefore a mode of action is permissible for the state and politics which, if need be, ignores existing law or prevailing morality. Such 'reasons of state' can deviate from the ethical norms which the individual reason, the individual conscience, has to follow. The ruler, who wisely in all things gives the appearance of gentleness, mercy and humanity, may and should offend against loyalty and honesty, mercy and humanity, for the sake of his rule.

Richelieu, who of course also acted under certain constraints in foreign and domestic policy, elevated reasons of state to be the basic principle of French foreign policy and practised an unscrupulous policy in the interest of France. Though he claimed it was dictated by reason, in fact it was orientated purely on power. Here treachery, intrigue and murder were as permissible as the suppression of minorities or an alliance with 'ideological opponents', with Protestant powers and even with the Islamic Turks. However, the **question** is: in such Realpolitik, are not **wars** a priori **pre-programmed** by the criteria of autonomous 'reasons of state'?

This is precisely what characterizes modernity: there is no longer a battle between Pope and emperor, as in the mediaeval paradigm; or between Catholics and Protestants, as in the Reformation paradigm; but now there is a **struggle for national hegemony in Europe**. The aim is to dominate, and in order to attain a dominant position, military conflicts will constantly be provoked and the sovereignty of other states will be unscrupulously violated. However, modern war is a **purely secular war**, waged without heed to the religious or confessional position of the opponent. War, now completely 'secularized', is more than ever regarded as basically unavoidable and in practice ineradicable and is waged with increasing expense and refinement. That being so, however, the **question** is how in such a Europe sovereign nations will avoid a war of annihilation involving all against all: the Thirty Years' War – possibly a prelude to even greater European wars, perhaps even a 'world war'.

Already in the fifteenth and sixteenth centuries, also in Italy, the idea of a genuine, permanent **balance of power** in Europe came into being (from the seventeenth century on this was then favoured above all by England, the coming leader as a maritime and colonial power). It became the dominant principle of the modern state system and thus a practical limit on national sovereignty. Moreover, this idea of a balance of power in Europe then succeeded in blunting individual conflicts, and over the centuries in thwarting the efforts of individuals – whether Philip II of Spain, Louis XIV of France, Napoleon I, or Wilhelm II of Germany (not to mention Hitler) – by alliances and changes of alliances ('*renversement des alliances*') between the other powers. The **question** is: could this idea of a 'concert of European powers' also prevent the competition and incessant wars between the nations? Despite countless European conferences or congresses and the demarcation of economic, military and political spheres of interest, **peace could not really be guaranteed**. Wasn't the Peace of Westphalia in 1648 itself a tremendous disappointment, since the second half of the seventeenth century was also full of war; the Peace of Westphalia – a model for further similarly unstable peace treaties (later even a 'Versailles')?

Many set their hope on a **new international law**. This was to be no longer canon law, Roman or Germanic law as in the Middle Ages and Reformation, but that international law the foundations of which were laid by legal theorists like Vitoria and Suárez, and which was developed on the basis of natural law, as we saw, by Jean Bodin, Richard Zouch, Hugo Grotius and Samuel von Pufendorf. But the '*deus legislator*' of the Spaniards was now hardly still necessary. Now, without any ethical and religious foundation, international law was to regulate relations between the nations and especially make the waging of war on land and water more tolerable and more humane. According to Pufendorf's realistic conception, international law consists partly of natural law dictated by reason and partly of customs usual among civilized peoples.

However, just how problematical these principles of modern politics were can be seen where they were pushed to the limit in the form of the sovereign nation state, reasons of state and the struggle for hegemony. And this happened first (centuries before they were finally brought into disrepute by Napoleon and, infinitely worse, by the Nazis and Socialism) under the absolutist regime of Louis XIV.

The modern power state: Louis XIV

Louis XIV[14] may never have really uttered the famous saying '*L'état, c'est moi*', but he acted on this principle, though as more recent historiography has brought out, his power in fact had its limits and the king constantly had to take into account the old 'estates' and customary law (property!). Giving a religious foundation and religious trimmings to his autonomy, by a reckless foreign policy Louis painfully disturbed the balance of

European power. No one could prevent him, for the claim of the national ruler had been heightened to an almost superhuman level. What since the Gregorian reform had been attributed uniquely to the absolutist mediaeval Popes was now, in a time when the Popes no longer had much political significance, attributed by the modern absolute state ruler to himself: 'God, who has appointed kings over men, wills that honour be shown to these as his representatives on earth; he alone has the right to judge them.' Thus Louis XIV, claiming for himself the Roman dictum *prima sedes a nemine iudicatur*.[15] Instead of 'one God – one Christ – one faith – one Pope' it was now '*un Dieu – une foi – une loi – un roi*'. Here were state and crown as a God-given dynastic possession and the unity of the state superelevated by the unity of faith!

After the death of Mazarin in 1661 the now twenty-three-year-old Louis – from his youth fearful of rebellions by the Fronde and the Paris mob – made himself his own prime minister. By being incorporated into a refined system of well-endowed court posts the aristocracy, robbed of its power, was misled over its political impotence; parliament was completely stripped of its power. The real power did not lie in the court with its 4,000 members, but with the king and a 'cabinet' (originally small room) consisting of a few highly qualified ministers, all from the middle class. **Louis' centralistic power state** was developed systematic- ally, the standing army equipped and the apparatus of taxation and administration modernized, supported by a finance minister named Colbert, who through a 'mercantile' trade policy (the state-controlled development of large-scale manufacturing and the promotion of exports coupled with restrictions on the import of finished goods by protective tolls) was able to provide the king with more and more finance. This was a system which despite everything was in many respects fragile, incohe- rent and prone to crises, directly effective only at the upper levels of the state, but with its militarism, bureaucracy and mercantilism it resulted in a thoroughgoing **social disciplining**.[16]

Louis cold-bloodedly planned and carried out **wars of conquest** in order to gain more territory and influence everywhere – even overseas. At first he was successful. And at the same time a new age dawned for the court culture and art of France, '*le grand siècle*', in the course of which France rose to become the **leading cultural nation** in Europe. Influenced by geometry, French classicism replaced the exuberance of baroque and now dictated taste even beyond France. Paris and the splendid chateau of Versailles (begun in 1661, finished in 1682) rather than Rome or Madrid was now the capital of culture; French and no longer Latin was the world language (and also the language of treaties). Corneille, Racine and Molière in literature; Poussin, Le Brun and

Mansart in painting and architecture; Lully, Rameau and Couperin in music, set the tone.

Everything – at least externally – went on in a highly ordered, symmetrical, indeed geometrical way: according to historical research, **geometry was the dominant characteristic of the era.**[17] Geometrical patterns provided orientation – from the state as a rationally constructed machine, through state buildings, fortifications and garden landscaping to drill and fencing, music and dancing. Attempts were even made to make the arts mathematical and adopt a scientific approach to life generally.

The 'Roi Soleil' with the omnipresent sun emblem was a politically powerful ruler, conscientious but intellectually rather superficial. Hardly a really religious man, he used **religion** brilliantly to **legitimize** his absolutism. For him the cultivation of the role of the ruler, making it charismatic and sacral, was no less important than modernization, centralization and bureaucratization. The disciplined course of the day (pompously ritualized, from the solemn rising to the solemn retiring to bed) even included a midday mass after the morning state council, but this did not prevent Louis going to one of his mistresses immediately afterwards, as he also did in the evening after supper.[18]

Louis' church policy aimed at a domesticated state church system, so he did not shrink even from conflict with Rome. His court bishop Bossuet, a leading Catholic theologian and preacher at this time, gave a virtuoso theological defence of the rights of the monarch directly appointed by God, responsible only to God, and all-powerful over his subjects, which was quite different from that of Hobbes. In the four 'Gallican Articles' he formulated the church-political self-understanding of the absolutist state (condemned in 1690 by Pope Alexander VII),[19] though ultimately without success. Louis XIV pursued a policy of confessionalizing, not for primarily religious grounds but equally for political reasons; as early as 1685 he repealed the Edict of Nantes and with the help of his dragoons sought the forcible conversion of the Reformed, so that more than a quarter of a million often educated and economically productive Huguenots emigrated with their know-how to Holland, Brandenburg-Prussia, England and even South Africa – to the detriment of France and its prestige in Europe.

The Sun King, obsessed with a greed for '*gloire*' for himself and '*grandeur*' for France, certainly ruled over the most populated, uniform and best-organized land in Europe. But his expensive armaments and his spendthrift character finally brought the state to the verge of bankruptcy, and his unnecessary conflicts and wars of conquest goaded all the other European powers to oppose him. Moreover the balance of power in Europe was in extreme danger. **Decline** followed as early as the 1680s, and was sealed in the thirteen-year War of the Spanish Succession, which fell in the last phase of Louis' rule (1701–1713). Insatiable in his lust for power, Louis had now also laid claim to the Spanish crown (for his nephew) and thus was again in bitter rivalry with the house of Habsburg. But gradually the people became weary of Louis' absolutist rule, and criticism of his regime grew louder and louder. France was forced back into the European balance of power.

However, at the beginning of the eighteenth century it was no longer the Catholic Habsburgs but the Protestant **maritime powers**, with strong finances and fleets, first Holland and then England, which proved to be France's most dangerous enemies. In both countries Parliament had prevented the total breakthrough of the royal absolutism which now gained the upper hand as far as Sweden, Poland and Russia. By voyages and trade, by prosperity and full state coffers (the Bank of England was also founded in 1694), Holland and England had created the foundations for their role in world history and their own 'golden age'. Since the 'Glorious (because bloodless) Revolution', England had been on the way to a constitutional monarchy and to a real **political alternative** to continental absolutism and soon became a model for the European Enlightenment. Finally, England was the leading power overseas and the arbitrator in Europe.

On his death bed, Louis XIV confessed that he himself had loved war too much and had been a spendthrift. Moreover the results of this policy were a decline in the population from 21 million in 1700 to 18 million in 1715, and the state household overdrawn by eighteen years' debts facing financial ruin and in the hands of private financiers, so that the people felt that Louis' death was a liberation and threw stones at his coffin. But neither his great-grandson Louis XV nor the next king, Louis XVI (who was to be guillotined eighty years later), had the power to change social structures which had already become untenable under Louis. This was a main cause of the Revolution. A French biographer, P.Goubert, rightly wrote of Louis XIV: 'Isolated in Versailles at a very early stage by his arrogance, an intriguer and a handful of priests and courtiers, he ignored and wanted to ignore the fact that this was an age of reason, science and freedom.'[20] An age of reason, science and freedom – what form was it taking?

3. The revolutions in science and philosophy

The revolution of modernity was primarily an **intellectual revolution**. Already a generation before Descartes and Galileo, in a synthesis of science, ethics and social reform, **Francis Bacon,** the English politician, philosopher and great pioneer (he died in 1626) had developed the utopian social model of a *Nova Atlantis*.[21] He argued that knowledge is power, and modern science should make it possible for all the needs of humanity to be satisfied without a collision: a constructive policy with the help of scientific technical experts, and thus a universal peace. In fact the **first great power of rising modernity is science.**

What Bacon proclaimed, but hardly laid the foundation for by empirical experiment, was initiated methodically by Galileo, Descartes and Pascal, followed by Spinoza, Leibniz and Locke, Newton, Huygens and Boyle. Are not the names of these geniuses (apart from Leibniz, barely a name from the lands in which the Reformation originated!) more representative of modernity, more expressive and to the present day more admirable than Louis XIV and all the names of the absolutist rulers of early modernity, which are now remembered only by historians? They were the ones who gained international significance and laid the foundation for the **new feeling of the superiority of reason,** which promised a quasi-geometrical certainty. And this superiority was to become the main characteristic of modernity. It stood behind both the scientific and the philosophical revolutions of the seventeenth century. The American economic theorist Stephen Toulmin therefore rightly speaks of a 'Counter-Renaissance' with a rational orientation in this century and of the vision of a 'cosmopolis' which now arose, i.e. of a society the rational order of which corresponded to the Newtonian picture of nature.[22]

The scientific revolution: Galileo – Newton

It was not a secularized scientist but a Catholic dean in royal Polish Prussia who, going back to an idea of Aristarchus of Samos, on the basis of his own observations, calculations and geometrical-kinetic reflections, laid the foundation for a truly revolutionary world-system: **Nicolaus Copernicus** (1473–1543). He studied above all in Italy and, as is well known, in his work *De revolutionibus orbium coelestium libri VI* (Six Books on the Circular Motions of the Heavenly Bodies)[23] proposed the heliocentric world system in place of the traditional geocentric world system of Ptolemy, which had proved increasingly unsuitable for predicting the positions of planets over long periods. This was a paradigm shift *par excellence*, first in physics, but then with effects on the whole view of the world and human metaphysics. The 'Copernican shift' became a proverb for various fundamental shifts which constitute modernity, a prime example of what a 'paradigm shift' means.

But the new model of the world, put forward purely theoretically and as a hypothesis by Copernicus and then confirmed and corrected, only appeared highly threatening to the traditional biblical picture of the world when the Italian mathematician, physicist and philosopher **Galileo Galilei** (1564–1642)[24] discovered with a telescope developed from a Dutch model the phases of Venus, four moons of Jupiter and the rings of Saturn, and found that the clusters of stars and the Milky Way consisted of individual stars. Here was an irrefutable confirmation of the Copernican model, according to which the earth goes round the sun, by a brilliant scholar who with the introduction of the quantitative experiment (the pendulum and the laws of gravity) became the **founder of modern science**. The basis was now laid for the demonstration of the laws of nature and for unlimited research into nature, which was to embrace increasingly new spheres. Of course Galileo himself recognized the threat posed by his researches to the biblical picture of the world. He presented his views on the relationship between the Bible and natural knowledge in a letter to the Benedictine B.Castelli[25] in 1613: if scientific knowledge holds, then a new interpretation of the Bible is due.

Galileo was confirmed a good two generations later in a big way by the no less brilliant English mathematician, physicist and astronomer Sir **Isaac Newton**. A professor at Cambridge, in 1687 he published his *magnum opus Philosophiae naturalis principia mathematica*,[26] in which he brought together his formulations of the three axioms of mechanics and his law of gravity, already discovered two decades earlier – all applied to the movement of the heavenly bodies (heavenly mechanics). At the same time he had discovered the nature of light and electricity and simultaneously with Leibniz had laid the foundation for infinitesimal and differential calculus. Whereas Descartes and Galileo provided just fragments, from these and other discoveries Newton rationally demonstrated a **convincing new world system**. Thus after Galileo Newton became the second founder of the exact natural sciences, the founder of classical theoretical physics, which was only to be modified at the beginning of the twentieth century by Einstein's theory of relativity.

And the church? The Inquisition

But how did the church react to this new picture of the world? What was its attitude to this Copernican 'shift of the entire constellation'? It is well known and significant that even Dean Copernicus delayed publication of his work almost up to his death – for fear of the Index and the stake. Was this perhaps a typically Roman Catholic anxiety about the new, above all about the new natural philosophy and natural sciences? No, the Reformers Luther and Melanchthon also rejected the work of Copernicus. As it had only a theoretical foundation, and had been presented only as a hypothesis, they thought that they could neglect it.

Moreover, Copernicus was only put on the list of forbidden books in 1616 – when the Galileo case became acute. **Religion** had now largely become the **power to persist**, the Catholic Church an institution which instead of being concerned about intellectual understanding, strictness and assimilation, called for censorship, the Index and the Inquisition.

That same year – three years after the letter to Castelli – the first great clash between Galileo and Rome took place. Whereas the Renaissance Popes were slow to be disturbed either by the discovery of new parts of the earth or the discoveries in the sphere of natural science, under the Popes of the Counter-Reformation the attitude of the Roman church also hardened in this respect:

– In 1600 the former Dominican **Giordano Bruno,** who had combined the Copernican model of the world with a pantheizing Neo-Platonic mystical Renaissance piety (and who in 1579 had even been expelled by the strict Protestant University of Tübingen after the Senate had refused him the *licentia docendi*[27]), was burned on the Campo de' Fiori in Rome.

– Already a year previously the anti-Aristotelian philosopher **Tommaso Campanella** had been condemned by the Inquisition. In prison he had then written his utopian *Città del Sole* (*The City of the Sun*, 1602),[28] and only managed to flee to France in 1645; the Jesuits tried to implement his ideal state with a comprehensive organization and no private property, ruled by authorities made up of wise men and priests, in the Indian reductions of Paraguay.

– In 1619 the Italian natural philosopher **Lucilio Vanini** was burnt at the stake in Toulouse because he had allegedly taught the identity of God and nature. Truly at that time it was fatal to fall into the hands of the Inquisition!

In 1632 **Galileo,** too, was now cited **before the Inquisition** and condemned on the basis of a prohibition allegedly pronounced in 1616. Apparently he did not make the legendary statement 'And yet it moves'. Nor, as is often asserted, was he subjected to torture. But in any case, the pressure was so great that as a loyal Catholic on 22 June 1633 he abjured his 'error'. Even then, however, he was still condemned to indefinite house arrest at his villa in Arcetri, where he remained among his pupils for eight years (he went blind after four years) and where he prepared the work on mechanics and the laws of gravity which was so important for the future development of physics.

Was Galileo's conflict with the church an unhappy chance? No, it was a **symptomatic precedent**, which poisoned at the roots the relationship between the new, rising natural sciences and the church and religion, especially since the attitude of Rome did not change later, but even hardened with the progress of science (and later especially of biological research, with Charles Darwin). The Galileo affair has often provided material for dramas – by the Marxist Bert Brecht, the Jew Max Brod and the Catholic Getrud von Le Fort – and now in our day a Pope whose judgments in matters of biology and the pill are as infallibly wrong as those of his predecessors in matters of astronomy and the heliocentric world has made himself look ridiculous by thinking that he could rehabilitate Galileo Galilei 350 years after his death. As if Galileo had not already been rehabilitated by Newton and the history of science![29]

This whole development confirms that official Catholic Church policy was fixated on the restoration of the mediaeval Counter-Reformation paradigm (P III), regardless of any losses (though of course at that time they could not yet be foreseen). So after the excommunication of the Protestants there was an almost silent **emigration of the natural scientists** from the church, a permanent conflict betwen science and the prevailing normative theology; moreover Italy and Spain, under the thumb of the Inquisition, did not produce any scientists. But even Rome could not stop the collapse of the mediaeval structure of the world with its disc of earth between heaven above and hell below; it could not stop the demystification of nature and the overcoming of mediaeval belief in the Devil, demons, witches and magic. And is it amazing that now not only scientific research but also philosophical thought and even political power went their own ways?

The scientific revolution: Descartes

The condemnation of Galileo in 1633, implemented in Catholic countries at the universities with all the means of the nunciatures, with informers and inquisitors, spread such an atmosphere of fear that the cool mathematician, scientist and philosopher **René Descartes** (1596–1650) postponed publication of his treatise *On the World or Treatise on Light*[30] indefinitely; in fact it was only published fourteen years after Descartes' death. Although Descartes originally did not want to publish anything further, he finally did publish his *Discourse on Method*,[31] which became the second linguistic classic of French prose after Calvin's *Institutes* and made no small contribution to the replacement of Latin as the language of scholars.

The claim by Bertrand Russell, one of the best-known mathematicians and philosophers of our time, that nothing significant happened in philosophy before the seventeenth century, is certainly one of his exaggerations. But it is no exaggeration to make **modern philosophy begin** with the Frenchman Descartes. In 1620 Descartes left Richelieu's Paris for the freer 'heretical' Holland, where he spent most of the rest of his life. That life ended in Protestant Sweden, where he died at the age of fifty-four of inflammation of the lungs (Queen Christiane, who used to summon him to philosophize at five o'clock in the morning, had called him there).

Here indeed was a new method. For the **certainty of mathematics,** which excludes any doubt, was to be the new **epistemological ideal** for the new age of calculation and experimentation and the new natural sciences. And no one embodies this ideal of unconditional mathematical and philosophical certainty more brilliantly than Descartes, the founder of analytical geometry and modern philosophy, whose Latinized name Cartesius became synonymous with *clarté*, clarity of thought with a geometric stamp. Here the genuinely modern element in Descartes' philosophical approach becomes evident: in a totally different way from the Renaissance, without any heed to former thought, to philosophical and theological traditions and schools, to state or church authorities, this philosopher wants to investigate freely what human beings really know and how far they can come to a truly well-founded judgment. The name Descartes stands for a **radical new foundation of philosophy and human knowledge by each individual.** Individuals are to master their lives in the surest, most reasonable responsibility for themselves. This is a thoroughly modern idea. And here scientific theory is no longer the highest aim in life, as it is in Aristotle and even in Thomas Aquinas, but – in a highly modern and functional way – the means of realizing a (rational) practice.

And how are individuals to get the rock of certainty under their feet? According to Descartes by the bold way of the *tabula rasa*: methodical, radical and universal doubt. For it is precisely by going through all doubt that human beings can attain the basic insight: as long as I am doubting I am thinking, and as long as I am thinking, I am: '*Cogito, ergo sum*': 'I think, therefore I am'. So **the fact of one's own existence is the foundation of all certainty.** From this Archimedean point Descartes raises all the basic questions of philosophy: the three great questions of the self, of God (proofs of God) and material things. Here he makes a sharp distinction between *res extensa* (extension, body, matter, the outside world), and *res cogitans* (thought, spirit, the self, the inner world) and thus lays the foundation for the modern (idealist) opposition of subject and object, human being and nature (understood mechanistically) – a dualism which is the presupposition for Newton's mechanistic model of the world.

With Descartes the Western consciousness reached an **epoch-making turning point** in a critical development: the **place of original certainty** has been **transferred** from God **to human beings.** That means that in modern times the move is no longer, as in the Middle Ages or the Reformation, from certainty about God to certainty about the self, but from certainty about the self to certainty about God. 'Here, we may say, we are at home, and, like the mariner after a long voyage in a tempestuous sea, we may now hail the sight of land; with Descartes the culture of modern times really begins to appear.' Thus Hegel was to exclaim almost two hundred years later in his *Lectures on the History of Philosophy*, when he came to speak of Descartes.[32] In fact, despite all resistance, Cartesianism became very much more than a school. It became a way of thinking, an attitude, a part of education generally. Its history largely becomes the history of philosophy. Not only do rationalism, psychologism and above all idealism on the right appeal to Descartes but – understandably, given Descartes' sharp division of body and soul as two substances – so too do empiricism, mechanism and indeed materialism on the left.[33] Moreover, 'modern' also became synonymous with striving for certainty, for strict unemotional rationality, for a great system of philosophy, nature and social science.[34]

Proofs of God and counter-proofs impossible: Kant

What was developed in the continental rationalism of Spinoza, Bayle and Leibniz and in the English empiricism of Hobbes, Locke and Hume finds its first great empirical rational synthesis in **Immanuel Kant**; 'Kant expresses the modern world in an intellectual structure.'[35] So it is not fortuitous that Kant spoke of a 'Copernican shift' in philosophy.[36] For the starting point of knowledge is no longer the given object which is pictured in the human understanding, which the understanding receives more or less passively. The starting point is the human understanding which (together with the senses) actively imposes its forms (categories) on what is given by the senses and thus constitutes the object of knowledge in the first place. Hence the self-knowledge of the human reason, the human capacity for knowledge in all its dimensions, more precisely the self-knowledge of the pure understanding and the pure reason in so far as with their 'pure' concepts and ideas they a priori constitute and regulate our experiences and their objects. That is the prior, 'transcendental' question put by Kant about the way in which we know objects, about the conditions of the possibility of any human knowledge at all. In this way the whole of reality is constructed from the human subject. But does that mean that Kant denied God?

Time and again the man from Königsberg, who composed not only scientific but also important political writings and works on the history of philosophy, has been accused of **criticism** in his three *Critiques* (*of Pure Reason*, 1781; *of Practical Reason*, 1788; and *of Judgment*, 1790),[37] and thus of agnosticism and veiled atheism. This is unjust. For it was Kant in particular – from his position between orthodoxy and freethinking, between Franco-German rationalism and the English empiricism and scepticism of David Hume – who sought to protect belief in God in a time of rising atheism against a 'gaping reason', indeed who wanted to bind reason by its own chains.

Behind Kant's criticism does not lie, as is so often assumed, resignation in matters of reason, but the conviction, ultimately founded on ethics and religion, that limits must be set to reason and that the limits of reason are not identical with the limits of reality. What reason does not know can exist. In the preface to the second edition of the *Critique of Pure Reason*, Kant himself remarks, 'I have therefore found it necessary to deny **knowledge**, in order to make room for **faith**.'[38] Even for the 'critical' Kant – like the French philosopher of culture, Jean-Jacques Rousseau, whom he so treasured (the only picture in Kant's study!) – faith is a truth of the heart, or, better, the conscience, before and beyond all philosophical reflection and demonstration. As Kant himself attests at the end of his *Critique of Pure Reason*, 'Belief in a God and in another world is so interwoven with my moral sentiment that as there is little danger of my losing the latter, there is equally little cause for fear that the former can ever be taken from me.'[39]

No wonder, then, that Kant, the man of the Enlightenment, at the same time went beyond the Enlightenment in his three critiques. For Kant set sharp **limits** to the naive omnipotence of **reason** specifically in the knowledge of the wholly other **God**, as he did to naive faith. It is clear that scientific **proofs of God** are **impossible**. No scientific knowledge can be gained of God's existence which is not in space and time and so is not the object of intuition, nor can any judgments be made about it, since these depend on intuition. According to Kant, the proofs of God have not only failed in fact but are theoretically quite impossible. Why? 'All our conclusions, all attempts to employ reason in theology in any merely speculative manner, are altogether fruitless and, by their very nature, null and void.'[40] Religion spreads its wings in vain in order through the power of thought to get beyond the world of appearances to 'things in themselves' (which are necessary for thought but cannot be seen) or even to get to the real God. Human beings cannot build towers which reach to heaven, but only homes, roomy enough and high enough for our affairs on the level of experience. Yet clearly the reverse is also the case: all proofs against the existence God have also failed. What is to be done?

Because of this, in questions of the knowledge of God Kant does not appeal to the 'theoretical' but to the **'practical' reason**, which manifests itself in human action: it is not concerned with scientific knowledge and critical investigation but with the moral action of human beings and the conditions for this possibility. Kant argues from the self-understanding of human beings as moral, responsible beings: it is not just a question of 'is', but of 'ought', not just a question of science, but of morality. Specifically in the *Critique of Practical Reason* Kant therefore no longer turns his gaze outwards or upwards to a beyond (a 'transcendent'), but back behind himself, as it were inwards, to the pre-existing condition of possibility (the 'transcendental'): God as the condition of the possibility of morality and happiness. Whereas Descartes understood God above all as perfect being and infinite substance, Spinoza understood God as the only substance or God-nature, and Leibniz understood God as the infinite monad, Kant took his starting point not from natural objects but from human beings as moral beings, and thence postulated God – not from theoretical but from practical necessity – as the supreme moral being and author of the world.[41]

Both the scientific revolution (Galileo–Newton) and the philosophical revolution (Descartes) inevitably had serious effects on European society, where for so many centuries the church authorities had dominated all thought. They led to a cultural revolution which finally also resulted in a political revolution.

4. The revolutions in culture and theology

'Cleopatra's nose; had it been shorter, the whole aspect of the world would have been altered':[42] Blaise Pascal, one of the great pioneer thinkers who also warned about the new age, was right: the course of world history is often governed by small matters. And yet it is governed not only by unique 'starry hours of humanity', as Stefan Zweig put it, but also by the shifts in the great 'entire constellations' and by no means by chance 'world-shaking transitions' (Goethe).

The word 'modern' becomes modern

The seventeenth and eighteenth centuries, too, saw no more and no less than the transition to a new entire constellation, to the paradigm of modernity. The word **'modern'** is itself an old one; it comes from late antiquity.[43] Only in the early French seventeenth-century Enlightenment is it used as a positive designation for a new sense of the times. It is now an expression of protest against the Renaissance cyclical view of history, related to antiquity which (for all its distancing of itself from the preceding Christian period of the dark 'Middle Ages') did not use 'modern' as a term to describe an era; the Rinascimento (cf. P III) was too 'backward' looking, too orientated on antiquity, for that. Only now, in the seventeenth century, as the result of confidence in autonomous reason, did it arrive at a new sense of superiority. This found expression in a polemic which lasted for around twenty years, the *Querelle des Anciens et des Modernes*, stemming from a 1687 session of the Académie française, founded by Richelieu, which has become famous.

It should be noted that for the first time in the history of Christianity in the seventeenth century the **impulses** for a new paradigm, a new basic model of the world, society, church and theology, primarily came **not from within theology and the church but from outside**: from a society which was rapidly becoming 'worldly', 'secular', and thus 'emancipating' itself from the supervision of church and theology. The mediaeval unity of thought was now definitively shattered; human beings came into the centre as individuals and at the same time the human horizon widened almost to infinity: geographically through the discoveries of new continents, physically through the telescope and microscope. And what the revival of classical studies was for the Renaissance, the rise of mathematics, the natural sciences and new philosophy was for the modernity which was now beginning.

This was a **breakthrough of an epoch-making extent**, no less a break than the Reformation. Up to the seventeenth century, Western culture, whether Catholic or Protestant, had been essentially shaped and pervaded by Christianity. But now an intellectual life was developing independently of the church and – especially as the Catholic Church was shutting itself in – increasingly against it. The Copernican shift was a scientific and philosophical revolution combined, which was to lead to a technological and then a political and finally industrial revolution.

It would not be difficult to show that, as in the case of Luther and the Reformation, so too with this paradigm shift at the beginning of modernity, particular laws manifest themselves. Indeed Thomas Kuhn made the Copernican shift the starting point for all his reflections on paradigm shifts. And so far as philosophy and theology, church and religion are concerned, I have already sketched out three features in connection with the two French mathematicians, scientists, inventors and philosophers – typical of modern times – Descartes and Pascal:[44]

– In the seventeenth century a deep **crisis** developed for the traditional Roman Catholic paradigm and the society based on it. This could not be coped with by scholastic theology or a reference to Augustinian, Reformation and Jansenist piety.

– A **new paradigm** which would have been basically acceptable even to theology and the church was becoming evident, already prepared for; here a mass of individual and social factors, both rational and irrational, were also involved in the paradigm shift.

– The **outcome** of the clash betwen old and new – especially given the resistance of the Catholic Church and the French crown – was quite **uncertain**. And it was to be decades before it showed any clear profile. But the signs of a new era were already clear at an early stage.

Turning against religion

I shall first sketch out in broad outline the general change in cultural climate and the marked religious cooling off. We noted that the new paradigm **announced** itself **in the seventeenth century** and became **established in the eighteenth century**. All too often there was a failure to see the revolutionary change coming, and social appearances were deceptive:

– In the seventeenth century, order, authority and discipline, church, hierarchy and dogma were still highly prized. But behind the brilliant façade of the state church they were unscrupulously misused by absolutist rulers and their devoted princes of the church to develop their own power and splendour.

– But in the eighteenth century, especially in Catholic France, these traditional values had already been largely rejected and ridiculed by the intellectual elite.

– In the seventeenth century, many educated people still thought like the great orator and court bishop Bossuet, the last prominent representative of a theology of history with an Augustinian stamp.

– But in the eighteenth century, they increasingly thought like the witty and sceptical polemicist and essayist Voltaire, who in his literary, philosophical and historical works rejected all positive religion, expressed his hatred of the church (*écrasez l'infâme*) and argued effectively for tolerance even towards the Protestants (Huguenots).

– In the seventeenth century, there was a marked rise of the middle class (merchants, financiers, industrialists, academics and the professions), not least by a progression through the rapidly growing bureaucracy up to ministerial level (by contrast, the rebellions of peasants exploited by higher taxes did not have any great effect).

– But in the eighteenth century, in Germany, while there was still a call for a 'good monarch' in the spirit of enlightened absolutism, who would guarantee the well-being of the state and its citizens on the basis of his patriarchal responsibility and rational insight (Frederick II of Prussia was an example), in France there was already a call for a constitution, a constitutional monarchy, and at the same time a separation of the powers on the English model as a presupposition for political freedom (thus Montesquieu, who died in 1755[45]). It was the middle class which with increasing energy opposed the wastefulness at court: the established mercantilistic economic system and above all the domination of the aristocracy and the senior clergy allied with them, which was not based on achievement but on birth alone.

For in contrast to the tolerant Protestant states, in France the Counter-Reformation reactionary paradigm was defended uncompromisingly and violently with censorship and the power of the police and the military, not only against the Protestants but also against stricter Catholic tendencies: against Pascal and the Augustinian ascetic Jansenists, and against mystical currents. In France, in practice Catholics now had a choice only between the official anti-Jansenist Jesuit Catholicism and the freethinking of Voltaire. This was a crazy alternative, which was to have fatal consequences.

Here things had not begun at all badly for religion. For in the seventeenth century the leading spirits in philosophy and science even in France were still interested in an accord with church teaching. Both Descartes and Pascal, and also Copernicus, Kepler, Galileo and Newton, the leading advocates of the new mathematical and mechanical sciences, not only believed in God but were confessing Christians. And even Voltaire, who popularized Newton's picture of the world on the continent, like d'Alembert and Diderot with their thirty-five-volume *Encyclopédie*[46] – the monumental work of the French Enlightenment, which as the **summa of modern knowledge** sought to bring together the Enlightenment criticism of state and church and give a rational explanation of human beings, nature and society – did not propagate the new mechanistic world view as atheists, but as deists. They believed in a creator and controller of the world machine (though he was very distant). There could have been an understanding, had the church side moved forward to a critical interpretation of the Bible in the light of the results of the new sciences and a more critical attitude to the *Ancien Régime*. But at least in Rome there was no thought of that.

The new belief in reason and progress

What is the motivating force, the drive which gives this intellectual and social movement its tremendous thrust? It is, as has already become clear, the power of autonomous reason:

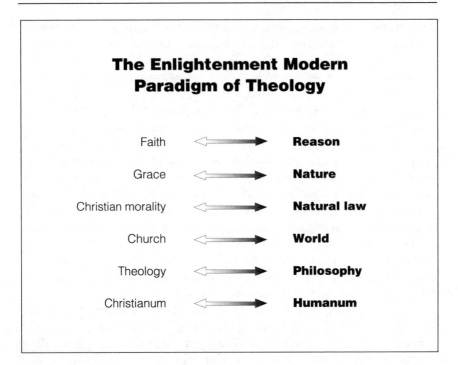

The Enlightenment Modern Paradigm of Theology

Faith	⟵⟶	**Reason**
Grace	⟵⟶	**Nature**
Christian morality	⟵⟶	**Natural law**
Church	⟵⟶	**World**
Theology	⟵⟶	**Philosophy**
Christianum	⟵⟶	**Humanum**

- For the mediaeval Roman Catholic paradigm the supreme authority was '*Ecclesia sive Papa*' (church = Pope), and for the Reformation paradigm it was the 'word of God'. However, for the paradigm of modernity the supreme authority is *ratio*, '*raison*', human '**reason**', the first guiding value for modernity.

What is man? Man must be seen as a natural being endowed with reason, who can trust in the fundamental possibility of knowledge through his reason and in his capacity to develop the conditions in which he lives. And the unprecedented dynamic of modernity is based on a third great value, trust in the rationality of human nature; a '*ratio*' which is not at all ecclesiastical, far less papal, as was proved in the case of Galileo – so different from that of Luther. '*Raisonnement*' (with a pragmatic intent) – the supreme human activity; to 'reason' (about oneself, society and history) – at that time was still by no means a taunt. '*Raison*' and thus moderation, balance, proportion: they should, they would, make possible a humane *savoir faire* and *savoir vivre*. In practice this also means that with this new faith in human **reason**, which becomes the **arbiter in all questions of truth**, modernity in the strict sense begins: all traditional authorities – whether Aristotle or Scholasticism, Pope or Bible – find themselves in a crisis, in a crisis over their credentials. What is reasonable, what is useful? In future only what is reasonable counts as true, useful and binding.

But – and people were clear about this above all in England – the reasonable is none other than the natural, human nature. No, law and constitution, economy and culture, even morality and religion are not to be built on what has grown up in history, on the traditional and the fortuitous, but on the **human nature which is common to all**, though of course this also allowed the reform of conditions in some circumstances. Instead of being on the oral, special, local, time-conditioned, the emphasis was now put on the written, universal, global, timeless.[47] Interest focussed on an autonomous natural law instead of on God's law and commandment. Instead of being on historical revelation and dogmatics, the emphasis was now on a natural religion which had been originally given, and which without any historical justification was assumed to be identical with the religion of reason. That means:

- In contrast to the Reformation and Counter-Reformation, the 'modern' entire constellation in the strict sense was orientated on the primacy of **reason** compared with faith; on the priority of **philosophy** (with its shift towards the human) over theology; on the priority of **nature** (the natural sciences, natural philosophy, natural religion, natural law) over grace; on the predominance of a **world** which was becoming increasingly secular over the church. In short, people now stressed the *humanum*, the universally human, rather than the *Christianum*, the specifically Christian. And the social model was no longer the pastor but the philosopher.

Granted, as we saw, a new attitude to life and the world, a reflection on human worth, which released people from the mediaeval order, had already taken place in the Italian Renaissance and in humanism. Art in particular was no longer locked into that mediaeval structure of order which was completely orientated on transcendence, but had become an end in itself: the aesthetic had a value of its own, manifested in secular theories of art, histories of art, art collections. But as I have emphasized, this came about with a retrospective look towards antiquity; *rinascimento*, re-birth, was the magic word.

Now, however, in the seventeenth century the intellectual elite began to think self-confidently, independently of authority and openly with a forward perspective: against the Renaissance in a **progressiveness** which was characteristic of modernity, which did not appeal to antiquity (Renaissance) or the Bible (Re-formation) but to self-sufficient human reason. Belief in the omnipotence of reason and the possibility of controlling nature was the foundation of the modern notion of progress.

In such a new awareness of themselves and their present, people could trust in their own progress and in progress generally. According to Voltaire, the principle of reason is not only the absolute criterion for the human disposition but also the motive force of human progress. This principle already distinguished the age of Louis XIV from the other three great cultural ages in European history: the Athens of Pericles, Rome under Augustus and the Florence of the Medicis; indeed it was superior to these, and because progress was constant could even be surpassed (however, even Voltaire did not think of revolution). In fact only now was there a quite central appeal to autonomous reason, with which human beings could increasingly dominate nature and even compensate for the loss of their central position in the universe. According to Pascal, both the weakness and the power of human beings lie in this experience of loss and gain: '*L'homme n'est qu'un roseau, mais c'est un roseau pensant*', 'The human being is only a reed, but he is a thinking reed.'[48]

One symptom (which indirectly is further confirmation of our periodization) is the fact that the secular **idea of progress**[49] so characteristic of modernity (once again in contrast to the Renaissance) similarly also takes shape in the seventeenth century, and in the eighteenth century is extended to all spheres of life – now the chronological pattern of all history. The whole **process of history** appears as **rationally progressive and progressing rationally**. Only now is there a new coinage, 'progress', emerging simultaneously with the word 'history'. It is a mechanical belief in progress which can be understood in both evolutionary and revolutionary terms. Later in the nineteenth century, at the climax of scientific, technical, industrial and political social development, belief in perpetual progress would become virtually the modern secular **substitute religion** (for both Liberals and Socialists), at the same time the indicator and factor of a political movement. There is no mistaking the fact that in the course of the development of modernity the tremendously optimistic belief in progress, which was given almost divine attributes like eternity, omniscience, omnipotence and absolute goodness, increasingly replaced belief in the one God. The realization of happiness already in this world – that was the aim. So:

• Instead of an unchanging, static, **eternal world order** with a hierarchical ordering (*ordo* as understood by Plato, Augustine and Thomas), instead of a Reformation two-realms doctrine of the kingdom of God and the kingdom of the world, there was now a new unitary view of world and history in the sense of a lasting **progress**: this is the second leading value of modernity.

This was to bring humankind an improvement of its situation, control of nature, and prosperity and happiness for the individual already in this life. The modern philosophers of history – Hegel, Marx and Comte – would shape a comprehensive secular view of the world and history and a theory of history under the leading idea of progress. But what form did Christianity take under these new conditions?

Toleration of religions – relativization of Christianity

After the Reformation and Counter-Reformation, after the age of confessionalism and the endless disputes and indescribable devastations caused by religion and confessions, after the Thirty Years' War around the middle of the seventeenth century, there was not only **religious exhaustion** but also – above all in the Protestant countries – a growing **religious toleration**. Toleration, which had even been utterly remote from the mind of the Reformers, now became almost a keyword of modernity. In the long run neither intolerant Tridentine Catholicism nor orthodox Protestantism, which in some respects was barely more tolerant, could stop freedom of thought from becoming established, not only in philosophy and the natural sciences, but also in politics and religion. The cost of intellectual intolerance was high. The Jews and Moors driven out of Spain were now developing business initiatives and prosperity in other cities – from Amsterdam to Istanbul. The Huguenots foolishly oppressed by Louis XIV were as successful in Prussia as they were in Holland and in England. The southern Catholic countries were in increasing danger of becoming scientifically and thus also technically and economically backward.

Now wars of religion were increasingly thought to be as inhuman and un-Christian as the burning of witches. Mediaeval and Reformation belief in the Devil, demons and magic, the trials and burnings of witches – first attacked, as we heard,[50] by the Jesuit Friedrich von Spee and then by the Protestant lawyer Christian Thomasius, the first professor to give lectures in German to large audiences (another sign of the times) – no longer fitted the new age of reason.

Here another development could no longer be overlooked. Just as telescopes could show astronomers that our earth is not a singular entity in the universe, so the news and reports of explorers, missonaries and merchants, which were becoming increasingly more precise, forced home the insight that the Christian religion was perhaps not such a unique phenomenon as had previously been believed. Indeed, the more intensive international communication became through the discovery of new lands, cultures and religions, the more evident the **relativity of**

European-style Christianity was. Now the Christian mission in Asia had serious repercussions on Christianity in Europe in a dialectic of a strange kind. Why?

The founder of the Catholic **China mission** at the end of the sixteenth century was the distiguished Jesuit **Matteo Ricci** (from 1583 in China and from 1601 in Peking). He had adapted wholly to the Chinese way of life in dress, language and behaviour: a Christian who behaved like a Confucian scholar![51] The very first Jesuits had reported to an amazed Europe the four-thousand-year-old, incomparably high, culture of China. But there was opposition in Rome and among the other orders to their pedagogical, diplomatic adaptation of Christianity, done with great boldness – often clearly for reasons of colonial or church policy or the policy of the order. The Jesuits were accused of selling out Christianity. It all led to a great dispute which then broke out as the **rites dispute**, when in 1634 Spanish Dominicans and Franciscans began to engage in mission in China.[52] The result was endless negotiations before the Roman Inquisition and vigorous discussions throughout Europe.

Meanwhile, despite everything, the mission in China had made no small progress: at any rate in 1670, i.e. around 100 years after Ricci's beginnings, there were said to be 273,780 Catholics, and the prospects for the future seemed good. In 1692 the most important emperor of the new Manchu dynasty, K'ang-hsi, had allowed the gospel to be preached throughout China by a new **edict of toleration**. Indeed, some Jesuits at the imperial court even had well-founded hopes for the conversion of this emperor, whom the mathematician, philosopher and diplomat Leibniz and many others in Europe regarded as the greatest ruler in the world. When the difficulties of the Jesuits in Rome over Chinese rites and names increased, Emperor K'ang-hsi sent an official response from the Chinese rites tribunal, which he had asked for, to the Pope. It arrived in Rome in 1701. It made clear that Confucius was not worshipped in China as a god but was venerated as a teacher; that ancestor worship was a commemoration and not a form of worship; and that the divine names 'T'ien' and 'Shang-ti' did not denote the physical heaven but the Lord of heaven and earth and all things.

But all this was of little use. In 1704 Pope Clement XI forbade the Chinese Christians to practise their rites under threat of excommunication; the same went for ancestor worship, the veneration of Confucius and the use of the two traditional names for God, Shang-ti ('Lord in the heights') and T'ien ('heaven'); only the newer Christian expression T'ien-chu ('Lord of Heaven') was allowed. But since the veneration of ancestors was virtually the foundation of the Chinese social structure and the Confucian ethos permeated all values, the consequence of this was that anyone who wanted to remain or become a Christian had to stop being Chinese. This was a fatal alternative, caused by a **mistaken papal decision of historic dimensions**, which moreover was to have catastrophic consequences for Christanity in China.[53]

The **Chinese reaction** to this Roman provocation began slowly under Emperor K'ang-hsi. 1717 saw the pronouncement of the verdict of the nine supreme courts of China: the expulsion of the missionaries, the prohibition of Christianity, destruction of the churches, compulsory abjuration of the Christian faith. The number of Catholics dropped rapidly, and they were mostly limited to peasants and fishermen – who lived in segregation and were despised. As a defence against opposition currents and Christianity, there was a dogmatizing of Confucianism within China on the Roman pattern – also with ominous consequences for future developments.

The rites dispute also did much to bring gloom to the first European to take seriously for philosophy the pluralistic structure of humanity, with races and cultures of equal worth, who strove for the reconciliation not only of the Christian churches (he had conversations with Bossuet) but also of Western and Eastern culture: the great ecumenist **Gottfried Wilhelm Leibniz**.[54] Just as the Christian missionaries instructed the Chinese in the gospel and in the new sciences, so in his view Chinese missionaries should teach natural religion, ethics and constitutional order in Europe. Only a few months before his death, Leibniz published a French *Treatise on the Natural Theology of the Chinese* (1716), in which with amazing empathy he attempted to harmonize the old terms Shang-ti and T'ien and also the more philosophical term T'ai-chi (the Great Ultimate) with a philosophical European understanding of God. According to him, God is omnipresent in the best possible system of his creation, which ultimately at any rate is not contradictory, the system of a 'prestabilized harmony'.

Leibniz's pupil and friend **Christian Wolff**, the most popular Enlightenment philosopher in Germany, was also interested in Chinese philosophy. A few years after Leibniz' death (in 1721), however, he had to leave the University of Halle and Prussian territory within forty-eight hours under threat of the death penalty, because he had provoked the wrath, not now of the Roman Inquisition but of the Protestant Pietists, with an all too positive lecture on the practical philosophy of the Chinese.[55]

Now Christianity clearly began to forfeit its universal position among the intellectual elites of Europe, after the clash with Islam had been carried on above all by military means and had been decided positively for Europe (the Turks were finally defeated before Vienna in 1683). And in Germany no one had grasped the problem more sharply than **Gotthold**

Ephraim Lessing (1729–1781). His great Enlightenment play *Nathan the Wise* (1779)[56] stages a dramatic conversation between the three world religions of Semitic origin and prophetic character, presented in vivid characters full of spirit and understanding: an enlightened Jew (Nathan, the first noble Jew in a German play), an enlightened Muslim (the distinguished Sultan Saladin) and an immature but ultimately enlightened Crusader, at the same time (with a simple monk) the opposite of that authoritarian church represented by the infamous papistical 'patriarch', which safeguards its claim to absoluteness by power politics and if need be with the stake, and keeps people under its thumb by refusing to allow them to come of age.

Lessing's work is more than a neutral drama about toleration; it is a utopian drama about reconciliation. It is about the political and religious utopia of a better future for humankind, symbolically reflected in the feast at the end of the play in which people of different faiths embrace one another: utterly in the spirit of Lessing's historical thought with its orientation on the future, there is a **vision** which is still, indeed again, inspiring today, **of a peace among the religions as the presupposition of peace in humanity generally!**

At least the notion of toleration continues in the European Enlightenment in the face of all confessionalism:

> Instead of the monopoly position of a single religion (*extra ecclesiam nulla salus*) as in the mediaeval paradigm, or the domination of two confessions (*cuius regio, eius et religio*), now there is the toleration of different Christian confessions and even different religions. Freedom of conscience, freedom of religious confession and religious practice stand right at the top of the list of human rights which are now increasingly being called for.

The Enlightenment as a cultural revolution

Instead of a call for Reformation, now everywhere the call for **Enlightenment** rang out. And as we heard,[57] in Germany, in the framework of the orthodox Protestant paradigm, prepared for by an individualistic, spiritualistic but dogmatically indifferent Pietism, according to Kant's famous definition Enlightenment was '**the emergence of human beings from a tutelage to which they had voluntarily acceded**': 'tutelage is the inability to make use of one's understanding without being guided by another. *Sapere aude!* Have courage to make use of your **own** understanding! That is the slogan of the Enlightenment.'[58]

To whom was this slogan of the Enlightenment addressed? **To the**

church authorities of all confessions who dominated all thought, and who although they had completely forfeited their credibility through disputes over faith and wars of faith still attempted to keep human beings in unworthy dependence. Therefore the Enlightenment sought to spread the light of reason, '*les lumières*', in a world darkened by church superstition and church prejudices. The overpowering influence of religion, church and theology characteristic of the European Middle Ages and even of the Reformation had become intolerable to an age of reason – not to mention all the business of monasteries, processions, pilgrimages and indulgences. What use now were all the old confessions and dogmas, the constant intervention of the church in state affairs, the supremacy of theology over the other disciplines in the universities? Didn't reason, which had become independent, prove more and more every day what it could achieve when it was not enslaved by church and theology and concentrated on a world to be mastered here instead of on a distant beyond?

As the Enlightenment sought to detach all human thought from its previous dependence on external authorities and to base it on intrinsically rational principles, it amounted to a **cultural revolution**. For in rebelling against the church authorities, in fact the Enlightenment was putting any authority in question – apart from that of reason. The Enlightenment presupposed, even though some people already doubted it at that time, that first, every human being is endowed with reason and thus has the capacity to make independent use of reason, and secondly, that reason as the supreme authority is objectively and immutably fixed. The consequences of this cultural revolution for Christianity were overwhelming: in contrast to the times of Luther, Calvin and Trent it was now no longer primarily religious, theological and ecclesiastical demands that were influencing political, economic, social and cultural processes. Quite the opposite, church organization, pietistic movements and theology were increasingly governed by political, economic, social and cultural factors.

That brings out a further characteristic of modernity: the **drifting apart of culture and religion** as the beginning of a process of 'secularization', threatening to Christianity, which was determining everything and was to prove to be a growing departure from the church and indeed Christianity. The Protestant theologian and social ethicist Ernst Troeltsch rightly speaks of a 'complete revolution in all areas of cultural life', with the tendency to give an 'immanent explanation of the world by means of universally valid knowledge and a rational ordering of life in the service of universally valid practical aims'.[59]

As we saw,[60] the foundations for this **process of secularization and emancipation** had been laid a long way back, in the high Middle Ages. With the help of Aristotle, Thomas Aquinas had allowed an independence – limited, to be sure, but real – of reason from faith, nature from grace, philosophy from theology, the state from the church. This highly unstable, natural-supernatural, two-level edifice had already been shaken by an unascetic humanism and a Renaissance which took a delight in this world when with an appeal to antiquity a new emphasis was put on the *humanum* and the autonomy of culture (art, literature). This was a development which was then checked by Luther's Reformation (and the Counter-Reformation) – to the fury of later secular spirits like Friedrich Nietzsche, until it came to light anew in the seventeenth century. Now, however, it was no longer faith in antiquity but – in a typically modern way – faith in reason. By its very nature the modern process of rationalization was at the same time a process of secularization.

Originally **secularization**[61] primarily denoted simply – in legal and political terms – the transference of church property into the secular sphere by individuals and states. But it now became increasingly clear that not only some church possessions but almost all the important spheres of human life – science, economics, politics, law, the state, culture, education, medicine, social welfare – were to be removed from the influence of the churches, theology and religion and put under the direct responsibility and at the direct disposal of human beings who themselves had become reasonable, of age, 'secular', worldly. So the world of human beings itself became a 'secular', worldly world.

Similarly, the word '**emancipation**' originally had a purely legal meaning, denoting the release of the child from parental authority or the slave from the power of the master. But then in a transferred political sense it denoted equal citizenship for all those who were in a state of dependence on others: Jews, peasants, workers, women, national, confessional or cultural minorities now had **self-determination** instead of being determined by others. Thus finally the word 'emancipation' came to mean the self-determination of men and women generally in the face of an authority which demanded blind obedience and a rule which was illegitimate: freedom from natural compulsion, from social compulsion and the self-compulsion of those who have not yet achieved their own identity.[62]

Now it became increasingly clear that human beings wanted above all to be human. Not superhuman, but not subhuman either. Almost at the same time as the earth ceased to be the centre of the cosmos, human beings learned to understand themselves as the centre of the human world which they had built. In a complex **process of 'demystification'** lasting for centuries, of which the great sociologist of religion Max Weber gave a pioneering analysis,[63] in this way human beings entered into their dominion: experiences, insights, ideas which had originally been gained from Christian faith and were bound up with it were now put at the disposal of human reason. The different spheres of life were less and less seen and given norms from the perspective of a world above. They were understood in terms of themselves, in terms of their own immanent laws. Human decisions and formative processes were increasingly guided by this and not by authorities beyond this world.

It is in fact amazing how rapidly a grip on the world could follow. Much, indeed almost all, that was previously attributed to God or to superhuman, other-worldly powers could now be brought under human control. Reason, freedom, being of age were the slogans. Human beings were masters of themselves and masters of nature – here was a self-definition (with all kinds of positive and negative consequences that could not yet be seen) which was to lead to **power over the world**.

There is no doubt about it; this was a cultural revolution which is still seen by parts of the official Catholic Church as a negative one. From the perspective of the secular world, it represented incomparable progress:

– Unprecedented **progress of the sciences**: philosophy and natural science changed. They no longer operated with dogmatic assumptions but with facts of experience. Historiography no longer remained a sub-division of rhetoric or ethics, but became a separate discipline.

– A completely **new social order**: religious toleration and freedom of belief were grounded in natural law; ideas like constitutional law, the abolition of the privileges of clergy and aristocracy arose; science and the arts, industry and trade were officially promoted; the schools were reformed.

– A **revaluation of the individual**: the innate rights of human beings were to be codified and put under state protection: the right to life, freedom and property and thus at the same time a social and political emancipation of citizens.

Theology – reconciled with the Enlightenment

Of course Christian theology, too, did not remain untouched by this cultural revolution. Indeed, here too the spirit of Enlightenment also led to a crisis, since now old plausibility structures within traditional theology were beginning to collapse. Here biblical scholarship played a key role; in the course of the critical historiography of the Enlightenment it broke with a tabu which even the Reformers had preserved: it **subjected scripture itself to historical-critical analysis**. The question suddenly became virulent: how much historical truth does the Bible really contain? And this basic question is radically different yet again from the one by which the Reformation had been driven: what religious truth does the

Bible contain compared with the traditions of the church? The truth-claim of the Word of God was all at once under discussion.

Like modern science and philosophy, so modern biblical criticism, too, had already begun in the seventeenth century. It remains associated with the name of **Richard Simon**. He was an Oratorian and contemporary of Descartes and Galileo who was largely unknown at the time. He had studied with the Jewish philosopher and biblical critic Baruch de Spinoza and a rabbi in Paris and was the first Christian author to show that the 'Five Books of Moses' (the Pentateuch) cannot come from one and the same author, but were compiled from different sources. The background to this is that the creation account in the book of Genesis had now proved to be the main obstacle to the acceptance of the new astronomy and physics. Historical-critical research and a definition of the nature of the biblical texts (the Bible is not a revealed textbook of physics, cosmology and biology!) were to contribute towards avoiding false clashes between faith and science. Here Richard Simon was seeking constructive solutions and had no intention of using his critical results to oppose church dogma.

But when Simon's *Histoire critique de l'Ancien Testament* (1678) appeared, it was immediately confiscated, at the request of the Bishop of Paris at court, Bossuet. The author himself was expelled from the Oratory. Simon continued to work indefatigably until his death and published his works in tolerant Amsterdam, but within the **Catholic Church** the spirit of critical biblical research had already been quenched before it could flourish. Moreover, to begin with Simon had no successor, so suspicious were those within the Roman Catholic paradigm of critical biblical scholarship from the start. They could cut themselves off from it because of its 'subversion' – at first, as always, successfully. The consequence was the **emigration of critical exegesis from the Church of Rome** and thus the emigration of the intellectual avant-garde in theology generally.

In **Protestantism** things were different. Here the Reformation principle continued, so that the new critical approach could finally be taken up and developed. In Germany with its mixed confessions, weakened for a long time in every respect by the confessional wars, the Enlightenment began very much later and took much more moderate forms than in Catholic France. We have already heard of the crisis of the Reformation Protestant paradigm (P IV), which in the meantime had hardened.[64] But whereas the orthodox and the Pietists largely persisted in the traditional paradigm, along with the majority of Protestant rulers, many theologians and churchmen now turned to the new, Enlightenment paradigm (P V).

Granted, in Germany the great mass of church people initially remained faithful to the traditional churches and their teaching. However, among the educated a departure from the old paradigm became evident, though because of the different historical situation it did not lead, as in France, to deism, atheism and materialism but to an enlightened form of Christian religion and finally to Idealism. Here the sponsor was not a mocker of religion like Voltaire, but **Gottfried Wilhelm Leibniz**. As we heard, he had striven for an enlightened reconciliation of the natural sciences with philosophy, of philosophy with theology, and indeed for an ecumenical mediation between Protestantism and Catholicism, finally even between European and Chinese thought. Leibniz does not stand for Enlightenment against religion but for Enlightenment in and with religion.

Still, that the new movement, historically the most powerful since the Lutheran Reformation, could not be stopped is already evident from the fact that Christian Wolff, the Enlightenment philosopher, expelled for his glorification of Confucius, could return to the University of Halle almost twenty years later under a new king, and that this new king – Frederick the Great – himself proved a decisive champion of the Enlightenment and had close contacts with Voltaire and other significant Frenchmen. He was able to show toleration not only to the French Huguenots but also to the Jesuits, ideologically at the opposite extreme, whose order had been abolished by the Pope under pressure from enlightened European governments.

However, the Enlightenment became established only slowly in the Protestant theology of Germany: the 'transitional theologians'[65] between the late orthodoxy of the seventeenth century and the new Enlightenment first of all wanted to be only 'rationally' orthodox, putting reason and revelation on the same level, and then in practice making reason superior to revelation; the theologians who followed Christian Wolff[66] did this quite openly and systematically, but still without attacking doctrine.

This **attack on dogma** was introduced by theologians who were deemed heretics and given the name '**neologians**'.[67] They did not deny revelation as such, but they kept quiet about this or that dogma, attacked another and reinterpreted a third. In short, they put the dogmas together and found the core of revelation: the religion of reason, based on God, freedom (= morality), immortality. Unexpectedly, here some things which already at an earlier stage were no longer very important became unimportant, superfluous: the divinity of Christ, his virgin birth, his death as satisfaction, his resurrection, ascension, coming again. The neologians did not dispense with these on the basis of great theories like a consistent Wolffianism. None of this any longer made sense to modern practical piety and moral effort directed at a better life. Enlightenment men and women did not feel any spiritual need for it: on the contrary, some of it had become burdensome and a hindrance to an emphasis on morality – one had only to think of original sin.[68]

So in Protestant Germany **Enlightenment theology** became established to a degree that was not possible for Catholic theologians tied to dogmas and above all to the magisterium. This theology rightly fought against every kind of obscurantism in theology, piety and church practice. Without the Enlightenment heretics and witches would still have been being burned and people tortured. So the great concerns of Enlightenment theology should not be despised. Unfortunately, however, they were often simplified, and degenerated into a flatly natural, optimistic and eudaimonistic religion for everyone, which took for granted an awareness of God and a natural moral law innate in all human beings along with the freedom of the will and the immortality of the soul – all for the purpose of sound morality, i.e. the formation of noble humanity.

So was this now to be the specifically **modern religion**? Are human beings good by nature and are moral virtues the presupposition for individual happiness? Instead of Luther's consciousness of sin, was there now to be the optimism of the great century? Was revelation a supplement to reason and Christianity the most advantageous of religions? Was Christ, or better Jesus, the wise teacher of morality, who brought to consciousness in a new and illuminating way what people already knew: a reasonable, natural human life? That is what many people in fact thought at that time: practice instead of theory, life instead of doctrine, morality instead of dogma. The true Christian faith is action, is working for the moral benefit of human beings and their happiness.

Now the call to return to the sources was made afresh, gently at first and then loudly, not only against the Reformation confessional writings which had been demystified with the help of a pragmatic view of history and a particular ideal picture of earliest Christianity, but also against holy scripture itself. And in this field the real decisions for modern theology were to be made.

The dawn of historical criticism of the Bible

Enlightenment exegesis first of all attempted to understand the texts simply in terms of themselves, undogmatically, though often the guideline was in fact a rationality understood in a basically Cartesian way. This rational biblical criticism – prepared for by Erasmus, Grotius and Hobbes, given a basis by Spinoza drawn from scientific and mathematical knowledge, and then consolidated by Bayle and Hume – now embarked on its victorious course right through Protestant theology.

On the new basis of Greek and Semitic philology; in the study of old codexes, textual traditions and the Jewish synagogue literature; in the historical thought which was slowly becoming established; and in its unmythological rationality, this modern scriptural exegesis had a very solid starting point. What could unhistorical reactionary Protestant biblicism with its verbal inspiration do in the face of it? Or a Catholic exegesis which was stuck in confessional polemic or in quoting and imitating the Fathers? It had become unstoppable. The **history of Jesus**, too, had to be explained by reason, contrary to all dogmatism. The battle was no longer over the church, as it was in the sixteenth and seventeenth centuries; in the century of indifferentism the dispute was over Jesus the Christ himself. The tendency of the early church and the Middle Ages towards a docetic dissolution of the historical Jesus had been reversed. 'The historical investigation of the life of Jesus did not take its rise from a purely historical interest; it turned to the Jesus of history as an ally in the struggle against the tyranny of dogma. Afterwards, when it was freed from this *pathos*, it sought to present the historic Jesus in a form intelligible to its own time.'[69]

Moreover it was German **historical biblical scholarship** which was to play the main role in the development of an enlightened paradigm of theology. Indeed, at the end of the nineteenth and beginning of the twentieth centuries, it was to establish this paradigm world-wide. The decisive presupposition was that the traditional view of an almost mechanical and magical **verbal inspiration** of the Bible, which was heavily influenced by Hellenistic notions but which had continued to be maintained by the Reformers and by Lutheran and Calvinist orthodoxy, was to be **abandoned** – in favour of a completely new universal hermeneutics which applied to both sacral and non-sacral texts.

The foundations for this typically modern hermeneutics were laid by **Johann Salomo Semler**, the most significant of the 'neologians', who claimed complete freedom for academic theology (though not for religion generally), and with his major *Treatise on the Free Investigation of the Canon* (1771–75) founded **historical-critical theology**. The initiator of modern undogmatic church history and the history of dogma, he also wanted to understand the Bible in an undogmatic way. So he simply ignored all inspiration and in a matter-of-fact way gave a historical demonstration of the origin of the biblical writings, which differ so much in character and value. In this way holy scripture became a collection of historical sources which, like secular sources, could only be understood properly by a historical approach. Philosophical and theological hermeneutics were embraced in a universal historical hermeneutics which now developed. Not all the historically-conditioned embellishments were to be accepted as the Word of God, but only those elements which served towards moral improvement.

Here Semler made the distinction between 'natural' ('rational') and 'positive' ('supernatural') religion which was so important for the subsequent period. In any case there could be no question of a complete Christianity at the beginning and a uniform doctrinal system in the Bible, as Protestant orthodoxy asserted. However, this did not mean that any individual and private doctrinal view could be made public religion without state assent. So Semler became involved in the greatest discussion to have broken out in German Protestantism since Martin Luther, finally against the one who had provoked it. Someone known to us here did an unknown a great honour.

Six months after Richard Simon's death, that acute Protestant 'lay theologian', and the most eloquent polemicist of classical German literature, **Gotthold Ephraim Lessing**, as court librarian at Wolfenbüttel, published *Fragments of an Unknown Author*, which had been written under the influence of the English Deists: *The Aims of Jesus and His Disciples*. The work came from the Hamburg professor of oriental languages **Hermann Samuel Reimarus**, who had discovered a mass of contradictions, human and all-too-human features in the disciples and even in Jesus himself in the New Testament sources. For Reimarus, the whole gospel of Jesus could be reduced to the message, 'Repent, for the kingdom of heaven is at hand.'[70] Here he had unerringly hit on the centre of Jesus' message. Time and again he warned against reading the present-day catechism into the Gospels. The biblical message had to be read in its original simplicity. 'Repent!': contrary to the Pharisees Jesus taught authentic morality and only authentic morality;[71] Reimarus praised it openly. There was no trace in Jesus himself of the revelation of new mysteries transcending reason (divine Sonship in the real sense, the Holy Spirit, the Trinity).[72] Nor was there anything about the abolition of the Mosaic ceremonial law.

Who was Jesus? According to Reimarus, none other than the political liberator of Israel and the Messiah of a worldly kingdom of heaven, and this led to a manifest fiasco: his death on the cross.[73] How did the disciples react? In the greatest disappointment of their lives they staged a great deception: the resurrection. Indeed, in their despair they seized on the second form of Jewish messianic hope then cherished in apocalyptic circles, for which the Messiah appears twice: first in humility (the reinterpretation of the death of Jesus as the atoning death of a spiritual redeemer from sin), and then in glory (on the clouds of heaven). Earliest

Christianity was nothing but a religion of a disappointed apocalyptic expectation of an imminent end, in the light of which all the Gospels were written – retrospectively.[74]

Even now we can understand the shock waves that such a historical-critical picture of earliest Christianity must have set off – after a good seventeen centuries of church preaching. Now the eyes of theologians and educated Christians had been opened even in Germany – in France, a few years before, the creed of Rousseau's Savoyard curate (in his novel *Émile*)[75] had caused a similar shock. What had become of the Christian message? Whereas some rejoiced and mocked, others protested and called for repudiation or censorship; preachers were at a loss, and some theological students gave up their studies. Lessing identified himself with Reimarus only with qualifications, and Semler attempted to refute the dead author sentence by sentence in an extensive work.

Indeed, here there was a real **revolution in theology**. But precisely as a result of it, in Germany there was serious historical-critical research into the Bible and especially the life of Jesus, which in time was to provide a historically assured and differentiated picture of Jesus. The dramatic story of the **quest of the historical Jesus** in the framework of the modern paradigm – 'from Reimarus to Wrede' – masterfully described by Albert Schweitzer in his theological phase – cannot be related here. But two bold Tübingen scholars, **David Friedrich Strauss** and **Ferdinand Christian Baur**, were to make a tremendous contribution in this area.

It was the young lecturer **David Friedrich Strauss** who in 1835 published his hypercritical book on the *Life of Jesus*,[76] which brought him immediate dismissal from church service and condemned him to the existence of a private scholar all his life. But the tasks had been posed for a century of research into the historical Jesus, at the end of which came an understanding of the initially contradictory relationship between the first three (Syn-optic) Gospels and their character as proclamation stories.[77]

At the same time the brilliant Protestant historian **Ferdinand Christian Baur**, inspired by Hegel's universal and dialectical view of history, had laid the foundations for a historical investigation of earliest Christianity, church history and the history of dogma which was no longer governed by dogmatic considerations and had no supernatural colouring, but was purely academic and scientific history.[78] The dispute with Baur's 'younger Tübingen school', which worked all too much with a priori Hegelian three-stage schemes, brought comprehensive clarification not only of the history of earliest Christianity but also of the history of dogma and theology generally. **Adolf von Harnack**'s three-volume history of dogma at the end of the century may be seen as a prime example of this.[79]

Thus nowhere is the **paradigm shift between Reformation and modernity** as manifest as in research into the Hebrew Bible and the New Testament. Thanks to the tremendous work initially of Protestant exegetes, the Bible has become the best-investigated book in world literature – verse by verse, word by word – and this is now also of supreme value in dialogue with other world religions. In comprehensive, detailed work, whole generations of scholars have struggled over every work, every sentence, indeed every word in textual and literary criticism, form and genre criticism, combined with the history of concepts, motifs and traditions.[80]

Here a new sense of what one may call 'inspiration' – no longer understood in a Hellenistic sense but in its original sense – has also become clear: the gospel of Jesus Christ as good news which is not to remain shut up in a book but to be preached again in a living way for each age: the **one word of God in all the fallible human words**. The gospel is not inspired infallible sentences but a message inspired by the Spirit of God and Jesus Christ and thus inspiring, which for non-believers remains a thoroughly problematical human word but for believers becomes the helping, liberating, saving Word of God. Here the strongest continuity between the modern paradigm of theology and the original Christianity becomes evident.

But of course it was impossible for historical-critical exegesis to provide what theology also needed in modernity, an overall vision, and the translation for a new time of the message which had now been elicited historically. Who would be the Origen, the Thomas Aquinas, the Luther of modernity? To survey these problems we now have to turn to the theologian who became the paradigmatic theologian of modernity and who therefore in the following chapter will be described as thoroughly as the earlier paradigmatic theologians.

5. Theology in the Spirit of Modernity: Friedrich Schleiermacher

A new period of church history may not have started with Friedrich Daniel Ernst Schleiermacher (1768–1834 – for all biographical details, once again see my *Great Christian Thinkers*), but with him it did come to theological maturity. Here the paradigm shift from the Reformation to **modernity** takes almost bodily form: Schleiermacher no longer lived, as Martin Luther still largely did, in a pre-Copernican mediaeval world of angels and devils, demons and witches, with a basically pessimistic and apocalyptic attitude, intolerant of other confessions and religions. It would never have occurred to him to have someone burned, as even Calvin had the anti-trinitarian Servetus burned, because of problems with a dogma of the early church. Far less did he have difficulties with modern science, with Copernicus and Galileo, like the Roman Popes imprisoned in the mediaeval paradigm: in the nineteenth century modern scientific works remained on the Index of books forbidden to Catholics, along with the Reformers and modern philosophy (from Descartes to Kant). Schleiermacher, who even as a professor still went to lectures on science, remained all his life convinced by Kant that there was a thoroughgoing regularity in nature: nature allowed no 'supernatural exceptions'. Supernaturalism in theology? That was not Schleiermacher's thing.

The embodiment of a paradigm shift

So in Schleiermacher we meet a theologian who is a **modern man** through and through. That means:

He knows and affirms the modern **philosophy** with which he had grown up and which had reached its challenging heights with Kant, Fichte and Hegel; as a classical philologist he had also gained the respect of classical scholars by his masterly translation of Plato.

He affirmed historical **criticism** and himself applied it to the foundation documents of the biblical revelation; in the great dispute over the fragments of Reimarus he would certainly have been on Lessing's side against Goeze, the chief pastor of Hamburg. At any rate, later he inaugurated historical criticism of the Pastoral Epistles with a critical study of I Timothy, which he said could not come from the apostle Paul; he attributed the writings of Luke to the community life of earliest Christianity and its oral tradition; he demonstrated the presence of a collection of sayings in the Gospel of Matthew; the writings of the New Testament were to be treated like any others; his hermeneutics (introduction to the understanding of texts) became a basic work for theological, philosophical and literary interpretations.

Above all he affirmed and loved modern **literature, art and social life** (which for him was an art). Indeed here he himself played an active part through his close links with the Berlin Romantic circles which were trying to get beyond the Enlightenment. So he was a theologian in the closest contact with writers, poets, philosphers, artists and political enthusiasts of every kind. Only now did his thought and writing achieve a broad horizon and finally succeed in combining the Romantic religion of feeling with scientific culture.

Furthermore, with his *Brief Account of Theological Study*[81] Schleiermacher was the first to show **theology its place in the modern university**. On a modern epistemological basis (not that of faith) he set the individual theological disciplines, which had fanned out in modernity, in an organic overall context and related them methodically and thematically to non-theological disciplines: philosophical theology (apologetics and polemics) formed the root, historical theology (exegesis, church history and dogmatics) was the body and practical theology (of which Schleiermacher is seen as the founder) the crown. Dogmatics, which used to dominate everything, is here seen incorporated into a system of disciplines of equal rank, ordered by function. In this way Schleiermacher more than any other gave theology its character as a modern discipline. Through his planning and organization, Schleiermacher, also a pioneer of the new educational system, not only gave Prussian **schools** their normative form but was also a co-founder of Berlin **University** and a decisive figure in establishing the **Berlin Academy of Sciences**. He was truly a theologian who in an astonishing way quite naturally took a place at the centre of modern life and played an active part in shaping it.

For religion in an age weary of religion

Schleiermacher was well aware of how ambivalent the picture of religion had become in his time, particularly among educated people, to whom he felt a special obligation. It hovered between affirmation and rejection, assent and mockery, admiration and contempt. So when on the occasion of his twenty-ninth birthday he was invited by those celebrating it to write a book by his thirtieth birthday (on the topic of how the cause of religion could be expressed in a new way), he took up the challenge. He addressed his book to the educated classes (he thought that one should preach to the uneducated), but explicitly above all to the educated among the **despisers of religion**, who were at least to know what they either despised, or did not know properly because of their prejudices.

Thus came into being his famous **first work**, *On Religion. Speeches to its Cultured Despisers*,[82] which appeared in Schleiermacher's thirty-first year, in 1799. Speeches: this word merely denotes the literary form which Schleiermacher chose. The text, which is often difficult to understand despite all the dithyrambic verve of his prose, and which for all its dependence especially on Fichte does not refer to anyone,[83] was never presented as 'speeches'. It was conceived from the start as a treatise, a thoroughly planned and structured rhetorical treatise in which (almost) everything is well related to the strategy of the argument.

So this book shows that Schleiermacher was a modern man through and through, but at the same time had remained in an amazing way a man of religion. Modern culture and religious conviction – Schleiermacher demonstrated in a challenging way that these need not be in contradiction. He wanted to bear witness to what he had struggled to discover himself: even today one could be modern **and** religious, critical **and** pious. And precisely in this way Schleiermacher became the teacher for nineteenth-century theology, a man of the spirit and modernity.

In fact all was not well with the cause of religion and theology at this time. Moreover in these years some of Schleiermacher's most famous contemporaries – Fichte, Schelling, Hegel and Hölderlin – had moved from theology into philosophy (or poetry). Certainly they had not given up 'religion' completely, but had incorporated it into their speculative metaphysical system – as philosophical thinkers who certainly cannot be said to have denied all religion (above all not the 'piety of thought' claimed by Hegel); however, the roots of their life and thought were genuinely philosophical. Many of Schleiermacher's new friends showed only an incomprehension of religion.

It needed someone of the stature of Schleiermacher to adopt a counter-position here that was worth taking seriously. Moreover, generally speaking there was no one on the church-theological scene who in these stormy times between Revolution and Restoration, Enlightenment and Romanticism, could ask the question 'What about religion?' as urgently, credibly and effectively as he could. 'It may be an unexpected and even a marvellous undertaking that any one should still venture to demand from the very class that have raised themselves above the vulgar, and are saturated with the wisdom of the centuries, attention for a subject so entirely neglected by them.' That is the way in which Schleiermacher begins, provocatively, his *Speeches*, which were initially published anonymously. He immediately adds that he, too, 'steeped in the wisdom of centuries', has in no way swung over into the pre-modern reactionary camp: 'With the cry of distress, in which most of them join, over the downfall of religion I have no sympathy, for I know of no age that has given religion a better reception than the present. I have nothing to do with the conservative and barbarian lamentation whereby they seek to rear again the fallen walls and gothic pillars of their Jewish Zion.'[84]

This makes it clear that Schleiermacher sees it as his almost prophetic mission, his divine calling, to bring religion to bear in a completely new way, for to him as a critical thinker religion, despite all his personal objections to particular doctrines, is anything but a 'neglected subject'; it is virtually the content and guiding light of his life. He wants to introduce it both to those contemporaries who have completely succumbed to the earthly and sensual and to those who speculate and moralize over empty ideas. The subject of religion is topical because it is given by the whole human situation and is therefore unavoidable.

All this depends on the question what one means by 'religion'. What, according to Schleiermacher, is **religion**? Is it that 'reasonable Christianity' which has been compiled of bits of metaphysics and morality? No. For the religious person, 'religion' is not a matter of systematizing and theorizing, as it is for the philosopher, nor is it a matter of formulae of faith and proofs, as it is for the orthodox dogmatician ('theologian of the letter'); for in the sphere of 'religion' it is not doctrine but life that has the priority. So religion is not simply a matter of being 'moral' in the spirit of Kant, or merely 'aesthetic' along the lines of Schiller, Goethe or Herder; for someone who is only moral or aesthetic is not yet pious, nor yet 'religious'. But in that case, who is 'religious'?

The peculiar feature of religion is a mysterious **experience**; it is **being moved by the world of the eternal**. So religion is about the heavenly sparks which are struck when a holy soul is touched by the infinite, a religious experience to which the 'virtuosi of religion' give direct expression in their speeches and utterances, and which is communicated by them also to ordinary people. To be more precise, religion seeks to experience the universe, the totality of what is and what happens, mediatively in **immediate seeing and feeling** (these categories come from Fichte): 'It is neither thinking nor acting, but intuition and feeling. It will regard the Universe as it is. It is reverent attention and submission, in childlike passivity, to be stirred and filled by the Universe's immediate influences.'[85]

One can also say that religion is a **religion of the heart**: in it human beings are encountered, grasped, filled and moved in their innermost depths and their totality – by the infinite which is active in all that is finite. No, religion is neither praxis nor speculation, neither art nor science, but a **'sense and taste for the infinite'**.[86] This living relationship to the eternal, the infinite, represents the original disposition of each individual 'I', but it must be aroused. Religious experiences are countless, and patience is called for. So in the religious consciousness the two limits, individuality and the universe, make contact. From a historical perspective this means that religion is:

– no longer as in the Middle Ages or even the Reformation a take-off, a flight into something beyond the world, supernatural;

– nor, as in Deism and the Enlightenment, a departure into something behind the world, metaphysical;

– rather, in a modern understanding it is the intimating, the seeing, the feeling, the **indwelling of the infinite in the finite**. The infinite in the finite, or God as the eternal absolute being that conditions all things – this, we can say, is the modern understanding of God and not (as Schleiermacher adds in the second edition at the end of the excursuses on the idea of God) 'the usual conception of God as one single being outside of the world and behind the world'.[87] Like Fichte, Schelling and Hegel, with philosophical strictness Schleiermacher rejects any anthropomorphizing of God. God in the modern understanding is the immanent transcendent primal ground of all being, knowledge and will.

We can see that in his bold enterprise Schleiermacher does not simply begin with some holy documents under the shell of which, in his view, the real **essence** of religion lies hidden. No, he wants 'to approach the matter from the other end and to begin with the clear-cut distinction between our faith and your ethics and metaphysics'.[88] So is there a contrast between religion on the one hand and morality and metaphysics on the other? This can only be understood against the background of the time. Schleiermacher was not dealing with an 'enlightened' atheism and materialism, as in the neighbouring France of the Revolution, but with a high-flown Idealism which had been produced by the Enlightenment in Germany: with an idealist metaphysics and morality. So Schleiermacher's concern had to be the **independence** of religion – even if the essence of religion has never existed anywhere in a pure and abstract form. He was concerned with the independence of religion **on the one hand from metaphysics**, i.e. philosophical speculation, and **on the other hand from morality**, i.e. moral effort. Indeed, wasn't it often the dispute over morality and especially metaphysics that made religion seem intolerant, spiteful, and persecuting instead of patient? Doctrinal statements, dogmas, concepts are not, however, religion but reflections on religion.

Now if this is the case, isn't the continuity of Protestant theology with the Reformation completely interrupted? Not necessarily.[89] For hadn't **Luther** already protested against the twofold alienation of **theology** by metaphysics and morality: against the transformation of theology into metaphysics by Aristotelian philosophy (a speculative ascent to God) and into Christian morality by a piety of works (speculation on one's own work)? **Schleiermacher** thinks similarly. He, too, attacks the alienation of **religion** by speculative thought and moralizing praxis. Religion or (as he will later say) piety is for Schleiermacher an utterly existential matter; it is the cause of the **feeling** which precedes and underlies all thought and action.

This feeling is not to be understood in a restricted psychological sense as Romantic enthusiastic emotion, but in a comprehensive, existential way as a sense of being encountered at the centre, as immediate religious self-awareness (Ebeling compares this function with that of the conscience in

Luther). Schleiermacher himself would later make this notion more precise, and withdraw the term 'intuition' of the universe, which was open to misunderstanding (with the senses, or spiritually? After all one can hardly see the universe as a whole), in favour of the term 'feeling'. As we shall see, he would speak more precisely in his *The Christian Faith* of religion as the **feeling of ultimate dependence**.

Question 1: Theology or philosophy?

Now if religion is the feeling of 'absolute dependence', isn't a dog the best Christian?[90] – thus one of the most malicious *bon mots* about Schleiermacher's thought, made by Georg Friedrich Wilhelm Hegel, from 1718 his Berlin colleague in philosophy as successor to Fichte. No, witty and spiteful as this *bon mot* is (Schleiermacher ignored Hegel's polemic), it misses the point, because it ignores not only the spiritual, holistic nature of 'feeling' but above all Schleiermacher's understanding of God with its emphasis on Christian freedom as compared with any religious servitude. So in 'feeling' Christians are not as 'dependent' on their God as dogs on their master. On the contrary.

Schleiermacher is concerned with the inner **freedom** of the moral person – the source of eternal youth and joy. Moreover, freedom is also a key word in the *Monologues*, the second major work which Schleiermacher published after the *Speeches* (as a New Year's gift at the beginning of 1800), in which he attempted to describe his religious view of life and the world in the form of a 'lyrical extract from a permanent diary'.[91] And in complete contrast to Hegel, already in the *Speeches* Schleiermacher is decidedly **against the state church**. For him, as a Reformed Christian, this is the source of all corruption. He called passionately for the separation of church and state on the French model, and in his fourth speech on religion virtually developed a programme for a radical reform of the church in which the parish communities would be replaced by personal communities (of the kind that he was later to have himself).

And yet aren't perhaps those critics right who point to the twilight nature of this theology, which has given itself over completely to modernity? Aren't they right when (like the young Karl Barth) they suspect Schleiermacher, who gave lectures not only on theology but also on the whole range of philosophy, of basically doing not theology but philosophy? In a much-admired late Postscript to a selection of Schleiermacher's writing in 1968 (fifty years after his *Romans* and in the year of his death), **Karl Barth again** raised this question, but remarkably enough in his old age he left it open:

– Is Schleiermacher's enterprise 'really a Christian **theology** orientated on

worship, preaching, instruction, pastoral care', which is merely in the 'inauthentic garb of a philosophy adapted to the people of its time'?
– Or is it an 'indifferently Christian **philosophy**' which has 'inauthentically concealed itself in the garb of a theology, Christian theology'?[92]

Along the lines of the early Barth, many representatives of 'dialectical theology' accused Schleiermacher of dissolving theology into philosophy ('philosophy of identity', 'Platonism', 'Gnosticism', 'pantheism' or 'Spinozism'), but in more recent times the Schleiermacher of the *Speeches* in particular has been defended as a theologian who developed 'an apology for Christianity presented with philosophical means',[93] whose theory of religion is indebted to a 'theological approach'.[94] By contrast, the view has been put forward that Schleiermacher must not be interpreted by means of 'notions of the confrontation and alternation of philosophy and theology'. Indeed, Schleiermacher's alternative is not one of philosophy or theology, but of philosophy or dogmatics.[95]

Taking all this into account, my answer to Karl Barth's question is that Schleiermacher's *Speeches* in no way present an indifferently Christian philosophy; from the beginning, these *Speeches* point in a hidden but unerring way to Christianity. However, this is not theology at least as Karl Barth did it, a theology which is dogmatic from the start (beginning with the Trinity) and in any case is ecclesiastical (obligated to church dogmas). But is Karl Barth's *Church Dogmatics* the only Christian theology? In his 1946 chapter on Schleiermacher he himself conceded that the anthropocentric 'reversal of the way of looking at things' need not necessarily mean that theology was now no longer theology, or had even become the enemy of theology': 'genuine, proper theology **could** be built up from such a starting point'.[96] No, there is no single way of doing theology. Schleiermacher, who had to study traditional dogmatics for his examination but abhorred it, deliberately chose another approach, with which he hoped to be able to reach the learned among the despisers of religion. This may appropriately be called the **fundamental theological** method, which works with universal leading insights and terms. In the subsequent period 'fundamental theology' was developed more by Catholic theologians than in Protestant theology, which contented itself with 'prolegomena to dogmatics'.

While recognizing the independence of the religious disposition, we must certainly discuss with Schleiermacher whether religion can so abruptly take leave of thought and action, theory and practice, metaphysics and morality, awareness of the truth and moral consciousness. Can there be a sense of truly being gripped by religion, void of any truth-content and dictates of the conscience? But we must immediately add that even Schleiermacher would not stop here. And it would become even clearer that the feeling of absolute dependence on the human side presupposes absolute causality from God's side, so that Christian theology cannot be said to have been delivered over to a secular philosophy.

Initially, it is important from a methodological perspective to see that Schleiermacher takes his readers from the place in the world where they stand and in the face of their misunderstandings attempts to work out the true understanding of religion generally. Here as far as possible he avoids any specifically theological conceptuality, or, where it cannot be avoided, he interprets it. So as substitutes for the word 'God', which is understood by his educated contemporaries in an anthropomorphic, pre-modern way, he prefers words like 'the universe', the 'infinite', the 'holy', concepts which he hopes will be more convincing to his modern contemporaries because they are less loaded. But in doing this doesn't Schleiermacher prove to be the advocate of an autonomous 'natural' religion, independent of any revelation?

The significance of the 'positive' in religion

Anyone who thinks that in his *Speeches* Schleiermacher is simply practising 'natural theology' (abhorred by many theologians since Karl Barth) should note that he makes it emphatically clear over against the whole theology of the Enlightenment that for him there is **no such thing as 'natural religion'**. This would in fact be rational with a moral orientation, so that everything beyond such a rational religion would have to be rejected as 'superstition'. No, for Schleiermacher such a natural or rational religion was an artificial product of philosophical reflection, without that life and immediacy which characterizes an authentic religion. So from the beginning, Schleiermacher is convinced that religion can be understood rightly only if it is not simply considered 'in general', but in the individual, living, concrete, religions. Schleiermacher calls these individual, concrete religions (Judaism, Christianity, Islam, etc.) positive religions.

Thus the *Speeches* end in a reflection on the 'positive' element in the religions. The basic notion is this. There is no 'Infinite' in itself, in pure abstraction. The Infinite can only ever be grasped in the finite: it empties and manifests itself in an infinite variety of forms. Any view of the universe is always an individual one, and none of these countless views can be excluded in principle. So 'religion' must individualize itself in different religions. As a result, anyone who wants to understand 'religion' must understand the different religions. The individual religions may have lost their original life and be identified with particular formulae, slogans and convictions; in the course of their long history they may have been distorted and deformed; nevertheless, they are authentic and pure individualizations of 'religion', if and to the extent that they make possible an experience of the Infinite in the human subject; in so far as they make a particular view of the Infinite their central point, their central view, to which everything in this religion is related.

Thus in his *Speeches* Schleiermacher took great pains not only to disperse all the prejudices of his modern contemporaries about religion generally, but also to make them open to the **'positive' element in the religions**, the positive ('given') in all religions. However, here we should note that for Schleiermacher the individual religions by no means all stand on the same level: he takes it for granted that what religion is has individualized itself most in Christianity. Christianity is thus relatively the best of all religions in human history. Christianity need not fear comparison with other religions.

Here we can only regret that Schleiermacher did not have more precise knowledge of the **non-Christian religions** (apart from Greek religion). Though he had also brought out an important aspect of 'religion' with his emphasis on religious experience, in later years he never had so broad a knowledge of the history of religions as, say, his later Berlin colleague and rival Hegel. In his lectures on the philosophy of religion Hegel treated the religions of humankind in a quite concrete way: as the great historical forms of the absolute Spirit revealing itself in the human spirit – beginning with the nature religions (the deity as a natural force and substance) in Africa, China, India, Persia and Egypt; through Judaism, Greek and Roman religion, the religions of spiritual individuality; to Christianity, which, as the highest form of religion, includes all previous forms in itself.

And yet there is no denying that no theologian was to give such a boost to the history, phenomenology and psychology of religion which was to develop so strongly: no theologian worked it out intellectually to such a degree as Schleiermacher. If there is still so much talk of **experience** in religious studies and theology this is essentially because of Schleiermacher, and if religion is no longer understood merely in private terms but as the affair of a **community**, this again is largely due to him. If Christianity can be understood as the best and supreme individualization of religion and so can be included in a comparison of religions, this too finds its legitimation, at least in principle, in Schleiermacher.

Question 2: Dissolution into anthropology?

But aren't those **critics** right who, following Emil Brunner, trace a line from Schleiermacher to mysticism,[97] and accuse him of wanting to replace the word of holy scripture which comes from outside with the speechless interiority of feeling; who indeed, according to Karl Barth, engaged in an **anthropologizing** and **subjectivizing of theology** and thus paved the way for Feuerbach's 'sublation' and dissolution of theology into anthropology?

The late **Karl Barth** also became cautious over this second question.

– In Schleiermacher does the human being feel, think and speak 'in relation to an Other which cannot be done away with', equivalent to a **subject** 'superior to his own being, feeling, knowing, willing and doing', in the face of whom 'worship, thanksgiving, penitence and petition are concretely possible, indeed called for?'

– Or in Schleiermacher do human beings feel, think and speak 'in and from a sovereign awareness of their own contemporaneity, indeed **oneness** with everything that could come into question as a subject, as something Other, different from them or even Another'?[98]

My answer to this question is: very much on the line from Descartes to Kant, Schleiermacher's theological reflection takes its **start from the subject** and personal experience, but this does **not** result in any **subjectivizing** and anthropologizing of theology. Already in his early works Schleiermacher explicitly emphasizes that without this 'religion' consisting in feeling, both thought and action would succumb to the pernicious desire to make the human being the centre of all things: 'in the whole universe seeing only the human being as the centre of all relationships, as the condition of all being and the cause of all becoming'.[99] In religion it is precisely the other way round. Religion wants 'to see the Infinite, its imprint and its description in the human being no less than in all other individuals and finite things'.[100] So there can be no question of any anthropocentricity in Schleiermacher, of any dissolution of theology into anthropology.

So the **suspicion of pantheism** which keeps being raised is also unjustified. Certainly, Schleiermacher wants to see the finite **in** the infinite and the infinite **in** the finite, but that is not to claim any 'oneness' of finite and infinite, nor to claim that God and the world are one and the same. Already at that time Schleiermacher energetically disputed that he was a pantheist. Despite all his study of Spinoza and his sympathy for him, all through his life he knew quite clearly where he differed from Spinoza, and moreover later claimed credibly that he had never for a moment been a follower of his. God is in all things, is in us. God and the world are related to each other, but they are essentially different. Granted, Schleiermacher wanted not only personalistic religions which attribute a peculiar consciousness to the Infinite to be recognized as religions, but also pantheistic religions, which do not. But at all events he resolutely rejected a God 'who would be only the genius of humankind'; such a conception of God was as alien to him as that of God as 'an individual totally distinct from humankind'.[101] He prefers to speak of the living God rather than the personal God.

So in principle, for Schleiermacher the real 'object' of religion is the infinite which appears in the finite, the divine life and action. Whether or not this is imagined in personal terms, what remains for the religious consciousness is a superior, supreme and ultimate power with which religious enthusiasts can feel at one in particular moments, but with which they are in no way substantially one. Just as Schleiermacher is no pantheist, so too he is no mystic of union, and in his *Monologues* (above all with the help of Fichte) he is clearly opposed to any Spinozan monism and determinism. So if we want to give his standpoint any label, panentheism would be better than pantheism. And it is from that perspective that we must also understand his new interpretation of fundamental theological concepts, concepts like miracle (without breaking the laws of nature), revelation (in human experience), prophecy and the effect of grace.

Now whether Schleiermacher's reinterpretation of basic theological concepts is satisfactory is another question. And though we cannot accuse him of anthropologizing and subjectivizing religion, the question of how Christian his theology is arises. Is he really a Christian theologian? Is he really doing Christian theology?

The uniqueness of Christianity

For Schleiermacher, the easiest way of finding access to the spirit of religions is to have a religion oneself. And this is certainly particularly important for someone who 'approaches the holiest in which the Universe in its highest unity and comprehensiveness is to be perceived':[102] Christianity. Nor can it be disputed, despite all criticism, that Schleiermacher made an essential contribution towards providing a constructive answer to the question of the **essence of Christianity** which had been posed by the Enlightenment. His view is that the essence of every religion must be seen in a 'basic vision', its 'vision of the Infinite'.[103] That is already true of Judaism and even more of Christianity.

So what is the central vision, the original being, the spirit of **Judaism**? This is a question which must be looked at briefly first. Like Hegel and other German Idealists, Schleiermacher was not very favourably disposed towards Judaism. For him, it did not offer the key to Christianity. Certainly Schleiermacher thought that Judaism had taught much, and that if one left aside the way in which politics, morality and ceremonial obscured the truly religious, it had been quite attractive in its 'beautiful childlike character'.[104] But what about its basic view, which shines through everywhere, its relationship to the Infinite? This was dominated by the idea of 'universal immediate **retribution**':[105] reward and punishment!

Here Schleiermacher understands the whole history of the Jewish people as a living conversation between God and human beings, a conversation in words and actions, in which prophecy and messianic faith have a special significance. But this living history had already died out at the time when with the end of the holy scripture in Judaism the dialogue of God with his people had also come to an end. So for Schleiermacher there is no doubt that to the present day Judaism is a dead religion, and we have to put up with that. However, we should not put up with Schleiermacher's distorted view of Judaism, which shows no sensitivity to the ongoing existence not only of the Jewish people generally, but also of the Jewish religion, albeit in the mediaeval rabbinic paradigm of the synagogue which was only broken open in Schleiermacher's time, at the end of the eighteenth century, by the influence of modernity (Moses Mendelssohn).[106] The only excuse for Schleiermacher that we might find is that in the Berlin of the time, modern and now assimilated Jews did not have any more positive a view of the past of their religion. And as early as 1799 Schleiermacher had indicated his opposition to Jews being accepted into the Protestant church, as many enlightened people wanted, provided that they accepted the basic truth of a natural religion of reason. His view was that they should be granted civil rights as Jews, independently of the Christian confession.

For Schleiermacher, of course, **Christianity** stands out clearly against the not very pleasant negative foil of Judaism – at least Christianity in its original form: 'The original intuition of Christianity is more glorious, more sublime, more worthy of an adult humanity, penetrates deeper into the spirit of systematic religion, and extends itself further over the whole Universe.'[107] Schleiermacher was convinced that the essence of religion can be seen purely and clearly only in Christianity.

But what is the central vision, the original essence, the spirit of **Christianity**, which can be defined despite all the historical distortions, despite all disputes over words and despite all the bloody holy wars? Schleiermacher sees the relationship between the finite and the infinite in Christianity as differing from that in Judaism. It is not determined by the idea of retribution but is a relationship between **corruption and redemption, enmity and mediation**. Christianity is polemical through and through, to the degree that it recognizes the universality of corruption and proceeds against the irreligion outside and inside itself. However, Christianity aims to penetrate to an ever greater holiness, purity and relationship to God: all that is finite is to be related everywhere and at all times to the infinite.

So Christianity represents religion to a higher potency, even if as a universal religion it should not exclude any other religion or any new religions. It does not have its origin in Judaism, but underivably and inexplicably in the one **emissary** on whom dawned the basic idea of universal corruption and redemption through higher mediation. What does Schleiermacher admire in Jesus Christ? Not simply the purity of his moral doctrine and the distinctiveness of his character, which combines power and gentleness; these are human features. The 'truly divine' in Christ is the 'glorious clarity to which the great idea he came to exhibit attained in his soul. This idea was, that all that is finite requires a higher mediation to be in accord with the Deity.'[108] What does this 'higher mediation' mean?

All that is finite needs the mediation of something higher for its redemption, and this 'cannot be purely finite. It must belong to both sides, participating in the Divine Essence in the same way and in the same sense in which it participates in human nature.'[109] Therefore he is not the only mediator but the unique mediator, of whom it is rightly said, 'No one knows the Father but the Son and the one to whom he wills to reveal it': 'This consciousness of the singularity of his religion, of the originality of his view, and of its power to communicate itself and to awake religion, was at once the consciousness of his office as mediator and of his divinity.'[110] It is beyond question that such a formulation of the significance of Jesus Christ even at that time made more than the orthodox frown.

Question 3: Dissolution into psychology?

From the beginning, Schleiermacher's **christology of consciousness** was sharply attacked: doesn't the revelation of God here become a mode of human knowing and feeling? Doesn't belief in Christ become an illuminating universal human possibility? Does Jesus Christ here still remain an objective historical entity which is distinct from pious feeling? Or is christology dissolved into psychology, a universal christological psychology instead of a concrete historical christology? And in all this isn't the deity of Christ ultimately left out of account? In his old age **Karl Barth** again put a critical question to Schleiermacher's christology (his third) – but here too he left it unanswered:
– Does the human being feel, think and speak 'primarily in relation to a

special, concrete reality which is thus definite and capable of definition, and only from that point, secondarily, in a process of generalization and abstraction in respect of the essence and meaning of that with which he finds himself in contact'?

– Or does the human being feel, think and speak 'primarily in relationship to a **universal** essence and meaning of reality which is elicited and established a priori, and only from that point, secondarily, with attention to its particular, concrete form which is definable and defined'?[111]

After the *Speeches* and *Monologues*, Schleiermacher clarified his christological position in a poetical-theological work *Christmas Eve*,[112] composed as a 'conversation', which appeared in 1805. A year previously Schleiermacher had been rescued from his exile in the small provincial town of Stolp by a call to the University of Halle as *extraordinarius* Professor of Reformed Theology and University Preacher. In his 'conversation', which is set at a family Christmas celebration with music, songs and food, in imitation of Plato's 'Dialogues', various conversation-partners, all of whom he presents sympathetically with inner understanding, show how differently they understand the experience of Christmas and the person of Christ.

There is the thoughful, reflective, unbelieving **Leonhard**, who practises radical historical criticism and understands the Christmas story symbolically. There is **Eduard**, a theologian of history who speculates in the style of Schelling; he idealizes the Christmas story in the light of the Johannine prologue and its incarnate Word, and understands Christ as the central human genre. And finally, probably closest to Schleiermacher, there is **Ernst** (Schleiermacher's third name), the theologian of experience, who, while he does not argue for the historicity of the Christmas story, does argue for its deep meaning as the appearance of the Redeemer, which is depicted here as an unsurpassable fact and as a binding religious reality: 'The story of the Redeemer remains the only universal feast of joy since for us there is no other principle of joy than redemption, and in the development of this, again the birth of the divine child is the first clear point, after which we expect no other and cannot postpone our joy any longer.'[113]

But at the end of the feast **Joseph** makes a late arrival; he refuses to give any interpretation of his own, and referring to his 'speechless joy'[114] invites the company to hand round the presents and join in joyful pious song. A 'Herrnhuter of a higher order'? Be this as it may, in the end the story is left open. Even now there is discussion as to which conversation-partner Schleiermacher identifies himself with, if he identifies himself with any of them. Schleiermacher's own answer comes in his 'dogmatics', *The Christian Faith*.

The Christian Faith: *a synthesis of tradition and modernity*

Schleiermacher's lectures in Halle and Berlin had now been sufficient preparation for him to write his theological *magnum opus*, which was to become the **most significant dogmatics of modern times**. However, he deliberately avoided the word 'dogmatics', and instead chose the title *The Christian Faith* – but now with the significant addition 'described consecutively in accordance with the Principles of the Protestant Church'.[115] If we use the *Speeches* once again as a comparison, what is immediately striking about the new work is its scholastic structure, which moreover had grown out of Schleiermacher's lectures and was used in lectures. It is divided into paragraphs, each introduced with a leading sentence (not always easy to understand) and then provided with long and sophisticated explanations. But this scholastic approach does not prove sterile. Rather, here we have a systematic theology with an artistic structure, which for its ingenious uniqueness and otherness can certainly be set alongside the *Summa* of Thomas Aquinas and Calvin's *Institutes*. It sought to be believing and pious, critical and rational, all at once – in its own way.

Anyone who patiently gets down to this work, the very language of which is difficult, cannot avoid increasingly admiring its grandiose internal architecture as time goes on. Under the **leading idea of redemption** (sin-grace) – forced right to the periphery in the Enlightenment – two **tripartite schemes** are worked together in the division and shaping of the material. There are three main sections, which describe 1. the Christian consciousness apart from sin and grace; 2. the consciousness of sin; 3. the consciousness of grace. And in turn each of these main parts contains three forms of dogmatic statements: first descriptions of human conditions, then concepts of divine properties, and finally statements about things in the world.

Schleiermacher, the master of both broad outline and fine detail, now finishes his work of art by fitting all the usual dogmatic 'doctrines' into this ninefold framework, at the same time largely maintaining the traditional order of themes in a way which is **modern and traditional**. For each doctrinal issue he quotes the Lutheran and Reformed confessional writings, earlier and contemporary dogmatics, and patristic and scholastic statements, to present an extensive account of the status quo; at the same time he also takes account of the criticism of the Enlightenment. Utterly honest intellectually, and with incomparable systematic power, undeterred as he was, he goes on to a critical and constructive stocktaking, examination and development of theology so far. It is immediately striking that contrary to the usual order, the doctrine 'of the divine Trinity' appears only at the end as a 'Conclusion', instead of at the beginning in the doctrine of God; Schleiermacher certainly did not mean this as a leave-taking, but it is hardly meant to be the crown of his systematic theology either.

Schleiermacher's modern *The Christian Faith* differs here both from mediaeval *Summas* and from any Reformation orthodox dogmatics, for which faith is primarily the holding of certain facts of revelation or truths of faith to be true.

By contrast, Schleiermacher's work:

– **has a strictly historical orientation**: for him – and this is said against both biblicism and rationalism – it is not the science of an (allegedly) timeless, unchanged Christian doctrine, but is 'the science which systematizes the doctrine prevalent in a Christian church at any one time' (§1;

– **has an ecumenical form**: the reference to a 'church' does not of course mean the authority of a magisterium but the confessional writings of the churches and their prime document, Holy Scripture. Here Schleiermacher did not think that the controversies between Lutheran and Reformed doctrine (unlike the opposition between Protestantism and Catholicism) were enough to split the church; he argued more than anyone else for the Lutheran-Reformed Union, introduced in Prussia at the Feast of the Reformation in 1817, with joint eucharistic celebrations. He understood his *Christian Faith* as a dogmatics of union;

– **is related to experience**: as is his wont, Schleiermacher begins from religious experience, the disposition or consciousness of Christians, the piety of the church community, in short from pious human consciousness (which, however, is collective and communal). The dogmatic statements certainly cannot be proved from scripture and tradition, but Schleiermacher can rightly claim to stand in the Christian tradition. For he explicitly does theology from the community of faith, from the church; not, though, to prove its faith but to make its innermost essence understandable in a critical and constructive way. So the two sayings of Anselm on the title page of his *The Christian Faith* are not just decoration from the tradition but express a consciousness of it. 'I do not attempt to know in order to believe, but I believe in order to know. For anyone who does not believe will not experience, and anyone who does not experience will not know.'[116]

In the programmatic **introduction** – often commented on as much as the body of the work itself – Schleiermacher again takes up important statements of his fundamental theology. They show that he still parts company not only with orthodoxy, but also with the Enlightenment identification of piety and the truth of reason. First of all the basic features of a theory of religion and the religious community are described (in the second edition called 'lemmas from ethics'), then the differences between the historical religions ('lemmas from the philosophy of religion'), and finally a definition of the essence of Christianity and of Protestantism ('lemmas from apologetics'). Some of the things that we know from the *Speeches* are made more precise here. On religion or – the word which is now preferred – '**piety**' we can read: 'Piety is intrinsically neither a knowing nor a doing but an inclination and determination of the feeling' (§8). The essence of religion or piety can thus be defined more precisely: 'The feature common to all pious stimulations, the essence of piety, is this, that we are aware of ourselves as being utterly dependent, in other words, that we feel dependent on God' (§9). The concept of the feeling of **absolute dependence** is thus a central concept of a general theory of religion in Schleiermacher, and not, as Hegel's criticism insinuates, the formula for the essence of 'Christianity'.

The key significance of Jesus as the Christ

So what, according to Schleiermacher's *The Christian Faith*, is the **essence of Christianity**? The famous definition runs: 'Christianity is a monotheistic faith, belonging to the teleological type of religion, and is essentially distinguished from other such faiths by the fact that in it everything is related to the redemption accomplished by Jesus of Nazareth' (§11).

If we are to understand this definiton of the essence of Christianity, which while simple is not all that simple to understand, we must remember four things:
– In the three stages of religious development presupposed by Schleiermacher, fetishism – polytheism – **monotheism** (universally advocated in the Enlightenment), Christianity stands on the top step not only as an 'aesthetic' religion (a religion of nature or destiny), but as a 'teleological' religion, i.e. one that is determined by a goal. It is thus an **ethical**, active religion, corresponding to human nature.
– The 'distinctive' feature of Christianity, which sets it apart from all other religions, does not lie in its natural rational character but in its **redemptive character**: for everything is governed by the basic opposition of sin and grace and precisely in that way related to the 'mediator' Jesus of Nazareth.
– Its **christocentricity** is already emphasized by the prominent position of christology in the 'Introduction': in Schleiermacher, christological statements stand at the point where in orthodox dogmatics there was a discussion of holy scripture. The central position of the person of Jesus Christ in Christianity is indispensable for Schleiermacher!

– The fundamental methodological starting point in the consciousness of faith is maintained: Schleiermacher does not begin from the objective story of Jesus of Nazareth, but from our pious Christian '**consciousness**', our consciousness of the church community, of redemption through the person of Jesus Christ.

That brings us back to Barth's question, which we had to postpone when discussing *Christmas Eve*: with the person of Jesus Christ is the pious consciousness related to a **particular**, concrete reality which thus is definite and capable of definition, or is this particular figure incorporated into a **universal** essence and meaning of history, and thus levelled down?

One difficulty about Schleiermacher's consciousness-christology was that the pious consciousness always only circles around itself, that it does not have any real object. This difficulty seems to me to be answered in *The Christian Faith*: Schleiermacher's christology is without doubt not just a postulate of the pious consciousness, nor the complex imagination of subjective faith. For we cannot overlook the fact that:

– Christian consciousness, Christianity generally, is inconceivable without the historical figure of Jesus of Nazareth as its **historical origin**.

– **At the centre of Christianity** is therefore not a universal idea of a moral doctrine, but a historical figure and his redemptive effect on human beings and history after him. The christocentricity of *The Christian Faith* (and the picture of Christ in Schleiermacher's sermons) is thus not the result of Schleiermacher's speculation, but a consequence of the history of Jesus Christ himself and what had followed from it.

– In Schleiermacher the historical figure does not remain an abstract 'saving event'; rather, his **history** can be **narrated**. Moreover it is no coincidence that Schleiermacher wrote a *Life of Jesus* which depicts Jesus of Nazareth with his unshakeable consciousness of God and his concern for suffering human beings. Certainly it is idealistic, all too orientated on the Gospel of John and the Greek ideal of 'noble simplicity and silent greatness', but nevertheless it is in no way simply in conformity with the ideals of the bourgeois society of Schleiermacher's time.[117]

At the same time, by taking up the criticism of the Enlightenment but applying it in accordance with religious and not purely rational criteria, in *The Christian Faith* Schleiermacher carried out a large-scale **demythologizing**: not only of the Old Testament narratives of a paradisal primal state of a first human couple, a primal fall and original sin, angels and devils, miracles and prophecies, but also of the New Testament narratives of Jesus' virgin birth, the nature miracles, resurrection, ascension and the prophecy of his return.

Despite all the demythologizing, the differences between Schleiermacher's christology and the Jesuology of the enlightened rationalists is clear. According to Schleiermacher, it follows from an analysis of the pious Christian consciousness,

– that Christ is the active one and human beings are recipients; it is Christ who overcomes the power of sin through his grace;

– that Christ makes possible a living communion with human beings and a new higher life in humankind;

– that the overall impact of Christ's ongoing personality is decisive for this rather than individual features (which are possibly dubious);

– that this historical personality bears within itself a primal perfection, so that it is not only a model which human beings are to imitate but a **primal image of the consciousness of God**, which grasps and forms them.

Thus the Redeemer as a historical person is the ground and cause of redemption. But how does this redemption come about in human beings? To summarize briefly what Schleiermacher worked out in his doctrine of redemption, redemption means being accepted into communion with Christ. The foundation of this new life is laid by **rebirth**, which consists of two elements: 'justification' (a changed relationship of human beings to God on the basis of faith and the forgiveness of sins) and 'conversion' (a changed form of life by moving from the community of sin into the community of grace through penitence and faith – though without the pietistic struggle over penitence). The life of rebirth is maintained and developed through **sanctification**: the good works of the reborn are natural effects of faith – despite all the sins which remain.

All the reborn gather in the community of believers, in the Christian **church**. This is grounded in the divine election and is united and lived out in all its members by that **communal spirit** who is none other than the **Holy Spirit** issuing from Christ and gaining power in believers. There can be no living communion with Christ without the indwelling of the Holy Spirit, and vice versa.

Question 4: And the christological dogmas?

In connection with the indwelling of the Holy Spirit we now take up the fourth critical question addressed by the old **Karl Barth** to Schleiermacher, which he again deliberately leaves open:

– Is the spirit which moves the feeling, speaking, thinking person 'an utterly **particular**, specific spirit, constantly distinguishing itself from all other spirits, a spirit which is really to be called "holy"'?

– Or is this spirit 'while individually differentiated, one that is **universally active**, but in individuals a diffuse spiritual dynamis'?[118]

In the second edition of his *The Christian Faith*, published in 1830, Schleiermacher considerably modified his remarks in this connection and made them more precise. So the answer must initially be given on the basis of what he said there in his epilogue on **the doctrine of the Trinity**:[119] that 'in Christ there was present nothing less than the Divine essence, which also indwells the Christian church as its common spirit', and that he means these expressions 'in no reduced or sheerly artificial sense' – as though there were only 'subordinate deities in Christ and the Holy Spirit'! Precisely 'this equating with each other of the divine and the human in Christ and the Holy Spirit and also the identification of the two with the divine being in itself' are for Schleiermacher 'what is essential for the doctrine of the Trinity'.[120] However, he distances himself from later church formulations in the hope that 'there must still be in store for this doctrine a transformation which will go back to its very beginnings'.[121]

What does this mean for the christological question in the narrower sense: for the question not only of Christ's function (his 'doings') but also Christ's **person**? Who was this Jesus Christ in the deepest sense? The old Herrnhuter was passionately concerned to answer this question. For a long time he laboured to find deeply religious new answers to old questions which at the same time would be clear and simple. Now, in *The Christian Faith*, he had an answer: Christ is **like** human beings! To what degree? 'In virtue of the identity of human beings.' Christ is **different** from all human beings! To what degree? 'By the constant potency of his God-consciousness, which was a veritable existence of God in him.'[122]

A **veritable existence of God** in Christ? Schleiermacher leaves no doubt here: whereas other people have only a general religious disposition and an 'imperfect and obscure' God-consciousness, Jesus' God-consciousness was 'absolutely clear, and determined each moment, to the exclusion of all else'.[123] This can be regarded 'as a continual living presence, and withal a real existence of God in him', in which at the same time his 'utter sinlessness' is given – and, as a presupposition of this, his lack of guilt from the beginning.[124] That means that in Christ 'the being of God' is there unbroken 'as the innermost fundamental power within him from which every activity emanates and which holds every element together'[125] (just as, to use an illustration, the intelligence as the basic force in human beings orders and holds together all other forces). The eternal Infinite is present in Jesus' consciousness with its unconditioned power and force yet without annihilating it; rather, it controls this consciousness and shapes the whole of Jesus' life so that he becomes an instrument, model and original. And this is decisive, for unless the

Redeemer has divine worth there can be no redemption, and vice versa. In this way the new living communion with Christ, the beginning of new life and the renewal of the disposition which is constantly necessary, are made possible – a process which takes place utterly through grace. That is the particular concern of Schleiermacher the theologian and above all Schleiermacher the preacher.

So has Schleiermacher answered the christological question? *Vere deus*? Truly God? Yes, Jesus is formed by the divine primal ground in a way unlike any other. Certainly God is present everywhere in the finite realm as the one who is active *par excellence*, but in Christ the God-consciousness is the principle which shapes the personality. His God-consciousness must be understood as a pure and authentic revelation, indeed as the true and authentic indwelling of the being of God in the finite. This is no supernatural miracle, and yet it is something quite unique and miraculous in this world dominated by sin. Here the believer does not postulate God's being, but becomes one with the divine which has a living influence on history with Christ – Schleiermacher's great concern since the *Speeches*.

Schleiermacher explained that with this interpretation of the divinity of Christ he was departing from 'that language of the Schools as used hitherto'[126] (the doctrine of the two natures). He was all the more aware of doing this, since, having given lectures on almost all the writings of the New Testament, he believed that his view could be grounded in the Bible; it was grounded 'upon the Pauline phrase "God was in Christ" and on the Johannine "the Word became flesh"'[127]! 'So Schleiermacher understood his own Christianity not as an imitation of an ethical ideal, which was the approach of the Enlightenment theology of the time, nor as an obedient acceptance of incomprehensible dogmatic doctrinal statements, but as a completely inward determination by the historical Jesus and the God present in him.'[128]

But is Schleiermacher on the other hand a naive 'pluralist'? Schleiermacher would oppose any pluralistic theology of religion which simply notes different 'saviours' in the world and in so doing thinks that it has solved the problem of the religions' claim to truth. He was convinced that Christ 'exclusively' has the being of God, so that only in connection with him can it be said that 'God has become' man.[129] 'The word became flesh' is for Schleiermacher 'the basic text of the whole of dogmatics'.[130]

There is one thing of which we may not accuse Schleiermacher, a modern theologian through and through, and many of those who followed him: that they squandered the 'substance' of Christianity, which they all wanted to keep, and handed it over to secularization. No, they took the utmost trouble to express the **essence of Christianity** in a new and credible way in a new time, and for the educated as well. For all the transformation, in the world of many confessions and religions they were still concerned with:

- belief in the one God: the infinite in the finite, the immanent-transcendent ground of all being, knowing and willing;
- discipleship of Jesus Christ: the man Jesus as the word of God, God's unique image, model and example, emissary, mediator and redeemer;
- the working of the Holy Spirit: the divine Spirit which emanates from Christ and gains power among believers and in the community.

Did Schleiermacher succumb to the spirit of modernity?

Of course from a present-day perspective dogmatic theologians can ask whether in his christological statements Schleiermacher reached **the level of the christological councils of the fourth and fifth centuries**. But Schleiermacher would reply that he thought that – in the perspective of the New Testament and the present – these conciliar christological statements had been superseded, **transcended**. Isn't Jesus of Nazareth an authentic human person? Instead of being from eternity a second divine person who entered into human existence? Instead of a truly human person with a human will, are there then to be two natures and two wills and contradictory theories about the divine and the human in Christ? And on top of that, three persons in one divine nature? Is all this biblical, original? Is it comprehensible and acceptable to modern men and women? There was good reason for Schleiermacher to put forward in his *The Christian Faith* the programmatic thesis: 'The ecclesiastical formulae concerning the person of Christ need to be subjected to continual criticism.'[131] Moreover, in an unparalleled piece of theological thinking he developed a modern christology not only beyond the two-natures doctrine of the early church, which was obviously time-conditioned, but also beyond the meagre Jesuology of the Enlightenment.

Of course Schleiermacher's doctrine, too, needs 'ongoing **critical treatment**' – as he himself would certainly agree. And this ongoing critical treatment – soon two centuries will have passed since Schleiermacher's epoch-making achievement – will have much to criticize. Which leads to the question: is Schleiermacher's so modern christology the christology for today? The following comments need to be made here.

First, in Schleiermacher's consciousness theology there is certainly room for the telling of the **story of Jesus**; after all, he himself gave lectures on the life of Jesus. To this degree he is open to a 'narrative theology'[132] (of the kind which today is unfortunately only called for in slogans rather than practised). Nevertheless, there is a danger in Schleiermacher's approach and the subordinate role of the Bible in *The Christian Faith* that our own experiences of redemption will control the telling of the story of Jesus all too much, instead of constantly not only being newly inspired by the story of Jesus but also being radically criticized and corrected by it. After all, the Christ of Christians is the abiding criterion and constant corrective of Christianity.

Secondly, the modern starting point from the human subject, from the **consciousness of the community of faith,** is to be affirmed in principle, even if one can find fault with Schleiermacher's definition of religion ('the feeling of absolute dependence') as an over-extension of the results of his analysis of the consciousness. But there is a danger which needs to be taken more seriously, that as a result of Schleiermacher's generally philosophical and theological remarks about religion and the definition of the essence of Christianity, in his 'Introduction' a prior decision has been taken as to 'what content is left for christology if it is to be different from anthropology'.[133]

Thirdly, Schleiermacher's idealistic interpretation of reality and harmonious basic mood hardly takes seriously the **real experiences of negativity** with the necessary urgency: the alienation and fragmentation of human beings; suffering, guilt and failure; and the contradictions and disasters of history. All this seems to be taken up and transcended in the unity of the divine plan of redemption. Schleiermacher also interpreted Jesus' unshakeable consciousness of God idealistically in the light of the Gospel of John, and thus largely got round and interpreted away the darkness of God and the tribulation, despite all the divine inwardness.

Fourthly, in his great systematic work Schleiermacher certainly described the prophetic, high-priestly and royal office of Jesus. But in so doing he did not give a central place to the **scandal of the cross** and the **hope of resurrection** which are fundamental to the New Testament writings. So he remained incapable of taking Jesus' abandonment by human beings and God really seriously (not to mention his flirtation with the hypothesis of a pseudo-death); in contrast to the Synoptic Gospels, he sees death and resurrection as the seamless transition of an ideal figure of cheerfulness and pure love from the physical to the spiritual present, which makes possible direct access to him for all those who live after him.[134]

All these are questions which have finally pushed this modern theology into the twilight: a theology of modernity which in some respects has succumbed to the spirit of modernity.

6. The revolutions in state and society

All the revolutionary movements in science and philosophy, in culture and theology, sketched out so far must of course be seen alongside the revolutions at the level of politics, state and society. Indeed in these areas the revolution even reached an unprecedented climax: the political breakthrough of modernity.

To begin with, the absolutist monarchs were still very glad to take up the demands of the Enlightenment – as though it were simply a matter of becoming detached from church ties; for a long time Enlightenment and absolutism went hand in hand and gave each other mutual support. However, this was fundamentally a misalliance. Enlightened monarchs like Frederick II of Prussia (or Joseph II of Austria) were thought exemplary, but because of this they embodied a 'kingdom of contradictions'.[135] For as time went on, the more socially consistent and politically concrete the formulation of the demands of the Enlightenment became, especially in France, the more they were also directed **against the absolutist monarchy**, which had robbed the aristocracy of its political power, secularized the church and domesticated the intellectuals. The cultural revolution of the Enlightenment was followed by political revolution. And the French Revolution was the revolution *par excellence*. In this book I cannot write its history, which is by no means coherent and clear, but we need to analyse its epoch-making significance for Christianity.

The Revolution: the nation as sovereign

There was still considerable puzzlement about the causes of the French Revolution even at its bicentenary in 1989.[136] However, what we have already heard in previous chapters about Louis XIV and his succesors, who continued to mismanage the Ancien Régime, and what we saw of the demands of the Enlightenment, are already enough to help us to understand the essential preconditions of the Revolution, which even for anti-revolutionaries like Goethe manifested itself as the 'consequence of a great necessity'. Just as the **church crisis** and the failure of the reform polices were the preconditions for the Reformation in Germany (with the dispute over indulgence as a catalyst), so the **economic and social crisis** of the 1770s was the precondition for the Revolution in France: waves of inflation, revolts over famine, mass unemployment and mass poverty. The catalyst was the bankruptcy of the state, which was now manifest and necessitated the convening of the Estates-General (which had not met since 1615) at Versailles on 1 May 1789. Here in the briefest time imaginable was the introduction to a political paradigm shift which no one (not even the pioneer thinkers Voltaire, Rousseau or the Encyclopaedists, who usually thought in terms of a king and a parliament with two chambers on the English model) expected in this radical form. We can only very rapidly recall the decisive factors and draw from them the necessary conclusions for Christianity.

Much as hatred and hostility against the church and the clergy had also accumulated in the Ancien Régime, the revolution was by no means primarily directed against the church. Why not? Because out of the 130,000 clergy, only the proverbial 'top ten thousand' defended their privileges. Like the German episcopate at the time of the Reformation, the French episcopate now without exception decided for the establishment. It allied itself with the Second Estate, the aristocracy, whereas the **lower clergy**, who by origin and social necessity belonged to the lower classes, **showed solidarity with the Third Estate**, the 98% of the non-privileged. The most significant reform work *What is the Third Estate?* (which was brought out again in German in 1968, the year of the student revolts), had in fact been written by an abbé, Emmanuel-Joseph Sieyès.[137] It made him the leading theoretician of the Third Estate, and with Count Mirabeau he was later to play a key role in the Constituent National Assembly and again later in Napoleon's *coup d'état*.

This abbé is representative of many: for social and religious reasons, a majority of the lower clergy had at first gone along with the decisive breakthrough towards the Revolution. They hoped that this release from the fetters of the Ancien Régime would bring about economic betterment and thus a deeper rooting of the church in the French people. After the opening of the Estates-General, because the two other estates were unwilling for reform, the Third Estate now constituted itself – against the historic constitutional law – as the **National Assembly**. It boldly claimed to be **the sole representative of the will of the nation** and the partner of the crown – the fundamental act of revolution. To emphasize the demand, a general strike on taxation was resolved upon (17 June 1789).

Now the Revolution developed explosive force: when the crown reacted with a demonstration of its power, the National Assembly made a formal declaration of intent in the ballroom of Versailles (10 June) to resist state authority (23 June) and finally to implement the **direct sovereignty of the people** (6/9 July), the theory and foundations of which had long been laid by philosophers (above all Rousseau). The National Assembly set itself up as the Constituent National Assembly and disputed the right of the monarchy to rule. Confidence was to be placed, not in the Enlightenment monarch, but in the people, the 'nation'. It was not the king who had sovereign power, but the National Assembly (the delegates) embodying the people.

- Instead of the mediaeval theocracy, embodied in the Pope (P III),
- instead of the Protestant authority, ruler or council (P IV),
- instead of the early modern enlightened absolutism,
- it was now **democracy** (P V), the people embodied in the National Assembly, which was sovereign. The **'nation'** was the third modern leading value.

However, the revolution was carried through only by the **violent actions of directed masses** – from now on typical of modern revolution – under the aegis of a programmatic ideology: *'liberté'* (political), *'égalité'* (social), *'fraternité'* (spiritual). It was the popular revolt and the storming of the Bastille on 14 July which compelled Louis XVI to recognize the Revolution and the National Assembly as the sovereign of France. Thus the symbol of absolute despotism had fallen, and 14 July later became the French national day. The subsequent armed revolt of the country masses in a collective panic (*'grande peur'*) led to the storming of the chateaux of the landowners and the destruction of archives and taxation records. On the instructions of Bishop Talleyrand (later to be foreign minister to the Directory, Napoleon and the Restoration), in the night of 4/5 August the National Assembly resolved to annul all feudal rights and special rights of estates, cities and provinces; the aristocracy and clergy 'voluntarily' renounced them. The seal was set on the **collapse of the Ancien Régime.** The history of events had as it were produced a structure of history.

The Rights of Man – the charter of modern democracy

Now the way was free for a new social order. Its foundation was laid by the **Declaration of the Rights of Man and of the Citizen** of 26 August 1789, composed after an American model by General Lafayette, the veteran of North America, with the collaboration of the American ambassador Thomas Jefferson. It is the central contribution of the Revolution, of which France is still rightly proud. What the Reformation is to German historical awareness, the Revolution is to the French. As has been demonstrated by François Furet, who indicated the need for a new orientation in research into the Revolution,[138] it extended far beyond the interests and strategies of a single class. And the Declaration on the Rights of Man in particular is not a 'bourgeois' declaration to mask the egotism of possession but is rather one of the great documents of modernity: the great **charter of modern democracy.**

The Charter of Modern Democracy

The National Assembly declares and recognizes, in the presence and under the auspices of the Supreme Being, the following rights of man and the citizen:

1. Men are born and remain free and equal in rights. Social distinctions can only be founded on general usefulness.

2. The aim of every political association is the preservation of the natural and inviolable rights of man. These rights are liberty, property, safety and resistance to oppression.

3. The principle of all sovereignty resides essentially in the nation. No body, no individual can exercise authority which does not derive expressly from it.

4. Liberty consists of being able to do anything which is not harmful to another person. Thus the exercise of the natural rights of every man is limited only by the need to ensure that other members of society enjoy these same rights. These rights can only be determined by law.

5. The law only has the right to forbid actions harmful to society. Anything which is not forbidden by law cannot be prevented, and no one can be compelled to do what is not ordained by law...

10. No one shall be harrassed for his opinions, even religious opinions, provided that they do not disturb public order as established by law.

11. Freedom of thought and expression is one of the most precious rights of man. Every citizen can therefore speak, write and print freely, subject to the responsibility for the abuse of such liberty in cases determined by law...

17. Property being an inviolable and sacred right, no one can be deprived of it...

Declaration of the Rights of Man and of the Citizen, 1789

This declaration makes a universal humanitarian claim extending beyond the class interests of the bourgeoisie. Indeed it formulates the **programme for a mission to humanity** far beyond the founding of the French nation state. Moreover, this declaration met with an unprecedented response all over Europe, and along with the North American Declaration of Independence which had already been promulgated brought about a distinct historical break: **the modern Enlightenment paradigm** (P V) had now manifestly also **become established in politics.**

Granted, even before the Revolution there had been a development towards the democratic state, a process of secularization and de-Christianization. But now all this had broken through overpoweringly in an unparalleled political, social and intellectual revolution. We should note that Catholic clergy, too, played a decisive part in the proclamation of the Rights of Man and the Citizen. Indeed, in the Constituent National Assembly there were voices calling for this first declaration of human rights on European soil to be passed 'in the name of God' and for a formulation of the duties of man. But to some it seemed too much to speak of the 'supreme legislator of the universe', while to others it seemed too little to speak only of 'nature'. So agreement was reached on the formula: 'in the presence and under the protection of the Supreme Being'.

Revolution against religion

The **status of religion** was unmistakably **different in France from North America.**
– In **North America** religion was not identified either with a state government or with a particular church. Rather, all the religious communities and even the rising political leadership a priori rejected a national state church. For whether they were rationalists like Jefferson, Franklin and Madison, who advocated a religion of reason, or 'pietists' in the tradition of John Wesley, who attached no special importance to dogmatic distinctions, they were all opposed to the advocates of a state church in their conviction that the **peaceful co-existence of faith communities in mutual tolerance** had to be guaranteed: the government was to be well disposed to religion and not hinder its free practice.
– In **France** things were quite different. There religion was identical with the church; the Catholic Church was the **state religion** and thus the most loyal support of and at the same time the chief beneficiary from the Ancien Régime. Anyone who rejected the Ancien Régime also had to be critical of the Catholic Church. So it was not the American Revolution (fundamental though that was to the political independence of the North American continent) but the **French Revolution** which as a so-called

revolution of the masses became a **turning point in world history** – with effects on Latin America, Turkey and India. So in the context of our paradigm analysis we must pay particular attention to this revolution in connection with Christianity.

After the forced move of the king from Versailles to Paris on 5/6 October 1789 the National Assembly, which had moved with him, now passed devastating **resolutions against the church**, the greatest, most powerful and richest corporation of the old system – first and above all to clean up the rotten state finances. It was this that first provoked counter-revolutionary movements, which for their part inflamed the mood of hostility towards the churches and religion among the revolutionaries.

– The **possessions of the church** were declared the property of the nation, and were auctioned or sold off in small lots: **clergy stipends** were reduced and taken over by the state treasury (2 November 1789).

– All monasteries and religious orders were dissolved and monastic vows were declared invalid and forbidden (13 February 1790).

– The absolutist structure of the French church was abolished and replaced by a 'Civil Constitution of the Clergy' (12 July 1790), and new dioceses were created to correspond to the boundaries of the departments (quite rationally covering the same areas – now there were 130 instead of 83). Pastors were chosen by all the citizens of the canton regardless of their religion; bishops were chosen by the state departmental administration; there was an advisory committee for bishops made up of priests and laity. On the whole this was a national church largely independent of Rome, in the spirit of the old Gallican freedoms.

Now there was the first massive revolt against these last radical measures among the clergy as well (often supported by the rural population).[139] But the effect on the other side was one of even greater radicalization. On the orders of the National Assembly, now every clergyman had to take an oath on the civil constitution (17 November 1790). Most of the bishops (who were aristocrats) and about half the lesser clergy refused to take the oath, because the Civil Constitution failed to recognize the authority of the Pope and the bishops. They forfeited their offices and were suspected of being counter-revolutionaries; of the 1100–1400 victims of the September massacre, around 300 were priests.

In the brief *Quod aliquantum* of 10 March 1791, Pope **Pius VI**, himself an aristocrat, declared the civil constitution invalid and with an appeal to divine revelation **repudiated 'the abominable philosophy of human rights'** (freedom of religion, conscience and the press, and the equality of all human beings) – albeit initially with the aim of 'protecting the rights of the church and the apostolic see from any attack'.[140] It was only when in the next year 40,000 priests who refused to give the oath were expelled from France – now, abroad, they acted with the emigré aristocrats as passionate opponents of the Revolution – indeed after countless priests and believers had been executed, church property desecrated and even Sunday abolished, that in 1793 a papal address finally rejected revolutionary principles unambivalently. From now on the Roman church emerged as the great enemy of the revolutionary transformation. Especially after France's war with neighbouring states, the persecution of priests and religious began in earnest.

The total break with the past

We need not be concerned here with the further turbulent and contradictory development of the French Revolution, the way in which it became increasingly radical, the waves of emigrations, the splits, intrigues, trials, executions and shifts in power – time and again in favour of the still more radical bourgeois Jacobins (lawyers, journalists and business people) who were now allied with the masses of urban poor, the petty-bourgeois and sub-bourgeois sansculottes (tradesmen, shopkeepers and workers). What is more important is how we assess these events in connection with Christianity.

From the beginning the **evaluations** of the Revolution were very different, depending on the political, social or ideological standpoint of the observer. For the optimistic revolutionary **Antoine de Condorcet**, who wrote his *Outline of a Historical Account of the Progress of the Human Spirit*[141] in Paris in 1794 and was to die in a revolutionary rising the same year, the Revolution was the culmination of progress. But to the traditionalist and papalist **Joseph de Maistre**, whom we have already met and whose *Contemplations of France*[142] had appeared in London in 1797, the Revolution seemed to be God's punishment for the godlessness of the French. Now year after year countless publications on the Revolution followed, including the large-scale accounts by Adolphe Thiers, Jules Michelet, Alexis de Tocqueville, Hippolyte Taine and Albert Mathiez. The works by non-specialist writers on the history of Revolution historiography alone are almost beyond counting.[143]

But the Revolution was neither the Chernobyl of French history, as the reactionary Catholic social historian Pierre Chaunu remarked, nor the rise and victory of the bourgeoisie, as has been claimed from the Socialist Jean Jaurès to the Communist Albert Soboul. Today the time of the '*en bloc* interpretation' of the Revolution as a time of the consistent class struggle of the bourgeoisie seems to be definitively over. The Revolution cannot either be condemned with a reference to the terrorist excesses of the sansculottes and their demands for emancipation or simply be glorified as the realization of the ideals of the Enlightenment and democracy despite the tremendous sacrifice. Certainly, under the rule of Robespierre the **guillotine** – the embodiment of a **death penalty** which was the same for all, technically perfect and thus utterly **modern** – took the lives of around 16,000 people in ten months.[144] And this bloody burden of the Revolution (though far exceeded by later revolutions or counter-revolutions) may not be justified as having been 'unavoidable', as it was earlier by Marxist historians (of course with Lenin and the Russian October Revolution in mind). Nor may it be put on the same level as the Holocaust, the industrial murder by the million of a whole people (including women and children), planned by a general staff on an industrial scale, as it was by right-wing opponents of the Revolution, who speak of ideologically conditioned genocide (*génocide franco-français*). Despite all the parallels, it was still a long way from the guillotine to the death camps and the gas chambers.

The same may be said of the **total war** which is seen as the embodiment of specifically **modern war** – namely a patriotic war involving the whole nation. The Jacobin regime won this war by a novel total mobilization ('*levée en masse*'): universal conscription, the abolition of the difference between soldiers and civilians, the rationing of food, and state control of the economy. But there is no overlooking the fact that this made the army increasingly important in society. The war of the Revolution which the Jacobin regime upgraded ideologically to a revolutionary war of freedom rapidly became a war of annexation which then provoked the opponents of the Revolution to yet more wars of liberation. And it was the two World Wars in the twentieth century which were first to demonstrate what terrible consequences the paradigm shift of modernity was to have for the waging of the war (war of the people, total war).

However, the radicalization of the Revolution is only in part a consequence of the wars of revolution. What François Furet has brought out is particularly important: the '**derailment**'('*derapage*') of the **Revolution**, in which the revolutionary process swept up the agents themselves, suspended the constitution, and released an uncontrollable dynamic, is by no means the product of pure chance. The Republican cult of reason and terror as a virtue (Robespierre) was not just caused by external factors (war, counter-revolution, a civil war in the west and south-east) but was **inherent in the revolutionary ideology and mentality**. The radicals had intended a total new beginning as never before: the utopia of a completely **new foundation for the social order and all its institutions, on reason alone**, a **rationalization** of the nation – regardless of all traditions, constitutions and institutions. The complicated traditional precepts and customs were to be replaced by simple laws derived from reason and natural law. The previous controlling institutions – absolute monarchy, aristocracy and the church – were to be swept away and an even more 'absolute' power than that of the king was to be established: the sovereignty of the people shared with no one, or more precisely the sovereignty of its assembly of delegates, which was no longer subject even to divine control. Indeed, finally democracy was elevated to the status of a new 'church' with its own forms of cult and faith: with Reason as goddess in place of God.

Indeed, the break could not be more radical, and even now – if we follow Furet – it is not clear how and why this **total break with the past** could come about. Mightn't it ultimately be connected with the fact that **France** had experienced **no Protestant Reformation** (P IV)? In the Reformation countries (in both the Old and the New Worlds), belief in God and religion remained credible despite all the criticism of religion and the churches. However, in religious terms, with its traditions, institutions and customs, the Catholic Ancien Régime still largely rested on **mediaeval foundations** (P III) which at the latest by the seventeenth century had completely lost credibility. Yet it was not the philosophical rationalism from Descartes to Voltaire that brought these rotten medi-aeval-feudalistic-clerical foundations crashing down, but only the phys-ical force of the political revolution. To be more precise, the philosophical insights, the scientific discoveries and the technical inventions gave the bourgeousie striving for political leadership the modern self-awareness that they needed. But it was the Revolution which first brought a radical end to the Middle Ages for French society. The Middle Ages were still preserved in the traditional French church until here, too, the Second Vatican Council introduced a new phase.

In May 1795, the liberal citizens gained a victory over the egalitarian lower classes, and the sansculottes were disarmed (the Prairial rebellion), a move already resolved on by the Jacobin club. There soon followed the proclamation of a constitution with a Directory, which manifested a clear withdrawal from social commitment and an absolutizing of private property. But in the face of the new invasion, internal opposition and state bankruptcy, the regime of the Directory soon found itself in crisis: this was the presupposition for the *coup d'état* by General **Napoleon Bonaparte** (18 Brumaire = 9 November 1799), who, while unsuccessful in Egypt, was victorious in Italy – organized along with Directory member Sieyès, the police minister Fouché and the foreign minister Talleyrand (a former clergyman). This military genius of acute intellect, iron will, indefatigable energy and boundless ambition, now First Consul, declared that the Revolution had been brought back to its principles and thus was 'at an end'.

Napoleon, not personally religious but an admirer of the organization of the Roman Church, concluded a concordat with the Pope (1801) and thus ended the experiment of a constitutional democratized church. He abolished the revolutionary calendar, crowned himself hereditary Emperor of the French in Notre Dame (1804) and King of Italy in Milan (1805), and with satellite states from Spain through Germany to Russia attempted to maintain his dictatorial absolutist military regime. Napoleon certainly continued to propagate the ideals of freedom, equality and brotherhood, but in fact he trampled them under foot. There was even a new conflict with Rome, which led to the imprisonment and deportation of the Pope to Fontainebleau (1812). But now, oppressed on all sides, Napoleon finally restored the papal state; two months later he had to abdicate (11 April 1814).

Even in France Robespierre was calumniated for his reign of blood, and hardly a square or a street was named after the lawyer from Arras. However, with Napoleon modern man seemed to have found his first secular myth. And even French historians hesitate between admiration and hatred. Despite the undisputable contribution by Napoleon towards the legal, administrative, financial and academic organization of France, some of which has survived to this day, and towards the abolition of the Ancien Régime in the rest of Europe (the Decision of the Deputation of the German Estates in 1803 and the dissolution of the Holy Roman Empire), for Napoleon nationalist expansion was clearly more important than the tasks of humanity. In other words, the **nationalist principle suppressed the humane principle.** And all the military campaigns and battles before Napoleon met his 'Waterloo' in 1815 cost hundreds of thousands of deaths!

That Italy (1861) and Germany (1871) then wanted to catch up with unifying the nation state is a consequence both of the nationalistic principle and of the independence of the new Slavonic nations in the Balkans (Serbia in 1878/82, Rumania 1878/81, Bulgaria 1878/1908 – now their churches were also independent of the Patriarchate of Constantinople). But there is no mistaking the fact that this nationalistic principle, worked out very much earlier, bequeathed modern Europe a pernicious **ideology**: that of **nationalism.** This declared the nation to be the supreme value, and constantly led to new bloody clashes between the nations, ultimately at the expense of France, which had long lost its credibility as the proclaimer and supporter of the revolutionary values of freedom, equality and brotherhood. Indeed, in the last decade of the nineteenth century nationalism culminated in **imperialism** and turned the system of European states into a world system. The USA extended to the Rio Grande and the Pacific, indeed to Hawaii and the Philippines; Russia

to Central and East Asia. France, Germany and above all England (in any
case already with a presence all over the world) divided Africa between
them; China and Japan had to open up to the European powers; and
Japan established its rule in East Asia. This nationalistic imperialistic
state system was the highly-explosive world political constellation on the
eve of the First World War. However, the special question which now
arises for us is: what did this political establishment of the modern
paradigm bring to Christianity?

What about Christianity?

There is still dispute about the 'cost-benefit analysis' of the French
Revolution. It is at least certain that the Revolution changed the pre-
industrial economic and social structure less than was assumed by the
traditional French historiography from Jules Michelet to Albert Soboul,
which was influenced by the Jacobin self-understanding. New French
specialist investigations have shown that the French Revolution was less
an economic-social revolution than, as I sketched out briefly, a **political
and social revolution,** though beyond question it now affected **religion
and the church** in a special way.

The Catholic Church of France (and soon also the church of other
'Catholic' states) paid a high price for its 'mediaeval' unwillingness and
inability to reform, which had lasted for centuries. There is no doubt that
the **church** was the **main victim of the Revolution** – even more than the
aristocracy, who were able to buy back some of their possessions later.
Having formed a state within the state, it lost not only its **secular power,**
which had extended to education, hospitals and welfare for the poor, but
also its enormous **property** and above all a considerable proportion of its
clergy: by emigration (around 4000), executions and deportations
(2,000–5,000), and resignations (also running into thousands). No
wonder that in the nineteenth century clergy with a liberal and political
commitment were more the exception. The great Gallican tradition of a
relatively independent French church had been destroyed. As time went
on, it was replaced more by a markedly anti-revolutionary Roman-
papalistic orientation with an episcopate and clergy which saw its only
refuge in Rome 'beyond the mountains' ('ultra-montanism').

However, this church could never again become what it was until
1789. An **epoch-making paradigm shift at least in its social environment**
also had deep effects on the church itself, whether or not it wanted this,
and did so even when after the Jacobin rule of terror there was a formal
declaration of the neutrality of the state in matters of religion, and the free
practice of religion was allowed within the framework of the new order.

One might think of the following fundamental changes which also had a direct or indirect effect on all the states in which the spirit of the French Revolution spread (often as a result of French armies).

1. The **culture of feudal society and the lower clergy**, dominated by the church and the clergy, with all its festivals and rites, symbols, regulations and patterns of behaviour, was now replaced by a **secularized democratic culture**. This saw itself legitimated by the principle of the sovereignty of the people and was based on human rights, of which the most effective agents were parliament and press, political clubs and sometimes also direct actions by the mass of the people. The main beneficiaries of the Revolution and the Directory and then the Empire were the middle classes, who had their base in property and education and not in a genealogy. Over the centuries they too had been kept from power in the church, where all the higher posts were occupied by the aristocracy; now a society of notables was made up of the well-to-do and the educated.

2. Partly by a planned strategy, the **Christian confessions** with their creeds, sacraments, legal ordinances and customs came to form a **national civil religion**.[145] Granted, the new calendar (year 1 beginning with the first day of the Republic, 22 September 1792) lasted only a few years; the 'Dekadi' (the tenth day as a feast day) was again replaced by Sunday and the repristinated old Roman anti-Christian cult, first of 'Reason' (as 'goddess') and then of the 'Supreme Being', survived the guillotining of Robespierre on 10 Thermidor of the year III (27 July 1794)[146] by only a few years. Even the cult of 'Théophilanthropie' favoured by the Directory could not maintain itself. But some other changes lasted and stamped people's mentalities:
– the Apostles' Creed was now replaced by the table of human rights;
– canon law was now replaced by the state constitution;
– the cross was now replaced by the tricolour (as a central public symbol);
– baptism, marriage and burial performed and registered by the pastor were now replaced by the state 'civil register' introduced by the civil authorities (which allowed divorce);
– the priesthood was replaced by teachers;
– the altar and the mass in the churches were now replaced by the altar of the Fatherland on which patriots had to sacrifice their lives;
– names of places, cities and states with a religious colouring now bore patriotic names (*liberté, concorde, constitution, nation, Voltaire, Rousseau*);
– the veneration of saints was replaced by the veneration of martyrs of the Revolution who had been made heroes (Marat);
– the Christian church festivals and patronal festivals with the 'Te Deum' now became public patriotic festivals with the 'Marseillaise';

– Christian ethics were now replaced with the Enlightenment ethics of the bourgeois virtues and social harmony.

3. Now **Catholic popular piety** was replaced by a blatant **de-Christianization**, which, although it had already taken a massive step forward under absolutism, was now established partly through planned government measures and partly also spontaneously under the influence of the sansculottes (the term already appears in the early nineteenth century). Of course there was already criticism of conditions in the church even before the Revolution, and of course popular piety in the communities was not suddenly 'abolished' or suppressed as it were by decree. Nevertheless, a clear break is unmistakable, with tremendous long-term effects. Here the numerous acts of *'vandalisme'* (this term now also became a slogan) against churches, the decorations of porches, representations of saints, shrines for relics and confessionals, were not so important, nor was the requisition of bells and precious church vessels or the decimation of the clergy. What was more decisive was the **alteration in the entire political constellation**: that osmosis between Christianity and the new culture which had time and again been possible in former paradigm shifts was not desired by the backward-looking hierarchy and especially by Rome in the case of the new Republican culture, and at the same time it was systematically prevented by the Revolutionaries through their Republican counter-culture. In Rome the Revolution was regarded as 'the end-result of a long chain of errors which began with Luther withdrawing the individual from the influence of the power of Rome' (and which was to continue in the errors of modernity down to Communism). The only way of curing it was thought to be 'the recovery of a Christian civilization, that is, of an essentially hierocratic order'. Thus the stocktaking by the Italian church historian Daniele Menozzi.[147] Nowadays this is called 're-evangelization'; in fact it is 're-Catholicizing', 're-Romanizing'.

So – in the framework of our paradigm analysis – what was the long-term result of the French Revolution? In France and in other 'Catholic states', which in spirituality and religion persisted in the mediaeval paradigm (P III) and initially rejected the paradigm shifts first of the Reformation (P IV) and then of modernity (P V), **two cultures**, opposite and deeply hostile to each other, **developed** (often along with a separation of church and state):

– the new militant **Republican laicist culture of the prevailing liberal bourgeoisie**: free-thinking, dynamic, progressive supporters of the Enlightenment and progress (P V);

– the deeply-rooted **Catholic-conservative**, clerical and royalist (later papalist) **counter-culture or sub-culture of the church** and of those dispossessed and disappointed by the Revolution: traditionalist, defensive, regressive, reactionary opponents of Enlightenment and progress (P III).

The march of the official **Catholic Church into a cultural ghetto** had begun, even if alongside the backward-looking right-wing Catholicism in France there was always a consciously modern, 'left-wing' Catholicism, which could not be quenched despite all the repression within the church. But in the great church ghetto after the Revolution people attempted to preach, teach and celebrate again as though nothing had happened, although such people were now clearly in the minority in society. After the reign of terror, they had again discovered a new conservative self-awareness, found promise in all the opponents of the Revolution, did not live badly on the gifts of the congregations and were also freed from many worldly burdens. The authority and structure of the church were consolidated again. However, its secular power remained reduced and its influence on society as a whole was limited: the split between two cultures

Modern Democracy (P V)	Roman System (P III)
End of the absolutist system	Conservation of the absolutist system
Disappearance of the estates	Preservation of the clerical estate
Rights of man and the citizen	Condemnation of the rights of man
Sovereignty of the people (representative democracy)	Exclusion of the people and clergy from electing bishops and the Pope
Division of authorities: legislative, executive, judicative	All authority in the hands of bishops and above all the Pope (primacy and infallibility)
Equality before the law	Two-class system of clergy and laity (*prima sedes a nemine judicatur*)
Free election of authorities at all levels	Nomination by the superior authority (bishops, the Pope)
Equality of Jews and those of other faiths	Catholic state religion (where this can be imposed)

had its effect everywhere, down to the schools, hospitals and social welfare. With the complete separation of the state and the church in 1905 – after the French hierarchy under Roman pressure had rejected what would have been a fair compromise – this development was sealed in France. The contrast between the paradigm of modern democracy (the foundations of which had been laid despite all the excesses of the Revolution) and the anti-democratic Roman system which had kept the mediaeval paradigm remained unmistakable right through the nineteenth and twentieth centuries, up to the Second Vatican Council.

Freedom, equality, fraternity: un-Christian?

Was there **a democratic alternative** for the Catholic Church at that time? There was for many clergy with a democratic leaning. One need think only of **Abbé Henri-Baptiste Grégoire**, later President of the Constituent Assembly and, as bishop, spiritual leader of the Constitutional Church, moved by the ideals of early Christianity and still a controversial figure within the church. He was a great champion of human rights, a Christianity tending towards republicanism, the equality of the lower classes of the population, the freedom of Jews and Blacks (in Haiti) and the vernacular in the liturgy. At the time, Grégoire's speech supporting the Civil Constitution of the Clergy persuaded sixty-two clergy deputies, including seven bishops, to take the oath. According to the most recent calculations, initially at any rate 52–55% of the French clergy were for the Civil Constitution – at least before the papal condemnations in March/April 1791 – though of course they differed greatly from region to region. 'So there were real chances for the organization of a Church of France which could reconcile religion and revolution.' This is the conclusion of the French political theorist and theologian Bernard Plongeron, who has painted a convincing portrait of this important pastor Grégoire, who was 'best placed to be the soul of this national renewal'.[148]

However, the reaction of Rome and the conservative part of the episcopate and clergy on the one hand and the anti-clerical radicalization of the Revolution on the other made a **reconciliation between church and democracy difficult**, though on Grégoire's prompting, after the Reign of Terror freedom of worship was again recognized on 21 April 1795 and a Gallican institutional church became possible, separate from the state and not a priori in opposition to Rome. However, many concerns which had been presented in both the national councils of the constitutional church in 1797 and 1801 would only be helped to a breakthrough by the **Second Vatican Council**: parliamentary proceedings, the collegiality of bishops, councils of priests, diocesan synods including laity, the liturgy in the vernacular. Only the principle of election in appointment to office (a 'revolutionary' reflection on the early church justified this by means of the election of the apostle Matthew) was not discussed even at Vatican II.

At any rate since Vatican II it can be said openly that **'freedom, equality and brotherhood'** – which for a long time were treated as slogans of the devil in the Catholic Church and in any case were only written formally into the French constitution in 1848 – have a **foundation in earliest Christianity**, though as we saw, at a very early stage this was overlaid by certain hierarchical power structures. Two things have become abundantly clear in our paradigm analysis: the earliest Christian ideals of freedom, equality and brotherhood (P I and P II), and the way in which they were already overlaid in the early church (P II) and even more in the mediaeval paradigm (P III). They were only partially restored to life even by the Reformation (P IV), but finally broke through powerfully in the French Revolution (P V). 'Freedom, equality and brotherhood': 'And Christians – some had thought of it in 1789 – have realized since then that the three words had a truly evangelical resonance.' That is how the French church historian Jean Comby concludes his remarks on those three 'principles for a nation and for a church'.[149]

The democratic slogans of the French Revolution need not a priori have been hostile to the church. The Catholic Church, and largely also the other churches, simply did not understand them, did not want to understand them then. Why not? Because they had moved so far from the original gospel freedom, equality and brotherhood. So in the light of the experiences of that time questions arise about a future **democratization of the church**, which in origin is neither an aristocracy nor a monarchy, but the 'people' of God, a community of believers in which all members share responsibility by appropriate decisions in freedom and solidarity. Precisely what does such a democratization mean? Certainly not a violent overthrow of the values and the leadership of the church, nor simply the rule of the people and thus human beings over Bible, revelation, God; a surrender of the eternal truth to the changing will of the people. Rather, democratization means a dynamic process of shaping as many people as possible in all the questions of church organization. In this way a form of life (not a form of rule) should be introduced at all levels of the church both in terms of disposition (with reference to principles, attitudes, style, modes of conduct) and structurally (in terms of forms of constitution, law and organization) which in solidarity (brotherliness and sisterliness), corresponds to the Christian message itself and at the same time to the modern sense of the greatest possible freedom and the best possible equality (equal rights).

Questions for the Future

The church of the future should no longer appear as the bulwark of reaction against democracy but in the spirit of its founder as a community in **'freedom, equality and brotherhood'**:

• The church a community of **free men and women**! Instead of this, may it appear as a controlling institution or even as a Grand Inquisitor? Mustn't freedom rather be expressed in the form taken by the church community, so that its institutions and constitutions never again have an oppressive or repressive character, establishing a rule of human beings over human beings? So the Christian church should be a sphere of freedom made possible in the light of the gospel and at the same time an advocate of freedom in the world.

• The church a community of those who are fundamentally **equal**! Instead of this, may it appear as a church of classes, races, castes or offices? Mustn't this equality influence the shaping of the church community, so that while the multiplicity of gifts and ministries is not levelled down by any mechanical egalitarianism, the fundamentally equal rights of members and groups which are so intrinsically different are guaranteed, and the structures of the constitution in no way encourage injustice and exploitation? So the Christian church should be a sphere of equal rights and at the same time an advocate of equal rights in the world.

• The church a community of **brothers and sisters**! Instead of this, may it be a system ruled in patriarchal fashion which with its paternalism and personality cult makes people regress and, whether legally or in practice, excludes or marginalizes the female sex (in holding office or being represented)? Mustn't the spirit of brotherliness and sisterliness be realized in the ordinances and social relations of the church community, so that the basically conflicting democratic demands for the greatest possible freedom and the best possible equality are reconciled in a brotherly and sisterly community of solidarity? So the Christian church should be a sphere of brotherhood and sisterhood and advocate that in the world.

But back to our paradigm analysis. If with the great slogans of the Revolution France dominated political developments throughout the nineteenth century, it did not remain the main political power. It was not France but Great Britain which became the leading world power in the nineteenth century. And this was connected with a historical development: even before the French Revolution, England had set in motion the revolution which produced the modern world economic system, indeed the new world civilization: the technological and industrial revolution.

7. The revolutions in technology and industry

France gave the modern world its political ideas, but as a result of the Revolution and the wars which followed it had been left behind economically. But England, which had already carried through its 'Glorious Revolution' and the parliamentarizing of the political system a century before the French Revolution, provided the economic stimuli and technical achievements: the steam engine, railways, factories. It initiated those technological and industrial revolutions which were to change the European world and thus Christianity no less deeply than the political revolution.

And yet, people asked at the time, isn't there a way back? A restoration of what went before? In the nineteenth century the history of Europe was caught up in a field of tension between permanence and change, legitimacy and revolution, restoration and reform. Of course it is impossible and indeed unnecessary here even to sketch out the course of this fullest of all centuries, which brought significant changes of astonishing vigour in all spheres, even within the church. Our concern is only to work out further basic features of the modern paradigm, though it is no longer possible to detect any coherent and uniform church development in it.

Back to the old: Restoration

The French Revolution itself, with its reign of terror, had already brought a rethinking and a decisive **correction of the irreligious Enlightenment** throughout Europe. And even before the Revolution there had been reactions against an extreme rationalism. Already during the eighteenth century, above all Jean-Jacques Rousseau's enthusiasm for feeling and nature and his pessimistic criticism of civilization and progress had made a great impression everywhere, as no less had the moral feeling of Lord Shaftesbury in England. Already during the period of *Sturm und Drang*, at least in Germany there had been a powerful outbreak of subjective feeling and a sense of piety. A new feeling arose for the original and the naive, for national traditions, for the historical development in the life of individuals and nations. We have heard of the great attempt to rehabilitate Christianity as a religion of humanity, as this was expressed in Schleiermacher (and also in Johann Gottfried Herder's philosophy of history). All this already pointed to the rise of early Romanticism.

But it was only after the terrors of the French Revolution and the

Napoleonic wars that the longing for the 'good old days' could break through generally. And now there was no lack of **attempts to restore the old paradigm both in the Protestant (P IV) and in the Catholic spheres (P III).** For the churches in particular (and not just for the Catholic Church), there was also a great temptation to exploit for church restoration the trend marked by the 'Holy Alliance' between the conservative states of Russia, Austria and Prussia, instigated by the far from holy Chancellor **Klemens Wenzel Count Metternich.** This was called **conservatism.** Already popular simply for fear of revolution, it asserted that certain pre-revolutionary orders had grown up historically and organically and indeed were 'divinely willed': the monarchical form of the state, a hierarchical society, the Roman Catholic Church, family and possessions might change over history, but in principle they were basic values which remained constant. In England **Edmund Burke,**[150] the skilful opponent of revolution, as a representative of this conservatism had affirmed a principle of preservation and improvement, but on the European continent it soon became sheer reaction. People like **Friedrich Gentz,** translator of Burke and adviser to Metternich – unwilling for reform – simply propagated the restoration of the Ancien Régime. Would the clocks be turned back in Europe?

After the victory over Napoleon and the Congress of Vienna in 1814/15 and in particular after the assassination of the poet Kotzebue, this is what happened. The Carlsbad treaties of 1819 are a political signal of restoration *par excellence*. Originally the 'Holy Alliance' was thought of as the obligation of the rulers towards a patriarchal Christian form of state. But under the aegis of the Austrian Chancellor Metternich, now state and church used all their power, all over Europe, in an attempt to suppress the new democratic freedoms and all the new intellectual stimuli, especially at the universities, by means of the old police measures and censorship. Now **restoration** was openly the slogan. Ideologically it was supported by constitutional theorists like the Swiss **Karl Ludwig von Haller,** who with his legitimistic work *The Restoration of Constitutional Law*[151] gave the era its name, along with the Prussian **Friedrich Julius von Stahl,** who held many offices and who in his *Philosophy of Law in Accordance with the Historical View*[152] opposed the revolutionary principle of the sovereignty of the people with the principle of princely legitimacy, in order to propagate as divine truth that all authority, the 'Christian state' and the unchangeable hierarchical order of the estates, existed by the grace of God – all with arguments from the Bible and the Reformers.

The **Roman Curia** also knew how to use this new, old spirit of the age. In 1815 it had received back almost in full the papal state which had been abolished by Napoleon and had immediately reintroduced the traditional monsignor economy there. In France Catholicism was now again a state religion, with the result that Royalist Catholic secret societies now took their turn in denouncing and persecuting ideological opponents. Restoration Catholic social theorists – with **Joseph de Maistre**, also **de Bonald**[153] – had propagated a return to the unshakeable authority of the Pope as early as 1797. Now they were extremely popular, above all as a result of de Maistre's book on the Pope,[154] in which he put forward what was then the novel ideology of infallibility, as we heard in connection with P III.

But the Protestant churches also took a course towards Restoration, though in a different way: they rediscovered their orthodox confession, or, better, their confessionalism. In the Church of England, too, there was a new move towards religion under the influence of Methodism on the one hand and in reaction to the French Revolution on the other; indeed there were the evangelical 'revivals' of which we heard in connection with the Reformation Protestant constellation (P IV). Finally, there was even an Anglo-Catholic movement orientated on the pre-Reformation period, though it was rejected by many people as coming too close to the Roman papacy (P III).

Together with a Neo-Pietism, a Lutheran **Neo-orthodoxy** took shape in Germany which in liturgy, theology, preaching and church order was orientated on the orthodox paradigm of the seventeenth century. This Protestant version of the Restoration was to reach its climax in the theological faculties and among the clergy of Germany in particular in the 1860s and 1870s (thus at the time of the Roman Syllabus and the First Vatican Council). At all events, the opportunity for a church union between Lutherans, Reformed and United which had dawned with the Enlightenment was missed, and no less fatefully that of greater independence from the state and the monarchy. Throughout the period these churchmen and theologians in principle condemned revolution as rebellion against God and proclaimed as solemnly that princes reigned by the grace of God as they proclaimed the duty of subjects to obey. So shouldn't liberal and progressive citizens be against the church, indeed anti-Christian?

These Protestant traditionalists didn't really grapple any more than did their traditionalist Roman Catholic fellow believers with a modernity which was now reaching its climax in the form of the modern atheism of Feuerbach, Schopenhauer, Marx and Nietzsche. Looking backwards, they hardly perceived how much the world had changed around them. Like the Popes, leading conservative Protestants rejected human rights and democracy and defended the glory of princely rulers. They, too, condemned most of the errors which were condemned in the papal Syllabus. Successfully?

Counter-revolutionary interludes

It has to be noted that the spiritual movements opposing the extremely rationalistic and irreligious Enlightenment which began towards the end of the eighteenth century were by no means all intent on going back behind the modern paradigm; they were often concerned with **movements within the modern paradigm**. One did not overcome the Enlightenment simply by going back behind it, but by pointing beyond it. That was true not only of English and French positivism (John Stuart Mill, Herbert Spencer and August Comte). It was already true of the Kantian critique of reason which, indeed, affirmed *Religion within the Limits of Reason Alone*, and not least by the post-Kantian Idealism of Fichte, Schelling and Hegel. It is true even more of classical German poetry (from Lessing and Wieland to Schiller and Goethe), which puts forward above all an aesthetic rather than a religious or primarily modern 'world-view'. Moreover, in the nineteenth century this largely found its way into higher education in Germany with its neo-humanistic ideal of education and a religious sense orientated more on an (idealized) Greek culture than on (all too real) Christianity. At least the Protestant churches had largely assimilated to the Enlightenment consciousness in their sermons and rituals, catechisms and hymns.

Even **Romanticism**, which arose in the 1790s, with its later transfiguration of the mediaeval social structure and repression of the Enlightenment, could only put a brake on the modern development; it could offer some wise corrections, but could not stop it. Romanticism began in a thoroughly progressive way with a small group of writers in Jena and Berlin interested in aesthetics (the early Fichte, the Schlegel brothers, Ludwig Tieck and Novalis): it emphasized feeling, imagination and the natural, and was interested in fairy tales and legends, the mythical and the mystical. But precisely because of this it eventually took a clear turn towards the religious, indeed the Catholic (aesthetic veneration of Mary and the saints), though often with Spinozan undertones of pantheism. Romanticism became a great international movement at the time of the Restoration (Chateaubriand's *Genius of Christianity*[155] had ushered it in in France in 1802), and there was a significant upsurge in religion (though again with a traditional confessionalist stamp).

But even this retrograde intellectual and political movement could neither shake nor absorb the new paradigm in the Catholic sphere. So we are forced to conclude that already from 1848 **Romanticism and Restoration** proved to be a **counter-revolutionary interlude**, although reaction once again conquered. Soon it was all up with the 'solidarity (readiness to intervene) of the thrones'. With their principle of legitimacy

– in favour of the re-established monarchy and the 'eternal' laws of human order – these could not throttle the forces of liberal democracy which had gained new strength and were primarily concerned with a constitutional and parliamentary form of state (with or without a monarchy) and democratic reforms.

The constitutional monarchy, a division of power with a parliament consisting of two chambers and the consolidation of basic rights on the English pattern, began to become established everywhere; the police state was replaced by the constitutional state, which protected the freedom and property of the individual and in which the state administration was bound by the law. However, there was a difference full of significance for the future, between the liberal Western powers of England and France and the conservative Central and Eastern states of Prussia, Austria and Russia (including the Ottoman empire). Yet even these could not dethrone the powers of modernity – science, technology, industry and democracy – again. On the contrary: in the nineteenth century industry was to establish itself in a revolutionary way, so that modern society took the form of an industrialized society. How did that come about?

Radical changes: technology and industry

Science was the proud mother of technology. The mathematicians, scientists and philosophers Descartes and Pascal had sought to put many of their ideas into practice technically. But they could not have had the remotest idea how much their new inductive science and mechanistic technology, building on mathematics and experiments, would inevitably change the world – human beings, their environment and also their world of faith – quite fundamentally.

To take just one example of the **technical revolution**: Benjamin Franklin had discovered the lightning conductor as early as the middle of the eighteenth century. What had seemed necessary for millennia now became increasingly superfluous: why should people still call on God in storm, thunder and lightning, once they had a lightning conductor on their roofs? And in this period there were yet other technical discoveries: the spinning machine, the mechanical loom, steam engines fired by coal . . . At the same time there were far-reaching innovations in modes of transport: the building of roads, bridges and canals, the development of the locomotive, the steamship, the telegraph, and in England, in 1825, of the first railway line.

All this was to change the face of the earth.[156] For it formed the basis of **new methods of production**: the smelting of iron by means of coke, steam power, and the division of labour. So the technical revolution developed consistently towards the mechanization of production and thus the transition from home industry to the making of machines and the running of factories. Masses of people found the conditions of their life and productivity completely changed in what is called the **industrial revolution,** a total revolution in economic affairs, social behaviour and mentality generally.

This industrial revolution was accompanied by a **population explosion** which was caused above all by better medical care and hygiene, but also by an **agricultural revolution** (rotation of crops, cultivation, machines, artificial fertilizer), intensified production of food (cultivation of potatoes and sugar beet) and increasing foreign trade. The pessimistic prognoses of the British national economist Thomas Malthus about an inevitable impoverishment of the masses (food production was hopelessly lagging behind population growth) seemed discredited, though the wages of farm workers were wretched and there were still famines when the crops failed. First introduced in textile production (cotton spinning) and coal mining (to produce steam power), the factory system became established, and with it industrial mass production all along the line.

All this had far-reaching consequences for human beings and the social structure as a whole. For now the mass of the population increasingly lived in the cities; and this **urbanization** brought new centres of concentration and real industrial landscapes. Manchester is an example: in 1650 the population was around 5,000; in 1760 around 17,000; in 1801 already more than 70,000; in 1851 around 218,000; and in 1901 around 544,000. Still farmworkers or shepherds the day before, now countless people became factory workers, usually out of necessity, having to stand by machines which were driven by inanimate energy and which imposed their laws on human beings. There were unprecedented quantitative changes to the whole structure of society which men, women and children mostly experienced quite helplessly and wretchedly as a qualitative change in their whole way of life and the whole meaning of life. Could traditional Christianity help these people who were often robbed of their former dignity, oppressed, wretched and on the rack?

Indeed **industrialization** represents an epoch-making revolution in the sphere not only of techniques, means of production, the generation of energy, transport and markets but also of social structures and mentalities. The great industrial 'lift off'[157] took place first in Great Britain, where industrialization was already in progress from the last quarter of the eighteenth century: moreover, because of its political and social conditions, its natural resources, its relatively mobile social structure and its monopoly in overseas trade (cotton!), Great Britain was also predestined to become the model for the industrial revolution. However, from England in the first third of the nineteenth century industrialization also embraced the Netherlands, Belgium, France, Switzerland and Germany only in the middle of the century and finally, from the last third of the century onwards, also Sweden, Italy, Russia and the rest of Europe; North America and Japan also followed.

The young industrial countries now experienced a rapid economic boom. Economic policy was liberalized, free trade was introduced, and restrictions which limited growth were dropped, so that in the second half of the nineteenth century a world economy with a division of labour and a free world market could develop. Furthermore, industrial techniques were now pursued on a scientific basis instead of simply empirically. They became **technology**, which had an effect particularly in the production of steel, now the key industry – a presupposition for the rapid development of the railway system, which made possible social interaction and communication in a way previously unknown. Of course a tremendous amount of capital had to be invested in this thrust towards industrialization – in the second phase above all in the areas of coal, iron, steel and machine-building. This led to the development of a banking system. So loan, investment and merchant banks were established not only in Great Britain, where there was plenty of capital, but throughout the rest of Europe.

No wonder that **Great Britain**, which had already become the leading power in world trade in the eighteenth century, could develop this position after the Napoleonic wars and the Congress of Vienna (1814/15). Granted, it lost the American War of Independence (1775–1783), but now it developed all the more energetically a new 'British Empire' which reached from Canada and Africa to Australia, India and Sri Lanka, Singapore and Hong Kong. At the same time internal reforms were implemented, despite all the resistance from the Church of England: complete political equal rights for Nonconformists, now in the form of Free Churches (1828); and Catholics (1829), who as a result of Irish immigration represented a growing minority and therefore one which could no longer be ignored.

The British position as the leading power still secured this empire. But soon after a European slump (1873) and a great depression, Great Britain was overtaken by Germany and the USA. Using new sources of energy like electricity and oil, in the last third of the nineteenth century both countries were able to intensify the competition considerably; it developed especially in the new industrial branches of electrotechnology, machine-building and the chemical industry (the motor and aviation industries were only to follow later). In other words, by the end of the nineteenth century the process of industrialization was beginning to take on global dimensions. The structures of a world economy were developing.

Thus it is clear that during the course of the nineteenth century **industry** – made possible by science and technology – along with democracy developed as the **fourth great force of modernity**. Hence the talk of an industrial society in which an aristocratic society relying on agriculture seemed largely to have been replaced by a bourgeois society. This **industrial society** presupposed another basic human attitude: the characteristic virtue of the modern entrepreneur, who now stood at the opposite pole to the factory worker, was in fact '*industrie*' (a loanword imported from France and soon also important in Germany) – that inventive diligence of the 'industrialist', often expressed as brutal individualism, who with his business activity created the intellectual and sociological preconditions for the transition from an agricultural to an industrial society which was quite decisively a competitive one. By division of labour, specialization, mechanization, rationalization and later automation of production, tremendous technological progress was achieved for the masses, in mining and in the energy and building sectors and finally also in the manufacturing industries. However, it also increasingly resulted in social revolutions and crises.

The shadow side: the wretched state of the proletariat

There had probably been no greater economic and social revolution in humankind than this industrial revolution since the beginnings of agriculture, the cities and the alphabet at the end of the neolithic age. However, the ensuing problems were extraordinary, and humankind is still tormented with them a century later. 'If the Industrial Revolution has not yet ended, but is continuing and now entering a second stage, that means that even the advanced industrial societies must cope with problems of social stratification and cultural and political renewal which are no less deep-seated than those preoccupying the so-called underdeveloped countries . . . As soon as the way towards industrialization has been taken, it is no longer possible to turn back or stop.'[158]

Today it has become clear to us that the much praised industrial revolution must not be understood only as a phase of economic growth. For all critical observers, **its social consequences** were certainly **not only positive**, even in the early phase. Granted, the real social product was increasing by leaps and bounds, with rising rates of investment and growth, both generally and per capita. Granted, it had proved possible to abolish the mass poverty which had arisen because of the agrarian revolution preceding industrialization, as a result of population growth and the liberation of the farmworkers. And given the over-population, in any case there would have been no way out without the process of industrialization and the growing possibilities of employment.

But the capitalistic industrial process gave rise to **new class conflicts**. Only now can one speak of a **proletariat** in a real sense rather than workers, i.e. a whole class of people who were affected above all negatively by the economic and social development, since they suffered from lower wages, longer hours, wretched working conditions and social uncertainty, practices which exploited children and women. In this way masses of people found themselves in a bleak situation, which occasionally led them to attack the machines and to other outbreaks of desperation. In short, the industrialization of living conditions created what we may call 'the social question'. Granted, increasing attempts were made to remedy the psychological and physical wretchedness of the early industrial proletariat caused by the *laissez-faire* approach of Manchester Liberalism, by higher wages and state social legislation. But there was no mistaking the fact that:

— In the long term the unequal development of the industrial sectors was consolidated and gave rise to a dubious difference between industrial countries and developing countries.

— As a result of democratic and industrial revolutions there was an erosion of the traditional value system and social system which at a very early stage led to reactions.

The new ideologies: Liberalism and Socialism

It has thus become clear that even Romanticism and political Restoration after the upheavals of the French Revolution could not stop the victorious progress of modernity. On the contrary:

— In the nineteenth century the **natural sciences** and also **medicine** made greater progress than ever. At the end of the century – the educated elites had largely become materialistic, agnostic and atheistic – not least with the help of Darwin's theory of evolution it was possible to dream of having solved 'the riddle of the universe' (to quote the title of the scientist Ernst Heckel's 1899 book).

— In parallel to the natural sciences, critical **historiography** had a no less rapid rise, a discipline which left nothing in the history of the world, the churches or theology unquestioned (apart from the dogmas immanent in its own discipline).

— And new **humane disciplines**, psychology and sociology, also announced themselves, with the claim that they could get to the bottom of the hitherto enigmatic laws of the human psyche (now people no longer liked talking about the 'soul') and human society (which was becoming more complex in every respect).

Indeed, the breathtaking progress of the sciences, above all in the second half of the century, made world politics, a world civilization, possible – against the background of a constantly rising world population and an ever-developing world economy. Couldn't one look to the future with great optimism? The foundation seemed to have been laid for unending progress.

On the other hand, the authoritarian reactionary politics of state and church in the period of the Restoration had resulted all over Europe not only in new revolutions but also in a process of **de-ecclesiasticization and de-Christianization**, first among the educated and then also among the workers. It had already assumed wide dimensions in the 1840s. As early as 1820/21 there had been social rebellion from Spain through Italy and Greece as far as Poland. Then whole **waves of revolution**, both times starting from Paris, swept over the European state, in 1830 (the July Revolution, the victory of the Liberal bourgeois over the Bourbons) and 1848 (the February Revolution), in which social protest and longings for freedom broke through with elemental force. National, democratic, Liberal and Socialist demands were intermingled, but neutralized one another. So for the moment reaction triumphed once again. But in the mass society which was now forming, the development towards more and more parliamentary systems was unstoppable. And at a very early stage the massive anti-clericalism which had come out in the revolutions shattered the dream of a church which again would rule over society. However, from 1848 it was not only the church but also the liberal bourgeoisie which feared revolution. Fear seized them that the protests of the lower classes (trade unions and factory workers) could lead to a 'red republic' of the kind which was then to emerge in the rebellion of the Paris communes after the capitulation in the Franco-German War of 1871.

These protest movements were now mostly backed by a new ideology: **Liberalism**. Constitutionally, this sought the protection of rights to personal freedom and a constitutional limitation of the power of the state over against any absolutist state power, and economically, the withdrawal of the state from the economic and social sphere and the recognition of freedom of business, trade, enterprises, competition and coalition. Its key witness is the enlightened Scottish theologian **Adam Smith** (died 1790), the founder of classical **national economics**. In his moral philosophical work[159] Smith attached supreme importance to the codified norms of justice (life, freedom, property, treaties), which kept self-interest in check. In his *magnum opus* on national economy,[160] however, he propagated justice and social harmony only on the basis of a free interplay of supply and demand, i.e. on the basis of unlimited economic competition within the framework of a self-regulated market ('invisible hand'), without any state intervention. In the reception of Smith's work, the principle of market economy almost completely displaced the ethical principle.

In this way Smith had given the developing bourgeois society a scientific economic interpretation of itself, but unwittingly had also contributed to an unrestricted domination of private capital and unrestrained Manchester capitalism. Granted, this was limited to England, but now constitutional and economic Liberalism established itself everywhere, backed by an educated and propertied middle class, which in France dominated the political system, in England was integrated into it and only in Germany still did not seem to have been politically emanicipated, because it still adapted too much to the aristocracy.

However, this middle class, which had elevated itself so successfully in industry, trade and finance, proved increasingly reserved over questions relating to the workers. Mindful of the destructive internal dynamics of revolution, it increasingly marked itself off from the 'Fourth Estate', especially after the workers, with better schooling and more political rights, went more and more on the offensive in proclaiming their own interests, followed their own leaders and also (with the help of middle-class intellectuals) developed their own ideology, **Socialism**. However, this Socialist workers' movement was by no means a unity from the begining. If we leave aside here the utopian early Socialists (from Saint-Simon to Proudhon), who were above all French, and the anarchists (Bakunin), who hardly made history, as is well known it was the 'scientific Socialism' of **Karl Marx** (died 1883) and **Friedrich Engels** (died 1895) which largely stamped the history of the workers' movement. As early as 1848, with their **Communist Manifesto**,[161] both proclaimed the world-view of a dialectical and historical materialism which took up critically the theory of Adam Smith (and his successor David Ricardo) and claimed that it had now analysed the laws of history once and for all on a scientific basis. The whole of human history had to be understood anew, time and again, on the basis of its economic sub-structure, as a history of dialectical class struggle which in the last late-capitalistic phases necessarily turns into a Socialist revolution because of the opposition of capital and labour, leads to the dictatorship of the proletariat, and ultimately issues in the classless society.

However, in organizational terms the Communists only partly dominated the workers' movement in the nineteenth century. In England at any rate the workers' parties had a more pragmatic orientation; only in continental Europe was this orientation directly an ideology, in so far as it aimed in a revolutionary Marxist or even an evolutionary democratic way at a removal of social abuses and a new just social order. The trade unions (of Socialist, Liberal or Christian origin) were often more important. But soon Socialism was to become an **international movement**. The first international workers' association, the 'First Internationale', was founded in London in 1864, with Karl Marx playing an active part; it took over from the *Communist Manifesto* the slogan 'Workers of the World, Unite!'. The middle classes caricatured this as a demon, although after the bloody defeat of the Paris commune rebellion in 1871 it soon collapsed again.

Whereas European history up to 1870 had been governed above all by the political struggle of the bourgeois for free constitutional and national state orders, from then on the social struggles of the proletariat against capitalism took on growing significance. In other words, the main issue was no longer just the **freedom** of the individual (the basic Liberal concern), but now increasingly **social justice** (the basic concern of Socialism) and thus a different, **more just order of society**.

In July 1889 (!) the 'Second Internationale' was founded in Paris, but in it the orthodox Marxists, the revolutionary Socialists and the Social Democrat revisionists were deeply divided not only over the question of 'social reform or revolution?' but also over the question of war, which from 1900 onwards was becoming explosive; in 1914 both the German and the French Socialists voted for war credits. However, in connection with Christianity we must more be concerned with the question: how did the churches react to the industrial revolution and social justice?

What about the churches?

If we look more closely at the reactions of the European churches to the process of industrialization in the nineteenth century – and there is a long bibliography on this industrial landscape which cannot be cited here – the situation seems almost impossible to take in. For the situation in Great Britain is very different from that in France, Belgium or Germany. Hence we owe a debt of gratitude to the Protestant church historian Martin Greschat of Giessen for venturing to transcend the usual national and confessional bounds of historical research, at least in the case of those industrial countries which were economically and culturally in a leading position, and offer a truly ecumenical account of the church and the industrial age which is fair to all sides and at the same time critical.[162] In it Greschat makes clear,

– that the revolution brought about by industrialization affected almost **all areas of human life,** far beyond the economic sphere;

– that the break with what was customary and taken for granted forced upon the church was a **shock** which still has effects today;

– that this shock also provoked a whole series of **new forms of church action** aimed at winning back not only the workers, whose detachment from the Christian tradition was most evident, but also other social classes;

– that with the industrial revolution **the whole of church life**, theology and personal piety **changed**.

Now along with the democratic upheaval following the French Revolution the churches saw themselves confronted with the industrial revolution, the effects of which on the paradigm shift of Christianity to modernity are our concern here. So what were the reactions of the churches of the leading European industrial nations to the industrial revolution? On the basis of Greschat's comments I want to distinguish the following reactions, which of course overlap in everyday life:

1. **Lack of perception**: most European churches took a long time to grasp the significance of the industrial revolution in any way. After all, they were living within their traditional paradigms in which they concentrated on themselves. They boasted that they were in possession of unchangeable 'eternal' truths, institutions and positions. So at first they did not notice that 'outside', a wholly new world, the modern paradigm, had become normative for masses of people. They did not notice that they themselves had been drawn into the undertow of the headlong development. Bishops of the Church of England (members of the House of Lords), like members of the Roman Catholic hierarchy and representatives of the Lutheran state church, at first defended the 'divinely-willed' order wherever they could – and the political and social injustice that went with it. And in industrially advanced England it took its own 'Waterloo' for the Church of England slowly to change its mind in the face of the tremendous indignation among the workers. On 16 August 1819 in Manchester, at St Peter's Fields (hence the name 'Peterloo'), a gigantic, disciplined workers' demonstration was broken up with bloodshed on the instructions of the City Council. Fatally, the Council also included two clergymen. So what had been possible in country areas for a long time now increasingly proved impossible in the urban concentrations which had grown up so dramatically: to keep the church out of the process of social transformation. But people were often paralysed by ignorance and helplessness. Still more preoccupied with questions from the Middle Ages or the Reformation, those in the churches found it difficult to find the time and strength to carry through the new interpretation for the times in the spirit of original Christianity which had now become necessary. There were similar difficulties in all the paradigms of Christianity (though these only emerged very much later in the Hellenistic-Byzantine-Russian paradigm P II).

2. **Charitable work and building up the church**: it took reports and disturbing brochures like those produced by the founder of the Salvation Army, William Booth, to show the churches how great was the mass misery in the industrial slums and how far advanced the progress of de-Christianization. Here we should not dismiss the numerous humanitarian actions of pastors and communities as social excuses: all the deep commitment, expressed in the provision of soup kitchens, the establishment of savings banks and the organization of many kinds of aid associations, for protecting the working conditions of women and children, and for reforms in housing, health and prisons (or as later in Germany for settlement work and protective legislation for workers). These were quite novel social actions done out of a Christian sense of responsibility, which helped many people in their desperate situation. But it also has to be conceded that these actions did not fundamentally change the existing social order; indeed it could not be changed fundamentally. For neither in the churches of Great Britain nor in those of the European continent was there any serious doubt about the justice of the existing social order. Indeed, once the worst social abuses had been removed, it was thought that there was no need to bother about more fundamental structural reforms. Wasn't it more important to build churches and chapels with which it was hoped that the alienation of the workers from the church and the drastic decline in attendance at worship could be remedied? The building of schools to educate the people went hand in hand with the building of churches – often with the best intentions, those of paternalistic bourgeois care.

3. **Church associations**: the association model made possible by the Declaration on the Rights of Man was typical of the nineteenth-century church in the industrialized states. There were more and more church associations of like-minded people, mostly laity (often led by clergy), in the form of associations, congregations, unions and societies. These associations were meant to help people in need and at the same time to reintegrate alienated, excluded or lapsed groups back into the church through a process of self-organization. A gigantic network of Catholic associations began to develop, especially in Germany (Pius, Vincent, Boniface Associations); the Catholic 'People's Association' was finally able to develop with great effectiveness into the largest Catholic association in the world with a wealth of initiatives of a religious, social and indirectly political kind.

But all the churches' proposals for social and political reform here were mainly aimed at incorporating the proletariat into the old social class structure. That is even true of **Wilhelm Emmanuel Ketteler**, who with his Advent sermons in Mainz in 1848 put the social question on the agenda of

German Catholicism and who, after being elected Bishop of Mainz in 1850, publicly made the church the advocate of the poor and suffering lower classes. It is also true of the ecumenically-minded **Johann Hinrich Wichern**, who initiated the 'Inner Mission' in German Protestantism and thus attempted to give a contemporary answer from the church to the new social challenges. For despite all the reforms of church social practice the self-understanding of the church, its truth and order, remained untouched by all this. Reforms were allowed only in incidental matters, externals, in means and forms, and not in essence and substance. But in the course of history it became increasingly evident that there was no longer any agreement in the church about the essence and substance of Christianity. The progressive erosion on the periphery was matched by the split within or the struggle for unity.

Moreover, the social movement in German Catholicism was finally overshadowed by the controversies over the definition of **papal infallibility in 1870**, the appropriateness of which was as vigorously and as unsuccessfully challenged by Ketteler as by the majority of the German and French episcopate, and which moreover led to the splitting off of the Old Catholic Church and the crisis over Modernism. Yet in their commitment, from the beginning Ketteler and the German episcopate, too, were primarily concerned with the church, with the freedom and independence of the Catholic Church from the absolutist state (and Protestant Prussia) and therefore with gathering and mobilizing believers – and only secondarily with social policy. In the time of Vatican I questions within the church and questions about a state church – above all the Pope and the papal state – again overshadowed the social problems; the question of papal infallibility overlaid that of society.

No wonder that there could only be a first **magisterial social doctrine** when the papal state had finally gone under and Pius IX, the reactionary Pope of infallibility, had died. Whereas Marx and Engels had proclaimed their *Communist Manifesto* as early as 1848, it was only in 1892 that the first papal social encyclical was published. This was by **Leo XIII**, who had already previously compelled the conservative French Catholics to be formally reconciled with their republic. The title of the encyclical was *Rerum novarum cupidi* ('Desirous of new things').[163] Critical on all sides, it affirmed the regulatory intervention of the state over against Liberalism and private property over against Socialism. Indeed for the first time, following Ketteler and the French social conservatives, this Pope developed an official 'social teaching of the church', though this again (like the second social encyclical **Quadragesimo anno** of Pius XI in 1931) was orientated on the retrograde model of an 'ordering by professional classes' (P III) with the determinative influence of the church.

4. **New interpretations of Christianity**: of course, in time there were social reforms in all the industrial countries; the only question for Christians was how far they should go. Taking up some impulses of the Enlightenment, it was mostly individuals or small groups who attempted not only to adapt but to redefine and practise Christianity with a view to the demands of the industrial age. This usually happened by paying more specific attention to a world which was changing so rapidly and markedly, and which in its social distress was very much in need of help. One might think of **Robert Owen**'s initiative over societies or **William Lovett**'s Chartist movement for universal suffrage. But given the enormous variety in social reality, these new theoretical and practical interpretations almost necessarily led to a pluralism in church order, theology and piety which in Protestantism – already a battlefield between Enlightenment rational advocates of freedom, justice and brotherhood (P V) and biblicistic-orthodox opponents of revolution (P IV) – easily led to the formation of further different and often mutually exclusive parties, groups and groupings. The proclamation of the gospel or social work – which was the true Christianity? Sometimes this process of reflection was almost seen as the dissolution of Christianity rather than as an expression of the power of a faith which even in such a changed social reality was time and again attempting to assume new forms.

However, one thing must make us suspicious: wherever there were new beginnings and spiritual dawns in the nineteenth century – and this applies not only to Roman Catholicism, which was not particularly pious about the state, but also to Protestantism and Anglicanism, which in part leant even more on the state and the monarchs – these were suspected, slowed down and often suppressed by the church authorities. Why? In stormy times the unity and coherence of the church seemed more than ever the supreme good, and appeared to require the exclusion of all views other than the religious view. That an infinite amount of energy was squandered on such disputes over the true Christianity within the church which was urgently needed for a credible proclamation of the gospel and for relevant praxis in the world was shown particularly in the confrontation with that new movement among the workers to which the future largely belonged:

5. **Confrontation with Socialism**: the test case for all the churches in the industrial societies was increasingly what attitude to take not only to Liberalism but also to **Socialism**, whether this had a Marxist revolutionary stamp (Communism) or was Social Democrat and evolutionary (revisionist). Of course the atheism associated with Marixsm was unacceptable to the churches; but because this very atheism had been caused largely by the churches (as I have explained at length

elsewhere[164]), it could have been the occasion for critical self-examination. But there was no more interest in theological self-criticism than in 'revolutionary' practical actions.

Granted, the Nonconformists in **England** had initially still given resolute support to social-political initiatives like the 'Anti-Corn Law League' of 1836 for the poorest of the poor. But later even they became increasingly assimilated, and emphasized their character as churches (indeed they were now mostly 'free churches') and the authority of their spiritual office over against the laity and also the need for order in the state, which made it easier to justify the adoption of capitalist methods by members who had gone up in the world. So all in all, here too there was no real structural reform, but ultimately an adaptation to the needs of the upper middle class, which led to a domestication and shallowness in English Nonconformity.

In **Germany**, too, the churches had moved so far from the workers that from the start the workers' party which grew between 1850 and 1875 under Ferdinand Lasalle, Wilhelm Liebknecht and August Bebel wanted to have nothing to do with them. Furthermore, atheistic and materialistic ways of thinking were spreading in a threatening way; there were numerous authors who exploited the results of both the critical historiography and the flourishing precise natural sciences which had grown up in the meantime, against the church and Christianity. One need think only of Darwin's theory of evolution, which caused an unparalleled shock wave, first in England and then throughout Europe, because it contradicted the biblical account of creation and allegedly degraded human beings.

Nor can it be disputed that although at least in German Protestant theology the high tide of orthodoxy was now receding, and under the impact of modern historiography people were turning towards freer theological views, in political and religious terms most of the leaders of the official churches were still primarily concerned with the church. To be specific: despite all the efforts at inner renewal and social action there was primarily a concentration on a church **programme of re-Christianization** to reintegrate into the class and corporate structure of the old social order those who had been alienated from the church (against the modern party state there was a call for a renewal of the professions and a demand for parliaments for them[165]). Thus the church was to hold together all social strata and classes in harmony and shape them spiritually by a disposition of love and mutual service. And although this idealistic enterprise of re-Christianization met with failure after failure among both the middle classes and the proletariat, and could not make any headway against the religious indifference and the rejection of the church, against agnosticism and atheism, those behind it just would not realize that with such a policy of reintegration into a former paradigm (whether P III or P IV) they were deceiving themselves (and at the end of the twentieth century the Pope who, as we heard, is again talking of a 're-evangelization' = 're-Catholicization' of Europe, still has not understood this).

To this degree I can only agree with Martin Greschat's final conclusion: 'So this theoretical and practical alternative to modernity, developed comprehensively by Catholicism and supported pragmatically by Protestantism, which also shared the responsibility for it, essentially insisted that the church must remain itself, that it must concentrate on its essence grounded in revelation, and from this origin pervade and guide society with its spirit.' And this meant: 'At most the churches accepted the reality of social change, and thus the modern world, only partially, never in principle. They saw the whole world being affected by it, but not themselves. This distance from reality gave the churches everywhere on the one hand the courage and good conscience with which they could largely see themselves as standing above the parties, above all conflicts. But the selfsame fact was also to a considerable degree the reason for the growing ineffectiveness of this theology and this courage within modern European industrial society.'[166]

Nowhere, perhaps, is it clearer that the traditional view advocated by the official church and theology that society must be governed by the church in decisive matters was no longer viable than in what has been wrongly abbreviated as the 'women's question'.

The new situation of women

If we look back on the revolutionary thrusts of modernity analysed above, we can make the following comments on the situation of women:

1. The **philosophical revolution** and the atmosphere of rationality which followed from it are doubtless responsible for the ending during the course of the seventeenth and eighteenth centuries of the witch-craze which was still virulent in the Reformation paradigm and which I have reported at length. At the same time, from the seventeenth century, in the upper classes, starting from France, there were '*femmes savantes*', highly educated women, who became the models for the aristocracy and the middle class: the salons of such ladies were meeting places for the cultured intelligentsia. But that still says little about the real equality of men and women in theory and practice. And how firmly cemented the traditional understanding of roles was is shown by the fact that even the **intellectual** philosophical or literary **elite** hardly made any difference here (some philosophers like Descartes, Spinoza, Leibniz and Kant were in fact

bachelors). For Kant, woman above all embodies 'the beautiful', while man embodies 'the exalted': 'laborious learning or painful brooding' would 'weaken the charm by which they (women) exert their great power on the other sex'.[167] Even for Rousseau, whose novel about education, *Émile*, was to influence educational theories so much in the subsequent period, the relationship between man and woman is one of control: the woman needs only as much education as is pleasing to the man. And in his famous 'Song of the Bell', which had such a tremendous influence on the middle classes of the nineteenth and twentieth centuries, Friedrich Schiller – here hardly differing from Goethe – assigned the woman once and for all a role in the silent inner room of the 'home', sending the man out alone 'into hostile life'. At any rate women could get themselves something of a modern education from the magazines and newspapers which were appearing at this time, and at the theatre.

It was the early **Romantic movement** which set **contrary accents** here, redefined the role of the sexes, fully affirmed the unity of spirituality and the senses in love, and recognized the happy relationship between man and woman in free self-fulfilment as a presupposition for a full life. Mention should be made here of **Friedrich Schlegel**, and also of **Friedrich Schleiermacher**, who did more than any other theologian to advance the theology of the sexes and emphasized the significance of the collaboration of male and female forces in the Christian community. But the weakness of all the Romantic new beginnings, which in any case hardly came out in public life in the atmosphere of the Restoration, was evident: the economic and legal conditions under which the mass of women lived in the rising industrial society remained unilluminated. Even the long book by **Johann Jakob Bachofen**, *Matriarchal Law* (1861),[168] taking up Schlegel and believing it possible to demonstrate historically a matriarchal form of society before the state, later replaced by a period of patriarchy, was in no way intended as support for the legal and political emancipation of women. Whatever may be thought of the hypothesis of an early matriarchy in this book, which for various reasons made many enemies, only later did historians and philosophers of culture become aware how much women had been kept back behind men in past millennia (even in the Bible), indeed how often they had been instrumentalized and dominated.

2. Both in America and in France the **political revolution** brought a declaration of the **Rights of Man** which 'really' should also have embraced women. But since in English and French '*homme*/man' can mean both 'human being' and 'male', these rights of man were very soon interpreted merely as the rights of males, especially where they were the right to vote, the right to property, coalition or speak in public. The

women involved in the French Revolution who were members of the newly formed revolutionary women's associations under the leadership of Olympe de Gouges and Rosa Lacombe composed their own 'Declaration of the Rights of Women and Citizenesses' as early as 1791. In it, article 10, for example, calls for the right of freedom to speak publicly, giving as the reason: 'Woman has the right to ascend the scaffold. She must equally have the right to ascend the (speaker's) tribune' (in England, Mary Wollstonecraft called for civil rights for women for the first time in 1792).[169] But the National Convention in Paris, utterly dominated by males, condemned such efforts. It wanted to be rid of the king of the country, but by no means to dethrone the king at home. So the legal dependence of the woman on the man, father or husband, was maintained, and women were only indirectly granted civil rights.

Thus on the whole women had to wait until the end of the First World War before they were given the vote in the leading industrial countries – the main demand of the early women's movement: in New Zealand (as early as 1893), Finland, Norway and Denmark this happened before the War, then in the Netherlands and the Soviet Union in 1917, Great Britain in 1918, in Germany in 1919, the United States in 1920 (France would only follow in 1944 and Switzerland in 1971!). However, we should note that even the constitutional establishment of equal rights by no means automatically brought equality in the sphere of the family or the workplace, and often it did not even result in the active collaboration of large numbers of women in parties, parliaments and governments – not to mention law courts, educational establishments and industry.

3. However, as early as the nineteenth century the **industrial revolution** had changed the status of women more deeply than any former historical developments, though initially more in a negative way. It was the new technological conditions of the production processes which necessitated the participation of women in the work. Spinning, knitting, weaving, stitching and other tasks moved outside the house in a quite unplanned way, into the factories and the cities. Consequently many women lost household tasks, sources of income and conversation, and with the growing need for labour were forced to become the cheaper and in some respects the more skilled rivals of men in factories. But this brought them into a new dependent relationship and often caused great distress, while the family as a group which had lived and worked together fell apart.

At the same time, though, efforts to give women an equal place alongside men began. However, it was not the churches which took the lead here, but Liberals and especially **Socialists**, who engaged in fundamental reflection on the situation of women in the conditions of production in an industrial society, analysed this closely and combined it with a passionate criticism of bourgeois society. Thus it is no chance that a section on the situation of women was already included in the **Communist Manifesto** of 1848. In their document Marx and Engels gave a sharp answer to the charge from bourgeois society that the Communists wanted to introduce a 'community of women': 'The bourgeois sees in his wife a mere instrument of production. He hears that the instruments of production are to be exploited in common, and, naturally, can come to no other conclusion than that the lot of being common to all will likewise fall to the women. He has not even a suspicion that the real point aimed at is to do away with the status of women as mere instruments of production. For the rest, nothing is more ridiculous than the virtuous indignation of our bourgeois at the community of women which they pretend is to be openly and officially established by the Communists. The Communists have no need to introduce community of women. It has existed almost from time immemorial. Our bourgeois, not content with having the wives and daughters of the proletarians at their disposal, not to speak of common prostitutes, take the greatest pleasure in seducing each other's wives. Bourgeois marriage is in reality a system of wives in common and thus, at the most, what the Communists might possibly be reproached with, is that they desire to introduce in substitution for a hypocritically concealed, an openly legalized community of women. For the rest, it is self-evident that the abolition of the present system of production must bring with it the abolition of the community of women springing from that system, i.e. of prostitution both public and private.'[170]

So Marx and Engels, taking up the ideas of L.H.Morgan and Bachofen, and explicitly defending the possibility of divorce without divorce proceedings, were concerned radically to change the status of women as 'mere instruments of production' and under the conditions of an industrial society in which work was shared to grant them equal rights and equal dignity with men.[171] Here the central idea of the Socialist interpretation of the emancipation of women was that the revolutionary liberation of the proletariat would almost automatically bring with it the liberation of women. Subsequently, one could also read this in August Bebel's (1840–1913) book on *The Woman and Socialism* (1883),[172] which with its dozens of editions was to shape the attitudes of Socialists and Communists on the women's question in the future. But even in the context of Socialism, including social democracy, it took a long time for people to lose their illusions that the social and the sexual revolutions were contemporaneous. After all, even the Socialists (down to the student movement of 1968) were quick to castigate social exploitation without considering the exploitation in their own families.

Of course the emancipation of women was also advanced from the **non-socialist** side. Thus as early as 1848 there was a women's congress in the USA which called for the recognition of women as citizens with equal rights. The movement for political emancipation in Great Britain began after 1860. It was the philosopher John Stuart Mill who put the first proposal for giving an active vote to women in Parliament in 1867. In Germany, the Universal German's Women Association was founded in 1865, and was predominantly concerned with questions of women's work and the education of women; now the daughters of the middle class were often under pressure to earn their living and thronged into the places of higher education. But here we are programatically interested more in the question of Christianity: how did theology and the church react to the new situation for women in the nineteenth century?

Have the churches thwarted or furthered the emancipation of women?

First of all, three general points may be made:
– The manifold women's movements which emerged in different countries at different times initially found hardly any support in the churches.
– In particular the *Communist Manifesto* of 1848 had hardly any effect on the churches in the first decades: its active working woman did not correspond to the traditional Christian model.
– The churches' efforts at women's emancipation, which began very much later, hardly reached the level of women working in industry, but remained limited to the middle class.

However, whereas in the framework of former paradigms it was still easier to talk about the status and role of 'women' in general, this becomes almost impossible within the framework of the modern paradigm, since national conditions take so many forms. The situation is still most uniform in the **Catholic-Romanic** countries, where the Roman church government very effectively extended its opposition to modernity to the efforts of women to achieve emancipation. Even Pope Leo XIII, who was more open than his predecessors, felt compelled as late as 1885 in the encyclical *Immortale Dei* to declare that 'the man is set over the woman', with a literal quotation from Augustine (cf. P III): women are to be subject to their husbands 'in chaste and faithful obedience, not for the satisfaction of lust but for the procreation of the human race and for life together in the family'.[173] Granted, in his social encyclical *Rerum novarum* of 1891, which has already been cited, the same Pope then not only condemned in general terms the unlimited exploitation of workers by employers who treated human beings as things, but also specifically condemned heavy manual labour for children and women. But the reason he gave for this was that the female sex was 'by nature fitted for home-work, and it is that which is best adopted at once to preserve her modesty and to promote the good bringing-up of children and the well-being of the family'.[174]

Thus tied to the natural law doctrine of antiquity and the Middle Ages (cf. P III), the Popes of the following period down to Pius XII still saw woman exclusively in terms of her 'natural disposition' as a mother, which now bound her to family and home. They could not perceive the thoroughgoing disadvantage, often oppression, suffered by women as a result of the pre-eminence of men which was the real challenge of modernity. As the Catholic social ethicist Stephan Pfürtner points out, 'A philosophy of essence and natural law derived the "essence of woman" from role relationships developed over history and from biological facts, and in turn made this the normative determination for female behaviour'; he sees the reason for this defective theory, which is highly pernicious in practice, in 'inadequate communication between theology and church government and the critical movements in the church and society of the time'. 'The pioneering ideas about emancipation from the bourgeois and socialist women's movement were hardly taken seriously in Catholicism, or largely repudiated.'[175] In fact it was **John XXIII** who was the first to bring about a change with the encyclical *Pacem in terris* and the Second Vatican Council, which also had a liberating effect on the Catholic women's associations, though the question of contraception (first left undecided and then decided in the negative) proved a permanent burden and a reason for millions of women to leave the church.[176]

The situation of women in **modern Protestant countries** is very much more complex, but increasing historical work is being done on it in most recent scholarship – in the face of all the silence over the role of women in Protestant church history, too. Moreover a collection of articles on the topic 'Women in Protestant History' which was published in the United States in 1985 appeared under the title *Triumph over Silence*.[177] This also applies to the German sphere, to which I must limit myself here for reasons of space, though in many respects it may serve as an example for other Protestant countries.[178]

Moves by individual emanicipated women at the beginning of the nineteenth century, Rachel von Varnhagen-Levin, Karoline von Günder-rode or Bettina von Arnim-Brentano, were at first hardly noticed; indeed within the church they met more with reserve and criticism. So it was no wonder that representatives of the early women's movement in Germany before 1848 (Fanny Lewand, Malwida von Meysenburg, Luise Otto) and the late women's movement (above all Helene Lange, the president of the newly founded 'Alliance of German Women's Associations', 1894) turned their backs on the church: 'Disappointed by Christianity, most of them never found their way back into a Christian congregation.'[179]

And yet the women's movement did not pass by the Protestant churches without any trace. Women involved in the church first became more active with the formation and development of the **Protestant Diakonia movement** (in addition to Hinrich Wichern, who has already been mentioned, Theodor Fliedner and Wilhelm Löhe were the leading figures). This not only gave women church office on the model of the early Christian community (as deaconesses): it also offerd girls from socially weakened families and families impoverished by the process of industrialization tasks in which they could develop their capabilities and take responsibility even if they were unmarried. Men and women could work together in such voluntary associations without the usual scheme of male superiority and female subordination. It was not least Schleiermacher and his understanding of religion which stood in the background where there was an understanding in the church which assigned an important place to the collaboration of men and women.

But even in the deaconess communities, Protestant male 'hierarchs' legally retained male pre-eminence in important decisions and in representation in the outside world. Here we can detect influences from the Catholic women's congregations which were dominated by male priests. In these circumstances, any interest on the part of the deaconesses (and the many pastors' wives) in equal rights for women in society was ruled out a priori. At first simply limited to charitable tasks (like the 'Association for the Care of the Poor and the Sick', founded by Amalie Sievekink in Hamburg in 1832), after the 1848 revolution this women's movement within Protestantism also dedicated itself to getting schooling and vocational training for girls and women in order to be prepared for functions in society and the state. It was the economist Dr Elisabeth Gnauck-Kühne, a sympathizer with Christian socialism, who then at a Protestant social congress in 1895 called for justice instead of mercy for women and made many men change their minds.

However, until very recently there has been far too little research into the more recent history of women who as Christians sought social responsibility in Germany, especially from the perspective of the women themselves. So in the Institute for Ecumenical Research of the University of Tübingen – as I already reported in connection with the patristic period (P II) – within the framework of the research project '**Women and Christianity**' we have investigated not only the situation of women in the first four Christian centuries but also the situation of Christian women in the nineteenth and twentieth centuries. A study by the historian Doris Kaufmann entitled *Women between Starting Point and Reaction. The Protestant Women's Movement in the First Half of the Twentieth Century*[180] is the result of this research. This study has produced important results particularly for our question, to which I want to refer here. For especially in the history of Protestant women, a disregard of the dominant thought-patterns, like the division of society into a public and a private sphere, the former thought of as the man's sphere of activity and the second as the woman's, has proved successful. One of the important results of the research in this project is that in particular within the framework of the church the boundaries between these areas, which were often thought of as separate, were often crossed, and women often 'invaded the public male sphere of the church'. This is particularly true of the **German Protestant Women's Alliance**, founded in 1899, which as a social movement involved in its contemporary environment was the main object of Doris Kaufmann's research.

It was possible to demonstrate that with reference to women's own exegesis of the biblical anthropology of the sexes and the definition of their tasks in this organization, women fought for new spheres of activity and responsibilities in church institutions and major Protestant organizations (e.g. the Inner Mission and later also world mission) – and did so **against** not inconsiderable **resistance within Protestantism and the church**. They indefatigably called for the right to vote in church and commune and for payment for community social work. And these Protestant women also attempted to change the relationship between the sexes (and the power that went with it) throughout society, by attacking the prevalent moral norms in the question of prostitution with reference to the demands of the gospel.

Moreover, this Protestant group (in party-political terms quite a conservative one), which aimed at a comprehensive redefinition of the place of women in the state, achieved **considerable successes** for all Protestant women against the background of the general inter-confessional women's movement, and was able to make an essential contribution towards their 'emancipation'. Granted, it was only after the revolution of 1918 (which they repudiated) that the Protestant women achieved the right to vote in church and commune which they had asked for. But even before 1918 they were able to establish their own places of education (Social Women's Schools), run their own social work projects (homes for women in danger, unmarried mothers), appear in politics and get the Protestant public used to women speakers and women members of Congress. This organization for the first time gave Protestant women loyal to the church the possibility of dedicating themselves to women's rights over and above their honorary work in the community and in welfare work, which was all that was customary up to the turn of the century, without having to leave the religious sphere. On the contrary, the German Protestant Women's Alliance attempted to make the Christian message itself the starting point of its commitment to women. In the 1920s these efforts were to bear fruit but also to bring disappointments; however, here I shall not be going beyond the end of the First World War.

Something else that Doris Kaufmann's investigation demonstrates for the history of the Protestant women's movement, even in the first half of the twentieth century, must also be mentioned: while **individual processes** of emancipation which began by claiming to take seriously the 'liberating force of the gospel for women' succeeded, such experiences of strength and the capacity to win through remained limited to Protestant women **at middle class-bourgeois and aristocratic levels.** Thus in its political and social action even the Protestant Women's Alliance ultimately could not cast off the interests of these classes — for all its proclamation of a women's solidarity with a Christian foundation going beyond the parties. The Protestant Women's Movement would not and could not achieve a general Christian social and political influence which transcended frontiers.

It was necessary to wait until after the Second World War, indeed until the 1960s and 1970s, for a new discussion to begin throughout society and the church about equal rights and partnership between men and women, taking into account the difference between the sexes. A new generation of women was growing up which more resolutely than former generations was insisting that being a Christian woman and social emancipation were no longer contradictory. The gospel contained sufficient stimuli to assure women not only of their own worth generally but also that their own rights to co-determination and participation in all spheres of church and society were no less than those of men. This new generation was to coin a new term for their awareness of themselves as Christian women: **'feminist theology'.** In other words, women no longer unquestioningly adopted the theological schemes of men, no longer practised their faith with experiences borrowed from men, but discovered the reality of their own experience and began to become subjects of their own theology. Here for the first time a theology was practised which took up what Elisabeth Moltmann-Wendel once described like this: 'There should be emphasis not only on the freedom from which one comes (justification) but also on the freedom to which one goes. That would mean openness to new roles and life-style, to a change in society and all kinds of co-operation. The human rights which come from justification still also have an unfulfilled future for many.'[181]

However, so many opportunities had been wasted by the church and theology, and the modern tendencies had been so little supported by the church governments, that thus far only a minority of women had been reached by the new Christian interpretation of the role of the woman in church and society, although it was women in particular who for a long time had provided much stronger local support for the institutional church than men. Not least in the women's question, it is evident today how far secularization has spread meanwhile in the modern world; it may have begun centuries ago, but most recently it has become a mass phenomenon.

The secularization, individualization and pluralization of religion

Intrinsically there need have been no crisis in Christianity: in the new age of reason the church could have had a quite constructive interchange with the rising forces of modernity – with the new philosophy, science and technology, with democracy and finally also with industrialization, instead of being aggressively opposed to it and identifying itself everywhere with the conservative strata of European society. We have already analysed the concepts of **secularization**, self-determination (emancipation) and control of the world (demystification) which emerged with the cultural revolution of the Enlightenment. The differentiation of certain spheres of social life from religion, giving them independence, made good sense and need not in any way have meant the disappearance of religion. The church could have let go of the spheres of philosophy, science, economics, politics, law, education and culture and allowed them to become independent without attempting to keep them under its mediaeval (or even Reformation) domination. A **'secularity'** (= 'affirmation of the world') in the light of Christian faith would have been possible. But since the Catholic Church above all did not recognize these opportunities, after the Enlightenment, with the French Revolution, for the first time in European history an aggressively anti-church, indeed anti-religious, view of the world broke through.

The completely **different experience of the United States with religion** showed that in the light of Christian faith, if one looked at it in terms of its beginnings, there was no objection in principle to the independence, the 'autonomy' of the secular sphere, from philosophy and science to art and culture, and that even in this world which had become 'secular' one could live as a believer and a Christian. On his visit to America in the 1830s Alexis de Tocqueville had already noted with amazement how great was the piety there, how very much better the denominations had been able to develop free of the state and how everyone could decide freely for his or her church. So here was a

Christianity practised freely in a pluralist church situation. Here were churches which financed themselves and had taken over not a few social functions in American society.

Europe, however, was dominated in the nineteenth century up to the First World War by the rationalistic humanistic world-view of the Enlightenment, not at all friendly to Christianity, which had broken through in the seventeenth century and established itself in the eighteenth. According to this, human history is constantly ascending, and moral progress matches scientific and technical progress. At the time of the French Revolution, not a few people assumed that Christianity would disappear under the avalanche of the secularization of all spheres of life. And in our century many sociologists from Auguste Comte to Max Weber thought it certain that religion would disintegrate as a result of the power of rationalization and demystification. Wasn't the awareness of the absence of God from the world constantly spreading? In the face of the **ever more powerful modern tendencies**, conservative Protestantism concentrated on the Bible, understood literally (fundamentalism, P IV), whereas Roman Catholicism, as we similarly saw, not only centralized and bureaucratized its organizational structures in a quite unprecedented way but also sacralized them (infallibility, P III). So on both sides an anti-modern defensive piety, often with a high emotional content, could develop.

Thus it is not surprising that the churches did not succeed in winning over their intellectual critics, far less penetrating the industrial proletariat of the cities which was now increasing with uncanny speed. Not only the bourgeois Liberals but also the proletarian Socialists mostly shared the enlightened rationalist ideology, which was indifferent, if not directly hostile, to Christianity. And not only political ideology, but also the natural sciences (above all Darwin's theory of evolution), favoured belief in reason and science, progress and democracy, nation and humanity, which now all too easily allied itself with religious indifference, agnosticism or even explicit atheism. So here secularization does not mean a secularity lived out in a Christian faith, but an ideological **secularism**, which despises traditional religion as an alienation of human beings from themselves and therefore fights both intellectually and politically against everything religious.

But even for believing Christians, Christianity was now no longer an all-determining factor, but one factor among others. In any case, instead of talking about Christianity, now people talked more often about religion, about the religions. But even religion (as an objective institution) or religious feeling (as a subjective attitude) no longer governed the whole of human life, but had become a special area in human society which could be more or less relevant for the individual. Together with science, law, politics and art, religion formed a 'sub-system' in the wider social structure. Explanations of nature, understandings of history, everyday life and language now had less and less of a religious stamp; they had become 'worldly', 'secular'. Now quite generally in European society a distinction was made between those who went to church, those open to religion, the indifferent and the secularized.

However, two factors compel us to make some distinctions in the general thesis of secularization. First, **secularization** has a **reverse side** which must not be overlooked. Formerly, despite notorious difficulties with religion, people felt themselves supported and borne up from infancy to old age by structures with a traditionally religious foundation, beginning from those of family life and the home, through those of work and festivals, to those of politics, the state and the church. And the churches in particular shaped everyday life with their patterns of interpretation and forms of life. But now people were increasingly becoming – as present-day educational theory puts it, following in the footsteps of existential philosophy – 'directors of their own lives': 'They experience themselves as being thrown upon themselves, they are themselves material and task. They see themselves challenged to choose; they can choose, they must choose, they must prove themselves to themselves and others in what they have chosen; they are obligated and responsible in what they have chosen.'[182] Yet only in our day is educational theory seriously reflecting on the consequences of this unprecedented **individualization** of life, which are not just positive: 'The situation of open possibilities of life provokes the question of the meaning of life.'[183] But a very much more difficult and fundamental question follows: **Where does one find a meaning of life** in a world which is secularized, 'demystified', and in which people often feel so alien and homeless? How can one prevent the de-ecclesiasticization and de-Christianization from finally being followed by a loss of religion and in the end by practical nihilism?

Secondly, according to recent investigations it is quite questionable whether Western society is caught up in an unstoppable process of secularization; at all events there can be no talk of a disappearance of religion.[184] Here all the prognoses of sociologists and politologists have gone wrong.[185] In fact religion continues to be an option for many people despite all the secularization and indifference. A large number of people even in Europe continue to be socialized by religion and the church. So even in European lands we seem to have less a demolition than a transformation of religion, a religious individualization and **pluralization**. Against the background of a social, cultural and aesthetic pluralism we now also have an ethical and religious pluralism: 'For the first time in the history of modern religion pluralism goes right down to the individual level and derives a new quality from that.' Thus the sociologist and theologian Karl Gabriel, who continues: 'Forced into a social form shaped by mass culture and the market, the religious traditions are directly accessible to individuals, are losing their character as destiny and are becoming the objects of individual selection and choice.'[186] Here both the individualization and the pluralization of religion can have both productive and destructive effects. Questions for postmodernity arise here.

Questions for the Future

• The **individualization of religion** gives people faced with often rigid religious institutions the possibility of making an independent choice, even in the religious sphere. It allows them to seek their own way to a fundamental happiness in life and promises them an autonomous, self-determined subjectivity.

Even if in the light of Christian faith we need not make any fundamental objections to personal experience, self-discovery, self-determination and self-fulfilment, isn't there a danger that self-fulfilment will lead to an overestimation of the self and to autistic self-centredness, because it is detached from responsibility for oneself and the world, from responsibility for fellow human beings and society, leading to a loss of solidarity, to isolation, or even to an assimilation to the general mood of the time? Is the slogan to be, 'Religious feeling, yes; religous commitment, no'?

• The **pluralization of religion** gives men and women new spiritual perspectives and religious possibilities after the abolition of the exclusive Christian monopoly position: an extension, enrichment and deepening of their own religious feelings through the insights, symbols, ethical demands and meditative practices of other religions and alternative movements.

Even if in the light of the Christian faith we need no longer make any fundamental objections to the de facto plurality of religions and systems of interpretation, where a choice of truths is on offer the result can be a random selection from what is available which carries no obligations. So isn't there a danger that on the free market of religious possibilities people will cobble together a private religion completely orientated on their needs, made up of authentically religious, para-religious and pseudo-religious elements: a highly unstable mixture of belief in God and occultism, belief in the resurrection and the doctrine of reincarnation, belief in providence and astrology?

So in the end doesn't Christianity become a mere quarry for a random world-view? In this way does 'God' remain the one who is not at our disposal, or does 'God' become an object to be manipulated for changing religious needs? Indeed, can the fragmentation or splintering of modern society be stopped by such pluralization?

8. The crisis of modernity

With this analysis of the great revolutionary thrusts, from the philosophical-scientific-technological revolution to the political and finally the industrial revolution, with the working out of the great leading ideas of reason, progress, nation and all their implications for society and the individual, we may regard the modern paradigm – its genesis, its constitutive elements and its effects on Christianity – to have been reconstructed for our purpose. And just as it was hardly necessary to describe the later phases of the other paradigms in detail, so too this is unnecessary in the case of the modern paradigm. There is no need to describe all the changes of diplomatic fronts and political alliances; all the countless wars of the modern great powers in Europe and on other continents; all the unprecedented progress of physics, chemistry, biology and medicine, and also of philology, history, the social sciences and the arts from the novel to opera; and finally the population growth, the development of the transport network, the extension of production, and also the ever more threatening ramifications of the social question, the growing international tensions and so much that was already in the making. Now we must turn to the **crisis** of modernity which became increasingly evident around the time of the First World War.

The conflicting results

Since modernity has become aware of itself, there have also been attempts to see clearly what it is: from the *Querelle des anciens et des modernes* through the progressive or conservative interpretations of the Revolution and the Restoration to the diagnoses of Georg Simmel and Max Weber, of Siegfried Kracauer and Walter Benjamin, of Theodor W.Adorno and Max Horkheimer, and lastly of Michel Foucault, Jean-François Lyotard, Jürgen Habermas, Antony Giddens and Stephen Toulmin, directly or indirectly provoked by the collapse marked by the First World War (and mostly very pessimistic).[187] Almost all of them were anticipated by the theologian **Karl Barth** with his radical criticism of modernity – there is a portrait of him in *Great Christian Thinkers*[188] – who initiated the postmodern paradigm of theology.

It is certain that after all the experiences of revolution, modernity now appears to thinking people in a different light from that in which it appeared to itself:

- There is still no disputing the magnificent achievements of modernity with its revolutions in science and philosophy, technology and industry, state and society; beyond question it has proved an unprecedented **innovatory thrust** for millions of people.
- But there are also critical questions which we cannot avoid putting to this modernity and its leading values of reason, progress, nation, etc., which resulted in an equally unprecedented existential **danger to humankind.**

The Enlightenment itself shattered some of its own basic assumptions, and the enlightened self-confidence became dissipated. Following Horkheimer and Adorno, this has been called the 'dialectic of the Enlightenment'.[189] We ought to call the results of modernity, which now seem to us to be largely ambivalent, the **dialectic of modernity** (including Liberalism **and** Socialism):

– There was progress in **scientific research** in all areas. But where was the contemporaneous **moral progress** which could have prevented the misuse of science (for example in physics, chemistry and biology)?

– A highly-efficient macro-technolology developed which spanned the world. But the **spiritual energy** which could have brought under control the risks of technology to be felt everywhere did not develop to the same degree.

– There was an **economy** which expanded and operated world-wide. But what are the resources of **ecology** for combatting the destruction of nature by industrialization, which is equally world-wide?

– In the course of a complex development **democracy** has slowly also been established in many countries outside Europe. However, what has not become established is a **morality** which can work against the massive power interests of the different men of power and power groups.

Today there may be said to be largely a consensus about the crisis of the modern paradigm and its leading value of reason, progress and nation (and I have reflected programmatically on this in my *Global Responsibility*). Faith in reason, progress and the great modern ideologies of nationalism, Liberalism and Socialism has been shaken.

Criticism of leading value I: reason

Today the modern absolutization of reason, **belief in reason**, seems to have been **shaken**. There is no doubt about it: a new foundation for philosophy on the basis of reason was unavoidable, and an enlightened rational criticism of the aristocracy and the church, state and religion, was urgently needed from the eighteenth century on, and finally also resulted in the self-critique of reason (Kant's *Critiques*). Even nowadays, only unreasonable people have fundamental objections to rationality and science. For even in the postmodern period of history, mathematical and scientific methods, along with the ideals of clarity, efficiency and objectivity, remain indispensable, in fields from nuclear physics to astrophysics, from microbiology to genetics and medicine.

But man does not live by reason alone. And the human spirit can do more than calculate and measure, analyse and rationalize. At the very foundation of modern philosophy the mathematician, physician and philosopher Blaise Pascal issued a warning against Descartes' overestimation of reason and his efforts to construct a universal science orientated on mathematics, arguing that not only reason, but willing and feeling, imagination and disposition, emotions and passions had rights of their own: there was **intuitive-holistic knowledge, sensing, feeling, experience** (Pascal's *'esprit de finesse'*)[190] as well as methodical rational thought (Descartes' *'esprit de géometrie'*).[191] And at the height of the Enlightenment, as is well known, Schleiermacher drew the attention of his Romantic friends to the fundamental importance of experiences, the cognitive significance of feelings, the dimension of inwardness. So criticism of modernity rightly asked and still asks: shouldn't methods and science be a means towards humanizing human beings instead of an end in themselves? Are mathematicizing, quantification and formalization adequate for covering the world of qualitative and specifically human phenomena, like laughter, music, art, sorrow, love in all their dimensions? Alongside the generalization of comprehensive statements isn't there that particular which is never completely to be grasped by reason: the immediate experience, the authentic experience, the happiness of the fulfilled moment? Mustn't questions of the human psyche and society, of law, politics and history, of aesthetics and religion also be treated with a method and a style which corresponds to a distinctive object, their object?

Reason (combined with the freedom of subjectivity), which increasingly made itself absolute and compelled everything to be legitimated by it, respecting no tradition, not incorporated into any cosmos and to which nothing was holy, subsequently destroyed itself. The self-confidence of reason – the presupposition for gaining power over the world – proved to be a delusion. Nowadays questions are being put to 'instrumental reason' from all sides by a holistic approach, and it in turn is being asked to legitimate itself. The supreme judge of yesterday is becoming today's defendant.[191] The reason which demystified everything seems itself to have been demystified. Even in the natural sciences, which for a long time saw the world as a well-oiled machine and thus willy-nilly laid the foundations for the exploitation and destruction of nature – after Einstein's general theory of relativity, Heisenberg's quantum mechanics and the discovery of elementary particles, which put in question the division between the observing subject and the observed object – a more holistic thought became established and thus there was a paradigm shift from the classical mechanistic physics of modernity.[192] To replace the domination of nature there is an urgent need for a 'new covenant'[193] of human beings with nature. Thus reason has lost its exclusive paradigmatic leading function; it must share it with nature. And what about progress?

Criticism of leading value II: progress

The modern absolutizing of progress, **belief in progress**, also seems to have been **shaken**. Granted, in the postmodern era of history, too, we can and may hope for further scientific and technological progress, on which the underdeveloped countries in particular are dependent. But the 'subdue the earth' in the biblical account of creation (Gen.1.28) means the consciously responsible use and cherishing of nature and not unscrupulous exploitation and progressive destruction. Critics of modernity rightly asked and ask: isn't the problematical achievement of modern man in particular, in exalting himself rationally above nature and using his capacities to gain control of it, responsible for the incalculable damage and the **destruction of the foundations of our natural life**? This destruction did not become a **problem** in ancient Israel or the New Testament period, in the Middle Ages or at the time of the Reformation, but **only in modernity**. In many cases what seemed to be 'progress' has turned into its opposite.

In fact eternal, omnipotent, universal progress, that great **God of modernity**, with its strict commandments 'You shall . . . more and more, better and better, faster and faster', has revealed its fatal **two-facedness**. Belief in progress has lost its credibility. The modern compulsion of modernity to get beyond itself seems to many people to be sinister. At the end of this century people generally have become aware of what pioneer thinkers had already understood at its beginning: economic 'progress', practised as an end in itself, has had devastating consequences of global dimensions. Scientists have often trivialized them by describing them as the 'side-effects' of scientific progress; economists have trivialized them as the 'external effects' of economic growth. But in reality they are first-order intrinsic effects (though chronologically they are second- and third-order), resulting in the destruction of the natural human environment and thus social destabilization on a large scale.

The price that we pay for this kind of progress is brought before our eyes daily by the media: the scarcity of resources, transport problems, pollution of the environment, destruction of the forests, acid rain, the greenhouse effect, the hole in the ozone layer, climatic change, the problem of waste disposal, the population explosion, mass unemployment, the collapse of civil order, the international debt crisis, Third World problems, excessive armaments, nuclear death . . . So the greatest triumphs and the greatest catastrophes of technology lie terrifyingly close together. Will an ever-growing humankind be able to cope with these problems which are multiplying daily? One need not be a Cassandra or a kill-joy to note that the present society intent on 'progress' is threatened with self-destruction – in the long term, or suddenly. The modern myth of progress itself seems to have been 'demystified'. Progress, too, has lost its undisputed paradigmatic leading function? And what about the nation?

Criticism of leading value III: nation

Since the First World War the modern absolutizing of the nation, that **nationalism** which arose with modernity, seems to have been **shaken**. At least in the European community, since the fearful reciprocal slaughtering of nations in the First and Second World War, it may be taken to have been superseded, even if national ambitions and rivalries still remain and the last twitchings of nationalism are evident in countries formerly under enforced Communist dictatorship. But the two typical major ideologies which ultimately came to overlay nationalism have also been compromised: **Liberalism**, which was unable to create any social justice, and **Socialism**, which muzzled individual freedom. So too were the antagonistic social systems of **capitalism and Communism**, bound up with them. Certainly not all the concerns of Liberalism and Socialism are in fact finished, least of all from a global perspective. For all too many people on our globe – in Africa, Latin America and Asia in particular – individual freedom and social justice remain unfulfilled promises.

But critics of modernity rightly make an important point. Both Liberalism and Socialism are outdated as ideologies providing a universal explanation and a universal solution. In any case these terms have become shells for all kinds of contents. In fact classical capitalism has corrected itself by adopting Socialist stuctural elements, while classical Socialism (Marxism) has proved incorrigible. The word 'Socialism' (it already had collectivist features) has long been replaced among far-sighted people with free 'Social Democracy', the term 'capitalism' (which always had connotations of individualistic exploitation) with 'social market economy'! Beyond the Socialist planned economy and the capitalist market economy, various forces are now working towards a market economy which is socially tolerable and ecologically regulated, in which a constant balance is sought between the interests of capital (efficiency, profit) on the one hand and social or ecological interests on the other. In practice, with the free welfare state in the industrial states guranteed by the state, we are moving towards a mixed system in which there are signs all over the industrialized states of a de-industrialization (in the direction of a service society). This too is a symptom that the world has entered a new paradigm, a **post-capitalist and post-socialist** and – in this sense – a **postmodern eco-social market economy.**

False reactions: ultramodernism, postmodernism and traditionalism

The dispute over the end of modernity is a dispute over the evaluation of modernity and thus also a dispute over the present and future of our globe. Notions which I have already sketched out in *Global Responsibility* must now also be introduced in this context.

1. **Ultramodernism** is no way out of the crisis of modernity. For given the development in world history that I have described, it makes little sense simply to propagate a heightening, intensification, modernization of modernity. The Enlightenment was quite unable to prevent the barbarism and unprecedented crimes against humanity with their numerous accomplices great and small. Nor was it reason, which was all too adaptable, that made resistance possible, but rather personal convictions: values, attitudes and criteria. However, the enlightened **ultramodernists** will not see that the times have changed. They have changed with the two World Wars, the Holocaust, the gulags and nuclear weapons, with the collapse of Fascism and Nazism, with the shattering of colonialism and Communism, with the crisis of capitalism and Socialism. There are still people who will not accept that the Socialist German Federal Republic was a total fiasco. Nor will they draw any conclusions from the fact that the end of religion and the death of God, announced time and again, have not taken place and that the widespread disregard of religion in the social sciences and social philosophy has proved to be a mistake.

It is amazing that so prominent a representative of this **ultramodernity** as the German philosopher **Jürgen Habermas** writes his polemic only against the 'postmodernity' of the French 'postmodernists', without reflecting on the change of epochs in our century or considering that the word 'postmodernity' (something of an emergency term until a more concrete word becomes established as a description for the new era) can have a reasonable meaning.[194] A progressive prejudice for the new (or what was new at the time) all too easily overlooks the way in which even modernism (novism) can become traditionalism and forgets that such a modernism can contribute little to the resolution of an epoch-making crisis. So we must ask: can reason be purged simply by reason? Can the basic deficiencies of modern science and the great damage done by technology simply be remedied by yet more science, yet more technology, as the 'unyielding men of the Enlightenment' (in a remarkable coalition with some technocrats and political pragmatists) think? Science and technology can contribute to the disintegration of a traditional ethic, but according to our experiences so far they cannot contribute a new one. And the 'traditional' discourse which presupposes an ideal, utopian communication society is hardly in a position by itself to be the basis of a new ethic.

Of course the question arises whether some of those who reject the term 'postmodern' for themselves, because (like the author of this book) they do not want to be 'postmodernists', are not **in fact Enlightenment postmodernists** after all. This may be true, for example, of the Munich sociologist Ulrich Beck, who first of all describes modern society in extraordinarily critical terms as a 'risk society'[195] which could end up in a great ecological, social and political catastrophe and then, to counter pessimism and fatalism, develops a theory of 'reflective moderniza-tion'[196] because the classical model of modernization no longer works, and yet further modernization puts in question the foundations of industrial society. Here in fact there is a step beyond modernity into a postmodernity (in the strict sense).

2. **Postmodernism**, too, is no way out of the crisis. For while 'postmodernism' proclaims an end to modernity, it only has 'radical pluralism' or relativism to offer as an alternative: truth, justice, humanity in the plural, with an appeal to J.-F. Lyotard[197] and Wolfgang Welsch.[198] But what is here described as 'postmodernity' is basically the character-istic of a **late modernity** which had manifestly disintegrated around the end of the century (P V). For are, say, arbitrariness, colourfulness, a mix of anything and everything, an anarchy of thoughts and styles, a principle of aesthetic and literary collage, a methodological 'anything goes', a moral 'anything that gives you pleasure', are these and suchlike going to

be able to overcome the dilemmas of modernity? Here the necessity of a lack of consensus is turned into the virtue of randomness. But modernity in all its contradictions is not really overcome like this; it is merely repeated yet again in a hyped-up form. At least to this degree, the conservative criticism of modernity[199] also applies to late modernity disguised as 'postmodernity'. Like a totalitarian unity without multiplicity, so too a relativistic plurality without unity is hardly the way to a better future.[200]

3. Finally, **anti-modernism**, too, is no way out of the crisis. For traditionalists, above all in the **Catholic Church**, simply want to retain the mediaeval Roman Catholic paradigm in which they had power and authority. So quite naturally they must be not only against the Reformation but even more against the Enlightenment. Their ideology of history, which is as self-righteous as it is simplistic, still claims that apostasy from the Pope and the church (with the Reformation) necessarily led to apostasy from Christ (in the eighteenth century) and God (in the nineteenth century) and thus finally to the fall into chaos (in the twentieth century). No wonder that prominent representatives of this **anti-modernity** feel more sympathy for the Middle Ages (P III) than for the Reformation and modernity. Certainly these anti-modernists use state-of-the-art modern technology, say, for propaganda, and accept 'post-modernity' in areas where it costs the church nothing, but in terms of mentality and argument they are still in the Middle Ages. They have a conservative prejudice for the old, the 'good old days', of a kind which one can also in fact find in all confessions and religions and even in politicians of different parties.

No wonder that such committed anti-modernists formally propagate a programmatic Counter-Enlightenment and church-political restoration which they disguise as 're-evangelization'. Whereas the postmodernists let pluralism degenerate into randomness, the antimodernists attempt to impose unity in the form of a clerical totalitarianism. The key political example here is **Poland**, where in the face of the majority of the Catholic (!) population an attempt was made to demonstrate what was really meant by the 'spiritual renewal of Europe'. The means used were a law on the media, restrictive laws on sexual morality (from the pill to abortion), a concordat, and replacement of civil marriage as far as possible by church marriage, the restriction of religious teaching in schools to the clergy, and the greatest possible influence for the 'church' (i.e. the hierarchy). The result, of course, was that a majority of people even in Poland soon got tired of such a policy of church supervision and voted out the parties concerned only four years after the great European revolution (in 1993). The main result of this has been that ever larger groups, above all the young generation, are turning away from this church and thus also from Christ and finally from God (because the church regarded God and Christ as its property). But secularization, individualization and pluralization have proved to be irreversible everywhere. Moreover the restoration of a premodernity at the end of modernity will fail, like earlier attempts, say those of the reactionary Romantics (there were also non-reactionary Romantics) in the nineteenth century, and will at best once again lead to a subculture and a Roman Catholic ghetto.

And what applied to Catholic traditionalism also, of course, applies to that **Protestant fundamentalism** which in a pre-Copernican and pre-Darwinian way would like to persist in the Reformation paradigm of the sixteenth century. Where the Catholic traditionalists flee from the 'onslaught' of modernity to the Pope as the 'infallible' pastor, Protestant fundamentalists flee to the Bible, the 'infallible' book.[201] And where the former attempt to impose their aims with 'Catholic' politics and the Inquisition, the latter do so with electronic media and apocalyptic, the threat of an imminent end to the world – which does not exclude alliances between fundamentalists and curialists (as we noted in connection with P IV).

Ultramodernism, postmodernism and traditionalism – all these, then, are hopelessly false reactions to modernity. But what is the positive aim to be? Here, first of all, is a basic answer. If Christianity is to survive its second millennium, it must:

- affirm the humane form of modernity instead of condemning modernity: there can be no Roman Catholic subculture! However, at the same time it must
- fight against the inhuman constraints and destructive effects of modernity: there can be no modernistic concessions and no sell-out of the substance of Christianity. So Christianity must
- transcend both positions in a new, differentiated pluralistic holistic synthesis, which can be called 'postmodern' in the good sense. I shall sketch this out quite briefly here.

9. Tasks for an analysis of postmodernity

The label is not decisive, but the subject-matter is. Whether or not we want to speak of 'postmodernity', there can be no disputing the fact that since the First and Second World Wars we have entered a **new era** (P VI), call it what one will.[202] Here I am using the term 'postmodern' as a heuristic term for discovering what distinguishes our era of history from those which have gone before.[203] **Postmodernity in the strict sense, which**

I hope to analyse more closely in a subsequent volume, seeks to describe the developments which really leave behind ('post-') them a modernity that has become questionable, without challenging the achievements of modernity in a pessimistic view of culture. There will be no going back here to a uniform interpretation of the world. Precisely within a paradigm which is really postmodern, there will inevitably be a multiplicity of heterogeneous schemes of life, patterns of action, language games, forms of life, conceptions of science, economic systems, social models and faith communities. This **multiplicity** does not exclude the quest for a fundamental **social consensus**. However, a quite specific aspect of the problems of modernity must be left out of account from the start.

Limiting the problems

In my paradigm analysis I have constantly had the **present** in mind, but have not yet analysed the particular profile of the present. I have tried to bring out as sharply as possible the historical presuppositions which are indispensable for an understanding of the present. Readers will themselves have felt how infinitely difficult it was in comparison with other eras to analyse modernity, so rich in content and excessively complex in the basic features necessary for a paradigmatic consideration. Unavoidably, here methodological limitations had to be imposed, not only on sectors covered (for example, there can be no treatment of modern art) but also on geographical areas, in order to concentrate on the dominant elements which govern the structures of the modern macro-constellation (P V).

In our approach it certainly became clear what an epoch-making significance the discovery, exploration, conquest and exploitation of the **'new' continents** had for European history (in the preliminary hermeneutical reflections on history relating to P IV). Here special importance was attached in particular to **North America**, which was developing most rapidly in religious, political, economic and social terms, to the American Revolution and the development of new forms of the church and a new picture of state and society; simply because of its common destiny with the Anglo-Saxon world and the way in which the Atlantic forms a 'bridge' to it, North America could not be completely omitted from our historically conditioned Eurocentric approach.

But the other non-European continents – **Latin America, Asia, Africa and Oceania** – had to be excluded from this specific analysis. For important as they all were and are from an economic, political, and in part also a cultural aspect, initially they had only peripheral significance for Christianity, which is our theme. After all, at first they were only the objects of a colonization and mission beginning from Europe, and not the subject of original Christian theology, spirituality and life-style. That happened only after the First and Second World Wars. It was above all the liberation movements in Latin America and partly also in Africa, and especially liberation theology, which for the first time provided effective stimuli not only for their own countries but also for the 'mother countries'.

In other words, neither in the past, nor even in the late nineteenth century, when the world was literally divided between the Great European powers, were these other continents (with North America well in the lead) individual agents in world politics with an autonomous role. This is only happening in the **present**, in the twentieth century. Indeed, this activation of the continents outside Europe in the sphere of Christianity and the church as well is a sure indication that Christianity has entered another entire constellation (P VI). This was already becoming evident at the end of the First World War. That war so shook the European rule of the world that after the Second World War it completely collapsed. All the former European colonies now gained their political independence from the European colonial powers in a relatively few years, in an unparalleled world-historical movement. So despite all the technological and economic dependence that remains, one can rightly call ours a **post-colonialist and post-imperialist age**. The paradigm of postmodernity is no longer a Eurocentric paradigm but a **polycentric paradigm** of different nations and religions.

It follows from this that in an account of the religious situation of our time the continents other than Europe (of course including North America) need separate treatment. However, this cannot be limited to present-day Christianity but must again begin with the first history of their Christianization, which in turn must be seen against the background of their non-Christian prehistory. This will be no small undertaking, but it will be a fascinating one; the 'end of history triumphalism' has flown as quickly as it came; we do not have to complain about 'tedium' in world history, but more about an overabundance of problems.

Central problem areas: ecology, the women's question, distributive justice, religion

Postmodernity, as I already attempted to sketch out provisionally in my *Global Responsibility*, means neither just romanticizing cosmetic operations in architecture and society nor just one theory of social, economic, political, cultural or religious organization. Rather, I apply the term 'postmodern' to everything that has taken shape in history in a **new world constellation** since the First and Second World Wars and which (as we are to hope and to work for) has a positive impetus towards a **new basic consensus** of integrating humane convictions which can be supported by non-believers and believers alike, indeed by the believers of every possible religion. If it is to survive, the democratic pluralist world society has to achieve this basic consensus. That is quite evident in four problem areas.

The modern development from the seventeenth century to the First World War left Christianity more problems than could be described here. But there are four problem areas where, first, the paradigm shift from modernity to postmodernity becomes particularly clear, and secondly, Christianity faces tremendous new tasks in the new era. They relate to **different dimensions of reality:**
– the cosmic dimension: human beings and nature;
– the anthropological dimension: man and woman;
– the sociopolitical dimension: poor and rich;
– the religious dimension: human beings and God.

Quite fundamental questions in respect of this arise for the coming era, not only for Christianity but also for the other prophetic religions. They are not posed here as cheap prescriptions, but as co-ordinates for orientation:

♊ † ☾ Questions for the Future

• Through science and technology modernity made immense progress in the **control of nature**.

But at the same time, by unrestrained exploitation of nature it undermined the foundations of human life: polluted air, polluted seas and lakes, poisoned earth, dying forests, threatened flora and fauna.

So for postmodernity, instead of an exploitative and destructive domination of nature, isn't a **partnership with nature** urgently needed? And what can the different religions, above all the prophetic religions, contribute in the postmodern paradigm on the basis of a cosmic religion to a change in planetary consciousness, to a new total synthesis of the scientific, technological and ethical religious spheres, to a peaceful symbiosis of all creatures and so to such an **ecological dimension**?

• Through the establishment of democracy modernity made unique progress in civil freedoms and **human rights**: freedom of conscience and of religion, freedom of assembly and of speech, freedom of the press.

But at the same time, by still retaining male superiority, modernity suppressed the rights of the other half of humankind. Only after the First World War was the vote given to women as well.

So for postmodernity, instead of discriminatory male privileges, isn't **equality for women** an urgent need everywhere? And what can the different religions, above all the prophetic religions, contribute in the postmodern paradigm on the basis of a feminist religious feeling to a change in global consciousness, to the realization of political and social human rights and so to the dimension of the **partnership** of man and woman?

• Through industrialization, modernity achieved tremendous progress in bringing **prosperity** to great masses, of a kind unprecedented in human history.

But at the same time, this led to a terrifying antagonism between the poor and the rich classes within modern society and, from a global perspective, between poor countries and rich countries.

So for postmodernity, instead of the North-South conflict, isn't international **distributive justice** for all peoples and individuals urgently necessary? And what can the different religions, above all the prophetic religions, contribute in the postmodern paradigm on the basis of a new liberating religious sense to a worldwide change in consciousness and to such a **social** dimension in the postmodern paradigm?

• Modernity, in its natural and humane sciences, was philosophically justified in concentrating on **reality as experienced**, and used unobjectionable methods when it necessarily left out of account God, who cannot be empirically detected or analysed like other objects.

But the modern natural and humane sciences have increasingly so generalized their results that hardly anything has been left for belief in an ultimate reality, and in the end, in practice belief in God has largely been replaced by belief in science. The methodologically justified limitation to our horizon of experience has often resulted in the arrogance of a sceptical agnosticism or an attitude of knowing better when confronted with meta-empirical questions.

So for postmodernity isn't a new openness to the whole, to the depths, of reality urgently necessary? In view of the modern loss of orientation, can the question of ultimate and primal meanings and criteria, values and norms, and thus of an ultimate ground of meaning, a priori be ruled out? So against the new horizon shouldn't there be a new openness to a **primal and ultimate spiritual reality** which we in the Jewish-Christian-Islamic tradition call God, and which, because it cannot be observed and analysed, also cannot logically be excluded or manipulated, but is credible and can be experienced indirectly? And what can the different religions, above all the prophetic religions, contribute in the postmodern paradigm on the basis of a multiconfessional religious sense to a change in planetary consciousness and to such an **ecumenical** dimension in the postmodern paradigm?

The first three areas of questions, too, are by no means only economic, political and social, but are of a deeply ethical and religious nature. And humankind must explicitly pose them in this age of transition between eras. However, if at the end of modernity there is again talk of religion, of the religions, and these religions have manifestly not gone under in modernity but despite all prognoses of their downfall have revived, often with new force, in traditional and unconventional forms, then for some analysts of the time a more threatening question arises. Will it not be the great **religions** which in the postmodern period again create, legitimate and inspire new **conflicts**?

Three opportunities for a new world order

We saw that in the framework of the modern paradigm, specifically in the course of the French Revolution, the **wars of the rulers** became **wars of the nations**. And with the end of modernity the wars of the nations became wars **of the ideologies**. Just consider:

– 1918 had already offered our century a **first opportunity** to replace the world of nationalistic modernity which had collapsed with the First World War with a new more peaceful global world order. However, this was prevented by the ideologies of Fascism, Communism, National Socialism and Japanism, all of which had their foundations in modernity. In retrospect they proved catastrophic false developments even for their supporters and set the whole world back by decades. Instead of a new world order there was world chaos.

– Then in 1945 (because of the obstruction caused by the Stalinist Soviet Union), the **second** opportunity for a new world order was missed. Instead of a new world order there was a division of the world.

– In 1989 all these reactionary ideologies (including that of a self-righteous anti-Communism) came to an end; the age of the great ideologies seems to be over. Again a new world order was propagated, though nothing was done towards realizing it. The wars (the Gulf War followed by the war in the Balkans) brought people back to earth. So has this **third** opportunity already been wasted? Instead of a new world order do we now have a new world disorder?

Some say that a new world disorder can be avoided provided that we do not act in an 'idealistic' way. For world order comes about only through a 'Realpolitik' which coolly calculates and implements national interests, unhampered by all too many 'moral feelings'. Thus the undoubtedly knowledgable and skilled politician and political theorist **Henry Kissinger**, who has already practised such 'Realpolitik' for many years and is now eloquently propagating them again in his most recent book,

Diplomacy.[203] Indeed this former Security Adviser and Secretary of State to President Nixon does not admire American politicians like Jefferson and Franklin, who aimed at a balance of ideals and interests, as much as European power politicians like Richelieu, Metternich and Bismarck. Kissinger ironically remarks: 'No other nation (than the United States) has ever based its claim to international leadership on its altruism.'[204] Moreover President Nixon, whom he advised, is praised as the first 'realistic' president since Theodore Roosevelt (the main representative of American expansionist policy!), while even now derogatory remarks are made about the peace movement against the Vietnam war.

But hasn't the 'Realpolitik' practised by the historical figures mentioned above also long faded into the twilight, as my account has clearly indicated? At any rate, Nixon's 'Realpolitik' led not only to a long overdue openness towards China but also to the prolongation of the Vietnam War by four years (at the cost of 20,492 American and around 160,000 South Vietnamese lives) and to its extension to Cambodia (with countless deaths).[205] The consequence was increasingly vigorous public protests, and paranoia in the White House – ending in Watergate and Nixon's impeachment . . . And finally didn't the moral tragedy of the two-tongued Western 'Realpolitik' in the Gulf and in Yugoslavia severely shake the political credibility of the USA, the EC and the United Nations, a policy which is unnecessarily prolonging the suffering of hundreds of thousands of people?

So we can follow Walter Isaacson, Kissinger's critical biographer, when on the one hand he emphasizes his 'respect' for Kissinger's 'brilliance as an analyst' but on the other expresses his 'reservations' about the 'lower priority' which Kissinger attaches to the 'values' which have made the American democracy such a powerful international force.[206] In view of the tension between moral ideals and national interests, Isaacson argues that Kissinger stands on the side of those 'realists' who strive for national interests, power and credibility against the 'idealists' who regard the dissemination of moral values as a decisive motive force for nations. But hasn't the American democracy in particular shown that it has always combined the pursuit of national interests with the propagation of values and ideals? Has American foreign policy ever been completely detached from moral values and ideals which are ultimately anchored in religion? So need interests and ideals necessarily be opposites? Indeed, isn't it in the interest of a realistic policy for this real world for it through ideas and visions to find a way out of the crises which it has itself produced?

A war of civilizations?

But won't wars also be inevitable in the future? Certainly, but the wars in a new world epoch will no longer be wars of ideologies, but primarily **wars of civilizations**. This at any rate is the thesis of the Director of the Institute of Strategic Studies at Harvard University, **Samuel P.Huntington**, which is being much discussed at present. It is developed in his striking article 'The Clash of Civilizations?'.[207] By **civilizations** Huntington, following **Arnold Toynbee**,[208] understands the 'cultural groupings' which extend beyond regions and nations. These are defined both by the objective elements of language, history, religion, customs and institutions and by the subjective self-identification of men and women. According to Huntington there are today eight 'civilizations' (with possible sub-civilizations): Western, Confucian, Japanese, Islamic, Hindu, Slavic-Orthodox, Latin American and African. So in the future we are to expect political, economic and military conflicts, say, between Islamic civilization and the West or Confucian-Asiatic civilization and the West, possibly combined with an 'Islamic-Confucian connection' of the kind that can already be seen in the constant flow of weapons from China and North Korea to the Middle East. 'The next world war, if there is one, will be a war between civilizations.'[209]

In the discussion which has taken place so far, especially in America,[210] Huntington has been accused of interpreting political and economic conflicts a priori as ethnic and cultural conflicts and giving them a religious charge (as the un-religious Saddam Hussein attempted retrospectively to do in the Gulf War, adopting a cynical tactic). Here a distinction must be made: of course most conflicts, from Berg Karabach through the Gulf War and Bosnia to Kashmir, are not primarily about civilization and religion but about territories, raw materials, trade and money, in other words are for economic, political and military interests. But Huntington is right: the ethnic and religious rivalries form the constant **underlying structures** for territorial disputes, political interests and economic competition, structures by which political, economic and military conflicts can be justified, inspired and intensified at any time. So while the great civilizations do not necessarily seem to me to be the **dominant paradigm** for the political controversies of the new world epoch, which Huntington thinks has replaced the Cold War paradigm and the First-Second-Third World scheme, it is the **deeper cultural dimension** to all antagonisms and conflicts between peoples which are always there and are in no way to be neglected.

But when it comes to this cultural dimension, we would do better to begin from the great **religions** (and their different paradigms) **instead of**

from civilizations, which are often difficult to define. In fact even Huntington is using the religions to define civilizations when he speaks of an Islamic, Hindu, Confucian or Slavic-Orthodox civilization. But I see two difficulties here:

– Can one separate **Orthodox Christianity** as a distinctive civilization from 'Western' Christianity, as Toynbee already did? A majority of Slavic-Orthodox East Europeans and indeed Russians will rightly protest that they are not part of the European 'West'; but as my whole account shows, Western and Slavic-Orthodox Christianity are by no means two completely different religions or civilizations, but 'only' two paradigms of one and the same Christianity (P II and P III). Certainly, these underwent separate developments in the second millennium, but a reconciliation in the future is in no way to be ruled out.

– Can one distinguish Western North American and **Latin American civilization** so sharply? On both continents, politics, economics and culture were given a Christian stamp, from Europe, at almost the same time – with the cruel elimination of the native Indio population. The difference is that for Latin America the Latin Catholic paradigm (P III) was to be normative, whereas the normative paradigm for North America was to be the Anglo-Saxon Protestant paradigm (P IV) and very soon the modern Enlightenment paradigm (P V).

However, Huntington must be said to be right on two decisive points:

• As Toynbee already noted, contrary to all superficial politicians and political theorists, who overlook the depth-dimension in world political conflicts, the **religions** are to be given a **fundamental role** in world politics: 'In the modern world, religion is a central, perhaps the central, force that motivates and mobilizes people . . . What ultimately counts for people is not political ideology or economic interest. Faith and family, blood and belief, are what people identify with and what they will fight and die for.'[211]

• Religions are not growing (as Toynbee thought) into a single unitary religion with Christian, Muslim, Hindu and Buddhist elements in the service of a single human society. It is much more realistic also to take into account their **potential for conflict** as rivals: 'Nation states will remain the most powerful actors in world affairs, but the principal conflicts of global politics will occur between nations and groups of different civilizations.'[212]

Indeed, it will strike anyone who is not blind to history that the modern state frontiers in Eastern Europe (and in part also in Africa) seem to pale in comparison with those **age-old frontiers** which were once drawn by peoples, religions and confessions: between Armenia and Azerbaijan, between Georgia and Russia, between the Ukraine and Russia, and also between the different peoples in Yugoslavia. According to Huntington, we shall also have to reckon in the **future** with **conflicts between civilizations**. 'Such conflicts also threaten in the future; indeed, we must fear that the most important conflicts of the future will occur along the cultural fault lines separating these civilizations from one another.'[213] Why? Not only **for geopolitical reasons**: because the world is becoming smaller and smaller, the interactions between people of different civilizations are becoming increasingly numerous, and the significance of the regional economic blocks is becoming increasingly important. But also for **reasons of** culture and **religious politics**: 1. because the differences between the civilizations are not only real but fundamental, often age-old and all-embracing, from the upbringing of children and the constitution of the state to the understanding of nature and God; 2. because many people are once again reflecting on their religious roots as a result of the cultural alienation and disillusionment with the West brought about by the process of economic and social modernization; 3. because human cultural characteristics and differences are less variable and dispensable than political and economic characteristics and differences (an Azerbaijani cannot become an Armenian and vice versa) and even more because religion divides men and women even more sharply and exclusively than membership of a people: 'A person can be half-French and half-Arab and simultaneously even a citizen of two countries. It is more difficult to be half-Catholic and half-Muslim.'[214] Particularly among peoples who are related in religion (what H.D.S.Greenway calls the 'kin-country syndrome'), e.g. between Orthodox Serbs, Russians and Greeks, religion plays a role which cannot be neglected.

Countries where large parts of the population come from different civilizations, like the former Soviet Union or former Yugoslavia, can disintegrate in such conflicts. Other countries like Turkey, Mexico and Russia, which are culturally to some degree a unity but are inwardly at odds over which civilization they belong to ('torn countries'), will be caused the greatest difficulties in any cultural reorientation that is necessary. And in view of the possibility of such conflicts between civilizations and religions, does not the future of humankind look extremely gloomy? How are we to react to this situation?

The alternative: peace between the religions

Not without justification, Huntington has been accused of a deep pessimism and even an irresponsible fatalism; if conflicts in the future are to be primarily conflicts between civilizations, then these are as it were given by nature and therefore even unavoidable; in that case the future of humankind will be constant, endless war. Indeed, in that case, in addition to the **'coming anarchy'** because of 'scarcity, crime, over-population, tribalism and disease' which the political journalist Robert D.Kaplan prognosticates in a striking and gloomy article in *Atlantic Monthly*,[215] there would ultimately and inevitably be a Third World War of civilizations which would necessarily lead to the end of our human race. Is there no alternative to this?

Huntington, too, is of the opinion that these **conflicts of civilizations** must be **avoided**. Not just by short-term strategies. In the longer term it is necessary to accommodate those non-Western civilizations which are preserving their traditional values and cultures and yet want to modernize themselves, and whose economic and military power will doubtless further increase. Huntington calls for this long-term strategy not only to maintain the economic and military power of the West in order to protect its own interests. Rather, his whole analysis culminates in a demand which is unusual for a political theorist (it was then taken up by Jacques Delors, the then President of the EC Commission[216]), 'to develop a deeper understanding of the basic religious and philosophical assumptions underlying the other civilizations and the ways in which people in those civilizations see their interest. It will require an effort to identify elements of commonality between Western and other civilizations.'[217] But there is only this one sentence . . .

This can be seen as support for this project on 'The Religious Situation of our Time' under the slogan 'No world peace without religious peace'. For in this project I am pursuing a strategy which is meant to prevent the 'clash of civilizations'. My starting point is: **'Without peace between the religions, war between the civilizations. No peace among the religions without dialogue between the religions. No dialogue between the religions without investigation of the foundations of the religions.'**

The analyses of the political theorist can partly be confirmed by those of the theologian, but at the same time they must be partly differentiated:

– If we recognize that Western and Eastern Christianity do not represent two religions/civilizations but two different constellations, albeit very different, **two paradigms** of the one Christianity (P II and P III), the convergence of, and mutual understanding between, which had already been considerably advanced by John XXIII, the Second Vatican Council and Patriarch Athenagoras of Constantinople, then we can also recognize that in particular an **ecumenical understanding between the churches** (in Yugoslavia, the Ukraine, between Rome and Moscow) could have prepared for understanding between the ethnic groups there (why should what was possible between French and Germans be impossible, say, between Serbs and Croats?).

– If we work out that even **two religions** like Christianity and Islam, which historically have been in constant confrontation, nevertheless have numerous features of faith and even more of ethics in common, then we need not give up hope that the tensions which have naturally always existed between religions and civilizations will not necessarily lead to a clash, even to a military collision. Peace is possible (why should not an agreement like that between Israelis and Palestinians also be possible between Armenians and Azerbaijanis, Indians and Pakistanis?).

– If **in each religion we attempt to work out the different paradigms** (the original, the ancient, the 'mediaeval', the modern paradigms) which, origins excluded, have all usually been preserved to the present day, we can see better how the fundamentalist option is nowhere the only one, but that in all the great religions (and quite especially in Judaism, Christianity and Islam) **several options** are on offer, at least some of which make understanding easier. In fact today every religion is unavoidably confronted with modernity, with modern science, technology, industry, democracy and culture generally.

The dispute in world history between power and morality

If Western **politicians, diplomats and lawyers** had a better knowledge of the other religions, they would be in a position not only to negotiate but also to carry on **dialogue**. In that case, at international negotiations and conferences like for example the most recent conference on human rights in Vienna they would not be embarrassed by the Chinese Communists, but could point out to them (and other autocratic Asian governments) that **human rights are not something exclusively Western**. For example, the concept of 'yen', the 'humanum', is quite a central concept of Chinese tradition which at the present time could very well be a basis for the human rights that are vigorously being called for all over Asia and Africa and in the long run cannot be suppressed by force.[218] Confucius was in fact already convinced that a government could most easily dispense with the military, if need be also with food, but least of all with the trust the people have in it.[219] And there is no disputing the fact that from China, Tibet, Burma and Thailand through Indonesian Westirian and the Philippians to Kenya and the Congo, human rights express something deeply longed for by subjects from their rulers. The 'dissidents' are by no means a tiny minority! Those millions whom the brave Nobel prizewinner Aung San Sun Kyi could mobilize in Burma through free elections could also be activated in China by a man like Wei Jingsheng if there were freedom of expression.[220]

However, clearly human rights for non-Western peoples will have a better foundation in their own ethnic religious traditions than simply in Western natural-law thinking. And if people in the West had a better knowledge of other religious and cultural traditions, they would understand why many Asians who are open to the West and affirm modernization are still **sceptical about the Western system of values.** Thus for example many Asians are unwilling to accept, say, unlimited individualism (with no concern for community) and absolute freedom (with all the phenomena of Western decadence connected with it); rather, as always, they attach importance to strong families, intensive education, strict work, frugality, unpretentiousness and national teamwork.[221]

But here the great and highly practical question arises: in the great **dispute between power and morality** in world history is not the ethical standpoint lost from the start, as the Machiavellians among the politicians and press commentators would constantly have us believe? Is the one who calls for the maintaining of certain humane 'values' also in foreign policy a naive 'preacher' and the one who constructs policy purely on 'interests' a cool 'strategist'? Are politics and morality as a rule compatible only as long as no important interests are affected? At all events, do not trade interests in particular prove stronger than politically moral postulate? It is remarkable that people still offer such allegedly realistic postulates when even the East European Communist dictatorships which operated so cynically with 'Realpolitik' finally had to capitulate to the moral postulates of their own population!

No, politics and morality are not a priori mutually exclusive, and what was right for example against the South African apartheid state cannot a priori be wrong against the Communist dictatorship in China. There is certainly a middle way between 'preaching' and 'Realpolitik', the way of a **political ethic of responsibility.** That means that a policy of human rights governed by an ethic of responsibility (say of the USA towards China) would have **to calculate coolly the real conditions under which it can be at all successful.** Specifically:

– A government advised by experts must right from the beginning consider realistically what instruments it has at its disposal for imposing demands for human rights; unfortunately, to have to withdraw idealistic demands under pressure encourages the political cynicism at home and abroad which there is a concern to overcome.

– The government must speak with one voice (the Treasury and the Trade Ministry may not speak a different language from the Foreign Ministry).

– The influential business community should not curry favour in trade negotiations with those who scorn human rights but similarly (in its own discreet way) insist on the need to observe moral criteria.

– In all unavoidable trade agreements the government should continually emphasize in public and in private that moral perspectives are and remain of prime importance to it and that without them real friendship between nations cannot be achieved.

– One government should draw the attention of the other to its own laws (which are often not observed: torture violates even Chinese law) and bring human rights to bear as universal (and not just Western) values and norms.

But does the West also practise the values which it often preaches to the 'rest of the world'? All this brings us to a last question which has not had its due in the discussion of Huntington so far, the question of an ethic, given the lack of orientation which is nowadays rampant everywhere.

Lack of orientation – a world problem

What should human beings hold on to – in all circumstances and everywhere? The **vacuum in orientation** is a world problem.

– Everywhere in the former **Soviet block** after the collapse of Communism and under the surface even in Communist **China**, still as oppressive as before, 'to cope with this moral and spiritual vacuum is a problem not only for China but for all civilizations'.[222]

– In the **United States**, where the population has increased by 41% since 1960 but violent crimes have increased by 560%, single mothers by 419%, divorces by 300%, children growing up in one-parent families by 300%,[223] and shootings are the second most frequent cause of death after accidents (in 1990 4,200 teenagers were shot);

– In **Europe**, where after the murder of a two-year-old child by two ten-year-olds in Liverpool even *Der Spiegel* complained in a cover story about the 'orientation jungle' and a lack of tabus unprecedented in cultural history: 'The youngest generation must cope with a confusion of values the extent of which is almost impossible to estimate. For them clear standards of right and wrong, good and evil, of the kind that were still being communicated by parents and schools, churches and sometimes even politicians in the 1950s and 1960s, are hardly recognizable any more.'[224]

What **Friedrich Nietzsche**, the most clear-sighted critic of modernity (though he did not overcome it), saw already arising in the nineteenth century, namely, man **'beyond good and evil'**, obligated only to his 'will to power',[225] the 'death of God' and overturning the 'whole of European morality', has become a fatal reality in the twentieth century: not only in figures of terror like Stalin and Hitler, not only in the Holocaust, the Gulag Archipelago and in two World Wars ending with atomic bombs, but also in everyday life, in the ever more frequent and unprecedented scandals involving leading politicians, businessmen and trade unionists in our industrial nations, or in the egocentricity, consumerism, violence and xenophobia of so many people, young people in particular.

If in a new world constellation which is coming into being, humankind on our planet is going to have any further guarantee of survival, there is urgent need for a **universal basic consensus on humane convictions**. A question which is thousands of years old is also unavoidable in our time. Why should one **do good and not evil**? Why do human beings not stand 'beyond good and evil'? Why are they not just obligated to their will to power, to success, riches, consumer goods, sex?[226] Fundamental questions are often the most difficult of all, and all over the world much about morals, laws and customs that had been taken for granted down the centuries because it was backed by religious authority is no longer automatically accepted. A worldwide dialogue, a global dialogue, has already been set in motion which should to lead to a consensus over shared values, standards and basic attitudes, to a world ethic.

For the fundamental question is: why should human beings — understood as individuals, groups, nations, religions — behave, not in a bestial way, merely ruled by their physical urges, but in a human, truly human, **humane** way? And why should they do this **unconditionally**, in other words in all circumstances? And why should **everyone** do this, and no class, clique or group, no state or party, be excepted? The question of an obligation which is both unconditional (categorical) and universal (global) is the basic question for any ethic in a society which is shaped by tendencies towards increasing scientific and economic globalization (one need think only of the international financial market or satellite television).

It should be evident that there is a fundamental problem here particularly for **modern democracy**, which has now also been adopted by Eastern Europe, about which we should not moralize in a self-righteous way but on which we should reflect self-critically. Given the way in which the free democratic constitutional state, which recognizes freedom of conscience and religion, understands itself, its world-view must be neutral, and tolerate different religions and confessions, philosophies and ideologies. Yet given all that, this state is supposed to decree meaning to life, no life-style. Isn't this quite manifestly the basis of the dilemma of any modern democratic state, whether in Europe, America, India or Japan?

People normally feel an unquenchable desire to hold on to something, to rely on something. In our technological world which has become so complex, and in the confusion of their private lives, they would like to have somewhere to stand, a line to follow; they would like to have criteria, a goal. In short, people feel an unquenchable desire to have something like a **basic ethical orientation**.

But all experiences show that human beings cannot be improved by more and more laws and precepts, nor of course can they be improved simply by psychology and sociology. In things both small and great we are confronted with the same situation: technical knowhow is not yet knowledge about meanings; rules are not yet orientations; and laws are not yet morals. Even the **law needs a moral foundation**! And security in our cities and villages cannot be bought simply with money (and more police and prisons). The ethical acceptance of laws (which provide the state with sanctions and can be imposed by force) is the presupposition of any political culture. What is the use to individual states or organizations, whether these be the EC, the USA or the United Nations, of constantly new laws, if a majority of people or powerful groups or individuals have no intention of observing them and constantly find enough ways and means of irresponsibly imposing their own or collective interests? *Quid leges sine moribus?* runs a Roman saying: what are laws without morals?

Towards a binding global ethic

Certainly all states in the world have an economic and legal order, but in no state in the world will this order function without an ethical consensus, without that ethical concern among its citizens by which the state with a democratic constitution lives. Already in the French Revolution there were those who wanted to have human duties formulated from the start alongside human rights. The international community has already created transnational, transcultural and transreligious legal structures (without which international treaties would in fact be sheer self-deception). But if a new world order is to exist, it needs a **minimum of common values, standards and basic attitudes**, an ethic which, for all its time-conditioned nature, is binding in all senses of the word on the whole of humanity, in short a global ethic.

It was the **Parliament of the World's Religions**, meeting in Chicago, which on 4 September 1993 passed a 'Declaration Toward a Global Ethic'[227] which for the first time in the history of religions formulated a minimal basic consensus relating to binding values, irrevocable standards and fundamental moral attitudes. This is a basic ethical consensus which:

– can be affirmed by all religions despite their 'dogmatic' differences and
– can also be supported by non-believers.

Now of course that does not mean that such a global ethic would make
the specific ethics of the different religions superfluous. The global ethic is
no substitute for the Sermon on the Mount or the Torah, the Qur'an, the
Bhagavadgita, the Discourses of the Buddha or the Sayings of Confucius.
On the contrary, it is precisely these age-old 'sacred texts', important to
billions of people, that can give a global ethic a solid foundation and make
it concrete in a convincing way. For while the global ethic has an external
perspective which is common to all religions, at the same time it has an
internal perspective which is specific to each religion.

– The world of the religions can be looked at as it were **from outside**: in
this external perspective (like that of religious studies), there are different
ways of salvation leading to the one goal, **many** true religions which can
mutually enrich and supplement one another, but which despite all their
'dogmatic' differences in ethics can demonstrate a minimum of common
values, standards and basic attitudes. The global ethic is to be discovered,
not invented.

– But at the same time (and without contradicting the first perspective),
the world of the religions can be looked at **from within**, for me from the
perspective of Christian faith. And in this internal perspective, for me as a
Christian (and of course the same is also true for Jews, Muslims, and all
the others) there is only the **one** true religion. For me that is Christianity,
in so far as it bears witness to the one true God, as this God has made
himself known in Jesus Christ – something which I attempted to describe
at the beginning as the 'essence of Christianity'. However, this one true
religion by no means excludes truth in other religions. Indeed, it is
particularly with regard to ethics that Christian faith also finds similar
elemental values, standards and basic attitudes in other religions, so that
Christian faith not only does not contradict a global ethic but supports
such an ethic from its specific perspective, giving it an unambiguous
foundation and making it more profound by making it more specific (cf.
the following two tables 'The Religions and a Global Ethic' and 'A Global
Ethic – Perspectives within Christianity').

The Religions
and a Global Ethic

Near Eastern-prophetic religions	Indian-mystical religions	Far Eastern-wisdom religions
Judaism	Hinduism	Confucianism / Taoism
Christianity	Buddhism	Japanese religions
Islam		

Nature and tribal religions

Religions of the native peoples in Africa, Asia, Oceania and America

A Global Ethic

Perspectives within Christianity

† **Christians** recognize Christ as the foundation, centre and criterion,

united with **Jews** and **Muslims** in faith in the one God of Abraham,

in co-operation with all men and women, **religious** and **non-religious**:

the **global ethic** as a duty and a hope!

Not an epilogue

This book is drawing to an end. But we are far from the end of the matter, which is an analysis of the religious situation of our time. I have paved the way to this through history and already opened the door on the present. So for the sake of the cause there can be no epilogue, no swansong, no postscript to this book, at best a look forward, a fore-word for the future.

A prospect

The historical analysis of the five previous macro-constellations of Christianity – the Jewish Christian apocalyptic, Hellenistic Byzantine, Roman Catholic, Reformation Protestant and Enlightenment modern paradigms – has brought us a deeper and sharper insight into the **past** of Christianity which is still present.

But precisely as a result of this historical and systematic diagnosis of the spiritual forces of a thousand-year-old history which still have an effect on the present we are constantly also directed to the **present**. After the paradigm shift which has taken place in our century from modernity to postmodernity we need a separate analysis to give us some idea of the different options there are for the **future**. I shall be making this in a second volume.

However, one thing is already certain: despite the present ecumenical 'low' we must hope and work to see that the new paradigm of Christianity is a post-confessional, **ecumenical paradigm** – otherwise the churches will become sects. The traces of the other 'confessional' paradigms will still be recognizable, but abolished and taken up in a new ecumenical synthesis of Christianity. In future this will no longer be characterized by three antagonistic confessions but by three complementary basic attitudes:

- Who is **Orthodox**? The analysis of P II made this clear. Those who are particularly concerned with 'right doctrine', true doctrine, specifically that **truth** which, because it is God's truth, must not be left to the whim of individuals (Christians, bishops, churches), but rather must be handed down creatively and lived out by being faithfully **transmitted** by the whole church to ever new generations.
- Who is **Catholic**? The analysis of P III has shown this. Those who are particularly concerned with the catholic, i.e. **whole**, universal, comprehensive church, specifically, with the **continuity** of faith and fellowship in faith in time and its **universality** in space.
- Who is **Evangelical**? The analysis of P IV was able to show this. Those who in all church traditions, doctrines and practices are particularly

concerned to refer constantly to the **gospel** (*euaggelion*, scripture), constantly intent on practical reform in accordance with the norm of this gospel.

But that has already made it clear that rightly understood, today basically 'Orthodox', 'Catholic' and 'Evangelical' attitudes are no longer by any means mutually exclusive. Today the born Orthodox or Catholic can be truly Evangelical, the born Protestant and Catholic can be truly Orthodox, the born Protestant and Orthodox can be truly Catholic in disposition. Aren't countless Christians all over the world – despite the resistance within the apparatus of the churches – in fact living out an authentic ecumenicity centred on the gospel? Today being a true Christian means being an ecumenical Christian.

The tasks for an ecumenical theology have remained, enormous tasks which have to be discussed in another volume. And individuals can easily become bewildered. For what are the challenges of the present and the possibilities in the future for Christianity in our time? I shall venture in what follows to identify these abiding tasks schematically, even if (despite considerable preliminary work) I am by no means certain that all that is indicated here can be carried through; only at the end of the way do we know what is really viable. So, with all the provisos, here is a **preliminary sketch** of the tasks still to be done (by me or others).

What are **the challenges of the present**? The following topics need to be discussed here:

Polycentric Christianity in a polycentric world

- Africa – a theological challenge
- Asia – successes and failures of Christianity
- Latin America – a continent between despair and hope
- North America – religious pluralism as an opportunity

What are the **possibilities for the future**? The following topics need to be discussed here:

Opportunities for a more Christian Christianity

- The rebirth of Eastern Orthodoxy
- The renewal of the Catholic Church
- The Reformation of the Reformation
- The opportunities for Christanity in the Third World

Perspectives for a more peaceful world ecumene

- Christianity and Judaism
- Christianity and Islam
- Christianity and Hinduism
- Christianity and Buddhism
- Christianity and Confucianism

New syntheses

- Religion and the cosmos (theology and the natural sciences)
- Religion and the psyche (theology and psychotherapy)
- Religion and the polis (theology and politics)
- Religion and culture (theology and aesthetics)

A religion for humankind

- Human beings and nature: cosmic religion
- Man and woman: holistic religion
- Rich and poor: liberating religion
- My religion and other religions: ecumenical religion

But already at the end of this book, some people will be asking: will Christianity still mean as much in the third millennium as it has done hitherto? Will it still have as much power and spirit? I now come back to the question I asked at the beginning: in the face of the challenges of the next post-Christian millennium, mustn't we despair of Christianity?

The mystery of Christianity

If at the end of this historical stocktaking we look back on the dramatic history of Christianity which has unfolded in different strands, if we once again remember what we have heard about the Jewish Christian apocalyptic, the Hellenistic Greek Russian, the Roman Catholic, the Reformation Protestant and finally the Enlightenment modern paradigms, surely at least it can be conceded that I have in no way concealed the deviations from the original foundation document, from the origin, from the originally good essence of Christianity; I have not concealed the gruesome aberrations and phenomena of decadence, the monstrous crimes and blasphemies of Christian representatives, but always addressed them clearly. There is no need here to mention once again the persecutions of the Jews and the heresy hunts, the 'holy' wars and the burning of witches, the wars of religion and all the other crimes committed in the name of Christianity. But at the same time I have attempted to make clear that the history of Christianity can in no way simply be told as a history of knaves and criminals, as a 'criminal history', but must be told in accordance with the facts, as a history in which the essence of Christianity keeps breaking through despite all the perversions.

And so there is a question which one cannot get out of one's head. Why has this Christianity kept surviving despite all the un-Christian elements in its history? For like a great river which has a modest beginning somewhere and has kept making new cuts through the emergent landscape, this religion has kept inserting itself into ever-new cultivated landscapes. In so doing it has experienced violent rejections and undergone revolutions, indeed has itself often caused new shifts in world history. But mustn't we also see here the stream of goodness, mercy, readiness to help, care, which flows from the source, from the gospel, through history? Granted: an infinite amount of debris, flotsam, silt and rubbish has been collected on the long way through the centuries. But has the water at the spring really become fully polluted, as many people say? In that case, how is it that the essence of Christianity did not get lost, but can be recognized time and again: Jesus Christ and his cause as an orientation, criterion, model for the concrete life of the individual and the community of faith, for relations with fellow human beings, human society and finally with God?

It is remarkable that time and again it was the **spirit of the Nazarene** which managed to establish itself even when persons, institutions and constitutions, failed, wherever there were not just words, but there was quite practical discipleship; for the truth of Christianity is not just knowledge of the truth but existential truth. So how is it that neither pagan emperors nor 'Christian' dictators, neither power-hungry Popes nor dark inquisitors, neither worldly bishops nor fanatical theologians have been able to quench this spirit? Why could the hierarchy never completely veil the diakonia, dogmatics never fully veil the discipleship of Christ? What is there about this spirit, that all down the centuries, in an unparalleled movement, it has continually motivated, indeed driven people to break down all the cultural, social, political, in short paradigmatic fortifications, and take seriously the earliest Christian ideal of a love for neighbours and others more distant? It is a strange historical mystery: monks and saints of the early church appear in it alongside court theologians and court bishops, Francis of Assisi alongside Innocent III and Boniface VIII, Martin Luther alongside Leo X, Catherine of Siena and Teresa of Avila alongside Grand Inquisitors, Blaise Pascal in the middle of French absolutism, Bishop Ketterer in a time when the social question was suppressed, Karl Barth, Dietrich Bonhoeffer and Alfred Delp in resistance to the Christianity of a bourgeois culture and National Socialism – not to mention figures in our day like John XXIII, Willem Visser't Hooft, Martin Luther King, Helder Camara and Mother Teresa.

All these known names simply stand as representatives of the countless unknowns whose names are not listed in any church history yet who nevertheless make up the hidden power of Christianity, its true spiritual history. They are representatives of that faith movement consisting of those countless unknowns down the centuries who have gone by the values, criteria and attitudes of the man from Nazareth, who have learned from them that the blessed are those who are poor before God, who do no violence, who hunger and thirst for righteousness, who are merciful, make peace and will be persecuted for righteousness' sake; who have learned from him to pay heed and to share, to be able to forgive and to repent, to be sparing, practise renunciation and offer help. To the present day they show that where Christianity really goes by its Christ and allows him to give it strength, it can offer a spiritual home, a place of faith, hope and love. Time and again they show in the everyday world that supreme values, unconditional norms, deepest motivations and highest ideals can be lived out, indeed that from the depths of belief in Christ suffering and guilt, despair and anxiety can also be overcome. No, this faith in Christ is no mere other-worldly consolation but a basis for protest and resistance against unjust situations here and now, supported and strengthened by an restless longing for the 'wholly Other'.

Granted, this often hidden history of Christianity is as uninteresting to criminologists and pathologists of Christianity as it is to certain journalists, hot-foot after the sensation of the day. After all, it is much easier to report on a scandal involving a bishop, or a papal visit, than on pastors in the parishes, wearing themselves out in the service of young and old, and still performing this service with a joyful heart and head held high. But it is precisely these men and women, whether ordained or not, who continue the cause of Jesus Christ. Indeed, as we saw, there have always been times when little of true Christianity was to be seen in the life and activities of hierarchy and theologians, but when nevertheless those countless, mostly unknown, Christians ('little people', but always including some bishops, theologians and particularly members of the parish clergy and religious orders) were there to keep alive the spirit of Jesus Christ.

And what kind of a spirit, what kind of a power is it that is at work everywhere? Is everything mere chance, mere fate, just a structural constellation? No. For believing Christians, beyond doubt more is involved here. For them it is clear that this effective spirit of Jesus Christ is not an unholy human spirit but the Holy Spirit, the spirit, the power and might of **God**: God's spiritual presence in the heart of believers and so also in the community of faith. This spirit sees to it that there is not just research, information and teaching about Christianity, but that Christianity is experienced with the heart and also really lived out and put into practice – for good or ill, since that is human nature, and in trust in this spirit of God. So Christians may be sure that Christianity has a future even in the third millennium after Christ, that this community of the spirit and faith has its own kind of 'infallibility'. However, this does not mean that some authorities in particular situations do not make mistakes or perpetrate errors, but rather, that despite all mistakes and errors, sins and vices, the community of believers will be maintained by the Spirit in the truth of Jesus Christ.

In a strange way one feels reminded of the famous advice of the Pharisee Gamaliel, a contemporary of Jesus, who was a Jewish teacher of the Law respected by all the people. At any rate according to the account in the Acts of the Apostles, after the arrest of the apostles he is said to have remarked to the 'supreme council' in Jerusalem about such Christians: 'If this plan or this undertaking is of men, it will fail; but if it is of God, you will not be able to overthrow them. You might even be found opposing God' (Acts 5.38f.).

Notes

Abbreviations

EncRel	*The Encyclopedia of Religion*, ed. M. Eliade (16 vols.), New York 1987
LThK	*Lexikon für Theologie und Kirche*, ed. J. Höfer and K. Rahner (10 vols.), Freiburg 1957ff.
RGG	*Die Religion in Geschichte und Gegenwart* (7 vols.), Tübingen ³1959
TRE	*Theologische Realenzykopädie*, ed. G. Krause and G. Müller (17 vols.), Berlin 1977ff.

Books by Hans Küng

Changing Church	*The Changing Church. Reflections on the Progress of the Second Vatican Council* (1964), London 1965
Church	*The Church* (1967), London and New York 1968
CR	*Christianity and Chinese Religions* (with Julia Ching) (1988), New York 1989 and London 1993
CWR	*Christianity and the World Religions. Paths of Dialogue with Islam, Hinduism and Buddhism* (with J. van Ess, H. von Stietencron and H. Bechert) (1984), London and New York 1985
Credo	*Credo. The Apostles' Creed Explained for Today* (1992), London and New York 1993
DGE	*Does God Exist? An Answer for Today*, London and New York 1980, reissued 1991
Fehlbar?	*Fehlbar? Ein Bilanz*, Zurich, Einsiedeln and Cologne 1973
GCT	*Great Christian Thinkers*, London and New York 1994
GR	*Global Responsibility. In Search of a New World Ethic* (1990), London and New York 1991
Incarnation	*The Incarnation of God. An Introduction to Hegel's Theological Thought as Prolegomena to a Future Christology* (1970), Edinburgh 1987
Infallible?	*Infallible? An Enquiry*, reissued with a new Foreword, London 1993
OBC	*On Being a Christian* (1974), London and New York 1976, reissued 1991

Structures	*Structures of the Church* (1962), London and New York 1965
Truthfulness	*Truthfulness. The Future of the Church*, London and New York 1968
TTM	*Theology for the Third Millennium* (1987), New York 1988 and London 1991

The Aim of This Book

1. For further detailed information cf. the relevant sections in the major **general histories:**
1. **World histories: L. Halphen and P. Sagnac** (eds.), *Peuples et civilisations. Histoire générale* (20 vols.), Paris 1926–37; **A. J. Toynbee**, *A Study of History* (12 vols.), Oxford 1934–61; **F. Valjavec** (ed.), *Historia Mundi* (10 vols.), Bern 1952–61; **M. Crouzet** (ed.), *Histoire générale des civilisations* (7 vols.), Paris 1953–7; **P.Renouvin** (ed.), *Histoire des relations internationales* (8 vols.), Paris 1953–8; **G. Mann** and **A. Heuss** (eds.), *Propyläen Weltgeschichte* (11 vols.), Berlin 1961–65; **H. Franke** et al. (eds.), *Saeculum Weltgeschichte* (7 vols.), Freiburg 1965–75; *Fischer Weltgeschichte* (36 vols.), Frankfurt 1966–81; **P. Boutruche** and **P. Lemerle** (eds.), *Nouvelle Clio. L'Histoire et ses problèmes*, Paris 1966ff.; **D. Hay** (ed.), *A General History of Europe* (12 vols.), new edition London 1987; **T. Schieder** (ed.), *Handbuch der europäischen Geschichte* (7 vols.), Stuttgart 1968–92.
2. **Church histories: J. Lortz**, *Geschichte der Kirche in ideengeschichtlicher Betrachtung*, Münster 1935, revised edition in 2 vols. [21]1962–64; **A. Fliche** and **V. Martin** (eds.), *Histoire de l'église depuis les origines jusqu'à nos jours* (21 vols.), Paris 1946–52; *Pelican/Penguin History of the Church* (7 vols.), Harmondsworth 1961–92; **H. Jedin** and **J. Dolan** (eds.), *History of the Church* (10 vols.), New York and London 1980–81; **K. D. Schmidt** and **E. Wolf**, *Die Kirche in ihrer Geschichte. Ein Handbuch*, Göttingen 1962ff.; **L. J. Rogier, R. Aubert** and **M. D. Knowles** (ed.), *Geschichte der Kirche* (5 vols.), Zurich 1971–75; **H. Gülzow** and **H. Lehmann** (eds.), *Christentum und Gesellschaft* (15 vols.), Stuttgart 1980ff. (four volumes have appeared so far); **M. Greschat** (ed.), *Gestalten der Kirchengeschichte* (12 vols.), Stuttgart 1981–85; **M. Mollat du Jourdin** and **A. Vauchez**, *Histoire du christianisme des origines à nos jours*, Paris 1990ff.
3. **Histories of dogma and theology: A. von Harnack**, *History of Dogma* (1900: 7 vols reissued as 3, 1961); **F. Loofs**, *Leitfaden zum Studium der Dogmengeschichte*, ed K. Aland (2 vols.), Halle 1951–53; **M. Schmaus** et al. (eds.), *Lehrbuch der Dogmengeschichte* (I–IV.2), Darmstadt 1959; **R. Seeberg**, *Lehrbuch der Dogmengeschichte* (Vols.I–IV.2), Darmstadt 1959; **J. Pelikan**, *The Christian Tradition. A History of the Development of Doctrine* (3 vols.), Chicago 1971–78.
In historical orientation I have been constantly helped by **K. Heussi**, *Kompendium der Kirchengeschichte*, Tübingen 1956, [12]1960, and **Der grosse Ploetz**, *Auszug aus der Geschichte von den Anfängen bis zur Gegenwart*, Würzburg [31]1991.

A. THE QUESTION OF ESSENCE

I. The Essence and Perversion of Christianity

1. Because, as I pointed out in the introduction, the conception presented in this book is the end-product of a long process of thought which has matured over decades, the structural elements on which it is based should be quite recognizable here. They should make it clear to the reader that the overall approach has been well tested. Consequently, in the notes from time to time I shall be referring to my earlier books. These references are not a ritual self-quotation but documentation of the course that has been described.

2. Cf. **T. B. Macaulay**, *On the Roman Catholic Church*. Macaulay published the text as early as 1840 in a review of an English translation of Ranke's *History of the Popes*.

3. Cf. **H. Küng**, *Judaism*, 2 A I 6, 'The fatal antisemitism of a Catholic, Adolf Hitler'.

4. **K. Adam**, *Das Wesen des Katholizismus*, Düsseldorf 1924, ^{12}1949, 17.

5. Id., 'Deutsches Volkstum und katholisches Christentum', *Theologische Quartalschrift* 114, 1933, 40–63: 41, 58.

6. Id., *Das Wesen des Katholizismus* (n.4), 249.

7. **H. de Lubac**, *Méditation sur l'Église*, Paris 1953.

8. **H. U. von Balthasar**, *Sponsa Verbi*, Einsiedeln 1961.

9. **G. von le Fort**, *Hymnen an die Kirche*, Munich 1924.

10. Cf. **H. Küng**, *Truthfulness*, A, 'Truthfulness: A Basic Requirement of the Church'.

11. Cf. **E. Drewermann**, *Kleriker. Psychogramm eines Ideals*, Olten 1989.

12. **F. Nietzsche**, *The Antichrist*, Complete Works, London 1911, 230f.

13. Cf. **K. Deschner**, *Kriminalgeschichte des Christentums* (4 vols.), Reinbek 1986–94, I, 11.

14. Ibid., I, jacket copy.

15. Cf. **H. Küng**, DGE, D, 'Nihilism – A Consequence of Atheism'.

16. Cf. **id.**, *Church*, C, 'The Fundamental Structure of the Church'.

17. Thus already in **id.**, *Structures*, Ch.VII, 'The Petrine Office in the Church and in Council'; cf. **id.**, *Church*, E II 3; **id.**, *Infallible?*, London ^{2}1994.

18. 'For the history of those whom I describe has made me their enemy', Deschner, *Kriminalgeschichte* (n.13), I, 53.

19. That both the content and form of Deschner's historiography are questionable in many ways was shown by a professional conference of historians and theologians, cf. **H. R. Seeliger**, *Kriminalisierung des Christentums? Karlheinz Deschners Kirchengeschichte auf dem Prüfstand*, Freiburg 1993 (cf. the important corrections to his treatment of Constantine, Julian, Athanasius, Ambrose, Augustine and Leo I and especially G. Denzler's contribution on the criticism of the papacy).

20. **H. Deschner**, 'Écrasez l'infâme oder Über die Notwendigkeit, aus der Kirche auszutreten', in **id.**, *Opus Diaboli. Fünfzehn unversöhnliche Essays über die Arbeit im Weinberg des Herrn*, Reinbek 1987, 115–29.

21. For what follows see **H. Küng**, *Church*, A, 'The Church as it is'.

22. Cf. the response by **K. J. Kuschel**, 'Ist das Christentum inhuman? Kritische Anmerkungen zu einer Streitschrift', *Herder Korrespondenz* 46, 1992, 222–6, to

F. Buggle, *Denn sie wissen nicht was sie glauben. Oder warum man redlicher-weise nicht mehr Christ sein kann. Eine Streitschrift*, Reinbek 1992, a book which lacks any historical-critical hermeneutics.

23. In my *Judaism*, as a Christian theologian in an ecumenical spirit I have attempted to bring out the 'essence' of *Judaism* which can be found in all the different epoch-making paradigms, with reference to numerous Jewish scholars, past and present.

II. 'Christianity' in Dispute

1. L.Feuerbach, *Vorlesungen über das Wesen der Religion* (given in Heidelberg in 1848/49), in *Gesammelte Werke*, ed. W. Schuffenhauer, Vol. VI, Berlin 1967, 30f.

2. For this section see H. Küng, DGE, C I, 'God – a human projection? Ludwig Feuerbach'.

3. L. Feuerbach, *The Essence of Christianity* (1841), translated by George Eliot, reissued New York 1957, 226–31; cf. Preface, xxxvii.

4. Ibid., 5.

5. Id., 'Notwendigkeit einer Reform der Philosophie' (1842), in *Sämtliche Werke*, ed. W. Bolin and F. Jodl, II, Stuttgart 1904, 218f.

6. A. von Harnack, *What is Christianity?*, reissued New York 1957 (original title *Das Wesen des Christentums*, Leipzig 1900; the title of the English translation obscures the point).

7. Id., *History of Dogma* (1885–1898), 7 vols. reissued as 3, New York 1971.

8. Id., *What is Christianity?* (n.6), 4.

9. K. J. Kuschel, *Born Before All Time? The Dispute over Christ's Origin*, London and New York 1992, 52.

10. Harnack, *What is Christianity?* (n.6), 6.

11. Cf. E. Troeltsch, 'What Does "Essence of Christianity" Mean?' (1903), in R. Morgan and M. Pye (eds.), *Ernst Troeltsch. Writings on Theology and Religion*, London 1977, 124–79.

12. Cf. id., *The Absoluteness of Christianity and the History of Religion* (1902), Richmond, Va. and London 1971.

13. Cf. H. Hoffmann, 'Die Frage nach dem Wesen des Christentums in der Aufklärungstheologie', in *Harnack-Ehrung*, Leipzig 1921, 353–65.

14. R. Schäfer, 'Christentum, Wesen des', in *Historisches Wörterbuch der Philosophie*, ed. J. Ritter, I, Darmstadt 1971, 1008–16: 1012.

15. Cf. H. Wagenhammer, *Das Wesen des Christentums. Eine begriffsge-schichtliche Untersuchung*, Mainz 1973.

16. Cf. ibid., esp. 121–3, 140–3. However, in view of the material which the author presents from Protestant theology, his claim that 'one cannot evaluate the formula "essence of Christianity" as a construction of Protestantism' (254, cf. 165), but that it rather has 'its home in the old Neo-Platonic and Gnostic-Hermetic stream of tradition' (165, cf.254) is not at all convincing. Because Wagenhammer's 'demanding theological stylization leads to summary assertions and steep theses' (thus the Kiel historian H. J. Birkner in his review in *Theologische Literaturzeitung* 102, 1977, 376–8: 377), despite its wealth of material and numerous careful detailed analyses this work contributes little

towards clarifying the question of the essence of Christianity. J. Werbick, *Vom entscheidend und unterscheidend Christlichen*, Düsseldorf 1992, who attempts to mark out the Christian way between Enlightenment and fundamentalism, is helpful here.

17. Cf. **Wagenhammer**, *Wesen des Christentums* (n.15), 50–4.

18. Cf. **J. Locke**, *The Reasonableness of Christianity, as Delivered in the Scriptures*, London 1695.

19. Cf. **J. Toland**, *Christianity not Mysterious: or, a Treatise Shewing, that there is Nothing in the Gospel Contrary to Reason, nor Above it: and that no Christian Doctrine can be Properly Call'd a Mystery*, London 1696, reissued New York 1978.

20. Cf. **M. Tindal**, *Christianity as Old as the Creation, or, The Gospel, a Republication of the Religion of Nature*, London 1730, reissued New York 1978.

21. Cf. **M. Schmaus**, *Vom Wesen des Christentums*, Augsburg 1947. Schmaus indeed emphasizes that 'the centre of Christianity is Christ' (185). But what does Schmaus's Christ include? Among many other problematical features also this: 'So Christ founded the papacy . . . The most far-reaching expression of the supreme leadership of the church by the Pope is papal infallibility. Though it was only established formally by the church through the Vatican Council in 1869, belief in it was nevertheless there from the beginning, though for a long time in an undeveloped form' (196f.)

22. Cf. **R. Guardini**, *Das Wesen des Christentums*, Würzburg ³1949. Guardini also impressively brings out the central significance of the person of Christ for Christianity, but from the start he commandeers it for his Roman Catholic understanding of the church, which *a priori* excludes any criticism of the church of Christ: 'Christ does not stand just anywhere, "absolutely", but has his place and is related to an order. The church is the continuing reality in history to which Christ is related; the sphere, rightly constructed, in which the essence of his figure can be seen and his word be heard fully . . . So taken in full, the formula runs: a content is Christian in so far as it is given by Christ in the church' (33).

23. Cf. Acts 11.26; cf. **E. Peterson**, 'Christianus', in *Frühkirche, Judentum und Gnosis*, Freiburg 1959, 64–87.

24. Cf. Gal.1.3.

25. **Ignatius of Antioch**, To the Magnesians 10.1.

26. **Id.**, To the Magnesians 10.3; cf. To the Romans 3.3; To the Philadelphians 6.1.

27. Cf. **A. Blaise**, *Dictionnaire latin-français des auteurs chrétiens*, Turnhout 1954, 556. Instead of the borrowed word *Christianismus*, in Latin the word *Christianitas* is used, which only over time developed a limited meaning.

28. Cf. **Josephus**, *Antiquities* 20.9.1 and 18.3.3.

29. **Pliny**, *Letter* 96.

30. **Tacitus**, *Annals* 15.44; cf. **J. B. Bauer**, 'Tacitus und die Christen (Ann.15.44)', *Gymnasium. Zeitschrift für Kultur der Antike und humanistische Bildung* 64, 1957, 497–503.

B. THE CENTRE

I. Basic Form and Original Motive

1. For what follows see **H. Küng**, OBC, B I 1, 'The Christ'.
2. Cf. ibid., C I 3, 'Emigration?' (the publications by H. Bardtke, O. Betz, F. F. Bruce, M. Burrows, G. R. Driver, A. Dupont-Sommer, H. Haag, J. Hempel, J. Jeremias, J. Maier, C. Rabin, K. Schubert, G. Vermes and Y. Yadin are important here).
3. Cf. **M. Baigent** and **R. Leigh**, *The Dead Sea Scrolls Deception*, London 1991 (the German title of which is *Verschlusssache Jesus* – a secret file on Jesus); **B. E. Thiering**, *Jesus and the Riddle of the Dead Sea Scrolls. Unlocking the Secrets of His Life Story*, San Francisco 1993; **R. Eisenman** and **M. Wise**, *The Dead Sea Scrolls Uncovered*, Shaftesbury 1992.
4. **J. B. Bauer**, 'Das "Elfenbeinturm" oder Forschung als Kommunikation', in K. Freisitzer et al. (eds.), *Tradition und Herausforderung. 400 Jahre Universität Graz*, Graz 1985, 423–30, points to the relativizing of analyses in the natural sciences.
5. Cf. **G. Grönbold**, *Jesus in Indien. Das Ende einer Legende*, Munich 1985 (this legend was propagated above all by N.Notowitsch in 1894 and has recently been revived by S. Obermeier and others).
6. Such trivial 'disclosure books' about Jesus are analysed critically by **J. Dirnbeck**, *Die Jesus-Fälscher. Ein Original wird entstellt*, Augsburg 1994.
7. For criticism of the sensationalizing Qumran literature cf. **J. H. Charlesworth** (ed.), *Jesus and the Dead Sea Scrolls*, New York 1992; **O. Betz** and **R. Riesner**, *Jesus, Qumran and the Vatican. Clarifications*, London and New York 1994; **K. Berger**, *Qumran und Jesus. Wahrheit unter Verschluss?*, Stuttgart 1993; **H. Stegemann**, *Die Essener, Qumran, Johannes der Täufer und Jesus. Ein Sachbuch*, Freiburg 1993. Cf. also the thematic volume on Qumran, *Bibel und Kirche* 48, 1993, no.1, and in it especially the contributions by J. A. Fitzmyer and H.-J. Fabry.

The Protestant (formerly Catholic) Heidelberg New Testament scholar **Klaus Berger** has recently attempted to make professional colleagues interesting with arrogant and ignorant outlines of theological publications in the *Frankfurter Allgemeine Zeitung* (including my *Great Christian Thinkers*). He has every reason to be more modest, seeing that he has dated an early mediaeval Jewish work to New Testament times. In 1989 Berger issued a 'wisdom work from the Cairo Geniza', already very well known through two partial editions (by A. E. Harkavy and S. Schechter, 1902–4), in a 'first edition', which is 'hardly a real advance on the publications by Harkavy and Schechter' – thus the Tübingen Protestant Old Testament scholar **Hans Peter Rüger**. In his own exemplary investigation and new edition of the text (*Die Weisheitsschrift aus der Kairoer Geniza. Text, Übersetzung und philologischer Kommentar*, Tübingen 1991, quotation p.2), the appearance of which Berger through his publishing house attempted to prevent by threats of a lawsuit, Rüger was able to demonstrate (1–19) that the 'superlinear punctuation' is 'not, as Berger remarks, Palestinian but the so-called simple Babylonian punctuation'; that the 'consonantal text of the manuscript has been misread' by Berger 'at many points'; that 'the Babylonian vowel signs have often been misunderstood'; that 'Berger's translation is not

always reliable'; that the work was not written, as Berger assumes, 'around 100
CE', but at the earliest after 'the end of the sixth century CE', and probably only
'in the twelfth century CE'; that Egypt as a place of origin (assumed by Berger) is
improbable; that 'the wisdom work from the Cairo Geniza is not', as Berger
assumes, 'perhaps a last attempt to combine realistic approaches of Hellenistic
philosophy with traditionally Jewish wisdom dualism', as Berger thinks, but must
be regarded as 'a product of mediaeval Jewish Platonism'. That the wisdom work
is not a text from around 100 but an early mediaeval rabbinic document was
already assumed by S. Schechter, and has meanwhile been confirmed by all
scholars who have been involved with it, both Christian and Jewish. Cf. especially
E. Fleischer, *The Proverbs of Sa'id ben Babshad*, Jerusalem 1990, 241–63, and G.
Veltri, *Theologische Rundschau* 57, 1992, 405–30. Berger's lack of scientific
perspicacity and his inability to give texts an adequate historical context and
interpretation disqualify this fluent writer as a reviewer of academic publications
by professional colleagues.
  8. For the specific differences between the Qumran community and the
community of Jesus' disciples, cf. **H. Küng**, OBC, C I 3. For Jesus there was no
separation from the world, no division of reality, no zeal for the law, no
asceticism, no hierarchical order and no religious rule.
  9. Cf. ibid., C VI 1, 'Limits to Demythologizing'.
  10. John 14.6.

II. The Central Structural Elements

  1. I Cor.12.4–6.
  2. Cf. **H. Küng**, CWR; id., CR. I find the conception of the typically prophetic
religion, as distinct from the Indian mystical or Chinese wisdom type, developed
in these two books confirmed in **G. T. Sheppard** and **W. E. Herbrechtsmeier**,
'Prophecy', *EncRel* XII, 8–14. After an analysis of five characteristics of prophets
they come to the conclusion: 'The founding prophets are distinct from others who
founded major religious traditions (such as Buddhism, Jainism, Confucianism,
and Taoismn). The founders of these traditions originating in India and China
were not divinely chosen messengers bearing a revealed message to humankind
but rather teachers and sages who had developed new philosophic insight and
practical discipline as a way of addressing religious problems' (10).
  3. Cf. the most recent study by **K.-J. Kuschel**, *Abraham. A Sign of Hope for
Jews, Christians and Muslims*, London and New York 1995. This is an
impressive study of the Abraham traditions in Judaism, Christianity and Islam
and a splendid plea for an Abrahamic ecumene.
  4. For the **Law** see **H. Küng**, *Judaism*, 1 B I 2, 'Sinai: Covenant and Law'; 3 B,
'Conflicts in Life and the Future of the Law'.
  5. Cf. Ex.19–Num.10.
  6. Cf. Ex.34.28; Deut.4.13; 10.4.
  7. Cf. Ex.20.2–17; Deut.5.6–21.
  8. For the **image of God in the Hebrew Bible**, after the earlier theologies of the
Old Testament by **W. Eichrodt, L. Köhler, O. Procksch, E. Jacob, G. von Rad** and
T. C. Vriezen see above all, **G.Fohrer**, *Theologische Grundstrukturen des Alten
Testaments*, Berlin 1972; **W.Zimmerli**, *Old Testament Theology in Outline*,

Atlanta 1978; **J.L.McKenzie**, *A Theology of the Old Testament*, New York 1974; **M.Rose**, *Der Ausschliesslichkeitsanspruch Jahwes. Deuteronomische Schultheologie und die Volksfrömmigkeit in der späten Königszeit*, Stuttgart 1975; **H.Vorländer**, *Mein Gott. Die Vorstellungen vom persönlichen Gott im Alten Orient und im Alten Testament*, Neukirchen 1975; **H. W. F. Saggs**, *The Encounter with the Divine in Mesopotamia and Israel*, London 1978; **C.Wester-mann**, *Elements of Old Testament Theology*, Atlanta 1982; **O. Keel** (ed.), *Monotheismus im alten Israel und seiner Umwelt*, Fribourg 1980; **S. Kreuzer**, *Der lebendige Gott. Bedeutung, Herkunft und Entwicklung einer alttestamentlichen Gottesbezeichnung*, Stuttgart 1983; **B.Andrade**, *Encuentro con Dios en la historia. Estudio de la concepción de Dios en el Pentateuco*, Salamanca 1985; **J.Vermeylen**, *Le Dieu de la promesse et le Dieu de l'alliance. Le dialogue des grandes intuitions théologiques de l'Ancien Testament*, Paris 1986; **A. D. Clarke** and **B. W. Winter** (ed.), *One God, One Lord in a World of Religious Pluralism*, Cambridge 1991. For the buried feminine aspects of the Jewish image of God see **O. Keel** and **C. Uehlinger**, *Göttinnen, Götter und Gottessymbole. Neue Erkenntnisse zur Religionsgeschichte Kanaans und Israel aufgrund bislang unerschlossener ikonographischer Quellen*, Freiburg 1992 (which is amply documented with illustrations, above all of seals). However (at least after the basic decision taken at the end of the sixth century BCE), these aspects were not accepted as a counterpart, partner, goddess for Yahweh. Cf. also **E. S. Gersten-berger**, *Jahwe – ein patriarchaler Gott? Traditionelles Gottesbild und feminist-ische Theologie*, Stuttgart 1988, and **M. S. Smith**, *The Early History of God. Yahweh and the Other Deities in Ancient Israel*, San Francisco 1990 (esp. Ch.III).

9. Cf. Isa.63.7–64.11.

10. Cf. Gen.1.27.

11. Cf. **H. Küng**, *Judaism*, 1 A II 7, 'The covenant with Noah: a covenant with humankind and the human order'.

12. Cf. **id.**, *Judaism*, 1 B I, 'The Central Structural Elements'.

13. More recent literature on the **historical Jesus** and New Testament christology includes: **G. Bornkamm**, *Jesus of Nazareth*, London and New York 1960; **O. Cullmann**, *The Christology of the New Testament*, London and Philadelphia ²1963; **N. Perrin**, *Rediscovering the Teaching of Jesus*, London and New York 1967; **E. Schweizer**, *Jesus Christ*, Atlanta and London 1989; **H. Braun**, *Jesus. Der Mann aus Nazareth und seine Zeit*, Stuttgart 1969; **C. H. Dodd**, *The Founder of Christianity*, London 1970; **F. Hahn**, *Christologische Hoheitstitel. Ihre Geschichte im frühen Christentum*, Göttingen 1974; **C. F. D. Moule**, *The Origin of Christology*, Cambridge 1977; **J. D. G. Dunn**, *Christology in the Making. A New Testament Inquiry into the Origins of the Doctrine of the Incarnation*, Philadelphia 1980; **J. Riches**, *Jesus and the Transformation of Judaism*, London 1980; **J. Blank**, *Der Jesus des Evangeliums, Entwürfe zur biblischen Christologie*, Munich 1981; **E.P. Sanders**, *Jesus and Judaism*, London and Philadelphia 1985; **W. Simonis**, *Jesus von Nazareth. Seine Botschaft vom Reich Gottes und der Glaube der Urgemeinde. Historisch-kritische Erhellung der Ursprünge des Christentums*, Düsseldorf 1985; **P. Fredriksen**, *From Jesus to Christ. The Origins of the New Testament Images of Jesus*, New Haven 1988; **M.de Jonge**, *Christology in Context. The Earliest Christian Response to Jesus*, Philadelphia 1988; **E. Richard**, *Jesus: One and Many. The Christological Concept of New Testament Authors*, Wilmington 1988; **J. Gnilka**, *Jesus von Nazaret. Botschaft und Geschichte*, Freiburg 1990; **J. D. Crossan**, *The Historical*

Jesus. The Life of a Mediterranean Jewish Peasant, San Francisco 1991; **N.A.Dahl**, *Jesus the Christ. The Historical Origins of Christological Doctrine*, Minneapolis 1991; **J.P.Meier**, *A Marginal Jew. Rethinking the Historical Jesus*, I, New York 1991; **R.Schnackenburg**, *Die Person Jesus Christi im Spiegel der vier Evangelien*, Freiburg 1993. Of course there are also chapters on the historical Jesus in the more recent systematic christologies of L. **Boff**, O. **González de Cardedal**, J. J. **González Faus**, W. **Kasper**, F.-W. **Marquardt**, J. **Moltmann**, K. H. **Ohlig**, W. **Pannenberg**, C. H. **Ratschow**, E. **Schillebeeckx**, P. **Schoonenberg**, J. L. **Segundo** and J. **Sobrino**. W. G. **Kümmel**, *Dreissig Jahre Jesusforschung (1950–1980)*, Königstein 1985, and A. J. **Hultgren**, *New Testament Christology. A Critical and Annotated Bibliography*, New York 1988, give surveys of scholarship.

    14. John 14.28.

    15. Luke 18.19.

    16. Cf. **K.-J. Kuschel**, *Born Before All Time. The Dispute over Christ's Origin*, London and New York 1992, 389–90.

    17. For the understanding of the cross cf. H. **Kessler**, *Die theologische Bedeutung des Todes Jesu. Eine traditionsgeschichtliche Untersuchung*, Düsseldorf 1970; H. **Cohn**, *The Trial and Death of Jesus*, London 1972; S. K. **Williams**, *Jesus' Death as Saving Event. The Background and Origin of a Concept*, Missoula, Montana 1975; W. H. **Kelber** (ed.), *The Passion in Mark. Studies on Mark 14–16*. Philadelphia 1976; M.-L. **Gubler**, *Die frühesten Deutungen des Todes Jesu. Eine motivgeschichtliche Darstellung aufgrund der neueren exegetischen Forschung*, Freiburg 1977; F. **Zehner**, *Das Leiden Christi nach den vier Evangelien. Die wichtigsten Passionstexte und ihre hauptsächlichen Probleme*, Vienna 1980; M. **Limbeck** (ed.), *Redaktion und Theologie des Passionsberichtes nach den Synoptikern*, Darmstadt 1981; D. **Flusser**, *The Last Days of Jesus in Jerusalem. A Current Study of the Easter Week*, Tel Aviv 1980; G.**Friedrich**, *Die Verkündigung des Todes Jesu im Neuen Testament*, Neukirchen 1982; J. D. **Crossan**, *The Cross that Spoke. The Origins of the Passion Narrative*, San Francisco 1988; K. **Grayston**, *Dying We Live. A New Enquiry into the Death of Christ in the New Testament*, Oxford 1990; G. **Barth**, *Der Tod Jesu Christi im Verständnis des Neuen Testaments*, Neukirchen 1992.

    18. For the problems associated with the **resurrection**, in addition to the books on Jesus and christologies already cited see the monographs by K. **Berger**, *Die Auferstehung des Propheten und die Erhöhung des Menschensohnes. Traditionsgeschichtliche Untersuchungen zur Deutung de Geschickes Jesu in frühchristlichen Texten*, Göttingen 1976; J. **Kremer**, *Die Osterevangelien. Geschichten um Geschichte*, Stuttgart 1977; F. **Zehrer**, *Die Auferstehung Jesu nach den vier Evangelien. Die Osterevangelien und ihre hauptsächlichen Probleme*, Vienna 1980; R.H.**Smith**, *Easter Gospels. The Resurrection of Jesus according to the Four Evangelists*, Minneapolis 1983; H.**Hendrickx**, *The Resurrection Narratives of the Synoptic Gospels*, London 1984; P.**Perkins**, *Resurrection: New Testament Witness and Contemporary Reflection*, New York 1984; H. **Kessler**, *Sucht den Lebenden nicht bei den Toten. Die Auferstehung Jesu Christi in biblischer, fundamentaltheologischer und systematischer Sicht*, Düsseldorf 1985; H.F.**Bayer**, *Jesus' Predictions of Vindication and Resurrection. The Provenance, Meaning and Correlation of the Synoptic Predictions*, Tübingen 1986; G. **O'Collins**, *Jesus Risen. An Historical, Fundamental and Systematic Examination of Christ's Resurrection*, New York 1987; P. **Hoffmann** (ed.), *Zur neutes-*

tamentlichen Überlieferung von der Auferstehung Jesu, Darmstadt 1988; **W. L. Craig**, *Assessing the New Testament Evidence for the History of the Resurrection of Jesus*, Lewiston, NY 1989.

19. Cf. **M. Hengel**, '"Setze dich zu meiner Rechten!" Die Inthronisation Christi zur Rechten Gottes und Ps 110,1', in M. Philonenko (ed.), *Le Trône de Dieu*, Tübingen 1994, 108–94.

20. Ibid., 191.

21. Cf. Isa.53.

22. For **New Testament ethics** cf. **K. H. Schelkle**, *Theologie des Neuen Testaments III, Ethos*, Düsseldorf 1970; **D. Wendland**, *Ethik des Neuen Testaments. Eine Einführung*, Göttingen 1970; **J. T. Sanders**, *Ethics in the New Testament. Change and Development*, Philadelphia and London 1975; **J.F.Collange**, *De Jésus à Paul. L'éthique du Nouveau Testament*, Geneva 1980; **B.Gerhardsson**, *The Ethos of the Bible*, Philadelphia 1981; **W. Schrage**, *The Ethics of the New Testament*, Edinburgh 1988; **R.F.Collins**, *Christian Morality. Biblical Foundations*, Notre Dame 1986; **R.Schnackenburg**, *Die sittliche Botschaft des Neuen Testaments* (2 vols.), Freiburg 1968; **S.Schulz**, *Neutestamentliche Ethik*, Zurich 1987; **E.Lohse**, *Theologische Ethik des Neuen Testaments*, Stuttgart 1988; **W.Marxsen**, *'Christliche' und christliche Ethik im Neuen Testament*, Gütersloh 1989; **H. Merklein** (ed.), *Neues Testament und Ethik*, Freiburg 1989; **H. Schürmann**, *Studien zur neutestamentlichen Ethik*, ed T. Söding, Stuttgart 1990.

23. Cf. Col.3.28–4.1.

24. Phil. 4.8.

25. Catalogue of virtues, Gal.5.22f.; catalogue of vices, Rom.1.29–31; I Cor.6.9f.; II Cor.12.20f.; Gal.5.19–21.

26. For what follows see **E. Käsemann**, *Commentary on Romans*, Grand Rapids and London [2]1982.

27. For the biblical **understanding of the Spirit**, in addition to the relevant lexicon articles (especially **E. Schweizer** in the *Theological Dictionary of the New Testament*) and sections in the New Testament theologies (especially **R.Bultmann**) see the following more recent works: **I. Hermann**, *Kyrios und Pneuma*, Munich 1961; **J. D. G. Dunn**, *Jesus and the Spirit. A Study of the Religious and Charismatic Experience of Jesus and the First Christians as Reflected in the New Testament*, London 1975; **B.Lindars** and **S. S. Smalley** (ed.), *Christ and Spirit in the New Testament*, Cambridge 1973; **M. E. Isaacs**, *The Concept of Spirit. A Study of Pneuma in Hellenistic Judaism and its Bearing on the New Testament*, London 1976; **E. Schweizer**, *Heiliger Geist*, Stuttgart 1978; **M.-A. Chevallier**, *Souffle de Dieu. Le Saint-Esprit dans le Nouveau Testament* (3 vols.), Paris 1978–91; **H.-J. Kraus**, *Heiliger Geist. Gottes befreiende Gegenwart*, Munich 1986. In addition there are numerous studies of the Holy Spirit in Paul and John. Systematic monographs on the Holy Spirit have been written by **H.U.von Balthasar, H. Berkhof, L. Bouyer, J.Comblin, Y.Congar, M.Dupny, F.X.Durwell, P.Evdokimov, B.J.Hilberath, J. Moltmann, H. Mühlen, C. Schütz, H. Thielicke, E.Timiadis** and **M. Welker**. For the questions in dispute between the Christian churches see the thematic volume of *Concilium* 128, 1979, edited by **J. Moltmann** and **H. Küng**, *Conflicts about the Holy Spirit*.

28. I Cor.15.45.

29. II Cor.3.17.

30. Phil.1.19; cf. Rom.8.9; Gal.4.6; II Cor.3.18.

31. Cf. Gen.1.2.
32. John 3.8.
33. John 16.13.
34. Cf. I Cor 12.28. On the **prophets after Christ** cf. **G.Dautzenberg**, *Urchristliche Prophetie. Ihre Erforschung, ihre Voraussetzungen im Judentum und ihre Struktur im ersten Korintherbrief*, Stuttgart 1975; **U.B.Müller**, *Prophetie und Predigt im Neuen Testament. Formgeschichtliche Untersuchungen zur urchristlichen Prophetie*, Gütersloh 1975; **P. S.Minear**, *To Heal and to Reveal. The Prophetic Vocation according to Luke*, New York 1976; **J.Panagopoulos** (ed.), *Prophetic Vocation in the New Testament and Today*, Leiden 1977; **E.E.Ellis**, *Prophecy and Hermeneutic in Early Christianity. New Testament Essays*, Tübingen 1978; **D.E.Aune**, *Prophecy in Early Christianity and the Ancient Mediterranean World*, Grand Rapids 1983; **W.A.Grudem**, *The Gift of Prophecy in the New Testament and Today*, Westchester, Ill. 1988; **A. Clark Wire**, *The Corinthian Women Prophets. A Reconstruction through Paul's Rhetoric*, Minneapolis 1990; **M. E. Boring**, *The Continuing Voice of Jesus. Christian Prophecy and the Gospel Tradition*, Louisville 1991.
35. Cf. Eph.2.20.
36. Cf. **H. Küng**, CWR, A I, 'Muhammad and the Qur'an: Prophecy and Revelation'.
37. Cf. **K.Jaspers**, *Die massgebenden Menschen*, Munich [4]1961.
38. Cf. **H. Küng**, CWR, A IV, 'Islam and the Other Religions. Jesus in the Qur'an'.
39. I Cor.2.2.
40. Cf. John 14.6.
41. Cf. John 6.35,48,51.
42. Cf. John 8.12.
43. Cf. John 10.7.
44. Cf. John 15.1,5.
45. Cf. John 10.11.
46. Cf. **E. Käsemann**, 'Liturgische Formeln im NT', in *RGG*[3] II, 993–6; **G. Bornkamm**, 'Formen und Gattungen im NT', in ibid., 999–1005. For the creeds see **O. Cullmann**, *The Earliest Christian Confessions*, London 1949; **K. H. Schelkle**, *Die Passion Jesu in der Verkündigung des Neuen Testaments*, Heidelberg 1949, 247–75; **J. N. D. Kelly**, *Early Christian Creeds*, London [3]1982.
47. Of the earliest and best known, I Cor.12.3.
48. E.g. I Cor.8.6.
49. E.g. I Cor 15.3–5; Rom.1.3f.
50. Cf. Matt.28.19; II Cor.13.13.
51. Cf. I Peter 3.18–20; cf. **H. Küng**, OBC, C V 1, 'Legends?'.
52. Cf. **id.**, *Credo*.
53. For the whole problem cf. **id.**, *Infallible?*, 118ff.
54. Cf. Mark 1.16–20; Matt.4.18–22.
55. Cf. Matt.7.21.
56. Cf. **J. Gründel** and **H.van Oyen**, *Ethik ohne Normen? Zu den Weisungen des Evangeliums*, Freiburg 1970; **A.Auer**, *Autonome Moral und christlicher Glaube*, Düsseldorf 1971; **D.Mieth**, 'Die Situationsanalyse aus theologischer Sicht', in *Moral*, ed. A.Hertz, Mainz 1972, 13–33; **W. Korff**, *Norm und Sittlichkeit. Untersuchungen zur Logik der normativen Vernunft*, Mainz 1973;

B.Schüller, *Die Begründung sittlicher Urteile. Typen ethischer Argumentation in der katholischen Moraltheologie,* Düsseldorf 1973; **F.Böckle,** *Fundamental-moral,* Munich 1977. For a survey of the more recent exegetical and ethical discussion cf. **R. Dillmann,** *Das Eigentliche der Ethik Jesu. Ein exegetischer Beitrag zur moraltheologischen Diskussion um das Proprium einer christlichen Ethik,* Mainz 1984.

57. For **discipleship of Jesus,** in addition to the exegetical literature see **D. Bonhoeffer,** *The Cost of Discipleship,* London and New York 1959; **K. Barth,** *Church Dogmatics* IV.2, Edinburgh 1958, §66.3; **E.Larsson,** *Christus als Vorbild,* Uppsala 1962; **A.Schulz,** *Nachfolgen und Nachahmen,* Munich 1962; **G. Bouwmann,** *Folgen und Nachfolgen im Zeugnis der Bibel,* Salzburg 1965; **H. D. Betz,** *Nachfolge und Nachahmung Jesu Christi im Neuen Testament,* Tübingen 1967; **M. Hengel,** *Nachfolge und Charisma,* Berlin 1968; **H. Merklein,** *Die Gottesherrschaft als Handlungsprinzip. Untersuchung zur Ethik Jesu,* Würzburg 1978.

58. Cf. **H. Küng,** OBC, C II.1, 'The changed awareness'.

59. **M. K. Gandhi,** cited in M. M. Thomas, *The Acknowledged Christ of the Indian Renaissance,* London 1969, 198.

60. For the **Sermon on the Mount,** in addition to the Jesus books mentioned, the New Testament theologies and commentaries on Matt.5.7, see the following more recent monographs: **W.D.Davies,** *The Setting of the Sermon on the Mount,* Cambridge 1964; **id.,** *The Sermon on the Mount,* Cambridge 1966; **G. Eichholz,** *Auslegung der Bergpredigt,* Neukirchen 1965; **H.-T Wrege,** *Die Überlieferungs-geschichte der Bergpredigt,* Tübingen 1968; **P. Pokorný,** *Der Kern der Bergpredigt. Eine Auslegung,* Hamburg 1969; **G.Miegge,** *Il Sermono sul monte. Commentario esegetico,* Turin 1970; **E. Schweizer,** *Die Bergpredigt,* Göttingen 1982; **H.Hendrickx,** *The Sermon on the Mount,* London 1984; **G.Strecker,** *Die Bergpredigt. Ein exegetischer Kommentar,* Göttingen 1984; **C.Bauman,** *The Sermon on the Mount. The Modern Quest for Its Meaning,* Macon, Ga 1985; **H. D. Betz,** *Studien zur Bergpredigt,* Tübingen 1985; **T.L.Donaldson,** *Jesus on the Mountain. A Study in Matthean Theology,* Sheffield 1985; **A. Kodjak,** *A Structural Analysis of the Sermon on the Mount,* Berlin 1986; **G. Lohfink,** *Wem gilt die Bergpredigt? Beiträge zu einer christlichen Ethik,* Freiburg 1988.

61. Cf. **H. Küng,** *Judaism,* 2 B II 3, 'A pious Pharisee?'.

62. Cf. Matt.5.18f.

63. Cf. **W. Trilling,** *Das wahre Israel. Studien zur Theologie des Matthäus-Evangelium,* Munich 1964, Ch. 9, 'Die Gesetzfrage nach Matt.5,17–20'.

64. Cf. Matt.5.39–41.

65. Cf. Luke 6.43f.; Matt.7.16,18.

66. Cf. **H. Küng,** *Judaism,* 2 B VII, 'Jewish Self-Criticism in the Light of the Sermon on the Mount?'.

67. Cf. Matt.5.41.

68. Cf. Matt.5.40.

69. Cf. Matt.5.39.

70. Cf, Ex.20.2–17; Deut 5.6–21.

71. Cf. Matt.5.20.

72. Cf. Rom.13.8–10.

73. **T. S. Kuhn,** *The Structure of Scientific Revolutions,* Chicago [2]1970, 175.

74. Cf. **H. Küng,** TTM, B II–IV C 1; **id.,** GR, Part C.

75. **S. Kierkegaard,** *Training in Christianity* (1850), London 1941, 39.

C. HISTORY

I. The Jewish Apocalyptic Paradigm of Earliest Christianity

1. **J. Le Goff, R. Chartier** and **J. Revel** (eds.), *La nouvelle histoire*, Paris 1978 (page references are to the German translation, *Die Rückeroberung der historischen Denkens*, Frankfurt 1990), here Le Goff, 28.

2. The Cambridge historian **P. Burke**, *The French Historical Revolution. The Annales School, 1929–89*, Cambridge 1990, gives sympathetic and critical information about the historiography of Marc Bloch and Lucien Febvre, then Fernand Braudels, and finally the 'third generation'.

3. Marc Bloch was imprisoned by the Gestapo and killed as a member of the Resistance in 1944.

4. Cf. **Le Goff**, *Die Rückeroberung* (n.1), 8.

5. Cf. ibid., 37, cf. 18.

6. Cf. **M. Weber**, *The Protestant Ethic and the Spirit of Capitalism*, London 1930. Cf. the conversation with Le Goff in *Die Zeit*, 12 April 1991.

7. Cf. **H. Jedin** and **J. Dolan** (eds.), *History of the Church* (10 vols.), London and New York 1980–81.

8. Cf. **A. Fliche** and **V. Martin**, *Histoire de L'Église. Depuis les origines jusqu'à nos jours* (12 vols.), Paris 1934–52.

9. Cf. **M. Mollat du Jourdin** and **A. Vauchez**, *Histoire du christianisme des origines à nos jours*, Paris 1990.

10. Cf. **H. Gülzow** and **H. Lehmann**, *Christentum und Gesellschaft*, Stuttgart 1980ff.; of the fourteen volumes planned, so far four have appeared.

11. The thematic volume of *Theologische Quartalschrift* 173, 1993, 4, edited by **J. Köhler**, *Theoriedefizite der Kirchengeschichte?*, with illuminating articles by **U. Altermatt, A. Holzem, A. Angenendt** and **G. de Rosa**, is symptomatic of the change which has also taken place in Catholic church historiography.

12. Fundamental historical categories like events, cycles, epochs, structures and times have been investigated by **K. Pomian**, *L'ordre du temps*, Paris 1984.

13. Cf. **Le Goff**, *Die Rückeroberung* (n.1), 39.

14. Ibid., 9.

15. Cf. **id.**, *History and Memory* (1977), New York 1993, Ch.I.

16. For the sociology of the **earliest community** cf. **M. Weber**, *Ancient Judaism*, Glencoe, Ill. 1952, especially the appendix, 'The Pharisees', and above all **G. Theissen**, *Studien zur Soziologie des Urchristentums*, Tübingen ³1989, especially Part II, 'Evangelien'. However, the picture of Jesus the 'itinerant preacher' may not have been developed by just one strand of tradition (essentially the logia source Q). For the further social and political context cf. **E. Stambaugh** and **D. L. Balch**, *The New Testament and Its Social Environment*, Philadelphia 1986. For the origin of the church cf. **H. Küng**, *Church*, B, 'The Coming Reign of God' (and the bibliography). Further theological works on the earliest community are: **P. V. Dias**, *Vielfalt der Kirche in der Vielfalt der Jünger, Zeugen und Diener*, Freiburg 1968; **id.**, *Kirche. In der Schrift und im 2.Jahrhundert*, Freiburg 1974; **G. Hasenhüttl**, *Charisma. Ordnungsprinzip der Kirche*, Freiburg 1969; **J. Becker et al.**, *Die Anfänge des Christentums. Alte Welt und neue Hoffnung*, Stuttgart 1987 (especially the contributions by **J. Becker, C. Colpe** and **K.**

Löning); **M. Hengel**, *The 'Hellenization' of Judaea in the First Century after Christ*, London and Philadelphia 1989; **L. Schenke**, *Die Urgemeinde. Geschichtliche und theologische Entwicklungen*, Stuttgart 1990; **J. Roloff**, *Die Kirche im Neuen Testament*, Göttingen 1993.

17. Cf. Acts 4.32; cf. 4.34f.; 2.44f.
18. Cf. Matt.5.3; Luke 6.20.
19. **B. Brecht**, *The Threepenny Opera*, London 1979, Act II, scene 6, pp.55f.
20. Cf. Matt.6.33.
21. Cf. Gal.2.10; Rom.15.26. Cf. **L. E. Keck**, 'The Poor among the Saints in Jewish Christianity and Qumran', *Zeitschrift für Neutestamentliche Wissenschaft* 57, 1966, 54–78. Whether as socially uprooted 'primitive Christian itinerant charismatics' rather than 'intentional missionaries' they were virtual 'outsiders' and 'confusingly similar to other dubious vagabonds' supported by 'local sympathizers', as **Theissen**, *Studien*, esp. 100f., presupposes, seems to me to be doubtful on the basis of the sources.
22. Cf. Acts 4.36f.; 5.1–11. If the gate from New Testament times excavated by **B. Pixner**, is the one called 'Gate of the Essenes' in Josephus and the local tradition going back to the first and second centuries of the first meeting place of Christians on Mount Zion (a Jewish-Christian synagogue?) is right, then Essenes and earliest Christians lived as it were side by side. Cf. B.Pixner, *Wege des Messias und Stätten der Urkirche. Jesus und das Judenchristentum im Licht neuer archäologischer Erkenntnisse*, Giessen 1991; **R. Riesner**, 'Das Jerusalemer Essenerviertel und die Urgemeinde', in the forthcoming Vol.II,26,2 of the handbook *Aufstieg und Niedergang der römischen Welt (ANRW)*.
23. Cf. Luke 5.11. Cf. **H. Braun**, *Jesus. Der Mann aus Nazareth und seine Zeit*, Stuttgart 1969, 104–13; **M. Hengel**, *Property and Riches in the Early Church*, London and Philadelphia 1974, Chapter 3, 'The Preaching of Jesus'.
24. Acts 4.32; cf. 4.34f.; 2.44f.
25. Cf. Acts 6.1–6.
26. Thus, carefully, on the sharing of possessions, **L. Schenke**, *Die Urgemeinde* (n.16), 90–4.
27. Cf. **H. Küng**, *Judaism*, I C III 8, 'The apocalyptists – warning and interpreting the time'; there are references there to works on apocalyptic by **O. Plöger, C. Rowland, D. Hellholm, G. W. E. Nickelsburg** and **M. E. Stone, J. J. Collins, M. Goodman**, and **P. D. Hanson**.
28. Cf. **H. Küng**, OBC, C II 1, 'Apocalyptic horizon'. There is a good survey of recent research in **K. J. Kuschel**, *Born Before all Time? The Dispute over Christ's Origin*, London and New York 1992, 217–21.
29. Cf. above B II 2, 'The central figure'.
30. Cf. Mark 9.1 par.; 13.30 par.; Matt.10.23.
31. Cf. Mark 13.4–6, 32 par.; Luke 17.20f.
32. That has again been recalled by **E. Käsemann**, 'The Beginnings of Christian Theology', in *New Testament Questions of Today*, London and Philadelphia 1969, 82–107.
33. Cf. Mark 13.
34. For the most recent attempt at a historical-psychological reconstruction see **C. Colpe**, 'Die älteste judenchristliche Gemeinde', in Becker, *Die Anfänge* (n.16), 59–79, and **Schenke**, *Die Urgemeinde* (n.16), 11–23.
35. Cf. Acts 2.22–36.
36. Cf. Acts 2.

37. The British exegete **J. D. G. Dunn**, *The Parting of the Ways. Between Christianity and Judaism and their Significance for the Character of Christianity*, London 1991, shows considerable sensitivity to 'the enduring Jewish character of Christianity', and much sound exegetical knowledge. Cf. also **H. Küng**, *Judaism*, 2 B III 4, 'What Jews and Christians continue to have in common'.

38. Cf. Acts 15.1; Gal.5.2f.

39. Cf. Matt.24.20.

40. Cf. Col.2.16.

41. Cf.Gal.2.12f.; Acts 21.20–26.

42. Cf. Matt.5.23; Acts 2.46; 3.1.

43. Cf. the illuminating analysis of early Christian piety by **L. W. Hurtado**, *One God, One Lord. Early Christian Devotion and Ancient Jewish Monotheism*, Philadelphia and London 1988.

44. Cf. **H. Küng**, *Church* C III 1, 'Members through baptism' (with bibliography).

45. John 3.22 differs (Jesus baptized), corrected in 4.2 (not he, but the disciples!).

46. Mark 16.15 is part of the added chapter; the attestation in John 3.5 is uncertain; the conclusion of Matthew in its trinitarian form goes back to a community tradition or praxis.

47. Cf. Mark 1.9–11 par.

48. Cf. Mark 1.4; for confirmation by Jesus cf. Mark 11.27–33.

49. Especially I Cor.12.13; Rom.6.3; cf. Acts 9.18.

50. Cf. Acts 2.38; 8.16; 10.48.

51. Cf. I Cor.1.13–15; Gal.3.27; Rom.6.3. Cf. **L. Hartman**, *'Auf den Namen des Herrn Jesus'. Die Taufe in den neutestamentlichen Schriften*, Stuttgart 1992.

52. Matt.28.19.

53. Cf. **H. Küng**, *Church*, C III 2, 'United in the fellowship of the Lord's Supper' (and bibliography).

54. Cf. Acts 2.46.

55. Cf. I Cor.11.23–25; Mark 14.22–25; Matt.26.26–29; Luke 22.15–20.

56. Cf. I Cor.11.23–25. This is clearly attested of Paul for the very beginning of his missionary activity in Corinth in the 40s, where he refers to a tradition which according to him goes back to the Lord himself.

57. After the classic investigation by **J. Jeremias**, *The Eucharistic Words of Jesus*, London and Philadelphia [2]1966, cf. now **E. Mazza**, *L'anafora eucaristica. Studi sulle origini*, Rome 1992.

58. Cf. I Cor.11.20.

59. *'Eucharistia'* is first used in the Didache (9.10) and in Ignatius and Justin.

60. Cf. I Cor.16.22.

61. Cf. **H. Küng**, *Church* B III, 'The Eschatological Community of Salvation'; C, 'The Fundamental Structure of the Church' (and bibliography).

62. Cf. **E. and F. Stagg**, *Woman in the World of Jesus*, Philadelphia 1978; **E. Moltmann-Wendel**, *The Women around Jesus*, London and New York 1982; **F. Quéré**, *Les femmes de l'Évangile*, Paris 1982; **J. Blank**, 'Frauen in den Jesusüberlieferungen', in G.Dautzenberg, H.Merklein and K.Müller (eds.), *Die Frau im Urchristentum*, Freiburg 1983, 9–91 (the book also contains contributions on the mother of Jesus and on women as witnesses to Easter); **B. Witherington**, *Women in the Ministry of Jesus. A Study of Jesus' Attitudes to Women and their Roles as reflected in His Earthly Life*, Cambridge 1984.

63. Cf. I Cor.7. Cf. the contribution by **H. Merklein** in *Die Frau im Urchristentum* (n.62), Chapter VII.

64. **E. Schüssler Fiorenza**, *In Memory of Her. A Feminist Theological Reconstruction of Christian Origins*, London and New York 1983, 135f.

65. Ibid., 138. For the limits to the 'argument from silence' cf. the critical comments by S. **Heine**, 'Brille der Parteilichkeit. Zu einer feministischen Hermeneutik', *Evangelische Kommentare* 23, 1990, 354–7.

66. **Schüssler Fiorenza**, *In Memory of Her* (n.64), 186.

67. **Ead.**, 140.

68. **Ead.**, 121.

69. Luke 4.32.

70. Cf. Mark 3.16; John 1.42.

71. Cf. Mark 8.29; 9.5; 10.28; 11.21.

72. Cf. Mark 3.16; Matt.10.2; Luke 6.14; Acts 1.13.

73. Cf. Mark 8.27–33.

74. Cf. Luke 22.27,31f.

75. Cf. I Cor.15.5; Luke 24.34.

76. The classic Protestant account of the **question of Peter** is O. **Cullmann**, *Peter. Disciple, Apostle, Martyr*, London and Philadelphia 1953. For the **new Catholic consensus** on the question cf. first the pioneering works by **A. Vögtle**, 'Messiasbekenntnis und Petrusverheissung. Zur Komposition Matt. 16,13–23 par.' (1957/58), reprinted in *Das Evangelium und die Evangelien. Beiträge zur Evangelienforschung*, Düsseldorf 1971, 137–70, and **B. Rigaux**, 'St Peter in Contemporary Exegesis', *Concilium* 1967/7, 72–86. Then especially the works of **J. Blank**, 'The Person and Office of Peter in the New Testament', *Concilium* 1973/3, 42–55; **R. Pesch**, 'The Position and Significance of Peter in the Church of the New Testament', *Concilium* 1971/4, 21–35; **W. Trilling**, 'Zum Petrusamt im Neuen Testament. Traditionsgeschichtliche Überlegungen anhand von Matthäus, 1 Petrus und Johannes', *Theologische Quartalschrift* 151, 1971, 110–33. The agreement between these three Catholic authors is brought out by **H. Küng**, *Fehlbar?*, 405–14. There is also some confirmation in **R. E. Brown, K. O. Donfried** and **J. Reuman** (eds.), *Peter in the New Testament. A Collaborative Assessment by Protestant and Roman Catholic Scholars*, Minneapolis 1973. Cf. also **A. Brandenburg** and **H.-J. Urban** (eds.), *Petrus und Papst. Evangelium, Einheit der Kirche, Papstdienst* (2 vols.), Münster 1977f.; **L. Sartori** et al., *Il servizio di Pietro. Appunti per una riflessione interconfessionale*, Turin 1978; **T. V. Smith**, *Petrine Controversies in Early Christianity. Attitudes towards Peter in Christian Writings of the First Two Centuries*, Tübingen 1985; **S. Benko**, *Pagan Rome and the Early Christians*, Bloomington 1984; **C. P. Thiede** (ed.), *Das Petrusbild in der neueren Forschung*, Wuppertal 1987; **M. Maccarrone** (ed.), *Il primato del Vescovo di Roma nel primo millennio: ricerche e testimonianze*, Rome 1989; **C. C. Caragounis**, *Peter and the Rock*, Berlin 1990; **W. R. Farmer** and **R. Kereszty**, *Peter and Paul in the Church of Rome. The Ecumenical Potential of a Forgotten Perspective*, New York 1990; **A. J. Nau**, *Peter in Matthew. Discipleship, Diplomacy, and Dispraise, with an Assessment of Power and Privilege in the Petrine Office*, Collegeville, Minn. 1992. Cf. also **R. Pesch**, *Simon-Petrus. Geschichte und geschichtliche Bedeutung des ersten Jüngers Jesu Christi*, Stuttgart 1980.

77. Cf. Matt.16.17–19.

78. Cf. Matt.16.17–19; Luke 22.31f.; John 21.1–19.

79. Cf. Acts 1–12.
80. Cf. Gal.2.9.
81. Gal.2.8.
82. Gal.2.8.
83. Cf. Gal.2.11f.; Acts 15.7.
84. Cf. I Cor.1–12.
85. Thus the Catholic exegete **J. Blank**, 'Neutestamentliche Petrustypologie' (n.76), 177.
86. Cf. I Clement 5.4.
87. Cf. **Ignatius**, To the Romans 4.3.
88. 'Papal Primacy and the Universal Church', in **R. E. Brown** et al., *Peter* (n.76), 149–86: 156. The most recent investigation by **O. B. Knoch** comes to the conclusion that the Letter of Clement expresses the conviction of the Roman community 'of possessing a unique authority, as the place of the activity and above all the death of the leading apostles Peter and Paul, in the preservation of the apostolic heritage, but not as the owner of a legal and authoritative precedence over all the other communities', 'Im Namen des Petrus und Paulus: Der Brief des Klemens Romanus und die Eigenart des römischen Christentums', in *Aufstieg und Niedergang der römischen Welt (ANRW), Geschichte und Kultur Roms im Spiegel der neueren Forschung*, II, 27.1, ed. W.Haase, Berlin 1993, 3–54: 12. For the tomb of Peter cf. **E. Kirschbaum**, *Die Gräber der Apostelfürsten. St Peter und St Paul in Rom*, Frankfurt 1957, ³1974. The additional chapter by **E. Dassmann** is important here; in it the assertions of the Roman archaeologist M.Guarducci are 'reduced to the level of reflections' by the objections of E.Kirschbaum: 'Thus the controversy is so far unresolved and will probably remain so in the future . . .' (243, 245).
89. **P. Hoffmann**, *Das Erbe Jesu und die Macht in der Kirche. Rückbesinnung auf das Neue Testament*, Mainz 1991, 43f. Hoffmann refers to **M. N. Ebertz**, 'Die Bürokratisierung der katholischen "Priesterkirche"', in P.Hoffmann (ed.), *Priesterkirche*. Düsseldorf 1987, 132–63.
90. Cf. Mark 6.3 par.; Matt.13.55.
91. Cf. Acts 12.1–3; cf. also I Thess.2.14f.
92. Cf. Mark 3.20f.
93. Cf. Mark 6.1–3.
94. Cf. I Cor.15.7; Gal.1.19.
95. For **James**, among the most recent publications see above all **M. Hengel**, 'Jakobus der Herrenbruder – der erste "Papst"?', in *Glaube und Eschatologie. FS W.G.Kümmel*, Tübingen 1985, 71–104; **E. Ruckstuhl**, 'Jakobus', *TRE* XVI, 485–7. There is an extensive account by **W. Pratscher**, *Der Herrenbruder Jakobus und die Jakobustradition*, Göttingen 1987.
96. Cf. **Josephus**, *Antiquities*, XX, 9,1.
97. Cf. Acts 21.28; 24.6.
98. Hengel, 'Jakobus' (n.95), 74.
99. Cf. **H. Küng**, *Judaism*, 2 B IV 5, 'The excommunication of the Christians'.
100. Thus **K. Wengst**, *Bedrängte Gemeinde und verherrlichter Christus. Der historische Ort des Johannes-Evangeliums als Schlüssel zu seiner Interpretation*, Neukirchen 1981; cf. **G. Reim**, *Studien zum alttestamentlichen Hintergrund des Johannesevangeliums*, Cambridge 1974. Cf. the theory of **M. Hengel**, *The Johannine Question*, London and Philadelphia 1989, esp. Ch.IV, argued at

length, that the Johannine corpus is the work of a single outstanding theologian who is head of a school.

101. Cf. John 7.2–10.

102. Cf. **H. Küng**, *Judaism*, 2 B IV 5, 'The excommunication of the Christians'.

103. **Wengst**, *Bedrängte Gemeinde* (n.100), 58; cf. also **R. E. Brown**, *The Community of the Beloved Disciple. The Life, Loves and Hates of an Individual Church in New Testament Times*, New York 1979.

104. Cf. **C. Dietzfelbinger**, 'Der ungeliebte Bruder. Der Herrenbruder Jakobus im Johannesevangelium', *Zeitschrift für Theologie und Kirche* 89, 1992, 377–403.

105. Cf. John 9.22; 12.42; 16.2.

106. John 19.38; cf. 9.22; 12.42.

107. **Dietzfelbinger**, 'Der ungeliebte Bruder' (n.104), 399.

108. Cf. John 14.6.

109. John 5.18.

110. John 10.33.

111. John 1.14.

112. **M. Theobald**, *Die Fleischwerdung des Logos. Studien zum Verhältnis des Johannesprologs zum Corpus des Evangeliums und zu I Joh*, Münster 1988, 490.

113. Cf John 1.4.

114. For this development cf. **L. Abramowski**, 'Der Logos in der altchristlichen Theologie', in C. Colpe et al. (eds.), *Spätantike und Christentum. Beiträge zur Religions– und Geistesgeschichte der griechisch-römischen Kultur und Zivilisation der Kaiserzeit*, Berlin 1992, 189–201.

115. **L. Goppelt**, *Theology of the New Testament*, ed. J. Roloff, Grand Rapids 1983, II, 297.

116. **H. Conzelmann**, *Outline of the Theology of the New Testament*, London and New York 1969, 343f.

117. Cf. **K.-J. Kuschel**, *Born Before All Time? The Dispute over Christ's Origin*, London and New York 1992.

118. Cf. ibid., 388–92.

119. In his *The Gospel of John* I, London 1982, 555f., the Catholic exegete **Rudolf Schnackenburg** rightly comments: 'Johannine Christology is not modelled on a set pattern of mythological speculation about a Redeemer descending from heaven and returning there again. It is rather the desire to establish clearly the Christian revealer's power to save that leads to the emphasis on his preexistence, so that now his "way" is seen more clearly to begin "above" and to return there once more.'

120. **Kuschel**, *Born Before All Time?* (n.117), 389.

121. Cf. John 10.30,38.

122. Cf. **K. H. Schelkle**, *Theologie des Neuen Testaments* II, *Gott war in Christus*, Düsseldorf 1973, 215.

123. Cf. **J. Gnilka**, *Johannesevangelium*, Würzburg 1983, 86.

124. Cf. **F. Mussner**, 'Ursprünge und Entfaltung der neutestamentlichen Sohneschristologie', in L.Scheffczyk (ed.), *Grundfragen der Christologie heute*, Freiburg 1976, 77–113, esp. 110.

125. John 14.9.

126. Cf. **Kuschel**, *Born Before All Time?* (n.117), 388.

127. Ibid., 389.
128. Ibid.
129. Cf. I Cor.3.11.
130. Cf. Phil.2.21: 'They all look after their own interests and not those of Jesus Christ'. Cf. I Cor.7.32–34, 'the affairs of the Lord'.
131. Cf. **Kuschel**, *Born Before All Time?* (n.117), 243–307.
132. Cf. Phil.2.6–11.
133. Cf. **Kuschel**, *Born Before All Time?* (n.117), 306.
134. Cf. Gal.4.4.
135. **B. van Iersel**, ' "Son of God" in the New Testament', *Concilium* 153, 1982, 37–42. This is confirmed by the most recent and so far the most thorough exegetical study, **J. Habermann**, *Präexistenzaussagen im Neuen Testament*, Bern 1990, 422.
136. Cf. Acts 2.22–36.
137. The original text I John 5.7f. speaks of spirit, of water (= baptism) and of blood (= eucharist) which 'agree' or 'are one' (both sacraments witness to the power of the one spirit). For interpretation cf. **R. Bultmann**, *The Johannine Epistles*, Hermeneia, Philadelphia 1973, 80f.
138. Cf. **Denzinger**, *Enchiridion*, no.2198.
139. Acts 7.55f.
140. II Cor.13.13.
141. Cf. John 14.16.
142. **Eusebius**, *Church History* III,27,3.
143. Ibid. III,5,3a.
144. After **M. Joël** and then **E. Schwartz, S. G. F. Brandon** and **J. Munck**; with qualifications above all **G. Lüdemann**, *Opposition to Paul in Jewish Christianity*, Minneapolis 1989: 'The Succession to the Earliest Community in Jerusalem. Analysis of the Pella tradition'. Most recently, in his dissertation **J. Verheyden**, *De vlucht van de Christenen naar Pella. Onderzoek van het getuigenis van Eusebius en Epiphanius*, Brussels 1988, has sought to prove by redaction-critical methods that Eusebius (on whom Epiphanius is dependent) wrote the note about Pella himself for theological (anti-Jewish) reasons.
145. With reference to the Jewish-Christian Pseudo-Clementines (*Recognitions* 37,39) and Luke 21 and following the historians **E. Meyer** and **M. Simon**, who argue for historicity, **J. Wehnert**, 'Die Auswanderung der Jerusalemer Christen nach Pella – historisches Faktum oder theologische Konstruktion?', *Zeitschrift für Kirchengeschichte* 102, 1991, 231–55, has pulled Vermeylen's arguments to pieces, hermeneutically, historically and exegetically. Cf. **C. Koester**, 'The Origin and Significance of the Flight to Pella Tradition', *The Catholic Biblical Quarterly* 51, 90–106 (discussion above all of Lüdemann).
146. **Wehnert**, 'Auswanderung' (n.145), 252.
147. **Eusebius**, *Church History* IV,5,14. For the complex question of the relatives of Jesus cf. **R. Bauckham**, *Jude and the Relatives of Jesus in the Early Church*, Edinburgh 1990. For the letter of Jude cited here cf. **R. Heiligenthal**, *Zwischen Henoch und Paulus, Studien zum theologiegeschichtlichen Ort des Judasbriefes*, Tübingen 1962.
148. I was given valuable information by Professor **James Robinson**, the New Testament scholar, a leading expert on Gnosticism and Director of the Institute for Christianity and Antiquity in Claremont, California, during a guest semester at our Institute for Ecumenical Research.

149. The Festschrift for **J. Daniélou**, who at a very early stage wrote a *Theology of Jewish Christianity*, London 1964 (Vol.1 of his *History of Early Christian Doctrine Before the Council of Nicaea*), *Judéo-Christianisme, Recherches de science religieuse* 60, 1972, 1–323, already gives an impression of the intensive detailed work of the most important scholars in this sphere. **H. J. Schoeps**, *Theologie und Geschichte des Judenchristentums*, Tübingen 1949, is a basic work on the history of Jewish Christianity. **A. F. J. Klijn** and **G. J. Reinink**, *Patristic Evidence for Jewish-Christian Sects*, Leiden 1973, provide quite complete material for the individual Jewish Christian groups which appear in the patristic (non-Gnostic) sources (Cerinthians, Ebionites, Nazoraeans, Symmachians, Elkesaites). **Klijn** has also produced the first comprehensive study of the Jewish-Christian Gospel tradition (with text and commentaries), *The Jewish Christian Gospel Tradition*, Leiden 1992. Cf. also **R. A. Pritz**, *Nazarene Jewish Christianity. From the End of the New Testament Period Until its Disappearance in the Fourth Century*, Jerusalem 1988. **G. Strecker**, 'Judenchristentum', *TRE* XVII, 310–25, reconstructs the historical development according to the most recent state of research; cf. **id.**, 'The Problem of Jewish Christianity', appendix I to W. Bauer, *Orthodoxy and Heresy in Earliest Christianity*, Philadelphia and London 1972, 241-85. **S.Légasse**, 'La polémique antipaulinienne dans le judéo-christianisme hétérodoxe', *Bulletin de Littérature Ecclésiastique* 90, 1989, 5–22, 85–100, reconstructs the individual Jewish-Christian doctrines from the perspective of anti-Paulinism. From an archaeological perspective cf. **B. Bagatti**, *Alle origini della chiesa* I, *Le comunità giudeo-cristiane*, Rome 1986 (Vol.II discusses the Gentile Christian communities). For the earlier literature see **F. Manns**, *Bibliographie du judéo-christianisme*, Jerusalem 1979. The material relating to both 'conservative' and 'liberal' Jewish Christianity is collected with didactic skill in **T. Carran**, *Forgetting the Root. The Emergence of Christianity from Judaism*, New York 1986.

150. However, the hypothesis of a Q community which is said to have heard nothing of Jesus' crucifixion seems to me to be more than improbable given the sensational event, the shortness of the distances and the numerous possibilities of communication. This is also true of the latest conjecture by **B. L. Mack**, *The Lost Gospel. The Book of Q and Christian Origins*, San Francisco and Shaftesbury 1993.

151. In addition to **Klijn**, cf. **W. R. Stegner**, *Narrative Theology in Early Jewish Christianity*, Louisville 1989.

152. Cf. **J. L. Martyn**, 'The Law-Observant Mission to Gentiles: The Background of Galatians', *Scottish Journal of Theology* 38, 1985, 307–24; **id.**, 'Paul and His Jewish-Christian Interpreters', *Union Seminary Quarterly Review* 42, 1988, 1–15.

153. Cf. Gal.1.6–9; 3.1–2,5; 4.17.

154. Cf. Gal.3.6–29.

155. Cf. **A. Acerbi**, *L'ascensione di Isaia: cristologia e profetismo in Siria nei primi decenni del II secolo*, Milan ²1989.

156. *Pseudo-Clementine Recognitions* 1,33–71. Cf. – after **H. Waitz**, **O. Cullmann** and **H.-J. Schoeps** – above all **G. Strecker**, *Das Judentum in den Pseudoklementinen*, Berlin 1957, ²1981.

157. This interpretation was worked out by **R. E. van Voorst**, *The Ascents of James: History and Theology of a Jewish-Christian Community*, Atlanta 1989, esp.163–80.

158. Cf. Jerome, *On Famous Men*, 3; cf. id., *In Jes.*40. 9–11. See also **Strecker**, 'Judenchristentum' (n.149), 312, 321.

159. This is referred to emphatically by **C. Colpe**, *Das Siegel der Propheten. Historische Beziehungen zwischen Judentum, Judenchristentum, Heidentum und frühem Islam*, Berlin 1990, 166f.

160. Cf. **Ignatius**, To the Magnesians 8–10.

161. Cf. **Irenaeus**, *Against the Heresies*, I,26,2; III,15,1; V,1,3.

162. Cf. **Justin**, *Dialogue with the Jew Trypho*, 48.3f.; 49.1.

163. **Epiphanius**, *Panarion* 29. There are also references in Jerome and Augustine.

164. Cf. **J. Hadot**, *La formation du dogme chrétien des origines à la fin du 4e siècle*, Charleroi 1990, 5f.

165. Cf. Mark 4.41; Luke 7.49; 8.25.

166. Cf. John 1.46.

167. **Strecker**, 'Judenchristentum', 323.

168. Cf. **Chrysostom**, *Sermons against the Jews*, Patrologia Graeca, Vol.48, 843–942.

169. I hope to go into this more closely in a later investigation. I found at least indirect confirmation in **F. Heyer**, *Die Kirche Äthiopiens*, Berlin 1971, 222f.; **E. Isaac**, *A New Text-Critical Introduction to Mashafa Berhan*, Leiden 1973 (from this important Ethiopian book the author infers two parties: Judaizing and Coptic-Monophysite Christianity).

170. Cf. **S. Weil**, 'Symmetry between Christians and Jews in India. The Cnanite Christians and the Cochin Jews of Kerala', in T. A. Timberg, *Jews in India*, New Delhi 1986, 182–94; **J. Kollaparambil**, *The Babylonian Origin of the Southists among the St Thomas Christians*, Rome 1992.

171. The Cologne Mani-Codex (inventory no.4780) was published in 1975/81 with a commentary by **A. Henrichs** and **L. Koenen**. There is now a standard edition by **L. Koenen** and **C. Roemer**, *Der Kölner Mani-Kodex. Abbildungen und diplomatischer Text*, Bonn 1985.

172. **A. Böhlig**, 'Preface', in **L. Cirillo** (ed.), *Codex Manichaicus Coloniensis. Atti del Simposio Internazionale 1984*, Cosenza 1986 (here the articles by J. Maier, K. Rudolph, G. Strecker, L. Cirillo, A. F. J. Klijn). For **Manichaeism** cf. above all **K. Rudolph**, *Gnosis*, Edinburgh 1984; **G. Widengren** (ed.), *Der Manichäismus*, Darmstadt 1977; **H. C. Puech**, *Sur le manichéisme et autres essais*, Paris 1979; **E. Rose**, *Die Manichäische Christologie*, Wiesbaden 1979.

173. Cf. **H. Küng**, CWR, A IV 2, 'Jesus as the servant of God'.

174. **A. Schlatter**, *Geschichte der ersten Christenheit*, Gütersloh 1926, 367f.

175. Cf. **A. von Harnack**, *Lehrbuch der Dogmengeschichte* II, Tübingen [4]1909, reprinted Darmstadt 1964, 529–38.

176. Cf. **Schoeps**, *Theologie* (n.149, taking up the work of C. Clement, T. Andrae and H. H. Schaeder), 342: 'Thus the fact that while Jewish Christianity disappeared in the Christian church, it conserved itself in Islam and that some of its impulses have lasted down to our day, proves to be a paradox of truly world-historical dimensions.'

177. **C. Buck**, Report to the American Academy of Religion, in *Abstracts AAR/SBL* 1983.

178. **Strecker**, 'Judenchristentum' (n.149), 323.

179. For this question cf. **C. Buck**, 'Exegetical Identification of the Sabi'un', *Muslim World* 73, 1982, 95–106; **G. Quispel**, 'The Birth of the Child. Some

Gnostic and Jewish Aspects', in *Jewish and Gnostic Man*, Eranos Lectures 3, Dallas 1986, 3–26. For the **Elkesaites** as Jewish Christian propagandists cf. – after **A. von Harnack** and the early monograph by **W. Brandt** (1912) – now **G. P. Luttikhuizen**, *The Revelation of Elchasai. Investigations into the Evidence for a Mesopotamian Jewish Christian Apocalypse of the Second Century and its Reception by Judeo-Christian Propagandists*, Tübingen 1985 (an apocalyptic book of revelation by a Mesopotamian Jew of the second century, originally written in Aramaic, was used a century later by Syrian Jewish Christians for religious propaganda in Christian churches in Palestine and Rome).

180. Cf. **J. Wellhausen**, *Reste arabischen Heidentums*, Berlin ²1927, 231–3.

181. Cf. **Colpe**, *Das Siegel der Propheten* (n.159), 237f.

182. Surah 33.40.

183. Cf. **Tertullian**, *Adversus Judaeos* VII, 12. The right reading is that of C. Colpe, *Signaculum omnium prophetarum*, not *prophetiarum* (prophesyings), as E. Kroymann conjectures (in *Corpus Scriptorum Ecclesiasticorum Latinorum*, Vol.70, and in *Corpus Christianorum*, Series Latina Vol.II.2, 1361 – in contradiction to p.1383, *prophetarum*).

184. **Colpe**, *Das Siegel der Propheten* (n.159), 28–34.

185. Ibid., 238.

186. Ibid., 169f.

187. Cf. **S.Pines**, 'The Jewish Christians of the Early Centuries of Christianity According to a New Source', *Proceedings of the Israel Academy of Sciences and Humanities* 2, 1968, 237–309. It was also Pines who drew Colpe's attention to the Sozomen text.

188. Cf. also **Colpe**, *Das Siegel der Propheten* (n.159), 171f.

189. **C. Schedl**, *Muhammad und Jesus*, Freiburg 1978, 565f.

190. Cf. **H. Küng**, CWR, A I 2, 'Muhammad: a Prophet? The Qur'an – God's Word?'

191. **Schlatter**, *Geschichte der ersten Christenheit* (n.174), 367f.

192. Cf. Rom.1.3–4; Acts 2.36; Phil.2.9–10; I Tim.3.16; I Peter 3.21; John 3.14. The Franciscan **E.Testa**, *The Faith of the Mother Church. An Essay on the Theology of the Judeo-Christians*, Jerusalem 1992, makes some interesting remarks about Jewish Christianity, but the detailed evidence is all too weak. Cf. e.g. on the Trinity: 'The Judeo-Christians believed in a Trinity of a subordinationist type: in only the Father as God most high, in the Son as an Angel, but as a divine being, in the Spirit/Ruah as an Angel/Mother' (225).

II. The Ecumenical Hellenistic Paradigm of Christian Antiquity

1. **T. S. Kuhn**, *The Structure of Scientific Revolutions*, Chicago ²1970, 175.

2. For a discussion of the use of the term 'paradigm' with reference to theology see **H. Küng** and **D. Tracy** (eds.), *Paradigm Change in Theology*, Edinburgh 1989.

3. For Antioch cf. **J. P. Meier** and **R. Brown**, *Antioch and Rome. New Testament Cradles and Catholic Christianity*, New York 1983; **J. E. Stambaugh** and **D. L. Balch**, *The New Testament in its Social Environment*, Philadelphia 1986.

4. Cf. Acts 11.19–26.

5. Acts 11.26.
6. Cf. **G. Theissen**, *Studien zur Soziologie des Urchristentums*, Tübingen [3]1989, 100f.
7. Cf. Gal.2.11–21.
8. Cf. **H. Küng**, *Judaism*, 2 B V 1 2, 'The controversial Paul', 'The sympathetic transformation'. For research on Paul cf. the early important articles by **R. Bultmann, K. Holl, H. Lietzmann, A. Oepke, R. Reitzenstein, A. Schlatter** and **A. Schweitzer**, collected by **K. H. Rengstorf**, *Das Paulusbild in der neueren deutschen Forschung*, Darmstadt 1965. For orientation on the state of research, which is almost impossible to keep up with, cf. the research reports by **H. Hübner**, 'Paulusforschung seit 1945. Ein kritischer Literaturbericht', in *Aufstieg und Niedergang der Römischen Welt. Geschichte und Kultur Roms im Spiegel der neueren Forschung*, ed. **W. Haase** and **H. Temporini**, II,25,4, Berlin 1987, 2649–80 (which also contains extended contributions on the most recent state of interpretation of individual Pauline letters); **O. Merk**, 'Paulus-Forschung 1936–1985', *Theologische Rundschau* 53, 1988, 1–81. For an introduction to the person and work of the apostle Paul, in addition to the Introductions to the New Testament see among the more recent critical works especially **M. Dibelius**, *Paul*, London 1953; **P. Seidensticker**, *Paulus, der verfolgte Apostel Jesu Christi*, Stuttgart 1965; **G. Bornkamm**, *Paul*, London and New York 1969; **E. Käsemann**, *Perspectives on Paul*, London and Philadelphia 1971; **O. Kuss**, *Paulus. Die Rolle des Apostels in der theologischen Entwicklung der Urkirche*, Regensburg 1971; **K. Stendahl**, *Paul among Jews and Gentiles*, Philadelphia and London 1977; **F. F. Bruce**, *Paul. Apostle of the Free Spirit*, Exeter 1977; **E. P. Sanders**, *Paul and Palestinian Judaism*, London and Philadelphia 1977; id., *Paul, the Law and the Jewish People*, Philadelphia and London 1983; id., *Paul*, Oxford 1991; **J. C. Beker**, *Paul the Apostle. The Triumph of God in Life and Thought*, Edinburgh and London 1980; **K. H. Schelkle**, *Paulus. Leben – Briefe – Theologie*, Darmstadt 1981; **G. Lüdemann**, *Paul Apostle to the Gentiles*, Philadelphia and London 1984; id., *Opposition to Paul in Jewish Christianity*, Minneapolis 1989; **W. A. Meeks**, *The First Urban Christians. The Social World of the Apostle Paul*, New Haven 1983; **H. Räisänen**, *Paul and the Law*, Tübingen 1983; **G. Theissen**, *Psychological Aspects of Pauline Theology*, Edinburgh 1987; **F. Watson**, *Paul, Judaism and the Gentiles. A Sociological Approach*, Cambridge 1986; **J. Becker**, *Paulus. Der Apostel der Völker*, Tübingen 1989; **E. Biser**, *Paulus. Zeuge, Mystiker, Vordenker*, Munich 1992; **P.-G. Klumbies**, *Die Rede von Gott bei Paulus in ihrem zeitgeschichtlichen Kontext*, Göttingen 1992.
9. Cf. **A. F. Segal**, *Paul the Convert. The Apostolate and Apostasy of Saul the Pharisee*, New Haven 1990. For **Paul from the Jewish side and in Jewish-Christian dialogue** cf. also among more recent literature **S. Sandmel**, *The Genius of Paul. A Study in History*, New York 1958; **H. J. Schoeps**, *Paul: The Theology of the Apostle in the Light of Jewish Religious History*, London 1961; **S. Ben-Chorin**, *Paulus. Der Völkerapostel in jüdischer Sicht*, Munich 1970; **M. Barth** et al., *Paulus – Apostat oder Apostel? Jüdische und christliche Antworten*, Regensburg 1977; **F. Mussner**, *Traktat über die Juden*, Munich 1979; **P. Lapide** and **P. Stuhlmacher**, *Paulus – Rabbi und Apostel. Ein jüdisch-christlicher Dialog*, Stuttgart 1981; **P. von der Osten-Sacken**, *Grundzüge einer Theologie im christlich-jüdischen Gespräch*, Munich 1982; id., *Evangelium und Tora. Aufsätze zu Paulus*, Munich 1987; **F. W. Marquardt**, *Die Gegenwart des Auferstandenen bei seinem Volk Israel. Ein dogmatisches Experiment*, Munich

1983; **E. Biser** et al., *Paulus – Wegbereiter des Christentums. Zur Aktualität des Völkerapostels in ökumenischer Sicht*, Munich 1984; **L. Swidler** et al., *Bursting the Bonds? A Jewish-Christian Dialogue on Jesus and Paul*, New York 1990.

10. Cf. I Cor.9.19–23; I Cor.8; Rom.14.

11. Cf. the study by **W. Thüsing**, Per Christum in Deum. *Studien zum Verhältnis von Christozentrik und Theozentrik in den paulinischen Hauptbriefen*, Münster 1965.

12. As is generally recognized by exegetes, the legitimation of the Gentile Christian communities which do not observe the Law is the sociological background to Paul's criticism of the Law.

13. Thus unfortunately also **E. L. Ehrlich** in his review of my *Judaism*, in *Die Weltwoche*, 13 February 1992. For the debate see **H. Häring** and **K.-J. Kuschel** (eds.), *Hans Küng. Neue Horizonte des Glaubens und Denkens. Ein Arbeitsbuch*, Ch. V, 'Dialog mit dem Judentum', Munich 1993 (only a very abbreviated version of this chapter appears in the English edition, *Hans Küng: New Horizons of Faith and Thought*, London and New York 1993).

14. Cf. **E. Käsemann**, 'Ministry and Community in the New Testament', in *Essays on New Testament Themes*, London 1964, 63–92. For *charisms* see further **M. Hengel**, *Nachfolge und Charisma. Eine exegetisch-religionsgeschichtliche Studie zu Mt 8, 21f. und Jesu Ruf in die Nachfolge*, Vienna 1968; **G. Hasenhüttl**, *Charisma. Ordnungsprinzip der Kirche*, Freiburg 1969; **U. Brockhaus**, *Charisma und Amt. Die paulinischer Charismenlehre auf dem Hintergrund der frühchristlichen Gemeindefunktion*, Wuppertal 1972; **J. Hainz**, *Ekklesia – Strukturen paulinische Gemeinde-Theologie und Gemeinde-Ordnung*, Regensburg 1972.

15. The differences between Palestinian and Pauline community order had already been investigated systematically by **E. Schlink**, *Der kommende Christus und die kirchlichen Traditionen*, Göttingen 1961, 160–95. For a discussion with E. Käsemann, H. Diem, E. Schlink and K.-H. Schelkle, cf. **H. Küng**, *Structures* VI, 3–5.

16. Cf. I Cor.12.28, significantly not repeated in 12.29; cf. also Rom.12.8.

17. I have already given an account of these highly complex relationships and developments on the basis of exegetical research in *Church*, E II 2, 'The diaconal structure'.

18. Cf. Phil.1.1.

19. I Cor.1.5,7.

20. Cf. Acts 20.28; here there are several bishops.

21. Cf. Didache 13–15, esp. 14.1f.; 15.1f.

22. Cf. Acts 11.27; 13.1–3; 21.10f.

23. I Thess.5.12.

24. Cf. I Cor.16.15f.

25. Gal.3.27f. There is already a 90-page bibliography on the question of **women in the New Testament**, which has recently been much discussed (cf. also C I 4, 'The significance of women'): **I. M. Lindboe**, *Women in the New Testament. A Select Bibliography*, Oslo 1990. In addition to the work by **E. Schüssler Fiorenza**, *In Memory of Her*, New York and London 1983, often cited in Chapter C I, cf. above all **O. Bangerter**, *Frauen im Aufbruch. Die Geschichte einer Frauenbewegung in der alten Kirche. Ein Beitrag zur Frauenfrage*, Neukirchen 1971; **E. M. Tetlow**, *Women and Ministry in the New Testament*, New York

1980; **R. Rieplhuber**, *Die Stellung der Frau in den neutestamentlichen Schriften und im Koran*, Altenberge 1986; **B. Witherington**, *Women in the Earliest Churches*, Cambridge 1988; id., *Women and the Genesis of Christianity*, Cambridge 1990; **B. Bowman Thurston**, *The Widows. A Women's Ministry in the Early Church*, Minneapolis 1989; **N. Baumert**, *Antifeminismus bei Paulus? Einzelstudien*, Würzburg 1992; id., *Frau und Mann bei Paulus. Überwindung eines Missverständnisses*, Würzburg 1992; **C. S. Keener**, *Paul, Women and Wives. Marriage and Women's Ministry in the Letters of Paul*, Peabody, Mass. 1992.

26. Cf. Rom.16.1–16.

27. For the titles *diakonos* and *prostatis* cf. **Schüssler Fiorenza**, *In Memory of Her* (n.25), 170–2.

28. Cf. Rom.16.7.

29. **U. Wilckens**, *Der Brief an die Römer*, Vol.III, Zurich 1982, 135.

30. Cf. I Thess.5.12; Rom.16.6,12.

31. Phil.4.2f.

32. Cf. Rom.16.3; I Cor.16.19; Acts 18.1; 18.18f.; 18.26.

33. Cf. I Cor.16.19; II Tim.4.19.

34. I Cor.11.5.

35. Eph.2.20.

36. **Schüssler Fiorenza**, *In Memory of Her* (n.25), 183.

37. Cf. **M. Küchler**, *Schweigen, Schmuck und Schleier. Drei neutestamentlichen Vorschriften zur Verdrängung der Frauen auf dem Hintergrund einer frauenfeindlichen Exegese des Alten Testaments im antiken Judentum*, Fribourg 1986.

38. Cf. I Cor.11.3.

39. Cf. I Cor.14.34f.

40. I Tim.2.11f.

41. Cf.Rom.16.7. **B. Brooten**, ' "Junia . . . hervorragend unter den Aposteln" (Rom.16.7)', in **E. Moltmann-Wendel** (ed.), *Frauenbefreiung. Biblische und theologische Argumente*, Munich 1978, 148–51, has made a detailed investigation of this. **V. Fabrega**, 'War Junia(s), der hervorragende Apostel (Röm 16,7), eine Frau?', *Jahrbuch für Antike und Christentum* 27/28, 1984/5, 47–64. Of the more recent commentaries on Romans, that by **U. Wilckens** has been open to the arguments advanced here (135).

42. Cf. **R. Albrecht**, *Das Leben der heiligen Makrina auf dem Hintergrund der Thekla-Traditionen. Studien zu den Ursprüngen des weiblichen Mönchtums im vierten Jahrhundert in Kleinasien*, Göttingen 1986, Ch.5.

43. Cf. John 19.25–27.

44. Cf. Mark 16.9–11; John 20.11–18.

45. Cf. **E. Moltmann-Wendel**, *The Women around Jesus*, London and New York 1982, Ch.3, 'Mary Magdalene'.

46. Cf. e.g.Titus 1.5,7.

47. Cf. I Thess.5.19.

48. For the New Testament **prophets** cf. above B II 3. For the **teachers** cf. **U. Neymeyer**, *Die christlichen Lehrer im 2.Jahrhundert. Ihre Lehrtätigkeit, ihr Selbsverständnis und ihre Geschichte*, Leiden 1989. For the significance of prophets and teachers in the church of that time and today cf. **H. Küng**, *Church*, E II, 'The diaconal structure'.

49. Here **H.von Campenhausen**, *Ecclesiastical Office and Spiritual Authority*

in the First Three Centuries, London and Philadelphia 1969, is still the standard work.

50. For the Roman urban community cf. **S. Benko**, *Pagan Rome and the Early Christians*, Bloomington 1984; **P. Lampe**, *Die stadtrömischen Christen in den ersten beiden Jahrhunderten. Untersuchungen zur Sozialgeschichte*, Tübingen 1987, ²1989.

51. For **Ignatius** cf. **H. Paulsen**, 'Ignatius von Antiochien', in M. Greschat (ed.), *Gestalten der Kirchengeschichte* I, Stuttgart 1984, 38–50 (with references there to the earlier accounts by H. W. Bartsch, T. Baumeister, K. Bommes, P. Meinhold, H. Paulsen, H. Schlier and T. Zahn).

52. Cf. **M. Hengel**, 'Jakobus der Herrenbruder – der erste "Papst"?', in *Glaube und Eschatologie. FS W. G. Kümmel*, Tübingen 1985, 71–104: 103.

53. Cf. I Clement 5.4.

54. Cf. already Rom.1.8.

55. Cf. **Ignatius**, To the Romans, IV.3.

56. Cf. ibid., Introduction.

57. Cf. **Irenaeus**, *Against the Heresies*, III,3,2f.

58. **P. Hoffmann**, *Das Erbe Jesu und die Macht in der Kirche. Rückbesinnung auf das Neue Testament*, Mainz 1991, 64f.

59. For Christianity in the Hellenistic-Roman period cf. in addition to the general church histories and lexicon articles the following more recent monographs: **A.von Harnack**, *The Expansion of Christianity in the First Three Centuries* (2 vols.), London 1904–5; **R. Bultmann**, *Primitive Christianity in its Contemporary Setting*, London 1956; **F. C. Grant**, *Roman Hellenism and the New Testament*, Edinburgh 1962; **A. D. Nock**, *Early Gentile Christianity and its Hellenistic Background*, New York 1964; id., *Essays on Religion and the Ancient World*, ed. Z. Stewart (2 vols.), Oxford 1972; **A. Toynbee** (ed.), *The Crucible of Christianity. Judaism, Hellenism and the Historical Background to the Christian Faith*, London 1969; **M. Simon**, *La civilisation de l'antiquité et le Christianisme*, Paris 1972; **R. A. Markus**, *Christianity in the Roman World*, London 1974; **T. Christensen**, *Christus oder Jupiter. Der Kampf um die geistigen Grundlagen des Römischen Reiches*, Göttingen 1981 (Danish original 1970); **M. Sordi**, *I Cristiani e l'Impero Romano*, Milan 1983; **S. Benko**, *Pagan Rome and the Early Christians*, Bloomington 1984; **R. MacMullen**, *Christianizing the Roman Empire (AD 100–400)*, New Haven 1984; **R. H. Nash**, *Christianity and the Hellenistic World*, Grand Rapids 1984; **M. Whittaker**, *Jews and Christians. Graeco-Roman Views*, Cambridge 1984; **R. L. Wilken**, *The Christians as the Romans Saw Them*, New Haven 1984; **J. Herrin**, *The Formation of Christendom*, Princeton and London 1987; **E. G. Weltin**, *Athens and Jerusalem. An Interpretative Essay on Christianity and Classical Culture*, Atlanta 1987. For the pagan and Jewish sources for early Christianity see the collections of texts by **C. K. Barrett**, *The New Testament Background. Selected Documents*, London 1965; **J. Leipoldt** and **W. Grundmann** (eds.), *Umwelt des Urchristentums* (2 vols.), Berlin 1966/67 (Vol.I describes the New Testament period and Vol.II contains relevant texts); **H. C. Kee**, *The New Testament in Context. Sources and Documents*, Englewood Cliffs, New Jersey 1984. For the beginnings of Christian art cf. **P. du Bourguet**, *Early Christian Art*, Amsterdam 1971.

60. **E. Gibbon**, *The History of the Decline and Fall of the Roman Empire* I.1, new edition Harmondsworth 1982, p.27.

61. Cf. **Pliny**, *Letter* 96. The most important texts by pagans on Christians are collected by **W. Den Boer** (ed.), *Scriptorum paganorum I–IV saec. de Christianis testimonia*, Leiden 1965. Cf. further **L. Herrmann**, *Chrestos. Témoignages paiens et juifs sur le christianisme au premier siècle*, Brussels 1970; **F. F. Bruce**, *Jesus and Christian Origins outside the New Testament*, London 1974.

62. For the **persecutions** cf. **R. M. Grant**, *The Sword and the Cross*, New York 1955; **E. R. Dodds**, *Pagan and Christian in an Age of Anxiety. Some Aspects of Religious Experience from Marcus Aurelius to Constantine*, Cambridge 1965; **W. H. C. Frend**, *Martyrdom and Persecution in the Early Church*, Oxford 1965; **P. R. E. Coleman-Norton**, *Roman State and Christian Church. A Collection of Legal Documents to AD 535*, I, London 1966; **J. Moreau**, *La persécution du Christianisme dans l'Empire romain*, Paris 1956; **J. M. Robinson** and **H. Koester**, *Trajectories through Early Christianity*, Philadelphia 1971; **P. Keresztes**, *Imperial Rome and the Christians* (2 vols.), Lanham, Md 1989.

63. The reports on research, 'Christliche Antike', published by the Graz patristic scholar **J. B. Bauer**, as successor to H. Rahner, in the *Anzeiger für die Altertumswissenschaft* (Innsbruck) for the years 1960, 1965, 1970, 1975 and 1991, give an admirable insight into the overwhleming amount of research devoted to Christian literature, church and society (I can refer to individual articles in the framework of this paradigm analysis only by way of exception).

64. The '**Apostolic Fathers**' are taken to include the Letters of Ignatius, Polycarp and Barnabas, the Didache (the Teaching of the Apostles, a first church order) and the apocalypse of the Shepherd of Hermas.

65. For **Justin**, in addition to the classical histories of dogma (A. von Harnack, F. Loofs, R. Seeberg), the more recent ones (J. Pelikan, C. Andresen) and the patrologies (B. Altaner, J. Quasten), cf. **C. Andresen**, *Logos und Nomos. Die Polemik des Kelsos wider das Christentum*, Berlin 1955, Part IV; **H. von Campenhausen**, *The Fathers of the Greek Church*, London 1963; **A. von Harnack**, *Geschichte der altchristlichen Literatur bis Eusebius*, Leipzig [2]1958, Part I.1, 99–114; II.1, 274–84; **H. Chadwick**, *Early Christian Thought and the Classical Tradition. Studies in Justin, Clement and Origen*, Oxford 1966; id., *The Early Church*, Harmondsworth 1967, Ch.4, 'Justin and Irenaeus'; **E. F. Osborn**, *Justin Martyr*, Tübingen 1973; id., *The Beginning of Christian Philosophy*, Cambridge 1981; id., *The Emergence of Christian Theology*, Cambridge 1993. I am most grateful to Profesor Eric Osborn of the University of Melbourne for valuable suggestions on this section.

66. Cf. **Justin**, *Apology*, I,46.

67. Ibid.

68. John 1.1f.

69. Cf. **Justin**, *Apology*, II,13.

70. John 1.9.

71. John 1.14.

72. Cf. **Justin**, *Apology*, II,13.

73. The American patristic scholar **R. L. Wilken** has analysed the arguments of the opponents of Christianity in *The Christians as the Romans Saw Them*, New Haven 1984. The most important historical articles since 1892 on **Julian the Apostate** have been collected in **R. Klein** (ed.), *Julian Apostata*, Darmstadt 1967. For Julian's cultural profile cf. **P. Athanassiadi-Fowden**, *Julian and Hellenism. An Intellectual Biography*, Oxford 1981. For the contemporary pros

and cons cf. **S. N. C. Lieu** (ed.), *The Emperor Julian Panegyric and Polemic.*
Claudius Mamertinus, John Chrysostom, Ephrem the Syrian, Liverpool 1986.
   74. This has already been convincingly worked out for Luke-Acts by
Bultmann's pupil **H. Conzelmann**, *The Theology of St Luke,* London 1960.
   75. Another Bultmann pupil felt that he had to convert to the Catholic Church
on the basis of this New Testament evidence, cf. **H. Schlier**, *Die Zeit der Kirche.*
Exegetische Aufsätze und Vorträge, Freiburg 1955, [2]1958.
   76. For the discussion see **H. Küng**, *Changing Church,* D 1, 'Early Catholicism
in the New Testament as a Problem of Controversial Theology'. The whole
problem is worked through by **H.-J. Schmitz**, *Frühkatholizismus bei Adolf von*
Harnack, Rudolph Sohm und Ernst Käsemann, Düsseldorf 1977.
   77. The pioneer in research into Gnosticism in the nineteenth century was the
Tübingen church historian F. C. Baur (1835). Its importance for church history
and the history of dogma was demonstrated by A. von Harnack and A.
Hilgenfeld, and then through the History of Religions School by W. Bousset, R.
Reizenstein and R. Bultmann. Basic recent studies are: **H. Jonas**, *Gnosis und*
spätantiker Geist, I, *Die mythologische Gnosis,* Göttingen 1934, [3]1964; II.1,
Von der Mythologie zur mystischen Philosophie, Göttingen 1954, [2]1966. The
best and briefest overall account of the nature, teaching, history and influence of
Gnosticism is **K. Rudolph**, *Gnosis,* Edinburgh 1984. Cf. further **E. Peterson**,
Frühkirche, Judentum und Gnosis. Studien und Untersuchungen, Freiburg 1959,
Darmstadt 1982; **N. Brox**, *Offenbarung, Gnosis und gnostischer Mythos bei*
Irenäus von Lyon. Zur Characteristik der Systeme, Salzburg 1966; id., *Erleuch-*
tung und Wiedergeburt. Aktualität der Gnosis, Munich 1989; **A. Böhlig**,
Mysterion und Wahrheit. Gesammelte Beiträge zur spätantiken Religionsge-
schichte, Leiden 1968; id., *Gnosis und Synkretismus. Aufsätze zur spätantike*
Religionsgeschichte (2 vols.), Tübingen 1989; **W. Eltester** (ed.), *Christentum und*
Gnosis, Berlin 1969; **M. Krause** (ed.), *Essays on the Nag Hammadi Texts in*
Honour of Alexander Böhlig, Leiden 1962; **E. Pagels**, *The Johannine Gospel in*
Gnostic Exegesis. Heracleon's Commentary on John, Nashville 1973; **ead.**, *The*
Gnostic Paul. Gnostic Exegesis of the Pauline Letters, Philadelphia 1975; **ead.**,
The Gnostic Gospels, London and New York 1979; **K. W. Tröger** (ed.), *Gnosis*
und NT. Studien aus Religionswissenschaft und Theologie, Berlin 1973; id. (ed.),
Altes Testament – Frühjudentum – Gnosis. Neue Studien zu "Gnosis und Bibel",
Gütersloh 1980; id., *Das Christentum im zweiten Jahrhundert,* Berlin 1988; **K.**
Rudolph (ed.), *Gnosis und Gnostizismus,* Darmstadt 1975; **A. Orbe**, *Cristología*
gnóstica. Introducción a la soteriología de los siglos II y III (2 vols.), Madrid
1976; **B. Aland** (ed.), *Gnosis. FS Hans Jonas,* Göttingen 1978; **K. Koschorke**, *Die*
Polemik der Gnostiker gegen das kirchliche Christentum. Unter besonderer
Berücksichtigung der Nag-Hammadi-Traktate "Apokalypse des Petrus" (NHC
VII.3) und "Testimonium Veritatis" (NHC IX.3), Leiden 1978; **B. Layton** (ed.),
The Rediscovery of Gnosticism. Proceedings of the International Conference on
Gnosticism at Yale, New Haven, Connecticut, March 28–31, 1978 (2 vols.),
Leiden 1980f.; id., *The Gnostic Scriptures,* Garden City, NY and London 1987;
P. Perkins, *The Gnostic Dialogue. The Early Church and the Crisis of*
Gnosticism, New York 1980; **C. Colpe**, 'Gnosis II (Gnostizismus)', in *Reallex-*
ikon für Antike und Christentum I, Stuttgart 1981, 538–69; **A. J. M. Wedder-**
burn (ed.), *The New Testament and Gnosis. Essays in Honour of R. McL.*
Wilson, Edinburgh 1983; **K. Berger** and **R. McL. Wilson**, 'Gnosis und
Gnostizismus', *TRE* XIII, 519–50; **W. Schmithals**, *Neues Testament und Gnosis,*

Darmstadt 1984; **J. Taubes** (ed.), *Religionstheorie und Politische Theologie,* Vol.II, *Gnosis und Politik,* Paderborn 1984; **C. W. Hedrick** and **R. Hodgson Jr** (eds.), *Nag Hammadi, Gnosticism and Early Christianity,* Peabody, Mass. 1986; **G. Quispel,** 'Gnosticism from Its Origins to the Middle Ages', *EncRel* V, 566–74; **J. Dart,** *The Jesus of Heresy and History. The Discovery and Meaning of the Nag Hammadi Gnostic Library,* San Francisco 1988. I am grateful to my Tübingen colleague the Gnostic specialist **Alexander Böhlig,** Professor of the Languages and Cultures of the Christian East, for reading through this chapter and for numerous suggestions.

78. Cf. **Irenaeus,** *The Unmasking and Refutation of False Gnosis,* above all Books I and II (usually cited as *Adversus haereses = Against the Heresies*). In addition there were a few Gnostic manuscripts in Coptic in the eighteenth/ nineteenth century.

79. First credit for academic study of the texts goes to the directors of the Coptic Museum in Old Cairo, the specialists J. Doresse, G. Quispel and H.-C. Puech. In the last forty years specialists from every possible country have published around 400 books, articles and reviews on the Nag Hammadi texts. Cf. **D. M. Scholer,** *Nag Hammadi Bibliography 1948–1969,* Leiden 1971 (continued from 1971 in the journal *Novum Testamentum*). Thanks to the indefatigable work of the Director of the Institute for Antiquity and Christianity in Claremont, California, **J. M. Robinson,** there is an eleven-volume facsimile edition of the thirteen Nag Hammadi codices which appeared in Leiden between 1972 and 1974. A one-volume translation into English has also appeared under Robinson's editorship, *The Nag Hammadi Library in English,* Leiden 1977, ³1988; Robinson's introduction provides an account of the confusing story of the finding of the texts. Cf. also **Pagels,** *Gnostic Gospels* (n.77), xiii–xxxvi.

80. Cf. **K.-J. Kuschel,** *Born Before All Time? The Dispute over Christ's Origin,* London and New York 1992, 135–40 (on Bultmann's understanding of Gnosticism) and 245–51 (on the relationship between the New Testament and Gnosticism).

81. For **Manichaeism** see the most recent summary account by **A. Böhlig,** 'Manichäismus', *TRE* 22, 25–45. Cf. **id.,** 'Mani und Platon – ein Vergleich', in A. von Tangerloo and S. Giversen (eds.), *Manichaica selecta,* Leuven 1991, 19–34.

82. This has been worked out above all by **R. Bultmann** in his various works, especially *Primitive Christianity* (n.59). Cf. also the publications by **E. Pagels** mentioned in n.77.

83. **Koschorke,** *Die Polemik der Gnostiker* (n.77), 237.

84. Cf. **K. W. Tröger,** 'Einführung. Zum gegenwärtigen Stand der Gnosis– und Nag-Hammadi Forschung', in id. (ed.), *Altes Testament* (n.77), 29.

85. Thus **Pagels,** *Gnostic Gospels* (n.77), xxxv.

86. This is the description which a number of participants in the 1966 Messina congress on the 'Origins of Gnosticism' put forward as theses. Quoted in **Rudolph,** *Gnosis* (n.77), 57.

87. Cf. **Jonas,** *Gnosis* (n.77), esp. Part I, and **Bultmann,** *Primitive Christianity* (n.59).

88. This is especially emphasized by **Pagels,** *Gnostic Gospels* (n.77), Ch.V.

89. **K. Rudolph** has analysed the extremely complicated Gnostic christologies in the framework of the Gnostic doctrine of redemption and redeemer, *Gnosis* (n.77), 113–70.

90. Ibid., 151.

91. Ibid., 154.

92. 'The Second Doctrine of the Great Seth' (Nag Hammadi Codex VII, 2), in James M. Robinson (ed.), *The Nag Hammadi Library*, Leiden ²1984, 329–38. For the motif of laughter in the history of Christianity see also, with reference to Gnostic material, the brilliant study by my Tübingen colleague Karl-Joseph Kuschel, *Laughter*, London and New York 1994.

93. Rudolph, *Gnosis* (n.77), 170.

94. Irenaeus, *Against the Heresies* III,17,4.

95. Cf. H. Küng, *Incarnation*, Ch.V.4, 'Christ Sublated in Knowledge'.

96. For the role of women in the sphere of Gnosticism cf. A. Jensen, *Gottes selbstbewusste Töchter. Frauenemanzipation im frühen Christentum?*, Freiburg 1992, 367–71.

97. Pagels, *Gnostic Gospels* (n.77), 202. The positive and negative aspects of the feminine in the various Gnostic writings are clearly expressed in the most recent relevant publications: cf. J. Jacobsen Buckley, *Female Fault and Fulfilment in Gnosticism*, Philadelphia 1988; K. L. King (ed.), *Images of the Feminine in Gnosticism*, Philadelphia 1988.

98. For an explanation cf. H. Küng, *Credo*.

99. For a long time Acts, James, Hebrews, III John and II Peter (presumably the latest writing in the New Testament) were also disputed. The Acts of Paul and Thecla were not included.

100. Cf. Irenaeus, *Against the Heresies* III,4,1; cf. II,2f. (on the Roman church).

101. I Peter 12.5; cf. Rev.1.6.

102. Mark 12.17.

103. Cf. Rom.13.1–7.

104. P. Brown, 'Antiquité tardive', in P. Ariès and G. Duby, *Histoire de la vie privée*, I, Paris 1985, 225–99.

105. H. Chadwick, *The Early Church* (n.65), 69.

106. Cf. id., 'Humanität', *Reallexikon für Antike und Christentum*, Stuttgart 1993, XVI, 663–71, esp.707f. W. Wischmeyer, *Von Golgatha zum Ponte Molle. Studien zur Sozialgeschichte der Kirche im dritten Jahrhundert*, Göttingen 1992, offers an important supplementary account of the conformity between church and Roman society and the decisive significance of the urban upper class for the growth of the church.

107. Cf. W. Bauer, *Orthodoxy and Heresy in Earliest Christianity* (1934), Philadelphia and London 1972.

108. The fair historical monograph by A. von Harnack, *Marcion. Das Evangelium vom fremden Gott* (1920), is still a model today. It is published with an appendix in *Neue Studien zu Marcion*, Darmstadt ³1960. More recent monographs have been written by J. Knox, *Marcion and the New Testament. An Essay in the Early History of the Canon*, Chicago 1942; E. C. Blackman, *Marcion and his Influence*, London 1948. Cf. also the brief summary by K. Beyschlag, 'Marcion von Sinope', in *Gestalten der Kirchengeschichte*, Stuttgart 1984, 69–81.

109. These works by Perpetua, Proba, Egeria and Eudokia have now been collected in one volume with introductions and notes by P. Wilson-Kastner et al. (eds.), *A Lost Tradition. Women Writers of the Early Church*, Washington 1981.

110. K. Thraede, 'Frau', in *Reallexikon für Antike und Christentum* VIII, Stuttgart 1972, 197–269: 240f. For women in antiquity including early

Christianity cf. **G. Duby** and **M. Perrot** (eds.), *Storia delle donne in occidente* I (ed. P.Schmitt Pantel), Rome 1990 (which contains a fine survey of women in early Christianity by **M. Alexandre**).

111. At the Institute for Ecumenical Research of Tübingen University, under my direction and with advice from Dr **Elisabeth Moltmann-Wendel**, a research project was undertaken on 'Women and Christianity', generously supported by the Volkswagen Foundation. It consisted of two part-projects: 'Sexuality, Marriage and Alternatives to Marriage in the First Four Christian Centuries' (under Dr **Anne Jensen**), and 'Being a Christian Woman in Twentieth-Century Church and Society' (under Dr **Doris Kaufmann**). The results of the research are now available in two monographs: **D. Kaufmann**, *Frauen zwischen Aufbruch und Reaktion. Protestantische Frauenbewegung in der ersten Hälfte des 2.Jahrhunderts*, Munich 1977; **A. Jensen**, *Gottes selbstbewusste Töchter. Frauenemanzipation im frühen Christentum?*, Freiburg 1992.

112. **A. von Harnack**, *The Expansion of Christianity in the First Three Centuries*, London 1904–5, II, 217–39, and the work of his pupil, **L. Zscharnack**, *Der Dienst der Frau in den ersten Jahrhunderten der christlichen Kirche*, Göttingen 1902, are still basic studies of the role of women in early Christianity. In this connection reference should be made to the important works (detailed bibiographies are given in the bibliography by A. Jensen) on the ordination of women in the early church (**R. Gryson**) or the refusal of ordination (**I. Raming**), and to the 'collections of sources' now available in different languages about the role of women in early Christianity (**O. Bangerter, J. Beaucamp, M. Ibarra Benlloch, J. Laporte, C. Mazzucco, C. Militello, S. Tunc**) and above all the pioneer work of American feminists (**E. Castelli, E. Clark, R. Kraemer, J. A. McNamara, R. Radford Ruether**).

113. Cf. **Jensen**, *Gottes selbstbewusste Töchter* (n.111), Ch.I, 'Frauen in den Kirchengeschichten: Die Entwicklung zur Männerkirche'.

114. Cf. ibid., Ch.II, 'Frauen im Martyrium: Mutige Bekennerinnen'.

115. Cf. ibid., Ch.III, 'Frauen in der Verkündigung: Charismatische Prophetinnen'.

116. Cf. ibid., Ch.IV, 'Erlösung durch Erkenntnis: Kluge Lehrerinnen'.

117. **Thraede**, 'Frau' (n.110), 244f.

118. For the most recent discussions cf. **B. Hübener** and **H. Meesmann** (eds.), *Streitfall feministiche Theologie*, Düsseldorf 1993.

119. Cf. Gal.3.28.

120. **Brown**, 'Antiquité tardive' (n.104), 256.

121. **Chadwick**, *Early Church* (n.65), 69.

122. For **Origen** cf. the earlier literature in **B. Altaner**, *Patrology*, London and New York 1960, 55. Cf. also **A. von Harnack**, *Der kirchengeschichtliche Ertrag der exegetischen Arbeiten des Origenes*, I–II, Leipzig 1918/19; id., *Geschichte der altchristlichen Literatur bis Eusebius*, ²1958, I.1, 332–405; II.2, 26–54; **J. Daniélou**, *Origen*, London and New York 1965; **H. de Lubac**, *Histoire et Esprit. L'intelligence de l'Écriture d'après Origène*, Paris 1950; id., *Recherches dans la foi. Trois études sur Origène, Saint Anselm et la philosophie chrétienne*, Paris 1979; **H. von Campenhausen**, *The Fathers of the Greek Church*, London 1963, Ch.4, Origen; **H. Crouzel**, *Théologie de l'Image de Dieu chez Origène*, Paris 1956; id., *Origène et la 'Connaissance mystique'*, Paris 1961; id., *Origène et la philosophie*, Paris 1962; id., *Origène*, Paris 1985; **M. Harl**, *Origène et la fonction révélatrice du Verbe incarné*, Paris 1958; **H. Kerr**, *The First Systematic*

Theologian. Origen of Alexandria, Princeton 1958; **R. P. C. Hanson**, *Allegory and Event. A Study of the Sources and Significance of Origen's Interpretation of Scripture*, London 1959; **P. Nemeshegyi**, *La Paternité de Dieu chez Origène*, Tournai 1960; **W. Jaeger**, *Early Christianity and Greek Paideia*, Cambridge, Mass. 1961; **G. Gruber**, *ZOE. Wesen, Stufung und Mitteilung des wahren Lebens bei Origenes*, Munich 1962; **K.-O. Weber**, *Origenes der Neuplatoniker*, Munich 1962; **R. Gögler**, *Zur Theologie des biblischen Wortes bei Origenes*, Düsseldorf 1963; **H. Chadwick**, *Early Christian Thought and the Classical Tradition. Studies in Justin, Clement and Origen*, Oxford 1966; **J. Rius-Camps**, *El dinamismo trinitario en la divinización de los seres racionales según Orígenes*, Rome 1970; **P. Kübel**, *Schuld und Schicksal bei Origenes, Gnostikern und Platonikern*, Stuttgart 1973; **W. Gessel**, *Die Theologie des Gebetes nach* De Oratione *von Origenes*, Paderborn 1975; **P. Nautin**, *Origène. Sa vie et son oeuvre*, Paris 1977; **L. Lies**, *Wort und Eucharistie bei Origenes. Zur Spiritualisierungstendenz des Eucharistieverständnisses*, Innsbruck 1978; id., *Origenes' Eucharistielehre im Streit der Konfessionen. Die Auslegungsgeschichte seit der Reformation*, Innsbruck 1985; id., *Origenes' "Peri Archón": eine undogmatische Dogmatik. Einführung und Erläuterung*, Darmstadt 1992; **U. Berner**, *Origenes*, Darmstadt 1981; **J. C. Smith**, *The Ancient Wisdom of Origen*, Lewisburg 1992. The most recent results of research into Origen (history, exegesis, philosophy and theology) can be found in the volume edited by **R. J. Daly** of documents from the Fifth International Origen Congress (*Origeniana quinta*, Louvain 1992), and will also appear in Vol.II.27,4 of *Aufstieg und Nidergang der römischen Welt (ANRW)*, ed. W. Haase and H. Temporini.

123. **C. Kannengiesser**, 'Origen, Augustine and Paradigm Changes in Theology', in **H. Küng** and **D. Tracy** (eds.), *Paradigm Change in Theology*, Edinburgh 1989, 113–29: 126.

124. **Origen**, *On the Principles*, Preface. The standard edition of the work, which is preserved above all in a Latin translation, is that of **P. Koetschau**, *Griechischen christlichen Schriftsteller der ersten drei Jahrhunderte* 22, Leipzig 1913. On the basis of this, **H. Görgemanns** and **H. Karpp** have produced a corrected Greek-Latin-German edition with notes, *Origenes, Vier Bücher von den Prinzipien*, Darmstadt 1976.

125. **Görgemanns** and **Karpp**, *Origenes. Vier Bücher von den Prinzipien* (n.24), 17.

126. Cf. **Origen**, *On the Principles*, Preface, 10.

127. Id., *Against Celsus* III,28.

128. Cf. **id.**, *On the Principles* IV, 2,4–6. The survey in **A. von Harnack**, *Geschichte der altchristlichen Literatur* I.1, 343–77, shows how powerful even the extant works of Origen on the Hexateuch, the historical, poetical and prophetic books of the Hebrew Bible and the New Testament are.

129. **Kannengiesser**, 'Origen' (n.123), 123.

130. **A. von Harnack**, *Dogmengeschichte* (abbreviated version), Tübingen ⁶1922, 154.

131. Cf. B II, 4, 'Shared short formulae of faith'.

132. **F. Loofs**, *Leitfaden zum Studium der Dogmengeschichte*, Halle ⁵1951, 97.

133. Cf. Acts 2.14–40.

134. Rom.1.3f.

135. **Ignatius**, To the Magnesians VI. 1.

136. **Id.**, To the Ephesians VII.2.
137. Cf. **Theophilus**, *Ad Autolycus* II, 15.
138. **Tertullian**, *Against Praxeas*, 12.6f.
139. For the history of the term cf. **H. Dörrie**, 'Hypostasis. Wort– und Bedeutungsgeschichte', in *Nachrichten von der Akademie der Wissenschaften in Göttingen aus dem Jahre 1955, philologisch-historische Klasse*, Göttingen 1955, 35-92; **H. Köster**, 'Hypostasis', in *Theological Dictionary of the New Testament*, Grand Rapids 1972, Vol.VIII, 572–89.
140. For the interpretation cf. **A. M. Ritter**, 'Dogma und Lehre in der Alten Kirche', in *Handbuch der Dogmen– und Theologiegeschichte*, ed. C. Andresen, I, Göttingen 1982, 99–283, esp.127–9.
141. I have made an earlier attempt to give a historical-systematic account of the main lines of christological development: **H. Küng**, *Incarnation*, Excursus I, 'The Way to Classical Christology'. These remarks were based above all on the early investigations of the history of dogma by **A. Grillmeier, A. Gilg, J. Liébaert** and **B. Skard**. Cf. the more recent investigations by **L. Bouyer**, *Le fils éternel. Théologie de la Parole de Dieu et Christologie*, Paris 1974; **M. G. Fouyas**, *The Person of Jesus Christ in the Decisions of the Ecumenical Councils. A Historical and Doctrinal Study with the Relevant Documents Referring to the Christological Relations of the Western, Eastern and Oriental Churches*, Addis Ababa 1976; **A. Grillmeier**, *Christ in Christian Tradition* I, Oxford [2]1975, II.1, Oxford 1987: **B. Studer**, *Dominus Salvator. Studien zur Christologie und Exegese der Kirchenväter*, Rome 1992.
142. There is a good summary of the teaching of Arius in **A. M. Ritter**, 'Arianismus', *TRE* III, 692–719.
143. Cf. **H.-G. Opitz** (ed.), *Urkunden zur Geschichte des arianischen Streites 318–328*, Berlin 1934f. **R. P. C. Hanson**, *The Search for the Christian Doctrine of God. The Arian Controversy 318–381*, Edinburgh 1988, is a more recent thorough study of the Arian dispute, which is continually being worked on by historians. For the wider historical context cf. **R. Lorenz**, *Das vierte Jahrhundert (Der Osten)*, Göttingen 1992.
144. In this formulation Arius was finally condemned at the Council of Nicaea (325), cf. **Denzinger**, *Enchiridion*, no.54. For the origin and interpretation of this disputed formula cf. the *Handbuch der Dogmen– und Theologiegeschichte*, ed. C. Andresen, Vol.I, Göttingen 1982, 144–51.
145. Cf. **F. Dinsen**, *Homoousios. Die Geschichte des Begriffs bis zum Konzil von Konstantinopel 381*, Kiel dissertation 1976.
146. The analysis by **M. Wiles**, 'The Philosophy in Christianity. Arius and Athanasius', in G.Vesey (ed.), *The Philosophy in Christianity*, Cambridge 1989, 41–52, is very illuminating.
147. Cf. **M. Tetz**, 'Athanasius von Alexandrien', *TRE* IV, 333–49; **C. Kannengiesser**, *Athanase d'Alexandrie, évêque et écrivain. Une lecture des traités Contre les Ariens*, Paris 1983.
148. **Athanasius**, *On the Incarnation of the Logos and his Bodily Appearing Among Us*, 54; cf. **C. Kannengiesser**, *Le Verbe de Dieu selon Athanase d'Alexandrie*, Paris 1990.
149. For **Nicaea**, in addition to the histories of the councils (above all C. J. von Hefele and J. Leclercq) and of dogma cf. especially **I. Ortiz de Urbina**, *Nicéa y Constantinoplá*, Vitoria 1969.
150. Cf. **Denzinger**, *Enchiridion*, no.54.

151. **K. Bringmann**, 'Tradition und Neuerung. Bemerkungen zur Religions-gesetzgebung der christlichen Kaiser des 4.Jahrhunderts', in *Reformatio et reformationes (FS L. Graf zu Dohna)*, Darmstadt 1989, 13–28: 21. Cf. also **Lorenz**, *Das vierte Jahrhundert* (n.143), 201f.

152. Cf. **H. Küng**, *Judaism*, 150–5.

153. Cf. **H. Schreckenberg**, *Die christlichen* Adversus-Judaeos-*Texte und ihr literarisches und historisches Umfeld (1–11.Jh.)*, Frankfurt 1982; **A. L. Williams**, *Adversus Judaeos. A Bird's Eye View of Christian Apologiae until the Renaissance*, Cambridge 1935; **S. G. Wilson** (ed.), *Anti-Judaism in Early Christianity*, Vol.II, *Separation and Polemic*, Waterloo 1986.

154. Cf. Cf. **H. Küng**, *Judaism*, 2 B IV, 'The History of an Alienation'.

155. **Melito of Sardes**, *Homily on the Passion*, ed. C. Bonner, London and Philadelphia 1940, no.94.

156. **G. Stemberger**, *Juden und Christen im Heiligen Land. Palästina unter Konstantin und Theodosius*, Munich 1987, 46.

157. Cf. the eight anti-Jewish sermons of **Chrysostom**, in *Patrologiae Graeca* 48, 843–92 – an arsenal for anti-Jewish witch-hunts.

158. Cf., in addition to histories of councils and dogmas, **Ortiz de Urbina**, *Nicéa y Constantinoplá* (n.149); **W. D. Hauschild**, *Die Pneumatomachen. Eine Untersuchung zur Dogmengeschichte des 4.Jhs.*, Hamburg dissertation 1967; **K. Lehmann** and **W. Pannenberg** (eds.), *Glaubensbekenntnis und Kirchengemein-schaft. Das Modell des Konzils von Konstantinopel (381)*, Freiburg 1982; **N. Silanes** et al., *El concilio de Constantinopla I y el Espíritu Santo*, Salamanca 1983.

159. Cf. **Denzinger**, *Enchiridion*, no.86; cf. **A. M. Ritter**, *Das Konzil von Konstantinopel und sein Symbol. Studien zur Geschichte und Theologie des Zweiten Ökumenischen Konzils*, Göttingen 1965. I shall go into the problems of the later Latin addition *filioque* (proceeding from the Father 'and the Son') in due course.

160. This is the hypothesis presented by **L. Abramowski**, 'Was hat das Nicaeno-Constantinopolitanum (C) mit dem Konzil von Konstantinopel 381 zu tun?', *Theologie und Philosophie* 67, 1992, 481–513, in a complex discussion.

161. In addition to the histories of councils and dogmas cf. **P. T. Camelot**, *Éphèse et Chalcédoine*, Paris 1962.

162. In addition to the earlier histories of councils and dogmas cf. above all **A. Grillmeier** and **H. Bacht**, *Das Konzil von Chalkedon* (3 vols.), Würzburg 1951–54; **Camelot**, *Éphèse et Chalcédoine* (n.161).

163. Cf. **Denzinger**, *Enchiridion*, no. 148.

164. Cf. **J. Alberigo** et al. (eds.), *Conciliorum oecumenicorum decreta*, Freiburg 1962, 28.

165. **A. von Harnack**, *Lehrbuch der Dogmengeschichte*, II, 397.

166. **J. Liébaert**, 'Christologie. Von der Apostolischen Zeit bis zum Konzil von Chalkedon (451)', in *Handbuch der Dogmengeschichte*, ed. M. Schmaus and A. Grillmeier, Vol.III, Freiburg 1965, 1–127: 127.

167. **K. Rahner**, 'Chalkedon – Ende oder Anfang?', in Grillmeier und Bacht, *Das Konzil von Chalkedon* (n.162), Vol.III, 3–49. And **L. Abramowski**, who in the third of her *Drei christologischen Untersuchungen*, Berlin 1981, has closely investigated *synapheia* and *asynchytos henosis* as a designation for trinitarian and christological unity, comes to the conclusion that we can regard the dialectic of the four famous adverbs 'as an extremely unsatisfactory result'; our

theological task today (is) the opposite: 'At any rate the man Jesus has remained for us; and the important thing is to talk of the binding character of his message and the authority of his person in the face of universal atheism in such a way that it becomes possible to speak of God in a new way' (109). For the place of Jesus in subsequent cultural history cf. **J. Pelikan**, *Jesus through the Centuries. His Place in the History of Culture*, New Haven 1985.

168. There is a thorough account of the non-Chalcedonian churches by the Coptic scholar **A. S. Atiya**, *A History of Eastern Christianity*, London 1968.

169. See Parts A and B of this volume.

170. Even historians of dogma who otherwise work with great scrupulosity seem to me to be all to anxious about orthodoxy when they should be giving a clear judgment on this development in the history of dogma – in contrast to their classical models (von Harnack, Loofs, Seeberg). **K. Beyschlag** certainly recognizes 'that the dogma of the Trinity today still' enjoys 'only pale unpopularity, if not complete incomprehension, even among theologians', but simply attributes this to the spirit of the time, without a touch of self-criticism. He even thinks that 'the dogma of the Trinity could bring about a refounding of the Christian worldview once created by Origen in which **God** is recognized as the embodiment of a universal Christian **culture** – but now in trinitarian fullness of being... ' (*Grundriss der Dogmengeschichte*, Vol.I, Darmstadt 1982, 275). Others, like **A. M. Ritter**, believe that they may speak of 'the most precious Christian deposit of revelation' where they should be explaining the 'meaning' of the dogma of the Trinity, but in the same breath concede that this dogma is 'liable to all kinds of misunderstandings' and 'even did not have any direct power of expression'. It is strange to talk about a 'most precious Christian deposit of revelation' which has no direct power of expression. Indeed, without noting the contradiction, the same historian of dogma continues: 'Deterring as a religous notion and ultimately asking too much of philosophical concepts, it (the dogma) seemed to make the 'mystery of the Trinity' (*mysterium trinitatis*) end up in the logical absurdity $3 = 1$.' Once he has become so clearly entangled in contradictions, even the appeal to Martin Luther which follows in the very next sentence cannot help (*Handbuch der Dogmen– und Theologiegeschichte*, Vol.I, Göttingen 1982, 213f.). It would have been more appropriate had the historian reflected critically on the New Testament and been more faithful to the Reformation slogan *sola scriptura*. All too little attention has so far been paid in the history of dogma to how, whether consciously or unconciously, for example 'adoptionist' or other scriptural texts have been bent and even changed in favour of the orthodox view; this has been systematically investigated for the first time by **B. D. Ehrman**, *The Orthodox Corruption of Scripture. The Effect of Early Christological Controversies on the Text of the New Testament*, Oxford 1993.

171. For the **history of the Byzantine empire and the Orthodox Church** cf. **G. Ostrogorsky**, *History of the Byzantine State*, Oxford 1956; **H. Berkhof**, *De kerk en de keizer, een studie over het ontstaan van de Byzantinistische en de theocratische staatgedachte in de vierde eeuw*, Amsterdam 1946; **G. Every**, *The Byzantine Patriarchate 451–1204*, London 1947; **W. de Vries**, *Der christlichen Osten in Geschichte und Gegenwart*, Würzburg 1951; id., *Orthodoxie und Katholizismus. Gegensatz oder Ergänzung?*, Freiburg 1965; **F. Dölger** and **A. M. Schneider**, *Byzanz*, Bern 1952; **G. Zananiri**, *Histoire de l'église byzantine*, Paris 1965; **H. G. Beck**, *Kirche und theologische Literatur im byzantinischen Reich*, Munich 1980; id., *Geschichte der orthodoxen Kirche in byzantinischen Reich*,

Göttingen 1980; **A. Michel,** *Die Kaisermacht in der Ostkirche (843–1204),* Darmstadt 1959; **J. Meyendorff,** *L'église orthodoxe hier et aujourd'hui,* Paris 1960; **id.,** *Orthodoxie et Catholicité,* Paris 1965; **K. Onasch,** *Einführung in die Konfessionskunde der orthodoxen Kirchen,* Berlin 1962; **A. Schmemann,** *The Historical Road of Eastern Orthodoxy,* London 1963; **T. Ware,** *The Orthodox Church,* Harmondsworth 1963; **J. M. Hussey** (ed.), *The Cambridge Mediaeval History,* Vol.IV, *The Byzantine Empire,* Parts I–II, Cambridge 1966f.; **S. Runciman,** *The Fall of Constantinople, 1453,* Cambridge 1965; **D. Obolensky,** *The Byzantine Commonwealth. Eastern Europe, 500–1451,* London 1971; **P. Kawerau,** *Das Christentum des Osten,* Stuttgart 1972; **id.,** *Ostkirchengeschichte,* Vols.I–IV, Louvain 1982–84; **F. G. Maier** (ed.), *Byzanz,* Frankfurt 1973; **A. Guillou,** *La civilisation byzantine,* Paris 1974; **D. A. Zakythinos,** *Byzantine Istoria 324–1071,* Athens 1972; **C. Mango,** *Byzantium. The Empire of New Rome,* London 1980; **W. Nyssen, H. J. Schulz** and **P. Wiertz** (eds.), *Handbuch der Ostkirchenkunde,* I, Düsseldorf 1984, Part 2, *Die geschichtliche Entwicklung der Ostkirchen;* **A. Ducellier,** *Byzance et le monde orthodoxe,* Paris 1986; **G. Dagron, P. Riché** and **A. Vauchez,** *Évêques, moines, et empereurs (642–1054),* Paris 1993.

I am grateful to Professor Dr **Fairy von Lilienfeld** and Professor Dr **Ludolf Müller,** two experts in Eastern Orthodoxy, for reading through Chapter C II 8–12 thoroughly and doing me a great service through their countless corrections of detail and constructive suggestions.

172. **Ostrogorsky,** *History of the Byzantine State* (n.171), 25.

173. **Schmemann,** *The Historical Road* (n.171), 199.

174. Cf. **P. Ariès** and **G. Duby,** *Histoire de la vie privée,* I, Paris 1985.

175. There is an impressive investigation of this for the period from Julian the Apostate to the fifth century in **A. Quacquarelli,** *Reazione pagana e trasformazione della cultura (fine IV secolare d.C),* Bari 1986.

176. **P. Brown,** 'Antiquité tardive', in Ariès and Duby, *Histoire* (n.104), I, 225–99: 265. Cf. **id.,** *The Making of Late Antiquity,* Cambridge, Mass. 1978.

177. **Id.,** 'Antiquité tardive' (n.176), 265.

178. Ibid., 265–763.

179. Cf. **R. A. Markus,** *The End of Ancient Christianity,* Cambridge 1990.

180. For the Christianized emperor ideology of Constantine cf. **F. Heim,** *La théologie de la victoire de Constantin à Théodose,* Paris 1992; **R. Leeb,** *Konstantin und Christus. Die Verchristlichung der imperialen Repräsentation unter Konstantin dem Grossen als Spiegel seiner Kirchenpolitik und seines Selbstverständnisses als christlicher Kaiser,* Berlin 1992.

181. Cf. **G. Ruhbach,** 'Die politische Theologie Eusebs von Caesarea', in id. (ed.), *Die Kirche angesichts der Konstantinischen Wende,* Darmstadt 1976, 236–58.

182. Cf. **F. Dölger,** *Regesten der Kaiserurkunden des Oströmischen Reiches von 565–1452* (5 vols.), Munich 1924–54.

183. **Id.,** in the preface to Michel, *Die Kaisermacht in der Ostkirche* (n.171).

184. Cf. the brief survey in **A. Raes,** 'Liturgie VI B': Einzeltypen', *LThK* VI, 1087–91; also **C. Detlef** and **G. Müller,** *Geschichte der orientalischen Nationalkirchen,* Göttingen 1981.

185. Cf. I Clement 40.6.

186. Cf. **Origen,** *Commentary on Jeremiah,* 11.3.

187. I Peter 2.10.
188. Cf. **H. Küng**, *Church*, E 1 2, 'The royal priesthood of all Christians'.
189. I owe this suggestion to Professor **Fairy von Lilienfeld**, who is probably the most competent expert on Eastern Orthodoxy in the Evangelical Church of Germany.
190. **H.-G. Beck**, *Byzantinisches Erotikon*, Munich 1986, 202f.
191. For **Eastern monasticism** cf. **I. Smolitsch**, *Russisches Mönchtum. Entstehung, Entwicklung und Wesen 988–1917*, Würzburg 1953; **K. S. Frank**, *Angelikos Bios*, Münster 1964; **id.**, *Grundzüge der Geschichte des christlichen Mönchtums*, Darmstadt 1975; **id.** (ed.), *Askese und Mönchtum in der alten Kirche*, Darmstadt 1975; **U. Ranke-Heinemann**, *Das frühe Mönchtum. Seine Motive nach den Selbstzeugnissen*, Essen 1964; **D. J. Chitty**, *The Desert a City. An Introduction to the Study of Egyptian and Palestinian Monasticism under the Christian Empire*, Oxford 1966; **B. Lohse**, *Askese und Mönchtum in der Antike und in der alten Kirche*, Munich 1969; **L. Bouyer**, *La vie de S. Antoine. Essai sur la spiritualité du monachisme primitif*, Bégrolles en Mauges [2]1977; **P. Canivet**, *Le monachisme syrien selon Théodoret de Cyr*, Paris 1977; **F. von Lilienfeld**, *Spiritualität des frühen Wüstenmönchtums*, Erlangen 1983.
192. Cf. **H. Küng**, CWR, C II 2.
193. **Clement of Alexandria**, *Stromata*, 1.15.
194. Buddha as Bodhisattva, Manichaean Bodisaf, Arabic Yudasaf, Georgian Jodasaph, Greek Joasaph, Latin Josaphat. The Buddha finally revered as a Christian saint. For the great Canadian scholar of religion **W. C. Smith**, *Towards a World Theology. Faith and the Comparative History of Religion*, London 1981, 9, this is one of the pieces of evidence for his thesis of 'the one religious history of humankind'.
195. Cf. **Lohse**, *Askese und Mönchtum* (n.191), chs.1 and 2.
196. Cf. the different evaluations of this phenomenon, which is so alien to us today, in **Ranke Heinemann** *Das frühe Mönchtum* (n.191), and **Frank**, *Angelikos Bios* (n.191).
197. For the following, with reference to the Apophthegmata Patrum (Sayings of the Desert Fathers), see **Brown**, *The Making of Late Antiquity* (n.176), 115–38.
198. Cf. Matt.19.16–24.
199. Cf. **P.Canivet**, *Le monachisme syrien*, Ch.VI, 'Les moines thaumaturges'.
200. Cf. the helpful survey of the faith and culture of the earliest Egyptian Christians by **E. Brunner Traut**, *Die Kopten. Leben und Lehre der ägyptischen Christen in Geschichte und Gegenwart*, Munich 1991, which is illustrated with many texts.
201. Thus the description of monasticism by the church historian **K. Baus**, 'Koinobitentum', *LThK* VI, 368.
202. Cf. Mark 1.12f.; this is developed at length in Matthew (4.1–11) and Luke (4.1–13).
203. Thus Matt.19.12f. of 'eunuchs (castrated) for the sake of the kingdom of heaven' (according to some exegetes a Matthaean addition).
204. Cf. I Cor.7 (esp.7.7); 9.5.
205. Among others, the Apophthegmata patrum, Abbas Dorotheos, Pseudo-Makarios, John Climacus, Barsanu phios and John were read (communication by F. von Lilienfeld).

206. For the **iconoclastic controversy** cf. **Ostrogorsky**, *History of the Byzantine State* (n.171), Ch.III, 'The Age of the Iconoclast Crisis (711–843)', 130–86; **L. Ouspensky and W. Lossky**, *Der Sinn der Ikonen*, Bern 1952; **J. Kollwitz**, 'Bild III', *Reallexikon für Antike und Christentum* II, Stuttgart 1954, 318–41; **H. J. Rothemund**, *Ikonenkunst. Ein Handbuch*, Munich 1954; **W. Felicetti-Liebenfels**, *Geschichte der byzantinischen Ikonenmalerei. Von ihren Anfängen bis zum Ausklange unter Berücksichtigung der Maniera Greca und der italobyzantinischen Schule*, Olten 1956; **id.**, *Geschichte der russischen Ikonenmalerei in den Grundzügen dargestellt*, Graz 1972; **E. Benz**, *Geist und Leben der Ostkirche*, Hamburg 1957, I, *Die orthodoxe Ikone*; **G. Lange**, *Bild und Wort. Die katechetischen Funktionen des Bildes in der griechischen Theologie des sechsten bis neunten Jahrhundert*, Würzburg 1969; **L. W. Barnard**, *The Graeco-Roman and Oriental Background of the Iconoclastic Controversy*, Leiden 1974; **C. von Schönborn**, *L'icône du Christ. Fondements théologiques élaboré entre le Ier et IIe Concile de Nicée (325–787)*, Fribourg 1976, revised German edition *Die Christus-Ikone. Eine theologische Hinführung*, Schaffhausen 1984; **S. Gerö**, *Byzantine Iconoclasm during the Reign of Leo III, with Particular Attention to the Oriental Sources*, Louvain 1973; **id.**, *Byzantine Iconoclasm During the Reign of Constantine V, with Particular Attention to the Oriental Sources*, Louvain 1977; **A. Bryer** and **J. Herrin** (eds.), *Iconoclasm. Papers given at the Ninth Spring Symposium of Byzantine Studies (University of Birmingham, March 1975)*, Birmingham 1977; **H.-G. Beck**, *Geschichte der orthodoxen Kirche im byzantinischen Reich*, Göttingen 1980, Ch.III, 'Das Zeitalter des Ikonoklasmus'; **J. Irmscher** (ed.), *Der byzantinische Bilderstreit. Sozialökonomische Voraussetzungen – ideologische Grundlagen – geschichtliche Wirkungen*, Leipzig 1980; **D. Stein**, *Der Beginn des byzantinischen Bilderstreites und seine Entwicklung bis in die 40er Jahre des 8.Jahrhunderts*, Munich 1980; **H. G. Thümmel** and **W. von Loewenich**, 'Bilder IV–V', *TRE* VI, 525–46; **H. G. Thümmel**, *Bilderlehre und Bilderstreit. Arbeiten zur Auseinandersetzung über die Ikone und ihre Begründung vornehmlich im 8. und 9. Jahrhundert*, Würzburg 1991; **id.**, *Die Frühgeschichte der ostkirchlichen Bilderlehre. Texte und Untersuchungen zur Zeit vor dem Bilderstreit*, Berlin 1992; **A. Grabar**, *L'Iconoclasme byzantin. Le dossier archéologique*, Paris 1984; **W. Nyssen, H.-J. Schulz** and **P. Wiertz** (eds.,) *Handbuch der Ostkirchenkunde, I.2, Die geschichtliche Entwicklung der Ostkirchen*; **A. Ducellier**, *Byzanz*, 288–98; **V. Cândea**, 'Iconoclasm', *EncRel* VII, 1f.; **J. Wohlmuth** (ed.), *Streit um das Bild. Das 2.Konzil von Nizäa (787) in ökumenischer Perspektive*, Bonn 1989; **H. D. Döpmann**, *Die Ostkirchen vom Bilderstreit bis zur Kirchenspaltung 1054*, Leipzig 1990; **L. Müller**, *Die Dreifaltigkeitsikone des Andréj Rubljów*, Munich 1990; **J. Pelikan**, *Imago Dei. The Byzantine Apologia for Icons*, Princeton 1990. **É. Coche de la Ferté**, *L'art de Byzance*, Paris 1982, gives an overall survey of Byzantine art with more than 1000 illustrations.

207. Cf. **Benz**, *Geist und Leben der Ostkirche* (n.206), 11.

208. Cf. **Ducellier**, *Byzanz* (n.171), 288–98.

209. **Gerö**, *Leo III* (n.206), 129.

210. Ibid., 127.

211. Cf. **C. Mango** in his introduction to the volume edited by Breyer and Herrin, 1–6. Mango thinks that one can even speak of iconoclasm as a 'Semitic movement' (6). Cf. also **Cândea**, 'Iconoclasm' (n.206), 1.

212. Cf. **Ostrogorsky**, *History of the Byzantine State* (n.171), 193.

213. Thus with far-reaching consequences for the present-day understanding of the church and art, **von Schönborn**, *Die Christus-Ikone*, in his conclusion, 226.

214. Cf. **Gerö**, *Leo III* (n.206), 129.

215. **Beck**, *Geschichte der orthodoxen Kirche* (n.206), 69f.

216. Cf. **Denzinger**, *Enchiridion*, 302–4, 306–8.

217. **Grabar**, *L'Iconoclasme byzantin* (n.206), 301f.

218. For the very complicated manufacture and complex symbolism of icons cf. especially **Ouspensky** and **Lossky**, *Der Sinn der Ikonen* (n.206), 11–56; P. **Evdokimov**, *L'art de l'icône. Théologie de la beauté*, Paris 1972; W. **Felicetti–Liebenfels**, *Geschichte der russischen Ikonenmalerei*, 1–12; L. **Ouspensky**, *La théologie de l'Icône dans l'Église Orthodoxe*, Paris 1980; G. **Distante** (ed.), *La legittimità del culto delle icone. Oriente e Occidente riaffermano insieme la fede cristiana*, Bari 1988. For historical criticism cf. **H. G. Thümmel**, 'Die Theorie der Ikone. Die ostkirchliche Bilderlehre', *Theologische Literaturzeitung* 16, 1991, 641–9.

219. Cf. **F. von Lilienfeld**, 'Hesychasmus', *TRE* XV, 282–9.

220. Cf. Matt.27.41; Heb.10.19.

221. Cf. **A. Jensen**, *Die Zukunft der Orthodoxie, Konzilspläne und Kirchenstrukturen*, Zurich 1986.

222. Cf. **von Harnack**, *Handbuch der Dogmengeschichte*, Vol.II, 490.

223. Cf. **Schmemann**, *The Historical Road* (n.171), 214.

224. Cf. **Ostrogorsky**, *History of the Byzantine State* (n.171), 213f.

225. **Michel**, *Die Kaisermacht in der Ostkirche* (n.171), 166: 'The *Epanagoge* represents a unique and vain attempt to secure the church her freedom in the Western sense, a "mere episode of contemporary conditioning" (H. F. Schmidt).'

226. Cf. **Schmemann**, *The Historical Road* (n.171), 220.

227. For the development of a **Slavonic-Byzantine Christianity**, in addition to the works on Byzantine history cf. above all **F. Dvornik**, *Byzantine Missions among the Slavs. SS. Constantine-Cyril and Methodios*, New Brunswick 1970; L. **Waldmüller**, *Die ersten Begegnungen der Slawen mit dem Christentum und den christlichen Völkern vom VI. bis VIII. Jahrhundert. Die Slawen zwischen Byzanz und Abendland*, Amsterdam 1976; **S. W. Swierkosz-Lenart**, *Le origini e lo sviluppo della cristianità slavo-bizantina*, Rome 1992; G. **Dagron**, P. **Riché** and A. **Vauchez**, *Bischöfe, Mönche und Kaiser*, Part IV. For the extremely complicated and changeable relationships between Byzantium and the Slavs cf. **Ducellier**, *Byzanz* (n.171).

228. There is much valuable information (despite the precarious date of publication!) on the struggle between Church Slavonic-Byzantine and Latin liturgy and tradition in the region of Bohemia, Moravia and Pannonia in E. **Winter**, *Tausend Jahre Geisteskampf im Sudetenraum. Das religiöse Ringen zweier Völker*, Salzburg 1938.

229. For the **history of Christianity in Russia**, in addition to the works on the Orthodox Church already cited (especially Meyendorff, Schmemann and Ware) see the collection of documents with commentary by P. **Hauptmann** and G. **Stricker** (eds.), *Die Orthodoxe Kirche in Russland. Dokumente ihre Geschichte 860–1980)*, Göttingen 1988 (henceforth *Dokumente*). Cf. also the monographs by **N. Zernov**, *The Russians and their Church*, London 1945; id., *The Russian Religious Renaissance of the Twentieth Century*, London 1963; **G. P. Fedotov**, *The Russian Religious Mind* (2 vols.), Cambridge, Mass. 1946/66; id. (ed.), *A Treasury of Russian Spirituality*, London 1950; **A. M. Ammann**, *Abriss der*

ostslawischen Kirchengeschichte, Vienna 1950; **H. Schaeder**, *Moskau das dritte Rom*, Darmstadt ²1957; **P. Kovalevsky**, *Saint Serge et la spiritualité russe*, Paris 1958; **N. Struve**, *Les Chrétiens en URSS*, Paris 1963; **J. Chrysostomus**, *Kirchengeschichte Russlands der neuesten Zeit* (3 vols.), Munich 1965–8; **K. Onasch**, *Grundzüge der russischen Kirchengeschichte*, Göttingen 1967; **M. Klimenko**, *Ausbreitung des Christentums in Russland seit Vladimir dem Heiligen bis zum 17. Jahrhundert. Versuch einer Übersicht nach russischen Quellen*, Berlin 1969; **H.-D. Döpmann**, *Die russische orthodoxe Kirche in Geschichte und Gegenwart*, Vienna 1977; **P. C. Bori** and **P. Bettiolo**, *Movimenti religiosi in Russia prima della rivoluzione (1900–1917)*, Brescia 1978; **J. W. Cunningham**, *A Vanquished Hope. The Movement for Church Renewal in Russia, 1905–1906*, New York 1981; **A. Poppe**, *The Rise of Christian Russia*, London 1982; **K. C. Felmy** et al. (eds.), *Tausend Jahre Christentum in Russland. Zum Millennium der Taufe der Kiever Rus'*, Göttingen 1988; **Pitirim von Volokolamsk** (ed.), *Die russiche orthodoxe Kirche*, Berlin 1988; **P. Bushkovitch**, *Religion and Society in Russia. The Sixteenth and Seventeenth Centuries*, Oxford 1992.

A whole series of further volumes of colloquies at various institutions appeared as part of the **millenary celebrations of the Russian church in 1988**: University of Tübingen (ed. R. D. Kluge and H. Setzer); University of Paris X-Nanterre (D.Obolensky et al.); University of London (ed. G. A. Hosking); University of Oregon (ed. A. Leong); Georgio Cini Foundation, Venice (ed. S. Graciotti); Institute for the Eastern Church, Regensburg (ed. A. Rauch and P. Imhof); UNESCO, Paris (ed. Y. Hamant); USSR Academy of Sciences, Moscow (ed. P. N. Fedoseyef). At the same time there were new accounts of the history of the Russian church by **M. Garzaniti, F. House** and **J.-C. Roberti**.

230. Cf. **L. Müller**, *Die Taufe Russlands. Die Frühgeschichte des russischen Christentums bis zum Jahre 988*, Munich 1987, 9–16. The most important documentary sources and those with narrative character from the beginning of the Russian church around 860 are also edited with a commentary in *Dokumente*, nos.1–25 – the account by the great patriarch Photius of the founding of the Russian church is particularly important. For the legend of Andrew in Byzantium, where in the time of Photius it was to serve as legitimation against the Roman appeal to Peter, cf. **F. Dvornik**, *The Idea of Apostolicity in Byzantium and the Legend of the Apostle Andrew*, Cambridge, Mass. 1958.

231. Cf. **Müller**, *Die Taufe Russlands* (n.230), 111–16.

232. Cf. **Fedotov**, *The Russian Religious Mind* (n.229), I, 412.

233. Metropolitans Hilarion (1051–1054) and Clement of Smolensk (1147–55).

234. For the **East-West schism** see the various articles by **V. Grumel** in *Échos d'Orient*, Paris 1933–40; **M. Jugie**, *Le schisme byzantin. Aperçu historique et doctrinale*, Paris 1941; **F. Dvornik**, *The Photian Schism. History and Legend*, Cambridge 1948; **id.**, *The Idea of Apostolicity in Byzantium and the Legend of the Apostle Andrew* (n.232); **id.**, *Byzance et la primauté romaine*, Paris 1964 (German ed. *Byzanz und der römische Primat*, Stuttgart 1966, to which page references are given); **Y. Congar**, *Neuf cents ans après. Notes sur le "Schisme oriental"*, Paris 1954; **S. Runciman**, *The Eastern Schism. A Study of the Papacy and the Eastern Churches during the XIth and XIIth Centuries*, Oxford 1955; **G. Denzler**, 'Das sogenannte Morgenländische Schisma im Jahre 1054', *Münchener Theologische Zeitschrift* 17, 1966, 24–66; **id.**, 'Das Morgenländischer

Kirchenschisma im Verständnis von Päpsten und ökumenischen Konzilien des Mittelalters', *Münchener Theologische Zeitschrift* 20, 1969, 104–17.

235. J. Meyendorff, 'Rom und die Orthodoxie – Autorität oder Wahrheit', *Catholica* 31, 1977, 352–68: 354.

236. Dvornik, *Byzanz* (n.234), 159f.

237. Ibid., 9.

238. Cf. Beck, *Geschichte der orthodoxen Kirche* (n.206), Ch.IV.1, 'Ignatios und Photios'.

239. Cf.Denziger, *Enchiridion*, 277.

240. For the *filioque* cf. L. Vischer (ed.), *Geist Gottes – Geist Christi. Ökumenische Überlegung zur Filioque-Kontroverse*, Frankfurt 1981.

241. Dvornik, *Byzanz* (n.234), 165.

242. Cf. Beck, *Geschichte der orthodoxen Kirche* (n.206), Ch.V.1, 'Kaiserliche Politik und Eigenwege der Patriarchen'.

243. The most recent thorough investigation by B. Roberg, *Das Zweite Konzil von Lyon* (1274), Paderborn 1990, describes this council of union as a 'wasted opportunity': 'The encounter with Orthodoxy which could and should have been the central theme of the council was not understood, let alone coped with as a task' (384). For the Council of Ferrara-Florence cf. J. Gill, *The Council of Florence*, Cambridge 1959; id., *Constance et Bâle-Florence*, Paris 1965; G. Alberigo (ed.), *Christian Unity. The Council of Ferrara-Florence 1438/39–1989*, Louvain 1991 (here above all the critical comments by H. Chadwick).

244. Ducellier, *Byzanz* (n.171), 12f.

245. A. Ducellier and his team have made a brilliant analysis of this through the various periods in all its economic, social, political, military and cultural complexity.

246. S. Runciman, *The Fall of Constantinople 1453*, Cambridge 1965.

247. Cf. the literature mentioned above on the history of Christianity in the Kiev period.

248. For the Russian church under Tatar rule see *Dokumente* nos.26–57 (with commentary by F. von Lilienfeld and E. Bryner).

249. Cf. *Dokumente*, nos. 28, 26.

250. G. Florovsky, *Ways of Russian Theology* I, Belmont, Mass. 1979, 3. Cf. also id., *Aspects of Church History*, Vaduz 1987, 186–91, for a degree of obscurantism in the Russian mentality.

251. Schmemann, *The Historical Road* (n.171), 305.

252. Ibid., 308.

253. For the role of the Metropolitan Isidore in connection with the Council of Ferrara-Florence and the election of metropolitans independent of Byzantium cf. *Dokumente*, nos. 58–66 (with commentary by F. von Lilienfeld and E. Bryner).

254. In fact Isidore was appointed by Eugene IV as *legatus a latere* for the 'provinces of Lithuania, Latvia and all Russia', and the 'cities, dioceses, districts and places of Poland', with full Roman authority 'to exterminate heresies, to increase and multiply the Catholic faith' and 'to preserve the authority of the Apostolic See' (cf. *Dokumente*, no. 60).

255. For the following events in the autocephalous Metropolis of Moscow and all Russia cf. *Dokumente*, nos.67–92 (with commentary by F. von Lilienfeld and E. Bryner).

256. Cf. *Dokumente*, no.67.

257. Cf. *Dokumente*, no.253.

258. For the Russian church under the first ten patriarchs (1589–1700) cf. *Dokumente*, nos.93–104 (with commentary by **P. Hauptmann**); **M. Batisweiler** et al. (eds.), *Der Ökumenische Patriarch Jeremias II. von Konstaninopel und die Anfänge des Moskauer Patriarchates*, Erlangen 1991 (with other articles on the history of the Moscow patriarchate).

259. Cf. *Dokumente*, nos.73 (Josif) and 75 (Vassian, a pupil of Nil's). Cf. **F.von Lilienfeld**, *Nil Sorskij und seine Schriften. Die Krise der Tradition im Russland Ivans III.*, Berlin 1963.

260. **H. Neubauer**, *Car und Selbstherrscher. Beiträge zur Geschichte der Autokratie in Russland*, Wiesbaden 1964, shows how constant reference was made to Byzantium in justification of the autocratic system, but how in other respects Realpolitik was practised at home and abroad. **H. J. Torke**, *Die staatsbedingte Gesellschaft im Moskauer Reich. Zar und Zemlja in der altruss-ischen Herrschaftsverfassung 1613–1689*, Leiden 1974, shows that the Russian autocracy is not to be identified with Asiatic despotism, but was also different from more liberal Western absolutism.

261. There is a balanced evaluation of Turkish rule, which is often seen in one–sidedly negative terms, in **T. H. Papadopoullos**, *Studies and Documents Relating to the History of the Greek Church and People under Turkish Domination*, Brussels 1952; **S. Runciman**, *The Great Church in Captivity. A Study of the Patriarchate of Constantinople from the Eve of the Turkish Conquest to the Greek War of Independence*, Cambridge 1968; **A. Ducellier**, *Byzanz* (n.171), in his final chapter (with J.-P. Arrignon) on the fate of Orthodox culture.

262. Cf. **E. Amburger**, *Geschichte des Protestantismus in Russland*, Stuttgart 1961.

263. Cf. **G. E. Zachariades**, *Tübingen und Konstantinopel. Martin Crusius und seine Verhandlungen mit der Griechisch-Orthodoxen Kirche*, Göttingen 1941; **EKD** (ed.), *Wort und Mysterium. Der Briefwechsel über Glauben und Kirche 1573 bis 1581 zwischen den Tübinger Theologen und dem Patriarch von Konstantinopel*, Witten 1958; **C. N. Tsirpanlis**, *The History and Ecumenical Significance of Jeremias II's Correspondence with the Lutherans (1573–1581)*, Kingston 1982; **D. Wendebourg**, *Reformation und Orthodoxie. Der ökumen-ische Briefwechsel zwischen der Leitung der Württembergischen Kirche und Patriarch Jeremias II. von Konstantinopel in den Jahren 1573–1581*, Göttingen 1986. There is also a detailed analysis of the theological questions in dispute in this thorough study.

264. **Wendebourg**, *Reformation* (n.263), 334.

265. In addition to the account by **G. A. Hadjiantoniou**, *Protestant Patriarch. The Life of Cyril Lucaris (1572–1638), Patriarch of Constantinople*, Richmond, Va. 1961, cf. above all the close historical analysis of **G. Hering**, *Ökumenisches Patriarchat und europäische Politik 1620–1638*, Wiesbaden 1968, which is based on the discovery of new sources.

266. This 'grand design' has been worked out by **P. Meyendorff**, *Russia, Ritual and Reform: The Liturgical Reforms of Nikon in the Seventeenth Century*, New York 1991. **C. Hemer**, *Herrschaft und Legitimation im Russland des 17.Jahrhunderts. Staat und Kirche zur Zeit des Patriarchen Nikon*, Frankfurt 1979, demonstrates convincingly that contrary to the prevalent opinion, Patriarch Nikon did not aim at the subordination of secular to spiritual power in principle.

267. Cf. **P. Hauptmann**, *Altrussischer Glaube. Der Kampf des Protopopen Avvakum gegen die Kirchenreformen des 17.Jahrhunderts*, Göttingen 1963; **N. Lupinin**, *Religious Revolt in the Seventeenth Century: The Schism of the Russian Church*, Princeton 1984.

268. Cf. **T. Riplinger**, *Die ukrainisch-bjelorussische Variante des byzantinisch-orthodoxen Paradigmas. Der Eigenweg der orthodoxen Kirche in polnisch-litauischen Staatsverband vom 14. bis zum 17.Jh. als Modell einer zeitgenössischen Erneuerung des orthodoxen Kirchentums* (MS). There is more in **I. Vlasovsky**, *Outline History of the Ukrainian Orthodox Church* (2 vols.), New York 1974–9; **I.Moncak**, *Florentine Ecumenism in the Kyivan Church*, Rome 1987; **A. Jobert**, *De Luther à Mohila. La Pologne dans la crise de la Chrétienté 1517–1648*, Paris 1974.

269. Instead of already in Byzantium 'from the creation of the world', with the year beginning on 1 September, now 'after the birth of Christ', with the year beginning on 1 January. The Gregorian calendar was not introduced by Peter either.

270. For the Russian Orthodox Church in the century of Peter the Great's church reform (1700–1801) see *Dokumente*, nos.105–45 (with commentary by **R. Stupperich**). Also, in addition to the numerous biographies of Peter the Great, on his church reform: **I. Smolitsch**, *Geschichte der russischen Kirche 1700–1917* (2 vols), Leiden 1964, Berlin 1990; **J. Cracraft**, *The Church Reform of Peter the Great*, London 1971; **A. V. Muller**, *The Spiritual Regulation of Peter the Great*, Seattle 1972.

271. Cf. *Dokumente*, no.115. **C. G. de Michelis**, *I nomi dell'avversario. Il 'papa-anticristo' nella cultura russa*, Turin 1989, points out that in this period the term **Antichrist** – in Russia always associated with the Pope – was transferred to Czar Peter (and the following Czars down to Stalin).

272. I also owe this important perspective to **F. von Lilienfeld**.

273. This is how **F.von Lilienfeld** translates it.

274. For the state church and the beginnings of renewal cf. *Dokumente*, nos.146–205 (with commentary by K. C. Felmy and G. Simon).

275. Cf. **L. Tolstoy**, *The Gospel in Brief* (Russian original), New York 1896; id., *What I Believe* (1884), London and New York 1921. The investigation by **L. Müller**, *Russischer Geist und evangelisches Christentum. Die Kritik des Protestantismus in der russischen religiösen Philosophie und Dichtung im 19. und 20.Jahrhundert*, Witten 1951, is very illuminating for the way in which modern Russian intellectuals, for whom the quest for truth is a heresy against the dogma of the church, have grappled with Protestantism.

276. Cf. **H. Küng**, *Literature and Religion*, New York 1994, 'F. M. Dostoievsky – Religion in Conflict with Religionlessness'.

277. Cf. **V. Solovyev**, *The Justification of the Good. An Essay in Moral Philosophy*, London 1918; cf. **L. Müller**, *Das religionsphilosophische System Vladimir Solovjevs*, Berlin 1956; **H. Gleixner**, *Vladimir Solov'evs Konzeption vom Verhältnis zwischen Politik und Sittlichkeit. System einer sozialen und politischen Ethik*, Frankfurt 1978; id., *Die ethische und religiöse Sozialismuskritik des Vladimir Solov'ev. Texte und Interpretation*, St Ottilien 1986.

278. Cf. **J. Oswalt**, *Kirchliche Gemeinde und Bauernbefreiung. Soziales Reformdenken in der orthodoxen Gemeindegeistlichkeit Russlands in der Ära Alexander II.*, Göttingen 1975. For the later renewal movement, the main concern of which was the emancipation of the church from state control, cf. **J. W.**

Cunningham, *A Vanquished Hope. The Movement for Church Renewal in Russia, 1905–1906*, Crestwood, NY 1981.

279. Cf. **Benz**, *Geist und Leben der Ostkirche* (n.206), chs.IX–XII; **Oswalt**, *Kirchliche Gemeinde und Bauernbefreiung* (n.278).

280. **G. Petrow**, quoted in Benz, *Geist und Leben der Ostkirche* (n.206), 132f. (unfortunately this text is not in *Dokumente*).

281. For the Russian Orthodox church in the Soviet state (since 1917) cf. *Dokumente*, nos.210–371 (with commentary by R. Rössler).

282. **V. I. Lenin**, '*Socialism and Religion*', *Collected Works*, Vol. 10, London 1982, 83f.

283. For **Orthodox theology and the Orthodox Church** cf. the recent monographs by **Benz**, *Geist und Leben der Ostkirche* (n.206); **S. Bulgakov**, *The Orthodox Church*, Clayton, Wis. 1964; **M.-J. Le Guillou**, *L'esprit de l'orthodoxie grecque et russe*, Paris 1961; **Ware**, *The Orthodox Church* (n.171); id., *The Orthodox Way*, New York 1979; **N. von Arseniew**, *Die russische Frömmigkeit*, Zurich 1964; **O. Clément**, *Byzance et le christianisme*, Paris 1964; **A. Schmemann**, *Introduction to Liturgical Theology*, London 1966; id., *Church, World, Mission. Reflections on Orthodoxy in the West*, Crestwood, NJ 1979; **R. Stupperich** (ed.), *Die Russische Orthodoxe Kirche in Lehre und Leben*, Witten 1966; **E. Timiadis**, *Lebendige Orthodoxie. Eine Selbstdarstellung der Orthodoxie im Kreise der christlichen Kirchen*, Nuremberg 1966; **G. Florovsky**, *Bible, Church, Tradition: An Eastern Orthodox View*, Belmont, Mass. 1972; id., *Creation and Redemption*, Belmont, Mass. 1976; id., *Ways of Russian Theology* (2 vols.), Belmont, Mass. 1979; **J. Meyendorff**, *Byzantine Theology. Historical Trends and Doctrinal Themes*, Fordham 1974; **V. Lossky**, *Orthodox Theology. An Introduction*, Crestwood, NY 1978; **A. Kallis**, *Orthodoxie: Was ist das?*, Mainz 1979; **V. Peri**, *La 'Grande Chiesa' Bizantina. L'ambito ecclesiale dell'Ortodossia*, Brescia 1981; **B. Sartorius**, *L'église Orthodoxe*, Paris 1973; **D. Staniloae**, *Orthodoxe Dogmatik* (2 vols., original in Rumanian), Gütersloh 1984/90; id., *Le génie de l'Orthodoxie. Introduction*, Paris 1985; **K. C. Felmy**, *Die Orthodoxe Theologie der Gegenwart. Eine Einführung*, Darmstadt 1990.

284. There is a historical and systematic survey of liturgy, sacraments, calendar, church music and iconography in the second volume of the *Handbuch der Ostkirchenkunde*, ed. W.Nyssen, H.-J. Schulz and P. Wiertz, Düsseldorf 1989.

285. **Benz**, *Geist und Leben der Ostkirche* (n.206), 175.

III. The Roman Catholic Paradigm of the Middle Ages

1. Protestant historians like Albert Hauck (died 1918), Heinrich Boehmer (died 1926), Hans von Schubert (died 1931) and Hermann Dörries (died 1977) also made important contributions to the evaluation of the Middle Ages.

2. Catholic theologians like Ignaz Döllinger (died 1890), Albert Erhard (died 1940), Franz Dölger (died 1940) and Joseph Lortz (died 1975) and their pupils made a decisive contribution towards overcoming this Roman Catholic fixation on the Middle Ages.

3. **A. Angenendt**, *Das Frühmittelalter. Die Abendändische Christenheit von 400–900*, Stuttgart 1990, 42. **H. Zimmermann**, *Das Mittelalter* (2 vols.), Brunswick 1975–79, is still helpful as a generally understandable introduction to

the history of the Middle Ages, with abundant bibliographies for this period, which is almost impossible to survey, as too is **H. Fuhrmann**, *Einladung ins Mittelalter*, Munich 1987.

4. This has been described by the great canon law historians Paul Hinschius (died 1898), Ulrich Stutz (died 1937) and H. E. Feine (died 1965).

5. During the nineteenth century German secular and church historians and historians of dogma never tired of demonstrating this.

6. Cf. **T. Klauser**, 'Der Übergang der römischen Kirche von der griechisch zur lateinischen Liturgiesprache', *Jahrbuch für Antike und Christentum*, Ergänzungsheft III, 1974, 184–94.

7. **H. von Campenhausen**, *The Fathers of the Latin Church*, London 1964, 35.

8. For **Augustine** (354–430) cf. the earlier literature in **B. Altaner**, *Patrology*, New York and London 1960, 102. In addition to the handbooks on the history of dogma, both the earlier ones (by A. von Harnack, F. Loofs, R. Seeberg) which are still important, and the more recent ones (by C. Andresen, K. Beyschlag, J. Pelikan, M. Schmaus and A. Grillmeier), cf. the following more recent monographs and general accounts: **É. Gilson**, *Introduction à l'étude de saint Augustin*, Paris 1929, ⁴1969; **H. I. Marrou**, *Saint Augustin et la fin de la culture antique*, Paris 1938, ⁴1958 (German edition *Augustinus und das Ende der antiken Bildung*, Paderborn 1981, to which page references are given); id., *Saint Augustin et l'Augustinisme*, Paris 1955, ⁸1973; **F. van der Meer**, *Augustinus de Zielzorger*, Utrecht 1947; **A. Zumkeller**, *Das Mönchtum des heiligen Augustinus*, Würzburg 1950, ²1968; **T. J. van Bavel**, *Recherches sur la christologie de saint Augustin. L'humain et le divin dans le Christ d'après saint Augustin*, Fribourg 1954; **J. J. O'Meara**, *The Young Augustine. The Growth of St Augustine's Mind up to his Conversion*, London 1954, ²1980; **R. W. Battenhouse** (ed.), *A Companion to the Study of St Augustine*, New York 1955; **M. Löhrer**, *Der Glaubensbegriff des hl.Augustinus in seinen ersten Schriften bis zu den Confessiones*, Einsiedeln 1955; **A. D. R. Polman**, *Het woord gods bij Augustinus*, Kampen 1955; **R. Schneider**, *Seele und Sein. Ontologie bei Augustin und Aristoteles*, Stuttgart 1957; **G. Strauss**, *Schriftgebrauch, Schriftauslegung und Schriftbeweis bei Augustin*, Tübingen 1959; **von Campenhausen**, *Fathers of the Latin Church* (n.7), ch. 6, 'Augustine'; **C. Eichenseer**, *Das Symbolum Apostolicum beim heiligen Augustinus, mit Berücksichtigung des dogmengeschichtlichen Zusammenhangs*, St Ottilien 1960; **C. Andresen** (ed.), *Zum Augustin-Gespräch der Gegenwart* (2 vols.), Darmstadt 1962/81; **P. Brown**, *Augustine of Hippo. A Biography*, London 1967; **A. Mandouze**, *Saint Augustin. L'aventure de la raison et de la grâce*, Paris 1968; **C. Boyer**, *Essais anciens et nouveaux sur la doctrine de saint Augustin*, Milan 1970; **R. A. Markus**, *Saeculum. History and Society in the Theology of St Augustine*, Cambridge 1970; **E. TeSelle**, *Augustine the Theologian*, London 1970; **J. Brechtken**, *Augustinus doctor caritatis. Sein Liebesbegriff im Widerspruch von Eigennutz und selbstloser Güte im Rahmen der antiken Glückseligkeits-Ethik*, Meisenheim 1975; **W. Geerlings**, *Christus exemplum. Studien zur Christologie und Christusverkündigung Augustins*, Mainz 1978; **R. E. Meagher**, *An Introduction to Augustine*, New York 1978; **W. Wieland**, *Offenbarung bei Augustinus*, Mainz 1978; **A. Schindler**, 'Augustinus', *TRE* IV, 645–98; **K. Flasch**, *Augustin. Einführung in sein Denken*, Stuttgart 1980; **A. Pincherle**, *Vita di Sant'Agostino*, Bari 1980; **H. Fries**, 'Augustinus', in H. Fries and G. Kretschmar (eds.), *Klassiker der Theologie*, I, Munich 1981, 104–29; **P. Muñoz Vega**, *Introducción a la síntesis de San*

Agustín, Quito 1981; **H. Chadwick**, *Augustine*, Oxford 1986; **P. Guilloux**, *El alma de San Agustín*, Madrid 1986; **M. Vannini**, *Invito al pensiero di Sant'Agostino*, Milan 1989. Numerous more recent monographs – by V. J. Bourke, A. Campodonico, N. Fischer, J. A. García-Junceda, A. di Giovanni, G. Santi, A. Schöpf – deal with Augustine's 'philosophy'. I am deeply grateful to my Graz colleague Professor Dr **Johannes B. Bauer** for a critical reading especially of the chapter on patristics and for valuable suggestions.

9. Cf. **S. Rose**, *The Place of Blessed Augustine in the Orthodox Church*, Platina 1983; **M. Azkoul**, *The Influence of Augustine of Hippo on the Orthodox Church*, Lewiston, NY 1990; he writes programmatically in the introduction: 'He is also responsible, in large measure, for the division between East and West; and, indeed, even for the Occident's loss of the patristic spirit . . . He is surely not the apex of the patristic tradition; in fact, he was the beginning of something new.'

10. **Marrou**, *Augustinus* (n.8), 489–95, is more specific; the quotation is on 495.

11. Cf. **B. Altaner**, 'Augustinus und die griechische Patristik', *Texte und Untersuchungen* 83, 1967, 316–31: 321.

12. For **Augustine's understanding of the church**, cf. F. **Hofmann**, *Der Kirchenbegriff des hl.Augustinus in seinen Grundlagen und in seiner Entwicklung*, Munich 1933; **J. Ratzinger**, *Volk und Haus Gottes in Augustins Lehre von der Kirche*, Munich 1954; **S. J. Grabowski**, *The Church. An Introduction to the Theology of St Augustine*, St Louis, Mo 1957; **É. Lamirande**, *L'Église céleste selon saint Augustin*, Paris 1963; id., *Études sur l'ecclésiologie de saint Augustin*, Ottawa 1969; **R. Crespin**, *Ministère et sainteté. Pastorale du clergé et solution de la crise donatiste dans la vie et la doctrine de saint Augustin*, Paris 1970; **Y. Congar**, *L'Église. De saint Augustin à l'époque moderne*, Paris 1970; **W. Simonis**, *Ecclesia visibilis et invisibilis. Untersuchungen zur Ekklesiologie und Sakramentenlehre in der afrikanischen Tradition von Cyprian bis Augustinus*, Frankfurt 1970; **P. Borgomeo**, *L'Église de ce temps dans la prédication de saint Augustin*, Paris 1972; **S.Folgado Florez**, *Dinamismo católico de la Iglesia en San Agustín*, Madrid 1977; **A. Giacobbi**, *La chiesa in S. Agostino*, Rome 1978; **F. Genn**, *Trinität und Amt nach Augustinus*, Einsiedeln 1986.

13. **Augustine**, *Sermo* 112.8. For the question of the use of force cf. E. L. **Grasmück**, *Coercitio. Staat und Kirche im Donatistenstreit*, Bonn 1964, esp.240–50.

14. **Brown**, *Augustine of Hippo* (n.8), 235.

15. Ibid., 240.

16. For Augustine's **anti-Pelagian doctrine of grace**, in addition to the relevant sections in **von Campenhausen** and **Brown**, see: H. **Jonas**, *Augustin und das paulinische Freiheitsproblem. Eine philosophische Studie zum pelagianischen Streit*, Göttingen 1930, [2]1965; A. **Mandouze**, *Saint Augustin. L'aventure de la raison et de la grâce*, Paris 1968; **J. P. Burns**, *The Development of Augustine's Doctrine of Operative Grace*, Paris 1980. Inspired by H. **Haag**, *Biblische Schöpfungslehre und kirchliche Erbsündenlehre*, Stuttgart 1966, U. **Baumann** produced the thorough ecumenical study *Erbsünde? Ihr traditionelles Verständnis in der Krise heutiger Theologie*, Freiburg 1980. H. **Häring** similarly produced a comprehensive systematic study of evil in the different phases of Augustine's theology, culminating in a resolute criticism of the doctrine of original sin, in his *Die Macht des Bösen. Das Erbe Augustins*, Zurich 1979, which

he developed also at the Institute for Ecumenical Research. For the history of the doctrine of original sin see the four-volume work by I. Gross, *Geschichte des Erbsündendogmas. Ein Beitrag zur Geschichte des Problems vom Ursprung des Übels*, Munich 1960–72.

17. The almost countless more recent monographs on original sin show what a burden Augustine's doctrine of **original sin** was on the whole of Latin theology: see e.g. those of P. F. Beatrice, I. Bertinetti, J. Bur, F. Dexinger, A.-M. Dubarle, E. Elorduy, D. Fernández, M. Flick and Z. Alszeghy, G. Freund, P. Grelot, E. Kinder, K. M. Köster, G. Matelet, H. Rondet, L. Scheffczyk, K. Schmitz-Moormann, P. Schoonenberg, A. Vanneste, P. Watté, K.-H. Weger et al.

18. Cf. **Augustine**, *De nuptiis et concupiscentia*, 1.24f.

19. All this influenced Augustine's biblical exegesis. For in contrast to most Greek and Syrian authors, Augustine understands the moment of shame after the first fall psychologically as clearly felt sexual shame – a punishment for sin. Thus the corruption of human nature inherited since Adam's fall manifested itself especially in the constant disruption caused by the sexual drive, which removes itself from the control of the will especially at the beginning and the climax of the act, but also in sleep and dreams (cf. Augustine, *Sermo* 151; *Contra Julianum Pelagianum*, above all book IV). It is not sexuality in itself which is the evil (as the Manichaeans thought), but the loss of control (thus Augustine). No, even the newborn child is not an innocent, but is rather a child born in sin which unconditionally needs liberation from original sin if it is not to be damned eternally. And this act of liberation is baptism, which must always be administered to the newborn child. And according to Augustine not only the young man but also the older man who is married has to fight against sexual desire and be concerned for 'chastity', combating the sexual fantasies which constantly arise. Let us be clear that never before had an ancient author given such a cool psychological analysis of sexuality.

20. Cf. **Augustine**, *Ep.* 217,V,16; *Enchiridion* XXIII–XXIX. For Augustine's **doctrine of predestination** cf. G. Nygren, *Das Prädestinationsproblem in der Theologie Augustins. Eine systematisch-theologische Studie*, Lund 1956. Also the selection of texts with commentary by J. Chéné, *La théologie de saint Augustin. Grâce et prédestination*, Lyons 1961. G. Kraus, *Vorherbestimmung. Traditionelle Prädestinationslehre im Licht gegenwärtiger Theologie*, Freiburg 1977, has produced a thorough account and balanced criticism of the ideas of predestination in Augustine, Thomas Aquinas, Luther, Calvin and Karl Barth – also in our Institute.

21. I Cor.4.7.

22. **Augustine**, *In primam epistolam Joannis* VII.8. Cf. **D. Dideberg**, *Saint Augustin et la première épître de saint Jean. Une théologie de l'agapè*, Paris 1975.

23. Cf. **K. E. Børresen**, *Subordination et Equivalence. Nature et rôle de la femme d'après Augustin et Thomas d'Aquin*, Oslo 1968, esp. ch.I,1–3.

24. For **Augustine's attitude to sexuality** before and after his conversion cf. **P. Brown**, *The Body and Society. Men, Women and Sexual Renunciation in Early Christianity*, London and New York 1988, 406–427. Augustine's theory of sex and sin was so important to him that at the age of seventy he sent a letter to Patriarch Atticus of Constantinople, John Chrysostom's successor (it has only been recently discovered), summing up his position as follows: 'An urge (he means the evil "urge of the flesh") which burns quite indiscriminately for objects allowed and disallowed; and which is bridled by the urge for marriage

(*concupiscentia nuptiarum*), that must depend on it, but that retrains it from what is not allowed . . . Against this drive, which is in tension with the law of the mind, all chastity must fight: that of the married couple, so that the urge of the flesh may be rightly used, and that of continent men and virgins, so that, even better, and with a struggle of greater glory, it should not be used at all. This urge, had it existed in Paradise . . . would, in a wondrous pitch of peace, never have run beyond the bidding of the will . . . It would never have forced itself upon the mind with thoughts of inappropriate and impermissible delights. It would not have had to be held upon the leash by married moderation, or fought to a draw by ascetic labour. Rather, when once called for, it would have followed the will of the person with all the ease of a single-hearted act of obedience' (quoted in **Brown**, *The Body and Society*, 423).

25. Cf. Rom.9–11; and **H. Küng**, *Judaism*, 3 B IV, 'The Future of the People of God'.

26. **Marrou**, *Augustinus* (n.8), 46.

27. Cf. above, C II 6, 'The shift under Constantine and the christological dispute'.

28. **Augustine**, *Confessions* III, VI (11); cf. *Soliloquies* I,i (1–6).

29. **Augustine**, *De Trinitate* I, III (5).

30. For Augustine's **doctrine of the Trinity** cf. M. Schmaus, *Die psycholog- ische Trinitätslehre des heiligen Augustinus*, Münster 1927, reprinted with an appendix 1967; **J.-L. Maier**, *Les missions divines selon saint Augustin*, Fribourg 1960; **A. D. R. Polman**, *De leer van god bij Augustinus*, Kampen 1965; **A.Schindler**, *Wort und Analogie in Augustins Trinitätslehre*, Tübingen 1965; **O. du Roy**, *L'intelligence de la foi en la Trinité selon saint Augustin. Genèse de sa théologie trinitaire jusqu'en 391*, Paris 1966; **D. Pintaric**, *Sprache und Trinität. Semantische Probleme in der Trinitätslehre de hl.Augustinus*, Salzburg 1983; **M. Smalbrugge**, *La nature trinitaire de l'intelligence augustinienne de la foi*, Amsterdam 1988.

31. Cf. **T. de Régnon**, *Études de théologie positive sur la Sainte Trinité* (3 vols.), Paris 1892–98, esp. I, 339f., 362; III, 162–5 (the Father as the principle of the Godhead).

32. **K. Rahner**, *Foundations of Christian Faith*, London and New York 1978, 135.

33. Cf. **Denzinger**, *Enchiridion*, no. 39; cf. **J. N. D. Kelly**, *The Athanasian Creed*, London 1964.

34. Cf. **Brown**, *Augustine of Hippo* (n.8), esp.ch.24.

35. Cf. **J. Moltmann**, *The Trinity and the Kingdom of God*, London and Minneapolis 1981. Sharp criticism of Moltmann has been expressed from both the German-speaking and the English-speaking world, cf. **K.-J. Kuschel**, *Born Before all Time? The Dispute over Christ's Origin*, London and New York 1992, 449–51. Similarly the Edinburgh theologian **J. P. Mackey**, 'Are There Christian Alternatives to Trinitarian Thinking?', in J. M. Byrne (ed.), *The Christian Understanding of God Today*, Dublin 1993, 66–75: 'What is wrong . . . is the projection of current ideas of human relationships into the divine being, resulting in an "immanent" Trinity which then, of course, becomes normative (and not merely inspiring) for the reconstruction of human relationships in civic and ecclesiastical societies' (67).

36. For Augustine's **City of God** cf. H. Scholz, *Glaube und Unglaube in der Weltgeschichte. Ein Kommentar zu Augustins De* civitate Dei, Leipzig 1911,

[2]1967; **E. Troeltsch**, *Augustin, die christliche Antike und das Mittelalter. Im Anschluss an die Schrift* De Civitate Dei, Munich 1915, reprinted Aalen 1963; **A. A. T. Ehrhardt**, *Politische Metaphysik von Solon bis Augustin* (2 vols.), Tübingen 1952; **J. Pintard**, *La sacerdoce selon Saint Augustin. Le prêtre dans la cité de Dieu*, Tours 1960; **R. A. Markus**, *Saeculum. History and Society in the Theology of St Augustine*, Cambridge 1970; **J. van Oort**, *Jeruzalem en Babylon. Een onderzoek van Augustinus'* De stad van god *en de bronnen van zijn leer der twee steden (rijken)*, The Hague 1986; **G. Lettieri**, *Il senso della storia in Agostino d'Ippona. Il saeculum e la gloria nel* De Civitate Dei, Rome 1988; **D. F. Donnelly** and **M. A. Sherman**, *Augustine's* De civitate Dei. *An Annotated Bibliography of Modern Criticism*, 1960–1990, New York 1991.

37. Thus according to Augustine both world history and the history of the individual now run in six periods, modelled on the pattern of the week of creation, which in world history becomes the world week. Since its creation the world has gone through six great ages. Thus for Augustine, the Bible itself already demonstrated the transitoriness of cultures, the reality of changes of era and 'paradigm shifts'. With Jesus Christ, the Lord of the City of God has appeared bodily in the world – the God-man as the climax of world history! Since then humankind has been living in the sixth day of the world week, in the end-time which will conclude with the Last Judgment. This is already announced in the downfall of the last world state, the Roman empire, which unmasked itself as a state of the devil in the persecution of Christians, but now has the merit of having secured a peace from which the City of God also profits. But Augustine remains mistrustful even of the Christian imperium, since pagan powers are still at work in it (cf. **F. G. Maier**, *Augustine und das antike Rom*, Stuttgart 1955). Augustine says hardly anything about the future of the Roman empire (whether West or East). By contrast, it is unshakably certain for him that the kingdom of God has an empirical form in this earthly time: the **Catholic Church**. It is the concrete embodiment and manifestation of the kingdom of God, but is not simply identical with the city of God, since the city of this world is still in fact at work in it. For Augustine, only God knows the elect.

38. Cf. above C II 2, 'The slow rise of the Bishop of Rome'.

39. For the **papacy**, in addition to the standard works on papal history by **E. Caspar, C. Falconi, J. Haller, L. von Pastor, L. von Ranke, J. Schmidlin, F. X. Seppelt** and **G. Schwaiger**, and the brief sketches of the history of the papacy by **A. Franzen** and **R. Bäumer, H. Fuhrmann, B. Schimmelpfennig, W. Ullmann**, and **H. Zimmermann**, cf. especially the series edited by **G. Denzler**, *Päpste und Papsttum*, Stuttgart 1971ff., which so far comprises 26 volumes (some important individual volumes are given special mention). Also the following monographs and general accounts with a historical orientation: **F. Heiler**, *Altkirchliche Autonomie und päpstlicher Zentralismus*, Munich 1941; **M. Maccarrone**, *Vicarius Christi. Storia del titolo papale*, Rome 1952; id. (ed.), *Il primato del vescovo di Roma nel primo millennio. Ricerche e testimonianze*, Vatican City 1991 (cf. especially the contributions by H. Fuhrmann and H. Zimmermann); **B. Tierney**, *Foundations of the Conciliar Theory*, Cambridge 1955; id., *Origins of Papal Infallibility, 1150–1360. A Study of the Concepts of Infallibility, Sovereignty and Tradition in the Middle Ages*, Leiden 1972; **W. Ullmann**, *The Growth of Papal Government in the Middle Ages*, London 1955; id., *A Short History of the Papacy in the Middle Ages*, London 1972; **F. Kempf**, 'Die päpstliche Gewalt in der mittelalterlichen Welt. Eine Auseinandersetzung mit

Walter Ullmann', in *Saggi storici intorno al Papato*, Rome 1959, 117–69; **G. Barraclough,** *The Medieval Papacy*, London 1968; **H. Zimmermann,** *Papstabsetzungen des Mittelalters*, Graz 1968; **id.,** *Das Papsttum im Mittelalter. Eine Papstgeschichte im Spiegel der Historiographie*, Stuttgart 1981; **F. Salvoni,** *Da Pietro al Papato*, Genoa 1970; **G. Denzler** (ed.), *Das Papsttum in der Diskussion*, Regensburg 1974; **G. Schwaiger** (ed.), *Konzil und Papst. Historische Beiträge zur Frage der höchsten Gewalt in der Kirche*, Munich 1975; **id.,** *Päpstlicher Primat und Autorität der Allgemeinen Konzilien im Spiegel der Geschichte*, Munich 1977; **M. Pacaut,** *La Papauté, des origines au concile de Trente*, Paris 1976; **K. A. Fink,** *Papsttum und Kirche im abendländischen Mittelalter*, Munich 1981; **M. Greschat** (ed.), *Gestalten der Kirchengeschichte XI–XII (Das Papsttum, I–II)*, Stuttgart 1985; **K. Schatz,** *Der päpstliche Primat. Seine Geschichte von den Ursprüngen bis zur Gegenwart*, Würzburg 1990. Cf. also the literature on the East-West schism, especially **F. Dvornik,** *Byzanz*, and the countless systematic and topical publications on the papacy.

40. Cf. **Eusebius of Caesarea,** *Church History* V, 24. The testimony of **Irenaeus** (*Adv.Haer.* III.3, 1–2) quoted by Vatican II also does not speak of any **legal** obligation of the other churches to agree with the Roman church. The Roman church (there is no mention of the Bishop of Rome) does not appear as having a legal primacy but as the prime guardian of the tradition because of its twofold succession (Irenaeus, too, relates it to Peter and Paul); in observing its faith people are also observing the faith of all the other churches.

41. Cf. **Ullmann,** *Short History of the Papacy* (n.39). In addition to the histories of the papacy, see also the perceptive account by **Heiler,** *Altkirchliche Autonomie* (n.39), Part II. The most important Roman documents can be read in **C. Mirbt** and **K. Aland** (eds.), *Quellen zur Geschichte des Papsttums und des römischen Katholizimus*, I, Tübingen [6]1967.

42. **H. Chadwick,** *The Early Church*, Harmondsworth 1967, 162.

43. Cf. **Y. Congar,** 'Titel, welche für den Papst verwendet werden', *Concilium* 11, 1975, 538–44 (never available in English), which sums up the wide-ranging research.

44. **Hofmann,** *Der Kirchenbegriff des hl.Augustinus* (n.12), 320f.

45. **Ratzinger,** *Volk und Haus Gottes in Augustins Lehre* (n.12), 180.

46. **Augustine,** 'But who can fail to be aware that the **sacred canon** of Scripture, both of the Old and New Testaments, is confined within its own limits, and that it stands so absolutely in a superior position to all later letters of the bishops, that about it we can hold no manner of doubt or disputation whether what is confessedly contained in it is right and true; but that all the **letters of bishops** which have been written, or are being written, since the closing of the canon, are liable to be refuted if there be anything in them which strays from the truth, either by the discourse of some one who happens to be wiser in the matter than themselves, or by the weightier authority and more learned experience of other bishops, or by the authority of councils; and further, that the **councils** themselves, which are held in the several districts and provinces, must yield, beyond all possibility of doubt (*sine ullis ambagibus cedere*), to the authority of plenary councils which are formed for the whole Christian world; and that even of the plenary councils, the earlier are often corrected (*saepe emendari*) by those which follow them when, by some actual experiment (*cum aliquo experimento rerum*), things are brought to light which were before concealed' (*On Baptism, Against the Donatists*, Book II, ch.3, in *Nicene and Post-Nicene Fathers* IV,

Buffalo 1887, 427). I have written to the same effect about the 'true (but not infallible) authority of the councils', on the basis of the excellent article by **H. J. Sieben** (which later appeared as a book, *Die Konzilsidee der alten Kirche*, Paderborn 1979), in the volume *Fehlbar?*, which I edited (414–22).

47. **Concilium Nicaenum** I, Canons VI–VII, in **J. Alberigo** et al. (eds.), *Conciliorum oecumenicorum decreta*, Freiburg 1962, 8.

48. Cf. **P.Stockmeier**, 'Leo I. der Grosse', in **M. Greschat** (ed.), *Das Papsttum* I (n.39), 56–69. For Leo's view of the primacy cf. **Ullmann**, *Short History of the Papacy* (n.39), 19–27. Cf. further **G. Corti**, *Il Papa vicario di Pietro. Contributo alla storia dell'idea papale* I, Brescia ²1966; **P. McShane**, *La Romanitas et le Pape Léon le Grand. L'apport culturel des institutions impériales à la formation des structures ecclésiastiques*, Tournai 1979; **M. M. Wojtowytsch**, *Papsttum und Konzile von den Anfängen bis zum Leo I. (440–61), Studien zur Enstehung der Überordnung des Papstes über Konzile*, Stuttgart 1981.

49. In addition to the letters of Pope Leo I see his various sermons on the anniversaries of his elevation to the throne of Peter, e.g. *Sermo* III,1–4; IV,2–4. Cf. **W. Ullmann**, *Gelasius I (492–496). Das Papsttum an der Wende der Spätantike zum Mittelalter*, Stuttgart 1981, esp. Ch.III, 'Die Petrinologie Leos des Grossen'.

50. Cf. Matt.16.18; Luke 22.32; John 21.15–17.

51. Cf. **A. Grillmeier** and **H. Bacht** (eds.), *Das Konzil von Chalkedon. Geschichte und Gegenwart* (3 vols.), Würzburg 1951–54, ²1959. For the substantive problem cf. **H. Küng**, *Incarnation*, especially Excursuses I–V.

52. It is unfortunately characteristic of the way in which Roman theology deals with historical truth that even the thirty-first edition of **H. Denzinger**'s *Enchiridion symbolorum definitionum et declarationum* (1854), edited by **K. Rahner** (1960), while bringing together all the material from early church history which supports a 'primacy of the Roman see' (above all, of course, from the very mouth of the Bishop of Rome), has completely suppressed Canon 28 of the Ecumenical Council of Chalcedon on New Rome, which is so important; Denzinger is a remarkably tendentious collection of texts! Unfortunately that is also true of the new thirty–seventh edition, 'improved' and 'expanded' by **P. Hünermann** in 1991, now in both Latin and German (and with 1706 pages of doctrinal documents). Since despite the tremendous and admirable work of editing and translation the tendency of Denzinger has not changed, Canon 28 of Chalcedon is still not thought worth including. Cf. by contrast the admirable edition *Conciliorum oecumenicorum decreta* by Alberigo et al., Freiburg 1962, pp.75f., which contains both the Greek and the Latin text of the long Canon 28 (cf. also p.71, Canon 17).

53. Cf. **Ullmann**, *Gelasius I* (n.49), esp. Chs.V–X. **Wojtowytsch**, *Papstum und Konzile von den Anfängen bis zu Leo I* (n.48), shows impressively that the Roman claim to power was always a Roman claim, which was not accepted during the first millennium even in the Western church.

54. At the First Vatican Council before the definition of infallibility (1870) this tendency understandably gave rise to vigorous discussions. Cf. **E. C. Butler**, *The Vatican Council. The story told from inside in Bishop Ullathorne's Letters*, London 1930, Ch.XIX: 'The Difficult Debate: The Opportunity for the Declaration of Infallibility'; **H. Küng**, *Infallible?*, II.3, 'Critical questions'; **id.**, *Fehlbar?* My critical questions are fully endorsed by **G. Kreuzer**, *Die Honoriusfrage im Mittelalter und in der Neuzeit*, Stuttgart 1975.

55. **Y. Congar,** *L'Ecclésiologie du Haut Moyen Age. De Saint Grégoire le Grand à la désunion entre Byzance et Rome,* Paris 1968, 159f.

56. Cf. **J. Langen,** *Das Vatikanische Dogma von dem Universal-Episcopat und der Unfehlbarkeit des Papstes in seinem Verhältnis zum Neuen Testament und der exegetischen Überlieferung* (4 vols.), Bonn 1871–76.

57. Cf. **E. Caspar,** *Geschichte des Papsttums von den Anfängen bis zur Höhe der Weltherrschaft,* I, Tübingen 1930, 115–30.

58. Text re-edited by **H. Fuhrmann,** *Das Constitutum Constantini (Konstantinische Schenkung),* Hanover 1958; cf. id., 'Constitutum Constantini', *TRE* VIII, 196–202.

59. Cf. **L. Valla,** *De falso credita et ementita Constantini donatione, deutsche Übersetzung aus der Reformationszeit,* ed. W.Setz, Basel 1981. Cf. **W. Setz,** *Lorenzo Vallas Schrift gegen die Konstantinische Schenkung. Zur Interpretation und Wirkungsgeschichte,* Tübingen 1975; also **D. Maffei,** *La donazione di Costantino nei giuristi medievali,* Milan 1964.

60. Cf. **E. Caspar,** *Geschichte des Papsttums* II, Tübingen 1933, 107–10: 'The pregnant version by the forger established itself victoriously: "*Prima sedes a nemine iudicatur*" subsequently became the formula for the papal primacy of jurisdiction' (110).

61. **H. Zimmermann,** *Papstabsetzungen des Mittelalters,* 5f.; cf. **H. Küng,** *Structures,* Ch.VII.3, 'Conflict Between the Pope and the Church'.

62. **Zimmermann,** *Papstabsetzungen des Mittelalters,* 6.

63. Luke 22.25f.

64. Cf. – after the foundations laid in **H. Küng,** *The Church,* E II 3, 'Infallible?' – id. (ed.), *Fehlbar?* (above all Chapter E).

65. Cf. **Arbeitsgemeinschaft ökumenischer Universitätsinstitute** (ed.), *Papsttum als ökumenische Frage,* Munich 1979.

66. Cf. **J. Martin,** *Spätantike und Volkerwanderung,* Munich 1987.

67. In the following survey of this cultural collapse I follow the excellent general description by **A. Angenendt,** *Das Frühmittelalter. Die abendländische Christenheit von 400 bis 900,* Stuttgart 1990, Part I, 3, Ch.1, 'Die Dekomposition der Alten Welt'.

68. Cf. **R. Schneider,** *Das Frankenreich,* Munich 1982; **G. Dagron, P. Riché** and **A. Vauchez,** *Evêques, moînes, et empereurs (642–1054),* Paris 1993 (by P. Riché).

69. **J. A. Jungmann,** 'Die Abwehr des germanischen Arianismus und der Umbruch der religiösen Kultur im frühen Mittelalter', in the collection of his works, *Liturgisches Erbe und pastorale Gegenwart,* Innsbruck 1960, 3–86: 3.

70. In addition to Angenendt's study, see also **J. A. Jungmann,** *Missarum Sollemnia. Eine genetische Erklärung des römischen Messe* (2 vols.), Vienna ²1949.

71. I Tim.2.5.

72. Cf. above C II 7, 'Symphony of empire and church'.

73. For **Gregory the Great,** in addition to the older literature and the relevant assessments in the classical histories of dogma, cf. **B. Altaner,** *Patrology,* London and New York 1960. Then, in addition to the relevant sections in the history of the papacy (esp.W. Ullmann) and the histories of the Middle Ages (especially A. Angenendt), see the following monographs: **O. M. Porcel,** *La doctrina monastica de San Gregorio Magno y la 'Regula Monachorum',* Madrid 1950; **J. P. McClain,**

The Doctrine of Heaven in the Writings of Saint Gregory the Great, Washington, DC 1956; **R. Rudmann**, *Mönchtum und kirchlicher Dienst in den Schriften Gregors des Grossen*, St Ottilien 1956; **C. Chazottes**, *Grégoire le Grand*, Paris 1958; **G. Dufner**, *Die 'Moralia' Gregors des Grossen in ihren italienischen Volgarizzamenti*, Padua 1958; id., *Die Dialoge Gregors des Grossen im Wandel der Zeiten und Sprachen*, Padua 1968; **V. Recchia**, *Gregorio Magno e la società agricola*, Rome 1978; **C. Dagens**, *Saint Grégoire le Grand. Culture et expérience chrétiennes*, Paris 1977; **D. Hofmann**, *Die geistige Auslegung der Schrift bei Gregor dem Grossen*, Münsterschwarzach 1968; **J. Richards**, *Consul of God. The Life and Times of Gregory the Great*, London 1980; **R. A. Markus**, *From Augustine to Gregory the Great. History and Christianity in Later Antiquity*, London 1983; **C. Straw**, *Gregory the Great. Perfection in Imperfection*, Berkeley 1988; **J. Modesto**, *Gregor der Grosse. Nachfolger Petri und Universalprimat*, St Ottilien 1989. There is a new bibliography by **R. Godding**, *Bibliografia di Gregorio Magno (1890/1989)*, Rome 1990.

74. Cf. **H. Fries** and **G. Kretschmar**, *Klassiker der Theologie I (Von Irenäus bis Martin Luther)*, Munich 1981.

75. Cf. **Greschat** (ed.), *Gestalten der Kirchengeschichte* (n.39), Vols. XI–XII.

76. Cf. **K. Fassmann** (ed.), *Die Grossen der Weltgeschichte*, II, Zurich 1972, 792–801, with a balanced assessment by H.-D. Altendorf.

77. **A. von Harnack**, *Dogmengeschichte* (abbreviated version), Tübingen ⁷1991, 33.

78. Ibid.

79. **U. Wickert**, 'Gregor I', in *RGG* II, 1837.

80. **R. A. Markus**, 'Gregor I', *TRE* XIV, 135–45: 137.

81. **von Harnack**, *Dogmengeschichte* (n.77), 332f.

82. Cf. **H. Hucke**, 'Gregor I', in *Das Grosse Lexikon der Musik*, ed. M. Honegger and G. Massenkeil, III, Freiburg 1980, 355f.

83. **Gregory the Great**, *Regula pastoralis* II,VI,22.

84. Id., *Epistola* XI, 64 (*Ad Augustinum Anglorum episcopum*).

85. Cf. id., *Epistola* I, 47 (*Ad Virgilium Arelatensem, et Theodorum Massiliensem episcopum*).

86. **Denziger** (ed.), *Enchiridion*, no.1828.

87. **Gregory the Great**, *Epistola* VIII, 30 (*Ad Eulogium episcopum Alexandrinum*).

88. **M. Luther**, *Supputatio annorum mundi* (1541, 1545), in *Werke*, Vol.53, Weimar 1920, 142: '*Gregorius magnus ultimus Episcopus Romanae Ecclesiae, sequentes sunt Papae, id est Pontifices Romanae Curiae.*'

89. **Ullmann**, *Short History of the Papacy* (n.39), 58.

90. Cf. **H. Stieglecker**, *Die Glaubenslehren des Islam*, Paderborn 1956–62.

91. Cf. **H. Pirenne**, *Mahomet et Charlemagne*, Paris 1937.

92. Cf. **D. B. Macdonald**, 'Djihad', in A. J. Wensinck and J. H. Kramers (eds.), *Handwörterbuch des Islam*, Leiden 1976, 112; **W. Ende**, 'Heiliger Krieg', in K. Kreiser and R. Wielandt (eds.), *Lexikon der Islamischen Welt*, Stuttgart 1992, 122. Further literature is given in connection with the Crusades.

93. Cf. **H. Küng**, *Judaism*, I B 1 'The Central Structural Elements'.

94. For a comparison between the Crusades and the *jihad* see **A. Noth**, *Heiliger Krieg und Heiliger Kampf in Islam und Christentum. Beiträge zur Geschichte und Vorgeschichte der Kreuzzüge*, Bonn 1966; **K. Armstrong**, *Holy War*, London 1988; **P. Willemart**, *Pour Jérusalem. Croisade et djihâd*,

1099–1187, Paris 1988; **E. Weber** and **G. Reynaud**, *Croisade d'hier, djihâd d'aujourd'hui. Théorie et pratique de la violence dans les rapports entre l'Occident chrétien et l'Orient mussulman*, Paris 1989. I want to go more closely into the problems of holy war, religion and violence in the third volume of my trilogy (on Islam).

95. For the further historical development cf. **H. Zimmermann**, *Das Mittelalter*, I, *Von den Anfängen bis zum Ende des Investiturstreits*, Brunswick 1975.

96. Cf. **A. de Vogüé**, 'Benedikt von Nursia', *TRE* V, 538–49; **K. S. Frank**, 'Benedikt von Nursia', in M. Greschat (ed.), *Gestalten der Kirchengeschichte*, Vol.III, Stuttgart 1983, 35–46; **B. Jasper**, *Die Regula Benedicti – Regula Magistri – Kontroverse*, Hildesheim 1975.

97. There are many biographies of **Charlemagne**, but there is no more recent generally recognized one which meets scholarly requirements. For the ecclesiastical-theological aspect of his activity cf. **É. Amann**, *L'époque carolingienne*, Paris 1947; **E. Ewig**, with his contributions in H. Jedin and J. Dolan (eds.), *History of the Church*, Vol.III, Chs.1–4, 10–23; **P. Classen**, *Karl der Grosse, das Papsttum und Byzanz. Die Begründung des karolingischen Kaisertums*, Sigmaringen 1888; **A. Angenendt**, *Das Frühmittelalter. Die abendlandische Christenheit von 400 bis 900*, Stuttgart 1990. New literature is also listed in **R. Schneider**, 'Karl der Grosse', *TRE* XVII, 644–9.

98. Cf. the precise analysis of the first coronation of the emperor by the Pope in **Ullmann**, *Short History of the Papacy* (n.39), 81–95.

99. Cf. **J. A. Jungmann**, *Missarum Sollemnia*, Parts 1 and 2 of which deal with the mass over the centuries and in the context of the church community, while Parts 3 and 4 discuss the course of the ritual with its individual elements.

100. **H. Hucke**, 'Gregorianischer Gesang', *Das grosse Lexikon der Musik*, 356–63: 357.

101. Ibid., 358.

102. Ibid., 362, with references to Hucke's own works and those of other researchers into Gregorian chant. Because Helmut Hucke and I were students together in Rome in 1954/55, I became familiar with the sensational reorientation of this branch of musical research from a very early stage.

103. **Jungmann**, 'Die Abwehr des germanischen Arianismus' (n.69), 21f.

104. After the basic research of **P. Anciaux, P. Galtier** and above all (after many preliminary studies) **B. Poschmann**, *Busse und Letzte Ölung*, Freiburg 1951, see now **H. Vorgrimler**, *Busse und Krankensalbung*, Freiburg ²1978; **K.-J. Klär**, *Das kirchliche Bussinstitut von den Anfängen bis zum Konzil von Trient*, Frankfurt 1991 (with a special emphasis on the mutual forgiveness of Christians not involving ministers).

105. There are collections of penitentiaries by **H. Wasserschleben** and **H. J. Schmitz**; cf. **C. Vogel**, *Les Libri paenitentiales*, Turnhout 1978; id., *Le pécheur et la pénitence au moyen âge*, Paris 1969.

106. **Vorgrimler**, *Busse und Krankensalbung* (n.104), 97.

107. **J. G. Ziegler**, *Die Ehelehre der Pönitentialsummen von 1200–1350. Eine Untersuchung zur Geschichte der Moral– und Pastoraltheologie*, Regensburg 1956, 169.

108. For what follows see the summary of historical research in **Angenendt**, *Das Frühmittelalter* (n.97), 345f. There is much material on the restrictions on the consummation of marriage and the demonization of the sexual in **Ziegler**, *Ehelehre* (n.107), Part IV.

109. For criticism of these views from the Catholic side see **S. H. Pfürtner,** *Kirche und Sexualität,* Hamburg 1972; **id.,** *Sexualfeindschaft und Macht. Eine Streitschrift für verantwortete Freiheit in der Kirche,* Mainz 1992; **G. Denzler,** *Die verbotene Lust.* 200 *Jahre christliche Sexualmoral,* Munich 1988.

110. Cf. **P. Hinschius** (ed.), *Decretales Pseudo-Isidorianae et Capitula Angilramni,* Leipzig 1863.

111. Cf. *Pseudoclementinen I, Homilien,* ed. B. Rehm, in Die griechischen christlichen Schriftsteller der ersten Jahrhunderte 42, 1953, 5–22.

112. Cf. **H. Fuhrmann,** *Einfluss und Verbreitung der pseudoisidorischen Fälschungen. Von ihrem Auftauchen bis in die neuere Zeit* (3 vols.), Stuttgart 1972–74; **id.,** 'Constitutum Constantini', *TRE* VIII, 196–202. The theologian **Y. Congar,** *L'ecclésiologie du haut moyen-âge. De Saint Grégoire le Grand à la deéunion entre Byzance et Rome,* Paris 1968, 226–32, is more perceptive in his analysis than many historians.

113. Cf. **H. Fuhrmann,** *Einladung ins Mittelalter,* Munich ³1988.

114. Ibid., 200.

115. Ibid., 202.

116. Ibid., 205.

117. The International Congress of Monumenta Germaniae Historia in Munich in 1986 on 'Forgeries in the Middle Ages' (cf. *Fälschungen im Mittelalter,* Hanover 1988, the proceedings of the congress) led to five volumes of around 750 pages, with more than 150 contributions; an index volume apppeared in 1990.

118. Remembering enjoyable discussions in the 1960s, which were also helpful to me, my then Tübingen colleague Horst Fuhrmann may perhaps understand the theological urgency of my historical and theological questions.

119. **Fuhrmann,** *Einladung* (n.113), 210.

120. Ibid., 214.

121. Ibid., 221.

122. Ibid., 219.

123. At the end of his book, **W. Speyer,** *Die literarische Fälschung im heidnischen und christlichen Altertum. Ein Versuch ihrer Deutung,* Munich 1971, draws attention to the 'modern criticism of authenticity', which 'above all shakes the church-political claims to power made both by the churches of Byzantium and Rome and by certain orders' (312).

124. **F. X. Seppelt,** *Geschichte der Päpste* II, Munich ²1955, 238.

125. Cf. **Fuhrmann,** *Einladung* (n.113), 220: 'Any closed system, any totalitarian society, examines above all differences in content from official doctrine; its formal and material correctness is ultimately secondary.'

126. Ibid., 196.

127. Cf. **H. Küng,** *Structures,* VII 6, 'Questions of Human Rights'.

128. **Congar,** *L'ecclésiologie du haut moyen–âge* (n.112), 230.

129. **Ullmann,** *Short History of the Papacy* (n.39), 109.

130. 'Saeculum obscurum': to give just two illustrations for no less than twenty popes between 896 and 963: Stephen VI (896/7) had his predecessor Formosus, who had only been buried for nine months, exhumed and set upon a throne in papal garments; Formosus was put on trial, had the finger of the right hand with which he had given the blessing hacked off, and was finally thrown into the Tiber. Thereupon Stephen himself was thrown into prison by a furious mob which invaded the Lateran, and was strangled by paid murderers. Or there was the reign of terror under the 'Senatrix' Marozia, who, tradition has it, was the

mistress of a Pope (Sergius III). She was the murderess of a second Pope (John X) and the mother of a third (her illegitimate son John XI), whom she kept captive in Castel Sant'Angelo until she herself was imprisoned on her third marriage by her legitimate son Alberic. He ruled Rome from 933 to 954 as '*Dux et senator Romanorum*', and the Popes of this time were his impotent tools.

131. Cf. **Zimmermann**, *Papstabsetzungen des Mittelalters* (n.39), Ch.V, appendices I and II.

132. For the Cluniac reform cf. **E. Sackur**, *Die Cluniacenser in ihrer kirchlichen und allgemeingeschichtlichen Wirksamkeit bis zur Mitte des 11.Jahrhunderts* (2 vols.), Halle 1892/94, Darmstadt [2]1971; **G. de Valous**, *Le monachisme clunisien des origines au XVe siècle. Vie intérieure des monastères et organisation de l'ordre* (2 vols.), Paris 1935, [2]1970; **A. Chagny**, *Cluny et son Empire*, Lyons [4]1949; **K. Hallinger**, *Gorze-Kluny. Studien zu den monastischen Lebensformen und Gegensätzen im Hochmittelalter* (2 vols.), Rome 1950–51; **E. Werner**, *Die gesellschaftlichen Grundlagen der Klosterreform im 11. Jahrhundert*, Berlin 1953; **A. Brackmann**, *Zur politischen Bedeutung der kluniazensischen Bewegung*, Darmstadt 1955; **G. Tellenbach** (ed.), *Neue Forschungen über Cluny und die Cluniacenser*, Freiburg 1959 (contributions by J. Wolasch, H.-E. Mager, H. Diener); **B. Bligny**, *L'Église et les ordres religieux dans le royaume de Bourgogne aux XIe et XIIe siècles*, Paris 1960; **H. E. J. Cowdrey**, *The Cluniacs and the Gregorian Reform*, Oxford 1970; **N. Hunt** (ed.), *Cluniac Monasticism in the Central Middle Ages*, London 1971; **N. Bulst**, *Untersuchungen zu den Klosterreformen Wilhelms von Dijon (962–1031)*, Bonn 1973; **J. Wollasch**, *Mönchtum des Mittelalters zwischen Kirche und Welt*, Munich 1973; **H. Richter** (ed.), *Cluny. Beiträge zur Gestalt und Wirkung der cluniazensischen Reform*, Darmstadt 1975; **R. G. Heath**, Crux imperatorum philosophia: *Imperial Horizons of the Cluniac Confraternitas, 964–110*, Pittsburgh 1976; **M. Pacaut**, *L'ordre de Cluny (909–1789)*, Paris 1986; **J. Köhler**, *Politik und Spiritualität. Das Kloster Hirsau im Zentrum mittelalterlichen Reformbewegungen*, Munich 1991.

133. The Oxford historian **H. E. J. Cowdrey**, *The Cluniacs and the Gregorian Reform*, seems to me largely to have clarified the question whether the Cluniacs anticipated certain principles and methods of the Gregorians (thus K. Hallinger and A. Brackmann) or did not (E. Sackur, G. Tellenbach), not least through the extremely eloquent and characteristic recognition of Cluny by Gregory VII at the Lenten Synod of 1080, which is usually neglected. In a first phase the papacy created extraordinary freedoms for Cluny (especially from the bishops of Macon and the bishops generally). Conversely, in the second phase Cluny's freedom was the decisive model for the freedom of the church which was to be fought for. Even if there is a broad spectrum of different attitudes among the Cluniacs, Cowdrey has established against the Tellenbach school (and especially H.-E. Mager): 'In all aspects of their work, whether as concentrated upon Cluny itself or as diffused amongst those who in any significant way drew their inspiration from it, it was the general rule that the Cluniacs collaborated whole-heartedly and intimately with successive Popes. In so doing, they were true to the purposes which the Cluny of Abbot Hugh set itself. Thus the reforming Popes were understandably at one in their praise of Cluniac monasticsm, and of its services to the Apostolic See and to the apostles to whom Cluny and the Papacy had a common dedication' (267).

134. According to Rev.2.6.

135. According to Acts 8.18–24.

136. Benedict IX (elected as an eighteen-year old, and morally corrupt) was deposed in Rome. Silvester III (anti-Pope, who resigned in favour of his godson John Gratian for compensation in the sum of 1,000 pounds of silver) was deposed in Sutri. Gregory VI (John Gratian, the third Pope in a year) had to declare himself deposed in Sutri and was banished.

137. Cf. **K.-H. Kandler**, 'Humbert a Silva Candida', in H. Fries and G. Kretschmar (eds.), *Klassiker der Theologie* I, Munich 1981, 150–64. For **Humbert** cf. further **G. Tellenbach**, *Libertas. Kirche und Weltordnung im Zeitalter des Investiturstreites*, Stuttgart 1936; **A. Michel**, *Die Sentenzen des Kardinals Humbert, das erste Rechtsbuch der päpstlichen Reform*, Leipzig 1943; **id.**, 'Die folgenschweren Ideen des Kardinals Humbert und ihr Einfluss auf Gregor VII', in *Studi Gregoriani per la storia di Gregorio VII e della riforma Gregoriana*, ed. G. B. Borino, Vol.I, Rome 1947, 65–92; **K. H. Kandler**, *Die Abendmahlslehre des Kardinals Humbert und ihre Bedeutung für das gegenwärtige Abendmahlsgespräch*, Berlin 1971.

138. For Hildebrand/Gregory VII (Gregorian reform), in addition to the relevant sections in the histories of the papacy cf. **L. F. J. Meulenberg**, *Der Primat der römischen Kirche im Denken und Handeln Gregors VII*, The Hague 1965; **F. Kempf**, 'The Gregorian Reform' and 'Changes within the Christian West during the Gregorian Reform', in H. Jedin and J. Dolan (eds.), *History of the Church* III, New York and London 1980, 351–403, 426–72; **G. Miccoli**, *Chiesa Gregoriana*, Florence 1966; **C. Schneider**, *Prophetisches Sacerdotium und heilsgeschichtliches Regnum im Dialog 1073–1077. Zur Geschichte Gregors VII und Heinrichs IV*, Munich 1972; **P. E. Hübinger**, *Die letzten Worte Papst Gregors VII*, Opladen 1973; **A. Nitschke**, 'Gregor VII', in *Die Grossen der Weltgeschichte*, ed. K. Fassmann, III, Zurich 1973, 268–81; cf. also Nitschke's articles in *Studi Gregoriani*, V and IX; **R. Morghen**, *Gregorio VII e la riforma della Chiesa nel secolo XI*, Palermo 1974; **H. Zimmermann**, *Der Canossagang von 1077. Wirkung und Wirklichkeit*, Wiesbaden 1975; **J. Vogel**, *Gregor VII. und Heinrich IV. nach Canossa. Zeugnisse ihres Selbstverständnisses*, Berlin 1983; **G. M. Cantarella** (ed.), *Il Papa ed il Sovrano. Gregorio VII ed Enrico IV nella lotta per le investiture*, Novara 1985; **P. G. Caron** et al., *La preparazione della riforma Gregoriana e del pontificato di Gregorio VII*, Fonte Avellana 1985. It is illuminating to see how **G. Tellenbach**, *Die westliche Kirche vom 10. bis zum frühen 12. Jahrhundert*, Göttingen 1988, works out the presuppositions and consequences of the 'shift in church history'. Numerous individual aspects of the history of Gregory VII and the Gregorian Reform are treated in the series of articles edited by **G. B. Borino**, *Studi Gregoriani per la storia di Gregorio VII e della riforma Gregoriana*, Rome 1947ff.

139. **Fuhrmann**, *Einladung* (n.113), 87.

140. **Y. Congar**, 'Der Platz des Papsttums in der Kirchenfrömmigkeit der Reformer des 11. Jahrhunderts', in J. Daniélou and H. Vorgrimler (eds.), *Sentire Ecclesiam. Das Bewusstsein von der Kirche als gestaltende Kraft der Frömmigkeit*, Freiburg 1961, 196–217: 196. I am grateful to the most significant ecumenical figure in France, Yves Congar, with whom I was allowed to work during the Second Vatican Council and then for decades in *Concilium*, the international theological journal, for drawing my attention at a very early stage to the significance of the revolution in the eleventh century. Cf. also his magisterial work *L'Église de saint Augustin á l'epoque moderne*, Paris 1970, esp. Ch.V on 'La réforme du XIᵉ siècle (saint Gregoire VII), tournant ecclésiologique'.

141. **Ullmann**, *Short History of the Papacy* (n.39), 140f.

142. **Congar**, 'Der Platz des Papsttums' (n.40), 215.

143. **E. Caspar** (ed.), *Das Register Gregors VII*, Vol.II, fasc.1–2, Berlin ²1955, 201–8, provides a critical edition of the original Latin version. There is a commentary in **K. Hofmann**, *Der 'Dictatus Papae' Gregors VII. Eine rechtsgeschichtliche Erklärung*, Paderborn 1933.

144. Cf. **Hofmann**, *Der 'Dictatus Papae'* (n.143), 14–24; **Y. Congar**, 'Der Platz des Papsttums', 204; **A. Fliche**, *La réforme grégorienne et la reconquête chrétienne (1057–1123)*, Paris 1950, 79.

145. Cf. **G. B. Borino**, 'Un'ipotesi sul "Dictatus Papae" di Gregorio VII', *Archivio della R.Deputazione Romana di storia patria* 67, 1944, 237–52. This argument follows **K. Hofmann**, 'Der "Dictatus Papae" Gregors VII. als Index einer Kanonessammlung?', in G. B. Borino (ed.), *Studi Gregoriani* I, Rome 1947, 51–7 (similarly S.Kuttner, P. Feine, P. E. Schramm, W. Ullmann, etc.).

146. Cf. **H. Fuhrmann**, 'Papst Gregor VII. und das Kirchenrecht. Zur Problem des *Dictatus Papae*', *Studi Gregoriani* XIII, Rome 1989, 123–50.

147. However, Gregory's thesis of a **personal sanctity of the Pope** on the basis of the merits of Peter failed to become established: presumably it could have been used all too easily against the legitimacy of a Pope. Instead of this, even in Rome the old doctrine was maintained that even a Pope could be heretical and moreover could be judged by the church. Gregory himself in fact spoke only of a Roman church free of error and not of a Roman Pope free of error.

148. That also applies to the new Latin-German edition of Denziger by **P. Hünermann** (³⁷1991), already mentioned, which quotes only seventeen lines (the confession of faith required of Berengarius of Tours) for the epoch-making figure Gregory VII, while giving John Paul II around 80 pages up to 1988!

149. This text is based on my own translation.

150. This is very well depicted in the portrait of Gregory by **A. Nitschke**, 'Gregor VII'.

151. For the **investiture dispute** see the German-Latin collection of sources by **F.-J. Schmale** and **I. Schmale-Ott** (eds.), *Quellen zum Investiturstreit* (2 vols.), Darmstadt 1978–84. Also **W.von den Steinen**, *Canossa, Heinrich IV. und die Kirche*, Munich 1957; **N. F. Cantor**, *Church, Kingship, and Lay Investiture in England 1089–1135*, Princeton, NJ 1958; **H.-G. Krause**, *Das Papstwahldekret von 1059 und seine Rolle im Investiturstreit*, Studi Gregoriani VII, Rome 1960; **H. Kämpf** (ed.), *Canossa als Wende. Ausgewählte Aufsätze zur neueren Forschung*, Darmstadt 1963; **O. Capitani**, *Immunità vescovili ed ecclesiologia in età 'pregregoriana' e 'gregoriana'. L'avvio alla restaurazione*, Spoleto 1966; **J. Deér** (ed.), *Das Papsttum und die süditalienischen Normannenstaaten 1053–1212*, Göttingen 1969; **J. Ziese**, *Historische Beweisführung in Streitschriften des Investiturstreites*, Munich 1972; **J.Fleckenstein** (ed.), *Investiturstreit und Reichsverfassung*, Sigmaringen 1973; **E. Werner**, *Zwischen Canossa und Worms. Staat und Kirche 1077–1122*, Berlin 1973; **H. Fuhrmann**, *Deutsche Geschichte im hohen Mittelalter von der Mitte des 11. bis zum Ende des 12.Jahrhunderts*, Göttingen 1978, ²1983; **M. Minninger**, *Von Clermont zum Wormser Konkordat. Die Auseinandersetzungen um den Lehnsnexus zwischen König und Episkopat*, Cologne 1978; **K. F. Morrison** (ed.), *The Investiture Controversy. Issues, Ideals, and Results*, New York 1978; **I. S. Robinson**, *Authority and Resistance in the Investiture Contest. The Polemical Literature of the Late Eleventh Century*, Manchester 1978; id., *The Papacy 1073–1198:*

Continuity and Innovation, Cambridge 1990; **R. Schieffer**, *Die Enstehung des päpstlichen Investiturverbots für den deutschen König*, Stuttgart 1981; **U.-R. Blumenthal**, *Der Investiturstreit*, Stuttgart 1982; **J. Vogel**, *Gregor VII. und Heinrich IV. nach Canossa. Zeugnisse ihres Selbstverständnisses*, Berlin 1983; **J. Laudage**, *Priesterbild und Reformpapsttum im 11.Jh.*, Cologne 1984; **id.**, *Der Investiturstreit. Quellen und Materialien*, Cologne 1989; **id.**, *Gregorianische Reform und Investiturstreit*, Darmstadt 1993; **K. Pennington**, *Popes and Bishops. The Papal Monarchy in the Twelfth and Thirteenth Centuries*, Philadelphia 1984; **B. Szabó-Bechstein**, *Libertas ecclesiae. Ein Schlüsselbegriff des Investiturstreits und seine Vorgeschichte (4.–11.Jh.)*, Rome 1985; **W. Goez**, 'Investiturstreit', *TRE* XVI, 237–47; **M. Stroll**, *Symbols as Power. The Papacy following the Investiture Contest*, Leiden 1991; **J. Miethke** and **A. Bühler**, *Kaiser und Papst im Konflikt. Zum Verhältnis von Staat und Kirche im späten Mittelalter*, Düsseldorf 1988; **C. Morris**, *The Papal Monarchy. The Western Church from 1050 to 1250*, Oxford 1989; **R. Somerville**, *Papacy, Councils and Canon Law in the 11th–12th Centuries*, Aldershot 1990; **S. Beulertz**, *Das Verbot der Laieninvestitur im Investiturstreit 1077–1123*, Hanover 1991. **W. Hartmann**, *Der Investiturstreit*, Munich 1993, gives a good survey of the present state of research.

152. This epoch-making controversy between Pope and king was reconstructed with historical accuracy in all its dramatic phases by the Tübingen historian of the papacy, **J. Haller**, *Das Papsttum. Idee und Wirklichkeit* II, Urach 1951, new edition Darmstadt 1962, in the brilliant chapter on Gregory VII, 365–430: 387. **Zimmermann**, *Der Canossagang* (n.151), clears up some important points on the basis of a scrupulous investigation of the sources.

153. **Fuhrmann**, *Einladung* (n.113), 83.

154. **F. X. Seppelt**, *Geschichte der Päpste* III, Munich 1956, 321.

155. I feel that this analysis of the **dominant** structures (there are of course always opposing factors) is confirmed by **Y. Congar**, *Die Lehre von der Kirche. Von Augustinus bis zum abendländischen Schisma*, Freiburg 1971, who writes this on the 'ecclesiological shift' in the eleventh century: 'For its part, Latin ecclesiology followed the course that we shall be indicating: the development of papal authority, legalism, clericalization, the challenge from the secular power which led the church to understand itself as a power' (60f.).

156. **M. Maccarrone**, 'I fondamenti "petrini" del primato romano in Gregorio VII', in *Studi Gregoriani* XIII, Rome 1989, 55–122: 122, ' . . .*beatum Petrum, apostolorum principem, esse omnium christianorum patrem et primum post Christum pastorem, sanctamque Romanam aecclesiam omnium aeccclesiarum matrem et magistram.*'

157. For **Innocent III** cf. the articles in *LThK* (**F. Kempf**), *EncRel* (**K. Pennington**), *TRE* (**G. Schwaiger**); also **C. E. Smith**, *Innocent III Church Defender*, Baton Rouge 1951; **F. Kempf**, *Papsttum und Kaisertum bei Innocenz III. Die geistigen und rechtlichen Grundlagen seiner Thronstreitpolitik*, Rome 1954; **id.**, 'Innocenz III', in M. Greschat (ed). *Das Papsttum I. Von den Anfängen bis zu den Päpsten in Avignon*, Stuttgart 1985, 196–207; **H. Tillmann**, *Papst Innocenz III.*, Bonn 1954; **H. Wolter**, 'The Papacy at the Height of its Power (1198–1216)', in H. Jedin and J. Dolan (eds.), *A History of the Church* IV, New York and London 1980, chs.18–24; **H. Roscher**, *Papst Innocenz III. und die Kreuzzüge*, Göttingen 1969; **M. Maccarrone**, *Studi su Innocenzo III*, Padua 1972; **C. R. Cheney**, *Pope Innocent III and England*, Stuttgart 1976; **M. Laufs**,

Politik und Recht bei Innozenz III. Kaiserprivilegien, Thronstreitregister und Egerer Goldbulle in der Reichs- und Rekuperationspolitik Papst Innozenz' III, Cologne 1980; **W. Imkamp**, *Das Kirchenbild Innozenz' III (1198–1216)*, Stuttgart 1983.

158. **Y. Congar**, 'Titel, welche für den Papst verwendet werden', *Concilium* 11, 1975, 538–44: 541 (never published in English); there is yet more here on the monopolizing of the titles.

159. Quotation from **Kempf**, 'Innozenz III.' (n.156), 197.

160. As 'Christ's representative', the 'king of kings, ruler of rulers, priest for ever after the order of Melchizedek', Innocent thought that he could rule and intervene everywhere – often rash in his claim to biblical legitimation. For example, he could see the divine throne of the Apocalypse (4.6–11) as the Holy See and the four beings around the throne as the four patriarchates, ready to serve like maids serving their mistress: 'How far such exegetical escapades impressed contemporaries can no longer be assessed, but certainly the basic principles which Innocent quite clearly laid down for the papal primacy of jurisdiction and energetically put into practice, came to have abiding significance, and were only freed from their one-sidedness by the Second Vatican Council', thus **F. Kempf SJ** (a church historian at the Gregoriana), *Innozenz III.*, 198.

161. **W. Inkamp**, *Das Kirchenbild Innocenz' III (1198–1216)*, Stuttgart 1983, 324.

162. Ibid.

163. For the Fourth Lateran Council see the decrees in **J. Alberigo** et al. (eds.), *Conciliorum oecumenicorum decreta*, Freiburg 1962, 203–47. For the history of the Lateran synods cf. **R. Foreville**, *Latran I, II, III et Latran IV*, Paris 1965; **Wolter**, 'Papacy' (n.157), Ch.22.

164. Cf. *Constitutiones*, 67–70.

165. Cf. **H. Küng**, *Judaism*, I C IV 8: 'Christian persecutions of the Jews and the "reasons" for them'. The anti-Judaism prompted by the election of Anacletus, who came from a Jewish family, as Pope, is illuminating; cf. **M. Stroll**, *The Jewish Pope. Ideology and Politics in the Papal Schism 1130*, Leiden 1987.

166. The *Decretum Gratiani* forms the first part of the *Corpus Iuris Canonici*, ed. **E. Friedberg** (1879), I, reprinted Graz 1955. For Gratian and classic canon law cf. **J. Gaudemet**, *La formation du droit canonique médiéval*, London 1980; **S. Kuttner**, *Gratian and the Schools of Law*, 1140–1234, London 1983, and the relevant sections in the canon law histories by **H. E. Feine** and **W. M. Plöchl**.

167. **Ullmann**, *Short History of the Papacy* (n.39), Ch.10, 'Central Government and the Papal Curia', 201–6, gives an impressive description of the tremendous degree of centralization and legalization.

168. There is still a separate canon law faculty alongside the philosophical and theological faculties at, say, the Pontifical Gregorian University (and a separate Canon Law Institute at the University of Munich, which has the right to award doctorates).

169. **Bernard of Clairvaux**, *De consideratione libri quinque ad Eugenium III*, Book IV, ch.3.

170. Cf. ibid.

171. Bishops well disposed to the Curia are dispensed from observing the age limit of seventy-five solemnly laid down by the Second Vatican Council, while conciliar bishops have to go at seventy-five.

172. Bernard's strong, centralistic Cistercian order (the first order in the strict sense to have 500 monasteries by the end of the twelfth century) had replaced as spiritual leader the highly aristocratic Cluny, which had developed throughout Europe into a rich, well-organized land-owning concern with the best agricultural land, but was less intent on direct political action than on spiritual, ascetic and mystical deepening (meditation on the cross). After the complete failure of the Second Crusade, to which Bernard of Clairvaux had issued a personal summons, and his death in 1153, there was a reaction against the domination of the clergy all over Europe.

173. After Barbarossa's defeat by the Lombards (the treachery of Henry of Louvain), **Alexander III** was able to establish himself as the rightful Pope in the face of Barbarossa, who wanted to regain the old position of the German emperor, and his three successive anti-Popes, though for many years he had to take refuge in France. He compelled the second most powerful ruler in Europe, Henry II of Anjou-Plantagenet, the ruler of England and the greater part of France, to submit to the penance of being scourged on the tomb of his deadly enemy, Archbishop Thomas à Becket of Canterbury, who had been murdered by Norman knights, in order to be released from the papal ban following from this 'murder in the cathedral'. After long years of banishment Alexander also regained control of Rome and in triumph celebrated the third ecumenical Lateran Synod of 1179, where in order to avoid future schisms he first of all decreed a two-thirds majority for papal elections (which is still required today). He reserved beatifications, which from the end of the tenth century had been within the Pope's competence, exclusively for the Popes. About a fifth of all the papal decretals before 1200 known to us fall in Alexander's pontificate. His almost 4,500 decretals put Gratian's theory of law into living, enforceable law. No wonder that this political Pope, too, was unpopular in Rome; he soon had to leave Rome again because of the anti-papal mood of hostility and died in Civitas Castellana.

174. **Kempf**, 'Innocenz III.' (n.156), 198. Kempf, who attributes a 'monistic impetus' at least to Gregory VII, then makes a great (but not very convincing) effort to combine in a 'unity in tension' Innocent's ambitions in world politics, which in contrast to Gregory's were real-political and diplomatic, with a 'wide-ranging recognition of the claim of worldly rulers to autonomy'; the dissertation by his pupil L. F. J. Meulenberg on Gregory VII, mentioned above, takes the same apologetic line, in acknowledged contradiction to the leading scholars A. Fliche, E. Voosen, G. Tellenbach, J. Haller, R. Morghen and W. Ullmann. Kempf's interpretation, presented on various occasions, was criticized at a very early stage by **H. Barion** in *Zeitschrift für Rechtsgeschichte*, Kanonistische Abteilung 46, 1960, 481-501. Cf. **J. Haller**'s long chapter on Innocent in *Das Papsttum. Idee und Wirklichkeit*, Vol. III, Urach 1952, new edition Darmstadt 1962, 296–480, and **H. E. Feine**, *Kirchliche Rechtsgeschichte. Die katholische Kirche*, Cologne [4]1964, 27–30. In the most recent report on research (1993), **Hartmann**, *Investiturstreit* (n.151), 96, maintains against Kempf Ullmann's assessment 'that Gregory VIII strove for a pre-eminence of the papacy in secular matters as well, and that this notion had an influence through Innocent III up to Boniface VIII'.

175. **Feine**, *Rechtsgeschichte* (n.174), 300. Innocent III in principle regarded all secular rulers as papal liegemen, whom he could appoint and, if necessary, also depose again. A man of towering intellect, who was never at a loss for a scholastic or legal argument, he was also able to justify and establish by decretals that while the Pope did not have a direct right to a say in the election of the German king, he

did in the bestowing of the dignity of emperor, which was an 'apostolic' grace and dependent on the fulfilment of certain conditions. In the dispute over the German throne, through skilful diplomacy he gained a concession from each of the combatants at the expense of the other, not only to secure the 'freedom of the church' from all political force but also to guarantee it – going far beyond the compromise of the Concordat of Worms.

176. The lamented symptoms of decay are often the subject of mediaeval parody, which usually comes from the clergy. Cf. **P. Lehmann**, *Die Parodie im Mittelalter*, Stuttgart ²1963, esp.25–93 ('Die kritisierende, streitende und triumphierende Parodie'). The twenty-four select parodies included in the appendix include the famous Gospel of Money.

177. Jer.48.10. In both form and content this prose verse falls outside the framework of the poem, and in the view of some exegetes is to be understood as an outbreak of emotion from a reader for whom the later hatred against Moab took such a sharp form. Cf. **A. Weiser**, *Das Buch des Propheten Jeremia*, 25.15–52.34, Göttingen 1966, 405f.

178. For the **Crusades** cf. **C. Erdmann**, *Die Enstehung des Kreuzzugsgedankens*, Stuttgart 1935, reprinted 1955; **S. Runciman**, *A History of the Crusades* (3 vols.), Cambridge 1951–54; **J. Richard**, *Le Royaume latin de Jérusalem*, Paris 1963; id., *Croisades et états latins d'Orient. Points de vue et documents*, Aldershot 1992; **K. M. Setton** et al. (eds.), *A History of the Crusades* (6 vols), Philadelphia 1955–89; id., *The Papacy and the Levant (1204–1571)* (4 vols.), Philadelphia 1976–84; **A. Waas**, *Geschichte der Kreuzzüge* (2 vols.), Freiburg 1967: **F. Gabrieli** (ed.), *Storici arabi delle crocciate*, 1957; **H. E. Mayer**, *Geschichte der Kreuzzüge*, Stuttgart 1965, ⁷1989; id., *Kreuzzüge und lateinischer Osten*, London 1983; **E. Sivan**, *L'Islam et la Croisade. Idéologie et propagande dans les réactions musulmanes aux Croisades*, Paris 1968; **J. Prawer**, *Histoire du royaume latin de Jérusalem* (original in Hebrew, 2 vols.), Paris 1969f.; **M. Purcell**, *Papal Crusading Policy. The Chief Instruments of Papal Crusading Policy and Crusade to the Holy Land from the Final Loss of Jerusalem to the Fall of Acre 1244–1291*, Leiden 1975; **T. P. Murphy** (ed.), *The Holy War*, Columbus 1976; **R. C. Schwinges**, *Kreuzzugsideologie und Toleranz. Studien zu Wilhelm von Tyrus*, Stuttgart 1977; **E. D. Hehl**, *Kirche und Krieg im 12. Jahrhundert. Studien zu kanonische Recht und politischer Wirklichkeit*, Stuttgart 1980; **R.** and **J. Riley-Smith**, *The Crusades. Idea and Reality, 1095–1274*, London 1981; **R. Penoud**, *Les hommes de la Croisade*, Paris 1982; **P. Rousset**, *La croisade. Histoire d'une idéologie*, Lausanne 1983; **B. Z. Kedar**, *Crusade and Mission. European Approaches towards the Muslim*, Princeton 1984; **E. Siberry**, *Criticism of Crusading 1095–1274*, Oxford 1985; **J. Riley-Smith**, *The First Crusade and the Idea of Crusading*, London 1986; id., *The Crusades. A Short History*, London 1987; **R. Chazan**, *European Jewry and the First Crusade*, Berkeley 1987; **A. Dupront**, *Du Sacré. Croisades et pélérinages, images et langages*, Paris 1987; **R. Delort** (ed.), *Les croisades*, Paris 1988: **J. A. Brundage**, *The Crusades, Holy War and Canon Law*, Hampshire 1991; **P. J. Cole**, *The Preaching of the Crusades to the Holy Land, 1095–1270*, Cambridge 1991; **S. Schein**, Fideles Crucis. *The Papacy, the West and the Recovery of the Holy Land, 1274–1314*, Oxford 1991; **J. Flori**, *La première croisade. L'Occident chrétien contre l'Islam*, Brussels 1992; **B. N. Sargent-Baur** (ed.), *Journeys Toward God. Pilgrimage and Crusade*, Kalamazoo, 1992. '*Militia Christi* e Crociata nei secoli XI–XIII' was also the

theme of a study week in Mendola (the proceedings were published: Milan 1992).
179. Cf. **Bernard of Clairvaux,** *De laude novae militae ad milites templi,* *Opera omnia,* Paris 1862, I, 921–40,
180. The French historian **J. Flori,** *La première croisade* (n.178), makes an important contribution to the history of the mentality of this time; in the part on 'Ideologies' (107–217) he works out carefully the different elements of the 'idéologie occidentale' which was now forming in controversy with Islam.
181. The **First Crusade** itself stems from the appeal of a Pope, Urban II. At the Synod of Clermont in 1095, in response to a request from the Byzantine emperor Alexius I Comnenus for support against the Turks, he called on the nobility and knights of France – young, strong men – to take a vow to go on pilgrimage with the aim of liberating both the Eastern Christians and the Holy Sepulchre of the Redeemer from the Muslims. Presumably the Pope himself was surprised that around 90,000 Crusaders (though only around eight per cent of these were nobles and knights) heeded his call; though decimated, amazingly they conquered Jerusalem on 15 July 1099. This was the only Crusade to achieve its military aim and found Crusader states: the kingdom of Jerusalem and the feudal states of Antioch, Odessa and Tripolis, which immediately became a bone of contention among the European powers.
182. This has been well brought out by **Riley-Smith,** *The First Crusade* (n.178).
183. In the Stedinger Crusade by the Archbishop of Bremen against his own peasants (to collect the church tithe), in the Crusades of the papacy against Emperor Frederick II and later against Frederick's son Conrad IV, and in the wars against the Hussites of Bohemia. Moreover, as **Schein,** *Fideles Crucis* (n.178), shows, the Popes for a long time continued to pursue the idea of a new Crusade to conquer the Holy Land (thus Clement V and the Council of Vienne, 1311/12).
184. Cf. **Siberry,** *Criticism of Crusading* (n.178).
185. Thus already during the Second Vatican Council the Vienna pastoral theologian **M. Pfliegler** summed up the German petition in a critical forerunner to the post-conciliar Catholic critiques of celibacy, *Der Zölibat,* which I published in the series Theologische Meditationen, Einsiedeln 1965; this was then followed by a whole series of books criticizing celibacy, including those of **F. Leist** (1968) and **A. Antweiler** (1969). The standard historical work on the question was written by the Catholic church historian from Bamberg, **G. Denzler,** *Das Papsttum und der Amtszölibat,* I–II, Stuttgart 1973/76, short version *Die Geschichte des Zölibats,* Freiburg 1993. This work not only quotes the church documents enforcing celibacy on the clergy in connection with the Gregorian reform, but also shows the tremendous discrimination against the wives of priests, who were still legitimate at the time; one needs only to read the taunts of Peter Damian (58–62), which may be said to be pathological, also to have a better understanding of the political agitation of his fellow cardinal, who later became Pope Gregory VII (64–74). But the countless testimonies to the resistance of the clergy to the Pope and the initially few bishops loyal to Rome, a resistance which was quite general in Germany but ultimately unsuccessful, is also important. Cf. also **A. L. Barstow,** *Married Priests and the Reforming Papacy. The Eleventh-Century Debates,* New York 1982. For the further context cf. **G. Denzler,** *Die verbotene Lust. 2000 Jahre christliche Sexualmoral,* Munich 1988.
186. Cf. **H. Grundmann,** *Ketzergeschichte des Mittelalters,* Göttingen 1963; also **S. Runciman,** *The Medieval Manichee. A Study of the Christian Dualist*

Heresy, Cambridge 1947; **O. Capitani** (ed.), *Medioevo ereticale*, Bologna 1977. Then there is an extensive specialist literature both on the Cathari (O. Aceves, L. Baier, J. Blum, A. Borst, A. Brenon, J. Duvernoy, H. Fichtenau, E. Griffe, J. Lucienne, R. Nelli, D. Roché, E. Roll, M. Roquebert, G. Rottenwöhrer, C. Thouzellier, G. Wild) and the Waldensians (G. Audisio, M. Firpo, G. G. Merlo, A. Molnar, M. Schneider, K. -V. Selge, C. Thouzellier, G. Tourn, V. Vinay). **E. Le Roy Ladurie**, *Montaillou*, Harmondsworth 1990, gives a vivid picture of the actual situation in a village in southern France on the basis of the proceedings of episcopal visitations.

187. Grundmann, *Ketzergeschichte* (n.180), G.31f.: 'For the first time here a community which had been condemned as a heretical sect was won back for the church, in that its religious aims were largely allowed and regulated by novel orders. This is a turning point in the attitude of the Curia to the religious movement and to heresy. Soon after that the Pope also succeeded in reconciling some groups of Waldensians with the church, and this shift also became the presupposition for the rise of the new mendicant orders.' Cf. also the study by **H. Grundmann**, *Religiöse Bewegungen im Mittelalter. Untersuchungen über die geschichtlichen Zusammenhänge zwischen der Ketzerei, den Bettelorden und der religiösen Frauenbewegung im 12. und 13. Jahrhundert und über die geschichtlichen Grundlagen der deutschen Mystik*, Berlin 1935, Darmstadt ²1961.

188. For the **Inquisition** in the Middle Ages, in addition to the histories of canon law by **H. E. Feine, J. Gaudemet** and **W. M. Plöchl** and the extensive specialist literature on the Inquisition in Spain, Italy and southern France, see **H. C. Lea**, *A History of the Inquisition of the Middle Ages* (3 vols.), New York 1887; **L. Förg**, *Die Ketzerverfolgung in Deutschland unter Gregor IX. Ihre Herkunft, ihre Bedeutung und ihre rechtlichen Grundlagen*, Berlin 1932; **J. Guiraud**, *Histoire de l'Inquisition au Moyen Âge* (2 vols.), Paris 1935–8; **J. Vincke**, *Zur Vorgeschichte der spanischen Inquisition*, Bonn 1941; **H. Maisonneuve**, *Études sur les origines de l'Inquisition*, Paris 1942, ²1960; **C. Reviglio della Veneria**, *L'inquisizione medievale ed il processo inquisitorio*, Turin ²1951; **E. van der Vekene**, *Versuch einer Bibliographie der Inquisition*, Luxembourg 1959; id., *Bibliotheca bibliographica historiae Sanctae Inquisitionis. Bibliographisches Verzeichnis des gedruckten Schrifttums zur Geschichte und Literatur der Inquisition* (3 vols.), Vaduz 1982–92 (7110 titles!); **A. S. Turberville**, *Medieval Heresy and the Inquisition*, London 1964; **J. R. Grigulevic**, *Ketzer – Hexen – Inquisitoren. Geschichte der Inquisition, 13–20 Jh.* (Russian original 1970) (2 vols.), Berlin 1976; **J. A. O'Brien**, *The Inquisition*, New York 1973; **E. Le Roy Ladurie**, *Montaillou* (n.186); **R. Kieckhefer**, *Repression of Heresy in Medieval Germany*, Philadelphia 1979; **A. Waingort Novinsky**, *A Inquisiçao*, Sao Paulo 1982; **G. Henningsen** and **J. Tedeschi** (eds.), *The Inquisition in Early Modern Europe. Studies on Sources and Methods*, Dekalb, Ill. 1986; **E. Peters**, *Inquisition*, New York 1988; **A. Dondaine**, *Les hérésies et l'Inquisition, XIIe–XIIIe siecles*, Documents et études, Aldershot 1990; **A. C. Shannon**, *The Medieval Inquisition*, Collegeville, Minn. 1991.

189. Text in **J. Alberigo** et al. (eds.), *Conciliorum oecumenicorum decreta*, 203–46, esp. *Constitutio 3: De haereticis* (209–11). For the Fourth Lateran Council cf. **H. Grundmann**, *Religiöse Bewegungen*, II.4, *Das Laterankonzil 1215*.

190. For the procedure of the present 'Sacred Congregation for the Doctrine of Faith' cf. the correspondence between the author and this Inquisition in **W. Jens** (ed.), *Um nichts als die Wahrheit. Deutsche Bischofskonferenz contra Hans Küng. Eine Dokumentation*, Munich 1976; **N. Greinacher** and **H. Haag** (eds.), *Der Fall Küng. Eine Dokumentation*, Munich 1980.

191. The Inquisition proceedings which are still provided for by law and also constantly take place are one of the main reasons why the Vatican may not subscribe to the European Council's Declaration on Human Rights. The Paris-Brussels journal *Golias*, ed. C. Terras, has an extremely informative 200 page dossier on the 'Nouvelle Inquisition' in its no.35, 1994, issue (including the names of 1000 'suspect' theologians from all over the world).

192. For **Dominic** and the poverty movement in the twelfth and thirteenth centuries see above all **P. Mandonnet**, *St Dominic and His Work*, London 1945, which is still valuable; cf. also **M.-H. Vicaire**, *Histoire de Saint Dominique* (2 vols.), Paris 1957; id., *Dominique et ces Prêcheurs*, Fribourg 1977. Texts on Dominic have been edited by **V. J. Koudelka**, *Die Verkündigung des Wortes*, Munich 1989.

193. **Grundmann**, *Ketzergeschichte* (n.86), G 37.

194. Cf. **H. Delder**, *Die Ideale des hl.Franziskus von Assisi*, Paderborn 1923.

195. Cf. **K. Esser**, *Anfänge und ursprüngliche Zielsetzungen des Ordens der Minderbrüder*, Leiden 1966; for the history of the Franciscan order cf. also **T. Lombardi**, *Introduzione allo studio del Francescanesimo*, Assisi 1975; id., *Storia del Francescanesimo*, Padua 1980.

196. Cf. **H. Feld**, 'Die Totengräber des heiligen Franziskus von Assisi', in E. Boshof (ed.), *Archiv für Kulturgeschichte* 68, Cologne 1986, 319–50; id., 'Franziskus von Assisi als Visionär und Darsteller', in W. Haug and D. Mieth (eds.), *Religiöse Erfahrung. Historische Modelle in christlicher Tradition*, Munich 1992, 125–53; id., *Franziskus von Assisi und seine Bewegung*, Darmstadt 1994, 189–214. I am grateful to Professor **Dr Helmut Feld** for reading this section of the book critically and contributing some improvements.

197. Cf. **P. Sabatier**, *Vie de Saint François d'Assise*, Paris 1894, definitive edition 1931.

198. **E. Benz**, *Ecclesia spiritualis. Kirchenidee und Geschichtstheologie der franziskanischen Reformation*, Stuttgart 1834, esp. Part III, Ch.IV.1: 'Die Umgestaltung der Franziskanerregel und des Franziskanerordens durch die römische Kirche'.

199. Francis of Assisi has prompted not only numerous less known biographers but also **G. K. Chesterton** and **J. Green** to write biographies; they have been followed in the spirit of a new liberating theology by **E. Balducci, L. Boff, A. Holl** and **R. Manselli**. The most recent scholarly accounts are dominated by **A. Rotzetter, W.-C. van Dijk** and **T. Matura**, *Franz von Assisi. Ein Anfang und was davon bleibt*, Zurich 1981, and above all **G. Wendelborn**, *Franziskus von Assisi. Eine historische Darstellung*, Leipzig 1977, along with a brief account by **U. Köpf**, 'Franz von Assisi', in M. Greschat (ed.), *Gestalten der Kirchengeschichte* III, Stuttgart 1983, 282–302.

200. Matt.10.8–10.

201. For Francis, however, this did not mean any real identification with social outsiders (lepers, the poor) or church outsiders. Cf. **Feld**, 'Franziskus von Assisi als Visionär' (n.196), 134–8: the decisive key experience is not the

encounter with the leper but the visionary experience before the crucifix in S. Damiano: he identifies himself with Christ.

202. **Francis of Assisi**, 'Hymn to the Sun'. There is a new critical edition of the text in **K. Esser** (ed.), *Die Opuscula des hl. Franziskus von Assisi*, Grottaferrata 1976, 128f.: 'Sora nostra morte corporale' (129).

203. Remarkably, though, relations with women were tabu (cf. the earlier rule no.12), despite his soul friendship with Clare, his most faithful disciple. However, from the beginning her women's community suffered much from church restrictions; cf. **Feld**, 'Die Totengräber' (n.196), 342–6.

204. **Francis of Assisi**, 'Testamentum', in Esser, *Opuscula* (n.202), 438–44: '*vivere secundum formam sancti Evangelii*' (439).

205. **Feld**, 'Die Totengräber' (n.196), 337–42.

206. Cf. ibid., 330–7.

207. For basic information see **L. Hödl**, 'Anselm von Canterbury', *TRE* II, 759–78; **M. A. Schmidt**, 'Anselm von Canterbury', in M. Greschat (ed.), *Gestalten der Kirchengeschichte* III, 123–47.

208. For example **K. Barth**, *Anselm. Fides Quarens Intellectum* (1931), London 1960.

209. Cf. **H. Küng**, GCT, Ch.4, 'Thomas Aquinas: University Science and Papal Court Theology'. The more recent literature on **Thomas Aquinas** is based on the careful researches of neo-Thomists like J. Berthier, P. Castagnoli, H. Denifle, F. Ehrle, M. Grabmann, P. Mandonnet and A. Walz. The best historical introduction to the work of Thomas is still that by the Frenchman **M. D. Chenu**, *Introduction à l'étude de saint Thomas d'Aquin*, Paris 1950 (revised German ed. *Das Werk des hl. Thomas von Aquin*, Graz 1960, to which page references are given); cf. also id., *Saint Thomas d'Aquin et la théologie*, Paris 1959. The American **J. A. Weisheipl**, *Friar Thomas d'Aquino. His Life, Thought and Works*, New York 1974, is a thorough critical biography based on the most recent state of scholarship. The most illuminating more recent theological introduction against a present-day horizon (and constantly taking Protestant theology into account) is that by the German theologian and former Dominican **O. H. Pesch**, *Thomas von Aquin. Grenze und Grösse mittelalterlichen Theologie. Eine Einführung*, Mainz 1988, ²1989. For further important new literature cf. **J. Pieper**, *Einführung zu Thomas von Aquin. Zwölf Vorlesungen*, Munich 1958; **S. Pfürtner**, *Luther und Thomas im Gespräch. Unser Heil zwischen Gewissheit und Gefährdung*, Heidelberg 1961; **J. B. Metz**, *Christliche Anthropozentrik. Über die Denkform des Thomas von Aquin*, Munich 1962; **M. Seckler**, *Das Heil in der Geschichte. Geschichtstheologisches Denken bei Thomas von Aquin*, Munich 1964; **E. Gilson**, *Le thomisme. Introduction à la philosophie de Saint Thomas d'Aquin*, Paris 1965, ⁶1983; **U. Kühn**, *Via caritatis. Theologie des Gesetzes bei Thomas von Aquin*, Göttingen 1965; **H. Vorster**, *Das Freiheitsverständnis bei Thomas von Aquin und Martin Luther*, Göttingen 1965; **L. Oeing-Hanhoff** (ed.), *Thomas Aquinas 1274/1974*, Munich 1974; **W. Mostert**, *Menschwerdung. Eine historische und dogmatische Untersuchung über das Motiv der Inkarnation des Gottessohnes bei Thomas von Aquin*, Tübingen 1978; **A. Zimmermann** (ed.), *Thomas von Aquin. Werk und Wirkung im Licht neuerer Forschungen*, Berlin 1988.

210. *Codex Iuris Canonici* (1917), canon 1366, 2.

211. The relationship between scripture 'and' ('*una cum*') tradition – co-ordination or subordination of tradition – which unfortunately was not finally

clarified even by Vatican II, is expressed in Canon 252.3 of the new CIC of 1983, but this does not contain any exclusive reference to Thomas Aquinas: 'There are to be classes in dogmatic theology which are always to be based upon the written word of God along with sacred tradition, in which the students may learn to penetrate ever more profoundly the mysteries of their salvation, with St Thomas as their teacher in a special way . . .'

212. Origen is not cited, nor of course are the Reformers and Orthodox and Protestant authors. John XXIII is only quoted five times (less than the Encyclical *Humani generis* = six times); Pius XII, by contrast, is quoted twenty-eight times.

213. Cf. **J. Le Goff**, *Les intellectuels au moyen age*, Paris 1957.

214. **Thomas Aquinas**, *Summa contra Gentiles*, I.2. Here Thomas cites Hilary, *De trinitate* 1, 37.

215. Cf. **E. Schillebeeckx**, 'Der Kampf an verschiedenen Fronten: Thomas von Aquin', in H. Häring and K.-J. Kuschel (eds.), *Gegenentwürfe, 24 Lebensläufe für eine andere Theologie*, Munich 1988, 53–67: 53–5.

216. Cf. **Bonaventure**, *De reductione artium ad theologiam*; English version with commentary, E. T. Healy (ed.), *Saint Bonaventure's* De reductione artium ad theologiam, New York 1939.

217. Cf. **Thomas Aquinas**, *Summa theologiae*, I q.1–26.

218. Cf. **id.**, *Summa theologiae*, I q.27–43.

219. This is about averting difficulties over Christian doctrinal truths, above all Trinity, incarnation, original sin, sacraments and resurrection.

220. **Id.**, *Summa contra Gentiles*, I.2.

221. For the prophetic preaching of **Joachim of Fiore** and the Franciscan movement cf. **H. Grundmann**, *Studien über Joachim von Fiore* (1927), Darmstadt 1966; **E. Buonaiuti**, *Gioacchino da Fiore. I tempi, la vita, il mesaggio*, Rome 1931; **E. Benz**, *Ecclesia spiritualis. Kirchenidee und Geschichtstheologie der franziskanischen Reformation*, Stuttgart 1934; **A. Crocco**, *Gioacchino da Fiore*, Naples 1960; **id.**, *Gioacchino da Fiore e il Gioachimismo*, Naples ²1976; **G. Wendelborn**, *Gott und Geschichte. Joachim von Fiore und die Hoffnung der Christentheit*, Vienna 1974; **H. Mottu**, *La manifestation de l'Esprit selon Joachim de Fiore. Herméneutique et théologie de l'histoire, d'aprés le 'Traité sur les Quatre Evangiles'*, Neuchâtel 1977; **B. McGinn**, *The Calabrian Abbot. Joachim of Fiore in the History of Western Thought*, New York 1985; **J. Moltmann**, 'Christian Hope – Messianic or Transcendent? A Theological Conversation with Joachim of Fiore and Thomas Aquinas', in id., *History and the Triune God*, London and Minneapolis 1991, 91–109. More recent monographs are specifically concerned with Thomas's polemic against Joachim (M. Gigante, J. I. Saranyana, W. Schachten) and others with the influence of Joachim (G. Hartvelt, H. de Lubac, R. B. Moynihan, M. Reeves, D. C. West).

222. **Thomas Aquinas**, *Summa theologiae* I–II, q. 106 a 4.

223. M. Seckler's thesis about Thomas's thinking on the theology of history, according to which the Christianized Neoplatonic egress-regress scheme contains a supportive 'Thoman formula of history and the world' (32), takes too little account of the fact that Thomas does not go essentially beyond the rudimentary historical thinking of his time. **Pesch**, *Thomas von Aquin* (n.209), 314, is right here: 'Thomas's theology of history consists in the fact that he does not have one in the usual sense.'

224. Cf. **Thomas Aquinas**, *Summa theologiae* I, q.65–74.

225. Cf. ibid., I–II, q.90–105.

226. Cf. ibid., q.35–45.

227. I am grateful to my colleague and specialist on Thomas Aquinas in the Institute for Ecumenical Research, Dr **Thomas Riplinger**, for having drawn my attention to this problem right at the beginning of my investigations of paradigms.

228. Cf. **Bonaventure**, *Itinerarium mentis in Deum*: English edition *The Mind's Journey to God*, trans. L. S. Cunningham, Chicago 1979.

229. Thomas shares with Origen and Augustine the view that the number of predestined is fixed in advance and is relatively small (most fall short). But he does not accept the restrictive interpretation that Augustine gives of God's universal will for salvation which is explicitly attested in the New Testament (cf. I Tim.2.4): God wills the salvation of all who will in fact be saved, or he wills salvation for people from all classes. Instead of this, he distinguishes between God's prevenient and subsequent will: 'God wills in advance that every human being shall be saved, but subsequently, in accordance with the requirement of his righteousness, he wills that some shall be damned' (*Summa theologiae*, I q.19, a.6 ad 1). For the whole problem cf. **G. Kraus**, *Vorherbestimmung. Traditionelle Prädestinationslehre im Licht gegenwärtigen Theologie*, Freiburg 1977, ch.2, 'Thomas Aquinas'.

230. **Chenu**, *Thomas von Aquin* (n.209), 49f.

231. Ibid., 51.

232. For the fate of this great Dominican, 'maître en théologie et en humanité', a theologian who showed solidarity with the Mission de France and the worker priests after the Second World War, see the devastating report by **F. Leprieur**, *Quand Rome condamne. Dominicains et prêtres ouvriers*, Paris 1989.

233. **Chenu**, *Thomas von Aquin* (n.209), 50.

234. Cf. above C III 2, 'Paradigm shift in the doctrine of the Trinity'.

235. Cf. the criticism in **H. Küng**, OBC, C VI 2, 'Slain for us'.

236. Cf. **Thomas Aquinas**, *Summa theologiae* I–II q.109–14.

237. Cf. **id.**, I–II, q.113.

238. Cf. **id.**, I–I, q.110 a.1; cf. q.116.

239. For the understanding of grace cf. **H. Küng**, *Justification*, ch.27, 'Grace as Graciousness'.

240. There is a long and wide-ranging discussion of these questions in **H. Küng**, DGE, A, 'Reason or Faith?'.

241. **Thomas Aquinas**, *Contra errores Graecorum*, II, chs.32–35; the forgeries are also frankly noted and discussed in the more recent Catholic commentaries, for example that by R. A. Verado (*Opuscula theologica*, Rome 1954), which has an excellent introduction. The researches by **F. H. Reusch**, *Die Fälschungen in dem Tractat des heiligen Thomas von Aquin gegen die Griechen*, Munich 1889, are basic here.

242. **Thomas Aquinas**, *Contra errores Graecorum*. II, ch.36. In this article, which is fundamental to papal doctrinal authority, Thomas bases himself on quotations from Cyril's *Liber thesaurorum*, which he takes from an anonymous *Libellus de processione Spiritus Sancti*, to a considerable degree made up of forgeries, inventions and false attributions. The quotations about the papacy – as we now know – are also forged: 'It is understandable that Thomas excerpted from the *Libellus* precisely those statements which were suitable as a basis for what he says about the primacy: but after what has been said, these are usually statements which have either been forged or interpolated with forgeries', **Reusch**, *Die Fälschungen* (n.241), 733.

243. Cf. **Thomas Aquinas**, *Summa theologiae*, II–II, q.1, a.10. On this cf. **Y. Congar**, 'Saint Thomas Aquinas and the Infallibility of the Papal Magisterium (*Summa theol.* II–II q.1 a.10)', *The Thomist* 38, 1974, 83–105, reprinted in id., *Thomas d'Aquin*, London 1984, VIII.

244. For Thomas's **political philosophy** cf. **T. Gilby**, *The Political Thought of Thomas Aquinas*, Chicago 1958; **P. Veysset**, *Situation de la politique dans la pensée de St Thomas d'Aquin*, Paris 1981; **M. Villey**, *Questions de saint Thomas sur le droit et la politique. Ou le bon usage des dialogues*, Paris 1987.

245. Cf. **Thomas Aquinas**, *Summa theologiae*, I–II, 95–7.

246. For the new phase of the Islamic-Christian controversy, which begins in the thirteenth century with the missionary activity of the Franciscans and Dominicans in Spain and the Near East, cf. the survey in **L. B. Hagemann**, *Christentum und Islam zwischen Konfrontation und Begegnung*, Altenberge 1983, 73–82.

247. **Chenu**, *Thomas d'Aquin* (n.243), 86–8.

248. For this work in the context of the dialogue between the religions cf. **L. B. Hagemann**, 'Missionstheoretische Ansätze bei Thomas von Aquin in seiner Schrift *De rationibus fidei*', in A. Zimmermann (ed.), *Thomas von Aquin*, 459–83.

249. For the current discussion cf. **N. Daniel**, *Islam and the West. The Making of an Image*, Edinburgh 1958; **A. T. Khoury**, *La controverse contre l'Islam*, Paris 1969; **id.**, *Les théologiens byzantins et l'Islam. Textes et auteurs (VIIIe–XIIIe)*, Paris ²1969; **id.**, *Polémique byzantine contre l'Islam (VIIIe–XIIIe s.)*, Leiden ²1972; **id.**, *L'Apologétique byzantine contre l'Islam (VIIIe–XIIIe s.)*, Altenberge 1875. – How dramatic a real dialogue with Islam could become was shown by a Christian scholar, Ali at-Tabari, who converted to Islam at the age of seventy and sought to justify his action by two apologetic works based on the Bible itself, with as literal a scriptural exegesis as possible. Cf. **O. H. Schumann**, *Der Christus der Muslime. Christologische Aspekte in der arabisch-islamischen Literatur*, Gütersloh 1972, expanded edition Cologne ²1982, 32–47.

250. Cf. **H. Küng**, *Judaism*, I C IV 8, 'Christian persecutions of the Jews and the "reasons" for them'.

251. Cf. **Thomas Aquinas**, *Summa theologiae*, I q.92, a.1–4.

252. Cf. ibid., II–II, q.177 a.2. **A. Mitterer**, 'Mann und Weib nach dem biologischen Weltbild des hl.Thomas und dem der Gegenwart', *Zeitschrift für katholische Theologie* 57, 1933, 491–556; **id.**, *Die Zeugung der Organismen, insbesondere des Menschen, nach dem Weltbild des hl.Thomas von Aquin und dem der Gegenwart*, Vienna 1947, already drew attention to Thomas's androcentrism and the way in which he often regards the woman as inferior.

253. Cf. **Thomas Aquinas**, *Summa theologiae*, I q.92, a.1.

254. For *occasionatus*, **A. Blaise** (ed.), *Lexicon latinitatis medii aevi*, Turnhout 1975, has '1. causé occasionellement, 2. imparfait, manqué'. Cf. also **A. Mitterer**, '*Mas occasionatus* oder zwei Methoden der Thomasdeutung', *Zeitschrift für katholische Theologie* 72, 1950, 80–103.

255. Cf. **Thomas Aquinas**, *Commentary on the Sentences*, IV d.25, q.2. qla 1, ad 4.

256. Cf. **id.**, *Summa theologiae*, Supplementum q.39, a.1.

257. At that time **lay preaching** was in any case a particularly provocative theme in view of the heretical movements. Thomas even explicitly opposes an office of preaching and teaching for **women**, a 'grace of the discourse of wisdom

and science', used by them *publice*, and does so with special arguments (cf *Summa theologiae*, II–II, q.177 a.2):
– Above all because of the condition that the female sex shall be subject to the man: teaching as a public office in the church is a matter for those set in authority (*praelati*) and not for subjects; these essentially include the woman because of her sex (and thus not just accidentally, like the simple priest, who is at any rate male);
– also for the sake of males, whose senses are not to be stimulated to lust by preaching women (lust = *concupiscentia* or *libido* has been a penetrating theme since Augustine!);
– finally, women in any case would not distinguish themselves in matters of wisdom to such a degree that they could be entrusted with a public task of teaching.

258. Cf. **K. E. Børresen**, *Subordination and Equivalence. The Nature and Role of Woman in Augustine and Thomas Aquinas*, Washington 1981; **ead.**, 'Die anthropologischen Grundlagen der Beziehung zwischen Mann und Frau in der klassischen Theologie', *Concilium* 12, 1976, 10–17 (never translated into English); **ead.**, *Image of God and Gender Models in Judaeo-Christian Tradition*, Oslo 1991; **K. E. Børresen** and **K. Vogt**, *Women's Studies of the Christian and Islamic Traditions. Ancient, Medieval and Renaissance Fore-mothers*, Dordrecht 1993. I am deeply grateful to Dr **Kari Børresen** of the University of Oslo for looking through this and other sections on women and for her valuable suggestions.

259. According to Børresen, too, there are significant **differences between Augustine and Thomas** over women. It is not just that Augustine gets by without a precise physiological theory and Thomas explicitly builds on the physiology of Aristotle, who is responsible for his remarkable statements about women. In addition, because of his less pessimistic attitude to the reality of creation, Thomas has a more positive attitude to sexuality throughout:
– Unlike Augustine, Thomas does not advocate a dualistic anthropology even for the original reality of creation (in paradise): the sensual feelings of the body are an essential part of human beings, and under the conditions of 'paradise' there could have been sexual intercourse even without sin: 'Consequently the natural satisfaction, as it would have been wholly governed by the reason, would have been even greater than the pleasure which is now associated with the sexual act' (**K. E. Børresen**, *Die anthropologische Grundlagen*, 12, referring to *Summa theologiae* I, q.98, a.1, 2).
– Unlike Augustine, Thomas has no almost compulsive anxiety about a sexuality allegedly corrupted by original sin, and its irrational character: he avoids the Augustinian identification of original sin with sexual desire (*concupiscentia, libido*): 'He breaks with this tradition in distinguishing between procreation (in which the father's seed works as an instrumental cause in passing on original sin) and desire, which normally accompanies sexual intercourse, but which does not represent any causal factor' (13, with reference to *Summa theologiae* I–II q.82. a.3; q.85, a.1).
– Unlike Augustine, Thomas does not simply see sexuality and its disorderly desire justified in marriage by the benefit of fertility (as though the ideal married love consisted in a continent love): 'Not only the intention of fertility but also the use of marriage as a means of salvation (from concupiscence) make the sexual act free from sin' (15, with reference to *Summa theologiae*, Supplementum q.41, a.3; q.42, a.2; q.49, a.5).

J. B. Bauer draws my attention to Thomas's insistence on the *ligatio rationis in concubitu conjugali*: *Summa theologiae*, I–II, q.34 a.1 ad 1; q.37, a 1. ad 2; q.72, a.2 ad 4; II–II, q.150 a.4 ad 3; q.153 a.2.

260. Cf. Y. Congar, 'Valeur et portée oecuméniques des quelques principes herméneutiques de Saint Thomas d'Aquin', *Revue des sciences philosophique et théologique* 57, 1973, 611–26; reprinted in id., *Thomas d'Aquin* (n.242), article IX.

261. It is more than questionable whether one can establish an intrinsic relationship of cause and effect between scholasticism and Gothic, between scholastic method and the principles of classical French cathedral architecture – thus E. Panofsky, *Gothic Architecture and Scholasticism*, Latrobe, Penn. 1951.

262. Cf. A. J. Gurjewitsch, *Das Weltbild des mittelalterlichen Menschen*, Munich 1980.

263. Cf. G. Duby (ed.), *Histoire de la vie privée*, II, *De l'Europe féodale à la Renaissance*, Paris 1985. Cf. also the analysis of feudalism by G. Duby, *Les trois ordres ou l'imaginaire du féodalisme*, Paris 1978.

264. Cf. J. Le Goff (ed.), *L'uomo medievale*, Rome 1987.

265. Cf. J. Bumke, *Höfische Kultur. Literatur und Gesellschaft im hohen Mittelalter* (2 vols.), Munich 1986.

266. Cf. R. Imbach, *Laien in der Philosophie des Mittelalters. Hinweise und Anregungen zu einem vernachlässigtem Thema*, Amsterdam 1989 (he discusses above all Lull and Dante).

267. Cf. A. de Libera, *Penser au Moyen Âge*, Paris 1991.

268. Cf. A. Borst, *Die Katharer*, Stuttgart 1953.

269. Cf. id., *Barbaren, Ketzer und Artisten. Welten des Mittelalters*, Munich 1988.

270. Cf. J. Le Goff, *La Naissance du Purgatoire*, Paris 1981.

271. Cf. P. Ariès, *Essais sur l'histoire de la mort en occident du moyen-âge à nos jours*, Paris 1975; id., *L'homme devant la mort*, Paris 1977; N. Ohler, *Sterben und Tod im Mittelalter*, Zurich 1990; and as a counterpart, P. Ariès, *L'enfant et la vie familiale sous l'ancien régime*, Paris 1960; S. Shahar, *Childhood in the Middle Ages*, London 1990.

272. Cf. above C III 4, 'What was preserved of the substance of faith'.

273. For a more recent introduction to the problems, with an abundant bibliography, cf. M. Mollat, *Les Pauvres au Moyen Âge. Étude sociale*, Paris 1978.

274. As an introduction (with reference to the Arabs and Islam) cf. H. Schipperges, *Die Kranken im Mittelalter*, Munich 1990 (with bibliography).

275. For women in the Middle Ages cf. T. Vogelsang, *Die Frau als Herrscherin im hohen Mittelalter. Studien zur consors regni Formel*, Göttingen 1954; M. Bernards, Speculum virginum. *Geistigkeit und Seelenleben der Frau im Hochmittelalter*, Cologne 1955; G. Koch, *Frauenfrage und Ketzertum im Mittelalter. Die Frauenbewegung im Rahmen des Katharismus und des Waldensertums und ihre sozialen Wurzeln (12–14.Jahrhundert)*, Berlin 1962; I. Raming, *Der Ausschluss der Frau vom priesterlichen Amt. Gottgewollte Tradition oder Diskriminierung? Eine rechtshistorisch-dogmatische Untersuchung der Grundlagen von Kanon 968 §1 des Codex Iuris Canonici*, Cologne 1973; J. M. Ferrante, *Woman as Image in Mediaeval Literature from the Twelfth Century to Dante*, New York 1975; E. Power, *Medieval Women*, Cambridge 1975; M. Bogin, *The Women Troubadours*, New York 1976; B. A. Carroll (ed.),

Liberating Women's History. Theoretical and Critical Essays, Urbana 1976; **F.** and **J. Gies**, *Women in the Middle Ages*, New York 1978; **A. Wolf-Graaf**, *Frauenarbeit im Abseits. Frauenbewegung und weibliches Arbeitsvermögen*, Munich 1981; **A. Kuhn** and **J. Rüsen** (eds.), *Frauen in der Geschichte* II, Düsseldorf 1982f.; **P. Ketsch**, *Frauen im Mittelalter. Quellen und Materialien*, I, *Frauenarbeit im Mittelalter*; II, *Frauenbild und Frauenrechte im Kirche und Gesellschaft*, Düsseldorf 1983; **A. M. Lucas**, *Women in the Middle Ages. Religion, Marriage and Letters*, Brighton 1983; **I. Ludolphy**, 'Frau' (V): Alte Kirche und Mittelalter', *TRE* XI, 436–41; **E. Ennen**, *Frauen im Mittelalter*, Munich 1984, [4]1991; **D. Herlihy**, *Mediaeval Households*, Cambridge, Mass. 1985; **M. C. Howell**, *Women, Production and Patriarchy in Late Medieval Cities*, Chicago 1986; **M. B. Rose** (ed.), *Women in the Middle Ages and the Renaissance. Literary and Historical Perspectives*, Syracuse 1986; **B. Frakele, E. List** and **G. Pauritsch** (eds.), *Über Frauenleben, Männerwelt und Wissenschaft. Österreichische Texte zur Frauenforschung*, Vienna 1987; **A. Kuhn**, 'Mittelalter', in *Frauenlexikon. Traditionen, Fakten, Perspektiven*, ed. A. Lossner, R. Süssmuth and K. Walter, Freiburg 1988, 749–60; **S. Shahar**, *Die Frau im Mittelalter*, Königstein 1988; **F. Bertini** et al., *Medioevo al femminile*, Bari 1989; **G. Duby** and **M. Perrot**, *Storia delle donne in occidente*, Vol.II (ed. C. Klapisch-Zuber), Rome 1990; **J. B. Holloway, C. S. Wright** and **J. Bechtold** (eds.), *Equally in God's Image. Women in the Middle Ages*, New York 1990; **C. Opitz**, *Evatöchter und Bräute Christi. Weiblicher Lebenszusammenhang und Frauenkultur im Mittelalter*, Weinheim 1990; **C. Walker Bynum**, *Fragmentation and Redemption. Essays on Gender and the Human Body in Mediaeval Religion*, New York 1991; **B. Lundt** (ed.), *Auf der Suche nach der Frau im Mittelalter. Fragen, Quellen, Antworten*, Munich 1991; **R. Pernoud**, *Leben der Frauen im Hochmittelalter* (French original), Pfaffenweiler 1991; **K. E. Børresen** and **K. Vogt**, *Women's Studies* (the survey of research by K. E. Børresen on pp.13–127 is particularly important here). The collection of sources edited by **E. Gössmann**, *Archiv für philosophie– und theologiegeschichtliche Frauenforschung* (4 vols. so far), Munich 1984–8, is especially worthwhile.

276. Cf. above C II 4, 'Were women emancipated by Christianity?'.

277. Cf. above C III 6, 'Private confession and rigorism in sexual morality'.

278. **J. Le Goff**, *L'imaginaire médiéval*, Paris 1985, 123.

279. One wonders, for example, what was the specific significance of the 'guardianship' under which women were put at that time, simply by virtue of their sex. What did this sexual supervision, first by the father and then by the husband, mean? Did it leave the women any legal rights and freedom of action? And what about a special Germanic form of marriage like 'Friedelehe', without a dowry, in which the husband had no mastery over his wife? What was the position among the Langobards (and perhaps also among the Franks and Anglo-Saxons)? Were women there still unable to administer, use and increase their property independently in the seventh century? Indeed, didn't a partnership between husband and wife predominate in the peasant households of the Middle Ages, so that a verdict is difficult because on the basis of the predominantly male sources we have better knowledge about the legal position of women in the Middle Ages than about their social status?

280. **Ennen**, *Frauen im Mittelalter* (n.275), 108.

281. Ibid.

282. **Kuhn**, 'Mittelalter' (n.275), 753f.

283. Cf. **Howell**, *Women* (n.275).

284. **Kuhn**, 'Mittelalter' (n.275), 758f.

285. Cf. **U. Baumann**, *Die Ehe – ein Sakrament?*, Zurich 1988.

286. Cf. **R. Kieckhefer**, *Repression of Heresy in Medieval Germany*, Philadelphia 1979, Ch.3, 'The War against Beghards and Beguines'. **P. D. Johnson**, *Equal in Monastic Profession. Religious Women in Medieval France*, Chicago 1991, notes a collapse in women's monastic culture from the twelfth century on.

287. **Ennen**, *Frauen im Mittelalter* (n.275), 245; cf. **M. Schmidt** and **K. E. Børresen**, 'Theologin (I–II)', in E. Gössmann et al. (eds.), *Wörterbuch der Feministischen Theologie*, Gütersloh 1991, 396–415.

288. Cf. the portrait by **E. Gössmann**, 'Hildegard von Bingen', in M. Greschat (ed.), *Gestalten der Kirchengeschichte* III, 224–37 (with bibliography).

289. For **mysticism**, cf. in addition to earlier works which are still important (above all the reprints of books by C. Butler, J. Bernhart and W. Preger): **L. Bouyer** et al. (eds.), *Histoire de la spiritualité chrétienne* (3 vols.), Paris 1960–66; **K. Ruh** (ed.), *Altdeutsche und altniederländische Mystik*, Darmstadt 1944; id., *Geschichte der abendländischen Mystik* (2 vols.), Munich 1990/93; **L. Cognet**, *Introduction aux mystiques rhéno-flamands*, Paris 1968; **F. W. Wentzlaff-Eggebert**, *Deutsche Mystik zwischen Mittelalter und Neuzeit. Einheit und Wandlung ihrer Erscheinungsformen*, Berlin ³1969; **A. M. Haas** and **H. Stirnimann**, *Das 'Einig Ein'. Studien zu Theorie und Sprache der deutschen Mystik*, Fribourg 1980; **J. Sudbrack** (ed.), *Zeugen christlicher Gotteserfahrung*, Mainz 1981; id., *Mystik. Selbsterfahrung – kosmische Erfahrung – Gotteserfahrung*, Mainz 1988; **G. Ruhbach** and **J. Sudbrack** (eds.), *Grosse Mystiker. Leben und Wirken*, Munich 1987; id. (ed.), *Christliche Mystik. Texte aus zwei Jahrtausenden*, Munich 1989; **R. Beyer**, *Die andere Offenbarungen. Mystikerinnen des Mittelalters*, Bergisch Gladbach 1989; **B. McGinn**, *The Foundations of Mysticism*, London and New York 1991; **P. Dinzelbacher**, *Mittelalterliche Frauenmystik*, Paderborn 1993.

290. For an introduction see **D. Mieth**, 'Meister Eckhart', in M. Greschat (ed.), *Gestalten der Kirchengeschichte* IV, Stuttgart 1983, 124–54 (with bibliography); cf. id., 'Gescheitert und doch furchtbar: Gründe und Hintergründe des Prozesses gegen Meister Eckhart (c.1260–1327/28)', in H. Häring and K.-J. Kuschel (eds.), *Gegenentwürfe. 24 Lebensläufe für eine andere Theologie*, Munich 1988, 81–95.

291. Cf. **O. Karrer**, 'Mystik' (IV), *LThK* VII, 734–41.

292. Cf. **F. Gils**, *Jésus Prophète d'après les Évangiles Synoptiques*, Louvain 1957; **R. Schnackenburg**, 'Die Erwartung des "Propheten" nach dem NT und den Qumran Texten', in *Texte und Untersuchungen* 73, 1959, 622–39; **F. Schnider**, *Jesus der Prophet*, Fribourg 1973.

293. John 14.9.

294. Cf. **F. Heiler**, *Prayer*, London and New York 1932, 135–7.

295. Cf. **K. Ruh**, 'Le miroir des simple âmes de Marguerite Porete' (1975), in *Kleine Schriften* II, Berlin 1984, 212–36; id., *Meister Eckhart, Theologe, Prediger, Mystiker*, Munich 1985, 95–114.

296. Cf. **E. Gössmann**, 'Die Geschichte und Lehre der Mystikerin Marguerite Porete (gest.1310)', in Häring and Kuschel (eds.), *Gegenentwürfe*, 69–79. Cf. further works on Porete in **K. E. Børresen** and **K. Vogt**, *Women's Studies*, 70–2.

297. For a study in greater depth cf. **H. Küng**, CWR, B I 2.

298. For the history of the veneration of Mary cf. **G. Miegge**, *The Virgin Mary*, London 1955; **W. Tappolet** (ed.), *Das Marienlob der Reformatoren. M. Luther, J. Calvin, H. Zwingli, H. Bullinger*, Tübingen 1962; **W. Delius**, *Geschichte der Marienverehrung*, Munich 1963; **H. Graef**, *Maria. Eine Geschichte der Lehre und Verehrung*, Freiburg 1964.

299. Cf. **Denzinger**, *Enchiridion*, no.111a; **G. Galbiati**, *Il Concilio di Efeso. Alle origini dei dogmi e del culto di Maria nel tormentato clima del Concilio di Efeso, tappa miliare per l'avento della mariologia*, Genoa 1977; **S. Benko**, *The Virgin Goddess. Studies in the Pagan and Christian Roots of Mariology*, Leiden 1993.

300. Cf. **K.-J. Kuschel** (ed.), *Und Maria trat aus ihren Bildern. Literarische Texte*, Freiburg 1990.

301. For the lack of biblical foundations for Marian dogmas cf. the article by the American Catholic exegete **J. McKenzie**, 'Die Mutter Jesu im Neuen Testament', in E. Moltmann-Wendel, H. Küng and J. Moltmann (eds.), *Was geht uns Maria an? Beiträge zur Auseinandersetzung in Theologie, Kirche und Frömmigkeit*, Gütersloh 1988, 233–40. **K. E. Børresen**, 'Maria in der katholischen Theologie', demonstrates that the two more recent dogmatic formulations about Mary are based on 'wrong anthropological presuppositions' (ibid., 72–87). This specialist in the history of dogma and theology puts forward 'the theory that these formulations lose their meaning and become literally incomprehensible as soon as their a prioris are no longer retained. If these mariocentric statements are no longer supported by the Augustinian doctrine of original sin handed down through the father's procreation or the classical doctrine of the immortal rational soul separate from the body, with its expectation of the risen body, they remain suspended in the void of sheer conjecture' (81). The volume mentioned above also contains contributions by internationally recognized professionals from Jewish and feminist, critical and traditional perspectives, quoted below, which give a survey of the state of present-day discussion on Mary.

302. **C. J. M. Halkes**, 'Maria – inspirierendes oder abschreckendes Vorbild für Frauen?', in Moltmann-Wendel et al. (eds.), *Was geht uns Maria an?*, 113–30: 114.

303. Cf. **E. Drewermann**, *Kleriker. Psychogramm eines Ideals*, Freiburg 1989, esp. II B 2 d.

304. **J. Moltmann**, 'Gibt es eine ökumenische Mariologie?', in Moltmann-Wendel et al. (eds.), *Was geht uns Maria an?* (n.301), 15–22: 15; cf. here also **S. Ben-Chorin**, *Die Mutter Jesu in jüdischer Sicht*, 40–50.

305. Luke 1.48.

306. Cf. also Mark 3.20f.

307. For the biblical evidence, in addition to the article by **J. McKenzie** cited above see the joint study by Protestant and Roman Catholic scholars: **R. E. Brown, K. P. Donfried, J. A. Fitzmyer** and **J. Reumann** (eds.), *Mary in the New Testament. A Collaborative Assessment by Protestant and Roman Catholic Scholars*, Philadelphia 1978.

308. **Halkes**, 'Maria' (n.302), rightly attaches importance to this from the feminist perspective.

309. Cf. **M. Warner**, *Alone of all Her Sex. The Myth and the Cult of the Virgin Mary*, London 1976.

310. For the question of the virgin birth cf. **H. Küng**, *Credo*, Ch. II, 'Jesus Christ; Virgin Birth and Divine Sonship'. For the question of the pre-

existence of Christ see above, C I 5, 'Pre-existence of the Logos in the Gospel of John'.

311. Cf. Luke 1.38; 2.34f.

312. Luke 1.

313. However, the New Testament does not once hint at a lover or even a wife of Jesus – the material for novels, musicals and writers of trivia; quite the contrary. **Elisabeth Moltmann-Wendel** (Tübingen) rightly highlights the repressed tradition of Jesus' friendship with Mary Magdalene over against the excessive stress on that of Jesus' mother Mary. I am grateful to her for a number of suggestions; she championed feminist concerns critically and constructively in the German-speaking world, earlier than others. See her 'Maria oder Magdalena – Mutterschaft oder Freundschaft', in ead., *Was geht uns Maria an?*, 51–9.

314. Gal.5.1.

315. II Cor.3.17.

316. Gal. 3.27f.

317. Cf. **C. Mirbt** and **K. Aland**, *Quellen zur Geschichte des Papsttums und des römischen Katholizismus* I, Tübingen ⁶1967, 457 (not included in Denziger!).

318. Cf. **Ullmann**, *Short History of the Papacy* (n.39), 266f.

319. Cf. **F. X. Seppelt** and **G. Schwaiger**, *Geschichte der Päpste*, IV, Munich ²1957, 53f.: 'So if the question whether Boniface was a heretic is to be answered in the negative, one cannot avoid the impression that his self-confidence and sense of power on occasion expressed themselves in forms which have a pathological character and which one can only interpret as a sign of megalomania. One thinks of that theatrical scene which has been handed down to us by the quite reliable report of a delegation from Aragon, when Boniface appeared before bishops and cardinals dressed alternately as Pope and emperor, and exclaimed, "I am Pope, I am emperor".'

320. Cf. **Denzinger**, *Enchiridion*, no.468. The papalist **Aegidius Romanus**, *De ecclesiastica potestate*, ed. R. Schola, Weimar 1929, provides the real ideological basis with many quotations. For Aegidius, all dominion on earth comes from the Pope.

321. Cf. **J. Huizinga**, *The Waning of the Middle Ages. A Study of the Forms, Life and Art in France and the Netherlands in the Fourteenth and Fifteenth Centuries*, London 1924.

322. The most recent account is that of **B. Guillemain** in Vol. VI of the *Histoire du christianisme des origines à nos jours*, edited by **M. Mollat du Jourdain** and **A. Vauchez**, under the title *Un temps d'épreuves (1274–1449)*, Paris 1990, Parts I.1 and III.1–2. The period is arbitrarily introduced with the Second Council of Lyons in 1274 and the church union which was agreed for a short period, and all the historical material is treated in three parts under three dogmatic categories (unity, sanctity and catholicity). Here one misses apostolicity, and thus the criterion of origin.

323. **Y. Congar**, *L'Église. De saint Augustin à l'époque moderne*, Paris 1970, ch.IX, brings out the conflict between the two spiritual trends – 'the one hierocratic and papalistic, the other favouring the church people and a lay society'.

324. Cf. **Dante Alighieri**, *De monarchia libri tres* (c.1310); modern edition London 1916.

325. Cf. **id.**, *The Divine Comedy* (composed 1307–1321), Harmondsworth 1969 (3 vols.), Inferno, Canto 19.

326. Cf. **Marsilius of Padua**, *Defensor pacis* (1324); modern edition ed. C. W. Nederman, Cambridge 1993.

327. Cf. **William of Ockham**, *Dialogus* (between 1332 and 1349); German edition, Dialogus. *Auszüge zur politischen Theorie*, ed. J. Miethke, Darmstadt 1992.

328. Cf. **B. Tierney**, *Origins of Papal Infallibility, 1150–1350. A Study on the Concepts of Infallibility, Sovereignty and Tradition in the Middle Ages*, Leiden 1972.

329. Paul VI's encyclical *Humanae vitae* on birth control (1968) was to show in a dramatic way how a Pope saw himself bound by the irreformable doctrines of his predecessors (irreformable, because they are infallible *e magisterio ordinario*) and became incapable of correcting an error.

330. Quoted and interpreted by **Tierney**, *Origins of Papal Infallibility* (n.328), 186–96.

331. Cf. **O. Prerovsky**, *L'elezione di Urbano VI e l'insorgere dello scisma d'occidente*, Rome 1960.

332. Cf. **H. Küng**, *Structures*, VII 3, 'Conflict Between the Pope and the Church'. In addition to death and resignation, mental illness (*amentia*), heresy and schism make up the five reasons for which a Pope may lose his office.

333. Cf. **F. Bliemetzrieder**, *Das Generalkonzil im grossen abendländischen Schisma*, Paderborn 1904.

334. Cf. **A. Hauck**, 'Die Rezeption und Umbildung der allgemeine Synode im Mittelalter', *Historische Vierteljahrschrift* 10, 1907, 465–82.

335. Cf. **M. Seidlmayer**, *Die Anfänge des grossen abendländischen Schisma. Studien zur Kirchenpolitik insbesondere der spanischen Staaten und zu den geistigen Kämpfen der Zeit*, Münster 1940.

336. Cf. **B. Tierney**, *Foundations of the Conciliar Theory*, Cambridge 1955. Tierney notes three great periods in the development of conciliar ideas: 1. Decretistic theories about the government of the church (1140–1220); 2. Papalism and canonist corporation doctrine in the thirteenth century; 3. The conciliar ideas in the fourteenth century. Cf. also **R. Bäumer** (ed.), *Die Entwicklung des Konziliarismus. Werden und Nachwirken der konziliaren Idee*, Darmstadt 1976; **H. Schneider**, *Der Konziliarismus als Problem der neueren katholischen Theologie. Die Geschichte der Auslegung der Konstanzer Dekrete von Febronius bis zur Gegenwart*, Berlin 1976; **C. M. D. Crowder**, *Unity, Heresy and Reform, 1378–1460. The Conciliar Response to the Great Schism*, London 1977; **A. C. Leopardi**, *Il conciliarismo. Genesi e sviluppo*, Bari 1978; **R. N. Swanson**, *Universities, Academics and the Great Schism*, Cambridge 1969; **G. Alberigo**, *Chiesa conciliare. Identità e significato del conciliarismo*, Brescia 1981; H. Schneider, who has investigated the discussion of the decrees of Constance down to the period of the Second Vatican Council, ends by stating: 'We still await an interpretation of the decrees of Constance which historically is completely satisfying' (339).

337. **Tertullian**, *De paenitentia* 13,6–7: ' . . .et ipsa representatio totius nominis magna veneratio celebratur'. For the further tradition from Athanasius to John XXIII, for whom the Second Vatican Council was 'la grande riunione del popolo cristiano', cf. **H. Küng**, *Structures*, III 2: 'It (= the ecumenical council) is a representation of the ecumenical council by divine convocation (= church).' In retrospect it is illuminating to see how in 1962 **J. Ratzinger** claims authorship of the thesis which I worked out in

my inaugural lecture in Tübingen (in 1960), 'The whole church appears as the one great council of God and the world' (although he had not previously called the church 'council'); but then, in a striking narrowness, he wants to reduce the collegiality of the church to the collegiality of the bishops, in order to overlook the collegiality both of the communities and of the church as a whole. So it is not surprising that he simply derives the infallibility of the church from the infallibility of the Word of God. Is it really so simple, as Ratzinger suggested at that time? 'For the church's fundamental infallibility follows quite naturally from the fact that it is the presence of the divine Word, and with it the divine truth in this world.' The transformation of the 'progressive' council theologian of 1962 to the 'regressive' Grand Inquisitor of the post–conciliar period, which many people find so remarkable, is not so completely incomprehensible in the light of such (and similar) remarks. For this 'pre-conciliar' controversy between Ratzinger and myself cf. *Structures*, VI 5, 'The representation of the offices and communities', 193–200.

338. As Martin V treated all three former supporters of candidates equally in his decrees after the Council of Constance (with a slight preference for the Pisa line, i.e. that of John XXIII), and neither a later Pope nor a council ever decided the question of the legitimacy of the three rival Popes, Angelo Roncalli in our century should really have called himself John XXIV.

339. For the history of the **Council of Constance**, cf. the literature in **K. A. Fink**, 'Konzil von Konstanz', *LThK* VI, 501–3; id., *Papsttum und Kirche im abendländischen Mittelalter*, Munich 1981 (especially Part I on the church constitution); **P. de Vooght**, *Les pouvoirs du concile et l'autorité du Pape au Concile de Constance. Le decret* Haec Sanctus Synodus *du 6 avril 1415*, Paris 1965. I am grateful to my former Tübingen colleague **Karl August Fink** and the Benedictine **P. de Vooght** for important suggestions towards clarifying this problem, which I took up in *Structures*, Chapter VII, and which are not superseded even by the most recent work by **W. Brandmüller**, *Das Konzil von Konstanz 1414–1418*, I, Paderborn 1991.

340. Granted, in his extended edition of Denzinger P. Hünermann quotes about fifteen pages of 'errors' of John Wyclif and Jan Hus (all questionnaires), but he, too, suppresses the central decrees of the council and quotes only one (incomplete) sentence from the decree *Haec sancta* (in small print); then, without taking any notice of the most recent scholarship, he repeats the anachronistic assertion that the extent to which the Pope confirmed the decree of the council is disputed. But it already follows from the bull *Inter cunctas* of 22 February 1418, which he quotes (nos.1247f.), that Pope Martin V called for recognition of all the decrees of Constance by the heretics (for interpretation see **F. X. Funk** and **P. de Vooght**, quoted by Küng, *Structures*, 246f.). All in all, this is yet further evidence that for all the historical effort in the latest editions, the *Enchiridion* of the Würzburg dogmatic theologian Heinrich Denziger is not an unprejudiced historical sourcebook (by contrast, see the *Enchiridion* of the councils by **J. Alberigo** et al., *Conciliorum oecumenicorum decreta*, Freiburg 1962, which has already been cited), but a product to serve Roman scholastic theology and church politics.

341. Here I am translating from the edition by **Alberigo**, 385.

342. Ibid., 414f.

343. **Fink**, 'Konzil von Konstanz' (n.339), 503. The work by **B. Hübler**, *Die Constanzer Reformation und die Concordate von 1418*, Leipzig 1867, is still

basic and is endorsed by the more recent researches of F. X. Funk, P. de Vooght and K. A. Fink.

344. **Ullmann,** *Short History of the Papacy* (n.39), 313.

345. Cf. H. Jedin, *A History of the Council of Trent*, I, London 1957, 66f.: 'With the Bull *Execrabilis* the restoration Papacy dealt the conciliar theory its first heavy blow. The result did not come up to expectations. In France and Germany it met with vigorous opposition and outside Rome it was not generaly accepted.' For the discussions at the time, especially those between Cajetan and J. Almain, see **O. de la Brosse,** *Le pape et le concile. Le comparaison de leurs pouvoirs à la veille de la Réforme*, Paris 1965.

346. **Denzinger,** *Enchiridion*, no.740.

347. Cf. **R. Bäumer,** 'Lateran-Synoden', *LThK* VI, 818: 'It was regarded by opponents of the Pope as not being a free council. It did not gain universal recognition, even at the Council of Trent,' **O. de la Brosse** et al., *Latran V et Trente*, Paris 1975.

348. Cf. **R. Bellarmine,** *De conciliis liber II*, cap. 17, in *Opera omnia*, Paris 1870, II.

349. Cf. **J. Michelet,** *Histoire de France*, VII, *Renaissance*, Paris 1835.

350. **J. Burckhardt,** *Die Kultur der Renaissance in Italien*, Basel 1860.

351. **J. Le Goff,** 'Pour un long Moyen-Âge', in *L'imaginaire médiéval*, 9–13: 8ff.

352. Cf. **S. Schüller-Piroli,** *Borgia, Die Zerstörung einer Legende. Die Geschichte einer Dynastie*, Olten 1963; **ead.,** *Die Borgia-Päpste Kalixt II. und Alexander VI.*, Vienna 1979; **ead.,** *Die Borgia Dynastie. Legende und Geschichte* (2 vols.), Munich 1980/82 (the Italian Cuban O. Ferrara, *El Papa Borgia*, Madrid [4]1952, had attempted a rehabilitation very much earlier which remarkably enough the author does not mention in her 1979 book). Although she is justified in working out the political significance of Alexander VI for Italian politics, some further comments need to be added. Of course a distinction must be made between legend and history, which must be the duty of every historian – and even the earlier historians did not completely neglect to do this. So there is nothing against saving the honour of Alexander, who like any human being had his good sides and qualities – expert knowledge of the law, administrative capacities, political dexterity and the gift of oratory; but even someone as well disposed to the papacy as Ludwig Freiherr von Pastor could not deny his corruption and perverseness. It may be pointed out that Alexander, with his abundant children, was unjustly accused of incest with his daughter Lucretia, that his son Cesare did not in fact murder his brother, etc., and that in Rome a 'black legend' was circulated, above all because he was a Spaniard and not an Italian and a Roman. But can it be said to be a rehabilitation if the Borgia Pope unscrupulously appropriated the 'papacy's reasons of state' and acted as immorally as any other Renaissance prince in pursuing his ends? An absolute politician and therefore a contemporary, indeed in his immoral individuality even a modern Pope, who was ahead of his time? Is all his nepotism and family politics, even the most cunning diplomacy and unscrupulous policy of alliances, to be justified, if this so political and so contemporary a Pope gained the freedom of the papal see by a policy of even-handedness? Leaving aside the moral standpoint, of course even the three marriages of the Pope's daughter Lucrezia can be justified along with providing for the other seven children which he had by different mistresses. Leaving aside the moral perspective . . . Be this as it may, this successor of Peter, murdered 'only

in the eleventh year of his eventful and successful papacy', as the author already notes with satisfaction in the preface to her book, is not demonized, as used to happen, but is now trivialized, so that he becomes a Pope for whom 'the moral conflict between his spiritual and worldly ties and interests remained hidden all his life', and who 'in almost unimaginable naivety was convinced that he was fulfilling his religious duties to the best of his ability' (*Borgia*, 145).

353. Cf. **H. Jedin**, *Katholische Reform oder Gegenreformation? Ein Versuch zur Klärung der Begriffe*, Lucerne 1946.

354. For the **Counter-Reformation** or Catholic reform cf. the accounts in the handbooks of history and the relevant lexicon articles (in particular that by **G. Maron** in *TRE*). The following are important for the context of the paradigm analysis: **J. Lortz**, *Die Reformation in Deutschland* (2 vols.), Freiburg 1940, new edition 1982; **L. Cristiani**, *L'Église à l'époque du concile de Trente*, Paris 1948; **K. Eder**, *Die Kirche im Zeitalter des konfessionellen Absolutismus (1555–1638)*, Freiburg 1949; **P. Janelle**, *The Catholic Reformation*, Milwaukee 1949; **G. Schreiber** (ed.), *Das Weltkonzil von Trient. Sein Werden und Wirken* (2 vols.), Freiburg 1951; **H. Daniel-Rops**, *L'Église de la Renaissance et de la Réforme*, II, *Une ère de renouveau: La Réforme catholique*, Paris 1955; **K. Bihlmeyer** and **H. Tüchle**, *Kirchengeschichte*, Vol.III, *Die Neuzeit und die neueste Zeit*, Paderborn [15]1956; **R. G. Villoslada** and **B. Llorca**, *La Iglesia en la época del Renacimiento y de la Reforma católica*, Madrid 1960, [2]1967; **L. Willaert**, *Après le concile de Trente. La Restauration catholique 1563–1648*, Paris 1960; **J. Delumeau**, *Naissance et affirmation de la Réforme*, Paris 1965; id., *Le Catholicisme entre Luther et Voltaire*, Paris 1971; **H. Jedin**, *Kirche des Glaubens – Kirche der Geschichte. Ausgewählte Aufsätze und Vorträge* (2 vols.), Freiburg 1966; **H. Jedin** and **J. Dolan** (eds.), *History of the Church* V, London and New York 1980; **E. W. Zeeden**, *Das Zeitalter der Gegenreformation*, Freiburg 1967; id. (ed.), *Gegenreformation*, Darmstadt 1973; id., *Konfessionsbildung. Studien zur Reformation, Gegenreformation und katholischer Reform*, Stuttgart 1985; **A. G. Dickens**, *The Counter Reformation*, London 1968; **R. De Maio**, *Riforme e miti nella Chiesa del Cinquecento*, Naples 1973; **M. Bendiscoli**, *Dalla Riforma alla Controriforma*, Bologna 1974; **M. R. O'Connell**, *The Counter Reformation 1559–1610*, New York 1974; **K. D. Schmidt**, *Die katholische Reform und die Gegenreformation*, Göttingen 1975; **H. Lutz**, *Reformation und Gegenreformation*, Munich 1979; **S. Zoli**, *La Controriforma*, Florence 1979; **P. Chaunu**, *Église, culture et société. Essais sur Réforme et Contre-Réforme (1517–1620)*, Paris 1981; **A. D. Wright**, *The Counter-Reformation. Catholic Europe and the Non-Christian World*, New York 1982; **M. Heckel**, *Deutschland im konfessionellen Zeitalter*, Göttingen 1983; **M. Hroch** and **A. Skybová**, *Die Inquisition im Zeitalter der Gegenreformation* (Czech original), Stuttgart 1985; **C. Brovetto** et al., *La spiritualità cristiana nell'età moderna*, Rome 1987; **J. W. O'Malley** (ed.), *Catholicism in Early Modern History. A Guide to Research*, St Louis 1988; **J. L. Bouza Álvarez**, *Religiosidad contrarreformista y cultura simbólica del Barroco*, Madrid 1990; **W. Seibrich**, *Gegenreformation als Restauration. Die restaurativen Bemühungen der alten Orden im Deutschen Reich von 1580 bis 1648*, Muñster 1991; **H. R. Schmidt**, *Konfessionalisierung im 16.Jahrhundert*, Munich 1992. In addition there have been various specialist investigations of the Counter-Reformation in individual European countries and regions.

355. Cf. **H. Jedin**, 'Catholic Reform and Counter-Reformation', in **id.** and **Dolan**, *History of the Church* (n.354), V, Part 2; **M. Venard** (ed.), *Le temps des*

confessions (1530–1620/30), Paris 1992, esp. Part I, Ch.5 (including a survey of the individual countries).

356. **L. von Pastor** devotes the impressive Vol.5 of his history of the papacy to the transitional Pope Paul III without describing him like his predecessors as a Pope 'in the age of the Renaissance' (which he already does in the title), or like his successors as a Pope 'in the age of the Catholic Reformation and Restoration'.

357. Text in **Mirbt** and **Aland** (n.317), *Quellen*, no.814.

358. Ibid., no.817; for the history of the Jesuit order cf. **J. E. Vercruysee**, 'Jesuiten', *TRE* XVI.

359. Text in **Mirbt** and **Aland** (n.317), *Quellen*, no.816.

360. Cf. **Paul VI**, bull, *Cum ex apostolatus officio*, 1559, text in in Mirbt and Aland, *Quellen*, no.842 (significantly, not a single document from Paul IV is included in Denziger).

361. For the **Council of Trent**, in addition to the Goerres edition of the acts of the council see the standard work by **H. Jedin**, *Geschichte des Konzils von Trient*, I–IV.2, Freiburg 1949–75 (only the first two volumes were translated into English, *History of the Council of Trent*, London 1957, 1962); cf. also **O. de la Brosse** et al., *Latran V et Trent*, Paris 1975; **R. Bäumer** (ed.), *Concilium Tridentinum*, Darmstadt 1979; **J. M. Rovira Belloso**, *Trento. Una Interpretación teológica*, Barcelona 1979; **A. Duval**, *Des sacrements au Concile de Trente*, Paris 1985; **J. Bernhard, L. Lefebvre** and **F. Rapp**, *L'époque de la Réforme et du concile de Trente*, Paris 1989.

362. The decrees on the faith are in **Denzinger**, *Enchiridion*, and in **J. Alberigo**'s collection on the council; the reform decrees are only in Alberigo.

363. Thus **Jedin**, *Katholische Reform oder Gegenreformation?* (n.353), 229f., 658.

364. **H. Lutz**, *Reformation und Gegenreformation* (n.354), notes: 'Not only in dogma, but also pastorally and organizationally, on many questions which Luther had put or taken over from Christian humanism the attitude adopted was a purely defensive one' (69). So we need to examine 'what terminological framework for the totality of old and new questions might perhaps have corresponded better to the working of Catholicism than Jedin's double concept'; Lutz cannot 'avoid the impression that some of the complex church and cultural changes do not fit properly into the model of Jedin's double concept' (155f.).

365. Cf. **Schmidt**, *Konfessionalisierung* (n.354), 67f.

366. Cf. **Denzinger**, *Enchiridion*, no.864 (canon 8 on baptism).

367. Cf. ibid., nos.792a–843; also **H. Küng**, *Justification*.

368. **Denzinger**, *Enchiridion*, no.783.

369. Ibid., 844.

370. Cf. above C II 3, 'Charismatic church in Paul'.

371. The number of **sacraments** depends on the **definition** of sacrament. Originally the term denoted a pledge of money, then an oath or the act of dedication; later in Christianity – in connection with the Greek *mysterion* – the mysteries of belief in the Trinity, the Incarnation, the work of Christ and individual facts of his life, the meaning of the Gospels or individual Christian cultic acts. It then depended, in particular, on the definition of the concept which concrete cultic acts were called sacraments and subsumed under the concept of sacrament: only baptism and eucharist or also ordination, anointing at a coronation, the dedication of nuns or marriage. The less the content of a concept is defined, the wider its extent, and vice versa: that is an old insight of Aristotelian

logic. So the more definite the concept of sacrament, the fewer sacraments there are: 30 (Hugo of St Victor), 12 (Peter Damian), 7 (Peter Lombard, the great Scholastics and then the Council of Trent), or 6 (Pseudo-Dionysius), 5 (the *Summa sententiarum*, the school of Anselm of Laon and William of Champeaux), 4 (the early mediaeval theologians, who in particularly counted baptism and chrism, body and blood), 3 (Isidore of Seville), 2 (a broad tradition from the early fathers to the Reformers.

372. For baptism and eucharist see **H. Küng**, *Church*, C III 1–2.

373. Cf. **H. Jedin**, *History of the Council of Trent* (n.361) II, 326: 'It is remarkable that no allusion whatever was made to the historical origin of the number seven. The Council contented itself with pointing to the analogies to be found in Scripture (Rev.1.16; 5.1; Ex.25.3, etc.), but overlooked the fact that the number was not to be found in the decisions of the Councils nor in patristic literature, and that more than a thousand years had elapsed before the identity of the sacramental rites in use from the days of the early Church with the two chief sacraments, Baptism and Eucharist, was recognized.'

374. Cf. **Denzinger**, *Enchiridion*, no.989.

375. Cf. **id.**, *Enchiridion*, 994–1000.

376. **Schmidt**, *Konfessionalisierung* (n.354), 25f.

377. Ibid., 41.

378. Of equal importance, but in a very different way, were the leaders of curial reform like Pius V and Carlo Borromeo, Cardinal Fisher and the English martyrs, the Jesuits Peter Canisius, Robert Bellarmine, Francisco Borgia, Aloysius Gonzaga, Stanislaus Kostka, the Spanish mystic John of the Cross, who was also a reformer of his order, John of God and Peter of Alcantara, and finally the French spiritualists like François de Sales and Vincent de Paul, Bérulle, Fénelon, Bourdaloue and Massillon, Pascal and in church scholarship Petavius, the Maurists and the Bollandists . . . a wealth of well-known names which stand for a large number of lesser-known ones.

379. Cf. the summary in **E. W. Zeeden**, *Das Zeitalter der Glaubenskämpfe 1555–1648*, Gebhardts Handbuch der deutschen Geschichte II, ⁹1970, 118–239.

380. Cf. the large illustrated volume by **Y. Bottineau**, *L'art baroque*, Paris 1986.

381. Cf. **H. Wölfflin**, *Renaissance und Barock. Eine Untersuchung über Wesen und Entstehung des Barockstils in Italien*, Munich 1888.

382. Cf. **H. Küng**, *Credo*, 8f., 18–20, 122–4, 158–61.

383. Cf. **Jedin** and **Dolan** (eds.), *History of the Church* (n.355), V, Ch.41, 'The Revival of Scholasticism'.

384. Cf. ibid., Ch.42, 'Der Rise of Positive Theology'; here there are more precise details on the works mentioned below.

385. Cf. **P. Sarpi**, *Istoria del Concilio Tridentino seguita dalla 'Vita del Padre Paolo' di Fulgenzio Micanzio* (2 vols), Turin 1974. It was available in Latin, French, English and German only ten years after its appearance in 1619.

386. The last complete edition by **F. Suárez**, *Opera omnia*, Paris 1856–61; Vols. V and VI, *De legibus* (almost 1200 pages), is especially important for legal philosophy and the philosophy of the state. So far, other than in histories of theology, no one has been led to write a complete account of **baroque scholasticism**.

387. Cf. **Congar**, *L'Église* (n.323), esp. chs. X–XIV, or from the Protestant side **F. Heyer**, *Die katholische Kirche von 1648 bis 1879*, Göttingen 1963.

388. **L. J. Rogier**, 'Die Kirche im Zeitalter der Aufklärung und Revolution', in id. et al., *Geschichte der Kirche* IV, Zurich 1966, 1–174: 29.

389. **R. Aubert**, 'The Catholic Church and the Revolution', in H. Jedin and J. Dolan (eds.), *History of the Church* VI, London and New York 1981, 3–84: 8.

390. For the age of Restoration, among the handbooks on church history cf. above all **J. Leflon**, *La crise révolutionnaire 1789–1846*, Paris 1951, and **R. Aubert, J. Beckmann, P. J. Corish** and **R. Lill**, *The Church Between Revolution und Restoration, History of the Church* VII, ed. H. Jedin and J. D. Dolan, London and New York 1981.

391. **F. X. Kaufmann**, *Kirche begreifen. Analysen und Thesen zur gesellschaftlichen Verfassung des Christentums*, Freiburg 1979; id., *Religion und Modernität. Sozialwissenschaftliche Perspektiven*, Tübingen 1989.

392. **K. Gabriel**, 'Die neuzeitliche Gesellschaftsentwicklung und der Katholizismus als Sozialform der Christentumsgeschichte', in K. Gabriel and F. X. Kaufmann (eds.), *Zur Sociologie des Katholizismus*, Mainz 1980, 201–25.

393. **K. Gabriel**, *Christentum zwischen Tradition und Postmoderne*, Freiburg 1992, 165.

394. An almost prime example of this development is Swiss Catholicism in the context of the rise of the liberal federal state as this has been analysed in an exemplary way by U. **Altermatt**, *Der Weg der Schweizer Katholiken ins Ghetto*, Zurich 1972; id., *Katholizismus und Moderne. Zur Sozial- und Mentalitätsgeschichte der Schweizer Katholiken im 19. und 20. Jahrhundert*, Zurich ²1991.

395. Cf. **R. Reinhardt** (ed.), *Tübinger Theologen und ihre Theologie. Quellen und Forschungen zur Geschichte der Katholisch-theologischen Fakultät Tübingen*, Tübingen 1977.

396. Cf. **id.**, 'Die Katholisch-theologische Fakultät Tübingen im ersten Jahrhundert ihres Bestehens. Faktoren und Phasen der Entwicklung', in id. (ed.), *Tübinger Theologen*, 1–42.

397. How little substantive basis there was to the proceedings against Hermes and how vulnerable they were in terms of formal law has been shown by the investigation of the Roman process by **H. H. Schwedt**, *Das römische Urteil über Georg Hermes (1775–1831). Ein Beitrag zur Geschichte der Inquisition im 19.Jahrhundert*, Freiburg 1980.

398. Cf. **Denzinger**, *Enchiridion*, nos.1700–1800.

399. Ibid., no. 1780.

400. Cf. **H. Küng**, *Infallible?*; id. (ed.), *Fehlbar?*.

401. Cf. **A. B. Hasler**, *Pius IX (1846–78), Päpstliche Unfehlbarkeit und 1.Vatikanisches Konzil. Dogmatisierung und Durchsetzung einer Ideologie* (2 vols.), Stuttgart 1977; id., *How the Pope Became Infallible*, New York 1981; G. **Thils**, *Primauté et infaillibilité du Pontife Romain à Vatican I. Et autres études d'ecclésiologie*, Louvain 1989.

402. For **Vatican I**, in addition to the early works of **J. Friedrich**, *Geschichte des Vatikanischen Konzils* (3 vols.), Bonn 1867–1887 (from an Old Catholic perspective), and **T. Granderath**, *Geschichte des Vatikanischen Konzils* (3 vols.), ed. K. Kirch, Freiburg 1903–1906 (from a curial perspective), cf. in particular **E. C. Butler**, *The Vatican Council. The Story told from Inside in Bishop Ullathorne's Letters*, London 1930, which gives a vivid account of the dramatic course of the council and individual interventions. This account could be

compared with the diaries of an Italian bishop and historian recently edited by L. Pásztor, *Il concilio Vaticano I. Diario di Vincenzo Tizzani (1869–1870)* (2 vols.), Stuttgart 1991f. Also the well-judged history of the council by the Louvain church historian R. Aubert, *Vatikanum I*, Paris 1964; id., *Le Pontificat de Pie IX*, Paris 1952. Cf. also C. Langlois, 'Unfehlbarkeit – eine neue Idee des 19.Jahrhunderts', in H. Küng (ed.), *Fehlbar?*, 146–60. It is impossible here to investigate different special aspects (revelation, foundation of faith, church and state) or persons (Döllinger, bishops).

403. Cf. Denzinger, *Enchiridion*, nos.1781–1820. Cf. C III 9 above, 'The power of reason and the turning point of theology'.

404. For antimodernism cf. R. Marlé (ed.), *Au coeur de la crise moderniste. Le dossier inédit d'une controverse. Lettres de M. Blondel, H. Bremond, F. von Hügel, A. Loisy . . .*, Paris 1960; P. Scoppola, *Crisi modernista e rinnovamento cattolico in Italia*, Bologna 1961; É. Poulat, *Histoire, dogme et critique dans la crise moderniste*, Paris 1962; id., *Modernistica. Horizons, physiognomies, débats*, Paris 1982; L. Bedeschi, *La Curia romana durante la crisi modernista. Episodi e metodi di governo*, Parma 1968; id., *Interpretazioni e sviluppo del modernismo cattolico*, Milan 1975; M. Ranchetti, *The Catholic Modernists. A Study of the Religious Reform Movement 1864–1907*, London 1969; O. Schroeder, *Aufbruch und Missverständnis. Zur Geschichte der reformkatholischen Bewegung*, Graz 1969; A. R. Vidler, *A Variety of Catholic Modernists*, Cambridge 1970; R. García de Haro, *Historia teologica del modernismo*, Pamplona 1972; O. Köhler, *Bewusstseinsstörungen im Katholizismus*, Frankfurt 1972; G. Maron, *Die römisch-katholische Kirche, von 1870 bis 1970*, Göttingen 1972; J. Greisch, K. Neufeld and C. Theobald, *La crise contemporaine. Du modernisme à la crise des herméneutiques*, Paris 1973; E. Weinzierl (ed.), *Der Modernismus. Beiträge zu seiner Erforschung*, Graz 1974; G. Schwaiger (ed.), *Aufbruch ins 20. Jahrhundert. Zum Streit um Reformkatholizismus und Modernismus*, Göttingen 1976; A. Hastings (ed.), *Bishops and Writers. Aspects of the Evolution of Modern English Catholicism*, Cambridge 1977; N. Trippen, *Theologie und Lehramt im Konflikt. Die kirchlichen Massnahmen gegen den Modernismus im Jahre 1907 und ihre Auswirkungen in Deutschland*, Freiburg 1977; B. Greco, *Ketzer oder Prophet? Evangelium und Kirche bei dem Modernisten Ernesto Buonaiuti (1881–1946)*, Zurich 1979; T. M. Loome, *Liberal Catholicism, Reform Catholicism, Modernism. A Contribution to a New Orientation in Modernist Research*, Mainz 1979; C. Tresmontant, *La crise moderniste*, Paris 1979; P. Colin et al., *Le Modernisme*, Paris 1980; G. Daly, *Transcendence and Immanence. A Study in Catholic Modernism and Integralism*, Oxford 1980; L. R. Kurtz, *The Politics of Heresy. The Modernist Crisis in Roman Catholicism*, Berkeley 1986.

405. Cf. H. Küng, *Judaism* 2 A II 5, 'A Pope who kept silent: Pius XII'.

406. According to Deut.6.4.

407. Cf. *Concilium* 11, 1975, Vol.10 (this issue was not translated into English).

408. W. Kasper, 'Bleibendes und Veränderliches im Petrusamt', ibid., 525–31: 529.

409. I already made this proposal for an ecumenical solution to the question of the primacy in *The Church*, I II 3.

410. Cf. Arbeitsgemeinschaft ökumenischer Universitätsinstitute (ed.), *Papsttum als ökumenische Frage*, Mainz 1979; R. Leuze, 'Papst, Papsttum (2.system-

atisch-ökumenisch)', in *Evangelisches Kirchenlexikon* III, Göttingen 1992, 1027–33.

411. All the documents on the controversy are in the relevant documentations: W. Jens (ed.), *Um nichts als die Wahrheit. Deutsche Bischofskonferenz contra Hans Küng. Eine Dokumentation*, Munich 1978: N. Greinacher and H. Haag (eds.), *Der Fall Küng. Eine Dokumentation*, Munich 1980.

412. However, Catholic theologians throughout the world (and, no less, Protestant fellow-travellers) who conform with the system have meekly gone along with Rome's attempt to silence critics (*damnatio memoriae*). Here is just one example. K. Schatz SJ has written a (moderately) apologetic account of the Roman primacy under the title *Der päpstliche Primat. Seine Geschichte von den Ursprüngen bis zur Gegenwart*, Würzburg 1990. From beginning to end he keeps quiet about the publications associated with my name, the critical questions (in particular about the Council of Constance and Vatican I) and the world–wide discussions. He follows the recipe for dealing with critical Catholic theologians (at that time de Lubac, Rahner, Bouillard, Congar et al.) which the then Prefect of Studies at the Pontifical Gregorian University, C. Boyer, SJ, gave me when I was a student, and which I have never followed: 'They should read such authors but never cite them.' The same author has also written a two-volume history of the council, *Vatikanum I, 1869–1870*, Paderborn 1992/3 (already in the preface there is a general verdict on the work of A. B. Hasler, to save having a serious discussion of this scholar, who died all too prematurely). We need not get too excited about the forthcoming third volume on the definition of the primacy and the infallibility of the Pope. However, a very recent positive example to the contrary is the volume by the Jesuit H. J. Sieben, *Katholisches Konzilsidee im 19. und 20.Jahrhundert*, Paderborn 1993. Here the author objectively and with fair references to my 'new approach' goes into a 'theology of the council' and also into my 'enquiry' about papal infallibility and the discussion to which it gave rise. The best history of the council is still the account by R. Aubert, which Schatz, too, describes as 'still not superseded' (Preface Vol.1).

413. According to a major survey by *Le Monde, La Vie* and *L'Actualité religieuse dans le monde*, carried out in 1994 by three leading sociologists of religion (G. Michelat, J. Sutter and J. Potel), in France, 83% of the population go by their conscience alone on moral questions and only 1% (one per cent!) by the teaching of the church. Cf. the summary by A. Woodrow of *Le Monde* in *The Tablet*, 21 May 1994. According to the *Allensbacher Jahrbuch der Demoskopie* 9, 1993, in Germany only 16% feel themselves bound by important decisions of the Pope (only 3% of those between 16 and 29), and 70% would set themselves above such decisions (86% of those between 16 and 29). Similar figures can also be got from other European countries (a dramatic decline in the authority of the church even in Poland), and in the USA and Canada.

414. An excellent investigation has now been made of 'evangelical Catholicity' by the Protestant theologian R. Becker, *Hans Küngs Modell einer 'evangelischen Katholizität' als der 'wahren Katholizität'*, Osnabrück dissertation 1994.

IV. The Protestant Evangelical Paradigm of the Reformation

1. Cf. the pioneering works by **B. Moeller**, *Reichstadt und die Reformation*, Gütersloh 1962; **id.**, *Deutschland im Zeitalter der Reformation*, Göttingen 1977, ²1981, and **E. W. Zeeden**, *Die Enstehung der Konfessionen. Grundlagen und Formen der Konfessionsbildung im Zeitalter der Glaubenskämpfe*, Munich 1965; **id.**, *Konfessionsbildung. Studien zur Reformation, Gegenreformation und katholischen Reform*, Stuttgart 1985. I am deeply grateful to the Reformation historian Prof. Dr **Friedhelm Krüger** of the University of Osnabrück for reading through Chapter C IV.

2. Cf. **H. Küng**, *Judaism*, 1 C II 2, 'The epoch-making achievements of David as king'.

3. Cf. **L. von Ranke**, *Deutsche Geschichte im Zeitalter der Reformation* (6 vols.), new edition by P. Joachimsen, Munich 1925/26.

4. For the **interpretation** of **Luther** cf. **A. Herte**, *Das katholische Lutherbild im Bann der Lutherkommentare des Cochläus* (3 vols.), Münster 1943; **J. Hessen**, *Luther in katholischer Sicht*, Bonn 1947; **E. W. Zeeden**, *Martin Luther und die Reformation im Urteil des deutschen Luthertums* (2 vols.), Freiburg 1950/52; **H. Stephan**, *Luther in den Wandlungen seiner Kirche*, Berlin ²1951; **H. Bornkamm**, *Luther im Spiegel der deutschen Geistesgeschichte. Mit ausgewählten Texten von Lessing bis zur Gegenwart*, Göttingen 1955, ²1970; **R. Stauffer**, *Le catholicisme à la découverte de Luther. L'évolution des recherches catholiques sur Luther de 1904 au 2ᵐᵉ concile du Vatican*, Neuchâtel 1966; **Wandlungen des Lutherbildes**, Würzburg 1966 (especially the contributions by E. Iserloh, W. von Loewenich, H. Jedin and F. W. Kantzenbach); **A. Hasler**, *Luther in der katholischen Dogmatik. Darstellung seiner Rechtfertigungslehre in den katholischen Dogmatikbüchern*, Munich 1968; **B. Lohse**, *Lutherdeutung heute*, Göttingen 1968; **W. Beyna**, *Das moderne katholische Lutherbild*, Essen 1969; **O. H. Porsch**, *Ketzerfürst und Kirchenlehrer. Wege katholischer Begegnung mit Martin Luther*, Stuttgart 1971; **H. F. Geisser** (et al.), *Weder Ketzer noch Heiliger. Luthers Bedeutung für den ökumenischen Dialog*, Regensburg 1872; **K. Lehmann** (ed.), *Luthers Sendung für Katholiken und Protestanten*, Munich 1982; **G. Maron**, *Das katholische Lutherbild der Gegenwart. Anmerkungen und Anfragen*, Göttingen 1982; **B. Moeller** (ed.), *Luther in der Neuzeit. Wissenschaftliches Symposion des Vereins für Reformationsgeschichte*, Gütersloh 1983.

5. For **Martin Luther** and the **Reformation in Germany**, in addition to important earlier works (especially by H. Grisar, R. Hermann, K. Holl, J. K. Köstlin and G. Kawerau, L. von Ranke and O. Scheel), cf. **G. Ritter**, *Luther. Gestalt und Tat*, Munich 1925, ⁶1959; **L. Febvre**, *Martin Luther. A Destiny*, New York 1929; **J. Lortz**, *Die Reformation in Deutschland* (2 vols.), Freiburg 1940, new edition 1982; **R. H. Bainton**, *Here I Stand. A Life of Luther*, New York 1950; **id.**, *The Reformation of the Sixteenth Century*, Boston 1952, ³1985; **K. A. Meissinger**, *Der katholische Luther*, Munich 1952; **E. H. Erikson**, *Young Man Luther. A Study in Psychoanalysis and History*, London 1958; **H. J. Iwand**, *Gesammelte Aufsätze* (2 vols.), Munich 1959/80; **F. Lau**, *Luther*, Philadelphia 1963; **M. Lienhard**, *Martin Luther. Un temps, une vie, un message*, Paris 1959, ³1991; **F. Lau** and **E. Bizer**, *Reformationsgeschichte Deutschlands bis 1555*, Göttingen 1964; **J. Delumeau**, *Naissance et affirmation de la Réforme*, Paris 1965; **R. Friedenthal**, *Luther. His Life and Times*, New York 1967; **H. Jedin** and **J. Dolan**, *History of the Church*, V, New York and London 1980; **R.**

Stupperich, *Geschichte der Reformation*, Munich 1967; **R. García-Villoslada**, *Martín Lutero* (2 vols.), Madrid 1973; **A. G. Dickens**, *The German Nation and Martin Luther*, London 1974; **R. Marius**, *Luther*, Philadelphia 1974; **H. Bornkamm**, *Luther. Gestalt und Wirkungen. Gesammelte Aufsätze*, Gütersloh 1975 (with a detailed criticism of Erikson's thesis); id., *Martin Luther in der Mitte seines Lebens. Das Jahrzehnt zwischen dem Wormser und dem Augsburger Reichstag*, ed. K. Bornkamm, Göttingen 1979; **P. Chaunu**, *Le temps des Réformes. Histoire religieuse et système de civilisation. La Crise de la chrétienté. L'Éclatement (1250–1550)*, Paris 1975; id., *Église, culture et société. Essais sur Réforme et Contre-réforme (1517–1620)*, Paris 1981; **H. A. Oberman**, *The Dawn of the Reformation*, Edinburgh 1987; id., *Luther, Man between God and the Devil*, New Haven 1990; id., *Die Reformation. Von Wittenberg nach Genf*, Göttingen 1986; **H. Lutz**, *Reformation und Gegenreformation*, Munich 1979; **E. Iserloh**, *Geschichte und Theologie der Reformation im Grundriss*, Paderborn 1980; id., *Kirche – Ereignis und Institution. Aufsätze und Vorträge*, Vol.II, *Geschichte und Theologie der Reformation*, Munster 1985; **P. Manns**, *Martin Luther. Ketzer oder Vater im Glauben?*, Hanover 1980; **M. Brecht**, *Martin Luther: His Road to Reformation*, Philadelphia 1985; id., *Martin Luther: Shaping and Defining the Reformation, 1521–1532*, Minneapolis 1990; id., *Martin Luther: The Preservation of the Church, 1532–1546*, Minneapolis 1993; **B. Lohse**, *Martin Luther. Eine Einführung in sein Leben und sein Werk*, Munich 1981, [2]1983; **W. von Loewenich**, *Martin Luther. Der Mann und das Werk*, Munich 1982; **J. M. Todd**, *Luther. A Life*, London 1982; **H. Junghans** (ed.), *Leben und Werk Martin Luthers von 1526 bis 1546* (2 vols.), Berlin 1983; **H. Löwe** and **C. J. Roepke** (eds.), *Luther und die Folgen. Beiträge zur sozialgeschichtlichen Bedeutung der lutherischen Reformation*, Munich 1983; **H. D. Rix**, *Martin Luther. The Man and the Image*, New York 1983; **G. Cogler** (ed.), *Martin Luther. Leben, Werk, Wirkung*, Berlin 1983; **G. Wendelborn**, *Martin Luther. Leben und reformatorisches Werk*, Berlin 1983; **J. M. Kittelson**, *Luther the Reformer. The Story of the Man and his Career*, Minneapolis 1986; **R. Schwarz**, *Luther*, Göttingen 1986; for Luther's life I have followed the work of the famous Luther scholar **R. W. Scribner**, *The German Reformation*, Atlantic Highland, NJ 1986, which sums up his earlier researches, and **H. Zahrnt**, *Martin Luther. Reformator wider Willen*, Munich 1986.

6. The first to bring this out in an unprejudiced way from the Catholic side was **Lortz**, *Die Reformation in Deutschland* (n.4), I, 1–144. **Chaunu**, *Le temps des Réformes* (n.5), esp. chs.IV–V, offers a more recent comprehensive account.

7. For **Luther's theology**, in addition to numerous important individual investigations e.g. on the doctrine of justification (A. Peters, O. H. Pesch, M. Seils, H. Vorster), cf. **J. Lortz**, *Die Reformation als religiöses Anliegen heute. Vier Vorträge im Dienste der* Una Sancta, Trier 1948; **H. Bornkamm**, *Luthers geistige Welt*, Gütersloh [2]1953; **R. Hermann**, *Gesammelte Studien zur Theologie und Reformation*, Göttingen 1960; id., *Gesammelte und nachgelassene Werke* (2 vols.), ed. H. Beintker et al., Göttingen 1967/81; **P. Althaus**, *The Theology of Martin Luther*, Philadelphia 1966; **B. A. Gerrish**, *Grace and Reason. A Study in the Theology of Luther*, Oxford 1962; **S. Pfürtner**, *Luther und Thomas im Gespräch*, Heidelberg 1963; **G. Ebeling**, *Luther*, London 1972; id., *Lutherstudien* (3 vols.), Tübingen 1971–85; **L. Pinomaa**, *Sieg des Glaubens. Grundlinien der Theologie Luthers*, revised and edited by H. Beintker, Göttingen 1964; **F. Gogarten**, *Luthers Theologie*, Tübingen 1967; **H. J. McSorley**, *Luthers Lehre*

vom unfreien Willen nach seiner Hauptschrift De Servo Arbitrio *im Lichte der biblischen und kirchlichen Tradition,* Munich 1967; **H. G. Koenigsberger** (ed.), *Luther. A Profile,* London 1973; **T. Beer,** *Der fröhliche Wechsel und Streit. Grundzüge der Theologie Luthers,* Leipzig 1974; **H. J. Iwand,** *Luthers Theologie,* ed. J. Haar, Munich 1974; **L. Grane,** Modus loquendi theologicus. *Luthers Kampf um die Erneuerung der Theologie 1515–1518* (Danish original), Leiden 1975; **R. Weier,** *Das Theologieverständnis Martin Luthers,* Paderborn 1976; **D. Olivier,** *La foi de Luther. La cause de l'Evangile dans l'Eglise,* Paris 1978; **O. H. Pesch,** *Hinführung zu Luther,* Mainz 1982; **G. Scharffenorth,** *Den Glauben ins Leben ziehen . . . Studien zu Luthers Theologie,* Munich 1982; **J. Atkinson,** *Martin Luther. Prophet to the Church Catholic,* Exeter 1983; **G. Brendler,** *Martin Luther. Theologe und Revolution,* Berlin 1983.

8. Cf. **H. Küng,** 'Katholische Besinnung auf Luthers Rechtfertigungslehre heute', in *Theologie im Wandel, Festschrift zum 150–jährigen Bestehen der Katholisch-Theologischen Fakultät an der Universität Tübingen 1817–1967,* Munich 1967, 449–68.

9. Cf. **H. Denifle,** *Die abendländischen Schriftausleger bis Luther über* Justitia Dei *(R 1, 217) und* Justificatio, Mainz 1905.

10. Cf. **O. H. Pesch,** 'Zwanzig Jahre katholische Lutherforschung', *Lutherische Rundschau* 16, 1966, 392-406. In his introduction to Luther's theology (1983) Pesch has followed through the controversy in an exemplary way.

11. Cf. **H. Küng,** *Justification.*

12. That the **doctrine of justification no longer divides the churches** has been confirmed:

(a) By the joint document of the Lutheran World Federation and the Roman Secretariat for Unity, *Das Evangelium und die Kirche* (Malta Report), 1972, in H. Meyer, H. J. Urban and L. Vischer (eds.), *Dokumente wachsender Übereinstimmung. Sämtliche Berichte und Konsenstexte interkonfessioneller Gespräche auf Weltebene 1931–1982,* Paderborn 1983, 248–71, esp. nos.26–30;

(b) By the document of the ecumenical working group of the Joint Ecumenical Commission 'Lehrverurteilungen-kirchentrennend?' (formed after John Paul II's visit to the Federal Republic of Germany in 1980): I. *Rechtfertigung, Sakramente und Amt im Zeitalter der Reformation und heute,* ed. K. Lehmann and W. Pannenberg, Freiburg 1986, esp. 35–75;

(c) By a report by the Vatican Council for Unity of 15 December 1992 which explicitly states 'that canons 1–32 on the decree on justification (of Trent) do not apply to Lutheran doctrine as set out in the confessional writings'. A 'far-reaching agreement' on eucharistic doctrine was also established. Cf. the report in *Herder Korrespondenz* 47, 1993, 176.

13. Cf. **M. Luther,** *On Good Works* (1520), LW (= Luther's Works, 55 vols., St Louis and Minneapolis 1955ff.) 32, 106ff.

14. Cf. **id.,** *To the Christian Nobility of the German Nation* (1520), LW 36, 11–126.

15. Cf. **id.,** *On the Babylonian Captivity of the Church* (1520), LW 36, 11–126.

17. **Id.,** *The Freedom of A Christian* (1520), LW 31, 333–77.

18. This is based on my own translation of Luther's concluding remarks in his speech: cf. the 'Colloquy with D. Martin Luther at the Reichstag at Worms', WA VIII, 814–87, esp. 838; the famous sentence 'Here I stand, I can do no other' is not authentic. For the historical context cf. **F. Reuter** (ed.), *Der Reichstag zu*

Worms von 1521. Reichspolitik und Luthersache, Worms 1971; here on Luther's stand especially **K.-V. Selge**, Capta conscientia in verbis Dei, *Luthers Widerrufs-verweigerung in Worms*, 180–207.

19. This is now also conceded from the Catholic side: cf. **W. Trilling**, 'Antichrist und Papsttum. Reflexionen zur Wirkungsgeschichte von 2 Thess 2, 1–10a', *Bonner Biblischer Beitrag 53*, 1980, 251–71.

20. Cf. **S. Pfürtner**, 'The Paradigms of Thomas Aquinas and Martin Luther. Did Luther's Message of Justification Mean a Paradigm Change?', in H. Kung and D. Tracy (eds.), *Paradigm Change in Theology*, Edinburgh 1989, 130–60.

21. Cf. **Ebeling**, *Luther* (n.7).

22. Cf. **id.**, 'Hermeneutik', *RGG* III, 242–62.

23. **U. Baumann**, *Die Ehe – Ein Sakrament?*, Zurich 1988, 29–44, esp. 33f., interprets this correctly.

24. Cf. **T. S. Kuhn**, *The Structure of Scientific Revolutions*, Chicago ²1970.

25. Cf. **H. Küng**, TTM, B II 5, 'How does Novelty Come into Being? Parallels from Natural Science and Theology'.

26. Cf. **Kuhn**, *Structure* (n.24), Ch.12, 'The Resolution of Revolutions'.

27. **Pesch**, *Hinführung zu Luther* (n.7), 44.

28. **H. Zahrnt**, 'Der Zeitgenosse', in H. J. Schultz (ed.), *Luther Kontrovers*, Stuttgart 1983, 26–40: 35.

29. Kuhn's book makes only passing mention of this decisive point, which brought him much criticism: in the natural sciences, too, there is the 'same bundle of data as before', but these are 'put into a new system of relations with one another' (85).

30. It is significant that Kuhn avoids this word until the very last pages of his book (cf. 170).

31. Cf. **L. Wittgenstein**, *Tractatus logico-philosophicus*, London 1922, 187.

32. Cf. **H. Küng**, DGE, E II, 'Fundamental mistrust or fundamental trust?', F IV.3, 'Belief in God as ultimately justified fundamental trust'.

33. Amazingly, even such an expert in the later Middle Ages as the former Tübinen Reformation historian **H. A. Oberman** underestimates the explosive force, say, of Erasmus's *Enchiridion militis Christianae* (Handbook for the Christian Soldier, 1503), which also became a theological bestseller in translation, and describes it as 'the most boring book in the history of piety' ('Luthers Reformatorische Ontdekkingen', in *Maarten Luther. Feestelijke Herdenking van zijn Vijfhonderdste Geboortedag*, Amsterdam 1983, 11–34: 31).
It is striking that Erasmus also does not get a good press from certain Catholic church historians who keep silent about his significance or give it a negative stamp. One only has to read the article on Erasmus in the Catholic *Lexikon für Theologie und Kirche* by the Catholic Münster Reformation historian **E. Iserloh** (III, 955–7), who as late as 1984/85 still thinks it important to present to the public a whole collection of second-rate anti-Lutheran controversial theologians under the title *Katholische Theologe der Reformationszeit* (2 vols., Münster 1984–85), of course without including Erasmus, who was at the peak of his fame immediately before the Reformation (he was called '*Doctor Universalis*', 'Prince of Learning' and 'Guardian of Honest Theology') and was without peer among 'Catholic theologians'. The way in which Iserloh deals with Erasmus (very much along the same lines as his teacher Joseph Lortz) is typical of a confessionalist Roman Catholic church historian: the obscure origins of Erasmus (in the end to be attributed to compulsory celibacy!) – he was the illegitimate child of a liaison

between the priest Roger Gerard and the daughter of a doctor, became an orphan around the age of fourteen, and was sent by his guardians into a monastery – are exploited in a psychological and moralizing way: 'The stain of his birth to which he never got used and the lack of family and home explain the unrest, suspicious evasion, anxiety to establish himself, sensitivity and need to make himself felt which are found so often in him.' So beware of this man! Thus preparations are made right from the cradle for the historian's dogmatic verdict, which is not worth quoting here. However, Erasmus has eventually received justice even from Catholic theologians – see the works of **F. X. Funk** and later **A. Auer** and **R. Padberg** et al.

34. Thus **C. Augustijn**, *Erasmus of Rotterdam*, Toronto and London 1991, 26. In the footsteps of the early brilliant biography of Erasmus written by **Johan Huizinga** in 1923, Augustijn, who is now perhaps the greatest expert on Erasmus, and is also a Dutchman, has incorporated into his biography German, French and English research, which are so contrasting – Erasmus the undecided anti-Lutheran, the rationalist early man of the Enlightenment, the classical humanist. The book can be followed confidently for the most important historical facts and circumstances.

35. Cf. **Erasmus of Rotterdam**, *Enchiridion* (1503), translation in M. Spinka (ed.), *Advocates of Reform*, Library of Christian Classics 14, London and Philadelphia 1953, 295–379.

36. Cf. **R. H. Bainton**, *Erasmus of Christendom*, New York 1969.

37. **Augustijn**, *Erasmus* (n.34), 48.

38. Cf. **Erasmus of Rotterdam**, *Encomium Moriae* (1511), modern edition *In Praise of Folly*, ed.H. Hudson, Princeton 1941.

39. Cf. **id.**, *Adagia* (1500, extended edition 1515), modern edition by M. M. Phillips, Cambridge 1964.

40. Cf. **id.**, *Querela pacis* (1518), modern edition *Our Struggle for Peace*, Boston 1950.

41. Cf. **id.**, *Institutio Principis Christiani* (1515), modern edition *The Education of a Christian Prince*, ed. L. K. Born, London 1936.

42. cf. **id.**, *Opera omnia*, Leiden edition V 140 C.

43. Cf. **F. Krüger**, *Humanistische Evangelienauslegung. Desiderius Erasmus von Rotterdam als Ausleger der Evangelien in seinen Paraphrasen*, Tübingen 1986.

44. **Id.**, *Opera omnia*, Amsterdam edition, IV.3, 753–6, 768–71.

45. Cf. **A. Renaudet**, *Études Erasmiennes (1521–52)*, Paris 1939.

46. Cf. **L. Bouyer**, *Autour d'Erasme. Études sur le christianisme des humanistes catholiques*, Paris 1955.

47. Cf. **F. Heer**, *Die Dritte Kraft. Der europäische Humanismus zwischen den Fronten*, Frankfurt 1959.

48. Ibid., 7. **F. Krüger**, *Bucer und Erasmus. Eine Untersuchung zum Einfluss des Erasmus auf die Theologie Martin Bucers (bis zum Evangelien-Kommentar von 1530)*, Wiesbaden 1970, has demonstrated for the Strasbourg Reformers the degree to which the legacy of Erasmus could persist among the humanistically inclined leaders of the Reformation.

49. Cf. **M. U. Edwards**, *Luther's Last Battles. Politics and Polemics 1531–46*, Ithaca 1983.

50. There is an interesting contrast in the evaluation of the Reformation between the mediaevalist **G. Tellenbach,** who emphasizes the continuity wih the

Middle Ages, and the Reformation historian **P. Meinhold**, who sees an almost modern reform programme for the rebuilding of society already realized in the Reformation, both in Vol.5 of the *Saeculum Weltgeschichte*, ed. H. Franke et al, Freiburg 1970, 206–8, 417–22. Cf. the balanced assessments of the Cambridge historian **R. W. Scribner**, *The German Reformation*, Atlantic Highland, NJ 1987, 55–63.

51. Cf. **E. W. Zeeden**, *Katholische Überlieferungen in den lutherischen Kirchenordnungen des 16.Jahrhunderts*, Münster 1959.

52. Historians' views differ widely over the pedagogical success of the Lutheran Reformation. For the negative thesis of G. Strauss and the counter-thesis of **J. Kittelson** et al. on the success of the Lutheran confessionalization see the account by **H. R. Schmidt**, *Konfessionalisierung im 16.Jahrhundert*, Munich 1992, 63–7.

53. Cf. **G. Franz** (ed.), *Beamtertum und Pfarrerstand 1400–1800*, Limburg 1972 (articles on the different German territories).

54. Cf. **M. Luther**, *Against the Roman Papacy, an Institution of the Devil* (1545), LW 41, 263–376.

55. It was **E. Troeltsch**, *The Social Teaching of the Christian Churches* (1912)(2 vols.), London 1931, who first attempted to legitimate the noncon-formists as a legitimate gospel movement by distinguishing between two types, 'sect' (a faith community based on a voluntary decision to join) and 'church' (a sacramental institution for salvation). **G. H. Williams**, *The Radical Reformation*, Philadelphia 1962, third revised edition Kirksville, Mo. 1992, gives a compre-hensive survey of '**enthusiasm**' and all the radical movements of the Reformation (Baptists, spiritualists and gospel rationalists). **H. Fast** (ed.), *Der linke Flügel der Reformation. Glaubenszeugnisse der Täufer, Spiritualisten, Schwärmer und Antitrinitarier*, Bremen 1962, offers an illuminating modernized collection of texts; cf. also **R. van Dülmen** (ed.), *Das Täuferreich zu Münster 1534–1535. Berichte und Dokumente*, Munich 1974.

56. **C. A. Pater**, *Karlstadt as the Father of the Baptist Movements. The Emergence of Lay Protestantism*, Toronto 1984, undertakes an evaluation of the often neglected Andreas Rudolff-Bodenstein from Karlstadt in Franconia.

57. Cf. **R. Wohlfeil** (ed.), *Der Bauernkrieg 1524–26. Bauernkrieg und Reformation*, Munich 1975 (esp. Wohlfeil's introduction and postscript).

58. Cf. **Luther**, *Admonition to Peace. A Reply to the Twelve Articles of the Peasants in Swabia*, LW 46, 3–43.

59. Cf. **Luther**, *Against the Robbing and Murdering Hordes of Peasants* (1525), LW 46, 45–55. In the first Wittenberg printing the work appeared as an appendix to Luthers *Admonition to Peace* . . . with the formulation 'Also against the Robbing and Murderous Hordes . . .' Luther had wanted to admonish the combatants to peace. It was only on his journey through Thuringia that he became so shocked by the peasants' revolt that he produced the 'Appendix' (against the 'others', i.e. rebellious peasants), probably while he was still travelling. Later the 'Appendix' was published separately and so was given a special pointedness, though without influencing the course of events, since Luther's writings only appeared when the rebellion had already been suppressed.

60. Cf. **F. Engels**, *The Peasant War in Germany* (1850), London 1927 (comparison between Luther and Müntzer, 68–73).

61. Cf. **E. Bloch**, *Thomas Münzer als Theologe der Revolution* (1921), Frankfurt 1962.

62. Reliable modernized collections of Müntzer's writings and letters have been edited by **G. Wehr** (1989), and **R. Bentzinger** and **S. Hoyer** (1990).

63. Cf. **T. A. Brady**, *Turning Swiss. Cities and Empire 1450–1550*, Cambridge 1985; his conclusion: 'Turning Swiss – a Lost Dream' (222–30).

64. Cf. **H. S. Bender**, *C. Grebel c.1498–1526. The Founder of the Swiss Brethren Sometimes Called Anabaptists*, Goshen, Ind. 1950.

65. The Hamburg historian, **H.-J. Goertz**, *Religiöse Bewegungen in der frühe Neuzeit*, Munich 1993 (with bibliography), has provided a history of the nonconformist religious movements from the Wittenberg movement (Carlstadt) to radical Pietism which is as informative as it is brief, and at the same time a fair survey and evaluation of the problems and tendencies of research.

66. Thus in his sociological interim survey **H.-J. Goertz**, *Die Täufer. Geschichte und Deutung*, Munich 1980, [2]1988; id., *Religiöse Bewegungen* (n.65), 86 (with references to the confirmation of this theory by other Baptist scholars like W. Klaassen, R. Klötzer, C. A. Snyder and J. M. Stayer).

67. Cf. **M. Luther**, 'Von den Schleichern und Winkelpredigern' (1532), WA 30, 510–27.

68. Cf. the account of research by **H. R. Schmidt**, *Konfessionalisierung im 16. Jahrhundert*, Munich 1992, Part B.

69. Cf. **H. Küng**, *Judaism*, I C V 2, 'Luther, too, against the Jews'.

70. For **Huldrych Zwingli**, in addition to earlier works by O. Farner and A. Rich cf. **W. Köhler**, *Huldrych Zwingli*, Leipzig 1943, new edition by E. Koch, 1983; **C. Gestrich**, *Zwingli als Theologe. Glaube und Geist beim Zürcher Reformator*, Zurich 1967; **M. Haas**, *Huldrych Zwingli und seine Zeit. Leben und Werk des Zürcher Reformators*, Zurich 1969; **G. W. Locher**, *Huldrych Zwingli in neuer Sicht. Zehn Beiträge zur Theologie der Zürcher Reformation*, Zurich 1969; id., *Die zwinglische Reformation im Rahmen der europäischen Kirchengeschichte*, Göttingen 1979; id., *Zwingli und die schweizerische Reformation*, Göttingen 1982; **F. Büsser**, *Huldrych Zwingli. Reformation als prophetischer Auftrag*, Göttingen 1973; **G. R. Potter**, *Zwingli*, Cambridge 1965; **W. H. Neuser**, *Die reformatorische Wende bei Zwingli*, Neukirchen 1977; **F. E. Sciuto**, *Ulrico Zwingli. La vita – il pensiero – il suo tempo*, Naples 1980; **U. Gäbler**, *Huldrych Zwingli. Eine Einführung in sein Leben und sein Werk*, Munich 1983; **H. Veldman**, *Huldrych Zwingli. Hervormer van kerk en samenleving*, Goes 1984; **A. Ziegler**, *Zwingli. Katholisch gesehen, ökumenisch befragt*, Zurich 1984; **J. V. Pollet**, *Huldrych Zwingli*, Fribourg 1985; id., *Huldrych Zwingli. Biographie et théologie*, Geneva 1988; id., *Huldrych Zwingli et le zwinglianisme. Essai de synthèse historique et théologique mis à jour d'après les recherches récentes*, Paris 1988; **W. P. Stephens**, *The Theology of Huldrych Zwingli*, Oxford 1986; id., *Zwingli. An Introduction to His Thought*, Oxford 1992; **P. Winzeler**, *Zwingli als Theologe der Befreiung*, Basel 1986; **B. Hamm**, *Zwingli's Reformation der Freiheit*, Neukirchen 1988.

71. Cf. **Neuser**, *Die reformatorische Wende bei Zwingli* (n.70).

72. Cf. **Locher**, *Die Zwinglische Reformation* (n.72).

73. Cf. **W. H. Neuser**, 'Zwingli und der Zwinglianismus', in C. Andresen (ed.), *Handbuch der Dogmen und Theologiegeschichte* II, Göttingen 1980, 167–238, esp. 167–76.

74. Cf. **H. Zwingli**, *Regarding the Choice and Freedom of Foods* (1522), German text in *Zwingli Hauptschriften*, I, ed. F. Blanke, O. Farner and R. Pfister, Zurich 1940, 5–57.

75. Cf. id., *Analysis and Reasons for the Concluding Discourses* (1523), German text in ibid., III–IV, Zurich 1947, 1952.

76. For Jean Calvin cf. F. Büsser, *Calvins Urteil über sich selbst*, Zurich 1950; F. Wendel, *Calvin*, London 1963; W. F. Dankbaar, *Calvijn, zijn weg en werk*, Nijkerk 1957, ²1982; E. Pfisterer, *Calvins Wirken in Genf. Neu geprüft und in Einzelbildern dargestellt*, Neukirchen 1957; J. MacKinnon, *Calvin and the Reformation*, New York 1962; A. Ganoczy, *Le jeune Calvin. Genèse et évolution de sa vocation réformatrice*, Wiesbaden 1966; W. Neuser, *Calvin*, Berlin 1971; T. H. L. Parker, *John Calvin. A Biography*, London 1975; W. J. Bouwsma, *John Calvin. A Sixteenth-Century Portrait*, Oxford 1988; R. S. Wallace, *Calvin, Geneva and the Reformation. A Study of Calvin as Social Reformer, Churchman, Pastor and Theologian*, Edinburgh 1988; A. E. McGrath, *A Life of John Calvin. A Study in the Shaping of Western Culture*, Oxford 1990.

77. J. Calvin, *Institutes of the Christian Religion* (1559 edition), ed. J. T. McNeill and F. L. Battles, Library of Christian Classics (2 vols.), IV, 2, 6, p.1048.

78. Dankbaar, *Calvijn* (n.76), 85.

79. Parker, *John Calvin* (n.76), XI.

80. On Calvin's thought cf. W. Niesel, *Die Theologie Calvins*, Munich 1938; T. H. L. Parker, *The Oracles of God. An Introduction to the Preaching of John Calvin*, London 1947; id., *Calvin's Doctrine of the Knowledge of God*, Edinburgh 1952, revised edition 1969; id., *Calvin's New Testament Commentaries*, London 1971; id., *Calvin's Old Testament Commentaries*, Edinburgh 1976; H. Schroten, *Christus, de Middelaar, bij Calvijn. Bijdrage tot de leer van de zekerheid des geloofs*, Utrecht 1948; T. F. Torrance, *Calvin's Doctrine of Man*, London 1949; id., *The Hermeneutics of John Calvin*, Edinburgh 1988; E. A. Dowey, *The Knowledge of God in Calvin's Theology*, New York 1962; H. Berger, *Calvins Geschichtsauffassung*, Zurich 1955; C. Calvetti, *La filosofia di Giovanni Calvino*, Milan 1955; J. F. Jansen, *Calvin's Doctrine of the Work of Christ*, London 1956; W. Krusche, *Das Wirken des Heiligen Geistes nach Calvin*, Göttingen 1957; R. S. Wallace, *Calvin's Doctrine of the Christian Life*, Edinburgh 1959; J. Moltmann (ed.), *Calvin-Studien 1959*, Neukirchen 1960; L. G. M. Alting van Geusau, *Die Lehre der Kindertaufe bei Calvin, gesehen im Rahmen seiner Sakraments– und Tauftheologie. Synthese oder Ordnungsfehler?*, Mainz 1963; K. Reuter, *Das Grundverständnis der Theologie Calvins unter Einbeziehung ihrer geschichtlichen Abhängigkeiten*, Neukirchen 1963; R. J. Mooi, *Het kerk – en dogmahistorisch element in de werken van Johannes Calvijn*, Wageningen 1965; E. D. Willis, *Calvin's Catholic Christology. The Function of the So-called* Extra Calvinisticum *in Calvin's Theology*, Leiden 1966; D. Schellong, *Das evangelische Gesetz in der Auslegung Calvins*, Munich 1958; id., *Calvins Auslegung der synoptischen Evangelien*, Munich 1969; H. Scholl, *Der Dienst des Gebetes nach Johannes Calvin*, Zurich 1968; id., *Calvinus Catholicus. Die katholische Calvinforschung im 20. Jahrhundert*, Freiburg 1974; H. Schützeichel, *Die Glaubenstheologie Calvins*, Munich 1972; T. Stadland, *Rechtfertigung und Heiligung bei Calvin*, Neukirchen 1972; W. Balke, *Calvijn en de doperse Radikalen*, Amsterdam 1973; F. Wendel, *Calvin et l'humanisme*, Paris 1976; W. S. Reid (ed.), *John Calvin, His Influence in the Western World*, Grand Rapids 1982; J. D. Douglass, *Women, Freedom, and Calvin*, Philadelphia 1985; M. Potter Engel, *John Calvin's Perspectival Anthropology*, Atlanta 1988; C. J. Sommerville, *The Secularization of Early Modern England. From Religious Culture to Religious Faith*, Oxford 1992.

81. Calvin, *Institutes* (1559) (n.77), I, 1, 1, p.35.
82. Calvin, *Institutio religionis christianae* (1536), I, in *Corpus Reformatorum* 29, Brunswick 1869, 42–55.
83. The German edition translated and edited by O. Weber, *Unterricht in der christlichen Religion*, Neukirchen 1955 (1057 pages + index), gives a rapid survey of the overall conception and details of the questions of the last edition of the *Institutes*.
84. Cf. G. Kraus, *Vorherbestimmung. Traditionelle Prädestinationslehre im Licht gegenwärtigen Theologie*, Freiburg 1977, IV: Johannes Calvin.
85. Remarkably enough, this *Consensus Genevensis de aeterna Dei praedestinatione* of 1552 prompted by Bolsec is missing even from the almost 1000–page edition by E. F. K. Müller, *Bekenntnisschriften der reformierten Kirche*, Leipzig 1903; it can be found in H. A. Niemeyer, *Collectio confessionum*, Leipzig 1840.
86. As we know, Bolsec took his vengeance on Calvin with a highly critical *Vie de Calvin* (1577); many of the charges can no longer be verified today. The debate between F. C. Roberts and P. C. Holtrop in *Perspectives. A Journal of Reformed Thought*, December 1993, 9–12, shows that the Bolsec affair can still spark off a vigorous controversy among Calvin supporters and Calvin scholars.
87. Calvin, *Institutes* (1559) (n.77), III, 21, 5, p.926.
88. For this complex of problems see the critical study by W. Gross and K.-J. Kuschel, '*Ich schaffe Finsternis und Unheil'. Ist Gott verantwortlich für das Übel?*, Mainz 1992, esp.85–90.
89. Cf. Ignatius of Loyola, *Spiritual Exercises* (1548), ed. T. Corbishley, London 1963. The most problematical part of the book is the end: the eighteen rules on 'The mind of the Church', especially rule 13.
90. Calvin, *Institutes* (1559) (n.77), III, 14, 18, p.785.
91. Cf. M. Weber, *The Protestant Ethic and the Spirit of Capitalism* (first version 1904/06), London 1930.
92. Cf. J.-F. Bergier, *Genève et l'économie européenne de la Renaissance*, Paris 1963; id., *Zu den Anfängen des Kapitalismus – Das Beispiel Genf*, Cologne 1972; id., *Wirtschaftsgeschichte der Schweiz. Von den Anfängen bis zur Gegenwart*, Zurich 1983, second updated edition 1990.
93. Id., *Zu den Anfängen des Kapitalismus* (n.79), 21.
94. Cf. McGrath, *Life of John Calvin* (n.71), ch.XI; A. Biéler, *La pensée économique et sociale de Calvin*, Geneva 1959; id., *L'Humanisme social de Calvin*, Geneva 1961; G. Miegge, L. Corsani and U. Gastaldi, *Protestantesimo e capitalismo da Calvino a Weber contributi ad un dibattito*, Turin 1983; G. Poggi, *Calvinism and the Capitalist Spirit. Max Weber's Protestant Ethics*, Amherst 1983.
95. Cf. G. Jellinek, 'Die Erklärung der Menschen- und Bürgerrechte' (1895, ⁴1927), in R. Schnur (ed.), *Zur Geschichte der Erklärung der Menschenrechte*, Darmstadt 1974 (with contributions to the discussion by E. Boutmy et al.); H. Lutz (ed.), *Zur Geschichte der Toleranz und Religionsfreiheit*, Darmstadt 1977 (especially the article by L. Moore).
96. For **Calvin's understanding of the church** cf. A. Ganoczy, *Calvin, théologien de l'église et du ministère*, Paris 1964; id., *Ecclesia ministrans. Dienende Kirche und kirchlicher Dienst bei Calvin*, Freiburg 1968; K. McDonnell, *John Calvin, the Church, and the Eucharist*, Princeton 1967; B. C. Milner, *Calvin's Doctrine of the Church*, Leiden 1970; L. Schümmer, *L'ecclésiologie de*

*Calvin à la lumière de l'*Ecclesia Mater. *Son apport aux recherches ecclésiologiques tenant à exprimer l'unité en voie de manifestation,* Bern 1981; **E. A. McKee,** *Elders and the Plural Ministry. The Role of Exegetical History in Illuminating John Calvin's Theology,* Geneva 1988.

97. Cf. **H. Höpfl,** *The Christian Polity of John Calvin,* Cambridge 1982, 103–27; cf. further **R. C. Hancock,** *Calvin and the Foundations of Modern Politics,* Ithaca 1989.

98. The basic documents of the Reformed churches – outside Geneva the Heidelberg Catechism and the Scottish, Belgic and Palatinate confessions or church orders are important – are available in a modern German edition by **W. Niesel** (ed.), *Bekenntnisschriften und Kirchenordnungen der nach Gottes Wort reformierten Kirche,* Zurich 1938; cf. also **P. Jacobs,** *Theologie reformierter Bekenntnisschriften,* Neukirchen 1959.

99. For **Calvin's understanding of the eucharist** cf. **R. S.Wallace,** *Calvin's Doctrine of the Word and Sacrament,* Edinburgh 1953; **H. Grass,** *Die Abendmahlslehre bei Luther und Calvin. Eine kritische Untersuchung,* Gütersloh 1954; **G. P. Hartvelt,** Verum corpus. *Een studie over een centraal hoofdstuk uit de avondmaalsleer van Calvijn,* Delft 1960; **J. Rogge,** Virtus und res. *Um die Abendmahlswirklichkeit bei Calvin,* Berlin 1965; **McDonnell,** *John Calvin* (n.96).

100. Cf. **R. Hooker,** *Of the Laws of Ecclesiastical Polity* (5 vols, 1593–97), new edition in two volumes, New Haven and London 1977, 1981.

101. This is illustrated in a multi-faceted collection of texts, **A. Duke, G. Lewis** and **A. Pettegree,** *Calvinism in Europe 1540–1610. A Collection of Documents,* Manchester 1992.

102. Cf. **G. W. Locher,** *Calvin. Anwalt der Ökumene,* Zollikon 1960.

103. **J. Foxe,** *Actes and Monuments of these Latter and Perillous Dayes* (1563), popular under the title *The Book of Martyrs* ([4]1583, new edition in 8 vols., New York 1965), a history of the English Reformation which is one-sided but full of facts, still remains basic for **the Reformation in England.** The more recent classic account has been written by **A. G. Dickens,** *The English Reformation,* London 1964. **C. Haigh** (ed.), *The English Reformation Revised,* Cambridge 1987 (the most important newer literature is on pp.1–33), has revised this picture, especially for the pre-Reformation period and the pace of the establishment of the Reformation in England. Later works include: **R. Cust** and **A. Hughes** (eds.), *Conflict in Early Stuart England. Studies in Religion and Politics 1603–1642,* London 1989; **D. Loades,** *Politics, Censorship and the English Reformation,* London 1991; **J. Spurr,** *The Restoration Church of England, 1646–1689,* New Haven 1991.

104. Haigh, *The English Reformation Revised* (n.103), 209.

105. For **Anglicanism** cf. **P. E. More** and **F. L. Cross** (eds.), *Anglicanism. The Thought and Practice of the Church of England. Illustrated from the Religious Literature of the Seventeenth Century,* London 1935; **J. W. C. Wand** (ed.), *The Anglican Communion, A Survey,* Oxford 1948; id., *Anglicanism in History and Today,* London 1961; **S. Neill,** *Anglicanism,* Harmondsworth 1958, Oxford [4]1977; id., 'Anglikanische (Kirchen-)Gemeinschaft', *TRE* II, 713–23. I am deeply grateful to Dr **John Bowden** (London) for reading through this section on Anglicanism.

106. The works of **Thomas Cranmer** have been edited by H. Jenkyns and J. E. Cox. For his life and work cf. **G. W. Bromiley,** *Thomas Cranmer Theologian,*

London 1956; J. Ridley, *Thomas Cranmer*, Oxford 1962; P. Brooks, *Thomas Cranmer's Doctrine of the Eucharist. An Essay in Historical Development*, London 1965; id., *Cranmer in Context. Documents from the English Reformation*, Cambridge 1989; G. R. Elton, 'Cranmer', *TRE* VIII, 226–9; M. H. Shepperd, 'Cranmer', *EncRel* IV, 137–8; M. Johnson (ed.), *Thomas Cranmer. A Living Influence for 500 Years*, Durham 1990.

107. Cf. J. I. Tellechea Idigoras, *Fray Bartolomé Carranza y el Cardenal Pole. Un navarro en la restauración católica de Inglaterra (1554–1558)*, Pamplona 1977; id., 'Carranza', *LThK* II, 957; id., *Fray Bartolomé Carranza. Documentos históricos*, Vols.Iff., Madrid 1962ff.

108. Cf. J. Jewel, *Apologia Ecclesiae Anglicanae* (1562); in English: *An Apologie, or aunswer in defence of the Church of England, concerninge the state of Religion used in the same*, London 1562, reprinted Amsterdam 1972.

109. Cf. Hooker, *Of the Laws of Ecclesiastical Polity* (n.100).

110. On John Knox cf. J. S. McEwen, *The Faith of John Knox*, London 1961; J. Ridley, *John Knox*, Oxford 1968; W. Stanford Reid, *Trumpeter of God. A Biography of John Knox*, New York 1974; D. Shaw (ed.), *John Knox. A Quatercentenary Reappraisal*, Edinburgh 1975.

111. Cf. F. J. Bremer, 'Puritanism', *EncRel* XII, 102–6 (bibliography).

112. Oliver Cromwell's letters and speeches have been edited by W. C. Abbot. The classical biography remains that by C. H. Firth, *Oliver Cromwell and the Rule of the Puritans in England*, Oxford 1900, new edition London 1947. For more recent literature cf. M. Ashley, 'Oliver Cromwell', *The New Encyclopedia Britannica* XVI, Chicago 1987, 875–9.

113. Cf. the collection of texts by classical Anglican authors in More and Cross, *Anglicanism* (n.105).

114. Cf. The Thirty Nine Articles of Religion, no.6 (the articles are to be found in the Anglican Book of Common Prayer).

115. The classic biography is that of R. W. Chambers, *Thomas More*, London 1935; it has been corrected in many respects by E. E. Reynolds, *The Field is Won. The Life and Death of Saint Thomas More*, Milwaukee 1968.

116. Cf. F. Baker, 'Methodist Churches', *EncRel* IX, 493–5.

117. Cf. id., 'Wesley Brothers', *EncRel* XV, 370f. (Dr Baker is also the editor of *The Works of John Wesley*, planned in 35 volumes). The five–volume standard biography is that by J. S.Simon; there are more recent biographies by F. Baker, H. Rack, M. Schmidt and C. E. Vulliamy.

118. Cf. G. F. Moede, *The Office of Bishop in Methodism. Its History and Development*, Zurich 1964; J. K. Mathews, *Set Apart to Serve. The Meaning and Role of Episcopacy in the Wesleyan Tradition*, Nashville, Tenn. 1985.

119. Anglican churches have entered into full communion (eucharistic fellowship and participation in the consecration of bishops) with the following churches: the Old Catholic Church of Europe, the Polish Catholic National Church in the USA, the Swedish and Finnish church, the independent church of the Philippines and the Reformed Syrian Mar Thoma Church in India. The Anglican provinces of South India, North India, Pakistan and Bangladesh have formed a new church union with other churches. But Anglican visitors to these churches have a claim to full membership, as the churches explicitly maintain the key points of the Anglican church.

120. G. Schaffernorth, 'Im Geist Freunde werden ... Die Beziehung von Mann und Frau bei Luther im Rahmen seines Kirchenverständnisses', in ead.,

Den Glauben ins Leben ziehen . . . *Studien zu Luthers Theologie*, Munich 1982, 122–202: 162.

121. Ibid., 174.

122. Ibid., 162.

123. **Luther**, 'Welche Personen verboten sind zu ehelichen' (1522), WA X/2, 263–6: 266.

124. Cf. **id.**, *To the Councilmen of All Cities in Germany, that they Establish and Maintain Christian Schools*, LW 45, 341–78.

125. Cf. **E. Reichle**, 'Reformation', in A. Lissner, R. Süssmuth and K. Walter (eds.), *Frauenlexikon. Traditionen, Fakten, Perspektiven*, Freiburg 1988, 927–34; **R. H. Bainton**, *Women of the Reformation*, Vol.I, *In Germany and Italy*; Vol.II, *In France and England*; Vol III, *From Spain to Scandinavia*, Minneapolis 1971–77, investigates the question in the European context.

126. Cf. C III 10, 'Women in the Middle Ages'.

127. Cf.**I. Ludolphy**, 'Frau (VI.Reformationszeit)', *TRE* XI, 441–3; **S. E. Ozment**, *When Fathers Ruled. Family Life in Reformation Europe*, Cambridge, Mass. 1983; **L. Roper**, *The Holy Household. Women and Morals in Reformation Augsburg*, Oxford 1989.

128. Cf. **J. Dempsey Douglass**, *Women, Freedom, and Calvin*, Philadelphia 1985.

129. Cf. **R. L. Graves** (ed.), *Triumph over Silence. Women in Protestant History*, London 1985.

130. Cf. **P. Crawford**, *Women and Religion in England 1500–1720*, London 1993.

131. Cf. **M. P. Hannay**, *Silent but for the Word. Tudor Women as Patrons, Translators and Writers of Religious Works*, Kent 1985.

132. **Crawford** (n.130) devotes a whole chapter to them.

133. Cf. **M. Kobelt-Groch**, *Aufsässige Töchter Gottes. Frauen im Bauernkrieg und in den Täuferbewegungen*, Frankfurt 1993.

134. Cf. the evaluation by the Catholic theologian **A. Jensen**, 'Im Kampf um Freiheit in Kirche und Staat: Die Mutter des Quäkertums, Margaret Fell', in H. Häring and K.-J. Kuschel (eds.), *Gegenentwürfe. 24 Lebensläufe für eine andere Theologie*, Munich 1988, 169–80.

135. **Crawford**, *Women and Religion* (n.130), 138.

136. Ibid., 139.

137. Ibid.

138. **Greaves** (ed.), *Triumph over Silence* (n.129), 12.

139. There are already numerous detailed investigations of the persecution of witches in particular regions (B. Ankarloo, Sweden; G. Bader, Switzerland: W. Behringer, South-east Germany; G. Bonomo, Italy; F. Byloff, Austria; P. F. Byrne, Ireland; G. Henningsen, Basque country; C. Larner, Scotland: A. Macfarlane, England; R. Mandrou, France; H. C. E. Midelfort, South-west Germany; E. W. Monter, France and Switzerland; J. Tazbir, Poland; R. Zguta, Russia). For Germany there is a survey of the present state of research by **G. Schormann**, *Hexenprozesse in Deutschland*, Göttingen 1981 (the same author has also written an admirable survey, 'Hexen', *TRE* XV, 297–304); cf. also the informative documentation by **W. Behringer** (ed.), *Hexen und Hexenprozesse in Deutschland*, Munich 1988, ²1933. Further more recent literature on this topic includes: **N. C. Cohn**, *Europe's Inner Demons. An Enquiry Inspired by the Great Witch-Hunt*, London 1975; **R. Kieckhefer**, *European Witch Trials. Their*

Foundations in Popular and Learned Culture, 1300–1500, London 1976; **H. Döbler**, *Hexenwahn. Die Geschichte einer Verfolgung*, Munich 1977; **M. Hammes**, *Hexenwahn und Hexenprozesse*, Frankfurt 1977; **C. Honegger** (ed.), *Die Hexen der Neuzeit. Studien zur Sozialgeschichte eines kulturellen Deutungsmusters*, Frankfurt 1978; **C. Ginzburg**, *I Benandanti. Stregoneria e culti agrari tra Cinquecento e Seicento*, Turin 1966; **E. Wissenlinck**, *Hexen. Warum wir so wenig von ihrer Geschichte erfahren und was davon auch noch falsch ist*, Munich 1986; **R. van Dülmen** (ed.), *Hexenwelten. Magie und Imagination vom 16.–20. Jahrhundert*, Frankfurt 1987; **G. Schwaiger** (ed.), *Teufelsglaube und Hexenprozesse*, Munich 1987; **H. Weber**, *Kinderhexenprozesse*, Frankfurt 1991.

140. **H. Haag**, *Vor dem Bösen Ratlos?*, Munich 1978, 164; cf. also **id.** and **K. Elliger**, *Teufelsglaube*, Tübingen 1974, Ch.4, 'Die Hexen'.

141. Cf. e.g. **Thomas Aquinas**, *Summa theologiae* II–II, q.93,a.2.

142. Cf. **J. Sprenger** and **H. Institoris**, *Malleus maleficarum* (1487); for the first time translated into German (in three parts) with an introduction by J. W. R. Schmidt, Berlin 1906, reprinted 1974. That the obscenities and perversions of which the witches were accused were to some degree a substitute satisfaction of sexual desires forbidden to Christians (and especially celibate priests) is not only a psychologizing hypothesis but is clearly demonstrated in this book: page after page there are discussions of 'whether witches can prevent the power to beget or the enjoyment of love' (I, 127–36), or 'whether witches bewitch male members by false illusions' (I, 136–45), and many examples are given 'of the manner in which they used to bewitch away male members' (II, 78–87).

143. The original Latin text of the bull is to be found in **C. Mirbt** and **K. Aland**, *Quellen zur Geschichte des Papsttums und des römischen Katholizismus* I, Tübingen ⁶1967, 282f.

144. **Schormann**, 'Hexen' (n.139), 303 (my italics).

145. **C. Honegger**, 'Hexen', in A. Lissner, R. Süssmuth and K. Walter (eds.), *Frauenlexikon*, 491–500: 498 (my emphasis).

146. Cf. **F. von Spee**, *Cautio criminalis, seu de processibus contra sagas* (1631); German edition: *Cautio criminalis oder Rechtliche Bedenken wegen der Hexenprozesse*, Weimar 1939.

147. Cf. the historical-theological analysis of these doctrinal disputes within Protestantism in **B. Lohse**, 'Dogma und Bekenntnis in der Reformation: Von Luther bis zum Konkordienbuch', in C. Andresen (ed.), *Handbuch der Dogmen –und Theologiegeschichte* II, Göttingen 1980, 1–164, esp. 102–38. There is no major complete account of Lutheran orthodoxy, any more than there is of baroque Scholasticism.

148. **Zeeden**, *Die Enstehung der Konfessionen* (n.1), 9f.

149. Ibid., 179.

150. Ibid.

151. There are explicit complaints in Protestant theology that the post-Reformation period of orthodoxy, often regarded as 'barren', has not been examined adequately by scholars for a long time – except for its theology. **Schmidt**, *Konfessionalisierung* (n.68), gives a good survey of the present state of scholarship. The volume edited by **M. Venard**, *Le temps des confessions (1530–1620/30)*, Paris 1992, offers much material both on the phenomenon of the confessions and on the life of Christians from a more French perspective.

152. The term comes from **G. Oestreich**, *Geist und Gestalt des frühmodernen Staats*, Berlin 1969, 187–97. For a definition of confessionalization as part of the

social disciplining of absolutism see the survey in **Schmidt**, *Konfessionalisierung* (n.68), 94–8 ('Sozialdisziplinierung – der Kampf gegen die Volkskultur', with bibliography).

153. For the **Lutheran confessional writings** cf. the standard edition, *Die Bekenntnisschriften der evangelisch-lutherische Kirche, herausgegeben vom Deutschen Evangelischen Kirchenausschuss im Gedenkjahr der Augsburgischen Konfession*, 1960, [10]1986. For the theology of the Lutheran confessional writings cf. **E. Schlink**, *Theologie der lutherischen Bekenntnisschriften*, Munich 1940, [3]1948; **F. Brunstäd**, *Theologie der lutherischen Bekenntnisschriften*, Gütersloh 1951; **H. Fagerberg**, *Die Theologie der lutherischen Bekenntnisschriften von 1539 bis 1537*, Göttingen 1965.

154. **Lohse**, *Dogma und Bekenntnis in der Reformation* (n.147), 163.

155. Cf. **J. Gerhard**, *Loci theologici* (1610–1622) (9 vols.), Tübingen 1639.

156. One need think only of the fruitful controversy with the Reformed Leiden systematic theologian **Johannes Cocceius** (Koch of Bremen), who no longer divided dogmatics by articles of faith (*loci*) but by the biblical covenants ('federal theology').

157. Cf. above, C III 12, 'Counter Reformation? Back to the mediaeval paradigm'.

158. For the **Reformed confessional writings** cf. above, C IV 6, 'Consistent Reformation, "Reformed" Protestantism'. For the development of the theology of Reformed orthodoxy (from the Calvinist Aristotelians through the Calvinist Ramists, disciples of Petrus Ramus, to the federal theology of Johannes Cocceius and the Synod of Westminster), cf. **W. H. Neuser**, 'Dogma und Bekenntnis in der Reformation: Von Zwingli und Calvin bis zur Synode von Westminster', in C. Andresen (ed.), *Handbuch der Dogmen– und Theologiegeschichte* II, 165–352, esp. 306–52.

159. Cf. **Zeeden**, *Entstehung der Konfessionen* (n.1), 181.

160. Cf. **H. Lutz**, *Reformation und Gegenreformation*, Munich 1982, 66.

161. Cf. **A. Feil**, *Metzler Musik Chronik vom frühen Mittelalter bis zur Gegenwart*, Stuttgart 1993, 171–3, with explanations on pp.174–300.

162. Ibid., 173.

163. **H. Lehmann**, *Das Zeitalter des Absolutismus. Gottesgnadentum und Kriegsnot*, Stuttgart 1980. Cf. the collection of texts by **W. Zeller** (ed.), *Der Protestantismus des 17. Jahrhunderts*, Bremen 1962.

164. Cf. **P. Nicolai**, *Freudenspiegel des ewigen Lebens* (1599), reprinted Soest 1963.

165. Cf. **J. Arndt**, *Vier Bücher vom wahren Christentum* (4 vols), Brunswick and Magdeburg 1606–10.

166. For the history and understanding of **Pietism** there are specialist publications on individual figures like Spener, Francke, Arnold, Zinzendorf and individual regions. See above all the history of Pietism which is now appearing under the editorship of **M. Brecht** and others, Vol.I, *Der Pietismus vom siebzehnten bis zum frühen achtzehnten Jahrhundert*, Göttingen 1993 (three further volumes will follow). Also **G. Küntzel** and **M. Hass** (eds.), *Die politischen Testamente der Hohenzollern nebst ergänzenden Aktenstücken* I–II, Leipzig 1911; **E. Hirsch**, *Geschichte der neueren Evangelischen Theologie im Zusammenhang mit den allgemeinen Bewegungen des europäischen Denkens*, II, Gütersloh 1951; **A. Langen**, *Der Wortschatz des deutschen Pietismus*, Tübingen 1954; **W. Zeller** (ed.), *Der Protestantismus des 17. Jahrhunderts*, Bremen 1962;

F. E. Stoeffler, *The Rise of Evangelical Pietism*, Leiden 1965; H. Weigelt, *Pietismus-Studien* I, Stuttgart 1965; F. W. Kantzenbach, *Orthodoxie und Pietismus*, Gütersloh 1966; H. Lehmann, *Pietismus und weltliche Ordnung in Württemberg vom 17. bis zum 20. Jahrhundert*, Stuttgart 1969; id., *Das Zeitalter des Absolutismus* (n.163); M. Schmidt, *Wiedergeburt und neuer Mensch*, Witten 1969; id., *Pietismus*, Stuttgart 1972; id., *Der Pietismus als theologische Erscheinung*, Göttingen 1984; J. Wallmann, *Philipp Jakob Spener und die Anfänge des Pietismus*, Tübingen 1970, ²1986; id., *Der Pietismus*, Göttingen 1990; H. Leube, *Orthodoxie und Pietismus. Gesammelte Studien*, Bielefeld 1975; M. Greschat (ed.), *Zur neueren Pietismusforschung*, Darmstadt 1977; id. (ed.), *Orthodoxie und Pietismus*, Stuttgart 1982; E. Beyreuther, *Geschichte des Pietismus*, Stuttgart 1967; id., *Frömmigkeit und Theologie. Gesammelte Aufsätze zum Pietismus und zur Erweckungsbewegung*, Hildesheim 1980; M. Scharfe, *Die Religion des Volkes. Kleine Kultur– und Sozialgeschichte des Pietismus*, Gütersloh 1980; T. Baumann, *Zwischen Weltveränderung und Weltflucht. Zum Wandel der pietistischen Utopie im 17. und 18. Jahrhundert*, Lahr 1991; E. M. Laine (ed.), *Der Pietismus in seiner europäischen und aussereuropäischen Ausstrahlung*, Helsinki 1992. M. Schmid and W. Janasch, *Das Zeitalter des Pietismus*, Bremen 1965, offer a helpful collection of texts.

167. Cf. K. Deppermann, 'Der englische Puritanismus', in Brecht et al. (eds.), *Der Pietismus* (n.165), 11–55.

168. Cf. E. C. McKenzie, *British Devotional Literature and the Rise of German Pietism* (2 vols.), St Andrews dissertation 1984.

169. Cf. J. van den Berg, 'Die Frömmigkeitsbestrebungen in den Niederlanden', in Brecht et al. (eds.), *Der Pietismus* (n.165), 57–112.

170. Cf. P. J. Spener, *Pia desideria: oder Hertzliches Verlangen Nach Gottgefälliger Besserung der wahren Evangelischen Kirchen sampt einigen dahin einfältig abzweckenden christlichen Vorschlagen* (1676), new edition by K. Aland, Berlin ³1964.

171. Cf. the precise analysis of these aspects of Brandenburg-Prussian policy relating to theology, canon law and church politics, state and power politics, in H. Lehmann, *Das Zeitalter des Absolutismus*, Ch.II.7, 'Territorialismus und Pietismus'.

172. Cf. K. Deppermann, 'August Hermann Francke', in M.Greschat (ed.), *Orthodoxie und Pietismus*, Stuttgart 1982, 241–60; also C. Hinrichs, *Preussentum und Pietismus. Der Pietismus in Brandenburg-Preussen als religiös-soziale Reformbewegung*, Göttingen 1917.

173. Pietism in **southern Germany** developed independently of Halle Pietism. The moderate and popular **Pietism of Württemberg** kept clear of extravagances (compulsive penance), maintained contact with academic theology, and thus found sympathy with the church government (permission for private assemblies for edification, 'hours'); the speculative biblicist Johann Albrecht Bengel and the theosophist Friedrich Christoph Oetinger were influential here. In the north-west, **Reformed Pietism,** influenced by English Puritanism and by the ascetic spirit of Calvin himself, had its sphere of influence under the control and leadership of the Utrecht professor Gisbert Voetius. The Reformed mystic Gerhard Tersteegen, in Mühlheim on the Ruhr, was an inspiration in all confessions.

174. Cf. G. Beyreuther, *Sexualtheorien im Pietismus*, Munich medical dissertation 1963, in *Werkausgabe*, Vol.II, *Zinzendorf*, Hildesheim 1975.

175. For the position of **women** in Pietism, with a fine evaluation of Count and Countess Zinzendorf, see **G. Scharffenorth** and **E. Reichle**, 'Frau VII (Neuzeit)', *TRE* XI, 446–50.

176. Cf. **G. Arnold**, *Unparteiische Kirchen- und Ketzer-Historie, vom Anfang des Neuen Testaments bis auf das Jahr Christi 1688* (4 vols.), Frankfurt 1699–1700, ²1729, reprinted Hildesheim 1967.

177. For the **revival movements** cf. **E. Hirsch**, *Geschichte der neuern evangelischen Theologie* III, Gütersloh 1951, Ch.33, on the division of Western European Protestant theology in opposite directions; **E. Staehelin**, 'Von der protestantische Orthodoxie zu den Erweckungsbewegungen', *Historia Mundi* VII, Bern 1957, 227–48; **O. Weber** and **E. Beyreuther** (ed.), *Die Stimme der Stillen. Ein Buch zur Besinnung aus dem Zeugnis von Pietismus und Erweckungsbewegung*, Neukirchen 1959; id., *Die Erweckungsbewegung*, Göttingen 1965; **É. G. Léonard**, *Histoire générale du Protestantisme*, Vol.III, *Déclin et Renouveau (XVIIIᵉ – XXᵉ Siècle)*, Paris 1964; **D. Lorz**, *'The Evangelization of the World in This Generation': The Resurgence of a Missionary Idea among the Conservative Evangelicals*, Hamburg 1970; **D. B. Rutman** (ed.), *The Great Awakening. Event and Exegesis*, Huntington, NY 1977; **U. Gäbler**, *Auferstehungszeit. Erweckungsprediger des 19.Jh.*, Munich 1991; **W. R. Ward**, *The Protestant Evangelical Awakening*, Cambridge 1992.

178. Thus the third volume of the major history of Pietism edited by **M. Brecht** and others will be devoted to the revivalist movements down to the present day.

179. For a provisional orientation cf. the classic investigation by **S. E. Ahlstrom**, *A Religious History of the American People*, New Haven 1972.

180. Cf. **C. G. Finney**, *Lectures on Revivals of Religion*, New York 1835, new edition by W. G. McLoughlin, Cambridge, Mass. 1960.

181. After 1780, revival movements finally developed in the churches of Scotland and England as well, opposing the rationalism and the growing secularization in church, theology and public life. This renewal movement had a very broad spectrum, ranging from the Anglican **Oxford Movement** (J. Keble, E. Pusey and J. H. Newman), which aimed at a Catholic, High Church piety, to the **Salvation Army** (William and Catherine Booth), which, uninterested in rites and sacraments, concentrated wholly on Christian social activity in line with the good news of Jesus, on the cure of drunkards, the education of orphans and the care of the poor and homeless in our great cities.

182. Cf. the survey in **G. A. Benrath** and **W. J. Hollenweger**, 'Erweckung, Erweckungsbewegungen', *TRE* X, 205–27.

183. For **fundamentalism** cf. especially the investigations by **M. E. Marty** and **R. S. Appleby** (eds.), *Fundamentalisms Observed*, Chicago 1991; *Fundamentalisms and the State. Remaking Polities, Economies, and Militance*, Chicago 1993, which have appeared as Parts I and III of the five-volume inter-religious study 'The Fundamentalism Project'. For American fundamentalism cf. **N. F. Furniss**, *The Fundamentalist Controversy, 1918–1931*, New Haven 1954; **E. R. Sandeen**, *The Roots of Fundamentalism. British and American Millenarianism 1800–1930*, Chicago 1970; **J. Barr**, *Fundamentalism*, London 1977; **G. M. Marsden**, *Fundamentalism and American Culture. The Shaping of Twentieth-Century Evangelicalism: 1870–1925*, New York 1980; **W. Joest**, 'Fundamentalismus', *TRE* XI, 732–8; **N. T. Ammermann**, *Bible Believers. Fundamentalists in the Modern World*, New Brunswick 1987; **R. J. Neuhaus** and **M. Cromartie** (eds.), *Piety and Politics. Evangelicals and Fundamentalists Confront*

the World, Washington, DC 1987; **D. Lecourt**, *L'Amérique entre la Bible et Darwin*, Paris 1992.

184. Text in **Sandeen**, *The Roots of Fundamentalism* (n.183), 273.

185. Cf. the examples in **Ebeling**, 'Hermeneutik', *RGG³*, 242–62: 251f.

186. Thus **M. E. Marty** in his introduction to the thematic volume of the international theological journal *Concilium* edited by J. Moltmann and me, on *Fundamentalism as an Ecumenical Challenge*, 1992/3, 'What is Fundamentalism? Theological Perspectives?', 3–13 (there are contributions in this volume from Jewish, Christian and Muslim authors).

187. Cf. **S. Tromp**, *De sacrae scripturae inspiratione*, Rome ⁵1953.

188. Cf. I John 5.7, and **Denzinger**, *Enchiridion*, no. 2198.

189. Cf. **P. Hebblethwaite**, 'A Fundamentalist Pope', and **H. Küng**, 'Against Contemporary Roman Catholic Fundamentalism', both in *Concilium* 1992/3, 88–96 and 116–25. How urgent the problem of fundamentalism has become in contemporary Catholicism is shown by the ever-increasing number of books being published on the subject: **J. Niewiadomski** (ed.), *Eindeutige Antworten? Fundamentalistische Versuchung in Religion und Gesellschaft*, Thaur 1988; **K. Kienzler** (ed.), *Der neue Fundamentalismus. Rettung oder Gefahr für Gesellschaft und Religion?*, Düsseldorf 1990; **T. F. O'Meara**, *Fundamentalism. A Catholic Perspective*, New York 1990; **H. Hemminger** (ed.), *Fundamentalismus in der verweltlichten Kultur*, Stuttgart 1991; **H. Kochanek** (ed.), *Die verdrängte Freiheit. Fundamentalismus in den Kirchen*, Freiburg 1991; **S. H. Pfürtner**, *Fundamentalismus. Die Flucht ins Radikale*, Freiburg 1991; **R. Schermann** (ed.), *Katholischer Fundamentalismus. Häretische Gruppen in der Kirche?*, Regensburg 1991; **J. Werbick** (ed.), *Offenbarungsanspruch und fundamentalistische Versuchung?*, Freiburg 1991.

190. **J. Neusner**, 'What is the Challenge of Contemporary Jewish Fundamentalism?', *Concilium* 1992/3, 49–52: 52.

191. For an **inter-religious comparison**, in addition to the volumes edited by Marty and Appleby the following investigations are important: **B. B. Lawrence**, *Defenders of God. The Fundamentalist Revolt against the Modern Age*, San Francisco 1989; **T. Meyer**, *Fundamentalismus. Aufstand gegen die Moderne*, Reinbek 1989; **id.** (ed.), *Fundamentalismus in der modernen Welt. Die Internationale der Unvernunft*, Frankfurt 1989; **M. Riesebrodt**, *Fundamentalismus als patriarchalische Protestbewegung. Amerikanische Protestanten (1910–28) und iranische Schiiten (1961–79) im Vergleich*, Tübingen 1990; **G. Kepel**, *La Revanche de Dieu. Chrétiens, juifs et musulmans à la reconquête du monde*, Paris 1991; **B. Misztal** and **A. Shupe** (eds.), *Religion and Politics in Comparative Perspective. Revival of Religious Fundamentalism in East and West*, London 1992.

192. Cf. **G. Hole**, 'Fundamentalism, Dogmatism, Fanaticism. Psychiatric Perspectives', *Concilium* 1992/3, 23–35.

193. Cf. **H. Küng**, *Judaism*, I A II 6, 'Adam and the universalism of the Hebrew Bible'.

194. Cf. **G. Müller-Fahrenholz**, 'What is Fundamentalism Today? Perspectives in Social Psychology', *Concilium* 1992/3, 14–22.

195. **K.-J. Kuschel**, *Abraham. A Sign of Hope for Jews, Christians and Muslims*, London and New York 1995, is a recent impressive example of such a theology. This book is the prelude to a comprehensive critical biblical theology of religions.

196. Cf. **Küng**, *Judaism*, 2 C II 5, 'Tradition and Reform in Conflict: Louis Jacob'.

197. I shall not go deeper into the topic in this historically orientated account of fundamentalism (there will be further discussion in Volume II of *Christianity*).

198. For the problems of Jewish fundamentalism cf. **Neusner**, 'What is the Challenge of Contemporary Jewish Fundamentalism?' (n.190), and **S. E. Karff**, 'What shall be the Answer to Contemporary Jewish Fundamentalism?', *Concilium* 1992/3, 53–8.

199. For the problems of Islamic fundamentalism cf. **E. Elshahed**, 'What is the Challenge of Contemporary Islamic Fundamentalism?', *Concilium* 1992/3, 61–69, and **M. S. Abdullah**, 'What Shall Be the Answer to Contemporary Islamic Fundamentalism?', *Concilium* 1992/3, 70–8.

200. **J. Moltmann**, 'Fundamentalism and Modernity', ibid., 109–15: 109.

201. Ibid., 114.

V. The Paradigm of Modernity, Orientated on Reason and Progress

1. There are countless works on specific questions of **modernity**, from architecture to Zeitgeist. However, even such highly respected lexicons as *LThK*, *RGG* and *TRE* are silent on modernity as such. **H. U. Gumbrecht**, 'Modern, Modernität, Modern', in O. Brunner et al. (eds.), *Geschichtliche Grundbegriffe* IV, Stuttgart 1978, 93–131, is important for the history of the concept. For the philosophical development of the concept cf. **R. Piepmeier**, 'Modern, die Moderne', in J. Ritter and K. Gründer (eds.), *Historisches Wörterbuch der Philosophie* VI, Darmstadt 1984, 54–62. **J. F. Wilson**, 'Modernity', *EncRel* X, 17–22, offers an analysis of the concept from the perspective of religious studies.

2. For what follows cf. **R. Bubner**, 'Paradigm Change: Some Continental Perspectives', in H. Küng and D. Tracy, *Paradigm Changes in Theology*, Edinburgh 1989, 242–54.

3. Cf. **H. Küng**, TTM, C I 2, 'The Question of Epochal Thresholds'.

4. Cf. C III 11 above, 'The Renaissance – a new paradigm?'.

5. Cf. my second, forthcoming volume on *Christianity*.

6. Of course **modernity** is usually treated in several volumes in all series and handbooks on world history, as it is in all histories of philosophy, science, economics and culture. It would make little sense to provide extended bibliographies on individual stages and sectors which are relatively well known to contemporaries. I feel it more important to give a compact overall view and a clear characterization of the modern paradigm than to accumulate facts and books. In historical orientation on facts generally I have been well served by *Der Grosse Ploetz. Auszug aus der Geschichte von den Anfängen bis zur Gegenwart* (1863), Freiburg ³¹1991, and on church history by **K. Heussi**, *Kompendium der Kirchengeschichte*, Tübingen ¹²1960.

7. Cf. e.g. **J. Kunisch**, *Absolutismus. Europäische Geschichte von Westfälischen Frieden bis zum Ende des Ancien Régime*, Göttingen 1986, especially the survey of research on pp.179–202. For the Peace of Westphalia cf. **H. Lutz**, *Reformation und Gegenreformation*, Munich 1979, 113–16.

8. Cf. **H. Lehmann**, *Das Zeitalter des Absolutismus. Gottesgnadentum und Kriegsnot*, Stuttgart 1980, III.1, on the causes, manifestations and consequences of the great crisis of the seventeenth century, gives a survey of the state of scholarship in this area and the results attained so far.

9. Cf. the report on research by **H. Duchhardt**, *Das Zeitalter des Absolutismus*, Munich 1989, 155–9 (there is also a good survey here of sources and literature in the different countries and individual areas).

10. Cf. **H. Küng**, *Judaism*, C V 4, 'Judaism on the threshold of modernity'.

11. Cf. **J. Bodin**, *Les six livres de la République* (1583), for a modern edition cf. *On Sovereignty*, ed. J. H. Franklin, Cambridge 1992.

12. Cf. **T. Hobbes**, *Leviathan or the Matter, Form and Power of a Commonwealth, Ecclesiastical and Civil* (1651), Harmondsworth 1981.

13. Cf. **N. Machiavelli**, *The Prince* (1532), Harmondsworth 1970. The apologists for the 'realist' Machiavelli come to grief in particular at Ch.18, 'How princes should honour their word', where politics in its 'autonomies' seems to be completely detached from ethical ties; nowhere does he merely assert, he seeks to give tactical instructions.

14. Cf. **V. L. Tapié**, 'Louis XIV', *Encyclopaedia Universalis* II, Paris 1985, 159–65.

15. Cf. above, C II 3, 'The Bishop of Rome's claim to power'.

16. Cf. **G. Oestreich**, *Geist und Gestalt des frühmodernen Staates*, Berlin 1969, 187–97.

17. **Duchhardt**, *Das Zeitalter des Absolutismus* (n.9), 75–8, gives a good summary of the results of research here.

18. For the course of this day cf. **P. Erlanger**, *Louis XIV*, Paris 1965, 334f.

19. Cf. **Denzinger**, *Enchiridion*, 1322–27.

20. **P. Goubert**, *Louis XIV et vingt millions de Français*, Paris 1966, 241f.

21. Cf. **F. Bacon**, *Nova Atlantis* (1627), modern edition *New Atlantis*, London 1897.

22. Cf. **S. Toulmin**, *Cosmopolis. The Hidden Agenda of Modernity*, New York 1990.

23. Cf. **N. Copernicus**, *De revolutionibus orbium coelestium libri VI* (1543), facsimile edition *On the Revolutions of the Heavenly Spheres*, London 1972.

24. Cf. **G. Galilei**, *Dialogue Concerning the Two World Systems* (1632), Berkeley 1967.

25. Cf. id., Letter to B. Castelli of 21 December 1613, in *Opere* V, Florence 1965, 281–8.

26. Cf. **I. Newton**, *Philosophiae naturalis principia mathematica*, London 1687, [3]1726, new edition in 2 vols, Cambridge, Mass. 1972.

27. Cf. **W. Jens**, *Eine deutsche Universität. 500 Jahre Tübinger Gelehrtenrepublik*, Munich 1977, 105f.

28. Cf. **T. Campanella**, *La città del Sole* (1602), Latin *Civitas solis* (1623), modern edition *City of the Sun*, Berkeley 1981.

29. **G. Denzler**, 'Der Fall Galilei und kein Ende', *Zeitschrift für Kirchengeschichte* 95, 1984, 223–33, rightly attacks the 'blind apologetics' which has still not died out in Catholic historiography over the case of Galileo – the most recent prime example is **W. Brandmüller**, *Galilei und die Kirche oder Das Recht auf Irrtum*, Regensburg 1982,

30. Cf. **R. Descartes**, *Le monde ou le traité de la lumière* (1664); for a modern English translation cf. 'The World, or Treatise on Light', in *The Philosophical*

Writings of Descartes, translated J. Cottingham, R. Stouthoff and D. Murdoch, Vol.1, Cambridge 1988, 81–98.

31. Cf. id., *Discourse on the Method for Rightly Conducting One's Reason and Feeling within the Sciences* (Leyden 1637), Harmondsworth 1970.

32. G. W. F. Hegel, *Lectures on the History of Philosophy*, III, London 1886, 217.

33. For an intensive discussion of René Descartes cf. H. Küng, DGE, A I, 'I think, do I therefore exist? René Descartes' (with a bibliography).

34. Cf. Toulmin, *Cosmopolis* (n.22), esp. Ch.3, 'The Modern Picture of the World'. For this reason I would differ from Toulmin, as I indicated in connection with P III: I would not call the Renaissance modernity, since, as Toulmin himself explains, some of its representatives (like Montaigne), while having a practical rationality, did not display the typical modern rationality.

35. J. Habermas, *Philosophical Discourse on Modernity*, Oxford 1990. However, the criticism in Toulmin, *Cosmopolis* (n.22), 277, should be noted: 'He (Habermas) describes as "modernization" the emancipation movement which began with the French Revolution and underwent a rationalization in Kant's universalistic theory of ethics . . . So for Habermas modernity is not characterized by a call to a rationalistic theory but in the obligation to an egalitarian praxis.'

36. Cf. Kant in his preface to the second edition of the *Critique of Pure Reason*, ed. N. Kemp Smith, London 1929.

37. Cf. id., *Critique of Pure Reason* (1781) (see n.36); *Critique of Practical Reason* (1788), London 1927; *Critique of Judgment* (1790), London 1978.

38. Id., *Critique of Pure Reason*, 29.

39. Ibid., 650.

40. Ibid., 528.

41. For an intensive discussion of Immanuel Kant cf. H. Küng, DGE, G III 2, 'More than pure reason: Immanuel Kant' (with bibliography).

42. B. Pascal, *Pensées*, London 1908, no.162.

43. For the history of the term cf. H. U. Gumbrecht, 'Modern', in *Geschichtliche Grundbegriffe. Historisches Lexikon zur politisch-sozialen Sprache in Deutschland* IV, Stuttgart 1978, 99–131. *Modernus* (from *modo*) = 'new' as opposed to *antiquus* = old.

44. Cf. H. Küng, DGE, A, 'Reason or Faith?'.

45. Cf. Montesquieu, *De l'ésprit des lois* (2 vols.), Geneva 1748, modern edition *The Spirit of the Laws*, Cambridge 1989.

46. Cf. M. Diderot and M. d'Alembert (eds.), *Encyclopédie, ou Dictionnaire raisonné des sciences, des arts et des métiers, par une Société de gens de lettres* (35 vols.), Paris 1751–80.

47. Cf. Toulmin, *Cosmopolis* (n.22), Part 1.

48. Pascal, *Pensées* (n.42), no.264.

49. Cf. R. Koselleck, 'Fortschritt', in *Geschichtliche Grundbegriffe* II, Stuttgart 1975, 351–423.

50. Cf. above C IV 8, 'Why the witch-craze?'

51. For what follows cf. H. Küng, DGE, G I 1, 'The many names of the one God'; id., CWR, IV 2.

52. Cf. L. von Pastor, *Geschichte der Päpste seit dem Ausgang des Mittelalters*, vol. XV, Freiburg ⁸1961, 284–354, 440f., 729–32.

53. Even a historian as well disposed to the pope as is Freiherr Ludwig von

Pastor does not comment on these events without a critical undertone: 'Only a decision of incalculable scope had been made with the prohibition of rites. The Chinese Christians were forbidden things which in their view were necessary for decency and a good way of life, and they were forbidden contrary to the declaration of the Emperor K'ang-hsi and the Chinese scholars' (Vol.XV, 309). In 1710 all this was confirmed and intensified by a new decree of the Roman Inquisition in the face of all the objections from the Chinese apostolic vicars and Jesuits; the threat of excommunication issued at the time against all authors of publications on rites and the dispute has still not been formally withdrawn even today.

54. Cf. J. **Ching** and **W. G. Oxtoby**, *Moral Enlightenment. Leibniz and Wolff on China*, Nettetal 1992.

55. Cf. **C. Wolff**, *Oratio de Sinarum philosophia practica*, Frankfurt 1726.

56. Cf. **G. E. Lessing**, *Nathan the Wise* (1779), English translation, New York 1972.

57. Cf. above, C IV 9, 'From the "inner light" to the "light of reason"'.

58. I. **Kant**, 'Beantwortung der Frage: Was ist Aufklärung' (1783), in *Werke* VI, 53–61: 53.

59. E. **Troeltsch**, 'Die Aufklärung' (1897), in *Gesammelte Schriften* IV, Tübingen 1925, 338–74; 339.

60. Cf. above, C III 9, 'The problematic separation of reason and faith'.

61. For **secularization** cf. F. **Gogarten**, *Verhängnis und Hoffnung der Neuzeit. Die Säkularisierung als theologisches Problem*, Stuttgart 1953; H. Cox, *The Secular City*, New York and London 1965; H. Lübbe, *Säkularisierung. Geschichte eines ideenpolitischen Begriffs*, Freiburg 1965; H. **Blumenburg**, *The Legitimacy of the Modern Age*, Boston, Mass. 1988; R. K. **Fenn**, *Toward a Theory of Secularization*, Ellington, Conn. 1978; D. **Martin**, *A General Theory of Secularization*, Oxford 1978; R. N. **Bellah** and P. E. **Hammond**, *Varieties of Civil Religion*, San Francisco 1980; H.-H. Schrey (ed.), *Säkularisierung*, Darmstadt 1981; H. Zabel, W. Conze and H. W. Strätz, 'Säkularisation, Säkulariserung', in *Geschichtliche Grundbegriffe* V, Stuttgart 1984, 782–829; H. Meyer, *Religionskritik, Religionssoziologie und Säkularisation*, Frankfurt 1988. More recent critical works on the thesis of secularization will be listed later.

62. Cf. **M. Greiffenhagen**, 'Emanzipation', *Historisches Wörterbuch der Philosophie* II, Darmstadt 1972, 448f.; id., 'Ein Weg der Vernunft ohne Rückkehr. Ist die Emanzipation in eine neue Phase getreten?', *Die Zeit*, 22 June 1973.

63. Cf. **M. Weber**, *The Protestant Ethic and the Spirit of Capitalism*, London 1930.

64. Cf. above, C IV 9, 'Confessionalism and traditionalism'.

65. The Lutherans J. F. Buddeus, C. M. Pfaff, the church historian J. L. Mosheim and his pupil J.P.Miller and the two Walchs (father and son), along with the Reformed Swiss S. Werenfels, J. F. Osterwald and the younger Turrettini were regarded as 'transitional theologians'.

66. I. G. Canz, J. Carpov and S. J. Baumgarten were regarded as 'Wolffians'; to them could be added a number of Catholics.

67. J. F. W. Jeremias, J. J. Spalding, F. Nicolai and C. F. Bahrdt were regarded as 'Neologians'; with some qualifications, the historians J. S. Semler, J. A. Ernesti and I. D. Michaelis went along with them.

68. Cf. **K. Barth**, *Protestant Theology in the Nineteenth Century*, London and Richmond, Va 1972, whose account of this, though one-sided, is well worth thinking about.

69. **A. Schweizer**, *The Quest of the Historical Jesus*, London [3]1950, 4; for further developments cf. especially 13–47.

70. **H. S. Reimarus**, *Von der Zwecke Jesu und seiner Jünger*, Brunswick 1778, §4.

71. Cf. ibid., §§5–7.

72. Cf. ibid., §§8–18.

73. Cf. ibid., §§29–30.

74. Cf. ibid., §31.

75. Cf. **J. J. Rousseau**, *Émile ou de l'éducation* (4 vols), Amsterdam 1762; there is a new edition with commentary by P.Richard, Paris 1951; modern English edition Harmondsworth 1991.

76. Cf. **D. F. Strauss**, *The Life of Jesus Critically Examined*, translated by George Eliot, London and Philadelphia 1973.

77. Around the end of the nineteenth century people were well informed not only about the different sources of the Pentateuch and the real history of the tribes of Israel (e.g. through Julius Wellhausen), but also about the chronological priority of the Gospel of Mark, which together with a source Q must have served as a basis for the main Gospels Matthew and Luke (= Synoptic question).

78. Cf. **F. C. Baur**, *Lehrbuch der christlichen Dogmengeschichte*, Stuttgart 1847, [3]1867; **id.**, *Geschichte der christlichen Kirche* (5 vols.), Tübingen 1853–63.

79. Cf. **A. von Harnack**, *Lehrbuch der Dogmengeschichte* (3 vols), Tübingen [4]1909, reprinted Darmstadt 1964.

80. The results of this research cannot be overlooked:

In research into the Gospels, **textual criticism** has established with the greatest possible accuracy the wording of the biblical writings in its earliest attainable form, by external and internal criticism, study of language and content, and the exploration of the history of the text.

Literary criticism has investigated the literary integrity of the writings. It has emphasized the difference in the legal, religious and social circumstances presupposed, in language, chronology and historical information, in theological and moral views. By distinguishing sources in the oral and written traditions it has clarified what may be the original material as opposed to later incorporations. It has defined the age, origin, audience and literary character of the New Testament writings. Using comparative procedures it has contrasted them with contemporary Jewish and Hellenistic literature and described their special characteristics.

Form and genre criticism have raised the question of the *Sitz im Leben* of the community and the individual, the literary genre, the framework of the smaller literary units and the original form, and thus have attempted to redefine the historical reliability and the content of the tradition.

Traditio-historical criticism has undertaken to illuminate the pre-literary process, has analysed the earliest hymns, liturgical fragments, legal statements, etc.; has connected them with worship, preaching, catechesis and community life; and has thus attempted to discover beginnings which are decisive for the rise of the church and the first study of its development.

81. Cf. **F. D. E. Schleiermacher**, *A Brief Outline of the Study of Theology* (1811), Richmond, Va 1966.

82. Cf. **id.**, *On Religion. Speeches to its Cultured Despisers* (1799), reissued with a preface by R. Otto, New York 1958.

83. **E. Hirsch**, *Geschichte der neueren evangelischen Theologie im Zusammenhang mit den allgemeinen Bewegungen des europäischen Denkens*, Vol.IV, Gütersloh 1960, esp. 500–20, has worked out Fichte's influence on Schleiermacher (in a one-sided way).

84. **Schleiermacher**, *On Religion* (n.82), 1,3.

85. Ibid., 277.

86. Ibid., 101.

87. Cf. ibid.

88. Ibid., 34.

89. Cf. **G. Ebeling**, 'Luther und Schleiermacher', in *Lutherstudien* III, Tübingen 1985, 405–27.

90. Cf. **G. W. F. Hegel**, 'Vorrede zu Hinrichs' Religionsphilosophie' (1822), in *Werkausgabe*, Vol.XI, Frankfurt 1970, 42–67, esp.58.

91. Cf. **F. Schleiermacher**, *Monologen. Eine Neujahrsgabe* (1800), KGA I.3, 1–61.

92. Cf. Barth's postscript to *Schleiermacher-Auswahl*, ed. H.Bölli, Munich 1968, 307.

93. Cf. **P. Seifert**, *Die Theologie des jungen Schleiermacher*, Gütersloh 1960, quotation p.15.

94. Cf. **F. Hertel**, *Das theologische Denken Schleiermachers untersucht an der ersten Auflage seiner Reden 'Über die Religion'*, Zurich 1965, esp.4–6. Both Seifert and Hertel relativize Fichte's influence (against Hirsch).

95. Cf. **H.-J. Birkner**, *Theologie und Philosophie. Einführung in Probleme der Schleiermacher-Interpretation*, Munich 1974, 43f. For this problem see also the discussion between **H. W. Frei, S. W. Sykes** and **R. T. Thiemann**, in **J. O. Duke** and **R. F. Streetman**, *Barth and Schleiermacher. Beyond the Impasse?*, Philadelphia 1984, 65–113.

96. **Barth**, *Protestant Theology in the Nineteenth Century* (n.68), 460.

97. Cf. **E. Brunner**, *Die Mystik und das Wort. Der Gegensatz zwischen moderner Religionsauffassung und christlichem Glauben dargestellt an die Theologie Schleiermachers*, Tübingen 1924.

98. Cf. **Barth**, Postscript (n.92), 308.

99. **Schleiermacher**, *On Religion* (n.82), 33.

100. Ibid.

101. Ibid., 101.

102. Ibid., 238.

103. Ibid., 235.

104. Cf. ibid., 239.

105. Ibid.

106. Cf. **H. Küng**, *Judaism*, I C V 6, 'The first modern Jew, Moses Mendelssohn'.

107. **Schleiermacher**, *On Religion* (n.82), 241.

108. Ibid., 246.

109. Ibid., 247.

110. Ibid.

111. **Barth**, Postscript (n.92), 308.

112. Cf. F. Schleiermacher, *Die Weihnachtsfeier* (1806), Berlin ²1826. English text: *Christmas Eve. A Dialogue on the Incarnation*, Richmond, Va 1967.

113. Ibid., 130.

114. Ibid., 146.

115. Cf. id., *The Christian Faith*, Edinburgh 1928.

116. Anselm of Canterbury, *Proslogion*, I; id., *De fide trinitatis et de incarnatione verbi* II.

117. Cf. F. Schleiermacher, *The Life of Jesus* (1832), reissued Philadelphia 1975.

118. Cf. Barth, Postscript (n.92), 309.

119. The following quotations are from *The Christian Faith* (n.115).

120. Ibid., 738f.

121. Ibid., 747.

122. Ibid., 385.

123. Ibid., 397.

124. Ibid.

125. Ibid.

126. Ibid.

127. Ibid.

128. D. Lange, 'Neugestaltung christlicher Glaubenslehre', in id. (ed.), *Friedrich Schleiermacher 1768–1834. Theologe – Philosoph – Pädagoge*, Göttingen 1985, 85–101: 101.

129. Schleiermacher, *The Christian Faith* (n.115), 397.

130. Cf. id., *Über die Glaubenslehre. Zweites Sendschreiben an Lücke*, KGA I, 10, 343.

131. Id., *The Christian Faith* (n.92), 389.

132. I myself have presented one in *On Being a Christian* (1974).

133. Cf. M. Junker, *Das Urbild des Gottesbewusstseins. Zur Entwicklung der Religionstheorie und Christologie Schleiermachers von der ersten zur zweiten Auflage der Glaubenslehre*, Berlin 1990, 210f.

134. Cf. D. Lange, *Historischer Jesus oder mythischer Christus. Untersuchungen zu dem Gegensatz zwischen Friedrich Schleiermacher und David Friedrich Strauss*, Gütersloh 1975.

135. Cf. T. Schieder, *Friedrich der Grosse. Ein Königtum der Widersprüche*, Frankfurt 1983.

136. For the **French Revolution and the church**, in addition to the general histories of the Revolution cf. A. Latreille, *L'Église catholique et la Révolution française. Le pontificat de Pie VI et la crise française (1775–1779)*, Paris 1946; C. Ledré, *L'Église de France sous la Révolution*, Paris 1949; M. Zywczynski, *Die Kirche und die Französische Revolution*, Leipzig 1953 (Polish original edition Warsaw 1951); H. Maier, *Revolution und Kirche. Studien zur Frühgeschichte der christlichen Demokratie (1789–1901)*, Freiburg 1959, ⁵1988; J. McManners, *The French Revolution and the Church*, London 1969; D. Menozzi, *Cristianesimo e Rivoluzione francese*, Brescia 1977; M. Vovelle, *Breve storia della rivoluzione francese*, Rome 1979; id., *La révolution contre l'Église. De la Raison à l'Être Suprême*, Brussels 1988; P. Christophe, *1789, les prêtres dans la révolution*, Paris 1986; T. Tackett, *Religion, Revolution, and Regional Culture in Eighteenth-Century France. The Ecclesiastical Oath of 1791*, Princeton 1986; P. Pierrard, *L'Église et la Révolution (1789–1889)*,

Paris 1988; **B. Plongeron** (ed.), *Pratiques religieuses. Mentalités et spiritualités dans l'Europe révolutionnaire (1770–1820),* Turnhout 1988; **J. Chaunu** (ed.), *Droits de l'église et Droits de l'Homme. Pie VI et les évêques français,* Limoges 1989; **P. Colin** (ed.), *Les catholiques français et l'héritage de 1789. D'un centénaire à l'autre 1889–1989,* Paris 1989; **V. Schubert** (ed.), *Die Französische Revolution. Wurzeln und Wirkungen,* St Ottilien 1989; **S. Desan,** *Reclaiming the Sacred. Lay Religion and Popular Politics in Revolutionary France,* Ithaca 1990; **G. Cholvy,** *La religion en France de la fin du XVIIIe à nos jours,* Paris 1991.

137. Cf. **E.-J. Sieyès,** 'Qu'est-ce que le tiers État', no place 1789. The three famous programmatic questions right at the beginning are: '1. What is the Third Estate? **Everything.** 2. What has it been in the political order so far? **Nothing.** 3. What does it want? **To be something.**'

138. Cf. **E. Weis,** preface to **F. Furet,** *Zur Historiographie der Französichen Revolution heute,* Munich 1989.

139. **R. Reichard** speaks of a 'conservative process of developing awareness which first gave the critics and opponents of the revolution a certain social basis in the masses', in connection with the investigation by **T. Tackett,** 'Die Stadteliten unter Priestereid von 1791', in R. Koselleck and R. Reichardt, *Die Französische Revolution als Bruch des gesellschaftlichen Bewusstsein,* Munich 1988, 579–605. In this connection reference should be made to the important series of German research into the Revolution which is to be edited by **R. Reichardt** and **E. Schmitt,** *Ancien Régime. Aufklärung und Revolution.*

140. Cf. **Pope Pius VI,** *Breve Quod aliquantum (10.3.1791),* together with the considérations *Breve Charitas (13.4.1791),* ed. M.-N.-S. Guillon, *Collection générale des brefs et instructions de Notre Très–Saint Père le Pape Pie VI* (2 vols.), Paris 1798 (translated in Chaunu, *Droits de l'Église*).

141. Cf. **A. de Condorcet,** *Esquisse d'un tableau historique des progrès de l'esprit humain,* Paris 1794.

142. Cf. **J. de Maistre,** *Considérations sur la France,* Basel 1797.

143. In his masterful survey of more than 200 years of historiography on the Revolution the Freiburg historian **E. Schulin,** *Die Französische Revolution,* Munich 1988, Part 1, convincingly shows how after the Second World War and the Vichy Regime the conservative trend of interpretation which had long been pronounced (and still has a home in the Académie Française) was little represented in public. In the post-war period the Socialist-Marxist interpretation held almost sole sway, represented at the Sorbonne from 1959 above all by **A. Soboul,** *The French Revolution 1787–1799* (1962), London 1974. But now in most recent times (even before 1989!) this has been replaced by the structuralist historical liberal school (based above all in the Sixth Section of the École Pratique des Hautes Études). Its great representative **F. Furet,** along with **D. Richet,** has produced the now normative account of the French Revolution: **F. Furet** and **D. Richet,** *La Révolution* (2 vols), Paris 1965/66; **F. Furet,** *Penser la révolution française,* Paris 1978; **id.** (ed.), *L'héritage de la révolution française,* Paris 1989.

144. Cf. **F. Furet** and **M. Ozouf,** *Dictionnaire critique de la Révolution Française,* Paris 1988, with reference to **D. Greer,** *The Incidence of the Terror during the French Revolution. A Statistical Interpretation,* Cambridge, Mass. 1935.

145. For what follows cf. above all the historical and statistical investigation by **Vovelle**, *La révolution contre l'église* (n.136), which gives a new view of the material.

146. The controversy which developed between A. Aulard and A. Mathiez around the turn of the century as to whether the transition from the cult of Reason to the cult of the Supreme Being is a repudiation and radical break or an almost imperceptible transition is not clearly resolved in **Vovelle**, *La révolution contre l'église* (n.136), 155–92, either.

147. **D. Menozzi**, 'The Significance of the Catholic Reaction to the Revolution', *Concilium* 201, 1989, 76–86: 82, 85. This issue, edited by C. Geffré and J. P. Jossua, is the best informed survey from a present-day theological perspective of the issues which give it its title: *1789: The French Revolution and the Church*.

148. **B. Plongeron**, 'The Birth of a Republican Christianity (1789–1801): Abbé Grégoire', ibid., 27–39: 33. However, the failure of certain members of the hierarchy to come to terms with the French Revolution is evident from the fact that even after 200 years (on 12 December 1989, the bicentenary celebration of the Revolution), the Archbishop of Paris, Cardinal Lustiger, refused to take part in the 'Céremonie Républicaine' of bringing Abbé Grégoire's body to the Pantheon.

149. **J. Comby**, 'Liberty, Equality , Fraternity. Principles for a Nation and for a Church', *Concilium* 201, 17–26: 25.

150. Cf. **E. Burke**, *Reflections on the Revolution in France* (1790), Harmondsworth 1982.

151. Cf. **C. L. von Haller**, *Die Restauration der Staats-Wissenschaft oder Theorie des natürlich-geselligen Zustands, der Chimäre des künstlich-bürgerlichen entgegengesetzt* (6 vols.), Winterthur 1816–34. Haller already writes programmatically in the preface: 'The legitimate thrones are restored; we also want to elevate to the throne legitimate science, that which stands in the service of the supreme Lord, to whom all creation bears witness that it is the true science' (Vol.I, iiif.).

152. Cf. **F. J. von Stahl**, *Die Philosophie des Rechts nach geschichtlicher Ansicht*, I–II.2, Heidelberg 1830–37.

153. Cf. **L.-G.-A. de Bonald**, *Théorie du pouvoir politique et religieux dans la société civile* (3 vols), Constance 1793.

154. Cf. **J. de Maistre**, *Du Pape*, Paris 1819: Chapter 1 of Book 1 already deals with infallibility in the spiritual order, which corresponds to 'sovereignty' in the worldly order.

155. Cf. **F. R. de Chateaubriand**, *The Genius of Christianity or, The Spirit and Reality of the Christian Religion* (5 vols), Baltimore 1856, reissued New York 1975.

156. For technological developments especially in England cf. **E. Hobsbawm**, *The Age of Revolution*, London 1962, Ch.9, 'Towards an Industrial World'; id., *Industry and Empire. An Economic History of Britain since 1750*, London 1969.

157. For discussion of this concept cf. **W. W. Rostow** (ed.), *The Economics of Take-off into Sustained Growth*, London 1963.

158. **C. M. Cipolla**, 'Die Industrielle Revolution in der Weltgeschichte', in K.Borchardt, *Die Industrielle Revolution in Deutschland*, Munich 1972, 7–21: 18f.

159. Cf. especially **A. Smith**, *The Theory of Moral Sentiments* (1769), ed. D. Daiches and A. L. Macfie, London 1976.

160. Cf. **A. Smith**, *An Inquiry into the Nature and Causes of the Wealth of Nations* (2 vols., 1776), ed. W. B. Todd, London 1976.

161. Cf. **K. Marx** and **F. Engels**, *The Communist Manifesto*, London 1888, reissued Harmondsworth 1967.

162. Cf. **M. Greschat**, *Das Zeitalter der Industriellen Revolution. Das Christentum vor der Moderne*, Stuttgart 1980 (with a bibliography on the industrial revolution in the various countries); **G. Besier**, *Religion – Nation – Kultur. Die Geschichte der christlichen Kirchen in den gesellschaftlichen Umbrüchen des 19.Jahrhunderts*, Neukirchen 1992.

163. **Leo XII**, *Rerum novarum cupidi* (1892), in *Acta Apostolicae Sedis* 23 (1890/91), 641–70, centenary edition London 1992.

164. Cf. **H. Küng**, DGE, C II E, 'Critique of the critique'.

165. 'The corporate order' was still the main value of the second social encyclical *Quadragesimo anno* (= forty years after *Rerum novarum*) of 1931, Pius XI's attempts to realize a 'class state' in Austria between 1934 and 1938, and corporate chambers in Portugal, Spain and Italy.

166. **Greschat**, *Das Zeitalter der Industriellen Revolution* (n.162), 236.

167. Cf. **I. Kant**, 'Beobachtungen über das Gefühl des Schönen und Erhabene' (1764), in *Werke* I, 821–84: 851f.

168. Cf. **J. J. Bachofen**, *Das Mutterrecht. Eine Untersuchung über die Gynaikokratie der alten Welt nach ihrer religiösen und rechtlichen Natur*, Stuttgart 1861.

169. 'Declaration of the Rights of Women and Citizenesses', text in **H. Schröder** and **T. Sauter**, 'Zur politischen Theorie des Feminismus. Die Deklaration der Rechte der Frau und Bürgerin von 1791', in *Aus Politik und Zeitgeschichte*, supplement to the weekly *Das Parlament* 48, 1977, 29–54: 51. Cf. **L. Doormann**, *Ein Feuer brennt in mir. Die Lebensgeschichte der Olympe de Gouges*, Weinheim 1993.

170. **Marx** and **Engels**, *Communist Manifesto* (n.161), 101.

171. Cf. **F. Engels**, *The Origin of the Family, Private Property and the State* (1884), Harmondsworth 1986.

172. Cf. **A. Bebel**, *Woman in the Past, Present and Future* (1879), London 1988.

173. **Leo XIII**, Encyclical *Immortale Dei* (1885), in E. Marmu (ed.), *Mensch und Gemeinschaft*, nos.833–907: 867.

174. **Leo XIII**, Encyclical *Rerum Novarum* (n.163), §42.

175. **S. H. Pfürtner**, 'Soziallehre, katholische', in *Frauenlexikon. Traditionen, Fakten, Perspektiven*, ed. A. Lissner, R. Süssmuth and K. Walter, Freiburg 1988, 1051–9: 1053.

176. According to a 1993 survey by the Allenbach Institute for Demoscopy on 'Women and Church', in the past ten years the percentage of Catholic women who claim a 'close connection' with their church has declined from 40% to 25% (however, the same thing has happened in the Protestant churches). The local church finds more sympathy: 43% of all Catholic women and 76% of women with an interest in the church say that they have had 'good experiences' in their parishes, and 69%/80% have 'a good opinion' of their pastors.

177. Cf. **R. L. Greaves** (ed.), *Triumph over Silence. Women in Protestant History*, Westport, Conn. 1985.

178. In what follows I am going by the excellent survey by **G. Scharffenorth** and **E. Reichle** in the articles 'Frau (Neuzeit)' and 'Frauenbewegung', *TRE* XI, 443–67, 471–81. There is also a good deal of material in **M. Perrot** (ed.), *Histoire de la vie privée*, Vol. IV, *De la Révolution à la Grande Guerre*, Paris 1987, especially chapters II and IV.

179. **E. Moltmann-Wendel**, 'Christentum und Frauenbewegung in Deutschland', in ead. (ed.), *Frauenbefreiung. Biblische und theologische Argumente*, Munich 1978 (a second, much revised edition of *Menschenrechte für die Frau*, Munich 1974), 13–77: 25.

180. Cf. **D. Kaufmann**, *Frauen zwischen Aufbruch und Reaktion. Protestantische Frauenbewegung in der ersten Hälfte des 20.Jahrhunderts*, Munich 1988.

181. **Moltmann-Wendel**, 'Christentum und Frauenbewegung' (n.179), 75. **Catharina Halkes**, 'Towards a History of Feminist Theology in Europe', in the *Jahrbuch der Europäischen Gesellschaft für die theologische Forschung von Frauen, Feministische Theologie im europäischen Kontext*, ed. A. Esser and L. Schottroff, Kampen 1993, 11–37, gives a survey of the most important events, publications and authors of early European feminist theology (1960–1975), from Gertrud Heinzelmann and Elisabeth Gössmann through Catharina Halkes, Elisabeth Schüssler-Fiorenza and Mary Daly to Kari E. Børresen and Ida Raming (to mention only the best known). The volume also contains a brief summary of the most important activities and publications since 1945 of the World Council of Churches, which with its consultations and publications – especially *Sexism in the 1970s* (1974) – has made a decisive contribution on the Protestant side to the breakthrough of feminist theological approaches.

182. **H. Thiersch**, 'Das Konfessionsmonopol und Sinnfragen in der säkularisierten Erziehung', in G. Klosinski, *Religion als Chance oder Risiko. Entwicklungsfördende und entwicklungshemmende Aspekte religiöser Erziehung*, Bern 1994, 42–53; 46. For the inevitability of choice in modern society cf. **P. L. Berger**, *The Heretical Imperative. Contemporary Possibilities of Religious Affirmation*, New York and London 1979; id., *A Far Glory. The Quest for Faith in an Age of Credulity*, New York 1992.

183. **Thiersch**, 'Das Konfessionsmonopol' (n.181), 46. These questions become more acute in an 'experience society'; cf. **G. Schulze**, *Die Erlebnisgesellschaft. Kultursoziologie der Gegenwart*, Frankfurt 1993.

184. This is shown by all the more recent empirical investigations into the end of the twentieth century, in the international sphere above all by the study carried out by 21 research centres in 16 countries, reported on by **A. M. Greeley**, *Religion around the World. An International Social Survey Programme Report*, Chicago 1993.

185. For the most recent discusion of the secularization thesis cf. **A. M. Greeley**, *Unsecular Man. The Persistence of Religion*, New York 1972; id., *Religious Change in America*, Cambridge, Mass. 1989; id., *Religion as Poetry* (forthcoming); **J.-P. Sironneau**, *Sécularisation et religions politiques*, The Hague 1982; **R. Stark** and **W. S. Bainbridge**, *The Future of Religion. Secularization, Revival and Cult Formation*, Berkeley 1985; **T. Molnar** and **A. de Benoist**, *L'éclipse du sacré. Discours et réponses*, Paris 1986; **S. Acquaviva** and **R. Stella**, *Fine di un'ideologia: la secolarizzazione*, Rome 1989; **J. K. Hadden** and **A. Shupe** (eds.), *Secularization and Fundamentalism Reconsidered*, New York 1989; **S. Martelli**, *La religione nella società post-moderna. Tra secolarizzazione e desecolarizzazione*, Bologna 1990; **L. Oviedo Torró**, *La secularización como*

problema. Aportaciones al análisis de las relaciones entre fe cristiana y mundo moderno, Valencia 1990; **O. Tschannen,** *Les théories de la sécularisation,* Geneva 1992.

186. **K. Gabriel,** *Christentum zwischen Tradition und Postmoderne,* Freiburg 1992, gives an excellent summary of the relevant sociological research in an analysis which is both empirical and fundamental (quotation, 150). The most recent sociological research on religion in Switzerland was carried out by **A. Dubach** and **R. J. Campiche** (eds.), *Jeder ein Sonderfall? Religion in der Schweiz,* Zurich 1992 (there are also clarifications by M.Krüggeler of the issue of the individualization of religion).

187. There is a discussion with some of these authors from a theological standpoint in **C. Geffré** and **J.-P. Jossua** (eds.), *The Debate on Modernity, Concilium* 1992/6.

188. Cf. **H. Küng,** GCT, Ch.VII, 'Karl Barth: Theology in the Transition to Postmodernity'.

189. Cf. **M. Horkheimer** and **T. Adorno,** *Dialectic of the Enlightenment. Philosophical Fragments,* London 1979.

190. Cf. **H. Küng,** *DGE,* A, 'Reason or Faith?'.

191. Cf. **M. Frank,** 'Zwei Jahrhunderte Rationalitäts-Kritik und die Sehnsucht nach einer "Neuen Mythologie"', in his volume of essays, Conditio moderna. *Essays, Reden, Programm,* Leipzig 1993, 30–50.

192. Cf. **F. Capra,** *The Turning Point,* London 1983.

193. Cf. **I. Prigogine** and **I. Stengers,** *Order out of Chaos. Man's New Dialogue with Nature,* London 1985. For the scientific background cf. **id.,** *Time, Chaos and the Quantum. Towards the Resolution of the Time Paradox* (forthcoming).

194. Cf. **J. Habermas,** *Theory of Communicative Action* (2 vols.), Oxford 1985, 1989; **id.,** *Moral Consciousness and Communicative Action,* Oxford 1990; **id.,** *Die Neue Unübersichtlickeit,* Kleine Politische Schriften V, Frankfurt 1985; **id.,** *Philosophical Discourse of Modernity,* Oxford 1990.

195. Cf. **U. Beck,** *Risikogesellschaft. Auf dem Weg in eine andere Moderne,* Frankfurt 1986.

196. Cf. **id.,** *Die Erfindung des Politischen. Zu einer Theorie reflexiver Modernisierung,* Frankfurt 1993.

197. Cf. **J.-F. Lyotard,** *The Postmodern Condition. A Report on Knowledge,* Manchester 1984 (in the closing remarks there is inappropriate polemic against Habermas' concern for a universal ethical consensus, 'an obsolete and suspect value' which Lyotard wants to abandon in favour of 'justice', 65–6). Cf. **M. Frank,** *Die Grenzen der Verständigung. Ein Geistergespräch zwischen Lyotard und Habermas,* Frankfurt 1988.

198. Cf. **W. Welsch,** *Unsere postmoderne moderne,* Weinheim ²1988, 4f. cf. 5, 'pluralism in principle'. There are further corrections in the Preface to the Third Edition (1991): the preservation and defence of plurality despite all the deep differences = 'postmodern conception'; curbing the superficial pluralism and eradicating plurality = 'a pseudo-postmodern conception' (xv).

199. Cf. **R. Spaemann,** 'Ende der Modernität', in *Moderne oder Postmoderne? Zur Signatur des gegenwärtigen Zeitalters,* ed. P. Koslowski, R. Spaemann and R. Löw, Weinheim 1986, 19–40.

200. No theologian has grappled more intensively and constructively with the problems of pluralism than the systematic theologian at the University of Chicago

Divinity School, **D. Tracy**, *Blessed Rage for Order. The New Pluralism in Theology*, New York 1975; **id.**, *The Analogical Imagination. Christian Theology and the Culture of Pluralism*, New York and London 1981; **id.**, *Plurality and Ambiguity. Hermeneutics, Religion, Hope*, New York and London 1987. For the debate between Tracy and G. Lindbeck cf. the contributions by **R. Lints** and **S. L. Stell** in *Journal of the American Academy of Religion* 61, 1993, 655–703.

201. That this is true not only of America is shown by the publications of the Conference of Confessing Communities in Germany, especially the 'Aufruf der Bekenntnisbewegung "Kein anderes Evangelium" zur Passions- und Osterzeit 1970', in **R. Bäumer, P. Beyerhaus** and **F. Grünzweig** (eds.), *Weg und Zeugnis. Bekennende Gemeinschaften im gegenwärtigen Kirchenkampf 1965–1980*, Bad Liebenzell 1980, 123–5, which is directed against the 'modernistic spirit of the time'.

202. For **H. Rothfels**, too, the leading Tübingen Professor of Modern History and founder of the *Vierteljahreshefte für Zeitgeschichte*, who returned from the US after the Second World War, 'modern history' begins with the end of the First World War.

203. **M. Schnell**, *Die Herausforderung der Postmoderne-Diskussion für die Theologie der Gegenwart*, Tübingen Dissertation 1994, has produced from our Institute for Ecumenical Research a comprehensive critical report of the discussion of postmodernity in the various spheres of culture and theology.

204. Cf. **H. Kissinger**, *Diplomacy*, New York and London 1994.

205. Cf. **N. Sheehan**, 'Nixon's "Peace" Strategy had a Heavy Price in Blood', *International Herald Tribune*, 30 April 1994; **A. Lewis**, '20492 Reasons Kissinger was Wrong', ibid., 7 June 1994.

206. Cf. **W. Isaacson**, 'How the World Works', *Time Magazine*, 2 May 1994. Cf. **id.**, *Kissinger, A Biography*, New York and London 1992, 766: 'But Kissinger's power-oriented realism and his banking on national interests faltered because it was too dismissive of the role of morality. The secret bombing and then invasion of Cambodia, the Christmas bombing of Hanoi, the destabilization of Chile – these and other brutal actions betrayed a callous attitude toward what Americans like to believe is the historic foundation of their foreign policy: a respect for human rights, international law, democracy, and other idealistic values. The setbacks Kissinger encountered as a statesman and the antagonism which he engendered as a person stemmed from the perceived amorality of his geopolitical calculations. Kissinger's approach led to a backlash against détente; the national mood shifted toward the moralism of Jimmy Carter and the ideological fervour of Ronald Reagan. As a result, not unlike Metternich, Kissinger's legacy turned out to be one of brilliance more than solidity, of masterly structures built of bricks that were made without straw.'

207. Cf. **S. P. Huntington**, 'The Clash of Civilizations?', *Foreign Affairs* 72, no.3, 1993, 22–49.

208. Cf. **A. Toynbee**, *The Study of History* (12 vols.), Oxford 1934–61.

209. **Huntington**, 'Clash of Civilizations' (n.207), 39.

210. Cf. the critical responses to Huntington by F. Ajami, R. L. Bartley, L. Binyan, J. J. Kirkpatrick, K. Mahbubani in *Foreign Affairs* 72, 1993, no.4 (September/October) and Huntington's 'Reponse' in no.5 (November/December), 186–94.

211. **Huntington**, 'Response' (n.210), 191f., 194.

212. **Id.**, 'Clash of Civilizations' (n.207), 22.

213. Ibid., 25.

214. Ibid., 27.

215. Cf. **R. D. Kaplan**, 'The Coming Anarchy', *The Atlantic Monthly*, February 1994, 44–76.

216. **J. Delors**, former President of the EC Commission, is also convinced that 'future conflicts will be sparked by cultural factors rather than economics or ideology'. And he warns: 'The West needs to develop a deeper understanding of the religious and philosophical assumptions underlying other civilizations, and the way other nations see their interests, to identify what we have in common' (quoted in **Huntington**, 'Response' [n.210], 194).

217. **Huntington**, 'Clash of Civilizations' (n.207), 49.

218. Cf. **Liu Shu-hsien**, 'Das Humanum als entscheidendes Kriterium aus der Sicht des Konfuzianismus', in H. Küng and K.-J. Kuschel (eds.), *Weltfrieden durch Religionsfrieden*, Munich 1993, 92–108; cf. also **S. Heilmann**, 'China, der Westen und die Menschenrechte', *China Aktuell*, February 1994, 145–51.

219. Cf. **Confucius**, *Analects*, 12.7.

220. Cf. **A.Mnouchkine, H. G. Berger** et al., *Der Prozess gegen den Schriftsteller Jingsheng*, ed. AIDA (International Association for the Defence of Persecuted Artists all over the World), Reinbek 1986; **Han Minzhu** (ed.), *Cries for Democracy. Writings and Speeches from 1989 Chinese Democracy Movement*, Princeton, NJ 1990.

221. Thus the diplomat and Director of the Institute of Policy Studies in Singapore, **T. Koh**, 'The 10 Values that Undergird East Asian Strength and Success', *International Herald Tribune*, 12 December 1993.

222. Cf. **Liu Binyan**, *Foreign Affairs* 72, 1993, no.4, 21.

223. Thus the reservations expressed by the Deputy Foreign Minister of Singapore, **K. Mahbubani**, in his response to Huntington in *Foreign Affairs* 72, 1993, no.4, 14.

224. Cf. *Der Spiegel*, 1993, no.9.

225. **H. Küng**, DGE, D I, 'The Rise of Nihilism: Friedrich Nietzsche'.

226. Cf. **W. J. Bennett**, *The Book of Virtues. A Treasury of Great Moral Stories*, New York 1994. This book, which advocates a 'reasonable mean between carte blanche for vandals and torture', put the former drugs representative of the American President on the best-seller list. Evidently it is again permissible to speak once again in public about responsibility, honesty, loyalty, courage, compassion, friendship, tenacity and self-discipline.

227. Cf. **H. Küng** and **K.-J. Kuschel** (eds.), *A Global Ethic. The Declaration of the Parliament of the World's Religions*, London and New York 1993.

List of Diagrams and Maps

A word of thanks

At the end of a book which has required unusual efforts, I feel unusual gratitude to all those who have contributed to the long toil. However, for those readers who (to judge by previous reviews) simply cannot understand how an individual can write such a large and complex book, let me once again spell out something which I felt went without saying. Like all my books, this book has not been thought out by a team, but by me, sentence by sentence – laboriously enough – and written down by hand. After that, though, it is constantly corrected by me and others.

Above all I must thank my colleague Dr Karl-Josef Kuschel, Privatdozent in the Catholic Theological Faculty in Tübingen and Deputy Director of the Institute for Ecumenical Research, who over past years has with deep commitment joined me in furthering the cause of a world ethic and understanding between the religions. The way in which he went through this book in a scholarly way, chapter by chapter, was indispensable to me and has resulted in countless improvements in content and style. I am also especially grateful to Frau Marianne Saur, who has time and again read through the different versions of the typescript to see that they were comprehensible; this was an important check. I am also grateful to my doctoral student and assistant in the project, Stephan Schlensog, who by virtue of his unusual twofold gifts was responsible both for checking the countless quotations and the extensive notes section and also for the graphic presentation of my schemes and the design and typesetting of the book. Because of this it was possible for me to work on the text to the last possible minute.

Finally, I must warmly thank all those who were responsible for the technical production of the countless versions of the text: Margarita Krause, succeeded by Franziska Heller-Manthey, but above all my personal secretary Eleonore Henn, without whose indefatigable commitment the Secretariat would not function. I am grateful to my doctoral student Mathias Schnell for obtaining the remarkably extensive literature needed, above all from the university library, for which no praise is too high, and for proof corrections. Thanks are due to Michel Hofmann for proof corrections and help in producing the index with its more than 2000 names. I am grateful to Piper Verlag, as already with my previous big book on **Judaism**, for its always smooth, collegial and professional collaboration: to the editorial department (Ulrich Wank), the production department (Hanns Polanetz), and of course also to the publishers themselves, Dr Klaus Piper and Dr Ernst Reinhard Piper.

Once again I cannot thank the Robert Bosch Jubilee Foundation and

the Daimler Benz Fund enough: it is through their generous support that
the research project 'No World Peace without Peace Between the
Religions' exists at all. They have made it possible for me to produce not
only the major study on *Judaism* (1991), but also the two small 'outriders'
to this book, *Credo. The Apostles' Creed Explained for Today* (1992),
and *Great Christian Thinkers* (1994). I hope that the final volume on
Islam will also be completed during the period of sponsorship.

I owe a special word of thanks, finally to three colleagues, who despite
many burdens of their own, with unusual collegiality and admirable
commitment have read through the whole manuscript and given me
valuable suggestions on historical matters: Professor Dr Johannes
B.Bauer, a specialist in patristics and ecumenics at the University of Graz;
Professor Dr Georg Denzler, a church historian at the University of
Bamberg; and finally Dr Thomas Riplinger, who in addition to reading
through the whole manuscript critically was an important help to me in
finding relevant literature, above all in the Tübingen university library. In
addition, various colleagues have read parts of the manuscript; I have
thanked them individually in the relevant chapters.

Hans Küng

Dominant Structural Elemen

1st/2nd centuries	11th century	16th

Apostles → **Councils** → **Pope** →

Earliest community | **Emperor** | Emperor

New Testament → **Church Fathers** → **Canon law** →

Apocalyptic | **Tradition** | **Scholasticism**

Jesus t
(God's Mes

P I | **P II** | **P III**

Jewish apocalyptic paradigm of earliest Christianity → *Ecumenical Hellenistic paradigm of Christian antiquity* → *Roman Catholic paradigm of the Middle Ages* →

of the Different Paradigms

ry   *17th/18th centuries*   *20th century*

Bible   **Reason**   **The one world**   **?**

Rulers/synods

Democracy   United Nations
Nation state   Peace movement
Technological progress   Women's movement
      Environmental movement

Confessions   **Science**   **Holistic thought**   **?**

**Protestant
orthodoxy**

**Historical-
critical
theology**

**Ecumenical
movement**

Unity of the churches
Peace between the religions
Ethic for humankind

Christ

(and Son)

P IV   **P V**   **P VI**

*rotestant evangelical
radigm
the Reformation*

*Paradigm of modernity
orientated
on reason and progress*

*Ecumenical
paradigm
of postmodernity?*